Dermato-
toxicology

Dermato-toxicology

fourth edition

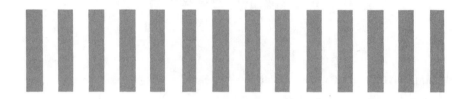

edited by

Francis N. Marzulli
Consultant in Toxicology
Bethesda, Maryland

Howard I. Maibach
University of California,
San Francisco, School of Medicine

●HEMISPHERE PUBLISHING CORPORATION
A member of the Taylor & Francis Group
New York   Washington   Philadelphia   London

DERMATOTOXICOLOGY, Fourth Edition

Copyright © 1991, 1987, 1983, 1977 by Hemisphere Publishing Corporation. All rights reserved. Printed in the United States of America. Except as permitted under the United States Copyright Act of 1976, no part of this publication may be reproduced or distributed in any form or by any means, or stored in a data base or retrieval system, without the prior written permission of the publisher.

Chapter 7, "Transdermal Delivery of Drugs: Nonclinical Regulatory Considerations," by Judi Weissinger, was written in the course of employment by the United States Government so that no copyright exists.

1 2 3 4 5 6 7 8 9 0   E B E B   9 8 7 6 5 4 3 2 1

This book was set in Times Roman by Hemisphere Publishing Corporation. The editors were Amy Lyles Wilson and Elizabeth Dugger; the production supervisor was Peggy M. Rote; and the typesetters were Deborah S. Hamblen, Lori Knoernschild, Darrell D. Larsen, and Cynthia B. Mynhier.
Printing and binding by Edwards Brothers.

A CIP catalog record for this book is available from the British Library.

Library of Congress Cataloging-in-Publication Data

Dermatotoxicology / edited by Francis N. Marzulli, Howard I. Maibach. — 4th ed.
    p. cm.
    Includes bibliographical references and index.

    1. Dermatotoxicology. I. Marzulli, Francis Nicholas. II. Maibach, Howard I.
    [DNLM: 1. Skin Diseases—etiology.   WR 140 D43518]
RL803.D47   1991
616.5—dc20
DNLM/DLC
for Library of Congress   90-15632
                                                                     CIP

ISBN 1-56032-055-9

contents

contributors

Susan M. Barlow, Ph.D.
Department of Health, Hannibal House, Elephant and Castle, Room 915, London SE1 6TE, United Kingdom

Margaret Bason, M.D.
Department of Dermatology, University of California, San Francisco, School of Medicine, Box 0989, Surge 110, San Francisco, California 94143-0989

Paul R. Bergstresser, M.D.
Department of Dermatology, University of Texas Southwestern Medical Center, 5323 Harry Hines Boulevard, Dallas, Texas 75235

B. M. E. von Blomberg, Ph.D.
Department of Pathology, Free University Hospital, De Boelelaan 1117, 1081 HV Amsterdam, The Netherlands

Robert L. Bronaugh, Ph.D.
Division of Toxicological Studies, Food and Drug Administration, 200 C Street, S.W., Washington, D.C. 20204

D. P. Bruynzeel, M.D., Ph.D.
Department of Dermatology, Free University Hospital, De Boelelaan 1117, 1081 HV Amsterdam, The Netherlands

Daniel A. W. Bucks, Ph.D.
Pharmetrix, 1330 O'Brien Drive, Menlo Park, California 94025

Michael P. Carver
Department of Human and Environmental Safety, Colgate-Palmolive Company, Piscataway, New Jersey

Steven W. Collier
Division of Toxicological Studies, Food and Drug Administration, 200 C Street, S.W., Washington, D.C. 20204

[†]K.D. Crow, M.D.
Wiltshire Area Health Authority, Swindon Health District, Princess Margaret Hospital, Okus Road, Swindon SN1 4JU, England

Ponciano D. Cruz, Jr., M.D.
Department of Dermatology, University of Texas Southwestern Medical Center, 5323 Harry Hines Boulevard, Dallas, Texas 75235

[†]Deceased.

John M. Davitt, Ph.D.
Division of Antiinfective Drug Products, Food and Drug Administration, 5600 Fishers Lane, Room 12-B-20, Rockville, Maryland 20857

John H. Epstein, M.D.
Department of Dermatology, University of California, San Francisco Medical Center, 3rd Avenue and Parnassus, San Francisco, California 94143

Claire A. Franklin, Ph.D.
Bureau of Human Prescription Drugs, National Department of Health & Welfare, 355 River Road, Tower B, Second Floor, Vanier, Ontario K1A 1B8 Canada

John M. Frazier, Ph.D.
Johns Hopkins University, School of Hygiene and Public Health, Department of Environmental Health Sciences, 615 North Wolfe Street, Baltimore, Maryland 21205–3343

Susi Freeman, M.D.
St. Vincent's Hospital, Skin and Cancer Foundation, 277 Bourke Street, Darlinghurst 20 10, Sydney, Australia

Gerard J. Gendimenico, Ph.D.
Dermatopharmacology, R. W. Johnson Pharmaceutical Research Institute, Route 202, Box 300, Raritan, New Jersey 08869

Robert B. Hackett, Ph.D.
Toxicology, Alcon Laboratories, Inc., 6201 South Freeway, Fort Worth, Texas 76134-2099

†Niels Hjorth, M.D.
Department of Dermatology, Gentofte Hospital, DK-2900 Hellerup, Copenhagen, Denmark

Daniel J. Hogan, M.D.
Department of Dermatology and Cutaneous Surgery, University of Miami, Box 016250 (R-250), Miami, Florida 33101

†Deceased.

Edward M. Jackson, Ph.D.
Research Services and Quality Assurance, The Andrew Jergens Company, 2535 Spring Grove Avenue, Cincinnati, Ohio 45214

Robert H. James, Ph.D.
Center for Devices and Radiological Health, Food and Drug Administration, HF2 134, 5600 Fishers Lane, Rockville, Maryland 20857

Kays Kaidbey, M.D.
IVY Laboratories (KGL Inc.), 3401 Market Street, Suite 226, Philadelphia, Pennsylvania 19104-3355

John Kao, Ph.D.
Department of Drug Metabolism, SmithKline Beecham Pharmaceuticals, 709 Swedeland Road, Box 1539, King of Prussia, Pennsylvania 19406

Georg Klecak, M.D.
Department of Biological and Pharmaceutical Research, F. Hoffman-La Roche & Company, Ltd., Dept. PF/TOX, Bdg. 73/101A, Ch-4002, Basle, Switzerland

Andrija Kornhauser, Ph.D.
Division of Toxicology, Food and Drug Administration, 200 C Street, S.W., Washington, D.C. 20204

Daniel Krewski, Ph.D.
Biostatistics & Computer Applications, National Department of Health and Welfare, Environmental Health Center, Room 107, Tunney's Pasture, Ottawa Ontario K1A OL2 Canada

Arto Lahti, M.D.
Department of Dermatology, University of Oulu, SF 902 20 Oulu, Finland

Lark A. Lambert
Division of Toxicology, Food and Drug Administration, 200 C Street, S.W., Washington, D.C. 20204

K. Lammintausta
Department of Dermatology, University of California, San Francisco, School of Medicine, Box 0989, Surge 110, San Francisco, California 94143-0989

Philip S. Magee, Ph.D.
BIOSAR Research Project, 141 Sealion Place, Vallejo, California 94591

Henry C. Maguire, Jr., M.D.
Departments of Medicine (Oncology) and Dermatology, Thomas Jefferson University, Jefferson Medical College, Philadelphia, Pennsylvania 19107

Howard I. Maibach, M.D.
Department of Dermatology, University of California, San Francisco, School of Medicine, Box 0989, Surge 110, San Francisco, California 94143-0989

Francis N. Marzulli, Ph.D.
Consultant in Toxicology; Past Association with Food and Drug Administration, University of California, San Francisco, and NAS/NRC. 8044 Park Overlook Drive, Bethesda, Maryland 20817.

S. L. Matchette
Center for Devices and Radiological Health, Food and Drug Administration, HF2 134, 5600 Fishers Lane, Rockville, Maryland 20857

Roger O. McClellan, Ph.D.
Chemical Industry Institute of Toxicology, Box 12137, Research Triangle Park, North Carolina 27709

T. O. McDonald, Ph.D.
Alcon Laboratories, P.O. Box 6600, Fort Worth, Texas 76101

James N. McDougal, Ph.D., Major, USAF, BSc
Toxic Hazards Division, Harry G. Armstrong Aerospace Medical Research Laboratory, Wright-Patterson Air Force Base, Dayton, Ohio 45433

Basil E. McKenzie, D.V.M., Ph.D.
Drug Safety Evaluation Division Worldwide, R. W. Johnson Pharmaceutical Research Institute, Route 202, Box 300, Raritan, New Jersey 08869

Torkil Menné, M.D.
Department of Dermatology, Gentofte Hospital, DK-2900 Hellerup, Copenhagen, Denmark

James A. Mezick, Ph.D.
Dermatopharmacology, R. W. Johnson Pharmaceutical Research Institute, Route 202, Box 300, Raritan, New Jersey 08869

Esther Patrick, Ph.D.
University of California, San Francisco, School of Medicine, Box 0989, Surge 110, San Francisco, California 94143-0989

William J. Powers, Jr., Ph.D.
Toxicology, Drug Safety Evaluation Division, R. W. Johnson Pharmaceutical Research Institute, Route 202, Box 300 Raritan, New Jersey 08869

S. Madli Puhvel, Ph.D.
Division of Dermatology, University of California, Los Angeles, School of Medicine, Los Angeles, California 90024

R. J. Scheper, Ph.D.
Department of Pathology, Free University Hospital, De Boelelaan 1117, 1081 HV Amsterdam, The Netherlands

Van Seabaugh, M.A.
Environmental Protection Agency, 1921 Jefferson Davis Highway, Arlington, Virginia 22202

Ellen K. Silbergeld, Ph.D.
Program in Toxicology, University of Maryland Medical School, Baltimore, Maryland 21210

Diana A. Somers, Ph.D.
Division of Environmental and Occupational
Toxicology, National Department of Health &
Welfare, Room 320, Environmental Health
Center, Tunney's Pasture, Ottawa, Ontario,
K1A OL2 Canada

E. George Thorne, M.D.
Dermatology, R. W. Johnson Pharmaceutical
Research Institute, Box 300, Raritan, New
Jersey 08869-0602

Frederick Urbach, M.D.
Dermatology, Temple University Medical
Practice, 220 Commerce Drive, Suite 120,
Fort Washington, Pennsylvania 19034

Wayne G. Warner, B.S.
Division of Toxicology, Food and Drug
Administration, 200 C Street, S.W.,
Washington, D.C. 20204

Judi Weissinger, Ph.D.
Pharmacology/Toxicology, Center for Drug
Evaluation and Research, Food and Drug
Administration, 5600 Fishers Lane, Rockville,
Maryland 20857

Ronald C. Wester, Ph.D.
Department of Dermatology, University of
California, San Francisco, School of
Medicine, Box 0989, Surge 110, San
Francisco, California 94143-0989

foreword

The field of toxicology is at an exciting juncture as the decade of the 1990s begins. It is an appropriate time to look at the past, consider the present, and anticipate the future for toxicology. Publication of the fourth edition of *Dermatotoxicology* provides an excellent opportunity for such reflection.

The roots of toxicology are ancient and undoubtedly predate recorded history. The earliest references to toxicology most often deal with poisons or potions. Other references call attention to the close relationship between poisons and remedies, in other words, the often quoted statement of Paracelsus: "All substances are poisons; there is none which is not a poison. The right dose differentiates a poison and a remedy." And some other references note poisonings related to occupation, in other words, the mad hatter syndrome from intake of mercury. The roots of toxicology, whether related to poisons, drugs, or agents encountered in the workplace or environment, usually had a descriptive orientation and most often concerned individuals rather than populations. An exposure to or intake of toxicants occurred and an effect was observed, usually of an obvious nature and within a short period of time. This kind of knowledge was readily applied to similar situations to avoid further poisonings, or in some cases, to assure that intended poisoning was carried out in an even more crafty way.

In this century, the field of toxicology has changed markedly. Descriptive toxicology and direct application to similar situations have been supplanted by the need to predict or estimate toxicity for different exposure situations than those for which actual observations exist. Increasingly, toxicologists have been called on to predict the potential nature and magnitude of adverse health effects at exposure levels much lower than those for which human observations are available and, in some cases, for materials for which human data do not exist.

The earlier concern for acute effects is now overridden by concern for diseases such as cancer that occur years after intake of a suspected toxicant. These diseases of concern, using cancer as an example, may be expected to occur at very low incidence in excess of the disease incidence occurring spontaneously, in other words, one cancer added to the base incidence of more than 200,000 cancer cases expected to occur from all causes in a population of a million individuals. Without question, emphasis has shifted from poisoning of individuals to individuals within a population. The exposure levels of concern are frequently orders of magnitude lower than that for which any human data exist, giving rise to the need for extrapolation. Furthermore, in many cases, human data are unavailable or insufficient, making it necessary to obtain information from studies using laboratory animals, tissues and macromolecules and conducted with exposure levels much higher than the exposure levels likely to be of concern for people. Thus, multiple extrapolations may be required—across species, downward in exposure level, in some cases, from subanimal systems to the intact mammal, and from a few individuals to large populations.

The earliest extrapolations were usually quite simplistic, involving the use of no observed effect levels and safety factors. Such approaches are most readily justified when dealing with health endpoints for which thresholds may exist. Even when thresholds exist, the situation becomes complicated when dealing with large populations that contain individuals of varying sensitivity. When dealing with induction of cancers, some types of which may not exhibit a demonstrable threshold between exposure and incidence, the extrapolation may be accomplished using mathematical models. Some of the models have been challenged as to the validity of the biological assumptions underlying their use. Unfortunately, it is quite likely that economic and logistical limitations on the size of populations that can be studied will probably preclude validation of most of the models by direct observations.

During the past two decades, it has become a tenet of faith of most toxicologists that increased confidence can be developed in the extrapolations noted above as we develop an improved understanding of the mechanisms of action of toxic agents. Some progress has been made in improving our knowledge of the mechanisms of action of toxicants; however, such information was not used in regulatory decisions in the 1970s and 1980s as often as one would have liked.

Looking to the future of toxicology, one of the critical issues is how to incorporate a better understanding of mechanisms of action of toxicants, as some might say—the relevant biology—into the various extrapolations as mentioned above that must be made as part of the process of controlling exposures to toxicants, thereby limiting the occurrence of adverse health outcomes. I submit that progress will be most notable when the experimentalist and regulator, after compiling and integrating the available data, identify the gaps in our knowledge which, if filled, would have the greatest impact on reducing the uncertainty in estimating health risks at relevant levels of human exposure.

Meeting these data needs will be a formidable challenge because it will focus attention on the need to understand mechanisms of action at exposure levels that are difficult, and perhaps not even possible, with traditional experimental approaches.

Success with this new toxicology, with an emphasis on reducing the uncertainty in our assessment of toxicant risks through an understanding of mechanisms of action at relevant exposure levels, will depend greatly on developing an improved capability for integrating data obtained from studies at various levels of biological organization ranging from macromolecules to cells to tissues and organs to intact mammals to populations of laboratory animals and, ultimately, to people. The explosion in our knowledge and capability at the molecular and cellular levels provides us with both opportunity and challenge. The opportunity relates to the immenseness of the knowledge and the power of the techniques. The challenge for toxicology is to integrate the information with a view to better understanding diseases that occur in intact individuals with complex modulating systems as members of large populations that may vary greatly in individual susceptibility to specific toxicants.

Of the various subspecialties of toxicology, none has received more pressure than dermatotoxicology for using approaches other than the study of whole animals as "alternatives" for assessing toxic effect of materials, in this case, materials applied to the skin. I hope that past emphasis on "alternatives" will shift to concern for integrating data obtained from complementary systems and a reduction, rather than elimination, of the use of laboratory animals. If this approach is not taken, lacking any data from laboratory animals, human populations may serve as the test system for validation of our estimates of toxicity derived from using cells, tissues, and computer models. This could have unfortunate consequences.

This fourth edition of *Dermatotoxicology* illustrates well the extent to which the field is at a juncture. The revisions of old chapters and the many new chapters clearly describe the current state of our knowledge of dermatotoxicology. The book is a careful blending of fundamental information on the mechanisms of action of toxicants on skin, practical information on the varied responses of skin to specific toxicants, and approaches to evaluating dermal toxicity. Equally as important, many of the chapters convey a sense of where the field is going. I am confident the book will be useful to a broad spectrum of readers; dermatotoxicologists, general toxicologists, occupational physicians, and regulatory authorities, all of whom are concerned with minimizing the occurrence of toxicant-induced skin disease.

Roger O. McClellan
Chemical Industry Institute of Toxicology

preface

Dermatotoxicology is defined as the science that deals with adverse skin effects and the substances that produce them. It also includes processes that may involve skin in some important manner, such as skin penetration.

The first edition of *Dermatotoxicology* was published in 1977. The second edition was brought out in 1983. It contained much new material. Chapters of the first edition relating to microbial flora, food additives, and an extensive coverage of chemicals that affect eccrine sweat glands and sebaceous glands were eliminated. The third edition of this text was published in 1987. It contained a new chapter on reproductive hazards of chemicals absorbed through the skin and updated material from the second edition. A chapter on pustulogenic chemicals from the second edition was eliminated (Tables of contents from the three previous editions can be found in the last Appendix.)

As in previous editions, the fourth edition of *Dermatotoxicology* provides information on theoretical aspects and practical test methods, including both *in vitro* and *in vivo* approaches. This edition displays increased attention to *in vitro* techniques in keeping with a worldwide movement for the development of suitable alternatives to animals when feasible. Good science must not be sacrificed solely to accomplish a replacement of animal investigations, however.

This edition deletes 18 chapters from the third edition, adds 17 new chapters, and updates the others. Arrangement of material in the fourth edition follows the plan of the third edition to a great extent. The rationale for this arrangement is discussed below.

Following this introductory preface material are 8 chapters on percutaneous penetration, also called percutaneous absorption. This is a natural starting point because a topically applied substance must first penetrate into the living skin in order to produce a physiologic or toxicologic effect. It must first pass through nonliving barrier tissues and be absorbed into underlying vasculature from which it passes into the circulatory system. Once absorbed, a skin-applied substance may affect the skin itself or other systemic organ systems.

Because of its location as the outermost organ with considerable area (about 1.7 sq. m.) and incomplete resistance to penetration, the skin plays an important role as a portal of entry into the body, along with ingestion, inhalation, and injection.

The outer skin is endowed with a nonliving, tough, keratinous, complex layer, the stratum corneum, whose lipid-aqueous nature and other chemical and physical properties make it resistant to penetration of substances in contact with it. Absorption of topically applied substances depends on the chemical nature of the compound, as well as the skin site, its area, state of hydration, intactness, duration of contact, and whether it is under cover. In addition, certain characteristics of the penetrant substance determine the actual amount that penetrates the skin. These include its molecular size, degree of dissociation, pH, volatility and its solubility in lipids and in water. Quantifying the amount of a substance that may be absorbed following skin contact, is the subject of the first six chapters. A variety of approachs is presented.

Percutaneous penetration, or transport through skin, sounds simple enough in concept. It is appropriate, however, to caution the uninitiated that despite certain similarities between *in vitro* and *in vivo* test systems (i.e., animals, humans, tissues), there is not a one-to-one relationship between results obtained with the various models that have been employed. This also applies to *in vivo* human systems, as compared with human exposures to skin contaminants under field conditions, where results must not be assumed to bear a one-to-one relation.

Certain substances that traverse the skin barriers are changed during this process. Thus skin, like liver, has a capacity to metabolize substances that pass through it en route to the general circulation. Steroidal substances such as testosterone and cortisone are important examples. Chapter 9 contains a more detailed description of the metabolic processes.

Some substances are cytotoxic and produce cellular injury as they penetrate skin. This effect, which produces a local inflammatory skin reaction characterized by erythema and edema, is known as irritant dermatitis, or simply skin irritation. Human and animal test methods and related extrinsic factors are discussed in Chapters 10 and 11.

Other substances, oftentimes irritant compounds, may, after repeated skin contact, develop a propensity to enhance the original inflammatory response. The skin is said to be hypersensitive or hyperreactive, an immunologically mediated process referred to as allergic contact dermatitis. Details of mechanisms involved, *in vitro,* animal and human tests are presented in Chapters 12–17.

Ultraviolet (UV) light has the capacity to energize chemicals that are said to be photoactive. Once light-activated, these chemicals can produce the equivalence of skin irritation and skin sensitization that is not produced in the absence of activating wavelengths. Psoralen-like compounds are a major source of chemicals that comprise this category. A national PUVA (psoralen-UVA) phototherapy program for serious cases of psoriasis provided an important stimulus for investigating sunlight-activated chemicals. UV radiation also has the capacity to penetrate the epidermis, where residing Langerhans cells become altered and modify immune function. This process has only recently been appreciated. Chapters 19–23 discuss various aspects of light related skin effects. Improvements in delivering and measuring light of various intensities and wavelengths suggested the need for a chapter on this subject (Chapter 18), which may be useful for those engaged in experimental work involving light radiation. New developments relating to the mechanics of photoallergy suggested the need for a detailed account of this process, which is featured in Chapter 24.

Repeated skin contact with a carcinogenic chemical may cause skin cancer at the site of contact. A different site may be involved if the carcinogen acts or is produced at a remote site. The most publicized cancer from skin contact is that reported by Sir Percival Potts a few centuries ago when he observed that chimney sweeps of England often developed scrotal cancer. This condition was related to a combination of poor hygiene, which allowed prolonged contact of carcinogen-laden soot with highly permeable scrotal tissue. Sunlight is probably even more important than chemicals as a source of skin cancer; however, light activated chemicals may also be carcinogenic. Cutaneous carcinogenesis with and without light is the subject of Chapter 25.

Chemicals that have special effects involving the sebaceous glands, and skin health are discussed in Chapters 26–28. The possibility that reproduction may be affected by skin contact with medicaments is the subject of Chapter 29.

In recent years, toxicologists, environmentalists, and others have gone beyond simple identification of toxic hazards. They now seek to quantitate risks associated with exposure. This development, although beset with controversy after a shaky start in the 1970s, has become an important aspect of toxicologic assessment. The dermal route, while not as prominent in importance in this regard as other routes, is beginning to achieve some attention and is discussed in Chapter 30.

Eye irritation traditionally has been included with dermatotoxicology and is discussed in Chapter 31.

Over the past several decades, the FDA has called on the scientific community to develop methods and tests that are appropriate to evaluate the safety of substances used in foods, drugs, and cosmetics that enter the marketplace. With arrival of newer regulatory agencies, other categories of substances were included, such as pesticides and commercial products not intended for human contact. Laws were enacted (Food, Drug and Cosmetic Act of 1938 and the 1960 revision of the Act) that require premarket testing to assess health hazard potential. These laws were enacted as a result of significant historic disasters (sulfanilamide, thalidomide). Guidelines for premarket safety evaluation have been promulgated. Progress in toxicology has gone hand-in-hand with a citizenry that is alerted to carcinogenic and toxicologic potential of chemicals to which they may be exposed.

The legitimate concern for human safety provides background for future concerns. As safety tests have been conducted largely on animals, a rising voice from animal rights groups has resulted in a push to supplant animals with nonanimal test models. Although scientists generally welcome the possibility of using cheaper, nonanimal methods that are adequately validated, they are rightly concerned about extremists who want all animal testing and research stopped immediately, prior to the development of adequate replacements. One effect of this political process has been a developing erosion of concern for human safety that was brought about by earlier human disasters. The recent abandonment of testing by certain cosmetic companies, in part as appeasement, in part as a money-saving device, is certainly cause for concern. The fourth edition of *Dermatotoxicology* provides an up-to-date assessment of progress in the development of skin and eye alternative test methods in Chapter 32.

Methods suggested by industry, the Organization for Economic Cooperation and Development (OECD), and regulating agencies for monitoring and evaluating the safety of topical drugs, cosmetics, and commercial products that accidentally contact skin, are the subject of Chapters 33, 34, and the appendixes.

The final chapter is of special interest to dermatologists and is a review of dermatologic drugs and various chemicals, both of which may produce systemic effects following contact with skin.

Francis N. Marzulli
Howard I. Maibach

preface
to the third editon

This edition contains most of the material from the two previous editions as well as new chapters, updated references, and other materials. Among the new chapters is one that provides introductory information on skin hypersensitivity. It precedes nine chapters on special aspects of this subject. We have also included a chapter on reproductive hazards from skin-absorbed chemicals, because of the increased concern about such effects.

Additionally, current interest in replacing the Draize test for evaluating eye irritation has directed our attention to a need to discuss the developments occurring in this area. Requests for methods of testing for contact hypersensitivity of the vagina have led to the inclusion of this subject as well. The induction of porphyria cutanea tarda by chemicals has also been included.

We would appreciate readers' comments and suggestions for future editions.

Francis N. Marzulli
Howard I. Maibach

preface
to the second edition

This edition updates many chapters of the first edition and eliminates certain topics found only in that edition (sweat and sebaceous gland toxicology, histologic and immunologic aspects of contact dermatitis, effects of drugs on cutaneous microbial flora, and cutaneous manifestations of food intolerance). The intent is to limit the size of this edition while increasing the scope of certain subjects.

We revised the order of presentation beginning with a brief description of the skin itself, its structure, function, and biochemistry. From this background information we proceed to a discussion of the barrier functions of skin and factors involved in dermal penetration with the thought that a topically applied substance must first penetrate the skin if it is to sensitize, irritate, or result in systemic effects. We present a more comprehensive treatment of this important subject with greater attention to practical and *in vitro* studies as well as theoretical considerations.

We follow this with an expanded section on skin sensitization, including a comparison of animal and human findings. Information on skin irritation has been updated.

We expanded our coverage of photobiology because of increasing recent interest and concerns in this area.

Finally, we introduce varied subjects of more than peripheral interest to many dermatotoxicologists, such as skin carcinogenesis, chloracne, pigmentation, eczema, urticaria, granulomas, hair, and sebaceous gland toxicology. Neurotoxic substances and toxicity from heavy metals are also discussed. Eye irritation is placed near the end of the book not because of a lack of importance but simply because the eye, though it shares many anatomic similarities with skin, is a separate and distinctly unique organ.

Test methods suggested by the Interagency Regulatory Liaison Group (IRLG) and Organization for Economic Cooperation and Development (OECD) are provided as appendixes for those toxicologists interested in regulatory agency guidelines. The IRLG is no longer a functioning group, however, and their guidelines are included for interest only.

Recent activities by animal welfare groups have resulted in a reappraisal of animal test methods with interest in using tissues or cell cultures in place of animals. The development of the Ames test for predicting carcinogenic potential was a leading stimulus to this type of effort. However, the Ames test has its limitations and toxicologists have been concerned for years about the applicability of animal tests to humans. But there is an ever great divergence between *in vitro* systems and humans. Tests involving complicated mechanisms, such as those that occur in immunology, require intact animals and become exceedingly difficult to replace by *in vitro* methods. The rabbit eye test for eye irritation has received wide adverse publicity by animal welfare groups. Yet, even with its limitations, the rabbit eye has an important capacity not shared by tissue cultures—it offers a time-frame for recovery and conjunctiva that are not unlike those of humans. If investigators treat the rabbit eye with the care used in human ocular experimentation this should substantially alleviate public concern for this issue.

In the future we may see a proliferation of *in vitro* test methods as pressures to replace animal testing develop. Only time will tell how useful they are.

Francis N. Marzulli
Howard I. Maibach

preface
to the first edition

Dermatotoxicology, a relatively new discipline, is defined as a science that deals with adverse skin effects and the substances that produce them. This volume represents a first attempt at consolidating recent developments in various aspects of skin research of interest and concern to researchers in dermatotoxicology.

Three key subdisciplines are skin irritation, skin sensitization, and skin penetration. Skin metabolism and skin carcinogenesis are related important subdisciplines. Pharmacologic aspects of skin are for the most part concerned with skin appendages such as the eccrine glands and the pilosebaceous apparatus.

A section on immunology is included as the basis of understanding allergic contact dermatitis. The science of immunology has undergone an explosion of new developments, some of which provide a better understanding of the complicated mechanisms that may be involved in skin sensitization. Eye irritation is included in this volume primarily because of a traditional linkage of eye and skin irritation.

Different in scope from those texts that deal with clinical dermatology or cosmetic science, this volume attempts to provide useful background, reference, and up-to-date state of the art information in areas such as skin irritation, skin sensitization, and skin penetration. The contents should be of special interest to those engaged in evaluating toxicologic safety; much of the impetus to the development of dermatotoxicology as a separate discipline derives from government regulations suggesting and sometimes demanding that certain products applied to the skin should be evaluated for toxic hazard prior to reaching the market place. This volume provides background information rather than specific test methodologies.

Because recent developments in some of these areas have been rapid and because of the time involved in the preparation of any such volume, some parts may be outdated by publication date. Certain chapters that were expected to have involved more extensive coverage were reduced in scope and others were eliminated in order to meet deadlines. We believe nevertheless that this represents a satisfactory beginning in this relatively new discipline and that it fulfills a need and provides a groundwork on which future authors can build.

We want to acknowledge the assistance in the review of manuscripts by Carl Bruch, John Lucas, Helen Reynolds, Joseph McLoughlin, Max Samter, Andrew Ulsamer, Robert Hehir, Van Seabaugh, Anne Wolven, Paige Yoder, William Markland, Leon Sanders, and Elizabeth Weisburger. We thank Mary Phillips, our editor at Hemisphere, for her valuable assistance in transforming our manuscript into a book.

Francis N. Marzulli
Howard I. Maibach

Dermato-
toxicology

1

percutaneous absorption: critical factors in transdermal transport

■ **Philip S. Magee** ■

INTRODUCTION

Transdermal transport and percutaneous absorption are technical terms for the penetration of human or animal skin by any applied chemical substance. The process is macroscopically simple with a common end point, namely, clearance from the dermis by the capillaries into the body's vascular system with subsequent beneficial or toxic results. However simple in appearance, the event is microscopically complex with many key factors relating to the physical, chemical, and biochemical constitution of the skin overlaid with the vast range of physicochemical behavior of the penetrant. Sorting out the skin and chemical factors for the purpose of estimating transport behavior is the primary thrust of this chapter.

There are two broad classes of chemicals having transdermal significance. One consists of dermally applied drugs where the objective is a local or systemic pharmacological response. Current research is divided between restraint (slow release technology) and enhancement (occlusion, permeation enhancers). The essence of the research vector is transdermal control. The other class involves accidental or deliberate (chemical warfare) exposure where the end point is toxicological hazard. This includes commercial and home and garden pesticides, polymer and paint chemicals, detergents and cleaning chemicals, and a broad range of heavy industrial chemicals for hundreds of important industries. It also includes unscheduled exposures to environmental accidents and mishandling of toxic waste disposal. With the exception of highly volatile chemicals, the principal organ exposed to these hazards is the skin. Research in this area is directed toward understanding transdermal flux rates and the toxico-logical consequences of penetration. At the practical end, such data contribute to risk assessment for industrial safety standards, shipping regulations, and worker reentry into sprayed croplands.

Obviously, development of accurate mathematical models for transdermal flux would greatly facilitate all related areas of research. The value of reliable estimates based on molecular structure cannot be overstated. In drug research, such estimates would signal the type and difficulty of delivery problems with untested drugs. In risk assessment, it would allow setting provisional safety standards and define priorities for toxicological studies. In general, the ability to set priorities with confidence can lead to enormous reduction in cost and time to deliver critical information.

This chapter will review the many reasons why quantitative structure-flux relations are difficult to generalize. Various levels of predictive confidence will be considered for "quantitative" relations, and the value of important qualita-tive relations will be stressed. It is wonderful to achieve sharply defined quanti-tative relations from precisely measured data, but not all data can be measured under controlled laboratory conditions. In many cases, medically evaluated data can only be categorized as $+$, $++$, $+++$, $++++$ (poor, fair, good, excellent), and in comparative clinical drug testing we may only know that drugs A to E are effective in the order $B > C > E > A > D$. Even in such cases, valuable insights at the semiquantitative or qualitative level can be achieved to help set research priorities and contribute to important medical decisions.

DERMAL STRUCTURES: POTENTIAL BARRIERS

Whole Skin

Whole human skin is described by Ridout and Guy (1988) as a multilay-ered heterogeneous organ composed of two main layers, dermis and epidermis, supported on varying amounts of subcutaneous fat. In the physical sense, the dermis forms the main bulk of the skin, supporting and binding the epidermal layer while providing strength and elasticity. It supports the embedded capillary system responsible for clearing drugs and chemicals that penetrate the upper avascular layers. It also supports hair follicles, sebaceous and sweat glands, and a neural network providing the skin with a delicate sense of touch. In contrast to a dermis thickness of 3–5 mm, the viable epidermis consists of several layers of proliferating nucleated cells with thickness ranging from 40 to 100 μm (0.04 to 0.1 mm). The "thickness" of the epidermal layer is strongly compromised locally by numerous invaginations of the dermis layer (Stuttgen, 1982). The uppermost layer, the stratum corneum, is thinner yet (10–20 μm) and consists of dead, keratinized cells with low water content (Schalla and Schaefer, 1982). This very thin layer is the primary barrier against most chemical invasions of the skin. Each of these layers is discussed in more detail in subsequent sections.

Our purpose at this point is to establish a physical picture and relate that image to experimental problems that complicate the development of general models. Physical variations can be extreme. No two patches of excised skin are identical, a factor carrying a guaranteed error for *in vitro* flux studies that is independent of experimental planning. Variations in skin permeability are well recognized (Idson, 1971; Wester and Maibach, 1983) and have been studied statistically by Southwall et al. (1984) and Magee (1983) in the penetration of standard chemicals through whole skin. The variance is inescapable and means that unreplicated studies on excised skin or on whole animals have little quantitative value. In human male studies of the dermal absorption of hydrocortisone, Maibach (1976) observed a 300-fold spread between the most resistant skin (foot arch) and the least (scrotum). In addition to regional variations, the skin can vary widely as a function of condition, race, sex, occupation, and age (Idson, 1971; Bronaugh et al., 1983; Behl et al., 1985). *In vitro* studies of sodium fluorescein penetration show that aged skin (71 ± 3 years) is about seven times more permeable than young skin (25 ± 2 years) (Christophers and Kligman, 1964). In a related study suggesting greater skin porosity with age, Kligman (1979) found a 2.5-fold greater rate of transepidermal water loss (TEWL) from a leg site on older subjects (66–81 years) compared to younger (19–26 years). Other age-related TEWL experiments are reviewed by Behl et al. (1985). The variance in these and other physical factors can be narrowed by careful selection of subjects or skin patches, coupled with sufficient replication of experiments.

Hydration is another critical factor affecting transdermal transport. As pointed out by Wester and Maibach (1985b), water can act as both vehicle and plasticizer in the stratum corneum. The stratum corneum *in vivo* is always partially hydrated but possesses enormous capacity to absorb additional water. Hydration is slow, and Scheuplein and Blank (1971) have shown continued swelling of immersed tissue for fully 3 d. The fully hydrated tissue contains five to six times its weight of strongly bound water, causing severalfold increase in the stratum corneum thickness (Scheuplein, 1966; Scheuplein and Morgan, 1967). *In vivo* hydration by natural moisture is induced by occlusion of the skin with a nonpermeable wrap or patch. Occlusion is frequently used in percutaneous experiments to minimize evaporative loss of an applied drug. Caution must therefore be exercised in comparing exposed applications with occluded, as the physical structure and aqueous content of the stratum corneum can be quite different. Occlusion also raises the tissue temperature, tending to accelerate the transport rate (Scheuplein and Blank, 1971). Additional consequences of hydration are reviewed by Wester and Maibach (1985b) and by Blank (1985).

Of remaining factors affecting transdermal transport in whole skin, delipidization is one of the more interesting. The hydrophobic nature of the skin surface is revealed in complete wetting by organic solvents (Rosenberg et al., 1973). Lipogenesis in skin is continuous, the sebaceous secretion forming an irregular film on the surface estimated to be 0.4–4 μm thick (Scheuplein and Blank, 1971; Tregear, 1966). Removing this layer by mild swabbing with acetone or ether has no effect on TEWL, but the layer could act as a barrier to polar molecules (Scheuplein and Blank, 1971). As reviewed by Menczel (1985), many different solvents have been used in skin delipidization experiments. With polar, water-miscible solvents such as acetone, the extracts are 30–40% lipids with 60–70% polar components. Less polar solvents are more selective for lipid extraction. Water permeation is strongly affected when acetone extraction is followed by hexane, removing almost the entire water vapor barrier (Onken and Moyer, 1963). The effect on drug penetration is variable. Fredriksson (1969) showed major variations in penetration of the AChE inhibitor sarin in delipidized (solvent treated) guinea pigs compared to water-treated controls. However, Bucks et al. (1983) found no significant effect in humans treated with 1,1,1-trichlorethane in experiments with topical hydrocortisone absorption.

Stratum Corneum

The structure of the horny layer (stratum corneum) has been concisely reviewed by Stuttgen (1982), and we will include with it some description of the outer surface lipids and the transitional cells of the underlying stratum granulosum. Elias and co-workers (1979) have separated these layers intact from the epidermis with staphyloccocal epidermolytic toxin, describing the intact sheet as the "barrier layer." The irregular surface layer of lipids discussed in the previous section was described as hydrophobic (lipophilic) based on wetting characteristics of organic solvents. Rosenberg et al. (1973) have refined the concept by measuring contact angles of solvent droplets on live and excised skin for a range of solvent properties. The work clearly shows that human skin, live or excised, has a hydrophobic surface with no evidence of polar interactions. Variations in the composition of surface lipids were studied by Wilkinson (1969). Squalene, free fatty acids, free sterols, and sterol esters were detected.

The stratum corneum proper consists of dead, partially desiccated, horny cells developed from keratinocytes migrating to the skin surface. Horny cells are composed of keratin filaments, 60–80 Å in diameter, embedded in an amorphous matrix composed of lipoprotein (Stuttgen, 1982; Scheuplein and Blank, 1971). Two types can be distinguished. Those closest to the surface have a network-like structure of keratin, being denser and less homogeneous than the lower (basal) cells. The strength and chemical inertness of keratin is attributed to the cystine disulfide bonds of the matrix protein and the insoluble membrane protein encasing the horny cells (Stuttgen, 1982; Matoltsy, 1976). The transition from keratinocytes of the stratum granulosum to the real horny cells of the stratum corneum (SC) occurs sharply from one layer to the next, with total renewal of the SC every 28 d. Electron photomicrographs show adjacent cells to be highly interlocked, as well as closely stacked (Scheuplein and Blank, 1971). The interdigitation of these elongated cells may contribute to the mechanical strength of the epidermis, which is provided largely by the stratum corneum. Also visible in the micrographs are the filled intercellular regions. These regions make up 10% or more of the SC volume and are filled with mixtures of both neutral and polar lipids (Elias et al., 1977; Grayson and Elias, 1982). The neutral lipids compose about 75% of the total (Elias et al., 1981) and consist of complex hydrocarbons, free sterols, sterol esters, free fatty acids, and triglycerides. The polar lipids contain phosphatidyl-ethanolamine, phosphatidylcholine, lysolecithin, ceramides, and glycolipids. Together, they constitute the primary barrier to TEWL, allowing humans and animals to live in a nonaqueous environment.

Viable Epidermis and Dermis Layers

While the stratum corneum is considered to be the rate-limiting barrier in most cases of percutaneous absorption, the lower layers can become barriers for some molecular structures. The stratum corneum is nonviable, tightly packed with partially desiccated cells, and possessed of limited metabolic activity (Stuttgen, 1982). By contrast, the supporting epidermis is actively proliferating, hydrated, and capable of an extraordinary range of metabolic activity (Tauber, 1982; Pannatier et al., 1978; Noonan and Wester, 1985). It is the most metabolically active layer of the skin, responsible for both detoxifying and sometimes intoxifying migrant molecules prior to uptake in the dermis vascular system. Thus, it forms both a physical aqueous barrier for very lipophilic compounds and a biochemical barrier in the sense of transforming the primary penetrant.

The epidermis varies greatly in thickness for reasons stated earlier and consists of several compact layers of rapidly proliferating cells (keratinocytes). As described by Ridout and Guy (1988), these cells ascend from the basal layer of the epidermal-dermal junction, generating fibrous proteins as they transform from normal living cells into the keratinized cells of the strata granulosum and corneum. In addition to a variety of cell types, the epidermis supports both the sweat and sebaceous glands (Tauber, 1982). The sebaceous glands are responsible for the outer layer of sebum on the skin, which may provide a minor contribution to the SC barrier as discussed by Scheuplein and Blank (1971). Considered together with the dermis, these layers provide facile transport to the vascular system for polar and moderately lipophilic penetrants. They can, however, function as barriers or retention layers for very lipophilic compounds resistant to oxidative metabolism.

The dermis is supported on a layer of subcutaneous fat and is essentially noncellular, consisting of a dense matrix of fibrous, collageneous connective tissue imbedded in a hydrous mass of mucopolysaccharide containing numerous vessels involved in thermoregulation of the body (Ridout and Guy, 1988; Schalla and Schaefer, 1982). It has been suggested by Scheuplein (1967) that the rich vascularity of the superficial layers of the dermis should drastically limit diffusion into the lower lying layers. This assumes the vascular system to be a perfect sink, a concept recently challenged by Guy and Maibach (1983), who argue that deeper penetration with tissue localization may be a more common event. The dermis is also richly ennervated with sympathetic nerve fibers responsible for regulating vasoconstriction and dilation, thus affecting the rate of xenobiotic clearance. Response to local effects in temperature receptors (e.g., vasoconstriction from cold) or from higher CNS centers (e.g., anger, fear, embarrassment) can lead to immediate effects in the dermis vascular system. In addition, stimulation of the sweat glands for whatever reason results in local formation of bradykinin, a potent polypeptide vasodilator (Berne and Levy, 1983). These interactive effects may alter the overall pharmacokinetics in some clinical cases but are unlikely to generate a rate-limiting barrier to percutaneous absorption. Clearance under most circumstances is fast relative to epidermal transport.

MOLECULAR STRUCTURE: PHYSICOCHEMISTRY

The many factors involving the skin are complemented by the almost unlimited variation in molecular structure and corresponding properties of deliberate and accidental penetrants. On the deliberate side are drugs, vehicles, and adjuvants (permeation enhancers) designed to penetrate the skin to produce desirable effects. The structural range is very large, but at least defined by therapeutic need and under experimental or clinical control. Accidental percutaneous absorption covers a much greater range of molecular structure, may express severe toxicological effects, and is under no control except for the manufacturer's warning label on commercial products. From household chemicals and pesticides through a vast range of chemicals used in hundreds of industries, the variation in molecular structure covers almost the entire range of organic chemistry. How can we get a "handle" on this much structural variation for the purpose of predicting behavior? The answer lies in our ability to define molecular descriptors for each structure that confine the molecule to a range of chemical and physical behavior.

The following sections describe measurable and calculable molecular properties that impact directly on transdermal transport. Such properties provide a means of classifying penetrants and, when developed into quantitative relations, a means for predicting behavior.

Bulk and Physical Properties

Volume and bulk parameters as described by Charton are essentially extensive in nature (Charton, 1983; Charton and Charton, 1979). All basically rank molecular size in some property, the most common being molecular weight (MW), volume (V_w), surface area (A_w), and a variety of experimental values such as molar refractivity (MR) and the Parachor (P). The last two are based on index of refraction and surface tension measurements, but have predominant contributions from molecular volume.

$$\text{MR} = \frac{n^2 - 1}{n^2 + 2} \left(\frac{M}{D} \right) \qquad P = \frac{M}{D - d} \gamma^{1/4}$$

$n = n_D$, index of refraction γ = surface tension, dyn/cm
M = molecular weight d = saturated vapor density
D = liquid density

Molecular weight is the most primitive measure of bulk, depending only on constitution. The descriptor has been used by Lien and co-workers (Lien and Wang, 1980; Lien, 1981; Lien et al., 1982) in the form of log(MW), which they attribute to the reciprocal dependence of the diffusion coefficient on the cube root of MW in the Sutherland–Einstein equation. In cases of diffusion through a variety of artificial membranes and also through corneal membranes, they find a negative dependence on log(MW) as the sole descriptor or in combination with other factors (Lien et al., 1982). In a study of the blood-brain barrier (rat), Levin (1980) has used MW to define an approximate upper limit for permeability. However, direct correlation of the brain capillary permeability coefficients for 27 compounds (log PC) was not related to MW ($r = 0.264$), but to log P(octanol/water) ($r = 0.904$) (Levin, 1980; Magee, 1984). An upper MW limit for percutaneous absorption has not been demonstrated and may exceed 15,000 (Wester and Maibach, 1985), based on the reported penetration of heparin (MW 17,000). However, observed penetration does not imply that practical molar quantities can be moved to the vascular system. For the blood-brain barrier, Levin (1980) found an upper practical limit of about 400. Considering the difficulty of transdermal steroid transport (MW 300–400), this may also be a reasonable limit for skin.

With respect to transdermal penetration, there are some indications of a correlative role for MW. One of the earliest is reported by Marzulli et al. (1965) in finding a nearly linear relation between steady-state penetration rate of isolated SC for simple organophosphates. Much later, Cooper and Kasting (1987) report a significant relation of MW with human skin diffusion coefficients for 29 varied drugs. However, they find an equivalent fit of the data against molecular volume (V_w). In addition, Guy and Hadgraft (1988) find that inclusion of MW improves an existing correlation between permeability coefficients (hairless mouse skin) of various chemicals with measured partition coefficients. The problem with MW as a descriptor is twofold. It is seldom a unique descriptor, being frequently colinear with MR and V_w for particular compound sets such as Marzulli's phosphates. Moreover, other than the implied relation with passive diffusion, it conveys no mechanistic information.

Bondi's volume (V_w) and molar refractivity (MR) are highly colinear and readily calculated from nearly additive fragments for any molecule or substructure (Bondi, 1964; Martin, 1978). These descriptors model London or dispersion forces (mutual induced dipole moments) and have been widely used to quantitatively describe binding problems (Coats et al., 1982; Goldblum et al., 1981; Magee, 1986). Bondi's surface area (A_w) is so highly colinear with V_w as to be redundant and is seldom used (Moriguchi et al., 1976). To the extent that transdermal transport involves strong binding in the stratum corneum or elsewhere, MR would be the most appropriate descriptor, as it is more frequently used by other investigators and is based on experimental measurements related to polarizability, the key mechanistic factor in London forces.

Physical properties relevant to skin transport are viscosity and volatility. Normally, both are experimentally determined, though volatility can be estimated as boiling point, heat of vaporization, or vapor pressure from contributing molecular fragments, and viscosity from empirical equation dependence (Rechsteiner and Grain, 1982). Both come into play when occlusion experiments are performed to reduce volatility losses of applied penetrants. Occlusion promotes hydration of the stratum corneum and higher skin temperatures, reducing viscosity of the penetrant and increasing the rate of absorption (Scheuplein and Blank, 1971). As pointed out by Gummer (1985), the Stokes–Einstein equation requires an increase in the diffusion coefficient for a decrease in viscosity. It is interesting to speculate that an increase in temperature will reduce viscosity of the SC interstitial lipids. However, recent work by two groups show that SC lipids require 60–80 °C to undergo thermal transition (Al-Saidan et al., 1987; Golden et al., 1987). Below this range, permeability coefficients of test chemicals remain constant.

Transport Properties

Unlike bulk properties, which measure the volume or size of molecular structure, transport properties are thermodynamic in nature. Partitioning between two immiscible phases is characterized by a free energy difference at equilibrium, namely, the energetic difference for creating the molecular cavity in each phase. The most commonly used descriptor for partitioning events is the distribution of a drug or chemical between *n*-octanol and water. An enormous amount of experimental work has led to thousands of measured partition coefficients between water and every reasonable organic phase. These have been catalogued by Hansch and Leo (1979), in the well-known Pomona Medicinal Chemistry Project database (Daylight Info Systems). The pioneering work in QSAR by Hansch over the past 25 years has led to general acceptance of octanol/water partitioning as a worldwide standard. Recent work on propylene glycol dipelargonate is extensive and shows that efforts to find a superior organic phase are still underway (Leahy et al., 1989). At this writing, however, the octanol/water system is dominant and used by most researchers.

As experimentally determined (Leo et al., 1971), the distribution coefficient represents the ratio of the phase concentrations as defined by *P*.

$$P = \frac{[C]/\text{octanol}}{[C]/\text{water}}$$

Ideally, these should be activities or extrapolated to infinite dilution, a condition closely approached when labeled compounds are used to measure distribution. With respect to the octanol/water system, log *P* = 0 defines equal distribution and an imaginary division between hydrophilic ($-\log P$) and lipophilic ($+\log P$) compounds. No such division exists as every organic/water phase has a different $\log P$ zero. Consequently, some compounds, such as p-nitrophenol, appear strongly lipophilic in octanol/water ($\log P = 1.91$) and strongly hydrophilic in cyclohexane/water ($\log P = -1.86$) (Seiler, 1974). The $\log P$ zero for a partitioning system has no intrinsic meaning. Log P is a continuum where even for "very hydrophilic" compounds, one is always more lipophilic than the other.

On the log P(octanol/water) scale, most systemic behavior in agriculture and medicine is observed in the range -0.5 to 3.5 with optimum behavior near $\log P = 2.0$ (Briggs et al., 1976; Magee, 1979). This applies only to passive diffusional transport. Compounds with log P much above 3.5 are kinetically slow in crossing aqueous barriers. Below $\log P = -0.5$, compounds tend to be kinetically trapped in aqueous phases, though some can move by active transport. The stratum corneum has no operating active transport mechanisms. Nevertheless, small very polar chemicals like dimethyl sulfoxide (DMSO) ($\log P = -1.35$) move rapidly through the skin, but not without considerable damage. Dimethyl sulfoxide causes swelling, distortion, and intercellular delamination of the stratum corneum (Chandrasekaran et al., 1977). Even acetone, which is legitimately in the systemic range ($\log P = -0.24$), causes delipidization with significant alteration of the barrier (Wester and Maibach, 1985a). Small polar compounds such as acetic acid, ethanol, acetone, and DMSO are considered amphiphilic in the sense of having miscibility with both water and many organics. Because of these barrier-altering effects, the systemic range for percutaneous absorption can be estimated as $\log P = -1.5$ to 3.5.

Ionization is another important factor affecting log P and related transport properties. Full ionization of a carboxylic acid or an aliphatic amine can shift log P from the neutral value by four orders of magnitude (-4.0 in the log) (Hansch and Leo, 1979; Leo et al., 1971). For carboxylic acids and strongly basic amines, log P is determined for the neutral compounds by partitioning between n-octanol and $0.1\ N$ HCl or $0.1\ N$ NaOH to suppress ionization. These compounds will ionize spontaneously in the mid-pH ranges (5–9) and behave quite differently than the neutral log P values predict. Weakly acidic compounds like phenols undergo partial ionization that depends on the electronic character of the ring substituents. In such cases, valid relations with log P can be corrected by including the substituent electronic effect (sigma minus) in the correlation (Scherrer, 1984). It is also valid to measure the actual distribution coefficient (log D) at a fixed pH and to use this in place of neutral log P modified by the electrical effect (Scherrer, 1984; Lee et al., 1985). While more concise mathematically, this method obscures the electronic effect in ionization.

Log P has been a remarkably successful correlation descriptor for hundreds of transport and nonspecific bindings where organic/aqueous phases are involved (Hansch and Dunn, 1972; Hansch and Clayton, 1973; Dunn et al., 1986). However, between a biphasic stratum corneum and an organic vehicle, a drug has several partitions between immiscible phases that do not involve water. Partitioning between different organic phases is not well studied and there is no guarantee that log P(octanol/water) will be an adequate descriptor. Magee (1985) is currently working on a variation of log P (S log P = log P/n, n = number of molecular units) that appears capable of describing phase preference for organic/organic distributions.

Guy et al. (1985b) have described a complicating factor in dermis transport, namely, radial transport. In all probability, radial transport begins in the stratum corneum and continues with increased penetration. Thus, a circular application on the skin can spread severalfold in area before reaching the capillary matrix in the dermis, with obvious concentration effects on the pharmacokinetics. The observation of radial transport suggests an analogy with paper and thin-layer chromatography where compounds diffuse radially during transport. The difference, of course, is that chromatographic transport is entirely lateral while skin transport is top to bottom. The analogy is interesting, however, as Magee (1986) has recently analyzed the energetics of adsorption-desorption processes in chromatography. It is certainly easy to visualize a thin-layer experiment on whole sheet SC or on powdered SC that could be analyzed in the same manner.

Binding

The chromatography analogy leads directly into the role that binding may play in transdermal transport. Binding can be specific, partially specific, or nonspecific in nature. Specific binding at enzymic sites can tax the full strength of QSAR science, invoking quantum chemical description, conformational analysis, and other factors that fully describe the event (Magee, 1989). This does not seem appropriate for binding in the stratum corneum and subsequent layers. For example, conformation does not appear to be important. In a recent study by Sidon et al. (1988), there was no discernible difference between dermal absorption of *cis*- and *trans*-permethrin in rhesus monkeys and rats. There is also no significant difference in the penetration of linoleic and linolenic acids (Schalla and Schaefer, 1985). The absence of these subtleties suggests the absence of highly specific binding sites for most penetrants. True nonspecific binding with various albumins correlates well with log P of the binding chemicals, showing no evidence of H-bond involvement (Vandenbelt et al., 1972; Dunn, 1973a, 1973b). As proteins form about 50% of the dry weight of cells and occur in enormous variety (*Escherichia coli* contains approximately 1100 proteins), the opportunities for donor and acceptor H-bonds with penetrants are immense (Flickinger et al., 1979). This is strongly expressed in the extreme range of experimental flux (Scheuplein et al., 1969) and percent absorption of closely related steroids (Wester and Maibach, 1985a). Sensitivity to H-bonding is the only reasonable explanation for the 100-fold differences observed in these steroids. Direct correlational evidence for strong H-bonding is presented in the section on Correlational Analysis. Epidermal and dermal retention effects (binding) are reviewed by Menczel et al. (1985), while Wester et al. (1987) provide direct evidence for binding of simple chemicals to powdered stratum corneum.

In summary, nonspecific binding in the skin layers analogous to that observed for binding to albumin is probable only for simple compounds that cannot hydrogen bond to organized protein structures. Hydrogen bonding is an operable mechanism of binding for those molecules having one or more donor or acceptor atoms, leading to oriented, partially specific binding. There is no evidence for reversible specific binding as a retention factor in transdermal transport. Specific binding is clearly involved in irreversible metabolic transformations as discussed in the next section.

Reactivity

Chemical. The case for uncatalyzed chemical reactivity in proteins is well established. The case for direct reactivity in the skin is a logical extension (Dupuis and Benezra, 1982). Reactive groups in proteins provide opportunities for many types of direct chemical reaction as shown in Table 1.

Strong acids and bases such as methanesulfonic acid or hydrazine are capable of destroying skin by direct cleavage of the peptide bond. Weaker acids and bases can modify skin by simple protonation of key groups accompanied by ion pairing. Ion pairs where both anionic and cationic partners are large are strongly associated with over 20 kcal/mole of binding energy in low-dielectric media (Isaacs, 1987). Aldehydes such as glutaraldehyde react with free amino groups in lysine or terminal amino acids to form Schiff bases, essentially irreversible at physiological pH. Also reactive toward free amino groups are isocyanates, isothiocyanates,

$$RCH{=}O \; + \; H_2NR' \; \xrightarrow{\text{neutral}} \; RCH{=}NR' \; + \; H_2O$$

anhydrides, thiolesters, reactive halides, and neutral sulfenylating agents. Neutral sulfenylating agents such as captan fungicide can react noncatalytically with

TABLE 1. Reactive Peptide Groups

Peptide group or structure	Reactants
Peptide bond	Strong acids, bases
Free amino groups, lysine, terminal amino acids	Aldehydes, alkylating agents, sulfenylating agents, conjugated reactants
Phenolic groups, tyrosine	Bromine, sulfenylating agents, isocyanates
Free carboxyl groups	Isocyanates
Sulfhydryl, cysteine	Conjugated reactants, alkylating agents, sulfenylating agents, isocyanates, oxidants
Disulfide, cystine	Cyanide ion, mercaptides, oxidants
Imidazole, histidine	Alkylating agents, isocyanates

amino, phenolic, imidazole, and sulfhydryl groups. The fastest reaction by far is with sulfhydryl, and these groups will be titrated first. Sulfhydryl groups from cysteine residues are abundant (2–3.6%) in the fetal epidermis of guinea pigs and rats (Singer et al., 1971). The percentage decreases somewhat after birth and dramatically by adulthood, presumably replaced by cystine disulfide bonds responsible for strength and chemical inertness in the SC keratin (Stuttgen, 1982). Sulfhydryl groups are also highly reactive to conjugated systems capable of supporting the Michael addition, such as acrylic esters and amides, vinyl sulfones, quinones, and doubly reactive compounds like acrolein. The addition reactions and direct nucleophilic displacements on reactive halides require a minor assist from a neighboring proton acceptor, abundant in proteins. In percutaneous experiments with methacrylamide in rabbits, 25–60% of the compound was protein bound after 24 h (Hashimoto and Tanii, 1985).

$$O_2N\text{-}C_6H_3(NO_2)\text{-}Cl + H_2NR' \xrightarrow{\text{neutral}} O_2N\text{-}C_6H_3(NO_2)\text{-}NHR' + HCl$$

$$RCSR'' + H_2NR' \xrightarrow{\text{neutral}} RCNHR' + R''SH$$
(with C=O)

$$\text{THP-}NSCCl_3 + HSR' \xrightarrow{\text{neutral}} Cl_3SSR' + THPI$$

$$H_2C=CHCH=O + HSR' \xrightarrow{\text{base}} R'SCH_2CH_2CH=O$$

$$C_6H_3(CH_3)_2\text{-}NHCCH_2Cl + HSR' \xrightarrow{\text{base}} C_6H_3(CH_3)_2\text{-}NHCCH_2Cl + HCl$$

Cysteine residues are easily converted to cystine disulfide links by many oxidants accidentally or deliberately applied to the skin. Among these are bromine, hydrogen peroxide, and benzoyl peroxide. In the semirigid matrix of the stratum corneum, oxidation could lead to thiyl radicals of moderate lifetime, though this has not been demonstrated.

$$\text{(C}_6\text{H}_5\text{)} - \overset{O}{\underset{}{C}} - O - \overset{O}{\underset{}{C}} - \text{(C}_6\text{H}_5\text{)} + 2RSH \xrightarrow{\text{neutral}} RSSR + 2 \text{(C}_6\text{H}_5\text{)} - COOH$$

$$2RSH + Br_2 \xrightarrow{\text{neutral}} 2RS^{\cdot} + 2HBr$$
(separated)

Cystine disulfide bonds are a major factor in the physical toughness of the stratum corneum and are chemically inert to a majority of reactive chemicals. They are vulnerable, however, to strong oxidants and to direct cleavage by cyanide ion (Kice, 1971).

$$RSSR + 2H_2O_2 \xrightarrow{\text{neutral}} RSO_2SR \xrightarrow{H_2O} RSO_3H + RSH$$

$$RSSR + CN^- \xrightarrow{\text{neutral}} RSCN + RS^-$$

The examples presented here do not represent the full range of uncatalyzed reactivity of chemicals toward skin, but merely suggest it. The focus of this section is to establish nonenzymatic reactivity as a major factor in the transdermal penetration of reactive chemicals and drugs. This provides a natural opening to skin metabolic activity as many metabolites are skin-reactive chemicals.

Biochemical. Skin metabolism has been reviewed by several groups (Tauber, 1982; Pannatier et al., 1978; Noonan and Wester, 1985) and treated in theory by others (Guy and Hadgraft, 1985b; Ando et al., 1977). Metabolism is intimately linked with allergic contact dermatitis (Dupuis and Benezra, 1982) and is a critical factor in dermally delivered prodrugs (Friend et al., 1988). As stated earlier, the viable epidermis is the major metabolic barrier to transdermal transport. The term "barrier" is used in the sense of reducing permeation of an applied chemical below that expected from its chemical potential. For example, aldicarb insecticide (temik) has an acute oral LD50 (rat) of 0.93 mg/kg, while the acute dermal is greater than 200 (Hartley and Kidd, 1983). Thus, the skin provides a nearly perfect metabolic barrier in the case of this AChE inhibitor. As the oral route forces a "first pass" through the liver, the skin can be very impressive as a metabolic organ. Some preprocessing may occur in the stratum corneum, which possesses a number of active enzymes derived from the horny cells and from sebum and microbiological growth in the SC (Stuttgen, 1982). However, the real capacity and metabolic variety exist in the viable epidermis. Metabolism is case sensitive, and the efficient degradation of aldicarb and many other toxic *N*-methylcarbamates does not imply generally greater activity in skin compared to liver. A case in point is the metabolic activation of ethyl parathion by mixed-function oxidase (mfo) oxidation to ethyl paraoxon, a lethal AChE inhibitor. Ethyl paraoxon is an ideal systemic (log $P = 1.98$), placing the toxicant on an equal basis after activation by the skin or liver. In addition, parathion is rapidly absorbed by the skin and no physical barrier is indicated. Dermal toxicity to rats (LD50 = 20–60 mg/kg) is about 25% of the oral toxicity (LD50 = 6–15), suggesting a similar fraction of mfo relative to the liver (Hartley and Kidd, 1983). Without belaboring the point, these examples show that skin can both activate and deactivate by enzymatic metabolism in parallel with the liver, providing a true first pass for many externally applied chemicals. The cited reviews show that skin and liver enzymes are similar, if not identical, in mixed-function oxidases, aromatic hydroxylases, dehydrogenases, ketoreductase, epoxyhydratase (epoxide hydrolysis), and various esterases. The skin also contains transferases for glucuronide and sulfate formation as well as glutathione conjugation. Activity varies from tenths of a percent to several percent and occasionally to near equivalence of liver activity for whole skin (Pannatier et al., 1978; Noonan and Wester, 1985). Activity in the epidermis (about 2.5% of whole skin) can equal or exceed that of the liver (Noonan and Wester, 1985).

Our purpose in this section is not to review skin metabolism, but rather to highlight it as an important factor and constant companion of transdermal transport. Some of the most interesting examples are those in which the metabolite is chemically reactive to skin structures. Many of these examples are associated with allergic contact dermatitis where biotransformation leads directly to irreversible chemical binding. While ordinary reactive chemicals (haptens) such as acrylates, quinones, or picryl chloride can react directly with skin to induce contact dermatitis, others (prohaptens) must be metabolically activated. A classic example is the metabolism of urushiol (poison ivy) to the cysteine-reactive *ortho*-quinone (Dupuis, 1979). Blocking the oxidation by methylation produces an inactive dimethoxy analog (Baer et al., 1966, 1970). Many other examples are cited by Dupuis and Benezra (1982).

Reaction with skin structures by directly active or metabolically activated chemicals will lead to physical changes that may obscure attempts to relate structure with flux. Even a related series of chemicals selected for a structure-flux study can give confusing results if the degree of parent structure metabolism varies inversely with the penetration rate. Structures penetrating most rapidly will undergo the least metabolism and/or irreversible binding. Long residence in the epidermal layer can also lead to greater enzyme induction and proportionately greater metabolism for slow moving penetrants. Inductions up to 30-fold have been observed in aromatic HC hydroxylase (Noonan and Wester, 1985). Of course, the skin can become saturated as reactive sites are used up and it is easy to imagine that initial and steady-state flux rates can be quite different for reactive penetrants. There is no question that pharmacokinetic models and correlations of molecular structure with flux are seriously complicated by both simple reactivity and metabolism.

TRANSPORT MODELS AND MECHANISMS

Models

The simplest model for transdermal transport is that of a rate-limiting epidermal barrier as described by Higuchi (1982). From a uniform matrix containing the drug, transport is limited by the stratum corneum, with the other skin layers acting as a perfect sink. This model came into early use because it works well for many uncomplicated drugs and chemicals in the systemic range (log $P = -1.5$ to $+3.5$). *In vitro* cell studies for transport across an excised patch of whole skin use a solvent on the dermis side to ensure perfect sink conditions. Reversible transport or accumulation in the dermis (slow clearance) is minimized experimentally. The concept of a simple monobarrier has led to a number of excellent transport studies with model membranes such as isopropyl myristate (IPM), tetradecane (Hadgraft and Ridout, 1987; Houk et al., 1987), and ethylene vinyl acetate copolymers (Friend et al., 1989). There is a strong similarity in the transport behavior of a series of phenols against IPM, tetradecane, and human skin (Houk et al., 1987), in support of a simple monobarrier model.

More sophisticated models have been developed for particular drugs (Wallace and Barnett, 1978; Ogiso et al., 1989; Guy and Hadgraft, 1985a; Chandrasekaran et al., 1978), for broad ranges of chemical behavior (Guy et al., 1985; Carver et al., 1989), to model ongoing metabolism (Guy and Hadgraft, 1985b) and to test for parallel pathways (Wallace and Barnett, 1978; Ogiso et al., 1989). Many theoretical treatments of pharmacokinetic models are in print (Guy and Hadgraft, 1983, 1985b; Albery and Hadgraft, 1979; Zatz, 1985; Kubota and Ishizaki, 1985). The principle features of these models are acceptance of multiple barriers and reversible transport. Simplifying assumptions are made in most skin absorption models to keep the kinetic expressions within reason. The absorption model of Guy and Hadgraft (1985b) considers concurrent metabolism and provides an excellent case for discussion. These are several points of interest. First, note that delivery from the vehicle through the stratum corneum is represented by a single rate constant, k_1. Reversibility is not considered even though partitioning between vehicles and isolated stratum corneum is well known (Bronaugh and Congdon, 1984; Anderson et al., 1988). Reversible transport is considered only between the viable epidermis and SC with the ratio k_1/k_3 representing the partitioning process. Transport of the applied drug (k_2, k_4) and transport of its metabolite (k_5/k_6) are treated as unidirectional. These assumptions are necessary to minimize the mathematical complexity of the model. By adjusting the rate constants experimentally, profiles can be developed that closely match observed behavior in this model (Guy and Hadgraft, 1985a, 1985b) and others (Carver et al., 1989; Guy et al., 1982, 1983).

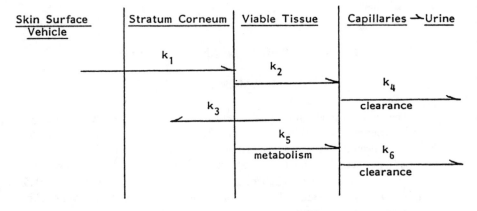

Percutaneous absorption is driven by concentration (Zatz and Dalvi, 1983) and is dependent on the thickness or volume of the tissue barriers. This is best represented by recasting the Guy and Hadgraft model into compartments where C_n and V_n represent the concentrations and tissue or vehicle volumes. Note that C_3 (concentration of applied chemical) and C_3' (metabolite concentration) are compartmented kinetically but occupy the same epidermal tissue, V_3. No reversibility of the polar metabolite into the SC is considered. In the final dermis/capillary compartment, C_4 represents the concentration derived from transport of C_3 and C_3'. Clearance is assumed to be fast relative to k_1, k_2, and k_3. The frequent success of these simplified models speaks well for the judgment of the investigators in emphasizing the probable rate determining steps. The amount of drug entering the stratum corneum at time t and the rate constant k_1 can be estimated by analyzing repeated tape strippings (Rougier et al., 1983, 1987; Tojo and Lee, 1989). This procedure provides experimental support for the pharmacokinetic models.

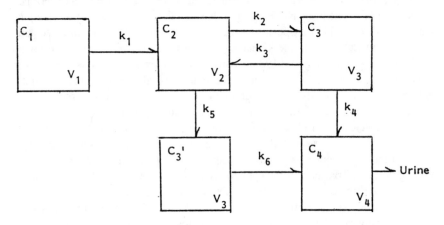

Steady-state conditions are probably not achieved *in vivo*. However, the slow approach to a steady state can be demonstrated *in vitro*, as a lag time intercept in plots of drug penetration versus time (Wallace and Barnett, 1978). Parallel pathways have also been suggested by *in vitro* studies (Wallace and Barnett, 1978; Ogiso et al., 1989), consistent with the biphasic structure of the stratum corneum (Michaels et al., 1975; Elias, 1983).

Mechanisms

Passive Transport. Penetration of a drug from the vehicle through the stratum corneum (k_1 in the model) may be passive or interactive. Fick's first law should apply or be closely approximated if the transport is purely diffusional. In one of its simplest forms,

$$dQ/dt = DK_p(C_d - C_r)/h$$

where dQ/dt is the rate of barrier penetration, D the diffusion constant, K_p the partition coefficient of drug between skin and vehicle, C_d the drug concentration in vehicle, C_r the drug concentration in receptor (sink), and h the barrier thickness. The rate of penetration dQ/dt is often expressed as a flux (J) in experimental units like $\mu g/cm^2 \cdot h$ (Michaels et al., 1975). As an equilibrium measure, the partition coefficient K_p will not vary much with moderate changes in temperature. However, the diffusion constant D is sensitive to temperature, and the rate of penetration increases accordingly. As a consequence, activation energies have been determined for water (Blank, 1985), various alcohols (Scheuplein and Blank, 1971; Rosenberg et al., 1973), ethyl ether, 2-butanone, 2,3-butanediol (Blank et al., 1967), a variety of phenols (Roberts et al., 1978), and three drugs of significant complexity (Ito et al., 1988).

Table 2 summarizes the data by ranking the log P(octanol/water) coefficient. There is clearly a drop in activation energy between log P = 1.90–2.10, suggesting one pathway for polar compounds, log P = −1.0 to 1.5, a transition from about 1.5 to 2.0, and a lower-energy path for more lipophilic compounds. These observations are valid when the stratum corneum is the rate-determining barrier and perfect sink conditions are established experimentally. Ito et al. (1988) have observed very high activation energies for two carboxylic acid drugs (indomethacin, $E\ddagger$ = 44.5; ibuprofen, $E\ddagger$ = 41.4) and for sulfanilamide ($E\ddagger$ = 30.4) using abdominal skin from the hairless rat. These values suggest an overriding effect of hydrogen bonding, independent of partitioning. Table 2 also contains some evidence of this for simple compounds. Thus, 2,3-butanediol and ethoxyethanol form stronger H-bonds than *n*-butanol, as does resorcinol versus phenol. The interplay of simple partitioning and H-bonding to protein structures is a feature common to all layers of the skin.

Recent work by Guy and co-workers shows substantial activation energies for simple interfacial transfer of nicotinic esters from water to *n*-octanol and from water to isopropyl myristate (Guy and Honda, 1984; Fleming et al., 1983). The interfacial transfer of methyl nicotinate from water to *n*-octanol has

TABLE 2. Activation Energies: Transdermal Transport

Compound	log P(o/w)	$E\ddagger$ (kcal/mol)	Reference[a]
Water	—	15	1
2,3-Butanediol	−0.92	>20	3
Ethanol	−0.30	16.4	2
2-Ethoxyethanol	−0.10	20 ± 2	3
2-Butanone	0.29	16 ± 2	3
n-Propanol	0.30	16.5	2
Ethyl ether	0.80	16 ± 2	3
Resorcinol	0.80	17.8	4
n-Butanol	0.88	16.7	2
Phenol	1.46	14.4	4
n-Pentanol	1.47	16.5	2
4-Methylphenol	1.94	13.7	4
3-Nitrophenol	2.00	13.3	4
n-Hexanol	2.03	10.9	2
2-Chlorophenol	2.15	9.6	4
n-Heptanol	2.49	9.9	2
4-Bromophenol	2.59	8.8	4
n-Octanol	2.97	8.7	2
2,4,6-Trichlorophenol	3.69	9.1	4

[a]References: 1, Blank (1985); 2, Scheuplein and Blank (1971); 3, Blank et al. (1967); 4, Roberts et al. (1978).

an enthalpy of activation equal to 10.3 kcal/mol at 20 °C. While most activation energies for multilayer transdermal transport are higher (Table 2), this value strongly suggests a special low-energy pathway for the higher alcohols and lipophilic compounds.

In general, membrane and soft tissue transport involving both organic and aqueous phases correlates well with experimental log P(octanol/water) values (Hansch and Dunn, 1972; Hansch and Clayton, 1973). Partitioning between the SC and viable epidermis can be defined by k_2/k_3 in the pharmacokinetic model, and indeed, this is found to correlate with log P for nine diverse chemicals (Guy et al., 1985a). Less obvious would be log P correlations for partitioning among the three nonaqueous phases of the vehicle and SC. That these organic/organic partitionings should correlate at least fairly well with log P(octanol/water) is supported by the following argument. Most organic/aqueous partitionings show good to excellent linear relations with log P(octanol/water) (Leo et al., 1971). Each represents the difference in free energy ($-RT \ln P$) of forming a cavity in water versus a cavity in the organic phase. As these are linear free energy relations, it is permissible to subtract two of them to generate a virtual partitioning between two organic phases as shown. While not achievable experimentally, this partition represents the free energy difference of forming cavities in *n*-octanol and chloroform and should clearly correlate with log P(octanol/water). Correlations of log P with partitioning among two or more organic phases are therefore

$$\log P(CHCl_3/H_2O) = 1.13 \log P(octanol/H_2O) - 1.34$$

$$n = 28 \quad r = 0.967$$

$$\log P(octanol/H_2O) - \log P(CHCl_3/H_2O) = \log P(octanol/CHCl_3)$$

anticipated. In support of this, many log P relations have been reported for stratum corneum partitioning (Wester and Maibach, 1985a; Bronaugh and Congdon, 1984; Anderson et al., 1988; Anderson and Raykar, 1989) and for skin permeability (Ridout and Guy, 1988; Houk et al., 1987; Tojo and Lee, 1989; Flynn, 1985; Jetzer et al., 1986; Roberts et al., 1977; Huq et al., 1986; Tojo et al., 1988b). These relations are discussed in more detail under Correlational Analysis.

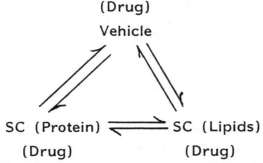

(Drug)

Vehicle

SC (Protein) ⇌ **SC (Lipids)**

(Drug)   **(Drug)**

Reversible binding of chemicals in the epidermal and dermal layers during penetration has been observed by many investigators and reviewed by Menczel et al. (1985). Such binding can be considered part of the barrier process and will generally correlate with log P for nonspecific association with dermal structures (Vandenbelt et al., 1972; Dunn, 1973a, 1973b). Binding of this type will retard penetration and increase the lag time to steady-state behavior (Tojo et al., 1988a), but will still follow Fick's law. Strong specific binding, however, or binding with reactivity (irreversible) will lead to non-Fickian behavior. Binding and retention of chemicals in the epidermal and dermal layers are naturally related, and many examples (Schalla and Schaefer, 1985; Menczel et al., 1985; Tojo et al., 1988a; Koch et al., 1988) have been cited.

Rate-Limiting Barriers

The stratum corneum is nature's principal barrier to catastrophic water loss and the ingress of foreign chemicals. However, the enormous range of chemical properties expressed by neutral or ionized molecules can overcome the default barrier and shift to a different transport mechanism. The stratum corneum offers at least two pathways for transport, either or both of which can be rate-limiting. A gradual shift from one pathway to the other can occur within a related series of compounds to complicate the structure-flux relation. If the series of compounds under study covers a broad enough range of log P values, the rate-limiting barrier can actually shift from the stratum corneum to the epidermal or dermal layers. This is clearly seen in studies by Behl and co-workers of C1–C8 alkanol permeation through hairless mouse skin (Behl et al., 1980, 1982). The regularity of the series breaks at n-octanol, which is clearly controlled by a different rate-limiting barrier, presumably the viable epidermis. Octanol has a log P(octanol/water) of 2.93, suggesting a barrier change some-what below this. Supporting evidence of a barrier change with increasing li-pophilicity comes from studies of phenols penetrating mouse and human skin (Jetzer et al., 1986; Roberts et al., 1977). Plots of the permeability coefficient against log P(octanol/water) are bilinear with a change in slope near log P = 2.3–2.4. This is consistent with normal behavior (SC limited) for n-heptanol (log P = 2.41). Very lipophilic compounds such as cypermethrin insecticide (log P = 5.39) and DDT (log P = 6.36) may penetrate the epidermal layers but do not penetrate whole skin (Scott and Ramsey, 1987; Grissom et al., 1987), being trapped in the dermis by an inability to diffuse through aqueous phases.

Parallel routes within the stratum corneum are easily detectable. Partition studies between SC and water of two phenols with log P = 1.63 and 1.95 show no difference between untreated and delipidized SC (Anderson and Raykar, 1989). This can only mean that these systemic compounds are partitioning exclusively into the protein domain of the SC. Referring back to Table 2, the sharp decrease in activation energy for alkanols occurs between n-pentanol (log P = 1.47) and n-hexanol (log P = 2.03), which presumably penetrates partly through the SC lipid barrier. The activation energy continues to drop with n-heptanol and n-octanol (log P = 2.93). This suggests that the SC lipid route becomes competitive around log P = 2.0 and fully functional above log P = 2.5 where the barrier gradually shifts from SC to viable epidermis. Elias et al. (1980) provide evidence that linoleic acid plays a key role in the lipid barrier function of SC.

Successive tape stripping has been known since 1940 to systematically remove layers of the stratum corneum (Wolf, 1940). In a recent study by Tojo et al. (1988b), the enhancement of penetration rate was plotted as a function of the number of strippings, n. The enhancement increased markedly with each strip-ping and then reached a plateau at a critical number, n_c (about 10). This obser-vation suggests a clearly defined boundary between the SC and viable epider-mis. Tape stripping studies by Feldman and Maibach (1965) produced some exceptionally interesting results with topically applied hydrocortisone. Despite a nearly ideal systemic log P = 1.61, the penetration rate only doubles after SC stripping. The authors suggested that both the SC and underlying layers served as skin barriers. This is contrary to expectations based solely on log P and points to the operation of multiple hydrogen bonds in binding hydrocortisone (2 C=O, 3 OH) in each layer.

In concluding this discussion of barriers, the reader should be aware of an exceptionally clear study of skin barriers by Marzulli (1962). Labeled tri-n-propyl and tri-*n*-butyl phosphates were studied on SC, full skin, stripped skin, dermis, and epidermis by a cell technique. Cumulative penetration is plotted against time to reveal the relations of each barrier for tri-*n*-propyl phosphate ($\log P = 1.87$). Stratum corneum and whole epidermis are nearly indistinguishable at steady state, while full skin, stripped skin, and dermis are increasingly permeable as expected. The plots obtained by Marzulli are for an ideal systemic, and it would be most interesting to see the progression of barrier behavior for penetrants with $\log P = 2.50$–4.00. Further studies in the same experimental style are clearly needed to define barriers as a function of penetrant properties. Strong hydrogen-bonding drugs like hydrocortisone, *para*-aminobenzoic acid (PABA), and sulfanilamide should be similarly studied.

CORRELATIONAL ANALYSIS

Stratum Corneum

The interaction of chemicals with the dominant barrier has been studied with the intact layer, with powdered SC, and on living subjects by tape stripping. The opportunity to describe behavior through plots or regression analysis is present whenever a series of compounds is measured by the same experimental methods. Measurements addressing mechanism include equilibrium binding (SC $\rightleftharpoons$ vehicle), nonequilibrium retention (*in vivo*), and steady-state flux. Barriers within the SC can be studied by comparing permeability data for natural SC and delipidized SC. With respect to drugs or chemicals, there are basically two types of experimental series, related and unrelated. Related compounds have a well-defined parent structure where physicochemical properties can be described in terms of varying chain length or substituents (Hansch and Leo, 1979). Unrelated compounds have no common skeletal structure and physicochemical properties must be based on measured or calculated values for the whole molecule (Rechsteiner and Grain, 1982).

Equilibrium partitioning and/or binding has been studied with whole SC (Wester and Maibach, 1985b; Raykar et al., 1988; Surber et al., 1989) and with powdered SC from adult foot calluses (Wester et al., 1987). Partitioning from water into whole SC is a slow diffusional process requiring 6–24 h for equilibrium at 37 °C (Raykar et al., 1988; Surber et al., 1989). The $\log P(\text{SC/water})$ reaches a maximum value around 6 hours for a series of steroids but requires longer for some phenols (Surber et al., 1989). Adsorption into powdered SC from water is much faster and essentially complete within 30 min at 37 °C (Wester et al., 1987). The very lipophilic polychlorobiphenyl (about 5 chlorines) is 96% partitioned into the SC within 30 min. There are only three compounds in this study, but the rank order of percent partitioned into SC— PCB (95.7), benzene (16.6), and 4-nitroaniline (2.5) is the same as the log $P(\text{octanol/water})$ rank: 6.51, 2.13, 1.39. A broader set of experimental chemicals would verify this relation with log P and permit the study of modifying effects, such as hydrogen bonding.

Raykar et al. (1988) studied a series of 11 hydrocortisone 21-esters by measuring SC/water partition coefficients for natural and delipidized stratum corneum. The esters cover a log P(octanol/water) range from 0.6 to 5.5. The relation of log P(SC/water) with log P(octanol/water) is smoothly curvilinear but when factored into protein and lipid domains, the relations are linear with slopes of 0.24 and 0.91, respectively. Lipid partitioning becomes important at approximately 3.0 on the log P(octanol/water) scale. A related study by Surber and Maibach on 14 different compounds having a log P range of -0.07 (caffeine) to 6.4 (etretin) was analyzed by Magee (Surber et al., 1989). The log P(SC/water) for 13 of the compounds gave a linear correlation with log P(octanol/water) with no evidence of curvature. The regression slope (0.253) agrees with that observed by Raykar and co-workers for partitioning of hydrocortisone esters into the SC protein domain (0.24). The outlier in the set is benzoic acid, which has a neutral log $P = 1.87$:

$$\log P(\text{SC/w}) = 0.253 \log P(\text{o/w}) + 0.860$$

$$T = 7.26$$

$$n = 13 \quad r = 0.909 \quad s = 0.263 \quad F = 52.46$$

and an ionized log P of about -2.0. Entering -2.0 in place of 1.87 for benzoic acid restores this compound to the set and improves the relation. It is clear that benzoic acid and other acids of similar or greater strength partition as the anion.

$$\log P(\text{SC/w}) = 0.274 \log P(\text{o/w}) + 0.775$$

$$T = 9.38$$

$$n = 14 \quad r = 0.938 \quad s = 0.264 \quad F = 87.93$$

In vivo retention in the stratum corneum can be measured by analysis of tape strips after a period of time. Rougier and co-workers (1983, 1987) have analyzed the stratum corneum (6 strippings) after 30 min of contact with 10 unrelated chemicals. In a most remarkable correlation ($r = 0.998$), they find a linear relation between SC absorption at 0.5 h and cumulative penetration at 96 h. Using a similar technique on human volunteers, Bucks and co-workers (1988) have studied the mass balances of four steroids under occluded and protected (nonocclusive) conditions. An extension of this work to 16 compounds (2 steroids, 12 phenols, 2 others) has been analyzed by Magee with surprising results (Bucks et al., 1990). The amount retained in the stratum corneum after 24 h (10 strippings) shows no correlation with log P(octanol/water), but correlates highly with the rank order of hydrogen bond donors (HBD) and acceptors (HBA). No other factors were detected.

$\log R = \log(\%$ retained in SC/24 h) — occluded study
(8 phenols, 2 polyesters) — no outliers

$$\log R = 0.850\text{HDB} + 0.581\text{HBA} - 2.11$$

$T = 3.51 \qquad\qquad 5.92$

$n = 10 \qquad r = 0.913 \qquad s = 0.480 \qquad F = 17.51$

$\log R = \log(\%$ retained in SC/24 h) — protected study
(2 steroids, 12 phenols) — 2 outliers deleted

$$\log R = 1.04\text{HBD} - 2.36$$

$T = 5.16$

$n = 12 \qquad r = 0.853 \qquad s = 0.485 \qquad F = 26.58$

$$\log R = 1.18\text{HBA} - 1.21$$

$T = 5.66$

$n = 12 \qquad r = 0.873 \qquad s = 0.452 \qquad F = 32.09$

In the protected study, HBA and HBD were highly colinear for these 12 compounds ($r = 0.893$) and could not be included together. This study clearly indicates that strong hydrogen bonding can override log P as a correlating factor. Donors (OH, NH) and acceptors (O, C=O) are roughly equivalent in forming H-bonds with the SC protein domain.

Steady-state permeability of SC was studied by Anderson et al. (1988) using the same 11 hydrocortisone esters from the SC partitioning experiments (Raykar et al., 1988). A log-log plot of the permeability coefficients versus their SC/water partition coefficients was fitted by a curvilinear regression. Inspection of the plotted points, however, suggests a bilinear relation with a change in transport mechanism near log P(SC/water) = 1.7, approximately where lipid domain partitioning becomes important (Anderson et al., 1988). In a related study of substituted p-cresols of log P(octanol/water) range $= -0.09$ to 1.95, the log P(SC/water) coefficients were identical in untreated and delipidized SC. These compounds fall on the same line with the hydrocortisone esters when the protein domain log P(SC/water) is plotted against log P(octanol/water), slope $= 0.27$ (Anderson and Raykar, 1989).

Much more precise work will be needed to fully understand partitioning into, binding in, and permeation of the stratum corneum. As a working hypothesis, partitioning into the protein domain is virtually exclusive for compounds with log P below 2.0. Competitive partitioning into the lipid domain occurs for more lipophilic compounds, and this may lead to bilinear or curvilinear log P relations. Hydrogen bonding in the protein domain can be an important modifier of behavior and may even dominate the mechanism.

Whole Skin

For a majority of chemicals, behavior in the stratum corneum will be mirrored in whole skin as Rougier and co-workers describe (1983, 1987). Thus, we can expect to find reports of log *P* correlations (Ridout and Guy, 1988; Wester and Maibach, 1985a; Houk et al., 1987; Bronaugh and Congdon, 1984; Michaels et al., 1975; Flynn, 1985; Jetzer et al., 1986; Roberts et al., 1977; Huq et al., 1986; Yano et al., 1986; Guy and Hadgraft, 1988) and correlations based on carbon count for homologous series (Wester and Maibach, 1985a; Flynn, 1985; Flynn et al., 1981; Durrheim et al., 1980). Homologous series are of little informational value in structure-flux relations as the carbon count is colinear with log *P*, molecular volume, polarizability, surface area, MW, and vapor pressure. As a working hypothesis, all of these relations can be considered to be log *P* relations. In support of this hypothesis, a plot of alkyl chain length versus partitioning of *n*-alkanols from 0.9% saline into full-thickness skin shows a change in mechanism between C6 and C7 (Flynn et al., 1981). This corresponds to log *P*(octanol/water) = 2.03 and 2.49, about where we now expect a change to occur. Penetration studies show a change in mechanism for *n*-alkanols between C7 and C8, again supporting the concept that chain length is analogous to log *P* (Behl et al., 1980, 1982).

Instead of reviewing another series of log *P* correlations, let us consider only those cases of particular interest where the chemical under study or the correlation has some feature of mechanistic interest. Those relations having a broad enough range in log *P* to show a change in mechanism are the most interesting. The observed changes can be bilinear with a sharp log *P* transition or curvilinear (parabolic approximation) where the optimum log *P* is the mechanistic midpoint. Both types are equally common throughout biochemical transport relations (Hansch and Clayton, 1973; Kubinyi, 1977).

Studies with complex hydrophilic compounds are rare and one wonders whether a simple log *P* relation will hold in regions outside of most experimental work. This question is partially resolved by Michaels et al. (1975) in permeation studies of human skin. An exceptionally broad range of unrelated compounds from fentanyl (log *P* = 3.49) to oubain (log *P* = −2.00) was studied. Oubain ($C_{29}H_{44}O_{12}$) and digitoxin ($C_{41}H_{64}O_{13}$, log *P* = 1.85) fit nicely on a plot of log(Flux)(cm/h × 10^3) versus log *P*(mineral oil/water). There appears to be a barrier change near estradiol (log *P* = 2.49). This study shows that both structurally complex and very hydrophilic compounds can conform to an existing log *P*–flux relation supported by much simpler compounds. There is an element of surprise here, as one might expect strong deviations for oubain and digitoxin due to multiple hydrogen bonding in the stratum corneum. This is not observed.

The treatment of skin as a membrane and its comparison with artificial membranes were reviewed by Nacht and Yeung (1985). Steady-state flux of salicylic acid, hydrocortisone, and water shows comparable flux for human skin and a variety of artificial membranes. Moreover, the transport behavior of compound series is remarkably similar. For a number of homologous series, Yalkowsky and Flynn (1973) and Kubinyi (1977) have shown analogous behavior for transport across synthetic and biological membranes, including human stratum corneum. Bilinear behavior with plateau or maxima is characteristic of most homologous series when log(responses) or log(flux) is plotted against chain length. Partitioning of alkanols from ethanol to *n*-nonanol into full-thickness hairless mouse skin is bilinear with a sharp increase in slope from C6 to C9. The higher slope corresponds to lipid domain partitioning and is very close to the slope for partitioning into polydimethylsiloxane as shown by Flynn et al. (1981). More recent work by Ridout and Guy (1988) and by Hadgraft and Ridout (1987) describes the use of isopropyl myristate (IPM) and tetradecane (TD) as *in vitro* models for skin lipids. While quantitative differences exist in shape and optima, the log-log plots of a series of phenol permeability coefficients versus octanol/water partitioning are quite similar for human skin, mouse skin, IPM, and TD. Jetzer and co-workers (1986) have shown closely analogous behavior for permeation of eight phenols through mouse skin, human skin, and silicone rubber. The permeability of mouse and human skin differ, but the barrier transition occurs at log $P = 2.4$ in both cases.

Both simple and complex phenolic compounds show optimal curvilinear or bilinear plots of log(% absorbed) or log(resistance) versus log P(octanol/water) (Houk et al., 1987; Roberts et al., 1977; Yano et al., 1986). Roberts et al. (1977) treat their data on 19 simple phenols penetrating human epidermis in a bilinear plot of log K_p(permeability) versus log P(octanol/water). The transition to a lower log K_p/log P slope occurs near log $P = 2.3$. Houk and co-workers (1987) have converted these data to skin transport resistance and describe a "parabolic" relation with log P. When the changes in slope are mild as in this case, the difference between a parabolic and bilinear description is basically a judgment call. The main difference here is that permeability versus log P is positively curved while transport resistance is negatively curved.

Magee (1990) has treated the permeability data of Roberts and co-workers by regression analysis using the parabolic approximation and testing for phenol ionization by including the electronic descriptor σ^-. Differential ionization of the 19 phenols is clearly indicated by the significant sigma correlation. Sigma minus is derived from the pK_a of phenols and correlation means that transport is occurring by two species, neutral and anionic. As log P for an anionic molecule lies 3–4 log units below the neutral log P, the correlation is an important part of the mechanism.

$$K_p = \text{permeability constant (cm/min} \times 10^5)$$

$$\log K_p = 2.38 \log P - 0.36 \overline{\log P^2} - 0.28 \Sigma\sigma^- - 1.89$$

$$T = 8.12 \qquad\qquad 5.92 \qquad\qquad 2.75$$

$$n = 19 \qquad r = 0.962 \qquad s = 0.171 \qquad F = 62.75$$

Finally, Yano and co-workers (1986) provide an instructive look at 8 salicylic derivatives and 10 diverse nonsteroidal antiinflammatory drugs. The measurements are performed on male volunteers (ventral forearm occluded with aluminum foil) with analysis of foil and skin rinse (ether) after 4 h. Immediate recovery from a second site is used as a reference and data are calculated as percent absorption. The experimental error is certainly higher than *in vitro* experiments, and distinguishing between parabolic and bilinear in plotting $\log(\%Abs)$ versus $\log P$ is not possible. The authors choose the parabolic approximation, and fairly well-defined optima are seen for both series. In full consistency with data from other studies, each plot shows optimal absorption (transport) at about $\log P = 2.3$. In fact, this and many other transdermal optima strongly resemble ordinary transport through membranes and soft tissue. For example, Hansch and co-workers (1967) find optimal behavior for hypnotic activity of barbiturates on rats, mice, and rabbits with $\log P_o$ (optima) ranging from 1.65 to 2.71 (average of 8 sets = 2.11). Regression of all eight data sets together weights the points equally ($n = 101$) and gives a calculated average $\log P_o = 2.21$ (Magee, 1979a).

One tempting conclusion from these comparisons is that transdermal transport and passive transport in soft tissue are mechanistically identical except for slow kinetics and a multiplicity of different barriers in skin.

SUMMARY AND CONCLUSIONS

Whole skin is viewed as a multilayered, heterogeneous organ with variability based on site, condition, age, gender, race, hydration, lipid content, and other factors. The stratum corneum is the principal barrier for TEWL and ingress of most xenobiotics. Its complex layers of interlocking, partially desiccated horny cells provide the main source of physical strength to the epidermis. The intercellular regions of the SC are filled with complex lipids defining a separate domain for chemical transport. Supporting the SC is the viable epidermis, a metabolic powerhouse that provides easy transport to the dermis capillary system for polar and moderately lipophilic compounds. Above $\log P = 2.5$ on the octanol/water scale, the epidermis provides increasing resistance to chemicals that partition poorly into aqueous phases.

The enormous range of chemicals deliberately or inadvertently applied to skin can be represented in terms of measurable or calculable molecular descriptors. Bulk descriptors such as MR correlate with London forces in strong binding events where polarizability and induced dipole moments come into play. The $\log P$(octanol/water) is the key descriptor for passive transport by partitioning, at least in the systemic range, which covers $\log P = -1.5$ to 3.5 for skin. Nonspecific binding to protein matter also correlates with $\log P$. However, strong H-bonding may be expressed by some penetrants and this can override the expected log *P* relation. Other than H-bonding in protein domains, there is no evidence for reversible, specific binding sites that recognize subtle differences in conformation or isomeric structures.

There is plenty of evidence for irreversible binding associated with chemical or metabolic.reactivity. Many protein structures undergo direct, uncatalyzed reactions with reactive chemicals. In addition, most metabolic processes available to the liver are operable in the viable epidermis with minor contributions from the SC. In combination with chemical reactivity, metabolism provides a real barrier to consummated transport of sensitive chemicals.

Most simple transport correlates nicely with log *P* and follows Fickian kinetics. Up to about log *P* = 2.0, transport through the protein domain is exclusive, with the parallel lipid route increasing in importance above 2.0. By about log *P* = 2.5, the entire rate-limiting barrier begins to shift from the SC to the viable epidermis. Highly lipophilic compounds like DDT may easily cross the SC through the low-energy lipid domain, but become trapped in the epidermis and dermis by an inability to cross aqueous phases.

The work of Raykar et al. (1988) clearly reveals the two domains of the SC in showing different partitioning slopes for the relation log *P*(SC/water) versus log *P*(o/w). For the hydrocortisone esters studied (log *P* = 0.6–5.5), lipid partitioning in the SC becomes important near log *P* = 3.0. In other experiments, we find that acids partition into the SC as the anion, while phenols partition in both neutral and ionic forms, controlled by the electronics of the ring substituents.

Most of the experimental work with different skins and chemicals is mutually supporting, though changes in mechanism may occur at somewhat different log *P* break points from one study to another. In general, behavior in the SC largely mirrors behavior in whole skin except for very lipophilic compounds. Moreover, repeated observations of optimal transport near log *P* = 2.3 strongly suggest that TD transport has much in common with ordinary passive transport through soft tissue.

REFERENCES

Albery, W. J. and Hadgraft, J. 1978. Percutaneous absorption: Theoretical description. *J. Pharm. Pharmacol.* 31:129.

Al-Saidan, S. M. H., Winfield, A. J. and Selkirk, A. B. 1987. Effect of preheating on the permeability of neonatal rat stratum corneum to alkanols. *J. Invest. Dermatol.* 89:430.

Anderson, B. D., Higuchi, W. I. and Raykar, P. V. 1988. Heterogeneity effects on permeability-partition coefficient relationships in human stratum corneum. *Pharm. Res.* 5:566.

Anderson, B. D. and Raykar, P. V. 1989. Solute structure-permeability relationships in human stratum corneum. *J. Invest. Dermatol.* 93:280.

Ando, H. Y., Ho, N. F. H. and Higuchi, W. I. 1977. Skin as an active metabolizing barrier I: Theoretical analysis of topical bioavailability. *J. Pharm. Sci.* 66:1525.

Baer, H., Dawson, C. R., Byck, J. S. and Kurtz, A. P. 1970. The immunochemistry of immune tolerance II. The relationship of chemical structure to the induction of immune tolerance to catechols. *J. Immunol.* 104:178.

Baer, H., Watkins, R. C. and Bowser, R. T. 1966. Delayed contact sensitivity to catechols and resorcinols. The relations of structure and immunization procedure to sensitizing capacity. *Immunochemistry* 3:479.

Behl, C. R., Flynn, G. L., Kurihara, T., Harper, N., Smith, W., Higuchi, W. I., Ho, N. F. H. and Pierson, C. L. 1980. Hydration and percutaneous absorption: I. Influence of hydration on alkanol permeation through hairless mouse skin. *J. Invest. Dermatol.* 75:346.

Behl, C. R., Barrett, M., Flynn, G. L., Kurihara, T., Walters, K. A., Gatmaitan, O. G., Harper, N., Higuchi, W. I., Ho, N. F. H. and Pierson, C. L. 1982. Hydration and percutaneous absorption III: Influences of stripping and scalding on hydration alteration of the permeability of hairless mouse skin to water and *n*-alkanols. *J. Pharm. Sci.* 71:229.

Behl, C. R., Bellantone, N. H. and Flynn, G. L. 1985. Influence of age on percutaneous absorption of drug substances. In *Percutaneous absorption*, eds. R. L. Bronaugh and H. I. Maibach, Chapter 14. New York: Marcel Dekker.

Berne, R. M. and Levy, M. N., eds. 1983. *Physiology*, pp. 605–607. St. Louis: C. V. Mosby.

Blank, I. H. 1985. The effect of hydration on the permeability of skin. In *Percutaneous absorption*, eds. R. L. Bronaugh and H. I. Maibach, Chapter 7. New York: Marcel Dekker.

Blank, I. H., Scheuplein, R. J. and Macfarlane, D. J. 1967. Mechanism of percutaneous absorption III. The effect of temperature on the transport of non-electrolytes across the skin. *J. Invest. Dermatol.* 49:582.

Bondi, A. 1964. van der Waals volumes and radii. *J. Phys. Chem.* 68:441.

Briggs, G. G., Bromilow, R. H., Edmonson, R. and Johnston, M. 1976. Distribution coefficients and systemic activity. The Chemical Society, Burlington House, London, special publication no. 29:129.

Bronaugh, R. L. and Congdon, E. R. 1984. Percutaneous absorption of hair dyes: Correlation with partition coefficients. *J. Invest. Dermatol.* 83:124.

Bronaugh, R. L., Stewart, R. F. and Congdon, E. R. 1983. Differences in permeability of rat skin related to sex and body site. *J. Soc. Cosmet. Chem.* 34:127.

Bucks, D. A. W., Maibach, H. I., Guy, R. H. and Magee, P. S. 1990. Dependance of epidermal retention on protein domain hydrogen-bonding. Unpublished study, PM529.

Bucks, D. A. W., Maibach, H. I., Menczel, E. and Wester, R. C. 1983. Percutaneous penetration of hydrocortisone in humans following skin delipidization by 1,1,1-trichloroethane. *Arch. Dermatol. Res.* 275:242.

Bucks, D. A. W., McMaster, J. R., Maibach, H. I. and Guy, R. H. 1988. Bioavailability of topically administered steroids: A "mass balance" technique. *J. Invest. Dermatol.* 91:29.

Carver, M. P., Williams, P. L. and Riviere, J. E. 1989. The isolated perfused porcine skin flap. III. Percutaneous absorption pharmacokinetics of organophosphates, steroids, benzoic acid and caffeine. *Toxicol. Appl. Pharmacol.* 97:324.

Chandrasekaran, S. K., Bayne, W. and Shaw, J. E. 1978. Pharmacokinetics of drug permeation through human skin. *J. Pharm. Sci.* 67:1370.

Chandrasekaran, S. K., Campbell, P. S. and Michaels, A. S. 1977. Effect of dimethyl sulfoxide on drug permeation through human skin. *Am. Inst. Chem. Eng. J.* 23:810.

Charton, M. 1983. Volume and bulk parameters. In *Steric effects in drug design. Topics in current chemistry 114,* eds. M. Charton and I. Motoc, Chapter 4. Berlin: Springer-Verlag.

Charton, M. and Charton, B. I. 1979. Significance of "volume" and "bulk" parameters in quantitative structure-activity relationships. *J. Org. Chem.* 44:2284.

Christophers, E. and Kligman, A. M. 1964. Percutaneous absorption in aged skin. In *Advances in the biology of skin,* ed. W. Montagna, Volume 6, p. 163. New York: Pergamon Press.

Coats, E. A., Shah, K. J., Milstein, S. R., Genther, C. S., Nene, D. M., Roesner, J., Schmidt, J., Pleiss, M. and Wagner, E. 1982. 4-Hydroxyquinoline-3-carboxylic acids as inhibitors of cell respiration. *J. Med. Chem.* 25:57.

Cooper, E. R. and Kasting, G. 1987. Transport across epithelial membranes. *J. Controlled Release* 6:23.

Daylight Chemical Information Systems, Inc., P.O. Box 17821, Irvine, CA 92713–7821. CLOGP program.

Dunn, W. J. III. 1973a. Binding of certain nonsteroid antiinflammatory agents and uricosuric agents to human serum albumin. *J. Med. Chem.* 16:484.

Dunn, W. J. III. 1973b. Specificity of binding to human serum albumin. *J. Pharm. Sci.* 62:1575.

Dunn, W. J. III, Block, J. H. and Pearlman, R. S., eds. 1986. *Partition coefficient. Determination and estimation.* New York: Pergamon Press.

Dupuis, G. 1979. Studies on poison ivy. *In vitro* lymphocyte transformation by urushiol-protein conjugates. *Br. J. Dermatol.* 101:617.

Dupuis, G. and Benezra, C. 1982. *Allergic contact dermatitis to simple chemicals. A molecular approach.* New York: Marcel Dekker.

Durrheim, H., Flynn, G. L., Higuchi, W. I. and Behl, C. R. 1980. Permeation of hairless mouse skin I: Experimental methods and comparison with human epidermal permeation by alkanols. *J. Pharm. Sci.* 69:781.

Elias, P. M. 1983. Epidermal lipids, barrier function, and desquamation. *J. Invest. Dermatol.* 80(Suppl.):44s.

Elias, P. M., Brown, B. E., Fritsch, P., Goerke, J., Gray, G. M. and White, R. J. 1979. Localization and composition of lipids in neonatal mouse stratum granulosum and stratum corneum. *J. Invest. Dermatol.* 73:339.

Elias, P. M., Brown, B. E. and Ziboh, V. A. 1980. The permeability barrier in essential fatty acid deficiency: Evidence for a direct role for linoleic acid in barrier function. *J. Invest. Dermatol.* 74:230.

Elias, P. M., Cooper, E. R., Korc, A. and Brown, B. E. 1981. Percutaneous transport in relation to stratum corneum structure and lipid composition. *J. Invest. Dermatol.* 76:297.

Elias, P. M., Goerke, J. and Friend, D. S. 1977. Mammalian epidermal barrier lipids: Composition and influence on structure. *J. Invest. Dermatol.* 69:535.

Feldmann, R. J. and Maibach, H. I. 1965. Penetration of C14-hydrocortisone through normal skin. *Arch. Dermatol.* 91:661.

Fleming, R., Guy, R. H. and Hadgraft, J. 1983. Kinetics and thermodynamics of interfacial transfer. *J. Pharm. Sci.* 72:142.

Flickinger, C. J., Brown, J. C., Kutchai, H. C. and Ogilvie, J. W. 1979. *Medical cell biology,* p. 33. Philadelphia: W. B. Saunders.

Flynn, G. L. 1985. Mechanism of percutaneous absorption from physicochemical evidence. In *Percutaneous absorption,* eds. R. L. Bronaugh and H. I. Maibach, Chapter 2. New York: Marcel Dekker.

Flynn, G. L., Durrheim, H. and Higuchi, W. I. 1981. Permeation of hairless mouse skin II. Membrane sectioning techniques and influence on alkanol permeabilities. *J. Pharm. Sci.* 70:52.

Flynn, G. L. and Yalkowski, S. H. 1972. Correlation and prediction of mass transport across membranes I: Influence of alkyl chain length on flux-determining properties of barrier and diffusant. *J. Pharm. Sci.* 61:838.

Fredriksson, T. 1969. Influence of solvents and surface active agents on the barrier function of the skin towards sarin. *Acta Dermato-Venereol.* 49:481.

Friend, D. R., Catz, P., Heller, J. and Okagaki, M. 1989. Transdermal delivery of levonorgestrel IV: Evaluation of membranes. *J. Pharm. Sci.* 78:477.

Friend, D., Catz, P., Heller, J., Reid, J. and Baker, R. 1988. Transdermal delivery of levonorgestrel II: Effect of prodrug structure on skin permeability *in vitro. J. Controlled Release* 7:251.

Goldblum, A., Yoshimoto, M. and Hansch, C. 1981. Quantitative structure-activity relationship of phenyl *N*-methylcarbamate inhibition of acetylcholinesterase. *J. Agric. Food Chem.* 29:277.

Golden, G. M., Guzek, D. B., Kennedy, A. H., McKie, J. E. and Potts, R. O. 1987. Stratum corneum lipid phase transitions and water barrier properties. *Biochemistry* 26:2382.

Grayson, S. and Elias, P. M. 1982. Isolation and lipid biochemical characterization of stratum corneum membrane complexes: Implications for the cutaneous permeability barrier. *J. Invest. Dermatol.* 78:128.

Grissom, Jr., R. E., Brownie, C. and Guthrie, F. E. 1987. *In vivo* and *in vitro* dermal penetration of lipophilic and hydrophilic pesticides in mice. *Bull. Environ. Contam. Toxicol.* 38:917.

Gummer, C. L. 1985. Vehicles as penetration enhancers. In *Percutaneous absorption,* eds. R. L. Bronaugh and H. I. Maibach, Chapter 43. New York: Marcel Dekker.

Guy, R. H. and Hadgraft, J. 1983. Physicochemical interpretation of the pharmacokinetics of percutaneous absorption. *J. Pharmacokinet. Biopharm.* 11:189.

Guy, R. H. and Hadgraft, J. 1985a. Kinetic analysis of transdermal nitroglycerin delivery. *Pharm. Res.* 5:206.

Guy, R. H. and Hadgraft, J. 1985b. Skin metabolism. Theoretical. In *Percutaneous absorption,* eds. R. L. Bronaugh and H. I. Maibach, Chapter 4. New York: Marcel Dekker.

Guy, R. H. and Hadgraft, J. 1988. Physicochemical aspects of percutaneous penetration and its enhancement. *Pharm. Res.* 5:753.

Guy, R. H., Hadgraft, J. and Maibach, H. I. 1982. A pharmacokinetic model for percutaneous absorption. *Int. J. Pharm.* 11:119.

Guy, R. H., Hadgraft, J. and Maibach, H. I. 1983. Percutaneous absorption: multidose pharmacokinetics. *Int. J. Pharm.* 17:23.

Guy, R. H., Hadgraft, J. and Maibach, H. I. 1985a. Percutaneous absorption in man: A kinetic approach. *Toxicol. Appl. Pharmacol.* 78:123.

Guy, R. H. and Honda, D. H. 1984. Solute transport resistance at the octanol-water interface. *Int. J. Pharm.* 19:129.

Guy, R. H. and Maibach, H. I. 1983. Drug delivery to local subcutaneous structures following topical administration. *J. Pharm. Sci.* 72:1375.

Guy, R. H., Maibach, H. I. and Hadgraft, J. 1985b. Radial transport in the dermis. In *Percutaneous absorption,* eds. R. L. Bronaugh and H. I. Maibach, Chapter 25. New York: Marcel Dekker.

Hadgraft, J. and Ridout, G. 1987. Development of model membranes for percutaneous absorption measurements. I. Isopropyl myristate. *Int. J. Pharm.* 39:149.

Hansch, C. and Clayton, J. M. 1973. Lipophilic character and biological activity of drugs II: The parabolic case. *J. Pharm. Sci.* 62:1.

Hansch, C. and Dunn, W. J. III. 1972. Linear relationships between lipophilic character and biological activity of drugs. *J. Pharm. Sci.* 61:1.

Hansch, C. and Leo, A. 1979. *Substituent constants for correlation analysis in chemistry and biology,* Chapter 4. New York: John Wiley and Sons.

Hansch, C., Steward, A. R., Anderson, S. M. and Bentley, D. 1967. The parabolic dependence of drug action upon lipophilic character as revealed by a study of hypnotics. *J. Med. Chem.* 11:1.

Hartley, D. and Kidd, H., eds. 1983. *The agrochemicals handbook.* Royal Society of Chemistry. Old Woking, Surrey: Unwin Brothers.

Hashimoto, K. and Tanii, H. 1985. Percutaneous absorption of C14-methacrylamide in animals. *Arch. Toxicol.* 57:94.

Higuchi, T. 1982. *In vivo* drug release from ointments and creams. In *Dermal and transdermal absorption,* eds. R. Brandau and B. H. Lippold, Figure 1, Chapter 5. Stuttgart: Wissenschaftliche Verlagsgesellschaft.

Houk, J., Hansch, C., Hall, L. L. and Guy, R. H. 1987. Chemical structure-transport rate relationships for model skin lipid membranes. In *In vitro toxicology approaches to validation,* eds. A. M. Goldberg and M. L. Principe, Poster 15. New York: Mary Ann Liebert.

Huq, A. S., Ho, N. F. H., Husari, N., Flynn, G. L., Jetzer, W. E. and Condie, L., Jr. 1986. Permeation of water contaminative phenols through hairless mouse skin. *Arch. Environ. Contam. Toxicol.* 15:557.

Idson, B. 1971. Biophysical factors in skin penetration. *J. Soc. Cosmet. Chem.* 22:615.

Isaacs, N. S. 1987. *Physical organic chemistry,* Table 1.16, p. 47. Essex, England. Longman Scientific & Technical.

Ito, Y., Ogiso, T. and Iwaki, M. 1988. Thermodynamic study on enhancement of percutaneous penetration of drugs by azone. *J. Pharmacobiodyn.* 11:749.

Jetzer, W. E., Huq, A. S., Ho, N. F. H., Flynn, G. L., Duraiswamy, N. and Condie, L., Jr. 1986. Permeation of mouse skin and silicone rubber membranes by phenols: Relationship to *in vitro* partitioning. *J. Pharm. Sci.* 75:1098.

Kice, J. L. 1971. The sulfur-sulfur bond. In *Sulfur in organic and inorganic chemistry,* ed. A. Senning, Volume 1, Chapter 6. New York: Marcel Dekker.

Kligman, A. M. 1979. Perspectives and problems in cutaneous gerontology. *J. Invest. Dermatol.* 73:39.

Koch, R. L., Palicharia, P. and Groves, M. L. 1988. Diffusion of (2-C14)diazepam across isolated hairless mouse stratum corneum/epidermal tissues. *J. Invest. Dermatol.* 90:317.

Kubinyi, H. 1977. Quantitative structure-activity relationships. 7. The bilinear model, a new model for nonlinear dependence of biological activity on hydrophobic character. *J. Med. Chem.* 20:625.

Kubota, K. and Ishizaki, T. 1985. A theoretical consideration of percutaneous drug absorption. *J. Pharmacokinet. Biopharm.* 13:55.

Leahy, D. E., Taylor, P. J. and Wait, A. R. 1989. Model solvent systems for QSAR. Part I. Propylene glycol dipelargonate (PGDP). *Quant. Struct.-Activity Relat.* 8:17.

Lee, G., Swarbrick, J., Kiyohara, G. and Payling, D. W. 1985. Drug permeation through human skin. III. Effect of pH on the partitioning behavior of a chromone-2-carboxylic acid. *Int. J. Pharmaceut.* 23:43.

Leo, A. J., Hansch, C. and Elkins, D. 1971. Partition coefficients and their uses. *Chem. Rev.* 71:525.

Levin, V. A. 1980. Relationship of octanol/water partition coefficient and molecular weight to rat brain capillary permeability. *J. Med. Chem.* 23:682.

Lien, E. J. 1981. Structure-activity relationships and drug disposition. *Annu. Rev. Pharmacol. Toxicol.* 21:31.

Lien, E. J., Alhaider, A. A. and Lee, V. H. L. 1982. Phase partition: Its use in the prediction of membrane permeation and drug action in the eye. *J. Parenter. Sci. Technol.* 36:86.

Lien, E. J. and Wang, P. H. 1980. Lipophilicity, molecular weight, and drug action: Reexamination of parabolic and bilinear models. *J. Pharm. Sci.* 69:648.

Magee, P. S. 1979a. Analysis of barbiturate hypnotic effect on rats, mice and rabbits. Unpublished study, PM155.

Magee, P. S. 1979b. Systemic and nonsystemic pesticides versus logP. Unpublished study, PM165.

Magee, P. S. 1983. Transdermal flux variance for 42 drugs (confidential studies). Unpublished study, PM221.

Magee, P. S. 1984. Rat brain capillary permeability. Unpublished study, PM249.

Magee, P. S. 1985. Virtual partitioning studies. Unpublished study, PM274–PM281.

Magee, P. S. 1986. Analysis of binding energetics in paper and thin-layer chromatography. *Quant. Struct.-Activity Relat.* 5:158.

Magee, P S. 1989. Interfacing statistics, quantum chemistry and molecular modeling. In *Probing bioactive mechanisms,* eds. P. S. Magee, D. R. Henry and J. H. Block, Chapter 3. Washington, D.C.: American Chemical Society.

Magee, P. S. 1990. Permeability of human epidermis to phenols: Correction for electronic effects. Unpublished study, PM530.

Maibach, H. I. 1976. *In vivo* percutaneous penetration of corticoids and unresolved problems in their efficacy. *Dermatologica* 152(Suppl.1):11.

Martin, Y. C. 1978. *Quantitative drug design. A critical introduction,* pp. 80–81. New York: Marcel Dekker.

Marzulli, F. N. 1962. Barriers to skin penetration. *J. Invest. Dermatol.* 89:387.

Marzulli, F. N., Callahan, J. F. and Brown, D. W. C. 1965. Chemical structure and skin penetrating capacity of a short series of organic phosphates and phosphoric acid. *J. Invest. Dermatol.* 44:339.

Matoltsy, A. G. 1976. Keratinization. *J. Invest. Dermatol.* 67:20.

Menczel, E. 1985. Skin delipidization and percutaneous absorption. In *Percutaneous absorption,* eds. R. L. Bronaugh and H. I. Maibach, Chapter 10. New York: Marcel Dekker.

Menczel, E., Bucks, D. A. W., Wester, R. C. and Maibach, H. I. 1985. Skin binding during percutaneous penetration. In *Percutaneous absorption,* eds. R. L. Bronaugh and H. I. Maibach, Chapter 3. New York: Marcel Dekker.

Michaels, A. S., Chandrasekaran, S. K. and Shaw, J. E. 1975. Drug permeation through human skin: Theory and *in vitro* experimental measurement. *Am. Inst. Chem. Eng. J.* 21:985.

Moriguchi, I., Kanda, Y. and Komatsu, K. 1976. van der Waals volume and the related parameters for hydrophobicity in structure-activity studies. *Chem. Pharm. Bull.* 24:1799.

Nacht, S. and Yeung, D. 1985. Artificial membranes and skin permeability. In *Percutaneous absorption,* eds. R. L. Bronaugh and H. I. Maibach, Chapter 29. New York: Marcel Dekker.

Noonan, P. K. and Wester, R. C. 1985. Cutaneous metabolism of xenobiotics. In *Percu-*

taneous absorption, eds. R. L. Bronaugh and H. I. Maibach, Chapter 5. New York: Marcel Dekker.

Ogiso, T., Ito, Y., Iwaki, M. and Atago, H. 1989. A pharmacokinetic model for the percutaneous absorption of indomethacin and the prediction of drug disposition kinetics. *J. Pharm. Sci.* 78:319.

Onken, H. D. and Moyer, C. A. 1963. The water barrier in human epidermis. Physical and chemical nature. *Arch. Dermatol.* 87:584.

Pannatier, A., Jenner, P., Testa, B. and Etter, J. C. 1978. The skin as a drug-metabolizing organ. *Drug Metab. Rev.* 8:319.

Raykar, P. V., Fung, M.-C. and Anderson, B. D. 1988. The role of protein and lipid domains in the uptake of solutes by human stratum corneum. *Pharm. Res.* 5:140.

Rechsteiner, C. E., Jr. and Grain, C. F. 1982. Boiling point. Vapor pressure. Liquid viscosity. In *Handbook of chemical property estimation methods,* eds. W. J. Lyman, W. F. Reehl and D. H. Rosenblatt, Chapters 12–14, 22. New York: McGraw-Hill.

Ridout, G. and Guy, R. H. 1988. Structure-penetration relationships in percutaneous absorption. In *Pesticide formulations,* eds. B. Cross and H. B. Scher, Chapter 10. Washington, D.C.: American Chemical Society.

Roberts, M. S., Anderson, R. A. and Swarbrick, J. 1977. Permeability of human epidermis to phenolic compounds. *J. Pharm. Pharmacol.* 29:677.

Roberts, M. S., Anderson, R. A., Swarbrick, J. and Moore, D. E. 1978. The percutaneous absorption of phenolic compounds: The mechanism of diffusion across the stratum corneum. *J. Pharm. Pharmacol.* 30:486.

Rosenberg, A., Williams, R. and Cohen, G. 1973. Interaction forces involved in wetting of human skin. *J. Pharm. Sci.* 62:920.

Rougier, A., Dupuis, D., Lotte, C., Roguet, R. and Schaefer, H. 1983. *In vivo* correlation between stratum corneum reservoir function and percutaneous absorption. *J. Invest. Dermatol.* 81:275.

Rougier, A., Lotte, C. and Dupuis, D. 1987. An original predictive method for *in vivo* percutaneous absorption studies. *J. Soc. Cosmet. Chem.* 38:397.

Schalla, W. and Schaefer, H. 1982. Mechanism of penetration of drugs into the skin. In *Dermal and transdermal absorption,* eds. R. Brandau and B. H. Lippold, Chapter 3. Stuttgart: Wissenschaftliche Verlagsgesellschaft.

Schalla, W. and Schaefer, H. 1985. Localization of compounds in different skin layers and its use as an indicator of percutaneous absorption. In *Percutaneous absorption,* eds. R. L. Bronaugh and H. I. Maibach, Figure 4, Chapter 22. New York: Marcel Dekker.

Scherrer, R. A. 1984. The treatment of ionizable compounds in quantitative structure-activity studies with special consideration to ion partitioning. In *Pesticide synthesis through rational approaches,* eds. P. S. Magee, G. K. Kohn and J. J. Menn, Chapter 14. Washington, D.C.: American Chemical Society.

Scheuplein, R. J. 1966. Analysis of permeability data for the case of parallel diffusion pathways. *Biophys. J.* 6:1.

Scheuplein, R. J. 1967. Mechanism of percutaneous absorption. II. Transient diffusion and the relative importance of various routes of skin penetration. *J. Invest. Dermatol.* 48:79.

Scheuplein, R. J. and Blank, I. H. 1971. Permeability of the skin. *Physiol. Rev.* 51:702.

Scheuplein, R. J., Blank, I. H., Brauner, G. J. and MacFarlane, D. J. 1969. Percutaneous absorption of steroids. *J. Invest. Dermatol.* 52:63.

Scheuplein, R. J. and Morgan, L. J. 1967. "Bound-water" in keratin membranes measured by a microbalance technique. *Nature (Lond.)* 214:456.

Scott, R. C. and Ramsey, J. D. 1987. Comparison of the *in vivo* and *in vitro* percutaneous absorption of a lipophilic molecule (cypermethrin, a pyrethroid insecticide). *J. Invest. Dermatol.* 89:142.

Seiler, P. 1974. Interconversion of lipophilicites from hydrocarbon/water systems into the octanol/water system. *Eur. J. Med. Chem.* 9:473.

Sidon, E. W., Moody, R. P. and Franklin, C. A. 1988. Percutaneous absorption of *cis-* and *trans*-permethrin in rhesus monkeys and rats: Anatomic site and interspecies variation. *J. Toxicol. Environ. Health* 23:207.

Singer, E. J., Wegmann, P. C., Lehman, M. D., Christensen, M. S. and Vinson, L. J. 1971. Barrier development, ultrastructure and sulfhydryl content of the fetal epidermis. *J. Soc. Cosmet. Chem.* 22:119.

Southwell, D., Barry, B. W. and Woodford, R. 1984. Variations in permeability of human skin within and between specimens. *Int. J. Pharm.* 18:299.

Stuttgen, G. 1982. Drug absorption by intact and damaged skin. In *Dermal and transdermal absorption,* eds. R. Brandau and B. H. Lippold, Chapter 2. Stuttgart: Wissenschaftliche Verlagsgesellschaft.

Surber, C., Maibach, H. I. and Magee, P. S. 1989. Partitioning of chemicals into whole human stratum corneum. Unpublished studies, PM468.

Tauber, U. 1982. Metabolism of drugs on and in the skin. In *Dermal and transdermal absorption,* eds. R. Brandau and B. H. Lippold, Chapter 8. Stuttgart: Wissenschaftliche Verlagsgesellschaft.

Tojo, K., Chiang, C. C., Doshi, U. and Chien, Y. W. 1988a. Stratum corneum reservoir capacity affecting dynamics of transdermal drug delivery. *Drug Dev. Ind. Pharm.* 14:561.

Tojo, K., Chien, Y. W., Chiang, C. C. and Keshary, P. R. 1988b. Effect of stratum corneum stripping on skin penetration of drug. *J. Chem. Eng. Jpn.* 21:544.

Tojo, K. and Lee, A. C. 1989. A method for predicting steady-state rate of skin penetration *in vivo. J. Invest. Dermatol.* 92:105.

Tregear, R. T. 1966. *Physical functions of the skin,* pp. 1–52. London: Academic Press.

Vandenbelt, J. M., Hansch, C. and Church, C. 1972. Binding of apolar molecules by serum albumin. *J. Med. Chem.* 15:787.

Wallace, S. M. and Barnett, G. 1978. Pharmacokinetic analysis of percutaneous absorption: Evidence of parallel penetration pathways for methotrexate. *J. Pharmacokinet. Biopharm.* 6:315.

Wester, R. C. and Maibach, H. I. 1983. Cutaneous pharmacokinetics: 10 steps to percutaneous absorption. *Drug Metab. Rev.* 14:169.

Wester, R. C. and Maibach, H. I. 1985a. Structure-activity correlations in percutaneous absorption. In *Percutaneous absorption,* eds. R. L. Bronaugh and H. I. Maibach, Chapter 8. New York: Marcel Dekker.

Wester, R. C. and Maibach, H. I. 1985b. Influence of hydration on percutaneous absorption. In *Percutaneous absorption,* eds. R. L. Bronaugh and H. I. Maibach, Chapter 18. New York: Marcel Dekker.

Wester, R. C., Mobayen, M. and Maibach, H. I. 1987. *In vivo* and *in vitro* absorption and binding to powdered stratum corneum as methods to evaluate skin absorption of environmental chemical contaminants from ground and surface water. *J. Toxicol. Environ. Health* 21:367.

Wilkinson, D. I. 1969. Variability in composition of surface lipids. *J. Invest. Dermatol.* 52:339.

Wolf, J. 1940. Das oberflachenrelief der menschlichen haut. *Z. Mikrosk. Anat. Forsch.* 47:351.

Yalkowsky, S. H. and Flynn, G. L. 1973. Transport of alkyl homologs across synthetic and biological membranes: A new model for chain length-activity relationships. *J. Pharm. Sci.* 62:210.

Yano, T., Nakagawa, A., Tsuji, M. and Noda, K. 1986. Skin permeability of various non-steroidal anti-inflammatory drugs in man. *Life Sci.* 39:1043.

Zatz, J. L. 1985. Percutaneous absorption. Computer simulation using multicompartmented membrane models. In *Percutaneous absorption,* eds. R. L. Bronaugh and H. I. Maibach, Chapter 13. New York: Marcel Dekker.

Zatz, J. L. and Dalvi, U. G. 1983. Evaluation of solvent-skin interaction in percutaneous absorption. *J. Soc. Cosmet. Chem.* 34:327.

2

physiologically based pharmacokinetic modeling

■ **James N. McDougal** ■

INTRODUCTION

Understanding and quantifying the penetration of chemicals into and through the skin is important in both pharmacology and toxicology. In nearly every case, the species of interest is the human species, although laboratory animals are often used as surrogates, particularly in the case of toxicological studies. Appropriate use of laboratory animals necessitates understanding differences between species so that the process of extrapolation to humans is meaningful. This is vital for *in vivo* animal studies, which are often more complex than *in vitro* animal studies. *In vivo* studies have the advantage of intact skin that has blood flow, is alive and responsive. Metabolism, nervous, and humoral responses are also present, and therefore living skin better reflects human exposure scenarios. Traditionally, the analysis of *in vivo* skin penetration in laboratory animals has involved estimation of the amount of chemical that has penetrated using either blood concentrations or the amount of chemical excreted after a dermal exposure. These methods are descriptive; applicability of the results is limited by the appropriateness of the specific experimental design and the similarities between the laboratory species chosen and humans.

Due to the recent increase in the availability of computer hardware and software, methods that are based on physiological and pharmacokinetic principles are now feasible alternatives for analysis of *in vivo* skin penetration. These physiologically based pharmacokinetic (PB-PK) approaches mathematically describe the dynamics of chemicals in the body in terms of rates of blood flow, permeability of membranes, and partitioning of chemicals into tissues. Characterizing absorption in terms of parameters that are measurable and species-specific facilitates extrapolations to the real species of interest, providing these parameters are known or can be determined for humans. This chapter describes physiologically based pharmacokinetic models, their use as a tool to quantify and understand the process of dermal penetration, and their suitability for dose, route, and species extrapolation.

WHY USE PB-PK MODELS?

One of the big advantages of dermal PB-PK models over traditional *in vivo* methods is the ability to accurately describe nonlinear biochemical and physical processes. Describing skin penetration based on blood concentrations or excretion rates as "percent absorbed" assumes all processes have a simple linear relationship with the exposure concentration. When nonlinear processes occur in the absorption, distribution, metabolism, or elimination of a chemical, describing absorption as "percent absorbed" is misleading. Dermal absorption may not be linear when there is binding or metabolism in the skin or when skin blood flow is a limiting factor. Many biochemical processes in the body are nonlinear: that is, the percent of chemical metabolized per hour at a low liver concentration may be much greater than the percent metabolized per hour at a high liver concentration. A quantitative description of saturable kinetics in the model may allow it to be predictive of blood or tissue concentrations from various doses. A complete mathematical description of dermal pharmacokinetics takes mass balance throughout the animal into account, and makes it possible to estimate fluxes (amount/time) and permeability constants (distance/time). These expressions of the penetration process are required to accurately predict penetration in other situations, such as different exposure area, time, or concentration, when nonlinear processes are present.

A properly validated dermal PB-PK description will provide more information from each experiment than is possible without it. For example, if it is the chemical concentration in an organ or tissue that is important, by understanding the quantitative relationship between blood concentrations and tissue concentrations, serial blood sampling may provide the estimate of the tissue dose that is required without the need for an invasive procedure to sample tissue concentrations. Another good example would be the estimation of rate of metabolism in the skin. Proper comparison of a PB-PK description of metabolite production after an intravenous infusion with the rates of metabolite production after application to the skin at several concentrations allows the metabolic parameters in the skin to be estimated.

In this age of increased concern over the use of animals in research, it is important to try to reduce animal use and get the most information from each animal that must be used. Before any experimentation, PB-PK models can often be used to form predictions that will help in designing experimental doses and sampling times, thus avoiding "range finding" experiments. During the experiment, PB-PK descriptions may allow the use of fewer animals because it may not be necessary to sacrifice animals at various time points to get tissue concentrations. After the study is complete, PB-PK models allow one to extrapolate results to other exposure areas, times, or concentrations, possibly eliminating the need to repeat an experiment under different conditions.

Another important reason for using physiologically based pharmacokinetic modeling of dermal absorption is to acquire the experience necessary to extrapolate to other species. Classical pharmacokinetic modeling assumes that the body can be adequately described by one to three compartments based on the shape of the semilogarithmic plot of plasma concentration versus time (Gibaldi and Perrier, 1982). The most common classical description is a two-compartment linear system where one compartment is the plasma and the other all remaining body water and the tissues. Using this type of model, the plasma concentration curve can be fit by a distributive phase (α) and a postdistributive phase (β). This type of model is useful in clinical situations for the changing dose or dose regimen. Classical modeling has occasionally been used in skin penetration studies (Cooper, 1976; Wallace and Barnett, 1978; Peck et al., 1981; Chandrasekaran et al., 1978; Birmingham et al., 1979; Guy et al., 1982; Kubota and Ishizake, 1986).

Figure 1 is a schematic representation of the classical two compartment pharmacokinetic model having a deep body compartment in quasi-equilibrium with the plasma. The first order transfer rates (K_{12}, K_{21}, K_{10}) are descriptive of a particular situation but do not allow extrapolation to other exposure conditions or species because their physiological basis is obscure. PB-PK models do allow extrapolation because of their physiological basis. It has been shown that a PB-PK model for the inhalation of styrene in rats can be predictive of blood and exhaled air concentrations of styrene in humans after scaling up the physiological and metabolic constants (Ramsey and Andersen, 1984). Extrapolation with a PB-PK model is only limited by the ability of the modeler to quantitatively describe the differences in the pharmacokinetic and physiological processes involved.

WHEN CAN PB-PK MODELS BE USED?

PB-PK models can be used in nearly any *in vivo* experimental situation in which the physiological and pharmacokinetic processes can be described adequately for the purposes of the scientific question to be answered. It is often not necessary to have an exhaustive description of the animal to be studied—only the simplest description that "works." It is possible to imagine a PB-PK model that describes blood flow, partition coefficients, and metabolic characteristics for each organ in a specific mammal, but a single scientific question that would require such an exhaustive description could not be imagined! Normally it is sufficient to lump all these organs into several compartments that have similar blood flows and partition coefficients. The requirement for quantitative under-

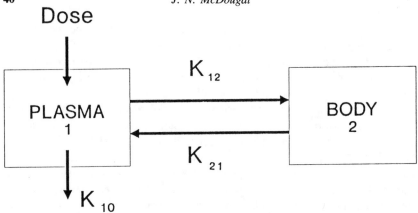

FIGURE 1 Classical pharmacokinetic model with two compartments and first-order transfer and elimination rates.

standing of these processes is both the strong point and the Achilles heel of PB-PK modeling. Quantitative descriptions are the strong point because of their basis in underlying principles, but they are the weak point because the level of understanding required is not easy to achieve. Often the initial description of a particular process is not adequate, but through experimentation and more careful description, based on sound pharmacokinetic and physiological principles, the fundamental understanding of the processes involved can be increased.

WHAT ARE THE COMPONENTS OF A PB-PK MODEL?

Simply speaking, a mammalian organism is comprised of diverse, sometimes metabolically active pools of fluid separated by membranes that prohibit, permit, or promote passage of the fluids and/or their dissolved contents. These fluids and membranes obey and can therefore be described by the physical laws of fluid dynamics, transport, and diffusion. Skin is one of the most important membranes because it separates and protects animals from their environment. The major fluids, which contribute 60% of body weight, are blood plasma, interstitial fluids, and intracellular fluids. Plasma, the most important fluid because of its continuous motion, transports the red cells, white cells, platelets, and soluble components in the blood. Interstitial fluid, which bathes cells with three times the volume of the plasma, is diffuse and separated from the plasma only by capillary walls. The comparatively static intracellular fluid is separated from the extracellular fluids by specialized cell membranes with sophisticated active transport systems. The membranes in the tissues that keep these fluids organized are protein-lipid structures of varying thicknesses, which may contain alterable apertures and carry metabolic enzymes. With this uncomplicated description as a basis, most pharmacokinetic processes can be simplified and described in terms of flows, volumes, solubilities, diffusion, and metabolic rates. When these physiological processes can be quantitated, a mathematical description can be constructed and compared with experiments to accurately describe the processes involved with physiologically based pharmacokinetic models (see reviews by Himmelstein and Lutz, 1979; Lutz et al., 1980; Gerlowski and Jain, 1983; Clewell and Andersen, 1989).

Tissue Compartments

The building block of a PB-PK model is the compartment. A compartment is a collection of fluids or tissues and/or organs with similar chemical concentrations that are grouped together because of physiological and pharmacokinetic characteristics rather than anatomical considerations (Lutz et al., 1980). Each lumped compartment receives inward flux, has a volume, and may incorporate binding or loss of chemical through outward flux or metabolism. Subcompartments may be necessary to accurately describe barriers to movement or sequestration of chemical. Figure 2 illustrates a lumped compartment.

Even this level of complexity is not always necessary to adequately describe the processes that are occurring. The transport of chemical across the thin capillary wall may be so rapid that the plasma and interstitial fluid have equivalent concentrations and therefore it may be possible to combine the plasma and interstitial fluid subcompartments into one extracellular fluid subcompartment. Diffusion across cellular membranes into the intracellular fluid may be so rapid that flow of the blood to the compartment is the rate-limiting factor affecting uptake of a chemical and therefore it may be possible to avoid subcompartments completely. The free concentration of chemical in the plasma, interstitial fluid, or intracellular fluid subcompartments will depend on whether binding or metabolism occurs in the subcompartment.

Simple PB-PK Model

Penetration of the skin is a process that lends itself to PB-PK modeling. Compartments are chosen based on an understanding of the pharmacokinetics of the chemical and the purpose for the model. Figure 3 shows a model with five simple compartments, which was designed for predicting blood concentrations from different exposure times and concentrations on the skin. Each compartment is well stirred, flow limited, and has no subcompartments. The description is of the venous equilibration type, without blood volume being specified because, in this description, blood is not a site for metabolism or binding.

The skin compartment envisioned has simple diffusion, is homogeneous, and is without subcompartments. The rapidly perfused compartment has high blood flow, has high affinity for the chemical, and represents kidney, viscera, brain, and other richly perfused organs. The slowly perfused compartment has low blood flow, has low affinity for the chemical, and represents muscle and other poorly perfused tissues and organs. The fat compartment has low blood flow, has high affinity for the chemical, and represents various types of fat.

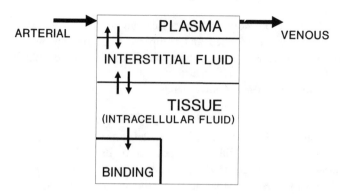

FIGURE 2 Diagrammatic description of a lumped compartment with three subcompartments and binding in the tissue subcompartment.

These expected transfer characteristics with the blood are important criteria in choosing the compartments. According to this description, the sole route of entry for the chemical is the skin, and elimination is by way of diffusion out of the skin followed by metabolism in the liver. Additional compartments would be required for a volatile chemical that could be lost through exhalation, for a chemical that could be eliminated in the kidney, or if concentration in a target organ (e.g., testis) was of particular interest.

Skin Compartment

A skin compartment is just a special subset of tissue compartments that, because it is the defined portal of entry and has definable anatomy and physiology, needs to be further elaborated. Figure 4 illustrates a skin compartment that contains most of the anatomical detail that may be important in skin penetration. Most of this detail will not be necessary for any particular chemical, but is described here for completeness.

Each subcompartment communicates in both directions with adjacent compartments, and each has a concentration, volume, and affinity for the chemical of interest. The surface subcompartment, although not strictly part of the skin, is crucial to making the PB-PK model functional. The surface area exposed, exposure concentration, amount applied to skin, and affinity of the chemical for the vehicle (if any) are all incorporated into this subcompartment. If evaporation is occurring or if the chemical is applied in a vehicle and the vehicle has a penetration rate of its own, terms characterizing these events must be incorporated into the description so the concentration in the surface subcompartment, which is the driving force for penetration, remains accurate.

The stratum corneum subcompartment represents the thin, densely packed, fully differentiated keratinocytes. This layer is the principal barrier to

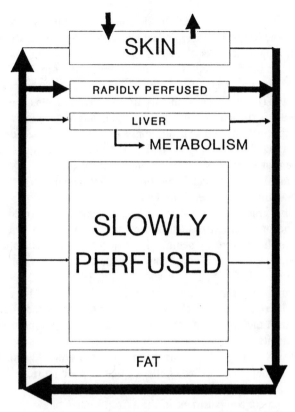

FIGURE 3 Diagrammatic representation of a PB-PK model with five simple compartments connected by blood flow. Compartment volumes and blood flow that they receive are approximately to scale.

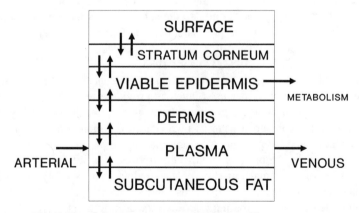

FIGURE 4 Diagrammatic representation of a skin compartment with six subcompartments and metabolism occurring in the viable epidermis.

penetration for most chemicals due to the completeness of its lipid-protein matrix (Marzulli and Tregear, 1961; Scheuplein, 1967; Mershon, 1975; Elias and Friend, 1975; Dugard and Scott, 1984). The stratum corneum has the potential to act as a reservoir for lipophilic chemicals and may provide binding sites. There is little, if any, metabolic activity and no active transport processes (Scheuplein, 1967) associated with this lifeless layer. In this description, the stratum corneum is treated as if it were homogeneous and well stirred. This is a gross oversimplification, and will not apply for all chemicals. For other types of chemicals it may be necessary to model the stratum corneum as the multilayered structure that it actually is (Blank and Scheuplein, 1964; Odland, 1983). Partial differential equations can be written to describe the skin if the concentration gradient within the skin is significant.

The viable epidermis subcompartment contains cells formed in the basal layer, which become keratinized and more compact as they migrate toward the surface to form the stratum corneum. The majority of the metabolic activity of the skin is found in this layer, and it may provide binding sites (Marzulli et al., 1969; Pannatier et al., 1978; Finnin and Shuster, 1985).

The dermis subcompartment provides structural support for the epidermal layers above. It consists of a thick fibrous matrix of elastin and collagen and is more porous than the other compartments. Chemicals may bind to these structural compartments as they transit through the skin. The collagen in the dermis constitutes approximately 77% of the dry mass of the skin (Odland, 1983). The upper part of the dermis contains capillaries that provide nutrients to the viable epidermis.

The plasma subcompartment in the skin provides blood flow to the dermis. Its vasculature is neurally regulated, provides nutrients and other essential chemicals to the skin, and affords a means for dissipation of body heat from the extremities. Pharmacokinetically, the plasma subcompartment receives chemicals that penetrate the skin, but it also receives chemicals from arterial blood. Chemicals from either point of entry to the skin leave via the venous blood. In this simplified description, the plasma subcompartment is between the dermis and the subcutaneous fat when it is actually imbedded in the papillary dermis (Braverman and Keh-Yen, 1983; Odland, 1983).

The subcutaneous fat subcompartment represents a layer of variable thickness, which is poorly perfused but may provide a reservoir for lipophilic chemicals. Its proximity to the plasma compartment raises the possibility that it could be a unique compartment in its own right, even though it is not between the skin surface and the plasma. Although the subcompartments make this skin compartment fairly complex for modeling purposes, it is still an obvious oversimplification of the actual intricacy of mammalian skin. Notably missing are appendages (sweat glands, hair follicles, and sebaceous glands), which have been suggested to be contributing pathways for absorption at early times with slowly diffusing charged chemicals (Scheuplein, 1967; Mershon, 1975).

Flux Equations

Flux equations are the key to an appropriate model; see Flynn and co-workers (1974) for an excellent review of mass transport. The rate of change of amount (expressed as a product of volume and concentration) in a subcompartment at any time is a balance between inward flux and outward flux:

$$V \frac{dC}{dt} = \text{influx}_{\text{total}} - \text{efflux}_{\text{total}} \tag{1}$$

where V is the volume, C is the free concentration (mass/volume), and influx and efflux are sums of the fluxes (mass/time) in each direction [Eqs. (2)–(4) below].

The general form for the equation describing unidirectional flux in a subcompartment where transportation of a chemical is occurring as a result of flow is

$$\text{Flux} = QC \tag{2}$$

where Q is flow (volume/time).

When the membrane between subcompartments (e.g., capillary or cell membrane) acts as a barrier to simple diffusion or when adjacent compartments such as the viable epidermis and dermis in Fig. 4 act like there is a membrane between them, the flux from outside to inside is described by the permeability-area cross-product and the concentration difference across the membrane:

$$\text{Flux} = PA(C_{\text{out}} - C_{\text{in}}) \tag{3}$$

where P is permeability (distance/time), A is area (distance^2), and C_{out} and C_{in} are the free concentrations at the outer and inner surfaces of the membrane (Flynn et al., 1974). The thermodynamic activity differential actually drives the transport process and, if the chemicals across the barrier are in different media, it is the effective concentration that must be used. Therefore, the concentration must be adjusted for partitioning between the media.

In some cases, movement across a membrane between subcompartments may not be by simple diffusion. If there is a saturable, active process involved, the description for flux would be

$$\text{Flux} = \frac{kVC}{K + C} \tag{4}$$

where k is the maximum transport rate (mass/volume·time), and K is the Michaelis constant (mass/volume).

Binding, Metabolism, and Excretion

The free concentration of chemical in a subcompartment can also be reduced by binding to proteins or cellular macromolecules, by several types of metabolic processes, and by excretion (Lutz et al., 1980; Gerlowski and Jain, 1983). Normally, these processes are either first-order, saturable, or some combination of the two. If the process is first-order, the general equation is

$$\text{Loss} = rCV \tag{5}$$

where loss has the same units as flux (mass/time) and r is a proportionality constant (time^{-1}). This description of loss will have the same form regardless of whether the first-order loss is due to irreversible binding, metabolism, or excretion.

When the binding, metabolism, or excretion is saturable, the loss can be described by an equation of the same form as Eq. (4) (Lutz et al., 1980; Gerlowski and Jain, 1983). The equation for saturable metabolism is

$$\text{Loss} = \frac{V_{\text{max}}C}{K + C} \tag{6}$$

where V_{max} is the maximum reaction velocity (mass/time).

Mass Balance Equations

Each lumped compartment. For subcompartments in Figure 2, Eqs. (7)–(9) (for plasma, interstitial fluid, and intercellular fluid in tissues, respectively) below conserve mass within the whole compartment:

$$V_p \frac{dC_p}{dt} = Q_t(C_a - C_v) + P_{is}A_{is}\left(\frac{C_{is}}{R_{is/ip}} - C_p\right) \tag{7}$$

$$V_{is}\frac{dC_{is}}{dt} = P_{is}A_{is}\left(C_p - \frac{C_{is}}{R_{is/p}}\right) + P_tA_t\left(\frac{C_t}{R_{t/is}} - C_{is}\right) \tag{8}$$

$$V_t \frac{dC_t}{dt} + P_tA_t\left(C_{is} - \frac{C_t}{R_{t/is}}\right) - rC_tV_t \tag{9}$$

where subscripts p, is, and t refer to the plasma, interstitial, and tissue (intercellular fluid) subcompartments, respectively (see Nomenclature), C_a is concentration in the arterial blood, C_v is the concentration in venous blood, and R is the partition coefficient between the media indicated by its subscripts. The concentration in the lumped compartment is the volume average of the concentration of the subcompartments:

$$C_i = \frac{C_p V_p + C_{is} V_{is} + C_t V_t}{V_p + V_{is} + V_t} \tag{10}$$

Each of the compartments shown in Figure 3 could require treatment as a diffusion limited lumped compartment as described above; however, the simplification shown in Eq. (18) below will adequately describe the pharmacokinetic behavior of the chemical.

Skin compartment. For skin subcompartments in Fig. 4, Eqs. (11)–(17) conserve mass within the whole compartment:

$$V_{sfc} \frac{dC_{sfc}}{dt} = P_{sc} A_{sc} \left(\frac{C_{sc}}{R_{sc/sfc}} - C_{sfc} \right) \tag{11}$$

$$V_{sc} \frac{dC_{sc}}{dt} = P_{sc} A_{sc} \left(C_{sfc} - \frac{C_{sc}}{R_{sc/sfc}} \right) + P_{ve} A_{ve} \left(\frac{C_{ve}}{R_{ve/sc}} - C_{sc} \right) \tag{12}$$

$$V_{ve} \frac{dC_{ve}}{dt} = P_{ve} A_{ve} \left(C_{sc} - \frac{C_{ve}}{R_{ve/sc}} \right) + P_d A_d \left(\frac{C_d}{R_{d/ve}} - C_{ve} \right) - \frac{V_{max} C_{ve}}{K + C_{ve}} \tag{13}$$

$$V_d \frac{dC_d}{dt} + P_d A_d \left(C_{ve} - \frac{C_d}{R_{d/ve}} \right) + P_p A_p \left(\frac{C_p}{R_{p/d}} - C_d \right) \tag{14}$$

$$V_p \frac{dC_p}{dt} = Q_{sk} (C_a - C_v) + P_p A_p \left(C_d - \frac{C_p}{R_{p/d}} \right) + P_{sf} A_{sf} \left(\frac{C_{sf}}{R_{sf/p}} - C_p \right) \tag{15}$$

$$V_{sf} \frac{dC_{sf}}{dt} = P_{sf} A_{sf} \left(C_p - \frac{C_{sf}}{R_{sf/p}} \right) \tag{16}$$

where the subscripts sfc, sc, ve, d, p, sf, and sk stand for surface, stratum corneum, viable epidermis, dermis, plasma, subcutaneous fat, and skin, respectively. The concentration in the skin as a whole is the volume average of the concentration of the subcompartments:

$$C_{sk} = \frac{C_{sc} V_{sc} + C_p V_p + C_{ve} V_{ve} + C_d V_d + C_{sf} V_{sf}}{V_{sc} + V_p + V_{ve} + V_d + V_{sf}} \tag{17}$$

It must be emphasized that these are theoretical descriptions of the process of skin penetration. These compartments have been chosen based on the current understanding of what may be the most important structural components involved. Exploration and understanding of these concepts will determine which are important subcompartments for each specific chemical to be studied.

Simplifying assumptions. For completeness, the hypothetical compartments in Figures 3 and 4 have been relatively rigorously described using the PB-PK approach to diffusion limitation in each subcompartment; however, until methods are developed to measure the permeability area cross-products (*PA*) for the subcompartment interfaces, many simplifications must be made to make the description useful for extrapolation. One simplifying approach has been to lump the *P* and *A* together into a single term, which has units of volume/time and is estimated or fit (Lutz et al., 1984; Miller et al., 1981; Angelo et al., 1984; Gabrielsson et al., 1985). A problem with both permeability-area cross-products and the combined term is lack of knowledge about how to scale this term so that it can be applied to another species. It has been assumed that the permeability term is constant physical process across species and the area can be scaled according to body weight (Gabrielsson et al., 1985).

There are several assumptions that have been used to collapse the subcompartments shown in Figs. 2, 3, and 4. When transfer across the cell membrane is the rate-limiting step, the plasma and interstitial subcompartments can be combined into a single extracellular compartment (Lutz et al., 1980; Gerlowski and Jain, 1983). When blood flow to the tissue is the rate-limiting step (i.e., blood flow much less than diffusion into the tissue), all subcompartments can be collapsed into a single well-stirred compartment where the rate of change in amount of chemical is related to blood flow and the difference between arterial blood and tissue blood concentrations (Lutz et al., 1977, 1984; Mintun et al., 1980; Andersen, 1981; Matthews and Dedrick, 1984; Clewell and Andersen, 1985; Andersen et al., 1987; Leung et al., 1988; Fisher et al., 1989), which is a consolidation of Eqs. (1) and (2):

$$V_i \frac{dC_i}{dt} = Q_i\left(C_a - \frac{C_i}{R_{i/b}}\right) \tag{18}$$

where the *i* subscript refers to any compartment and $R_{i/b}$ is the partition coefficient between the tissue and blood. It has also been assumed that the concentration of chemical in tissue is in equilibrium with mixed venous blood. The second concentration term, tissue concentration divided by the tissue to blood partition coefficient, is substituted for the concentration in venous blood, assuming the following at equilibrium:

$$R_{i/b} = \frac{C_i}{C_v} \tag{19}$$

where C_v is the concentration in venous blood leaving the tissue.

Full PB-PK model. When differential equations are written for the skin and body compartments, they need to be connected in such a way that total mass in the whole organism is conserved. The mass balance in the liver compartment is the same except for the addition of saturable metabolism [Eq. (6)]:

$$V_1 \frac{dC_1}{dt} = Q_1 \left(C_a - \frac{C_1}{R_{1/b}} \right) - \frac{V_{max}(C_1/R_{1/b})}{K + (C_1/R_{1/b})} \tag{20}$$

where C_1 is concentration in the liver. The simple skin compartment in Fig. 3 can be described as a well-stirred compartment with simple diffusion:

$$V_{sk} \frac{dC_{sk}}{dt} = Q_{sk} \left(C_a - \frac{C_{sk}}{R_{sk/b}} \right) + P_{sk} A_{sk} \left(C_{sfc} - \frac{C_{sk}}{R_{sk/sfc}} \right) \tag{21}$$

The first term on the right side of the equation describes the effect of blood flow; the second term is the gain of chemical from the skin surface.

The concentration of chemical in mixed venous blood is the average of all the amounts leaving a compartment:

$$C_v = \frac{\Sigma_i (Q_i C_i)}{Q_c} \tag{22}$$

where Q_c is cardiac output (total blood flow).

Parameters of a Model

The parameters that are required for the model will depend on the compartments that have been chosen based on pharmacokinetics, although it is important to know that the parameters are available or can be determined because they may be the limiting factors in the structure of the model. Physiological parameters for rats with a model for volatile lipophylic chemicals (McDougal et al., 1986) are shown in Table 1.

It is important that the blood flows account for the total cardiac output. The sum of the volumes of the compartments only accounts for 91% of the

TABLE 1. Physiological Parameters from a PB-PK Model for Rats

Lumped compartment	Blood flow (% cardiac output)	Volume (% body weight)
Rapidly perfused	56	5
Liver	20	4
Slowly perfused	10	65
Fat	9	7
Skin	5	10

TABLE 2. Partition Coefficients for Some Organic Chemicals

Chemical	Muscle/air	Fat/air	Liver/air	Blood/air
Styrene	46.7	3476	140.7	40.2
m-Xylene	41.9	1859	92.0	46.0
Toluene	27.7	1021	82.8	18.0
Perchloroethylene	20.0	1638	69.9	19.9
Benzene	10.3	499	17.8	17.8
Halothane	4.5	182	7.6	5.3
Hexane	2.9	159	12.0	2.3

body weight. The other 9%, which is not accounted for, is nonperfused tissue such as fur, crystalline bone, cartilage, and teeth.

Chemical-specific parameters of a model are partition coefficients, binding coefficients, and metabolic rates. Partition coefficients describe the ratio of chemical concentrations in different materials at equilibrium. They reflect the solubility of a chemical in biological fluids and tissues and are essential components of physiologically based models. Some of the partition coefficients determined by Gargas and co-workers (1989) that have been used for a PB-PK model of dermal absorption of organic vapors (McDougal et al., 1990) are shown in Table 2. These partition coefficients were measured by determining, at equilibrium, the ratio of concentrations between the blood or tissue and air. Tissue/blood partition coefficients can be estimated by dividing the tissue/air partition coefficient by the blood/air partition coefficient.

Metabolic constants describe the rate of loss of chemical from a lumped compartment, although they may have been determined for a whole animal or a representative tissue. Table 3 shows saturable (V_{max} and K_m) and first-order (K_{fo}) metabolic constants from McDougal and co-workers (1990). Most of these metabolic constants for rats were determined *in vivo* by gas uptake techniques (Gargas et al., 1986), but they can also be determined *in vitro* (Reitz et al., 1988; Sato and Nakajima, 1979; Dedrick et al., 1972).

TABLE 3. Metabolic Constants for Some Organic Chemicals

Chemical	V_{max} (mg/kg/h)	K_m (mg/l)	K_{f0} (kg^{-1} h^{-1})
Styrene	8.4	0.4	0.0
m-Xylene	4.2	0.4	2.0
Toluene	4.7	1.0	0.0
Perchloroethylene	0.0	0.0	0.3
Benzene	3.3	0.6	0.0
Halothane	7.0	0.2	0.0
Hexane	6.0	0.4	3.4

Computer Simulations

PB-PK models are sets of time-dependent, nonlinear simultaneous differential equations such as those described above. Most common computer programming languages, such as FORTRAN, Basic, and C, could be used to solve these differential equations simultaneously, although the ease at which it could be done would be greatly improved with add-on integration routines and plotting packages. Continuous system simulation languages such as Advanced Continuous Simulation Language (ACSL) and SimuSolv, which were designed for engineering simulations, make the process of coding, debugging, modifying, and running a PB-PK model much easier. ACSL has a version which is available for personal computers (Mitchell and Gauthier Associates, 73 Junction Square Drive, Concord, Mass.). SimuSolv (Dow Chemical Company, Midland, Mich.) adds optimization routines that interface with ACSL. These simulation languages are interactive and allow easy data entry, on-line changes of model parameters, and plotting of the results. These simulation languages have been the most important factor influencing the increased use of PB-PK models.

HOW DO YOU DEVELOP PB-PK MODELS?

PB-PK models are unlike "canned" computer programs that can be used for various purposes once they are written. They are radically different from such multipurpose programs as statistical routines, spreadsheets, and databases because the structure of a PB-PK model is dependent on the interaction of a specific chemical with a specific species. The result of using a PB-PK model for a chemical other than that for which it was intended would be like using an Ohio state tax preparation package to prepare a California state tax return. Each unique chemical-species interaction requires that the salient physiological and pharmacokinetic principles be understood and quantitatively described. Development of a PB-PK model is an iterative process that requires insight, trial and error, and careful laboratory investigation. PB-PK models can and should be developed before the first laboratory experiment. As knowledge is gained in the laboratory, each new understanding should be quantitatively described in the model. Simulation and experimentation should be accomplished concurrently. Simulation prior to experimentation will allow appropriate data to be collected. Experimentation will confirm or increase the understanding that is quantified in the model. The key is understanding at the appropriate level, as opposed to description on a superficial level.

Choose Compartments

Decisions about the form of the skin compartment are related to the behavior of the chemical in the skin. Lag time (the time before steady state penetration rate is achieved) is the single most important determining factor. If lag time prior to achieving steady state absorption is short (i.e., 15 min), a simple well-stirred homogeneous skin compartment (Fig. 3) may be an adequate description. If the lag time is longer, which is more common, it will be necessary to include part or all of the skin subcompartments shown in Fig. 4. Distribution of the chemical in the skin will determine which compartments are important to describe explicitly. Many of the methods that have been developed to study the skin will be useful for increasing the understanding required for an appropriate mathematical description. These include *in vitro* methods for metabolism and penetration, laser Doppler velocimetry, tape stripping, and ultrastructural analysis by light or electron microscopy.

Deciding which compartments, in addition to a skin, to include in a model requires knowledge of the pharmacokinetics of the chemical of interest. Depending on the chemical, pharmacokinetic information may be available from the literature or it may need to be determined in the laboratory before determining the structure of the model. Compartments must be included in a model to represent the major organs of metabolism and excretion. For example, a chemical that is primarily eliminated in the urine by an active process would require a kidney compartment, but a chemical that is eliminated primarily by exhalation would require a lung compartment. Metabolism studies with radiolabeled chemicals or other analytical methods, such as gas chromatography or high-performance liquid chromatography, will provide the kinetic data required to chose the important compartments for loss of parent chemical. Additional lumped compartments must be included to account for distribution of the chemical in the animal. A lipophilic chemical would require a fat compartment or compartments while a chemical that does not distribute to the fat would not. Distribution studies with radiolabeled or nonlabeled chemicals provide the details necessary for appropriate choices of compartments. New analytical methods such as positron emission tomography or nuclear magnetic residence imaging may appear promising to provide valuable distribution information in the whole animal. Organs in which the chemical has similar distribution may be lumped together if the organs have similar blood flow. Blood to organs can be determined from the literature or from microsphere techniques. Other compartments that may be desired in the model would be representative of target organs for toxicity or therapeutic effect.

Decisions about the form of a lumped compartment and the requirement for subcompartments depend on the relationship between blood flow to the compartment and solubility of the chemical in the compartment. Deciding whether the limiting factor in transfer of chemical from blood to the compartment is flow or diffusion is not always simple to determine experimentally (Riggs, 1963). It is probably best to assume blood flow is the limiting factor unless there is evidence otherwise or flow limitation does not adequately describe the behavior of a compartment. The most important principle in PB-PK modeling is to use the simplest description that adequately describes the behavior of the chemical.

Determine Physiological Parameters

Species-specific physiological parameters, such as blood flow and volumes of organs, are often available in the physiology handbooks or reviews (U.S. EPA, 1988; Fiserova-Bergerova and Hughes, 1983; Gerlowski and Jain, 1983; Snyder et al., 1974) or from published PB-PK models (Adolf, 1949; Dedrick, 1973; Lutz et al., 1980; Ramsey and Andersen, 1984). It is necessary to make decisions about which physiological parameters to use from the literature because there will undoubtedly be a range of values available. Avoid the temptation to change the physiological parameters to fall outside this normal range to obtain agreement between prediction and observation. If this temptation is not resisted, the result will be the loss of the ability to extrapolate. The physiological parameters in a PB-PK model for any species should be robust and not change when a different chemical is modeled, unless there is sound evidence that the chemical specifically causes changes, such as in blood flow. When prediction and observation do not agree there are two explanations: either the results of the experiment are not accurate or the model assumptions are inadequate. Once experimental calculations have been checked, the best approach is to determine if the structure of the model is adequate. In some cases, an important compartment has been overlooked or a diffusion limitation has been described as a flow limitation.

Determine Chemical Parameters

Metabolic constants, partition coefficients, and binding coefficients are much less available in the literature than the physiological parameters, and they must often be determined experimentally. Metabolic constants can be determined in many ways, both *in vitro* and *in vivo*. Methods used specifically for PB-PK modeling are the tissue homogenate methods of Dedrick and co-workers (1972) and *in vivo* gas uptake methods for measuring metabolism of volatile chemicals (Gargas et al., 1986). Partition coefficients for volatile chemicals in blood and tissue homogenates can be determined by the vial equilibration technique (Gargas et al., 1989). Partition coefficients for nonvolatile chemicals can be determined by measuring tissue and blood concentrations after continuous dosing to achieve equilibrium. Binding, which is distinguished from partitioning because it is not linearly related to concentration, can be determined by various methods (Dedrick and Bischoff, 1986; Lin et al., 1982). The same caveat about changing physiological parameters to fit the data applies to the chemical parameters. Halving the blood/air partition coefficient because it fits the experimental results better may solve an immediate problem at the expense of the general applicability of the model.

Validate Model where Absorption is Absent

Before a PB-PK model can be used to describe the process of absorption through the skin, it is necessary to gain some confidence in the quantitative description of pharmacokinetics when absorption is absent. The model should successfully simulate blood concentrations, tissue concentrations, or expired breath after intravenous exposures at several concentrations. Urinary or fecal excretion could also be used for validation, but they are not optimum because sampling times are critical. Ideally, prolonged intravenous infusions at several concentrations and intravenous boluses at several concentrations should be used to make sure that the physiological and pharmacokinetic parameters chosen will adequately describe the processes of distribution, metabolism, and excretion for a wide range of concentrations. An alternative approach would be to achieve the same confidence with subcutaneous infusions using minipumps (J. M. Gearheart, personal communication).

Validate Model with Dermal Absorption

When the parameters not involved in absorption are fixed, then the model can be used to understand the process of absorption through the skin. Parent chemical distribution in the body after absorption through the skin and hepatic metabolism will follow the same principles independent of the absorption process. When these processes are understood and quantified, the rate of absorption through the skin can be determined based on blood, tissue, breath, or excreta concentrations. Permeability constants can be determined by using the model to determine total chemical absorbed as long as the concentration on the skin and the surface area are known (McDougal et al., 1986). Figure 5 shows predicted blood concentrations for several organic chemicals when rats were exposed to carefully controlled vapor concentrations during whole-body exposures (McDougal et al., 1989).

Extrapolation to Humans

The ability to extrapolate from laboratory species to humans is one of the most important reasons for using PB-PK models. Ramsey and Andersen (1984) have shown that a physiologically based pharmacokinetic model for inhalation of styrene vapors in rodents can predict the pharmacokinetic behavior of inhaled styrene in humans by changing the blood flows, organ volumes, and partition coefficients to those of humans. The same principles could be used to extrapolate dermal absorption studies to humans if differences in skin structure are taken into account. It will be possible to quantitate the species differences in blood flow, differences in stratum corneum, and epidermal and subcutaneous fat thickness and composition, as well as the effect of the type and number of appendages on skin penetration in various species.

It has recently been shown that organic vapor penetration rates determined in rats using a PB-PK model are two to four times greater than penetration rates in humans calculated from the literature based on the total absorbed after whole-body exposures (McDougal et al., 1990). The consistency of these comparisons suggests that differences in permeability may be due to physical differences in the skin. Using this as an example, it is important to understand

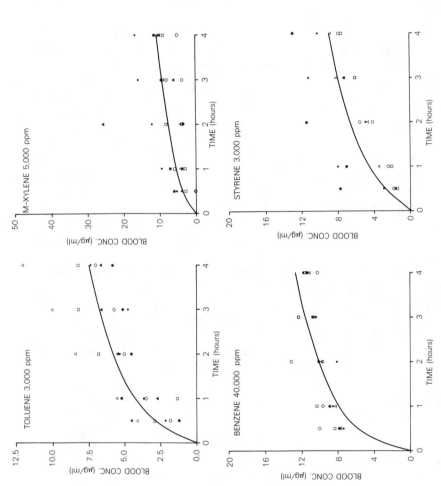

FIGURE 5 Comparisons of achieved blood concentrations (different symbol for each rat) and model predictions based on the best fit curve for each data set.

55

some of the approaches and limitations involved in extrapolation to humans. It is not possible to directly extrapolate, with any confidence, the published PB-PK model for organic vapors in rats to the published human studies. This is because the human studies were based on urinary output and/or exhaled breath and the rat studies were based on blood concentrations. It would be fairly easy to make the rat model capable of predicting exhaled breath and urinary output by adding urinary output and validating the rat model for these routes of excretion.

Once the rat model accurately predicted experimental results in the rat for urinary output and exhaled breath, the rat model could be used to address the human data by changing the physiological, pharmacokinetic, and biochemical parameters in the model to those of the human. For example, alveolar ventilation rates, blood flows, organ volumes, and urine volumes would need to be changed to those of the human. Partition coefficients, metabolic rates, and urinary excretion rates would need to be found or determined for each chemical of interest and changed in the model. With the published rat description, permeability constants were determined with confidence because the model was validated with a route where absorption was absent, that is, inhalation. If the scaled-up rat model did not predict the dermal exposures in humans, it could be because the permeability constant in humans is different (as suspected) or because the physiological or pharmacokinetic parameters used for humans were incorrect. It would be necessary to make sure that these parameters were correct with a route of absorption other than dermal.

Providing the rest of the description was correct, any inaccuracy in the prediction would be due to differences in permeability constant in the skin, and the permeability constant could be estimated by determining the constant required to fit the data. If the simple skin compartment [Eq. (21)] was descriptive for this chemical in the rat it would most likely be descriptive of the same chemical in the human. Other types of chemicals that penetrate more slowly than organic vapors may require that the skin be broken into some or all of the subcompartments described in Eqs. (11)–(16). In such a case, the subcompartments would also require that the structural differences in the skin be understood and quantitated.

When the Model Fails

Paradoxically, models are often most useful when they fail to adequately describe the experimental data. During the process of developing a more adequate description of the pharmacokinetic processes involved, a lot of insight can be gained that will apply to other situations and increase the understanding of the skin specifically and pharmacokinetics in general. It is the physiological foundation of the description that forces an investigator to design experiments to determine where the description is inaccurate. When frustration occurs, it is important to remember that the behavior of chemicals in living systems is not arbitrary. Chemicals and biological systems interact in accordance with physicochemical principles, which once understood are very reasonable and reliable. PB-PK modeling is an iterative process that requires theory and observation to come closer together until the final result is achieved.

Future of PB-PK Skin Models

PB-PK modeling can be applied to the effect of vehicles on penetration rates and penetration enhancement by understanding and quantitating the processes involved. Improved skin compartments can be developed and validated that include some of the subcompartments shown in Fig. 4 to be predictive of penetration rates of chemicals that have more complicated absorption profiles. Skin models can be used to extrapolate exposure standards based on other routes to dermal exposures. This understanding can be used to determine the effect of liquid chemicals on their own penetration rates by causing changes in the skin. Pharmacodynamic models that relate an effect, such as irritation, inflammation, or carcinogenesis, to the skin concentration can be developed.

CONCLUSION

Physiologically based pharmacokinetic models provide tremendous capacity to increase the understanding of dermal absorption. The ability to extrapolate between *in vivo* exposure conditions, doses, and species allows laboratory animal studies to provide a wealth of information applicable to human exposure situations. The ability to apply quantitative descriptions to processes occurring in the skin is limited only by our ability to understand the processes involved.

NOMENCLATURE

C	Concentration (mass/volume)
V	Volume
A	Area (distance^2)
Q	Flow (volume/time)
P	Permeability (distance/time)
K	Michaelis constant (mass/volume)
k	Maximum transport rate (mass/volume·time)
r	Proportionality constant (time^{-1})
R	Partition coefficient (unitless, ratio of concentrations)
V_{max}	Maximum velocity (mass/time)

Subscripts

a	arterial
b	blood
c	cardiac output
d	dermis
e	extracellular

fo	first order
i	*i*th tissue
is	interstitial
p	plasma
sc	stratum corneum
sf	subcutaneous fat
sfc	surface
sk	skin
t	tissue
v	venous
ve	viable epidermis

REFERENCES

Adolf, E. F. 1949. Quantitative relations in the physiological constitutions of mammals. *Science* 109:579–585.

Andersen, M. E. 1981. A physiologically-based toxicokinetic description of the metabolism of inhaled gases and vapors: Analysis at steady state. *Toxicol. Appl. Pharmacol.* 60:509–526.

Andersen, M. E., Clewell III, H. J., Gargas, M. L., Smith, F. A. and Reitz, R. H. 1987. Physiologically based pharmacokinetics and the risk assessment process for methylene chloride. *Toxicol. Appl. Pharmacol.* 87:185–205.

Angelo, M. J., Bischoff, K. B., Pritchard, A. B. and Presser, M. A. 1984. *J. Pharmacokin. Biopharm.* 12:413–436.

Birmingham, B. K., Greene, D. S. and Rhodes, C. T. 1979. Systemic absorption of topical salicylic acid. *Int. J. Dermatol.* 18:228–231.

Blank, I. H. and Scheuplein, R. J. 1964. The epidermal barrier. In *Progress in Biological Sciences in Relation to Dermatology*, eds. A. Rook and R. H. Champion, pp. 246–261. London: Cambridge University Press.

Braverman, I. M. and Keh-Yen, A. 1983. Ultrastructure of the human dermal microcirculation. IV. Valve-containing collecting veins at the dermal–subcutaneous junction. *J. Invest. Dermatol.* 81:438–442.

Chandrasekaran, S. K., Bayne, W. and Shaw, J. E. 1978. Pharmacokinetics of drug permeation through human skin. *J. Pharm. Sci.* 67:1370–1374.

Clewell III, H. J. and Andersen, M. E. 1985. Risk assessment extrapolations and physiological modeling. *Toxicol. Ind. Health* 1:111–131.

Clewell III, H. J. and Andersen, M. E. 1989. Improving toxicology testing protocols using computer simulations. *Toxicol. Lett.* 49:139–158.

Cooper, E. R. 1976. Pharmacokinetics of skin penetration. *J. Pharm. Sci.* 65:1396–1397.

Dedrick, R. L. 1973. Animal scale-up. *J. Pharmacokin. Biopharm.* 1:435–461.

Dedrick, R. L. and Bischoff, K. B. 1968. Pharmacokinetics in applications of the artificial kidney. *Chem. Eng. Prog. Symp. Ser.* 84. 64:32–44.

Dedrick, R. L., Forrester, D. D. and Ho, D. H. W. 1972. *In vitro–in vivo* correlation of drug metabolism-deamination of 1-β-D arabinofuranosylcytosine. *Biochem. Pharmacol.* 21:1–16.

Dugard, P. H. and Scott, R. C. 1984. Absorption through skin. In *Chemotherapy of Psoriasis,* ed. H. P. Baden, pp. 125–144. Oxford: Pergamon Press.

Elias, P. M. and Friend, D. S. 1975. The permeability barrier in mammalian epidermis. *J. Cell Biol.* 65:180–191.

Finnen, M. J. and Shuster, S. 1985. Phase 1 and phase 2 drug metabolism in isolated epidermal cells from adult hairless mice and in whole human hair follicles. *Biochem. Pharmacol.* 34:3571-3575.

Fiserova-Bergerova, V. and Hughes, H. C. 1983. Species differences on Bioavailability of inhaled vapors and gases. In *Modeling of Inhalation Exposure to Vapors: Uptake, Distribution and Elimination*, ed. V. Fiservoa-Bergerova, vol. 2, pp. 97-106. Boca Raton, Fla.: CRC Press.

Fisher, J. W., Whittaker, T. A., Taylor, D. H., Clewell III, H. J. and Andersen, M. E. 1989. Physiologically based pharmacokinetic modeling of the pregnant rat: A multiroute exposure model for trichloroethylene and its metabolite, trichloroacetic acid. *Toxicol. Appl. Pharmacol.* 99:395-414.

Flynn, G. L., Yalkowsky, S. H. and Roseman, T. J. 1974. Mass transport phenomenon and models: Theoretical concepts. *J. Pharm. Sci.* 63:479-509.

Gabrielsson, J. L., Johansson, P., Bondesson, U. and Paalzow, L. K. 1985. Analysis of methadone disposition in the pregnant rat by means of a physiological flow model. *J. Pharmacokin. Biopharm.* 13:355-372.

Gargas, M. L., Andersen, M. E. and Clewell III, H. J. 1986. A physiologically based simulation approach for determining metabolic constants from gas uptake data. *Toxicol. Appl. Pharmacol.* 86:341-352.

Gargas, M. L., Burgess, R. J., Voisard, D. E., Cason, G. H. and Andersen, M. E. 1989. Partition coefficients of low-molecular-weight volatile chemicals in various liquids and tissues. *Toxicol. Appl. Pharmacol.* 98:87-99.

Gerlowski, L. E. and Jain, R. K. 1983. Physiologically based pharmacokinetic modeling: Principles and Applications. *J. Pharm. Sci.* 72:1103-1127.

Gibaldi, M. and Perrier, D. 1982. *Pharmacokinetics.* New York: Marcel Dekker.

Guy, R. H., Hadgraft, J. and Maibach, H. I. 1982. A pharmacokinetic model for percutaneous absorption. *Int. J. Pharm.* 11:119-129.

Himmelstein, K. J. and Lutz, R. J. 1979. A review of the application of physiologically-based pharmacokinetic modeling. *J. Pharmacokin. Biopharm.* 7:127-137.

Kubota, K. and Ishizaki, T. 1986. A calculation of percutaneous drug absorption—I. Theoretical. *Comput. Biol. Med.* 16:17-19.

Leung, H-W, Ku, R. H., Paustenbach, D. J. and Andersen, M. E. 1988. A physiologically based pharmacokinetic model for 2,3,7,8-tetrachlorodibenzo-*p*-dioxin in C57BL/6J and DBA/2J mice. *Toxicol. Lett.* 42:15-28.

Lin, J. H., Sugiyama, Y., Awazy, S. and Hanano, M. 1982. *In vitro* and *in vivo* evaluation of the tissue-to blood partition coefficient for physiological pharmacokinetic models. *J. Pharmacokin. Biopharm.* 10:637-647.

Lutz, R. J., Dedrick, R. L. and Zaharko, D. S. 1980. Physiological pharmacokinetics: An *in vivo* approach to membrane transport. *Pharmacol. Ther.* 11:559-592.

Lutz, R. J., Dedrick, R. L., Matthews, H. B., Eling, T. E. and Anderson, M. W. 1977. A preliminary pharmacokinetic model for several chlorinated biphenyls in the rat. *Drug Metab. Dispos.* 5:386-395.

Lutz, R. J., Dedrick, R. L., Tuey, D., Sipes, I. G., Anderson, M. W. and Matthews, H. B. 1984. Comparison of the pharmacokinetics of several polychlorinated biphenyls in mouse, rat, dog, and monkey by means of a physiological pharmacokinetic model. *Drug Metab. Dispos.* 12:527-535.

Marzulli, F. N. and Tregear, R. T. 1961. Identification of a barrier layer in the skin. *J. Physiol.* 157:52-53p.

Marzulli, F. N., Brown, D. W. C. and Maibach, H. I. 1969. Techniques for studying skin penetration. *Toxicol. Appl. Pharmacol. Suppl.* 3:76-83.

Matthews, H. B. and Dedrick, R. L. 1984. Pharmacokinetics of PCBs. *Annu. Rev. Pharmacol. Toxicol.* 24:85-103.

McDougal, J. N., Jepson, G. W., Clewell III, H. J., MacNaughton, M. G. and Andersen, M. E. 1986. A physiological pharmacokinetic model for dermal absorption of vapors in the rat. *Toxicol. Appl. Pharmacol.* 85:286–294.

McDougal, J. N., Jepson, G. W., Clewell III, H. J., Gargas, M. L. and Andersen, M. E. 1990. Dermal absorption of organic chemical vapors in rats and humans. *Fundam. Appl. Toxicol.* 14:299–308.

Mershon, M. M. 1975. Barrier surfaces of skin. In *Applied Chemistry at Protein Interfaces*, pp. 41–73. Washington, D.C.: American Chemical Society.

Miller, S. C., Himmelstein, K. J. and Patton, T. F. 1981. A physiologically based pharmacokinetic model for the intraocular distribution of pilocarpine in rabbits. *J. Pharmacokin. Biopharm.* 9:653–677.

Mintun, M., Himmelstein, K. J., Schroder, R. L., Gibaldi, M. and Shen, D. D. 1980. Tissue distribution kinetics of tetraethylammonium ion in the rat. *J. Pharmacokin. Biopharm.* 8:373–409.

Odland, G. F. 1983. Structure of skin. In *Biochemistry and Physiology of the Skin,* ed. L. A. Goldsmith, vol. 1, pp. 3–63. New York: Oxford University Press.

Pannatier, A., Jenner, P., Testa, B. and Etter, J. C. 1978. The skin as a drug-metabolizing organ. *Drug Metab. Rev.* 8:319–343.

Peck, C. C., Lee, K. and Becker, C. E. 1981. Continuous transepidermal drug collection: Basis for use in assessing drug intake and pharmacokinetics. *J. Pharmacokin. Biopharm.* 9:41–57.

Ramsey, J. C. and Andersen, M. E. 1984. A physiologically based description of the inhalation pharmacokinetics of styrene in rats and humans. *Toxicol. Appl. Pharmacol.* 73:159–175.

Reitz, R. H., Mendrala, A. L., Park, C. N., Andersen, M. E. and Guengerich, F. P. 1988. Incorporation of in vitro enzyme data into the physiologically-based pharmacokinetic (PB-PK) model for methylene chloride: Implications for risk assessment. *Toxicol. Lett.* 43:97–116.

Riggs, D. S. 1963. *The Mathematical Approach to Physiological Problems: A Critical Primer.* Cambridge, Mass.: MIT Press.

Sato, A. and Nakajima, T. 1979. A vial-equilibration method to evaluate the drug-metabolizing enzyme activity for volatile hydrocarbons. *Toxicol. Appl. Pharmacol.* 47:41–46.

Scheuplein, R. J. 1967. Mechanism of percutaneous absorption. II. Transient diffusion and relative importance of various routes of skin penetration. *J. Invest. Dermatol.* 48:79–88.

Snyder, W. S., Cook, M. J., Nasset, E. S., Karhhausen, L. R., Howells, G. P. and Tipton, I. H. 1974. *Report of the Task Group on Reference Man.* Oxford: Pergamon Press.

U.S. Environmental Protection Agency. 1988. *Reference Physiological Parameters in Pharmacokinetic Modeling.* U.S. Environmental Protection Agency, Office of Health and Environmental Assessment, Office of Research and Development, Washington, D.C., EPA/600/6-88/004.

Wallace, S. M. and Barnett, G. 1978. Pharmacokinetic analysis of percutaneous absorption: Evidence of parallel pathways for methotrexate. *J. Pharmacokin. Biopharm.* 6:315–325.

3

in vitro percutaneous absorption

■ **Robert L. Bronaugh** ■ **Steven W. Collier** ■

INTRODUCTION

In vitro techniques are now widely used in the assessment of percutaneous absorption of potentially toxic chemicals. A major advantage of *in vitro* systems is that they allow for absorption measurements through human skin of chemicals too toxic to test ethically in human subjects. Absorption rates and skin metabolism can be measured more accurately in the *in vitro* system because sampling is performed directly beneath the barrier layer. Skin metabolism can be studied in viable skin without interference from systemic metabolic processes. Finally, absorption measurements are obtained much more easily from diffusion cells than from analysis of biological specimens from clinical studies. As with *in vivo* studies, the accuracy of *in vitro* measurements depends on the use of proper methodology.

IN VITRO METHODOLOGY

Diffusion Cell Design

Although many different designs have been utilized for diffusion cell studies, there are really only two basic types: the one-chambered and the two-chambered cell. Each type of cell has its own place in percutaneous absorption studies.

Variations of the two-chambered cell have been used for years to create conditions in which the diffusion of a compound in solution can be measured from one side of the membrane to the other (Scheuplein, 1965). An infinite dose (one that is large enough to maintain constant concentration during the course of an experiment) is added to one side of the membrane and its rate of diffusion across a concentration gradient into a solution on the opposite side is determined. Usually the solutions on both sides of the membrane are stirred to ensure uniform concentrations. Studies comparing permeation through skin to Fickian diffusion through a membrane are performed in this fashion. The two-chambered cell is useful for studying mechanisms of diffusion through skin and for measuring absorption from drug delivery devices when compounds are applied to skin at an infinite dose and a steady-state rate of delivery is desired.

The exposure of skin to permeating substances usually occurs under conditions that are different from those created in the two-chambered cell. Some substances, such as drug and cosmetic products, are intentionally applied to skin in creams or lotions. Other chemicals, often of toxicological interest, come in contact with skin in a wide variety of vehicles in our environment. Often the amount of penetrating substance on the surface of the skin is relatively small, and as permeation proceeds, a steady-state rate of absorption is not attained (finite dosage). In these examples, absorption of the chemicals through skin can only be studied in a one-chambered cell. The surface of the skin in this type of cell is open to the environment, so that thin layers of material can be applied in vehicles relevant to *in vivo* exposure. The skin is not excessively hydrated by continued exposure to an aqueous solution, as it is in the two-chambered cell. The chamber beneath the skin serves as a container for the receptor fluid that is continually stirred; samples are taken through a side-arm for subsequent determination of rates of absorption. If desired, infinite doses can also be applied to the skin in the one-chambered cell for determination of steady-state absorption kinetics. Finite dose techniques and the design of a static diffusion cell are described by Franz (1975).

A flow-through cell system (Bronaugh and Stewart, 1985) was introduced to automate sample collection from a one-chambered cell. It also facilitates the maintenance of skin viability because the physiological receptor fluid is continually replaced. The receptor fluid is pumped beneath the skin through a chamber with a volume of only 0.13–0.26 ml (depending on skin surface area of diffusion cell). This small volume allows the receptor contents to be rapidly and completely flushed out with flow rates of 1.5 ml/h or greater. Similar values have been obtained with flow-through and static cells in terms of the amount of material absorbed and the time course of absorption (Bronaugh and Stewart, 1985).

Special attention may be necessary in measuring the permeability of highly volatile compounds when the skin is not occluded to prevent evaporation. The short walls on the tops of some diffusion cells can protect the skin surface from air currents, and it has been suggested that this protection may be responsible for differences between *in vivo* and *in vitro* results (Bronaugh and Maibach, 1985; Bronaugh et al., 1985). Diffusion cells have been designed to collect evaporating material above the surface of the skin (Spencer et al., 1979; Reifenrath and Robinson, 1982). These cells have proven particularly useful in studies of the effectiveness of mosquito repellents and in studies of volatile compounds that require mass balance determinations.

Preparation of Skin

A membrane used in an *in vitro* study should simulate as closely as possible the barrier layer in skin. The barrier layer refers to the thickness of skin a compound must diffuse through *in vivo* before being taken up by blood vessels in the upper papillary dermis, and then entering the systemic circulation. The thickness of the barrier layer, which includes the whole epidermis and a small portion of the dermal tissue, varies, depending on the type of skin used, but is generally in the range of 100 μm for human skin.

If additional dermal tissue is present on the skin membrane used in a diffusion experiment, the effects of this tissue on absorption depend on the solubility of the chemical. A water-soluble substance will diffuse readily through the aqueous dermal tissue and its absorption will be affected only minimally by the presence of additional tissue. However, hydrophobic compounds will diffuse through this tissue very slowly and therefore will appear to be absorbed much more slowly than those observed in *in vivo* studies.

The use of full-thickness skin is really justifiable only when animal skin that is already very thin is used, such as that of the mouse (400 μm) (Behl et al., 1984) or rabbit. With the skin of other animals, such as the rat (800–870 μm) (Yang et al., 1986), guinea pig, monkey, and pig, full-thickness skin is almost 1 mm thick, and human skin can be several millimeters thick (Loden, 1985). Therefore, some means should be used to prepare a membrane that accurately reflects the barrier layer in thickness. As mentioned above, this is particularly important when hydrophobic compounds are examined. The use of the dermatome is the best way to prepare biological membranes for percutaneous absorption studies. Unlike other methods, a dermatome can be used with hairless or haired skin, and it can be used without adversely affecting the viability of the membrane.

Elevation of temperature has been used for a number of years to loosen the bond between the epidermis and dermis for the preparation of epidermal sheets. Baumberger et al. (1942) placed full-thickness human skin on a hot plate for 2 min at a temperature of 50 °C and found that the epidermis could easily be removed from the dermis by using blunt dissection. Heated water (60 °C) is used more commonly for this separation because of better temperature control, which leads to more reproducible results (Scheuplein, 1965; Bronaugh et al., 1981). Heat separation of skin is useless, however, for preparing a membrane for absorption studies with haired skin. The hair shafts remain in the dermis, causing holes to be created in the epidermal membrane as it is pulled from the dermis. Therefore, only the skin from hairless animals can be separated by this procedure. A different length of exposure to heat may be required for separation of animal skin.

The effect of heat on the viability of skin is of concern in absorption/metabolism studies. The enzymatic hydrolysis of diisopropyl fluorophosphate in human skin appeared to be inactivated during the heat separation procedure (Loden, 1985). However, separation of epidermis from dermis using 55 °C heat for 30 s reduced aryl hydrocarbon hydroxylase activity only 10–15% (Mukhtar and Bickers, 1981).

Epidermis has been separated from dermis after soaking full-thickness human and animal skin in different chemical solutions. Exposure times are usually measured in hours; therefore, viability of skin is probably lost.

The effects of 2 M solutions of various salt anions and cations on separation of the epidermis was investigated with human skin (Felsher, 1947). The epidermis was separated by acids and bases at pH values that caused swelling of the collagen. The most potent anions were bromide, thiocyanate, and iodide ions, whereas acetate, sulfate, and citrate ions were ineffective in causing separation.

The advantage of chemical separation is that it appears to be effective in separating the epidermis from the dermis of haired animals under certain conditions. The barrier properties remain unaltered because the hair shaft comes out of the dermis during separation and stays in place in the epidermis. Scott and co-workers (1986) reported that after soaking skin from 28-day-old Wistar rats in 2 M sodium bromide for 24 h, epidermal membranes could be separated from the dermis. However, this procedure was ineffective with skin of older rats (7–8 wk of age).

A few studies are reported in the literature concerning the separation of epidermis and dermis by incubation of skin in enzyme preparations. The protease dispase produced an epidermal sheet that could be peeled easily from the dermis of human skin after a 24-h incubation at 4 °C (Kitano and Okada, 1983). A crude bacterial collagenase at a concentration of 0.1 or 0.2% was effective in the preparation of epidermal sheets after a 3-h incubation at 37 °C. (Hentzer and Kobayasi, 1978). Unlike dispase separation, most of the cells were nonviable following separation, but differences in temperature of the incubations may have been responsible. The use of the enzymes pancreatin and trypsin for epidermal–dermal separation has also been described (Omar and Krebs, 1975).

Receptor Fluid

The selection of the receptor fluid has become an increasingly important decision as investigators strive to create *in vitro* conditions that can adequately duplicate the *in vivo* situation. For measuring the absorption of water-soluble compounds, the use of normal saline or an isotonic buffer solution may be sufficient. Recently it was demonstrated that some chemicals are metabolized significantly during the percutaneous absorption process (Kao et al., 1984). The viability of skin can be maintained for 24 h in a flow-through diffusion cell by using a physiological buffer as the receptor fluid (Collier et al., 1989a). Metabolism and percutaneous absorption can be measured simultaneously as discussed below in the Metabolism section. The combined information gives a more complete picture of absorption because the actual permeating species are identified.

Many members of important classes of chemicals, such as fragrances, pesticides, and petroleum products, are highly lipophilic and readily enter and diffuse through the stratum corneum. The measurement of percutaneous absorption by *in vitro* methods of these water-insoluble compounds requires special techniques and is a frequent source of experimental error. When hydrophobic compounds are applied *in vivo,* they are taken up by blood perfusing the skin directly below the epidermis. When these compounds are applied to skin *in vitro,* they are absorbed into the skin but will not freely partition from it into a saline or aqueous buffer solution. Analysis of the receptor fluid suggests that little or no penetration of skin is taking place. We examined a number of receptor fluids for their ability to facilitate partitioning from skin and thus give permeation results comparable to the *in vivo* absorption of several fragrance ingredients (Bronaugh and Stewart, 1984). The absorption of [^{14}C]cinnamyl anthranilate and [^{3}H]cortisone from a petrolatum vehicle was measured through rat skin (Table 1). Cortisone, the control compound, had enough water solubility that its permeation was not limited by partitioning into the receptor fluids. If a receptor fluid enhanced the absorption of cortisone (in addition to the fra-

TABLE 1. Effect of Diffusion Cell Conditions on the Absorption of Cinnamyl Anthranilate (Cortisone Control)[a]

Receptor fluid	Cinnamyl anthranilate % absorbed (5 days)	Cortisone permeability constant × 10^5 (cm/h)
Normal saline (4), whole skin	5.0 ± 0.3	3.8 ± 0.7
1.5% Volpo 20 (4), whole skin	5.4 ± 0.9	—
Normal saline (4)	5.8 ± 0.4	7.1 ± 0.5
1.5% Volpo 20 (10)	15.5 ± 1.2	6.1 ± 0.5
6% Volpo 20 (8)	27.9 ± 1.8	7.0 ± 0.5
20% Volpo (8)	18.3 ± 1.8	9.3 ± 0.9
Rabbit serum (4)	8.3 ± 0.6	6.8 ± 0.8
3% Bovine serum albumin (4)	12.1 ± 1.2	5.4 ± 0.2
50 : 50 Methanol : water (4)	27.1 ± 2.0	17.2 ± 0.5
1.5% Triton-X (4)	17.9 ± 1.1	10.8 ± 0.5
6% Triton-X (4)	38.4 ± 2.9	14.5 ± 0.3
6% Pluronic F68 (4)	7.3 ± 1.3	9.8 ± 0.6

[a]Values are the mean ± SEM of the number of determinations in parentheses. For most experiments, a 350-μm section from the surface of whole rat skin was prepared with a Padgett electrodermatone. Compounds were applied to skin in a petrolatum vehicle. *In vivo* absorption of cinnamyl anthranilate was 45.6%.

grance ingredient), the increase in absorption was considered to be due to an alteration of the barrier properties of the skin by the receptor fluid. Although rabbit serum or a serum albumin solution would be desirable from a physiological standpoint, those substances were less effective in enhancing absorption than the nonionic surfactants and organic solvents used. The most effective receptor fluid that could be used without apparent damage to the skin was the nonionic surfactant polyethylene glycol 20 oleyl ether (Volpo 20, Croda Inc., New York, N.Y.). A suitable receptor fluid must be selected cautiously to avoid alteration of the barrier properties of skin. Agents that enhance partitioning of hydrophobic test compounds may also remove lipid-soluble constituents of skin. A water solubility of less than approximately 10 mg/l (in combination with good lipid solubility) would indicate a potential problem in a diffusion cell with a standard aqueous receptor fluid (Bronaugh and Stewart, 1984).

Recently, we found it necessary to take a different approach in our studies of the absorption/metabolism of hydrophobic compounds. The use of a lipophilic receptor fluid can destroy metabolic activity of skin. Alternatively, percutaneous absorption can be measured if the material absorbed into skin and remaining there at the end of the experiment is included as part of the absorbed compound (Bronaugh et al., 1989a). If an epidermal membrane is used and if the receptor fluid is stirred and contains protein (4% bovine serum albumin), then the artificial dermal reservoir is eliminated and the receptor fluid contents more accurately reflect rates of skin permeation of hydrophobic compounds (Bronaugh et al., 1989b).

Mixing of Receptor Contents

In most diffusion systems receptor contents can be mixed by some kind of automatic stirring device in the receptor fluid. In a flow-through cell with a small receptor volume (less than 0.5 ml), agitation from the fluid flowing through the cell can provide adequate mixing. As mentioned above, we recently observed that for water-insoluble compounds an increased partitioning of the test compound into receptor fluid occurs when receptor contents are mixed with a small stirring bar. Presumably the same effect could be achieved by increasing the flow rate of the receptor fluid; however, this would dilute the receptor fluid levels of absorbed material and possibly make analytical methods more difficult.

SKIN METABOLISM AND PERCUTANEOUS ABSORPTION

It has now been established that skin is capable of a variety of biotransformational processes (Pannatier et al., 1978; Bickers, 1980; Kappus, 1989). Although the activity of many enzymatic processes, particularly oxidative ones, is much lower in skin than in liver (Bronaugh et al., 1989a), reductive processes and N-acetyltransferase have been reported as relatively active in skin (Kawakubo et al., 1988; Fuchs et al., 1989). The importance of metabolism during percutaneous absorption depends on the structure and biological activity of the penetrating compounds and metabolite(s). For benzo[a]pyrene (B[a]P), metabolism in the skin is necessary for activation to a proximate skin carcinogen. For other compounds little or no metabolism may take place, and so for them skin metabolism may not be toxicologically important.

The predominant experimental techniques for cutaneous enzyme activity have been the use of epidermal homogenates (Alvares et al., 1973; Andersson et al., 1982; Cheung et al., 1985; Kulkarni et al., 1987) and epidermal cells in culture (Coomes et al., 1983). The use of isolated cells or subcellular fractions to study cutaneous metabolism *in vitro,* although advantageous for some specific enzymatic studies, does not attempt to model the *in vivo* situation. The architecture of the intact organ controls water and ionic gradients (Warner et al., 1988a, 1988b), and pH effects (Cohen and Iles, 1975) appear to affect its metabolism and differentiation. Intact skin may be a more useful model for estimating metabolic rates and processes encountered *in vivo* and has been used by a few researchers for skin metabolism studies (Kao et al., 1984; Collier et al., 1989a; Riviere et al., 1986). The measurement of metabolism during the percutaneous penetration process requires a suitable system for measuring percutaneous absorption and maintaining skin viability, a sensitive analytical methodology for penetrant and metabolite measurement, and a suitably prepared skin membrane. *In vivo,* the extent of cutaneous metabolism is difficult to differentiate from systemic metabolism. Frequently the rates of cutaneous metabolism are low when compared to liver, and the measurement of metabolites is sometimes precluded by the quantity of blood that must be collected. When venous effluents are collected for analysis, the contribution of skin metabolism is confounded with that of plasma metabolism. Carefully designed and validated *in vitro* skin models can unambiguously provide metabolic data.

For percutaneously absorbed compounds with biologically active metabolites (toxic or therapeutic), metabolic rates determined during percutaneous absorption provide the intermediate kinetic data for linking pharmacokinetic parameters, such as rates of absorption, with pharmacodynamic effects. Cutaneous metabolism exhibits the same types of complexities as hepatic metabolism. The relative activities of different processes in a metabolic scheme determine the spectrum of metabolites. Saturability of cutaneous metabolic pathways may be common for moderately and quickly absorbed compounds. To investigate some of these relationships, specific activities for aryl hydrocarbon hydroxylase and ethoxycoumarin deethylase in skin were determined (Storm et al., 1990) (Table 2). B[a]P readily absorbs percutaneously (Bronaugh and Stewart, 1986). It is metabolized only slightly in the skin; however, this is sufficient to exert its topical carcinogenicity. B[a]P is very lipophilic and resists partitioning into aqueous receptor fluids of *in vitro* systems. The more polar metabolites of B[a]P are able to partition into receptor fluid, where the most metabolites were recovered in *in vitro* diffusion-cell studies. Figure 1 shows the cumulative metabolic disposition of B[a]P in Sencar mouse and hairless guinea

TABLE 2. Specific Activity of Microsomal Enzymes in Skin[a]

Species	Aryl hydrocarbon hydroxylase (pmol/min/mg protein)	Ethoxycoumarin deethylase (pmol/min/mg protein)
Hairless guinea pig	2.51 ± 0.35^b	3.8 ± 2.7^c
Human	0.24 ± 0.08^b	Not detectable
Sencar mouse	3.35 ± 0.07^b	10.4 ± 1.4

[a]Values are the mean $\pm$ SEM of three or four determinations. Hairless guinea pig and human skin were from 200-μm sections; mouse skin was full thickness.
[b]Significantly different from both other species (LSD test, $p < .01$).
[c]Less than Sencar mouse (t-test, $p = .06$).

pig skin from these studies and the rates of metabolism based upon the appearance of metabolites in the receptor fluid fractions. 7-Ethoxycoumarin and 7-hydroxycoumarin are much more hydrophilic compounds that readily partition into the receptor fluid. By quantitating parent and metabolite at different times during 7-ethoxycoumarin penetration, the relationship between rate of penetration and extent of metabolism can be elucidated. Ethoxycoumarin deethylase is active in human skin but at a very low level, and it is very easily saturated. The higher activity in mouse and guinea pig skin is reflected by the inability of 7-ethoxycoumarin to saturate the deethylase by percutaneous penetration (Fig. 2). Determination of these relationships can be useful, for example, in optimizing the formulation of topically applied products and reducing the uncertainty in risk assessment from percutaneous exposure to toxic compounds.

Dynamic *in vitro* skin diffusion systems that maintain tissue viability have a unique utility in dermatoxicological investigations. The proper use of such systems and the proper interpretation of the data they provide are necessary for accurate experimental conclusions. In these studies, the use of thick skin preparations is not only undesirable from a percutaneous diffusional perspective but also might limit duration of viability by limiting diffusion of perfusate and dissolved oxygen to viable epidermis. Skin utilizes most glucose anaerobically, producing lactate. The maintenance of viability in static cells is complicated by cumulative depletion of glucose from the receptor fluid and the necessity of a buffer capacity large enough to maintain physiological pH values. Adequate measures must be taken to ensure the microbiological integrity of the diffusion-cell system to differentiate between mammalian cell and bacterial metabolism. The apparatus must be sterilized before each study. The receptor fluid must also be sterilized, and because viable primary skin tissue cannot be sterilized, antibiotics must be used. Serum use might be justified in the study of lipophilic compound penetration and metabolism to provide a more lipophilic receptor fluid; however, the variability of serum and its intrinsic ability to metabolize some compounds is of concern. The use of bovine serum albumin for this purpose instead of whole serum represents a less costly and better defined alternative. When determining the contributions of cutaneous metabolism in an absorption study, as is standard practice for any biochemical study, suitable blanks must be performed to correct for any nonenzymatic changes in the parent compound.

Intact viable dermatome skin sections from mice, rats, hairless guinea pigs, and humans have been used in flow-through diffusion cells to study the penetration and metabolism of estradiol, testosterone (Collier et al., 1989a), acetyl ethyl tetramethyltetralin (AETT), butylated hydroxytoluene (BHT) (Bronaugh et al., 1989a), B[a]P, 7-ethoxycoumarin (Storm et al., in press), and azo

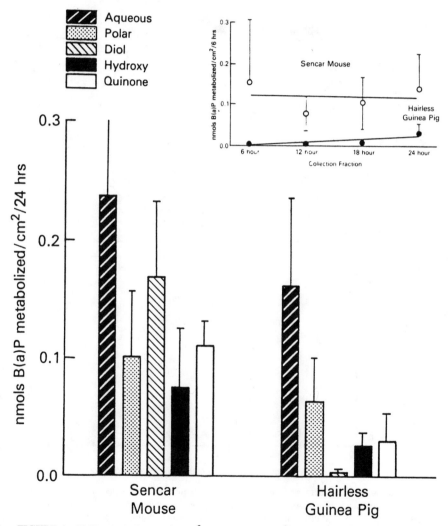

FIGURE 1 B[a]P metabolized [nmol/cm^2/24 h and nmol/cm^2/6 h (inset)] by Sencar mouse and hairless guinea pig skin in flow-through diffusion cells. Values are means $\pm$ SEM of four or five determinations.

R. L. Bronaugh and S. W. Collier

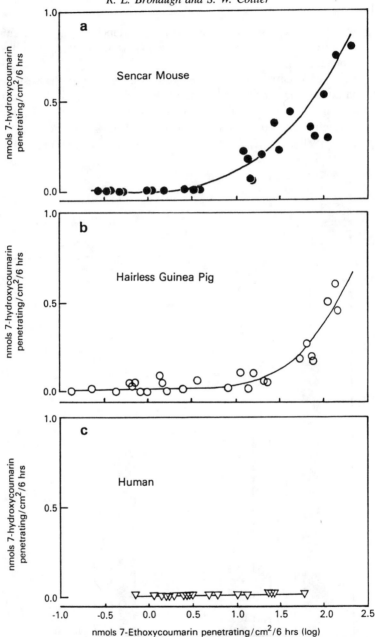

FIGURE 2 Relationship between rate of 7-ethoxycoumarin (7-EC) percutaneous penetration and 7-EC cutaneous metabolism in (*a*) Sencar mouse, (*b*) hairless guinea pig, and (*c*) human skin. Values represent individual determinations of rate of 7-EC penetration (log) and simultaneous rate of 7-hydroxycoumarin penetration for each 6-h collection period after application of 7-EC in 10 μl acetone at doses ranging from 5 to 250 μg/cm^2.

colors (Collier et al., 1989b). The extent of metabolism of a percutaneously absorbed compound cannot be assumed to be negligible. By suitably preparing and maintaining viable skin *in vitro*, the investigator can readily assess percutaneous absorption and the effects of cutaneous metabolism on topically absorbed compounds.

REFERENCES

Alvares, A. P., Kappas, A., Levin, W. and Conney, A. H. 1973. Inducibility of benzo[a]pyrene in human skin by polycyclic hydrocarbons. *Clin. Pharmacol. Ther.* 14:30–40.

Andersson, P., Edsbäcker, S., Ryerfeldt, Å. and Von Bahr, C. 1982. In vitro biotransformation of glucocorticoids in liver and skin homogenate fraction from man, rat, and hairless mouse. *J. Steroid Biochem.* 16:787–795.

Baumberger, P. J., Suntzeff, V. and Cowdry, E. V. 1942. Methods for the separation of epidermis from dermis and some physiologic and chemical properties of isolated epidermis. *J. Natl. Cancer Inst.* 2:413–423.

Behl, C. R., Flynn, G. L., Kurihara, T., Smith, W. M., Bellantone, N. H., Gataitan, O. and Higuchi, W. I. 1984. Age and anatomical site influences on alkanol permeation of skin of the male hairless mouse. *J. Soc. Cosmet. Chem.* 35:237–252.

Bickers, D. R. 1980. The skin as a site of drug and chemical metabolism. In *Current Concepts in Cutaneous Toxicity,* eds. V. A. Drill and P. Lazar, pp. 95–126. New York: Academic Press.

Bronaugh, R. L. and Maibach, H. I. 1985. Percutaneous absorption of nitroaromatic compounds: In vivo and in vitro studies in the human and monkey. *J. Invest. Dermatol.* 84:180–183.

Bronaugh, R. L. and Stewart, R. F. 1984. Methods for in vitro percutaneous absorption studies. III: Hydrophobic compounds. *J. Pharm. Sci.* 73:1255–1258.

Bronaugh, R. L. and Stewart, R. F. 1985. Methods for in vitro percutaneous absorption studies. IV: The flow-through diffusion cell. *J. Pharm. Sci.* 74:64–67.

Bronaugh, R. L. and Stewart, R. F. 1986. Methods for in vitro percutaneous absorption studies. VI. Preparation of the barrier layer. *J. Pharm. Sci.* 75:487–491.

Bronaugh, R. L., Congdon, E. R. and Scheuplein, R. J. 1981. The effect of cosmetic vehicles on the penetration of *N*-nitrosodiethanolamine through excised human skin. *J. Invest. Dermatol.* 76:94–96.

Bronaugh, R. L., Stewart, R. F., Wester, R. C., Bucks, D., Maibach, H. I. and Anderson, J. 1985. Comparison of percutaneous absorption of fragrances by humans and monkeys. *Food Chem. Toxicol.* 23:111–114.

Bronaugh, R. L., Stewart, R. F. and Storm, J. E. 1989a. Extent of cutaneous metabolism during percutaneous absorption of xenobiotics. *Toxicol. Appl. Pharmacol.* 99:534–543.

Bronaugh, R. L., Collier, S. W. and Stewart, R. F. 1989b. In vitro percutaneous absorption of a hydrophobic compound through viable hairless guinea pig skin. *Toxicologist* 9:61.

Cheung, Y. W., Li Wan Po, A. and Irwin, W. J. 1985. Cutaneous biotransformation as a parameter in the modulation of the activity of topical corticosteroids. *Int. J. Pharm.* 26:175–189.

Cohen, R. D. and Iles, R. A. 1975. Intracellular pH: Measurement, control, and metabolic interrelationships. *CRC Crit. Rev. Clin. Lab. Sci.* 6:101–143.

Collier, S. W., Sheikh, N. M., Sakr, A., Lichtin, J. L., Stewart, R. F. and Bronaugh,

R. L. 1989a. Maintenance of skin viability during in vitro percutaneous absorption/metabolism studies. *Toxicol. Appl. Pharmacol.* 99:522–533.

Collier, S. W., Storm, J. E. and Bronaugh, R. L. 1989b. Structure-related differences in the metabolic fate of aniline during azo color metabolism in Sencar mouse skin. *Toxicologist* 9:164.

Coomes, M. W., Norling, A. H., Pohl, R. J., Müller, D. and Fouts, J. R. 1983. Foreign compound metabolism by isolated skin cells from the hairless mouse. *J. Pharmacol. Exp. Ther.* 225:770–777.

Felsher, Z. 1947. Studies on the adherence of the epidermis to the corium. *J. Invest. Dermatol.* 8:35–47.

Franz, T. J. 1975. On the relevance of in vitro data. *J. Invest. Dermatol.* 64:190–195.

Fuchs, J., Mehlhorn, R. J. and Packer, L. 1989. Free radical reduction mechanism in mouse epidermis skin homogenates. *J. Invest. Dermatol.* 93:633–640.

Hentzer, B. and Kobayasi, T. 1978. Enzymatic liberation of viable cells of human skin. *Acta Dermatol. Venereol. (Stockh.)* 58:197–203.

Kao, J., Hall, J., Shugart, L. R. and Holland, J. M. 1984. An in vitro approach to studying cutaneous metabolism and disposition of topically applied xenobiotics. *Toxicol. Appl. Pharmacol.* 75:289–298.

Kappus, H. 1989. Drug metabolism in the skin. In *Pharmacology of the Skin. II,* eds. M. W. Greaves and S. Shuster, pp. 123–163. New York: Springer-Verlag.

Kawakubo, Y., Manabe, S., Yamazoe, Y., Nishikawa, T. and Kato, R. 1988. Properties of cutaneous acetyltransferase catalyzing *N*- and *O*-acetylation of carcinogenic arylamines and *N*-hydroxyarylamine. *Biochem. Pharmacol.* 37:265–270.

Kitano, Y. and Okada, N. 1983. Separation of the epidermal sheet by dispase. *Br. J. Dermatol.* 108:555–560.

Kulkarni, A. P., Nelson, J. L. and Radulovic, L. L. 1987. Partial purification and some biochemical properties of neonatal rat cutaneous glutathione *S*-transferases. *Comp. Biochem. Physiol.* 87B:1005–1009.

Loden, M. 1985. The in vitro hydrolysis of diisopropyl fluorophosphate during penetration through human full-thickness skin and isolated epidermis. *J. Invest. Dermatol.* 85:335–339.

Mukhtar, H. and Bickers, D. R. 1981. Drug metabolism in skin. *Drug Metab. Dispos.* 9:311–314.

Omar, A. and Krebs, A. 1975. An analysis of pancreatic enzymes used in epidermal separation. *Arch. Dermatol. Res.* 253:203–212.

Pannatier, A., Jenner, P., Testa, B. and Etter, J. C. 1978. The skin as a drug-metabolizing organ. *Drug Metab. Rev.* 8:319–343.

Reifenrath, W. G. and Robinson, P. B. 1982. In vitro skin evaporation and penetration characteristics of mosquito repellents. *J. Pharm. Sci.* 71:1014–1018.

Riviere, J. E., Bowman, K. F., Monteiro-Riviere, N. A., Dix, L. P. and Carver, M. P. 1986. The isolated perfused porcine skin flap (IPPSF). I. A novel in vitro model for percutaneous absorption and cutaneous toxicology studies. *Fundam. Appl. Toxicol.* 7:444–453.

Scheuplein, R. J. 1965. Mechanism of percutaneous absorption. I. Routes of penetration and influence of solubility. *J. Invest. Dermatol.* 45:334–346.

Scott, R. C., Walker, M. and Dugard, P. H. 1986. *In vitro* percutaneous absorption experiments: A technique for the production of intact epidermal membranes from rat skin. *J. Soc. Cosmet. Chem.* 37:35–41.

Spencer, T. S., Hill, J. A., Feldmann, R. J. and Maibach, H. I. 1979. Evaporation of diethyltoluamide from human skin in vivo and in vitro. *J. Invest. Dermatol.* 72:317–319.

Storm, J. E., Collier, S. W., Stewart, R. F. and Bronaugh, R. L. 1990. Metabolism of xenobiotics during percutaneous penetration: Role of absorption rate and cutaneous enzyme activity. *Fundam. Appl. Toxicol.*

Warner, R. R., Myers, M. C. and Taylor, D. A. 1988a. Electron probe analysis of human skin: Element concentration profiles. *J. Invest. Dermatol.* 90:78–85.

Warner, R. R., Myers, M. C. and Taylor, D. A. 1988b. Electron probe analysis of human skin: Determination of the water concentration profile. *J. Invest. Dermatol.* 90:218–224.

Yang, J. J., Roy, T. A. and Mackerer, C. R. 1986. Percutaneous absorption of benzo[a]pyrene in the rat: Comparison of in vivo and in vitro results. *Toxicol. Ind. Health* 2:409–416.

4

in vivo percutaneous absorption

■ Ronald C. Wester ■ Howard I. Maibach ■

INTRODUCTION

Percutaneous absorption is a primary focal point for dermatotoxicology and dermatopharmacology. Local and systemic toxicity depend on a chemical penetrating the skin. The skin is both a barrier to absorption and a primary route to the systemic circulation. The skin's barrier properties are impressive. Fluids and precious chemicals are reasonably retained within the body, while at the same time hundreds of foreign chemicals are restricted from entering the systemic circulation. Many pharmacologists and physicians have been frustrated in their attempts to deliver drugs to and through the skin.

Even with these impressive barrier properties, the skin is a primary body contact with the environment and the route by which many chemicals enter the body. In most instances the toxicity of the chemical is slight and/or the bioavailability (rate and amount of absorption) of the bioactive chemical is too low to cause an immediate response. However, some chemicals applied to the skin have proved to be toxic. In addition, potentially toxic chemicals that come in contact with the skin continue to be discovered.

This chapter deals with the methods used to study *in vivo* percutaneous absorption and the many factors affecting it. The interpretation of such studies should be restricted to the limits of the study design. The methodology and supportive information discussed here should help formulate good study design.

METHODS USED TO DETERMINE *IN VIVO* PERCUTANEOUS ABSORPTION

Skin Stripping: Short-Term Exposure

The cellophane tape stripping method determines the concentration of chemical in the stratum corneum at the end of a short application period (30 min) and by linear extrapolation predicts the percutaneous absorption of that chemical for longer application periods. The chemical is applied to skin of animals or humans and after the 30-min application time the stratum corneum is blotted and then removed by successive tape applications. The tape strippings are asssayed for chemical content. Rougier, Lotte, and co-workers have established a linear relationship between this stratum corneum reservoir content and percutaneous absorption using the standard urinary excretion method. The major advantages of this method are (1) the elimination of urinary (and fecal) excretion to determine absorption and (2) the applicability to nonradiolabeled determination of percutaneous absorption because the skin strippings contain adequate chemical concentrations for nonlabeled assay methodology. This is an exciting new system for which more research is needed to establish limitations (Rougier et al., 1983, 1986; Dupuis et al., 1986).

Skin Flaps

The methodology is to surgically isolate a portion of skin (pig) so that a singular blood supply is created to collect blood containing the chemical that has been absorbed through skin. The skin flap can be used to study percutaneous absorption *in vivo* or *in vitro*. The absorption of chemicals through skin and metabolism within the skin can be determined by assay of the perfusate. The isolated perfused porcine skin flap (IPPSF) is an alternative *in vitro* animal model used by Riviere et al. (1986, 1987). The skin sandwich flap (SSF) is an island flap that has split-thickness skin grafted to its subcutaneous surface directly under the superficial epigastric vasculature. In this setting, the dermis of the donor skin and subcutaneous tissue of the host flap grow together, sandwiching the vessels supplying the flap, the superficial epigastric vessels. Two additional steps allow this sandwich to be converted to an island sandwich flap, which is isolated on its vasculature and transferred to the rat's back by a series of surgical procedures. The juncture on the femoral vessels supplying and draining the flap can be readily visualized with an incision in the groin and is accomplished routinely. The exposed vein draining the flap tolerates multiple venipunctures. The SSF can be constructed with either human, pig, or rat skin as the donor skin (Pershing and Krueger, 1989).

Systemic Bioavailability (Blood and Excreta)

Percutaneous absorption *in vivo* is usually determined indirectly by measuring radioactivity in excreta following topical application of the labeled compound. In human studies, plasma levels of the test compound are extremely low following topical application, often below assay detection level, so it is necessary to use tracer methodology. The labeled compound, usually carbon-14 or tritium, is applied to the skin. The total amount of radioactivity excreted in urine (or urine plus feces) is then determined. The amount of radioactivity retained in the body or excreted by some route not assayed (CO_2, sweat) is corrected by determining the amount of radioactivity excreted following parenteral administration. This final amount of radioactivity is then expressed as the percent of the applied dose that was absorbed (Feldmann and Maibach, 1969a). The equation used to determine percutaneous absorption is

$$\text{Percent absorbed} = \frac{\text{total radioactivity excreted following topical administration}}{\text{total radioactivity excreted following parenteral administration}} \times 100$$

Determination of percutaneous absorption from urinary radioactivity excretion does not account for metabolism by skin. The radioactivity in urine is a mixture of parent compound and metabolites. Plasma radioactivity can be measured and the percutaneous absorption determined by the ratio of the areas under the curve for plasma concentration versus time following topical and intravenous administration (Wester and Noonan, 1978). Radioactivity in blood and excreta can include both the applied compound and metabolites. If the metabolism by skin is extensive and different from that of other systemic tissues, then this method is not valid because the pharmacokinetics of the metabolites are not representative of the parent compound. However, in practice, this method has given results similar to those obtained from urinary excretion (Wester et al., 1981).

The way to determine the absolute bioavailability of a topically applied compound is to measure the compound by specific assay in blood or urine following topical and intravenous administration. This is difficult when plasma concentrations after topical administration are low. However, as more sensitive assays are developed, estimates of absolute topical bioavailability will become a reality. A comparison of the above methods was performed by using [^{14}C]nitroglycerin in rhesus monkeys (Table 1). The difference between the estimate of absolute bioavailability (56.6%) and that of [14]C (72.7–77.2%) is the percent of compound metabolized in the skin as the compound was being absorbed. For nitroglycerin this is about 20% (Wester et al., 1981).

Surface Disappearance

Another approach used to determine *in vivo* percutaneous absorption is to measure the loss of radioactive material from the surface as it penetrates the skin. Recovery of an ointment or solution following skin application is difficult because total recovery from the skin is never assured. With topical application by a transdermal delivery device, the total unit can be removed from the skin and the residual amount of drug in the device can be determined. The difference

TABLE 1. Bioavailability of Topical Nitroglycerine Determined from Plasma Nitroglycerin, Plasma ^{14}C, and Urinary Excretion of $^{14}C^a$

Method	Mean bioavailability (%)
Plasma nitroglycerin AUC^b	56.6 ± 2.5
Plasma total radioactivity AUC^b	77.2 ± 6.7
Urinary total radioactivity^c	72.7 ± 5.8

^{a}See Wester et al. (1981) for details.
^{b}Absolute bioavailability of nitroglycerin and ^{14}C:

$$\text{Percent} = \frac{\text{AUC (ng·h/ml)/topical dose}}{\text{AUC (ng·h/ml)/iv dose}} \times 100$$

^{c}Percent = (total ^{14}C excretion following topical administration)/(total ^{14}C excretion following iv administration) × 100.

between the applied and the residual dose is assumed to be the amount of drug absorbed. One must be aware that the skin may act as a reservoir for unabsorbed material.

Biological Response

Another *in vivo* method of estimating absorption is to use a biological/pharmacological response (McKenzie and Stoughton, 1962). Here, a biological assay is substituted for a chemical assay and absorption is estimated. An obvious disadvantage to the use of a biological response is that it is only good for compounds that will elicit an easily measurable response. An example of a biological response would be the vasoconstrictor assay in which the blanching effect of one compound is compared to that of a known compound. This method is perhaps more qualitative than quantitative.

Other qualitative methods of estimating *in vivo* percutaneous absorption include whole-body autoradiograpy and fluorescence. Whole-body autoradiography will give an overall picture of dermal absorption followed by the involvement of other body tissues with the absorbed compound.

PARAMETERS THAT AFFECT *IN VIVO* PERCUTANEOUS ABSORPTION

Drug Concentration, Surface Area, and Time

When a compound comes in contact with skin the amount of absorption will depend on many parameters. Foremost among these parameters are concentration of applied dose, surface area, and contact time. As the concentration of applied dose increases, the efficiency of absorption (percent) can change. However, a more relevant point is that as the amount applied per unit area is increased the total amount absorbed into the body may increase (Wester and Maibach, 1976; Scheuplein and Ross, 1974). The other parameter closely associated with dose is surface area. Increasing the area of surface on which the dose is applied increases the amount absorbed (Noonan and Wester, 1980). Therefore, the greatest potential for percutaneous absorption can occur when a high concentration of compound is spread over a large part of the body. Percutaneous absorption also increases with skin contact time. Figure 1 shows the gradual increase in percutaneous absorption of malathion in humans with increased skin contact time.

Skin Site of Application

Variation in absorption occurs depending on the anatomic site of application. This is true for both humans (Feldmann and Maibach, 1967; Maibach et al., 1971) and animals (Wester et al., 1980b). Table 2 shows the effect of anatomical region on *in vivo* percutaneous absorption of parathion and malathion in humans (Wester and Maibach, 1989a). Similar results exist for hydrocortisone (Feldmann and Maibach, 1967). The data are of obvious practical significance in that increased total absorption is found for head, neck, and axilla, where both cosmetic and environmental exposure are greater. Preliminary results indicate that the vulva (not mucosa) shows greater absorption than forearm skin but less absorption than scrotal skin. Similar anatomic variation

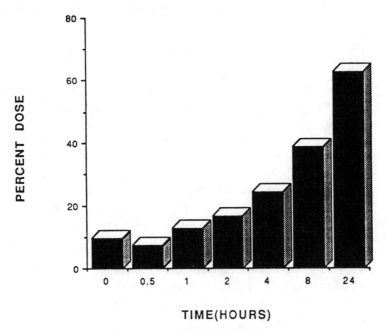

FIGURE 1 Time course for percutaneous absorption of malathion in man. Systemic absorption increases with chemical residence time on skin.

TABLE 2. Effect of Anatomical Region on *In Vivo* Percutaneous
Absorptions of Pesticides in Humans

Anatomical region	Dose absorbed (%)	
	Parathion	Malathion
Forearm	8.6	6.8
Palm	11.8	5.8
Foot, ball	13.5	6.8
Abdomen	18.5	9.4
Hand, dorsum	21.0	12.5
Forehead	36.3	23.2
Axilla	64.0	28.7
Jaw angle	33.9	69.9
Fossal cubitalis	28.4	
Scalp	32.1	
Ear canal	46.6	
Scrotum	101.6	

has been shown for pesticides (Maibach et al., 1971). With the wide variety of chemical moieties examined (steroids, pesticides, and antimicrobials) the general pattern of regional variation holds. One exception was carbaryl, which was extensively absorbed from the forearm, although other sites were not significantly higher. This suggests that carbaryl is extensively absorbed from all body sites.

Occlusion

Percutaneous absorption is increased if the site of application is occluded. Occlusion is a covering of the application site, either intentionally as with bandaging or unintentionally as by putting on clothing after applying a compound topically. A vehicle such as an ointment can also have occlusive properties. Occlusion results in a combination of many physical factors affecting the skin and the applied compound. It changes the hydration and temperature of the skin, and these physical factors affect absorption. It also prevents the accidental wiping off or evaporation (volatile compound) of the applied compound.

Exposure to humans is usually to uncovered skin areas (head, face, neck, hands, arms), although pesticides will get under clothing. In animal studies, it is necessary to protect the skin site of application so that the animal does not ingest the dose (pseudo-oral results). Yet occluding the site will enhance skin absorption beyond that relative to humans. Therefore, the use of nonocclusive protective covers is recommended for animal studies.

Skin Condition

There are skin conditions other than hydration and temperature that affect percutaneous absorption. The most obvious is loss of barrier function of the stratum corneum through disease or damage. Skin also changes with age. The genesis of the stratum corneum occurs during gestation and is probably concluded by birth (Singer et al., 1971). Preterm infants probably do not have a fully developed stratum corneum and therefore may have increased skin permeability (Nachman and Esterly, 1971). The skin of the elderly also undergoes change and this may influence absorption. Virtually any type of change in skin condition, especially in the barrier function of the stratum corneum, whether natural or inflicted, may change the percutaneous absorption of the skin.

Shown in Fig. 2 are the results of removal of the stratum corneum with cellophane tape stripping, occlusion with plastic film, removal of the epidermis with cantharidin, and the combination of stripping and occlusion (Feldmann and Maibach, 1965). Stripping the skin with tape until it glistens removes the stratum corneum and causes damage to the upper layers of the epidermis; this is a model for damaged and diseased skin. Stripped skin shows a fourfold increase in penetration of hydrocortisone. Occluding the hydrocortisone with a plastic film during the first 24 h causes a 10-fold increase in absorption over that of unoccluded skin. Recent work (unpublished) at our laboratory indicates that trapping of water under the occlusive layer is necessary for this increased penetration. Removal of the epidermis by topical application of a cantharidin solution leaves a denuded skin site, which absorbs 15 times more hydrocortisone than untreated skin. The greatest absorption was obtained by stripping followed by a 24-h occlusion, yielding penetration 20 times the value for normal skin.

It is commonly stated that the stratum corneum is the major barrier to percutaneous penetration. This is generally true for intact skin. Fortunately, when the stratum corneum is damaged the other layers function as barriers to penetration, as evidenced by these data; none of the damages inflicted on the skin caused 100% absorption. Presumably, each epidermal cell membrane, the basement membrane, and other cellular structures must also have barrier properties.

Vehicle

Percutaneous absorption of a drug from a vehicle depends on the partitioning of the drug between the vehicle and the skin and the solubility of the drug in the vehicle. In addition to drug solubility, factors such as drug concentration and pH may influence the interaction between vehicle, drug, and skin. The vehicle may change the integrity of the skin and this will influence absorption. An example would be an occlusive vehicle, which would alter skin hydration. Vehicles can contain an agent such as urea that will enhance percutaneous absorption, or the vehicle itself will enhance absorption. The best example of the latter is dimethyl sulfoxide (DMSO), which readily permeates skin and causes enhanced absorption. In most cases the vehicle disappears quickly, and its destination is not determined. The increase in absorption observed with DMSO may be due to changes in the horny layer, shown by significant decreases in electrical resistance after treatment. Others have attempted to en-

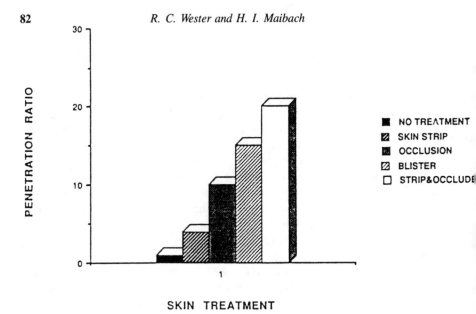

SKIN TREATMENT

FIGURE 2   Hydrocortisone absorption through modified skin in human.

hance penetration by employing bases with lower solvency for the active compound than the skin lipids. With lower solubility in the carrier it is expected that the compound would preferentially diffuse into the skin. This effect was not observed with mineral oil and propylene glycol, which are poor hydrocortisone solvents but produced no significant change in penetration (Anjo et al., 1980).

Multiple Dose Application

Figure 3 summarizes the *in vivo* percutaneous absorption of single (day 1) versus multiple (8-day) skin applications in humans. For malathion (Wester et al., 1983) and the steroids hydrocortisone, testosterone, and estradiol (Bucks et al., 1989) there is no difference in percutaneous absorption between single and repeated application. Repeated skin application in animals in which topical toxicity is determined is another story. Table 3 shows that when animal skin is washed with soap and water between repeated applications, skin absorption is enhanced. Washing skin in humans has no apparent effect. Also, multiple application in animals without skin wash has no effect.

Figure 4 shows the percutaneous absorption of hydrocortisone following a single application of 40 $\mu g/cm^2$ and the same amount applied in divided doses. The total amounts absorbed per 24-h application are different. Absorption from one application of the high concentration was greater than absorption from the same concentration applied in equally divided doses (Wester et al., 1977b, 1980b). This suggests that the absorption from subsequent applications was influenced by the first topical application.

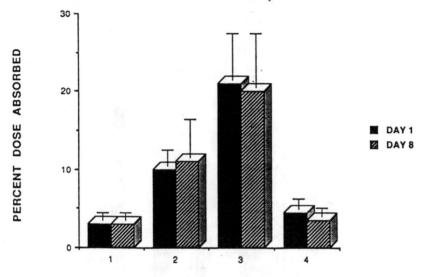

(1)HYDROCORTSONE (2)ESTRADIOL (3) TESTOSTERONE (4)MALATHION

FIGURE 3 Percutaneous absorption in human for single dose application and when the chemical is applied in a continual series for 8 days.

There is a correlation between frequency of application, percutaneous absorption, and toxicity of applied chemical. Wilson and Holland (1982) determined the effect of application frequency in epidermal carcinogenic assays. Application of a single large dose of a highly complex mixture of petroleum or synthetic fuels to a skin site increased the carcinogenic potential of the chemical compared to a smaller or more frequent application (Table 4). The carcinogenic toxicity correlated well with the results of Wester et al. (1980b) (Fig. 4), where a single applied dose increased the percutaneous absorption of the material compared to smaller or intermittent applications.

TABLE 3. Percutaneous Absorption with Multiple-Dose Animals, Human, and Skin Wash

Chemical	Species	Wash	Absorption	Reference
Malathion	Human	Yes	Same	Wester et al. (1983)
Malathion	Guinea pig	Yes	Enhanced	Bucks et al. (1989)
Malathion	Guinea pig	No	Slight	Bucks et al. (1989)
Hydrocortisone	Human	Yes	Same	Bucks et al. (1989)
Hydrocortisone	Rhesus	Yes	Enhanced	Wester et al. (1980a)
Benzoyl peroxide	Guinea pig	Yes	Enhanced	Bucks et al. (1989)
Benzoic acid	Rhesus	No	Same	Bucks et al. (1989)
Parathion	Rhesus	No	Same	Bucks et al. (1989)
Salicylic acid	Rhesus	No	Same	Bucks et al. (1989)
Estradiol	Human	Yes	Same	Bucks et al. (1989)
Testosterone	Human	Yes	Same	Bucks et al. (1989)

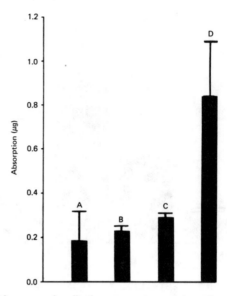

FIGURE 4 Effect of frequency of application on percutaneous absorption of hydrocortisone from ventral forearm of rhesus monkey. Ordinate is micrograms absorbed. Bar A, 13.3 $\mu g/cm^2$ applied once at 9:00 a.m. Bars B and C, 40 $\mu g/cm^2$ applied in divided doses of 13.3 $\mu g/cm^2$ at 9:00 a.m., 2:30 p.m., and 9:00 p.m. The site of application was washed between divided doses for C, but not for B. Bar D, 40 $\mu g/cm^2$ applied at 9:00 a.m.

Metabolism

A single chemical entity is applied to the skin, but what enters the systemic circulation is that chemical entity and its metabolites. Percutaneous first-pass metabolism is defined as the metabolism of the compound as it is absorbed through the skin. This is about 16–20% for topical nitroglycerin (Wester et al., 1981) and about 100% for benzoyl peroxide (Nacht et al., 1981).

In both *in vitro* and *in vivo* percutaneous absorption studies, amounts and rates of absorption are determined from radioactivity counting. The implication is that the rates and amounts represent the applied compound, whereas in fact

TABLE 4. Shale Oil-Induced Incidence of Epidermal Tumors

Shale oil	Dose (mg)	Frequency (per week)	Total dose per week (mg)	Number of animals with carcinogenic tumors
OCSO No. 6	10	4×	40	2
	20	2×	40	4
	40	1×	40	13
PCSO II	10	4×	40	11
	20	2×	40	17
	40	1×	40	19

they represent the applied compound and its metabolites. Unless the applied parent compound is measured by a specific assay, the lack of metabolites cannot be assumed.

In the preceding section the capacity of the skin to change or respond to the applied compound was discussed. This also applies to skin metabolism and the subsequent percutaneous absorption. Skin metabolic enzymes, like other metabolic enzymes, can be induced. For example, chronic administration of coal tar products can change the metabolic activity of skin. This or other inducing products can be applied as part of the treatment course or added in the vehicle used to deliver a particular compound.

Race

Wester et al. (1990) examined the effect of race on percutaneous absorption. Figure 5 shows that with the test chemicals benzoic acid, caffeine, and acetylsalicylic acid there was no difference in skin absorption for Caucasians, Blacks, and Asians.

Skin Decontamination

Decontamination of a chemical from the skin is commonly done by washing with soap and water. It has been assumed that washing will remove the chemical. However, recent evidence suggests that many times the skin and the body are unknowingly subjected to enhanced penetration and systemic

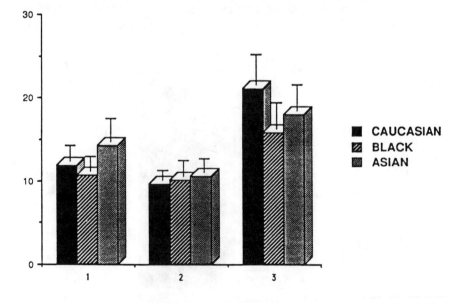

FIGURE 5 Percutaneous absorption in human volunteers with Caucasian, Black, and Asian skin.

absorption/toxicity because the decontamination procedure does not work or may actually enhance absorption (Wester and Maibach, 1989b). What is certain is that soap and water wash will remove chemical from the stratum corneum (Fig. 6). However, *in vivo* percutaneous absorption is a dynamic process, and decontamination capacity becomes reduced with time (Fig. 7). As chemicals are absorbed into the skin (and on into the body) they cannot be removed by skin surface wash.

COMPARATIVE *IN VIVO* STUDIES

The basic data for *in vivo* human percutaneous absorption, to which animal models are compared, were obtained by Feldmann and Maibach (1969a, 1969b, 1974). In these clinical studies a specific concentration of radioactive compound was applied to a specific nonoccluded anatomic site and the subjects were requested not to wash the area for 24 h.

Bartek et al. (1972) undertook a comparative study of percutaneous absorption in rats, rabbits, miniature swine, and humans. The methodology used with animals was similar to that used with humans, except that in animals the compounds were applied to the back and the skin was shaved. Radioactive compounds were applied to the skin in the same manner that had been used with humans. A nonoccluding device was used to keep the animal from removing the applied compound.

Haloprogin, a topical antifungal agent, was completely absorbed in the rat and the rabbit. Penetration through the skin of pigs and humans was similar and

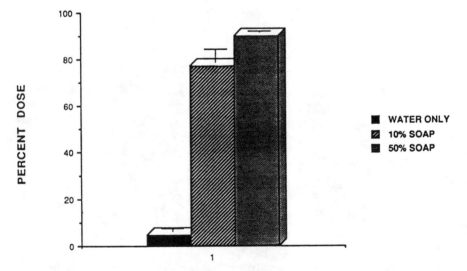

FIGURE 6   Ability of soap to partition alachlor from powdered human stratum corneum into rinse water.

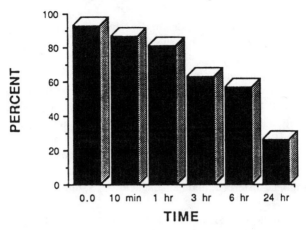

TIME

FIGURE 7   Removal of PCBs from rhesus monkey skin with soap and water. As time progresses, less PCBs are removed because they are being absorbed into the skin and into the body.

much slower than it was through rat and rabbit skin. Penetration of acetylcysteine was minimal in all species. Cortisone, a minimal penetrant through the skin of humans and miniature swine, was well absorbed in the rat and rabbit. Caffeine readily penetrated the skin of all species. With butter yellow (dimethylaminoazobenzene), penetration through rabbit skin was much greater than through the skin of the other three species. Testosterone penetration was greatest in the rabbit, followed closely by the rat and then the pig, which was closest to humans. The results of this study showed rabbit skin to be the most permeable to topically applied compounds, followed closely by rat skin. In contrast, it appears that the permeability of the skin of the miniature swine is closer to that of human skin. Clearly, percutaneous absorption in the rabbit and rat would not be predictive of that in humans. It is not known whether the subtle differences seen between pig and human skin were due to methodology (site of application, shaving) or the skin itself. However, in general the pig appears to be a good predictor of percutaneous absorption in humans.

Bartek and La Budde (1975) also studied the percutaneous absorption of pesticides in the rabbit, pig, and squirrel monkey and compared the results with the absorption observed in humans. The compounds were applied to the backs of animals and compared with application to the human ventral forearm. DDT was a minimal penetrant in humans, whereas in the rabbit and pig penetration rates were considerably greater. Absorption in the squirrel monkey was very low; however, the value reported was uncorrected with parenteral control data. Penetration of lindane, parathion, and malathion in the rabbit exceeded that in the other species. With lindane, penetration in the squirrel monkey was closer to that in humans, whereas with parathion, penetration in the pig was closest to that in humans. Penetration of malathion was similar in the squirrel monkey and the pig and could be predictive of that in humans. It appears that the *in vivo* percutaneous absorption of pesticides in the rabbit was again much greater than in humans, whereas penetration in the pig and squirrel monkey was closer to that in humans.

Several comparisons of percutaneous absorption in the rhesus monkey and in humans have been made (Wester and Maibach, 1975a, 1975b, 1976, 1977; Wester and Noonan, 1980; Wester et al., 1979). The methodology and site of application (ventral forearm) were the same for both species. The site of application was lightly clipped in the monkey. A direct comparison of unshaven and lightly clipped skin showed no difference in absorption (Wester and Maibach, 1975a). The *in vivo* percutaneous absorption and dose response for hydrocortisone, testosterone, and benzoic acid were similar for rhesus monkeys and humans.

Hunziker et al. (1978) studied the percutaneous absorption of ^{14}C-labeled benzoic acid, progesterone, and testosterone in the Mexican hairless dog and compared the absorption with that observed in humans. Total absorption and maximum absorption rates were greater in humans than in the hairless dog. Surface counting experiments showed that benzoic acid and progesterone persisted on the dog skin far longer than on human skin.

In several of the preceding studies the percutaneous absorption of testosterone was determined. In these studies the same topical concentration (4 μg/cm^2) and method of analysis (determination of urinary ^{14}C excretion) were used. Table 5 summarizes the results. Absorption of testosterone in the rat and rabbit was high compared to that in humans. Absorption in the pig was approximately twice that in humans, and the rhesus monkey was closest to humans. The site of application for the rat, rabbit, and pig was the back, whereas for the rhesus monkey and human the site of application was the ventral forearm. Percutaneous absorption of testosterone in the rhesus monkey and human varies with site of application. What proportions of the variation in the above comparison are due to species and to site of application are not known. However, the comparison points out that when a difference is found, it could be a sum of the many variables in the study.

The comparative *in vivo* data that have been reviewed demonstrate that percutaneous absorption in the pig and monkey (rhesus and squirrel) is similar to that in humans, whereas in the rat, and especially in the rabbit, skin penetra-

TABLE 5. Percutaneous Absorption of Testosterone in Several Species

Species	Percent of dose absorbed	Ratio
Human	13.2	1.0
Rhesus monkey	18.4	1.4
Pig	29.4	2.2
Guinea pig	34.9	2.6
Rat	47.4	3.6
Rabbit	69.6	5.3

tion is greater than that observed in humans. The skin of the Mexican hairless dog has significantly different permeability characteristics than human skin. This is illustrated in Figure 8 for DDT percutaneous absorption.

For dermatotoxicology, predicting human skin absorption for health risk assessment should require an animal model relevant to man for percutaneous absorption. Despite the cited literature, absorption in the rat is chosen because of the animal's low cost and availability (Zendzian, 1989). The disparity between rat and a more relevant animal model, the rhesus monkey, is illustrated in Table 6 for dinoseb (Wester et al., 1989).

This discussion does not mean that a suitable animal model has been developed. In fact, old models are continually being evaluated and new models are being pursued. Andersen et al. (1980) determined the percutaneous absorption of hydrocortisone, testosterone, and benzoic acid in the guinea pig. Absorption of hydrocortisone and benzoic acid was similar to that in humans, but testosterone was absorbed to a greater extent in the guinea pig. The absorption value for testosterone was closer to the human value if the excretion of radioactivity in urine and feces was measured rather than that in urine alone. If a large proportion of the radioactivity is excreted in feces, a more accurate estimate of the percutaneous absorption can be obtained by determining the radioactivity excretion in both urine and feces. Another animal model available for percutaneous absorption studies is the hairless mouse, with and without a thymus. With thymus-deficient hairless mice, skin from other species (including humans) can be transplanted and the percutaneous absorption through the transplanted skin determined (Kruger and Shelby, 1981).

IN VIVO AND *IN VITRO* PERCUTANEOUS ABSORPTION

Franz (1975) evaluated the permeability of 12 organic compounds *in vitro* in excised human skin and compared the results with those obtained previously by Feldmann and Maibach in living humans. Care was taken to ensure that the *in vitro* conditions closely followed those used *in vivo,* although it was necessary to use human abdominal skin for the *in vitro* studies. Also, the doses employed ranged from 4 to 40 $\mu g/cm^2$, with the assumption that the percent of applied dose absorbed would not be dose dependent. Quantitatively, the *in vitro* and *in vivo* data did not agree. The *in vitro* method was of value to the extent that it tended to distinguish compounds of low permeability from those of high permeability. However, there are notable differences, suggesting that the *in vitro* method alone would not always be a reliable or accurate predictor of percutaneous absorption in living humans. A more recent presentation by Franz (1979) suggested that many of the differences in the above studies were due to technical reasons. Future work in this area may prove the *in vitro* method to be predictive of *in vivo* absorption.

Table 7 contains a comparison of paraquat permeability constants for human and other animal skin samples determined by *in vivo* and *in vitro* methodol-

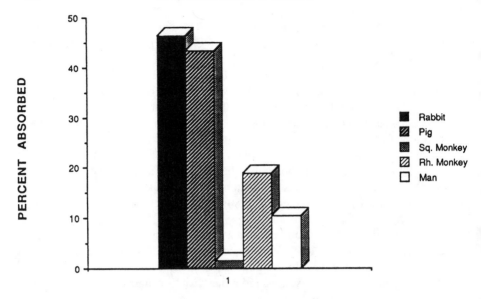

ACETONE VEHICLE

FIGURE 8   Comparative percutaneous absorption of DDT in various animal models and in human.

ogy. There was a multithousandfold difference in permeability between human skin and different animal skins (Wester and Maibach, 1985).

Table 8 shows that absorption of triclocarban in a standard *in vitro* static system was 0.13 ± 0.05% of applied dose through human adult abdominal skin. *In vivo* in humans, the absorption was 7.0 ± 2.8%. The difference was due to insolubility of triclocarban in the small volume of saline in the reservoir of the static system. By changing to a continuous flow system, the volume of saline was greatly increased, the solubility of triclocarban was no longer the

TABLE 6. *In Vivo* Percutaneous Absorption of Dinoseb in Rhesus Monkey and Rat

Applied dose ($\mu g/cm^2$)	Skin penetration (%)	Dose accountability (%)
	Rat	
51.5	86.4 ± 1.1	87.9 ± 1.8
128.8	90.5 ± 1.1	91.5 ± 0.6
643.5	93.2 ± 0.6	90.4 ± 0.7
	Rhesus monkey	
43.6	5.4 ± 2.9	86.0 ± 4.0
200.0	7.2 ± 6.4	81.2 ± 18.1
3620.0	4.9 ± 3.4	80.3 ± 5.2

TABLE 7. *In Vivo* and *In Vitro* Absorption of Paraquat through Human and Laboratory Animal Skin

Species	Paraquat permeability rate (μg/cm^2)	Paraquat permeability constant (cm/h $\times$ 10^5)
In vivo		
Human	0.03	—
In vitro		
Human	0.5	0.7
Rat	—	27.2[a]
Hairless rat	—	35.3[a]
Nude rat	—	35.5[a]
Mouse	—	97.2[a]
Hairless mouse	—	1065[a]
Rabbit	—	92.9[a]
Guinea pig	—	196[a]

[a]Significantly different from human.

limiting factor in absorption, and *in vitro* absorption approached that of *in vivo* absorption (Wester et al., 1985).

Thus we see from the above comparative *in vivo* and *in vitro* studies that *in vitro* percutaneous absorption may not be substantiated by *in vivo* data.

PERCUTANEOUS ABSORPTION IN THE NEONATE

Little is known about percutaneous absorption in the infant. Yet it is in the infant where the greatest toxicological response has been seen following topical administration.

Percutaneous absorption in the newborn rhesus monkey was assessed (Wester et al., 1977a). The study showed that absorption of testosterone in the full-term newborn was the same as that in the adult. With one other newborn rhesus, a topical dose of 40 μg/cm^2 testosterone was applied to the ventral forearm and the area was occluded with Saran wrap and adhesive tape for 24 h. Percutaneous absorption was 14.7%, which was twice the value for nonoccluded absorption.

The study showed that a high percentage of a steroid can be absorbed

TABLE 8. *In Vitro* and *In Vivo* Percutaneous Absorption of Triclocarban

System	Percent dose absorbed
Static system (23 °C)	
Human adult abdominal skin ($n = 8$)	0.13 $\pm$ 0.05
Continuous flow system (23 °C)	
Human adult abdominal system ($n = 12$)	6.0 $\pm$ 2.0
Human, *in vivo*	7.0 $\pm$ 2.8

through the skin of an infant. It also suggested an interesting relation between the skin surface area of a newborn and the systemic availability of the applied compound. Once the compound (and/or metabolites) is absorbed, it is available systemically. In the newborn the ratio of surface area (square centimeters) to body weight (kilograms) is three times that in the adult. Therefore, given an equal application area of skin in the newborn and adult, the systemic absorption seen in the newborn can be much more when based on kilograms of body weight. After topical application of the same strength of compound to both the adult and the newborn, the systemic availability in the newborn is 2.7 times that in the adult (Table 9). With a different ratio of skin surface to body weight, the therapeutic ratio is probably lower in the newborn than in the adult when the compound is applied topically. This increased systemic availability in the newborn would also be related to any differences in systemic metabolism between the newborn and the adult.

PHARMACOKINETICS OF PERCUTANEOUS ABSORPTION

Most of the preceding discussion of pharmacokinetics has focused on bioavailability from a percutaneous route of administration. Bioavailability can be defined as the rate and extent to which the administered drug ingredient or therapeutic moiety is absorbed from a drug formulation and becomes available at the site of drug action and/or reaches the general circulation. Other pharmacokinetic parameters are the distribution, metabolism, and excretion of the applied chemical. Distribution can be in the layers of skin or in all tissues of the body through the general circulation. Metabolism can be a two-way street. A toxic chemical can be detoxified by metabolism. Skin and other tissue enzymes can also be induced. The enzymes can then form toxic metabolites. The rate of excretion is important, for it also determines the steady-state concentration of chemical within the body. Therefore, with percutaneous absorption we focus on the bioavailability potential of a chemical. However, the potential toxicity or effective therapeutic dose may depend on the total pharmacokinetics of the chemical.

TABLE 9. Systemic Availability in Newborn and Adult
following Topical Application

Parameter	Adult[a]	Infant[b]
Surface area (cm^2)	17,000	2200 (13% of adult)
Topical dose (mg)	100	13 (13% of adult)
Patient weight (kg)	70	3.4 (neonate)

[a]Systemic dose = (100 mg × 0.2)/(70 kg) = 0.28 mg/kg; 0.2 represents 20% of compound absorbed.
[b]Systemic dose = (13 mg × 0.2)/(3.4 kg) = 0.76 mg/kg.

DISCUSSION

In vivo percutaneous absorption is a complex biological process. The skin is a multilayered biomembrane that has certain absorption characteristics. If the skin were a simple inert membrane, absorption parameters could easily be measured and they would be fairly constant provided there was no change in the chemistry of the membrane. However, skin is a dynamic living tissue, and its absorption parameters are susceptible to constant change. Factors such as occlusion, vehicles, and skin condition can rapidly change the absorption characteristics. Also, the skin will change through its own growth patterns. With percutaneous absorption, the skin would not be viewed as an inert membrane but as a dynamic living biomembrane with unique properties.

Animals are used in experiments with substances that cannot be used in humans. No one animal, with its complex anatomy and biology, will simulate the penetration in humans for all compounds. We found that rhesus monkeys and miniature domestic pigs yield the best correlation with human penetration. Physical studies and *in vitro* models yield useful information about the mechanism of penetration and its theoretical implications, but they have not duplicated human *in vivo* rates or total penetration. Therefore, the best estimate of human percutaneous absorption is determined by *in vivo* studies in humans or animals.

The key to good data is the design at the start of the study. The interpretation of results should not go beyond the limits of the study. We have summarized many aspects of percutaneous absorption. Each of these should be carefully considered. The results will lead to a better understanding of percutaneous absorption.

REFERENCES

Andersen, K. E., Maibach, H. I. and Anjo, D. M. 1980. The guinea pig: An animal model for human skin absorption of hydrocortisone, testosterone and benzoic acid. *Br. J. Dermatol.* 102:447–453.

Anjo, D. M., Feldmann, R. J. and Maibach, H. I. 1980. Methods for predicting percutaneous penetration in man. In *Percutaneous Absorption of Steroids,* eds. P. Mauvais-Jarvis, C. F. H. Vickers, and J. Wepierre, pp. 31–51. New York: Academic Press.

Bartek, M. J. and La Budde, J. A. 1975. Percutaneous absorption *in vitro.* In *Animal Models in Dermatology,* ed. H. Maibach, pp. 103–120. New York: Churchill-Livingstone.

Bartek, M. J., La Budde, J. A. and Maibach, H. I. 1972. Skin permeability *in vivo:* Comparison in rat, rabbit, pig and man. *J. Invest. Dermatol.* 58:114–123.

Bucks, D. A. W., Maibach, H. I. and Guy, R. H. 1989. *In vivo* percutaneous absorption: Effect of repeated application versus single dose. In *Percutaneous Absorption,* 2d ed., eds. R. Bronaugh and H. Maibach, pp. 633–651. New York: Marcel Dekker.

Dupuis, D., Rougier, A., Roguet, R. and Lotte, C. 1986. The measurement of the stratum corneum reservoir: A simple method to predict the influence of vehicles on *in vivo* percutaneous absorption. *Br. J. Dermatol.* 115:233–238.

Feldmann, R. J. and Maibach, H. I. 1965. Penetration of ^{14}C hydrocortisone through normal skin: The effect of stripping and occlusion. *Arch. Dermatol.* 91:661-666.

Feldmann, R. J. and Maibach, H. I. 1967. Regional variation in percutaneous penetration of ^{14}C cortisone in man. *J. Invest. Dermatol.* 48:181-183.

Feldmann, R. J. and Maibach, H: I. 1969a. Absorption of some organic compounds through the skin in man. *J. Invest. Dermatol.* 54:339-404.

Feldmann, R. J. and Maibach, H. I. 1969b. Percutaneous penetration of steroids in man. *J. Invest. Dermatol.* 52:89-94.

Feldmann, R. J. and Maibach, H. I. 1974. Percutaneous penetration of some pesticides and herbicides in man. *Toxicol. Appl. Pharmacol.* 28:126-132.

Franz, T. J. 1975. Percutaneous absorption. On the relevance of *in vitro* data. *J. Invest. Dermatol.* 64:190-195.

Franz, T. J. 1979. The finite dose technique as a valid *in vitro* model for study of percutaneous absorption in man. Presented at the Annual Scientific Seminar, Society of Cosmetic Chemists, May, Dallas, Texas.

Hunziker, N., Feldmann, R. J. and Maibach, H. I. 1978. Animal models of percutaneous penetration: Comparison in Mexican hairless dogs and man. *Dermatologica* 156:788-798.

Kruger, G. G. and Shelby, J. 1981. Biology of human skin transplanted to the nude mouse. I. Response to agents which modify epidermal proliferation. *J. Invest. Dermatol.* 76:506-510.

Maibach, H. I., Feldmann, R. J., Milby, T. H. and Serat, W. F. 1971. Regional variation in percutaneous penetration in man. *Pestic. Arch. Environ. Health* 23:208-211.

McKenzie, A. W. and Stoughton, R. B. 1962. Method for comparing percutaneous absorption of steroids. *Arch. Dermatol.* 86:608-610.

Nachman, R. L. and Esterly, N. B. 1971. Increased skin permeability in pre-term infants. *J. Pediatr.* 79:628-632.

Nacht, S., Yeung, D., Beasley, J. N., Jr., Anjo, D. M. and Maibach, H. I. 1981. Benzoyl peroxide: Percutaneous penetration and metabolic disposition. *J. Am. Acad. Dermatol.* 4:31-37.

Noonan, P. K. and Wester, R. C. 1980. Percutaneous absorption of nitroglycerin. *J. Pharm. Sci.* 69:365-366.

Pershing, L. K. and Krueger, G. G. 1989. Human skin sandwich flap model for percutaneous absorption. In *Percutaneous Absorption,* 2d ed., eds. R. Bronaugh and H. Maibach, pp. 397-414. New York: Marcel Dekker.

Riviere, J. E., Bowman, K. F., Monteiro-Riviere, N. A., Dix, L. P. and Carver, M. P. 1986. The isolated perfused porcine skin flap (IPPSF). *Fundam. Appl. Toxicol.* 7:444-453.

Riviere, J. E., Bowman, K. F. and Monteiro-Riviere, N. A. 1987. On the definition of viability on isolated perfused skin preparations. *Br. J. Dermatol.* 116:739-741.

Rougier, A., Dupuis, D., Lotte, C., Roguet, R. and Schaefer, H. 1983. *In vivo* correlation between stratum corneum reservoir function and percutaneous absorption. *J. Invest. Dermatol.* 81:275-278.

Rougier, A., Dupuis, D., Lotte, C., Roguet, R., Wester, R. C. and Maibach, H. I. 1986. Regional variation in percutaneous absorption in man: Measurement by the stripping method. *Arch. Dermatol. Res.* 278:465-469.

Scheuplein, R. J. and Ross, L. W. 1974. Mechanism of percutaneous absorption. V. Percutaneous absorption of solvent deposited solids. *J. Invest. Dermatol.* 62:353-360.

Singer, E. J., Wegmann, P. C., Lehman, M. D., Christensen, M. S. and Vinson, L. J.

1971. Barrier development, ultrastructure, and sulfhydryl content of the fetal epidermis. *J. Soc. Cosmet. Chem.* 22:119–137.

Wester, R. C. and Maibach, H. I. 1975a. Percutaneous absorption in the rhesus monkey compared to man. *Toxicol. Appl. Pharmacol.* 32:394–398.

Wester, R. C. and Maibach, H. I. 1975b. Rhesus monkey as an animal model for percutaneous absorption. In *Animals Models in Dermatology,* ed. H. Maibach, pp. 133–137. New York: Churchill-Livingstone.

Wester, R. C. and Maibach, H. I. 1976. Relationship of topical dose and percutaneous absorption in rhesus monkey and man. *J. Invest. Dermatol.* 67:518–520.

Wester, R. C. and Maibach, H. I. 1977. Percutaneous absorption in man and animal: A perspective. In *Cutaneous Toxicity,* eds. V. Drill and P. Lazar, pp. 111–126. New York: Academic Press.

Wester, R. C. and Maibach, H. I. 1985. *In vivo* animal models for percutaneous absorption. In *Percutaneous Absorption,* eds. R. Bronaugh and H. Maibach, pp. 251–266. New York: Marcel Dekker.

Wester, R. C. and Maibach, H. I. 1989a. Regional variation in percutaneous absorption. In *Percutaneous Absorption,* 2d ed., eds. R. Bronaugh and H. Maibach, pp. 111–119. New York: Marcel Dekker.

Wester, R. C. and Maibach, H. I. 1989b. Dermal decontamination and percutaneous absorption. In *Percutaneous Absorption,* 2d ed., eds. R. Bronaugh and H. Maibach, pp. 335–342. New York: Marcel Dekker.

Wester, R. C. and Noonan, P. K. 1978. Topical bioavailability of a potential anti-acne agent (SC-23110) as determined by cumulative excretion and areas under plasma concentration time curves. *J. Invest. Dermatol.* 70:92–94.

Wester, R. C. and Noonan, P. K. 1980. Relevance of animal models for percutaneous absorption. *Int. J. Pharmacol.* 7:9–110.

Wester, R. C., Noonan, P. K., Cole, M. P. and Maibach, H. I. 1977a. Percutaneous absorption of testosterone in the newborn rhesus monkey: Comparison to the adult. *Pediatr. Res.* 11:737–739.

Wester, R. C., Noonan, P. K. and Maibach, H. I. 1977b. Frequency of application on percutaneous absorption of hydrocortisone. *Arch. Dermatol.* 113:620–622.

Wester, R. C., Noonan, P. K. and Maibach, H. I. 1979. Recent advances in percutaneous absorption using the rhesus monkey model. *J. Soc. Cosmet. Chem.* 30:297–307.

Wester, R. C., Noonan, P. K. and Maibach, H. I. 1980a. Percutaneous absorption of hydrocortisone increases with long-term administration: *In vivo* studies in the rhesus monkey. *Arch. Dermatol.* 116:186–188.

Wester, R. C., Noonan, P. K. and Maibach, H. I. 1980b. Variations in percutaneous absorption of testosterone in the rhesus monkey due to anatomic site of application and frequency of application. *Arch. Dermatol. Res.* 267:229–235.

Wester, R. C., Noonan, P. K., Smeach, S. and Kosobud, L. 1981. Estimate of nitroglycerin percutaneous first-pass metabolism. *Pharmacologist* 23:203.

Wester, R. C., Maibach, H. I., Bucks, D. A. W. and Guy, R. H. 1983. Malathion percutaneous absorption following repeated administration to man. *Toxicol. Appl. Pharmacol.* 68:116–119.

Wester, R. C., Maibach, H. I., Surinchak, J. and Bucks, D. A. W. 1985. Predictability of *in vitro* diffusion systems: Effect of skin types and ages on percutaneous absorption of triclocarban. In *Percutaneous Penetration,* eds. R. Bronaugh and H. Maibach, pp. 223–226. New York: Marcel Dekker.

Wester, R. C., McMaster, J., Bucks, D. A. W., Bellet, E. M. and Maibach, H. I. 1989. Percutaneous absorption in rhesus monkeys and estimation of human chemical exposure. In *Biological Monitoring for Pesticide Exposure: Measurement, Esti-*

mation, and Risk Reduction, eds. R. Wang, C. Franklin, R. C. Honeycutt and J. C. Reinert, pp. 152–157. ACS Press.

Wester, R., Rougier, A., Lotte, C. and Maibach, H. 1990. Influence of race on percutaneous absorption in human subjects. *Pharm. Res.* 7:5–187.

Wilson, J. S. and Holland, L. M. 1982. The effect of application frequency on epidermal carcinogenesis assays. *Toxicology* 24:45–54.

Zendzian, R. P. 1989. Skin penetration method suggested for environmental protection agency requirements. *J. Am. Coll. Toxicol.* 8:829–835.

5

percutaneous absorption and skin decontamination of PCBs

■ Ronald C. Wester ■ Howard I. Maibach ■

INTRODUCTION

A cumulative total of 1.4 billion pounds of PCBs was marketed in the United States. PCB production was banned by EPA in 1978; however, approximately 160 million pounds was in use in the electric utility industry in 1981 (EPRI, 1985) and continues in use today. PCBs are extensive in the environment due to disposal and they strongly resist biodegradation. Thus, through work on transformers and capacitors, and through environmental contact (casual or active cleanup), human skin is exposed to PCBs. This chapter discusses the percutaneous absorption of PCBs *in vivo* and *in vitro* from the vehicles in transformers and capacitors, mineral oil, and trichlorobenzene, and the ability of soap and water and solvents to decontaminate PCBs from skin. *In vitro* partition systems and *in vivo* skin decontamination in rhesus monkeys illustrate the dynamic time lapse between initial skin contact, ability to remove PCBs from skin, and irreversible removal (skin absorption).

This chapter was adapted, in part, from material published in the *Journal of Toxicology and Environmental Health,* and is reprinted with permission from the editor.

We thank Electric Power Research Institute, Palo Alto, California, for support, and Drs. Walter Weyzen and Gordon Newell for their intellectual assistance.

METHODOLOGY

Percutaneous Absorption

Skin absorption was determined by ^{14}C cumulative excretion following intravenous and topical administration of [^{14}C]PCBs to rhesus monkeys and guinea pigs (Wester and Maibach, 1975, 1976; Wester et al., 1983). Percent topical dose absorbed was determined using the following relationship:

$$\text{Percent dose absorbed} = \frac{\text{total } ^{14}C \text{ urinary } + \text{ fecal excretion following topical administration}}{\text{total } ^{14}C \text{ urinary } + \text{ fecal excretion following iv administration}} \times 100$$

The [^{14}C]-42% PCB (PCB-42) (0.128 mCi/mg) and [^{14}C]-54% PCB (PCB-54) (0.098 mCi/mg) were obtained from Amersham Corp. The 42% and 54% refer to the percent chlorine in the PCB. These can be considered representative of commercial PCBs.

Adult healthy female rhesus monkeys from the University of California at San Francisco and at the California Primate Research Center, Davis, were used. Following intravenous administration, monkeys were placed in metabolic cages where urine and feces were collected daily for 30 days. For topical administration, monkeys were placed in specially designed metabolic chairs (Primate Products, Woodside, Calif.) for the first 24 h (the duration of topical exposure prior to washing). These chairs had thoracic arm restrainers that separated the site of application (abdomen) from the animal's mouth, hands, and feet. The chair also had a belly plate below the application site. This separated the site from the animal's feet, plus any topical PCBs that might fall from the skin by exfoliation landed on the belly plate and not in the urine and feces collections area. Thus, the site of application was isolated from contaminating the urine and feces. After 24 h, the skin application site was washed with soap and water, and the animals were placed in metabolic cages for continued urine and feces collection.

The intravenous dose of [^{14}C]-PCB-42 (32.7 μg in 200 μl propylene glycol) and [^{14}C]-PCB-54 (47.4 μg in 100 μl propylene glycol) was a bolus injection into the cephalic vein. Topical application was to the rhesus monkey abdominal skin after light clipping of hair, which does not affect percutaneous absorption (Wester and Maibach, 1975).

The topical application was formulated in a 10-μl solution and applied to a 10-cm^2 skin area. [^{14}C]-PCB-42 was administered at a concentration of 4.1 μg/cm^2 in mineral oil and 4.0 μg/cm^2 in trichlorobenzene. [^{14}C]-PCB-54 was administered at a concentration of 4.8 μg/cm^2 in mineral oil, 4.78 μg/cm^2 in trichlorobenzene, and 4.1 or 19.3 μg/cm^2 in acetone.

Guinea pigs were isolated in metabolic cages and administered [^{14}C]-PCB-42 and [^{14}C]-PCB-54 both iv and topically (4.6 μg/cm^2 PCB-42 and 5.2 μg/cm^2 PCB-54). Urine and feces were collected for 16 days (Wester et al., 1983).

In vitro percutaneous absorption was done with recently obtained human cadaver skin (not frozen), which was dermatomed to a thickness of 0.25–0.3 μm. Skin was mounted in continuous flow diffusion cells with a flow rate of 5 ml/h for the saline reservoir fluid (Skelly et al., 1987).

PCBs at concentrations of 1–2 μg/cm² were applied in mineral oil or trichlorobenzene and the diffusion system was run for 17 h. Radioactivity was determined in accumulated reservoir fluid by direct scintillation counting. The skin was then separated into a surface plus stratum corneum fraction, and into an epidermis plus dermis fraction. Radioactivity in the skin fractions was determined by dissolving the skin in Soluene (Packard), then mixed with PCS (pseudocumene cocktail solubilizer) scintillation fluid (Packard) and counted. Each diffusion cell was rinsed with PCS scintillation fluid to determine residual radioactivity in the system. This total accountability allowed determination of mass balance.

Radioactivity in urine and plasma were determined by liquid scintillation counting using PCS fluid. Radioactivity in whole blood was determined by oxidation (Packard TriCarb model 4640), followed by liquid scintillation counting.

Skin Decontamination

The *in vitro* model utilizes the partition coefficient of the potential decontaminant and powdered human stratum corneum (Wester et al., 1987). Callus from human adult soles of feet were obtained and cut into small pieces. The pieces were ground together with dry ice and then freeze-dried to form a powder. Using standard sieves, callus powder that passed through a 40-mesh sieve but stopped by 80-mesh sieve was used. [14C]PCB in mineral oil (2 μg PCB/4 ml) was added to the powdered stratum corneum (2 mg). This mixture set for 15 min, then 1 ml decontaminant was added and everything was mixed. The mixture set for intervals of 0, 1, 10, 60, 240, and 480 min. The mixture was then centrifuged and decontaminant was removed for 14C assay.

For *in vivo* studies rhesus monkeys were isolated in metabolic chairs. The abdominal skin was marked with a series of 1-cm² areas. [14C]-PCB-42 in trichlorobenzene or mineral oil was applied to each marked area. Dosing was 2 μl vehicle/cm² containing 4 μg/cm² PCBs. After an initial 15-min interval, skin was washed 5 successive times with soap and water (20% Ivory liquid v/v with water) or the solvents trichlorobenzene, mineral oil, or ethanol applied to a cotton-tip swab. Carbon-14 analysis was by scintillation counting (Fig. 1).

RESULTS

In Vivo Percutaneous Absorption

Table 1 gives the *in vivo* disposition of PCB-42 following intravenous and topical administration to rhesus monkeys. With iv administration, 39.4 ± 4.9%

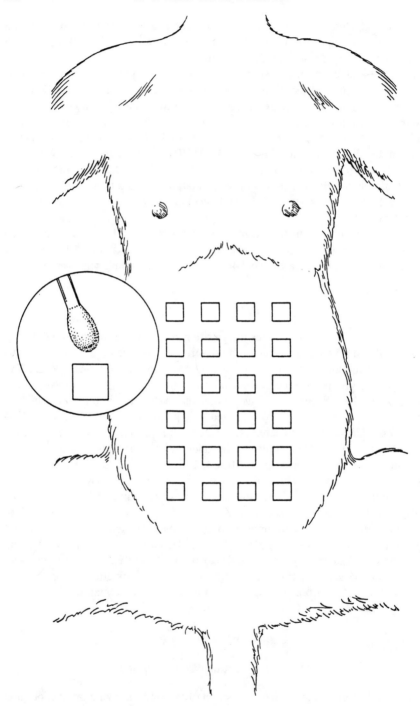

FIGURE 1 Layout of 1-cm^2 grids on rhesus monkey abdomen that are washed with a cotton-tip swab laden with appropriate solvent at appropriate times.

TABLE 1. *In Vivo* Disposition of PCB-42 Following Intravenous and Topical
Administration to Rhesus Monkeys

	Route of administration[a]					
Cumulative excretion (days)	Intravenous in propylene glycol		Topical in mineral oil		Topical in trichlorobenzene	
	Urine	Feces	Urine	Feces	Urine	Feces
1–10	34.6 ± 6.5	—	5.2 ± 1.8	1.4 ± 1.1	5.8 ± 0.9	2.6 ± 1.4
11–20	3.1 ± 1.0	—	1.2 ± 0.8	1.1 ± 2.2	0.6 ± 0.3	0.4 ± 0.1
21–30	1.7 ± 0.6[b]	—	0.7 ± 0.6	1.7 ± 1.9	0.0 ± 0.0	0.5 ± 0.4
Total	39.4 ± 5.9[b]	16.1 ± 0.8[b]	7.1 ± 3.2	4.2 ± 3.7	6.5 ± 1.1	3.5 ± 1.0
Total dose	55.5 ± 5.1		11.3 ± 4.7		10.0 ± 2.1	

[a]Mean percent ± standard deviation for 4 monkeys.
[b]Total is for 34 days.

administered dose was excreted in urine and 16.1 ± 0.8% was excreted in
feces over the 30-day period (55.5 ± 5.1% total dose disposition). Most
of the urinary ^{14}C excretion occurred in the first 10 days. Following topical
application in mineral oil or trichlorobenzene, 11.3 ± 4.7 and 10.0 ± 2.1%
total dose, respectively, were excreted over the 30-day period. The majority of
the ^{14}C excretion was urinary and occurred in the first 10 days.

Table 2 gives the *in vivo* disposition of PCB-54 following intravenous and
topical administration to rhesus monkeys. With intravenous administration,
26.7 ± 7.5% of the dose was excreted in 30 days. The major route of [14]C
excretion was fecal, and the majority of this was in the first 10 days. With

TABLE 2. *In Vivo* Disposition of PCB-54 Following Intravenous and Topical
Administration to Rhesus Monkeys

	Route of administration[a]					
Cumulative excretion (days)	Intravenous in propylene glycol		Topical in mineral oil		Topical in trichlorobenzene	
	Urine	Feces	Urine	Feces	Urine	Feces
1–10	5.2 ± 1.7	13.8 ± 3.5	1.1 ± 0.5	1.2 ± 1.2	1.6 ± 0.7	0.8 ± 0.5
11–20	1.2 ± 0.5	2.8 ± 1.6	0.2 ± 0.1	0.6 ± 0.6	0.7 ± 0.4	0.1 ± 0.1
21–30	0.6 ± 0.2	3.1 ± 1.6	0.05 ± 0.07	2.4 ± 1.9	0.4 ± 0.1	0.3 ± 0.3
Total	7.0 ± 2.2	19.7 ± 5.8	1.3 ± 0.6	4.2 ± 1.9	2.7 ± 1.0	1.2 ± 1.6
Total dose	26.7 ± 7.5		5.5 ± 2.2		3.9 ± 0.9	

[a]Mean percent ± standard deviation for 4 monkeys.

topical administration in mineral oil or trichlorobenzene, 5.5 ± 2.2 and 3.9 ± 0.9% total doses, respectively, were excreted over the 30-day period.

The *in vivo* percutaneous absorption of PCB-42 and PCB-54 was calculated from the ratio of urinary and fecal excretion following intravenous and topical application. Table 3 shows that with PCB-42, percutaneous absorption in the rhesus monkey was 20.4 ± 8.5% from mineral oil, 18.0 ± 3.8% from trichlorobenzene, and 21.4 ± 8.5% from acetone vehicle. With PCB-54, percutaneous absorption was 20.8 ± 8.3% from mineral oil and 14.6 ± 3.6% from trichlorobenzene. In guinea pigs with acetone vehicle, 33.2 ± 6.3% of the PCB-42 and 55.6 ± 2.6% of the PCB-54 were dermally absorbed.

Blood ^{14}C concentrations following intravenous and topical administration of PCB-42 and PCB-54 to rhesus monkey were near detection level; therefore, the only conclusion that can be reached is that low levels of radioactivity were detectable over the 30-day period.

In Vitro Percutaneous Absorption

Table 4 gives the *in vitro* percutaneous absorption of PCB-42 and PCB-54 applied in mineral oil and trichlorobenzene vehicles. Percutaneous absorption (that which diffuses into the reservoir fluid) was less than 1%. The majority of the radioactivity was in the surface plus stratum corneum skin layer and the epidermis plus dermis skin layer. System wash was 1–15%, giving total recovery approaching 100% for all but PCB-42 in trichlorobenzene.

The lower mass balance for PCB-42 in trichlorobenzene prompted further study, where PCB-42 in mineral oil and in trichlorobenzene was placed on glass slides and left exposed to air for 17 h. The percent dose remaining was 95.9 ± 1.8% for PCBs in mineral oil and 40.3 ± 14.5% for PCBs in trichlorobenzene. This suggests that the low recovery may be due to volatility (Atlas et al., 1986).

In Vitro Decontamination

Table 5 gives the *in vitro* decontamination of PCB-42 from human powdered stratum corneum. Values (mean ± SD) are given for soap and water, mineral oil, ethanol, and water, from a few minutes to 8 h. PCBs would not partition from stratum corneum into water ($<1\%$). With soap and water an

TABLE 3. *In Vivo* Percutaneous Absorption of PCBs

	Percent dose absorbed			
	Rhesus monkey			Guinea pig,
PCB	Mineral oil	Acetone	Trichlorobenzene	acetone
42%	20.4 ± 8.5	21.4 ± 8.5	18.0 ± 3.8	33.2 ± 6.3
54%	20.8 ± 8.3	^{a}	14.6 ± 3.6	55.6 ± 2.6

^{a}Not determined.

TABLE 4. *In Vitro* Percutaneous Absorption of PCBs

Entity	PCB-42 MO[a]	PCB-42 TCB[b]	PCB-54 MO[a]	PCB-54 TCB[b]
	PCB and formulation (mean % ± SD)			
Percutaneous absorption	0.20 ± 0.02	0.16 ± 0.09	0.07 ± 0.0	0.06 ± 0.00
Surface/stratum corneum	70.0 ± 17.1	22.0 ± 8.0	23.8 ± 5.6	20.8 ± 5.9
Skin (epidermis and dermis)	29.8 ± 10.0	29.4 ± 5.6	49.4 ± 9.7	85.8 ± 20.3
System wash	13.9 ± 7.1	1.1 ± 0.4	14.6 ± 4.1	1.3 ± 1.1
Total recovery	113.9 ± 27.4	52.6 ± 12.3	87.8 ± 9.9	109.3 ± 18.4

[a]MO, mineral oil.
[b]TCB, trichlorobenzene.

average 33% PCBs partitioned from stratum corneum. Mineral oil removed 66.7% PCBs and ethanol removed an average 85%. Table 6 gives similar results for 54% PCBs, where mineral oil (74%) and ethanol (85%) were better decontaminants of powdered stratum corneum than soap and water. Trichlorobenzene was used as a decontaminant, but it dissolved the powdered stratum corneum and thus could not produce a partition coefficient. It should be noted that when the mixtures set for hours, the partitioning of PCBs out of powdered stratum corneum increased. This is probably due to lipids in the powdered stratum corneum leaching into the decontaminants and taking the PCBs with them.

In Vivo Decontamination

Table 7 gives PCB-42 removal *in vivo* from rhesus monkey skin with 5 successive washes following a 15-min skin application time. Soap and water,

TABLE 5. *In Vitro* Decontamination of PCB-42 from Human Powdered Stratum Corneum

Time	Soap and water	Mineral oil	Ethanol	Water
	Percent dose partitioned into decontaminant			
0 min	28.4 ± 5.9	63.3 ± 7.6	81.3 ± 6.1	
1 min	26.5 ± 3.5	48.8 ± 3.9	80.0 ± 6.1	<1%
10 min	31.5 ± 3.6	62.1 ± 3.5	80.2 ± 2.1	
1 h	34.8 ± 2.5	64.8 ± 2.3	85.7 ± 3.8	
4 h	38.3 ± 2.5	75.6 ± 1.8	92.2 ± 0.4	
8 h	40.2 ± 3.9	85.7 ± 5.2	92.1 ± 2.5	
Average	33.3	66.7	85.2	

TABLE 6. *In Vitro* Decontamination of PCB-54 from Human Powdered Stratum Corneum

Time	Percent dose partitioned into decontaminant		
	Soap and water	Mineral oil	Ethanol
0 min	12.5 ± 2.9	55.4 ± 12.0	78.2 ± 7.2
1 min	27.3 ± 4.5	54.6 ± 8.8	78.0 ± 2.2
10 min	28.3 ± 12.3	63.1 ± 8.2	82.1 ± 12.6
1 h	30.0 ± 9.4	90.6 ± 8.2	92.3 ± 5.9
4 h	37.9 ± 10.5	95.7 ± 4.5	93.2 ± 5.1
8 h	40.2 ± 3.9	85.7 ± 5.2	92.1 ± 2.5
Average	28.8	74.2	85.5

trichlorobenzene, and mineral oil were able to remove all of the PCB-42 on the skin. This complete removal took two to three successive washes. Ethanol was not very effective, removing only 63% of the PCBs in five successive washes.

Table 8 gives the *in vivo* skin decontamination of PCB-42 for time periods beyond the initial 15-min application time. Through an elapsed time of 1 h no differences were seen. However, at 3 h the amount of PCB-42 removed has decreased, and this decreased ability to remove PCB-42 continues at 6 h and 24 h. By 24 h only about 25% of the PCBs can be recovered from the surface of the skin.

Table 9 gives the *in vivo* skin decontamination of PCB-42 applied in mineral oil over a 24-h time period. Soap and water were able to remove about 70% of the PCBs over a 3-h period. This decreased to 50% at 6 h and only 30% of the PCBs could be removed at 24 h. Mineral oil was more efficient in removing the PCBs following the initial 15-min period (the PCBs were in mineral oil on the skin). This decontamination ability quickly disap-

TABLE 7. PCB-42 Removal from Rhesus Monkey Skin with Successive Washes Following Initial 15-Minute Application Time[a]

Successive wash number	Percent dose removed			
	Soap and water	Trichlorobenzene	Mineral oil	Ethanol
1	62 ± 13	79 ± 12	64 ± 5	51 ± 7
2	19 ± 9	14 ± 4	21 ± 6	8 ± 2
3	7 ± 2	5 ± 1	10 ± 2	2 ± 1
4	3 ± 1	3 ± 1	5 ± 1	1 ± 0
5	2 ± 1	1 ± 1	3 ± 2	1 ± 1
Total	93 ± 7	102 ± 7	102 ± 9	63 ± 4

[a]Application vehicle is trichlorobenzene.

TABLE 8. *In Vivo* Skin Decontamination of PCB-42 Applied in Trichlorobenzene

Time interval of washing post-application of PCBs	Percent applied dose removed[b]			
	Soap and water[c]	Trichlorobenzene	Mineral oil	Ethanol
0.0[a]	93 ± 7	102 ± 7	63 ± 4	102 ± 9
10 min	87 ± 10	86 ± 9	68 ± 5	95 ± 6
1 h	81 ± 11	92 ± 8	72 ± 8	79 ± 11
3 h	63 ± 17	74 ± 12	49 ± 3	74 ± 8
6 h	57 ± 26	58 ± 15	52 ± 7	56 ± 12
24 h	26 ± 13	25 ± 19	26 ± 7	36 ± 8

[a]Following 15-min skin application interval.
[b]Mean ± SD for 4 rhesus monkeys.
[c]20% (v/v) Ivory liquid soap/water.

peared in 10 min. By 24 h only 45% of the PCBs could be recovered off the surface of skin.

DISCUSSION

PCBs are probably rapidly and extensively absorbed through the skin, and then are generally distributed throughout the body and slowly eliminated. Percutaneous absorption of PCB-42 in rhesus monkey using acetone vehicle was 21.4% of applied dose; percutaneous absorption of both PCB-42 and PCB-54 whether applied in mineral oil or trichlorobenzene was also about 20%. Since absorption is approximately the same for the vehicles acetone, mineral oil, and trichlorobenzene, the applied vehicle probably had little effect on skin absorp-

TABLE 9. *In Vivo* Skin Decontamination of PCB-54 Applied in Mineral Oil

Time interval of washing post-application of PCBs	Percent applied dose removed[b]	
	Soap and water[c]	Mineral oil
0.0[a]	71 ± 18	90 ± 10
10 min	71 ± 27	68 ± 19
1 h	71 ± 33	63 ± 28
3 h	68 ± 13	64 ± 15
6 h	51 ± 30	65 ± 22
24 h	30 ± 14	45 ± 40

[a]Following 15-min skin application interval.
[b]Mean ± SD for 4 rhesus monkeys.
[c]20% (v/v) Ivory liquid soap/water.

tion ($p > .05$). Slightly higher percutaneous absorption was shown in the guinea pig.

The excretion of PCBs is also of relevance in terms of human health hazard evaluation. Total disposition of PCB-42 in rhesus monkey in 30 days was $55.5 \pm 5.15\%$ and that of PCB-54 was $26.7 \pm 7.5\%$ of intravenous doses. Slow urinary and fecal excretion were still occurring during the 21- to 30-day period, and low levels of ^{14}C in blood were detectable, suggesting that disposition was still an ongoing process. However, for PCB-42 approximately one-half the dose and for PCB-54 the majority of the dose had not been excreted at 30 days. It remains to be determined why the PCB-54 is more resistant to body removal. The difference perhaps could be metabolic.

The *in vitro* skin absorption did not correlate with the *in vivo* data. Water reservoir fluid for chemicals not soluble in water creates non-sink conditions, and the chemicals cannot diffuse from the skin into the reservoir fluid. This was shown for trichlorocarbanilide (Wester et al., 1985) and probably is also true for PCBs. A 6% Oleth 20 was used to improve solubility (Bronaugh, 1985), but had no effect on improving PCB *in vitro* absorption.

In vitro and *in vivo* models to study potential decontamination are presented. The *in vitro* partitioning suggested that soap and water would not be effective and that the solvent ethanol would be effective. *In vivo* the opposite was true. *In vivo* skin decontamination involves a rubbing component as well as a "solvent" component. The soap and water detergent will help loosen "flakes" of surface stratum corneum and wash/rub the cells away, taking any absorbed PCBs with it. Ethanol as a solvent may help drive the PCBs further into the skin. The remarkable ability of soap and water with the natural *in vivo* process of rubbing to remove PCBs from skin is shown in Figs. 2, 3, and 4. Since soap and water would be the most abundantly available washing system, use of other solvents does not seem justified.

Figures 3 and 4 also illustrate the elapsed time between initial PCB skin contact and attempted PCB removal. The process of percutaneous absorption is a time event, and as the PCBs penetrate further into skin, removal becomes irreversible. After 24 h of skin contact only about 25% of initial PCB contamination can be removed by skin washing.

The *in vivo* absorption and excretion data presented here cannot be used alone; they must now be utilized with animal (and human) data to refine risk assessment. It then becomes necessary to put this skin absorption data in perspective with existing PCB information. First, the current Toxicological Profile for Selected PCBs (1987) concludes that there are no quantitative data on dermal exposure to PCBs. This paper combined with the previous publications (Wester et al., 1983, 1987, 1990) now offers quantitative data that show dermal absorption of PCBs to be a primary route into the body. An update on mortality of workers exposed to PCBs in the past (Brown, 1987) reports serum PCB levels in the 50–1500 ppb range, yet mortality from all causes was lower than expected. For current electric utility personnel, PCB plasma values were 5 ± 4

PCB-42 REMOVAL WITH SOAP AND WATER

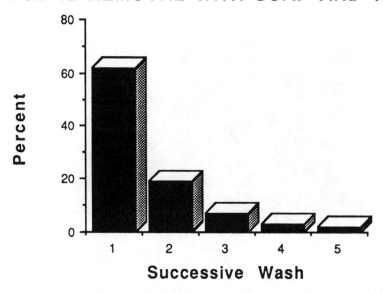

FIGURE 2 Ability of successive soap and water washes to remove 42% PCBs from rhesus monkey skin after a 15-min PCB exposure.

PCB-42 REMOVAL WITH SOAP AND WATER

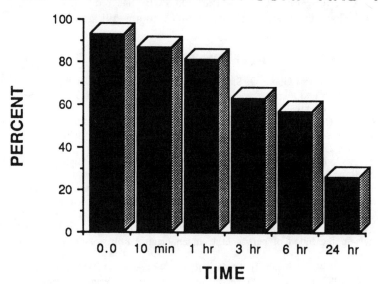

FIGURE 3 Ability of soap and water to remove 42% PCBs, in trichlorobenzene solution on skin, as skin contact time increases to 24 h of exposure.

PCB-42 REMOVAL WITH SOAP AND WATER

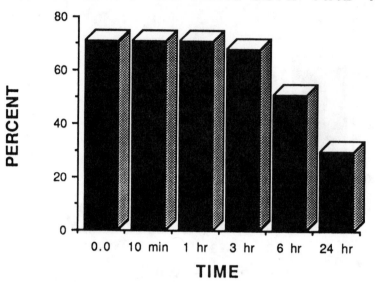

FIGURE 4 Ability of soap and water to remove 42% PCBs, in mineral oil solvent on skin, as skin contact time increases to 24 h of exposure.

ppb for preemployment and 4 ± 4 ppb for current employment (Sahl et al., 1985). Therefore, it seems that caution around PCBs has reduced exposure. However, PCBs have taken environmental refuge and are still a concern.

REFERENCES

Atlas, E., Bidleman, T. and Giam, C. S. 1986. Atmospheric transport of PCBs to the oceans. In *PCBs and the Environment*, ed. J. S. Waid, vol. 1, pp. 79–100. Boca Raton, Fla.: CRC Press.

Bronaugh, R. 1985. Determination of percutaneous absorption by *in vitro* techniques. In *Percutaneous Absorption*, eds. R. Bronaugh and H. Maibach, pp. 267–279. New York: Marcel Dekker.

Brown, D. P. 1987. Mortality of workers exposed to polychlorinated biphenyls—An update. *Arch. Environ. Health* 42:333–339.

EPRI. 1985. *Health Effects Assessment of PCBs,* vol. 1. *Critical Review and Evaluation of Toxicity Information on PCBs and Related Compounds.* Palo Alto, Calif.: Electric Power Research Institute.

Sahl, J. D., Crocker, T. T., Gordon, R. J. and Faeder, E. J. 1985. Polychlorinated biphenyls in the blood of personnel from an electric utility. *J. Occup. Med.* 27:639–643.

Skelly, J. P., Shah, V. P., Maibach, H. I., Guy, R. H., Wester, R. C., Flynn, G. I. and Yacobi, A. 1987. FDA and AAP report of the workshop on Principles and Practices of *In vitro* Percutaneous Penetration Studies: Relevance of Bioavailability and Bioequivalence. *Pharm. Res.* 4:265–267.

Toxicological Profile for Selected PCBs. 1987. Agency for Toxic Substances and Disease Registry, Oak Ridge National Laboratory No. 1425-1425-A1.

Wester, R. C. and Maibach, H. I. 1975. Percutaneous absorption in the rhesus monkey compared to man. *Toxicol. Appl. Pharmacol.* 32:394–398.

Wester, R. C. and Maibach, H. I. 1976. Relationship of topical dose and percutaneous absorption in rhesus monkey and man. *J. Invest. Dermatol.* 67:519–520.

Wester, R. C., Bucks, D. A. W., Maibach, H. I. and Anderson, J. 1983. Polychlorinated biphenyls (PCBs). Dermal absorption, systemic elimination, and dermal wash efficiency. *J. Toxicol. Environ. Health* 12:511–519.

Wester, R. C. and Maibach, H. I. 1985. *In vivo* animal models for percutaneous absorption. In *Percutaneous Absorption,* eds. R. Bronaugh and H. Maibach, pp. 251–266. New York: Marcel Dekker.

Wester, R. C., Maibach, H. I., Surinchak, J. and Bucks, D. A. W. 1985. Predictability of *in vitro* diffusion systems. Effect of skin types and ages on percutaneous absorption of triclocarbon. In *Percutaneous Absorption,* eds. R. Bronaugh and H. Maibach, pp. 223–226. New York: Marcel Dekker.

Wester, R. C., Mobayen, M. and Maibach, H. I. 1987. *In vivo* and *in vitro* absorption and binding to powdered stratum corneum as methods to evaluate skin absorption of environmental contaminants from ground and surface water. *J. Toxicol. Environ. Health* 21:367–374.

Wester, R. C., Maibach, H. I., Bucks, D. A. W., McMaster, J., Mobayen, M., Sarason, R. and Moore, A. 1990. Percutaneous absorption and skin decontamination of PCBs. In vitro studies with human skin and in vivo studies in the rhesus monkey. *J. Toxicol. Environ. Health* 31:235–246.

6

percutaneous absorption of hazardous substances from soil

- Ronald C. Wester ■ Daniel A. W. Bucks ■
- Howard I. Maibach ■

INTRODUCTION

Hazardous substances can cause adverse effects in humans only if exposure occurs. Soil has recently been recognized as a potentially important medium of exposure. Skin absorption is now recognized as a port of entry into the human body for environmental hazardous substances. The soil is a medium with which human skin has constant contact. This can be work-related (farming; waste hazard disposal), recreational (gardening), or a child's delight (beach; sand box).

A major dilemma in establishing regulatory limits for environmental pollutants is the establishment of environmental standards or limits for chemical concentrations in soil at industrial and residential sites. Factors and assumptions used to predict the bioavailability of a chemical from soil significantly affect the establishment of a virtually safe dose or acceptable daily exposure level of a compound in soil. The two major concerns in setting relevant contamination levels are public safety and cost/feasibility of cleanup. Public safety depends upon the inherent toxicity of the hazardous chemical and the bioavailability (rate and extent of systemic absorption). The cost of remediation varies dramatically with the level to which soil must be decontaminated, and excessive remediation means that limited resources will be spent without providing additional protection of public health. For example, Paustenbach et al. (1986) reported the cost of removing and disposing of soil containing more than 1 ppb 2,3,7,8-tetrachlorodibenzo-p-dioxin (TCDD) at the Castlewood site in Missouri to be $17,000,000. However, if the level for cleanup at that site were set at 10 ppb,

111

the cost would drop to $6,000,000, and minimal action would be required at 100 ppb TCDD. The authors state that other sites, such as Times Beach, Mo., show an even more dramatic relationship between the cost of cleanup and the degree of remediation.

DDT

DDT residues can still be detected in California soils some 13 years after the last use of DDT. Every one of 99 sites sampled in 32 counties showed detectable levels ranging from trace amounts to 15 ppm (Wester et al., 1990). DDT can be absorbed through human skin (Feldmann and Maibach, 1974).

The soil used in this study has been designated as Yolo County soil sample 65-Calif-57-8 (26% sand, 26% clay, 48% silt). DDT-contaminated soil was prepared at levels of 10 ppm of compound to soil, and 0.04 g soil/cm^2 skin area. Table 1 and Fig. 1 give the *in vitro* percutaneous absorption of DDT from soil and acetone vehicle into human skin. DDT readily penetrated human skin when applied in acetone vehicle. Significantly less DDT penetrated human skin from soil. DDT would not readily partition from human skin into plasma in the receptor phase. Skin surface wash removed most of the remaining chemical. Total chemical accountability was greater than 80% (Wester et al., 1990).

Figure 2 shows the *in vivo* percutaneous absorption of DDT in rhesus monkey. An average of 18.9 ± 9.4% DDT was absorbed from acetone vehicle, and significantly less (p = .04), 3.3 ± 0.5%, was absorbed from soil (Wester et al., 1990). Absorption of DDT in humans from acetone vehicle (Feldmann and Maibach, 1974) is included.

Hawkins and Reifenrath (1984) studied DDT skin absorption *in vitro* using pig skin. DDT readily penetrated into skin (47 ± 7%) but not into receptor fluid (0.2 ± 0.2%). Bronaugh et al. (1989), using rat skin, reported similar proportions of 48 ± 3% in skin and 0.6 ± 0.2% in the receptor fluid. Wester et al. (1990a) found less DDT (18 ± 13%) in human skin but agree that little DDT will partition into aqueous receptor fluids. *In vivo* percutaneous absorption of DDT reported as percent of applied dose was 46.3 ± 1.4% (rabbit), 43.4 ± 7.9% (pig), 1.5 ± 2.0% (squirrel monkey), and 10.4 ±

TABLE 1. *In Vitro* Percutaneous Absorption of DDT from Soil into Human Skin

Vehicle	Skin	Plasma receptor fluid	Surface wash	Total
		Percent applied dose		
Soil	1.0 ± 0.7	0.04 ± 0.01	95.6 ± 18.2	96.6 ± 18.4
Control acetone	18.1 ± 13.4	0.08 ± 0.02	63.7 ± 12.8	82.0 ± 9.8

Note. 24-h skin application time.

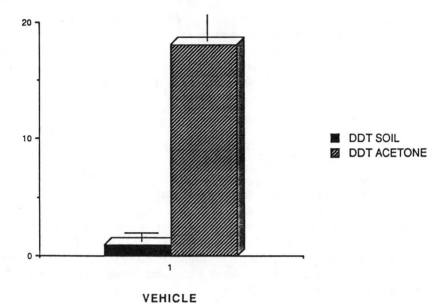

FIGURE 1   *In vitro* DDT percutaneous absorption from soil on human skin.

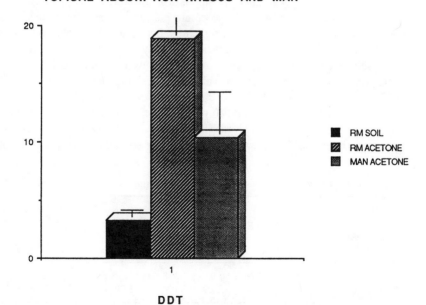

FIGURE 2   *In vivo* DDT percutaneous absorption from soil in rhesus monkey and human.

3.6% (human) (Bartek and LaBudde, 1975; Feldmann and Maibach, 1974). Data for absorption of DDT in rhesus monkey were not significantly different ($p > .05$) from humans for the acetone formulation application. The general conclusion for absorption of DDT from soil is that it will occur, but that the absolute amount will be less than if the DDT chemical only was deposited on skin. The best estimate for DDT chemical absorption in human skin is 10–20% for 24-h exposure.

BENZO[a]PYRENE

The first, and historically most important, carcinogen isolated from coal tar was benzo[a]pyrene. It is the smallest and therefore most easily synthesized unsubstituted polycyclic aromatic hydrocarbon that will produce tumors. The epoxide diol of benzo[a]pyrene is the ultimate carcinogen responsible for the adducts of benzo[a]pyrene with DNA (Scribner, 1985). Benzo[a]pyrene in contact with skin is absorbed into the metabolically active epidermis and converted to these metabolites, which produce the tumors (Noonan and Wester, 1987, 1989; Wester and Maibach, 1985).

Table 2 and Fig. 3 give the *in vitro* percutaneous absorption of benzo[a]pyrene from soil and acetone vehicle into human skin. Benzo[a]pyrene readily penetrated human skin when applied in acetone vehicle. Significantly less benzo[a]pyrene penetrated human skin from soil. Benzo[a]pyrene would not readily partition from human skin into plasma in the receptor phase. Skin surface wash removed most of the remaining chemical. Total chemical accountability was 77–93%. Figure 4 gives the *in vivo* percutaneous absorption of benzo[a]pyrene in rhesus monkeys. An average of 51.0 ± 22.0% benzo[a]pyrene was absorbed from acetone vehicle, and significantly less ($p = .015$), 13.2 ± 3.4%, was absorbed from soil (Wester et al., 1990).

Bronaugh and Stewart (1986) reported the *in vitro* percutaneous absorption of benzo[a]pyrene through rat skin to be 3.7% using normal saline as the receptor phase and 56.0% when the surfactant solubilizer 6% PEG-20 oleyl

TABLE 2. *In Vitro* Percutaneous Absorption of Benzo[a]pyrene from Soil into Human Skin

Human skin source	Percent applied dose			
	Skin	Plasma receptor fluid	Surface wash	Total
Soil	1.4 ± 0.9	0.01 ± 0.004	91.2 ± 13.2	92.7 ± 13.1
Control acetone	23.1 ± 9.7	0.09 ± 0.02	53.0 ± 17.1	76.89 ± 14.7

Note. 24-h skin application time.

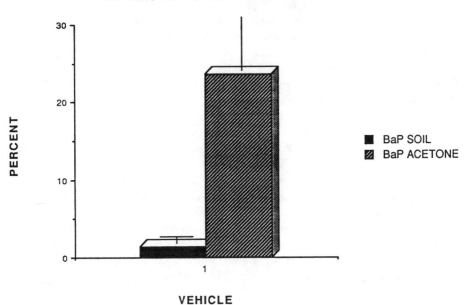

FIGURE 3 *In vitro* benzo[a]pyrene percutaneous absorption from soil on human skin.

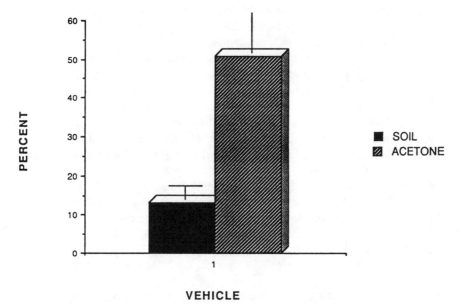

FIGURE 4 *In vivo* benzo[a]pyrene percutaneous absorption in rhesus monkey.

ether was added to the receptor phase. Yang et al. (1989) determined benzo[a]pyrene percutaneous absorption *in vitro* through rat skin (using PEG-20 oleyl ether) to be 38.1%. Wester et al. (1990a) reported that *in vitro* percutaneous absorption of benzo[a]pyrene through human skin with human plasma as receptor fluid (and no surfactant solubilizer) was 0.09%. Kao (1989) reported benzo[a]pyrene *in vitro* percutaneous absorption to be 1.9% in rat skin and 2.7% in human skin. Thus, the amount of 23.7% in human skin (Wester et al., 1990b) represents that amount which the surfactant solubilizer placed in the receptor fluid. *In vivo,* benzo[a]pyrene percutaneous absorption was 48.3% (Bronaugh and Stewart, 1986) and 35.3% (Yang et al., 1989) in the rat compared to 51% in the rhesus monkey.

Yang et al. (1989) reported that percutaneous absorption of benzo[a]pyrene from soil matrix *in vitro* was 8.4%, giving a reduction ratio of 8.4%/38.1% = 0.2. *In vivo* the ratio was reduced to 9.2%/35.3% = 0.26. In Wester et al. (1990b) the soil reduction ratio *in vitro* was 1.4%/23.7% = 0.06, and *in vivo* it was 13.2%/51.0% = 0.26. Therefore both studies suggest that percutaneous absorption of benzo[a]pyrene from soil is about 25% of that from other more conventional vehicles.

LEAD

Roels et al. (1980) conducted an environmental study concerning blood lead (Pb) levels among 11-year-old children attending schools situated less than 1 and 2.5 km from a primary lead smelter. Age-matched control children from a rural and an urban area were contemporaneously examined. Samples analyzed for lead were hand rinses, blood, air, and soil. The hand rinses were collected by slowly pouring 500 ml of 0.1 N NHO$_3$ over the palm of one hand while the fingers were slightly spread. As expected, lead exposure based upon blood lead levels decreased with distance from the smelter. Inhalation of airborne lead was the major source of slightly increased lead levels in adults, whereas children demonstrated an increased blood lead level resulting from soiled hands. The authors conclude that in a lead smelter area, the enforcement of a permissible limit for airborne lead alone may not necessarily prevent an excessive exposure of children to environmental lead, since past emission of lead and possible transport of lead-containing dirt (e.g., through road transport) will maintain a high level of lead in soil-dust and dirt irrespective of the current concentration of atmospheric lead. Using the data published by Roels et al. (1980) we estimate the mass of soil per area of skin adhering to the children as 2.3 ± 0.3 mg soil/cm^2 hand (assuming an area of 70 cm^2 for the child's palm and fingers and the rinsing procedure completely removes the dirt; Table 3). This value agrees with Driver et al. (1989), who reported soil adherence to be 0.2–2 mg soil/cm^2 skin depending upon soil type and particle size.

TABLE 3. Mass of Soil per Unit of Area Adhering to Children[a]

Location	Soil (Pb μg/g)	Hand (μg Pb)	Soil/hand (mg/cm^2)
Rural	114	17	2.1
Urban	112	20.4	2.6
2.5 km	466	62.2	1.9
<1 km	2560	436	2.4
Mean			2.3
SD			0.3

[a]Adapted from Roels et al. (1980).

TCDD (DIOXIN)

Poiger and Schlatter (1980) studied the effect of solvents and adsorbents on the *in vivo* percutaneous penetration of TCDD using the hairless rat animal model (sex and site of application not published). The percutaneous penetration of TCDD from soil, methanol, activated carbon-water paste, petrolatum, polyethylene glycol 1500, or polyethylene glycol 1500-water was examined under aluminum foil occluded conditions. TCDD topical exposure levels ranged from 6.5 to 43 ng/cm^2. Soil was sieved to < 160 μm, then ground in a mortar prior to formulation with TCDD. Each formulation was applied over 3-4 cm^2 for 24 h. Percutaneous penetration was assessed by measurement of radioactivity in the liver 24 h postapplication of compound. The relative dermal bioavailability of TCDD from the above formulations was assessed by comparison of liver TCDD levels at 24 h from dosing. This type of analysis reported by these authors indicated that adsorption of TCDD to activated carbon completely prevented its percutaneous penetration. Our statistical analysis of their data indicated a significant difference ($p < .01$, ANOVA) in TCDD penetration from the MeOH, petrolatum, and soil formulations. TCDD penetration from MeOH was significantly greater ($p < .05$, Newman-Keuls test) than from petrolatum or soil formulations. There was no significant difference ($p > .05$, Newman-Keuls test) between soil and petrolatum formulations. In addition, a significant difference ($p < .01$, ANOVA) in TCDD penetration from the polyethylene glycol 1500, polyethylene glycol-15% water, and soil formulations was observed. Newman-Keuls test results indicated that TCDD penetration from soil was significantly less ($p < .05$) than from polyethylene glycol 1500 or polyethylene glycol-15% water formulations, but there was no significant difference ($p > .05$) in TCDD penetration from the polyethylene glycol 1500 and polyethylene glycol-15% water formulations. The authors conclude that TCDD penetration is highly dependent on the formulation in which it is applied and that mixing TCDD with soil or activated carbon results in reduced compound.

Shu et al. (1988) determined TCDD bioavailability from Times Beach, Mo., soil in the presence and absence of used crankcase oil. Tritiated TCDD was added to the soil and mixed by passage through the 40-mesh screen three times. In studies employing crankcase oil, the used oil was first added to the soil to achieve 0.5 or 2.0% (w/w) prior to [³H]TCDD addition. *In vivo* dermal bioavailability of soil-bound TCDD was estimated using male Sprague-Dawley and hairless (Naked ex Backcross and Holtzman strain) rats. A 12-cm² area of the back was the site of application. Haired rats were lightly clipper-shaven prior to dosing. The TCDD contaminated soil was applied by gentle rubbing. The site of application was covered with a nonocclusive perforated aluminum eye protector whose edges were covered with foam, backed with adhesive, and affixed in place with masking tape. The relative dermal bioavailability of TCDD from the above formulations was assessed by comparison of liver TCDD levels at 24 h from dosing, and therefore the rate or total extent of TCDD percutaneous penetration is not known. However, relative differences in percutaneous penetration between the various treatment modalities should not be affected. The data indicated that variations in TCDD dose (10 compared to 100 ppb TCDD in soil) and oil concentration (0, 0.5, and 2.0%) did not affect the relative percent applied dose penetrating skin. A 4-h exposure resulted in about 60% of an applied dose penetrating from a 24-h exposure. There was no significant difference in TCDD percutaneous penetration from soil between lightly clipper-shaven rats and hairless rats. Unfortunately the authors did not do the control study involving TCDD penetration in the absence of soil.

Using the data from Poiger and Schlatter (1980), Kimbrough et al. (1984) of the Centers for Disease Control (CDC) have stated: "one ppb of 2,3,7,8-TCDD in soil is a reasonable level at which to begin consideration of action to limit human exposure for contaminated soil." Subsequently, Kissel and McAvoy (1989) reexamined the CDC risk assessment using a fugacity-based dermal exposure model incorporated in a physiologically based pharmacokinetic model. Their results suggest that CDC's dermal risk assessment is not conservative and predict dermal bioavailabilities well in excess of that assumed by the CDC.

Brewster et al. (1989) have studied the *in vivo* dermal absorption of [³H]TCDD using male F344 rats. Radiolabeled TCDD was applied at six dose levels (0.00015, 0.001, 0.01, 0.1, 0.5, and 1.0 μmol/kg) from an acetone solution to the intracapular region of the back (total surface area of application not reported). The site of application was covered with a stainless steel perforated cap. The percentage of applied dose absorbed (defined as the difference between the administered dose and the amount in the application site) declined with increasing dose while the absolute total mass (μg/kg) absorbed increased nonlinearly with dose. Absorption of TCDD ranged from approximately 40% of the applied dose when applied at 0.001 and 0.00015 μg/kg to approximately 18% at the 0.1, 0.5, and 1.0 μg/kg dose levels. Major tissue depots included liver, adipose tissue, skin, and muscle. The investigators conclude:

> [Our] results indicate that the dermal absorption of these compounds is incomplete and that systemic toxicity following acute dermal exposure to levels found in

the environment is unlikely. . . . Although the potential for systemic toxicity after acute environmental exposure to these chemicals is low, chronic low-level dermal exposure to these compounds . . . could result in bioaccumulation of [TCDD] body burdens sufficient to induce toxicity.

Evident from the statements from the several laboratories cited above is the lack of consensus on the dangers of topical TCDD exposure. Further research to determine a potential safe level of TCDD exposure from soil is warranted.

BENZENE AND TOLUENE

Skowronski et al. (1988, 1989) studied the *in vivo* percutaneous penetration of benzene and toluene when applied as pure chemical and when incorporated with sandy or clay soils. Male Sprague-Dawley rats were dosed on 13 cm^2 of lightly shaved costoabdominal skin. The application site was occluded with a glass cap. Chemicals were applied for 48 h. Percutaneous penetration was assessed by urinary excretion of radiolabel.

The authors showed that the percutaneous penetration of benzene was significantly higher ($p < .05$) when applied as the pure chemical (86%) compared to application with either soil and penetration was significantly higher ($p < .05$) from sandy soil (64%) compared to clay soil (80%). The authors conclude that percutaneous penetration of a chemical from soil can approach levels observed when applied as pure compound.

DISCUSSION

Exposure assessment of an area with chemical-contaminated soil is linked to considerations of excess risks of developing specific adverse health effects as a result of the total cumulative dose an individual receives. The total cumulative dose is a function of several factors, including:

1. Concentration(s) of contaminant(s) in the soil
2. Location of and access to contaminated areas
3. Type(s) of activity(ies) in contaminated areas
4. Duration of exposure
5. Specific exposure mechanisms
6. Soil type and moisture content
7. Amount of soil adhering to skin
8. Skin site and total area of exposure
9. Time of exposure (acute and chronic)

Accumulation of compound in plants and the half-life of the compound in the soil are additional important factors in the determination of relevant cleanup levels and methodology to be employed. Dose rate may be an important factor in acute exposure assessment. The potential of increased risk from receiving high doses at susceptible life stages may be offset or exceeded by repair mechanisms operative at times of lesser dose. Clearly, the above mandates further study.

In general, the above investigations have revolved around a specific site with investigators employing many different techniques, methodologies (in vitro or in vivo), surface concentrations, and volumes of application to animals and/or humans. Of concern to all is the extrapolation of results obtained using animal models to estimate human body burden following topical exposure. Animal skin is usually more permeable than human. When rank ordered, rat skin is more permeable than monkey or human, and monkey skin closely approximates the permeability of human (Wester and Maibach, 1975, 1983). Therefore, in studies employing rodents, one expects the result to overestimate percutaneous penetration in humans. Furthermore, we believe that results obtained using in vitro systems must be substantiated in vivo before use in establishing regulatory guidelines because of the wide range in results one can obtain employing different in vitro methodologies.

In many cases, one must realize that experimental conditions employed in some of the above investigations do not mimic actual environmental exposure situations, and therefore the results reported may not be relevant to estimate potential human body burden following topical exposure. Results to date indicate that soil does not enhance chemical percutaneous penetration. However, under certain experimental conditions, levels of chemical absorption from soil may approach those following topical application of pure chemical.

Hopefully this chapter will stimulate discussion between the regulatory committees, industrial personnel, and academicians. A consensus on guidelines should be followed in conducting relevant studies to answer the questions raised.

REFERENCES

Bartek, M. J. and LaBudde, J. A. 1975. Percutaneous absorption. In *Animal Models in Dermatology,* ed. H. Maibach, pp. 103–120. New York: Churchill Livingstone.

Brewster, D. W., Banks, Y. B., Clark, A.-M. and Birnbaum, L. 1989. Comparative dermal absorption of 2,3,7,8-tetrachlorodibenzo-p-dioxin and three polychlorinated dibenzofurans. *Toxicol. Appl. Pharmacol.* 97:156–166.

Bronaugh, R. L. and Stewart, R. F. 1986. Methods for in vitro percutaneous absorption studies. VI: Preparation of the barrier layer. *J. Pharm. Sci.* 75:487–491.

Bronaugh, R. L., Stewart, R. F. and Storm, J. E. 1989. Extent of cutaneous metabolism during percutaneous absorption of xenobiotics. *Toxicol. Appl. Pharmacol.* 99:534–543.

Driver, J. H., Konz, J. J. and Whitmyre, G. K. 1989. Soil adherence to human skin. *Bull. Environ. Contam. Toxicol.* 43:814–820.

Feldmann, R. J. and Maibach, H. I. 1974. Percutaneous penetration of some pesticides and herbicides in man. *Toxicol. Appl. Pharmacol.* 28:126–131.

Hawkins, G. S., Jr. and Reifenrath, W. G. 1984. Development of an in vitro model for determining the fate of chemicals applied to skin. *Fundam. Appl. Toxicol.* 4:5133–5144.

Kao, J. 1989. The influence of metabolism on percutaneous absorption. In *Percutaneous Absorption*, eds. R. Bronaugh and H. Maibach, pp. 259–282. New York: Marcel Dekker.

Kimbrough, R. D., Falk, H., Stehr, P. and Fries, G. 1984. Health implications of 2,3,7,8-tetrachlorodibenzodioxin (TCDD) contamination of residential soil. *J. Toxicol. Environ. Health* 14:47–93.

Kissel and McAvoy. 1989. Reevaluation of the dermal bioavailability of 2,3,7,8-TCDD in soil. *Hazardous Waste Hazardous Mater.* 6:231–240.

Noonan, P. K. and Wester, R. C. 1987. Cutaneous biotransformations and some pharmacological and toxicological implications. In *Dermatotoxicology,* eds. F. Marzulli and H. Maibach, pp. 71–93. Washington, D.C.: Hemisphere.

Noonan, P. K. and Wester, R. C. 1989. Cutaneous metabolism of xenobiotics. In *Percutaneous Absorption,* eds. R. Bronaugh and H. Maibach, pp. 53–75. New York: Marcel Dekker.

Paustenbach, D. J., Shu, H. P. and Murray, F. J. 1986. A critical examination of assumptions used in risk assessments of dioxin contaminated soil. *Reg. Toxicol. Pharm.* 6:284–307.

Poiger, H. and Schlatter, C. 1980. Influence of solvent and adsorbents on dermal and interstitial absorption of TCD. *Fundam. Comment. Toxicol.* 18:477–481.

Roels, H., Buchet, J. P., Lauwerys, R. R., Bruaux, P., Claeys-Thoreau, F., Lafontaine, A. and Verduyn, G. 1980. Exposure to lead by the oral and the pulmonary routes of children living in the vicinity of a primary lead smelter. *Environ. Res.* 22:81–99.

Scribner, J. D. 1985. Chemical carcinogenesis. In *Environmental Pathology,* ed. N. K. Mottet, pp. 17–55. New York: Oxford University Press.

Shu, H., Teitelbaum, P., Webb, A. S., Marple, L., Brunck, B., Del Rossi, D., Murray, F. J. and Paustenbach, D. 1988. Bioavailability of soil-bound TCDD: Dermal bioavailability in the rat. *Fundam. Appl. Toxicol.* 10:335–343.

Skrowronski, G. A., Turkall, R. M. and Abdel-Rahman, M. S. 1988. Soil adsorption alters bioavailability of benzene in dermally exposed rats. *Am. Ind. Hyg. Assoc. J.* 49:506–511.

Skrowronski, G. A., Turkall, R. M. and Abdel-Rahman, M. S. 1989. Effects of soil on percutaneous absorption of toluene in male rats. *J. Toxicol. Environ. Health* 26:373–384.

Wester, R. C. and Maibach, H. I. 1975. Percutaneous absorption in the rhesus monkey compared to man. *Toxicol. Appl. Pharmacol.* 32:394–398.

Wester, R. C. and Maibach, H. I. 1983. Cutaneous pharmacokinetics: 10 steps to percutaneous absorption. *Drug Metab. Rev.* 14:169–205.

Wester, R. C. and Maibach, H. I. 1985. Dermatotoxicology. In *Environmental Pathology,* ed. N. K. Mottet, pp. 181–194. New York: Oxford University Press.

Wester, R. C., Maibach, H. I., Bucks, D. A. W., Sedik, L., Melendres, J., Liao, C. and DiZio, S. 1990. Percutaneous absorption of DDT and benzo[a]pyrene from soil. *Fundam. Appl. Toxicol.* 15:510–516.

Yang, J. J., Roy, T. A., Krueger, A. J., Neil, W. and Mackerer, C. R. 1989. In vitro and in vivo percutaneous absorption of benzo[a]pyrene from petroleum crude-fortified soil in the rat. *Bull. Environ. Contam. Toxicol.* 43:207–214.

7

transdermal delivery of drugs: nonclinical regulatory considerations

■ **Judi Weissinger** ■

INTRODUCTION

Prior to phase 1 clinical study, drugs are studied by the intended route of administration to establish evidence of effectiveness, understand the mechanism of action, evaluate the potential human risk, and establish a clinical study dose range. General guidelines exist that describe the types of nonclinical studies that can be used to pharmacologically and toxicologically characterize a drug and to predict its safety for entrance into phase 1 trials. A careful evaluation of the results of these studies usually provides some prediction of the effects to be expected, both desired and adverse, when the drug is administered to man (Weissinger, 1989).

Most drugs when applied to the skin for topical or systemic use are poorly absorbed, and if absorbed, exhibit varying bioavailability (Shah and Skelly, 1988). It is nonetheless sometimes desirable to administer therapeutic preparations transdermally:

1. To prolong the therapeutic effectiveness of drugs with short half-lives by decreasing the dosing frequency (e.g., testosterone, scopolamine, nitroglycerin)
2. To administer drugs that are poorly or inconsistently bioavailable orally (e.g., testosterone, insulin)

Thanks are due to the Pharmacology/Toxicology Transdermal Delivery Committee members and to Dr. D. Bruce Burlington for their scientific and editorial suggestions.

3. To bypass the effects of first-pass clearance or liver enzyme induction which may preclude systemic availability (e.g., estrogen, nitroglycerin)
4. To allow for continual therapeutic effects by producing steady state sustained levels (e.g., scopolamine, clonidine)
5. For convenience and comfort (e.g., fentanyl, clonidine, insulin)
6. To allow for rapid cessation of therapy if needed (e.g., estrogen for cyclical therapy in postmenopausal women every 21 days)

Transdermal delivery systems have been developed to bypass some of the therapeutic difficulties encountered when a drug has a short half-life, poor oral bioavailability, or first-pass metabolism (Shaw and Chandrasekaran, 1978).

The four regulatory categories of preclinical situations arising from the varying degrees of knowledge of the safety and effectiveness of the transdermal delivery system (TDS) or the drug, either a new chemical entity (NCE) or already approved, may be visualized as in Table 1. A detailed discussion of the pharmacology/toxicology considerations for product development in categories I–IV is the subject of the latter half of the chapter.

There are similarities in this diverse group of drugs chosen for transdermal administration. In general, the drugs that are good candidates for use with transdermal delivery systems are potent (do not need more than 10–100 mg to get a therapeutic dose), are nonirritating locally, have low molecular weights (<1000), and are highly soluble in both oil and water with partition coefficients approximately equal to 1 (Weissinger, 1990). In general, transdermal delivery systems are most desirable when nonirritating to the skin, composed of inert substances, and highly viscous. The transdermal delivery system, not the skin, controls the delivery (rate of entry) of the drug into the system (Knepp et al., 1987). In the case of adhesive systems, the skin is the rate-limiting membrane.

PHARMACOLOGIC/TOXICOLOGIC CONSIDERATIONS

Model

Any time an animal model is chosen for transdermal pharmacology and toxicology studies to predict potential safety in humans, the similarity of the animal skin with respect to absorption, irritation, hypersensitivity, and biotransformation capabilities is important. Several publications have compared animal skin to human skin, using various drugs as indices of permeability (Bartek et al., 1972). Rat and rabbit skin have been shown to be more permeable than human skin. Pig skin is often the most comparable. Percutaneous absorption and epidermal barriers in the adult rhesus are similar to the adult human. *In vitro* models of human skin are being studied and significant contributions to the development of TDSs are anticipated.

There are several factors that affect penetration other than the species

TABLE 1. Categories of Preclinical Situations

	New chemical entity	Approved drug	No drug (but intended for NDA[a] approval)
New transdermal delivery system	I	III	II
Approved transdermal delivery system	I	IV	
Alternate route of administration		IV	

[a]NDA, new drug application.

differences—the anatomic site (back skin more permeable), temperature (increase more permeable), humidity (increase more permeable), nature of the vehicle (and occlusion), and disease and nutrition states. Age may also affect absorption, as neonates often absorb greater amounts of drug than adults given equal application area of skin (Groth et al., 1983; Webster et al., 1977). The contribution of these variables to the conditions for approval are normally studied in clinical trials but could be considered preclinically where appropriate.

Absorption

Three major questions arise in defining the usefulness of transdermal delivery. Will the drug partition from a TDS to the skin? Will a drug diffuse through the stratum corneum? Will the drug get into the systemic circulation?

In vitro studies have been considered to address these bioavailability questions using isolated stratum corneum from surgical or autopsy patients. *In vivo* absorption can be quantitated either directly from plasma or tissue levels or on the basis of the percent of dose that is excreted in the urine for a period of time after application of a known amount to the skin (correcting for excretion by other routes). In addition to pharmacokinetic parameters, level of therapeutic or toxic response may also be a quantitative parameter of absorption.

If any component of the TDS or the penetration accelerant is absorbed, then toxicity tests should be performed. Soaps and glues have been shown to enhance cutaneous penetration of chemicals in contact with the skin. If detergents or adhesives that affect the absorption profile are proposed for use, then these should be used in the initial nonclinical and clinical absorption studies.

Dermal Irritation

Irritation at the site of application should be studied in animals. Rabbits usually have the most sensitive skin. When clonidine was demonstrated to be mildly irritating in animals, the clinical evidence indicates that the animal studies were a valid predictor because 10–38% of the patients with clonidine TDS exhibited slight to moderate irritation at the application site (Weber et al., 1984). In testing situations where hair must be clipped, this mechanical irritation should be separated from any produced by the product. If there is a possibility the product may get in the eye via topical use, primary eye irritation studies in rabbits may also be necessary.

Hypersensitivity

Very little is known about the hypersensitivity potential of most orally and parenterally administered compounds (Monkhouse and Huq, 1988). Erythema should be characterized as either local irritation or allergic erythema. Animals may be tested for 10–14 days with the product or system, and then, after a 10- to 14-day recovery interval, administered the TDS via the same site. Guinea pigs and rabbits are often ideal for these studies.

Biotransformation at the Site of Administration

The skin is not a passive barrier that merely restricts the diffusion of chemical agents into the body. It is a viable, metabolizing membrane that can metabolize an assortment of substances before they become systemically available. Metabolic capabilities may vary at different areas of the body. Noonan and Webster (1985), in reviewing the cutaneous metabolism of drugs, showed comparability with the liver metabolism in hydroxylation, reduction, hydrolyses, sulfate and glucuronide conjugation, and oxidation. They also showed similarity in the inducibility of enzymes, and saturability of the system that occurs with rapid absorption. It is still evident, however, that certain animals may metabolize a drug more or less rapidly than humans. *In vitro* studies using human skin may be useful in assessing biotransformation.

REGULATORY CONSIDERATIONS

New Chemical Entity: Category I

For a new chemical entity, whether an approved or novel TDS is proposed, the following considerations apply.

The general guidelines for new chemical entities should be followed to preclinically characterize a drug intended for administration using a TDS (Goldenthal, 1968). The route of administration for several critical studies, such as single and repetitive administration, the chronic toxicity, the reproductive toxicity, and the carcinogenicity should be the same as the intended clinical route. Considerations should be given to usefulness of any comparative information that would be gained with additional testing via iv or oral routes of administration. Some chemicals may be more toxic dermally administered than orally because of a change in biotransformation pattern. Hexachlorophene, a highly toxic chemical, is extensively metabolized by the liver but unmetabolized when applied to the skin, and may be absorbed unchanged into the bloodstream.

Usually, if biotransformation occurs in the skin it is assumed to deactivate or detoxify chemicals through metabolism. In the case of transdermal testosterone, an active metabolite, dihydrotestosterone, is produced by enzymes in the scrotal sac (FDA, 1988). After TDS administration of testosterone, blood levels in patients and volunteers showed much individual variation in testosterone levels (Bals-Pratsch et al., 1986). Measurement of the dihydrotestosterone patterns in patients and volunteers showed similar patterns. Therapeutically skin metabolism may or may not be significant, but it is important to be aware of its occurrence to make that judgment.

Irritation and hypersensitivity should be characterized in an animal model such that predictions can be made of these adverse reactions in humans.

Considerations in Conducting Preclinical Studies to Characterize New Transdermal Delivery Systems: Category II

The object of the TDS is to deliver the drug into the body at a controlled rate such that variations in skin permeability are overcome. As described previously, the rate-limiting step may be the TDS, or the skin in the case of adhesives. The TDS and its components, raw materials, and intermediates are usually characterized preclinically in short-term animal studies. The TDS final product and the accelerants are subject to similar toxicology considerations as new chemical entities. The biotransformation and complete toxicity profile of the TDS is generally necessary if the components are in any way absorbed.

Absorption. Absorption of components may be studied as for a new chemical entity. Toxicity of the finished TDS due to oral absorption may be studied by oral administration to dogs of multiple TDSs, checking for recovery of the intact system and monitoring any adverse effects. With this information, the contribution of the system to oral toxicity observed when combined with drug may be defined. This is useful because there have been reports of oral ingestion of discarded systems by children (Corneli et al., 1989).

Irritation. The finished product should be studied initially in acute irritation and repeat dose (21-day) primary irritation studies. If irritation is observed, the backing, the control membrane, the contact adhesive, and the penetrant enhancer should be similarly studied to identify the component responsible for irritation.

Approved Drug with New TDS: Category III

The pharmacologic/toxicologic considerations may vary when an approved chemical entity is proposed for use with a novel TDS (new system for use with an approved drug). Repeat-dose transdermal administration and pharmacokinetics are needed to check the availability, maintenance of steady state, rate and extent of delivery, and reproducibility of system, and to compare the kinetics of the drug to administration by the approved route. If these are comparable, irritation and hypersensitivity may be considered for evaluation clinically.

Irritation. Primary irritation studies would be conducted applying the drug or placebo in the TDS to two places on the body of each animal, that is, two spots on back. Acute irritation and repeat-dose irritation studies should be conducted.

Hypersensitivity. This study is similar to the repeat-dose irritation study, but after 2 weeks of administration of drug-filled and placebo-filled systems and a 2-week untreated recovery interval, administration is repeated using the TDS at the same site. Skin is observed for erythematous reactions and any evidence of allergic reaction systemically (anaphylaxis, increased histamine, etc.).

Contact sensitization should also be evaluated. If penetration through the stratum corneum is assisted with 2.5% lauryl sulfate, the study design should include the use of a 48-h patch and 10–11 days of recovery followed by repeat administration. Drug and placebo may be studied in the same animal and the results compared.

Biotransformation and toxicological profile. All biotransformation should be compared to biotransformation by the approved route to enable the application of previous data to safety evaluation. If the transdermal delivery system is proposed to bypass liver or gastrointestinal metabolism, elimination is similar for similar products, and an equal or lesser amount of parent compound is circulating, depending upon the activity of the metabolites, some existing data could be useful. In other words, elimination of first-pass effect or biotransformation in the skin will alter the metabolic profile, and that alteration should be described.

Previous Approval: Category IV

The pharmacologic and toxicologic considerations where both the delivery system and the chemical entity have previously been approved depend upon the adherence of the characteristics of the system to the predictions. Where the pharmacology and toxicology of a parenterally administered approved chemical entity is well characterized, new preclinical toxicology studies may not be needed. Pharmacokinetics and tissue distribution should be evaluated to optimize size selection of TDS with product and are useful as evidence that the system is delivering the intended dose in a predictable fashion (Schmitt et al., 1981). Also, studies comparing performance of the system in the dose range proposed using successive applications, different body locations, and change in the contact layer of the system are important. Steady-state blood levels should be evaluated with respect to response and to other parenteral routes. The effect of any changes in administration, distribution, biotransformation, and excretion on skin enzymes systems and inducibility should be considered in determining whether additional pharmacology/toxicology studies are needed.

Systemic toxicity is usually previously well characterized. Toxicologically, the unknown factors are local toxicity from dermal application, hypersensitivity with dermal application, and alterations in toxicity profile based upon route of administration. If (1) the irritation and hypersensitivity issues are satisfactorily addressed, (2) absorption can be predicted and controlled such that unexpected peaks do not occur with application (as determined by a pharmacokinetic and tissue distribution study), and (3) the alternate route of administration does not produce unique metabolites or substantially more potent derivatives to the system than have been tested, prediction of a safe initial dose for initiating clinical studies may be made. Where some of these issues are not satisfied, scientific rationale may be submitted to the Food and Drug Administration Center for Drug Evaluation and Research (FDA/CDER) for consideration and review to propose that these issues be addressed with dose escalation in phase 1 and 2 studies in human volunteers. The dose would be expected to be substantially reduced and escalation intervals modified. In the interest of expediency, animal models may be more useful to answer these questions.

If carcinogenicity has not been evaluated, the duration of use will be important in determining the need for such studies. The route of administration may make a difference in considering skin carcinogens or photocarcinogens, and carcinogenicity studies may be requested. If the reproductive toxicity has been evaluated, it may be altered with dermal administration. Less reproductive toxicity may be observed as less drug is absorbed or less active metabolites made, or it may be more toxic if lack of metabolism produces higher quantities of parent drug or skin metabolism produces higher levels of a toxic metabolite. These topics should be considered, and any conclusions reached should be presented to and discussed with the CDER along with supporting data before making assumptions that these studies are not needed.

Considerations for accelerants. Skin penetration, specifically stratum corneum penetration, occurs through a polar or lipid path (Cooper, 1985). Drugs that are absorbed through the polar pathway have enhanced penetration if surfactants, which increase protein structural changes, are included in the preparation. Drugs that are absorbed via the lipid pathway have enhanced penetration in the presence of solvents that increase lipid fluidization. The dominant pathway for a given drug can be evaluated by ascertaining the degree of absorption at various pH values above and below the pK_a. If the drug is better absorbed in the unionized form, the lipid pathway predominates; if it is better absorbed in the ionized form, the polar pathway predominates.

If an accelerant is used to increase permeability, then the penetrant must be characterized pharmacologically and toxicologically. If accelerants change skin permeability, then pharmacokinetic profiles must be recalculated and reevaluated and the extent that the change is related to a toxicity of the drug must be determined. If the accelerant changes the TDS in some way such that the components are now bioavailable, then the TDS may need to be reevaluated. If the accelerant is absorbed, it must be characterized pharmacologically and toxicologically as a new chemical entity. For an already approved accelerant that is chemically and physically stable in the proposed system, has no pharmacologic activity of its own, and is nonabsorbed and nontoxic, only irritation and hypersensitivity may be needed to characterize a given system with a given drug.

SUMMARY

Four regulatory categories have been presented addressing the pharmacology/toxicology studies that might be appropriate under each situation. The studies that may be used to address the pharmacologic and toxicologic concerns for initiation of phase 1 studies and NDA approval depend upon the information available from previous approvals for drugs, delivery systems, penetration enhancers, and adhesives. Nonclinical pharmacology and toxicology information is necessary for all novel drugs, novel delivery systems, novel adhesives, and novel penetration enhancers. The pharmacokinetics and the local and systemic effects need to be characterized for drugs previously approved in the delivery system proposed. The choice of an appropriate *in vitro* or animal model for conducting preclinical studies should be made considering the similarity to humans and intact integument, and the knowledge of the cutaneous characteristics of the species.

The Pharmacology/Toxicology Transdermal Delivery Committee is developing definitive points to consider, further addressing nonclinical considerations and the details of the study design, which studies compose an appropriate battery, and which studies can be conducted using either the drug or the delivery system and which must be conducted on the finished product. This guidance resulting from their interaction will be based upon sound scientific rationale and will be applicable to most product classes.

REFERENCES

Bals-Pratsch, M., Kruth, U., Yoon, Y. and Nieschlag, E. 1986. Transdermal testosterone substitution therapy for male hypogonadism. *Lancet* 2:943–946.

Bartek, M., La Budde, J. and Maibach, H. 1972. Skin permeability in vivo: comparison in rat, rabbit, pig, and man. *J. Invest. Dermatol.* 58:114–123.

Cooper, E. 1985. Vehicle effects on skin penetration. In *Percutaneous Absorption,* eds. R. L. Bronaugh and H. I. Maibach, pp. 525–529. New York: Marcel Dekker.

Corneli, H., Banner, W., Vernon, D. and Swenson, P. 1989. Toddler eats clonidine patch and nearly quits smoking for life. *J. Am. Med. Assoc.* 261:42.

FDA. 1988. Presentation in Open Endocrine and Metabolic Advisory Committee Discussion, February 26, 1988.

Goldenthal, E. 1968. Current views on safety evaluation of drugs. *FDA Papers,* 13–18.

Groth, H., Vetter, H., Knuesel, J. and Vetter, W. 1983. Allergic skin reaction of transdermal clonidine. *Lancet* 2:850–851.

Knepp, V., Hadgraft, J. and Guy, R. 1987. Transdermal drug delivery—Problems and possibilities. *CRC Rev. Ther. Drug Carrier Systems* 4:13–37.

Monkhouse, D. and Huq, A. 1988. Transdermal drug delivery—Problems and promises. *Drug Dev. Ind. Pharm.* 14:183-209.

Noonan, P. and Webster, R. 1985. Cutaneous absorption of xenobiotics in transdermal drug delivery systems in the United States. In *Percutaneous Absorption,* eds. R. L. Bronaugh and H. I. Maibach, pp. 65-85. New York: Marcel Dekker.

Schmitt, L., Shaw, J., Carpenter, P. and Chandrasekaran, S. 1981. Comparison of transdermal and intravenous administration of scopolamine. *Clin. Pharmacol. Ther.* 29:282.

Shah, V. and Skelly, J. 1987. Regulatory consideration in transdermal drug delivery systems in the U.S. In *Transdermal Controlled Systemic Medications,* ed. Y. W. Chien, pp. 399-410. New York: Marcel Dekker.

Shaw, J. and Chandrasekaran, S. 1978. Controlled topical delivery of drugs for systemic action. *Drug. Metab. Rev.* 8:223-233.

Weber, M., Drayer, J. and McMahon, F. 1984. Transdermal administration of clonidine. *Arch. Intern. Med.* 144:1211-1213.

Webster, R., Noonan, P., Cole, M. and Maibach, H. 1977. Percutaneous absorption of testosterone in the newborn rhesus monkey: Comparison to adult. *Pediatr. Res.* 11:737-739.

Weissinger, J. 1989. Nonclinical pharmacologic and toxicologic considerations for evaluating biologic products. *Reg. Toxicol. Pharmacol.* 10:255-263.

Weissinger, J. 1990. Pharmacology and toxicology of novel drug delivery systems: Regulatory issues. *Drug Safety* 5 (suppl): 107-113.

8

transdermal drug delivery systems: an academic view

■ Daniel J. Hogan ■ Howard I. Maibach ■

INTRODUCTION

Research over the last decade has demonstrated that drug delivery through the skin is feasible for many simple potent drug molecules (<1000 daltons) via transdermal drug delivery systems (Guy et al., 1987). Currently six drugs are marketed in these systems (estradiol, nitroglycerin, clonidine, scopolamine, fentanyl, and isosorbide dinitrate), and research on the transdermal delivery of other drugs is continuing (Brown and Langer, 1988; Shaw et al., 1987a). These therapeutic systems are custom made for each drug as drugs vary in their potency, half-life, clearance, percutaneous absorption, cost, etc. (Shaw et al., 1987a). These devices are discs that generally consist of a backing membrane, impermeable to the drug, a reservoir containing the drug, and a rate-controlling membrane attached to the skin with an adhesive such as medical-grade acrylate-based copolymer (Wick et al., 1989) (Fig. 1). The clonidine and scopolamine dosage forms are multilaminates; the estradiol and nitroglycerin dosage forms use a semisolid or liquid drug reservoir (Shaw et al., 1987a). The simplest systems are essentially adhesive tape with incorporated drug. A dermal patch delivery system containing 21% salicylic acid in an adhesive patch composed of karaya, polyethylene glycol-300, propylene glycol, and quaternium-15 is marketed for the local treatment of warts. This device is applied overnight and releases approximately 50% of its content of salicylic acid in 1 h and 90% by 8 h.

D. J. Hogan and H. I. Maibach

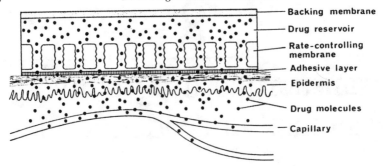

FIGURE 1 Cross-section of transdermal drug delivery system. (From Hogan, D. J. and Maibach, H. I. 1990. "Adverse dermatologic reactions to transdermal drug delivery systems." *J. Am. Acad. Dermatol.* 22:812).

Advantages of Transdermal Drug Delivery Systems

Transdermal drug delivery systems allow the continuous and sustained administration of drugs through the skin. Gastrointestinal and hepatic first-pass metabolism are avoided (Guy et al., 1987). Gastric discomfort is less than that experienced with oral administration for many medications (Shaw et al., 1987a). More even and predictable serum drug levels may be achieved. Steady-state plasma concentrations of a drug are achieved without the high peak levels associated with oral therapy (Guy et al., 1987). The avoidance of high peak levels may help minimize the side effects of certain drugs. The frequency of drug administration may be reduced with transdermal drug delivery. Multiday continuous drug delivery is possible even for short-half-life drugs (Shaw et al., 1987a).

Disadvantages of Transdermal Drug Delivery Systems

Relatively low plasma concentrations of a drug are achieved using transdermal drug delivery. The skin is an excellent barrier for some compounds, and only a low percentage of many topically applied drugs will be absorbed percutaneously (Guy et al., 1987). The expense of transdermal drug delivery is only justified for drugs for which conventional administration has severe disadvantages (Shaw et al., 1987a).

Transdermal drug delivery should improve patient compliance, but dermatological side effects may interfere with this novel drug delivery system. Table 1 summarizes the incidence of dermatitis in patients using the most commonly employed devices.

GENERAL EFFECTS OF TRANSDERMAL DRUG DELIVERY SYSTEMS ON THE SKIN

Nonimmunologic

Effect of occlusion. Transdermal drug delivery systems are designed for application to the skin for 12 h to 7 days (Brown and Langer, 1988). Discs should not be re-applied to the same site. Long-term occlusion inevitably causes sweat and water vapor to accumulate beneath the patch. Evaporation of this water is inhibited. Sweat ducts may also become occluded by this sustained occlusion and heat (Hurkmans et al., 1985). Sweat may break through sweat duct walls and induce a pruritic intraepidermal inflammatory reaction (miliaria rubra). Such reactions are limited to the application site (Hurkmans et al., 1985). These common reactions resolve within a day. The experimental incorporation of hydrogels that absorb water helped minimize cutaneous irritation from a transdermal drug delivery system in one study (Hurkmans et al., 1985).

Occlusion creates an ideal climate for overgrowth of bacteria and yeast. Pretreatment with chlorhexidine helped minimize bacterial overgrowth under discs that contained gels that did not absorb water (Hurkmans et al., 1985).

Irritant contact dermatitis. Irritant contact dermatitis may occur with any transdermal drug delivery system. Individuals vary in their susceptibility to irritant contact dermatitis. Those with atopic dermatitis or other active dermatitis are most susceptible. The greater the period of occlusion, the greater the risk of irritant contact dermatitis. Repetitive application of therapeutic patches to a site increases the risk of irritant contact dermatitis and allergic contact dermatitis.

Transient erythema. The removal of a therapeutic system affixed to the skin with a pressure-sensitive adhesive may cause transient erythema (Fisher, 1984).

Burns from microwave ovens. One report describes a man who received a second-degree burn on his chest at the site of a nitroglycerin disc from

TABLE 1. Contact Dermatitis in Series of Patients Using Transdermal Drug Delivery Systems

Drug	First author	Year	Number of patients treated with device	Percent contact dermatitis, irritant/ allergic	Positive oral challenge
Clonidine	Groth	1985	35	11%/31%	0/4
	Groth	1983	29	?/38%	ND[a]
	Horning	1988	20	?/50%	0/2
	Physician's Desk Reference	1988	101	25%/5%	ND
			673	?/19%	ND
					1/217
	Maibach	1987	3079	?/12.5%	1/29
Estradiol	Utian	1987	448	24%/?	ND
Nitroglycerin	Kapoor	1985	30	10%/0%	ND
Scopolamine	Homick	1983	11	27%/0%	ND
	Gordon	1989	164	0/10%	ND
	Shupak	1989	65	0/4.4%	ND

[a]ND, not done.

a microwave oven that had a leak (Murray, 1984). It was suggested that the metallic element of the disc was heated by the microwave radiation. A subsequent study found it unlikely that exposure of the most common transdermal drug delivery systems to microwave diathermy fields or low level leakage radiation from microwave ovens would cause burns in users (Mosley et al., 1990).

Inadvertent transfer of medication. Transfer of medication to another site. Several reports describe anisocoria due to scopolamine therapeutic systems. Scopolamine may be transferred to the eye from the medication disc via the patient's fingers (Carlston, 1982; McCrary and Webb, 1982). Patients who insert and remove contact lenses should be particularly careful when handling scopolamine discs (Carlston, 1982).

Person-to-person transfer. Occasionally drug delivery systems may become dislodged inadvertently. One report describes the inadvertent transfer of a clonidine disc from a parent to a child (Reed and Hamburg, 1986). The child developed systemic symptoms. Loss of adhesion of a transdermal system for testosterone to scrotal skin occurred frequently during the initiation of this treatment in a clinical trial (Bals-Pratsch et al., 1986). The longer the period of application, the greater the loss of skin adhesion by transdermal devices (Wick et al., 1989).

Immunologic

Allergic reactions to drug delivery systems are usually caused by one or more compounds in the adhesive layer or by the drug itself (Neiboer et al., 1987). Cutaneous irritation from prolonged occlusion may facilitate sensitization to constituents of a disc (Neiboer et al., 1987). The longer the period of occlusion, the greater the cutaneous irritation induced. These conditions simulate the "maximization procedure" devised by Kligman to predict the capacity of a chemical to provoke allergic contact dermatitis (Kligman, 1966).

Scopolamine. Scopolamine, the first drug approved for transdermal drug delivery (Brown and Langer, 1988), is marketed for the prevention and treatment of motion sickness (Anonymous, 1989; Brown and Langer, 1988; Homick et al., 1983; Shaw et al., 1987a). In contrast to the other drugs marketed in transdermal drug delivery systems, the discs are applied to the postauricular area rather than to the trunk (Anonymous, 1989a). The absorption of topically applied medications is greater through the skin of the postauricular area than through truncal skin (Scheuplein and Fronaugh, 1983; Shaw et al., 1987a).

Allergic contact dermatitis. There are at least 22 published cases of allergic contact dermatitis to scopolamine drug delivery systems (Gordon et al., 1989; Shupak et al., 1989; Trozak, 1985; van der Willigen et al., 1988). These reactions occur in up to 10% of users (Gordon et al., 1989). Cross-reactions to atropine have not been reported in patients with allergic contact dermatitis to scopolamine (Trozak, 1985).

Allergic contact dermatitis to scopolamine cream and allergic keratoconjunctivitis to scopolamine have also been reported (Trozak, 1985). Patients suspected of allergic contact dermatitis to scopolamine should be patch tested to 1% scopolamine in petrolatum or water (Fisher, 1984).

Irritant contact dermatitis. Skin irritation may occur with both the placebo and active scopolamine patches. The incidence of skin irritation increased with the duration of occlusion and was maximal at the longest period of occlusion studied, 72 h (Homick et al., 1983).

Delerium and other distal effects from transdermal scopolamine. Transdermal scopolamine is not recommended for use in children (Anonymous, 1989a). Delirium has been attributed to transdermal scopolamine in children and the elderly. Patients may not remember that these patches are medications (MacEwan et al., 1985). The presence of a patch may only be discovered on physical examination.

Transdermal scopolamine has been reported to precipitate glaucoma (Fraunfelder, 1982; Hamill et al, 1983). This device should not be used by those predisposed to glaucoma.

Clonidine. Transdermal drug delivery systems of clonidine are available in the United States for the treatment of hypertension (Anonymous, 1988). They are more expensive than oral clonidine and considerably more expensive than thiazide diuretics (Horning et al., 1988). The most common reason for discontinuing treatment with clonidine discs is local severe skin reactions (Horning et al., 1988). Numerous reports document allergic contact dermatitis to transdermal clonidine (Anonymous, 1985; Grattan and Kennedy, 1985; Groth et al., 1983, 1985; Horning et al., 1988; Maibach, 1987; White and Guidry, 1986). The incidence of sensitization is up to 50% (Horning et al., 1988). These systems are designed to be applied for a week: several days longer than the application period for transdermal drug delivery systems for other drugs (Brown and Langer, 1988). It has been suggested, but not documented, that shortening the period between changes of the patches from 7 to 3 days may help decrease the incidence of sensitization, which is higher in women and lower in blacks (Anonymous, 1985, 1988).

Rebound hypertension has been reported in elderly hypertensive patients who discontinue transdermal clonidine. One report suggested that allergic contact dermatitis to clonidine impaired the percutaneous absorption of transdermal clonidine, which led to the development of rebound hypertension in a patient (White and Guidry, 1986). Allergic contact dermatitis to nitroglycerin in transdermal patches was reported to lead to exacerbation of angina that improved when the patient switched to oral nitrates (Carmicheal and Foulds, 1989). Most patients with allergic contact dermatitis to transdermal clonidine developed dermatitis within the first 26 weeks of treatment (Maibach, 1987). An occasional patient with allergic contact dermatitis to transdermal clonidine has developed a generalized eruption (Maibach, 1987). Most patients with allergic contact dermatitis to clonidine challenged with oral clonidine experience no flare of dermatitis (Grattan and Kennedy, 1985; Horning et al., 1988; Maibach, 1987). The high incidence of allergic contact dermatitis to transdermal clonidine may limit its usefulness in the treatment of hypertension (Anonymous, 1985; Groth et al., 1985; Mougeolle, 1988). Patients suspected of having developed allergic contact dermatitis to clonidine should be patch tested to 9% clonidine in petrolatum (Maibach, 1987). One case of allergic contact dermatitis to polyisobutylene in the clonidine disc has been reported (Groth et al., 1983, 1985).

Nitroglycerin. Nitroglycerin's instability (half-life of only 3 min) stimulated the development of its transdermal drug delivery system (Shaw et al., 1987a). Erythema under a nitroglycerin (glyceryl trinitrate) disc is common since this drug is a vasodilator (Fisher, 1984). There are case reports of allergic contact dermatitis to nitroglycerin in ointments and in transdermal drug delivery systems used to treat angina (Fischer and Tyler, 1985; Harari et al., 1987; Hendricks and Dec, 1979; Kapoor et al., 1985; Rosenfeld and White, 1984; Topaz and Abraham, 1987). It is of interest that one of the first cases developed allergic contact dermatitis to nitroglycerin only after he switched from nitroglycerin ointment to a nitroglycerin patch (Rosenfeld and White, 1984). Repetitive application of nitroglycerin patches to the same site has been emphasized as a risk factor for the development of sensitization to nitroglycerin (Fischer and Tyler, 1985). Multifocal areas of allergic contact dermatitis to nitroglycerin in a transdermal drug delivery system with extensive postinflammatory hypermelanosis has also been reported (Harari et al., 1987). Nitroglycerin should be patch tested at a concentration of 0.2 mg nitroglycerin/ml water (Rosenfeld and White, 1984). One report found that patients allergic to topical nitroglycerin could continue to use nitroglycerin ointment if, on removal of nitroglycerin ointment, they applied a potent topical corticosteroid cream, 0.05% fluocinonide, to the site of application (Hendricks and Dec, 1979). Patients with a history of allergic contact dermatitis to nitroglycerin usually do not develop dermatitis if treated with oral glyceryl trinitrate (Harari et al., 1987; Rosenfeld and White, 1984).

Estradiol. Concern for the hepatotoxicity of oral estradiol was one of the factors that stimulated the development of a transdermal drug delivery system for estradiol (Shaw et al., 1987a). The most common adverse reaction to transdermal estradiol during clinical trials was erythema and cutaneous irritation at the application sites. This occurred in 17% of the women treated and caused 2% to discontinue treatment (Anonymous, 1989b). Ethanol is present in the formulation as an enhancer of percutaneous penetration of estradiol (Brown and Langer, 1988). No experimental sensitization or phototoxic reactions to estradiol in a transdermal drug delivery system were obtained in a small number of volunteers (Utian, 1987). Skin irritation to transdermal estradiol is said to be more common in warm or humid climates, which accentuate the effects of cutaneous occlusion (Anonymous, 1987). Allergic contact dermatitis has been attributed to the adhesive for this device and to hydroxypropylcellulose, which is the major component of the drug reservoir of the transdermal estradiol patch

(McBurney et al., 1989; Schwartz and Clendenning, 1988). It appears that there are other potential allergens in the drug reservoir (McBurney et al., 1989). Allergic contact dermatitis to the estradiol in these patches has not been reported.

THE FUTURE

Transdermal drug delivery systems for coumarin, isoproterenol HCl, indomethacin, alpha-melanotropin [(Nle4,D-Phe)alpha-MSH], meperidine, nicotine, testosterone, PHNO (a dopamine agonist), timolol, verapamil, azatadine, and other antihistamines may be available in the near future (Bals-Pratsch et al., 1986; Chien et al., 1988; Dietz et al., 1986; Dorr et al., 1988; Hendricks and Dec, 1979; Lang, 1989; Patel and Vasavada, 1988; Ritschel and Barkhaus, 1988; Ritschel et al., 1989; Sekine et al., 1987; Shaw et al., 1987a, 1987b). Unlike other transdermal drug delivery systems, the system for testosterone is applied to scrotal skin, which has the highest rate of percutaneous absorption for steroids (Bals-Pratsch et al., 1986). In contrast to the therapeutic system for estradiol, which is designed to deliver micrograms of estradiol, the transdermal system for testosterone is designed to deliver milligrams of testosterone (Bals-Pratsch et al., 1986). Transient local pruritus has been reported in a few of the men treated with the placebo delivery system for testosterone (Bals-Pratsch et al., 1986).

Improved predictive tests for the potential development of allergic contact dermatitis to drugs in these systems is needed. Standard predictive tests in guinea pigs and conventional clinical trials had indicated that clonidine was not a contact allergen, but many users of clonidine in transdermal drug delivery systems developed allergic contact dermatitis to clonidine (Shaw et al., 1987b). Better definition of the relationship between length of occlusion and risk of sensitization is indicated.

The incorporation of agents such as propylene glycol (Ritschel and Nayak, 1987) in transdermal drug delivery systems to enhance percutaneous penetration of drugs may increase the range of drugs that can be delivered by these systems, but dermatologic reactions to these enhancers of percutaneous absorption could limit their usefulness. The role of topical corticosteroids in the suppression of dermatitis to transdermal drug delivery systems needs to be better defined, especially for patients who require continued treatment with a therapeutic device. Improved patient education to minimize reapplication of these devices to the same site would help reduce the risk of sensitization.

REFERENCES

Anonymous. 1985. Discussion in problems during long-term treatment. In *Low Dose Oral and Transdermal Therapy of Hypertension,* eds. M. A. Weber, J. I. M. Drayer, and R. Kolloch, pp. 66–70. Darmstadt: Steinkopff Verlag.

140   D. J. Hogan and H. I. Maibach

Anonymous. 1987. Transdermal estradiol overall safety profile, Panel discussion III. *Am. J. Obstet. Gynecol.* 156:1338–1341.
Anonymous. 1988. Catapress-TTS. In *Physicians' Desk Reference*, ed. B. Huf, pp. 719–721. Oradell, N.J.: Medical Economics.
Anonymous. 1989a. Transderm-V, CIBA-GEIGY. In *Compendium of Pharmaceuticals and Specialities*, 24th ed., ed. C. M. Krogh. Ottawa: Canadian Pharmaceutical Association.
Anonymous. 1989b. Estraderm, CIBA. In *Compendium of Pharmaceutical and Specialities*, ed. C. M. Krogh, pp. 379–381. Ottawa: Canadian Pharmaceutical Association.
Bals-Pratsch, M., Yoon, Y. D., Knuth, U. and Nieschlag, E. 1986. Transdermal testosterone substitution therapy for male hypogonadism. *Lancet* 2:943–946.
Brown, L. and Langer, R. 1988. Transdermal delivery of drugs. *Annu. Rev. Med.* 39:221–229.
Carlston, J. A. 1982. Unilateral dilated pupil from scopolamine disk. *J. Am. Med. Assoc.* 48:31.
Carmicheal, A. J. and Foulds, I. S. 1989. Allergic contact dermatitis from transdermal nitroglycerin. *Contact Dermatitis* 21:113–114.
Chien, Y. W., Xu, H. L., Chians, C. C. and Huang, Y. C. 1988. Transdermal controlled administration of indomethacin. I. Enhancement of skin permeability. *Pharm. Res.* 5:103–106.
Dietz, A. J., Carlson, J. D. and Beck, C. L. 1986. Effect of transdermal azatadine on reducing histamine-induced wheal area. *Ann. Allergy* 57:38–41.
Dorr, R. T., Dawson, B. V., al-Obeidi, F., Hadley, M. E. and Levine, N. 1988. Toxicologic studies of a superpotent alpha-melanotropin, (Nle4,D-Phe7)alpha-MSH. *Invest. New Drugs* 6:251–258.
Fischer, R. G. and Tyler, M. 1985. Severe contact dermatitis due to nitroglycerin patches. *Southern Med. J.* 78:1523–1524.
Fisher, A. A. 1984. Dermatitis due to transdermal therapeutic systems. *CUTIS* 34:526–531.
Fraunfelder, F. T. 1982. Transdermal scopolamine precipitating narrow-angle glaucoma (letter). *N. Eng. J. Med.* 307:1079.
Gordon, D. R., Shupak, A., Doweck, I. and Spitzer, O. 1989. Allergic contact dermatitis caused by transdermal hyoscine. *Br. Med. J.* 298:1220–1221.
Grattan, C. E. H. and Kennedy, C. T. C. 1985. Allergic contact dermatitis to transdermal clonidine. *Contact Dermatitis* 19:225–226.
Groth, H., Vetter, H. Knuesel, J. and Better, W. 1983. Allergic skin reactions to transdermal clonidine. *Lancet*:850–851.
Groth, H., Vetter, H., Knuesel, J., Baumgart, P. and Vetter, W. 1985. Transdermal clonidine in essential hypertension: Problems during long-term treatment. In *Low Dose Oral and Transdermal Therapy of Hypertension*, eds. M. A. Weber, J. I. M. Drayer, and R. Kolloch, pp. 60–65. Darmstadt: Steinkopff Verlag.
Guy, R. H., Hadgraft, J. and Bucks, D. A. W. 1987. Transdermal drug delivery and cutaneous metabolism. *Xenobiotica* 17:325–343.
Hamill, M. B., Suelflow, J. A. and Smith, J. A. 1983. Transdermal scopolamine deliver system (TRANSDERM-V) and acute angle-closure glaucoma. *Ann. Ophthalmol.* 15:1011–1012.
Harari, Z., Sommer, I. and Boleslaw, K. 1987. Multifocal contact dermatitis to nitroderm TTS 5 with extensive postinflammatory hypermelanosis. *Dermatologica* 174:249–252.
Hendricks, A. A. and Dec, W. 1979. Contact dermatitis due to nitroglycerin ointment. *Arch. Dermatol.* 115:853–855.

Homick, J. K., Kohl, R. L., Reschke, M. F., Degioanni, J. and Cintron-Trevino, N. 1983. Transdermal scopolamine in the prevention of motion sickness; Evaluation of the time course of efficacy. *Aviat. Space Environ. Med.* 54:994–1000.

Horning, J. R., Jr., Zawada, E. T., Summons, J. L., Williams, L. and McNulty, R. 1988. Efficacy and safety of two-year therapy with transdermal clonidine for essential hypertension. *Chest* 93:941–945.

Hurkmans, M., Bodde, H. E., Van Driel, L. M. J., Van Doorne, H. and Junginger, H. E. 1985. Skin irritation caused by transdermal drug delivery systems during long-term (5 days) application. *Br. J. Dermatol.* 112:461–476.

Kapoor, A. S., Dang, N. S. and Reynolds, R. D. 1985. Sustained effects of transdermal nitroglycerin in patients with angina pectoris. *Clin. Ther.* 7:674–679.

Kligman, A. M. 1966. The identification of contact allergens by human assay. III. The maximization test: A procedure for screening and rating contact sensitizers. *J. Invest. Dermatol.* 54:994–1000.

Lang, A. E. 1989. Additional comments on Parkinson's disease. *Can. Med. Assoc. J.* 140:513–514.

MacEwan, G., William, R., Noone, R. A. and Joseph, A. 1985. Psychosis due to transdermally administered scopolamine. *Can. Med. Assoc. J.* 133: 4331–4332.

Maibach, H. 1987. Oral substitution in patients sensitized by transdermal clonidine treatment. *Contact Dermatitis* 16:1–8.

McBurney, E. I., Noel, S. B. and Collins, J. H. 1989. Contact dermatitis to transdermal estradiol system. *J. Am. Acad. Dermatol.* 20:503–510.

McCrary, J. A., III and Webb, N. R. 1982. Anisocoria from scopolamine patches. *J. Am. Med. Assoc.* 243:353–354.

Mosley, H., Johnston, S. and Allen A. 1990. The influence of microwave radiation on transdermal delivery systems. *Br. J. Dermatol.* 122:361–364.

Mougeolle, J. M. 1988. Allergies medicamenteuses: cas particulier des systemes therapeutiques transdermiques. *Nouv. Dermatol.* 4(7:suppl.):511–512.

Murray, K. B. 1984. Hazards of microwave ovens to transdermal delivery system. *N. Eng. J. Med.* 310:721.

Neiboer, C., Bruynzeel, D. and Boorsma, D. M. 1987. The effect of occlusion of the skin with transdermal therapeutic system on Langerhans cells and the induction of skin irritation. *Arch. Dermatol.* 123:1499–1502.1.

Patel, R. A. and Vasavada, R. C. 1988. Transdermal delivery of isoproterenol HCL: An investigation of stability, solubility, partition coefficient, and vehicle effects. *Pharm. Res.* 5:116–119.

Reed, M. T. and Hamburg, E. L. 1986. Person-to-person transfer of transdermal drug-delivery systems: A case report. *N. Engl. J. Med.* 314:1120.

Ritschel, W. A. and Barkhaus, J. K. 1988. Use of sorption promoters to increase systemic absorption of coumarin from transdermal drug delivery systems. *Arzneimittelforschung* 38:1774–1777.

Ritschel, W. A. and Nayak, P. M. 1987. Evaluation in vitro and in vivo of dimeticone transdermal therapeutic systems. *Arzneim. Forsch.* 37:302–306.

Ritschel, W. A., Sathyan, G. and Denson, D. D. 1989. Transdermal drug delivery of meperidine. *Methods Find. Exp. Clin. Pharmacol.* 11:165–172.

Rosenfeld, A. S. and White, W. B. 1984. Allergic contact dermatitis secondary to transdermal nitroglycerin. *Am. Heart J.* 108:1061.

Scheuplein, R. J. and Fronaugh, R. L. 1983. Percutaneous absorption. In *Biochemistry and physiology of the skin,* ed. L. A. Goldsmith, pp. 1255–1295. New York: Oxford University Press.

Schwartz, B. K. and Clendenning, W. E. 1988. Allergic contact dermatitis from hydroxypropyl cellulose in a transdermal estradiol patch. *Contact Dermatitis* 18:106–107.

Sekine, T., Machida, V. and Nagai, T. 1987. Gel ointment of verapamil for percutaneous absorption. *Drug. Des. Deliv.* 1:245–252.

Shaw, J. E., Cramer, M. P. and Gale, R. 1987a. Rate-controlled transdermal therapy utilizing polymeric membranes. In *Transdermal Delivery of Drugs,* eds. A. F. Kydonieus and B. Berner, pp. 102–116. Boca Raton, Fla.: CRC Press.

Shaw, J. E., Prevo, M. E. and Amkraut, A. A. 1987b. Testing of controlled-release transdermal dosage forms. *Arch. Dermatol.* 123:1548–1556.

Shupak, A., Gordon, C. R., Spitzer, O., Mendelowitz, N. and Melamed, Y. 1989. Three-years' experience of transdermal scopolamine: Long-term effectiveness and side-effects. *Pharmatherapeutica* 5:365–369.

Topaz, O. and Abraham, D. 1987. Severe allergic contact dermatitis secondary to nitroglycerin in a transdermal therapeutic system. *Ann. Allergy* 59:365–366.

Trozak, D. J. 1985. Delayed hypersensitivity to scopolamine delivered by a transdermal device. *J. Am. Acad. Dermatol.* 13:247–251.

Utian, W. H. 1987. Transdermal estradiol overall safety profile. *Am. J. Obstet. Gynecol.* 156:1336–1338.

van der Willigen, A. J., Oranje, A. P., Stolz, E. and van Joost, T. 1988. Delayed hypersensitivity to scopolamine in transdermal therapeutic systems. *J. Am. Acad. Dermatol.* 18:146–147.

White, T. M. and Guidry, J. R. 1986. Rebound hypertension associated with transdermal clonidine and contact dermatitis. *Western J. Med.* 145:104.

Wick, K. A., Wick, S. M. and Hawkinson, M. S. 1989. Adhesion-to-skin performance of a new transdermal nitroglycerin adhesive patch. *Clin. Ther.* 11:417–424.

9

skin metabolism

■ John Kao ■ Michael P. Carver ■

INTRODUCTION

The skin, being the most external organ in the body, is constantly exposed to a variety of hazardous environmental agents, and it is also a surface upon which drugs, cosmetics, and miscellaneous chemicals are intentionally applied. While the skin is an effective barrier, it is becoming increasingly apparent that it is not a complete barrier. In fact, the skin is recognized as an important portal for the entry of chemicals into the systemic circulation. Furthermore, with the increasing awareness that adverse health effects can result from topical exposure, skin absorption, as reflected by the extensive literature on the subject, has become an important aspect of both toxicology and pharmacology.

Until recently, studies in skin toxicology were concerned mainly with developing methods for producing and evaluating skin irritation and allergic reactions in both animal and human skin. Adjunct to these studies, research activities in dermal absorption were concerned primarily with physicochemical and biophysical factors that influence skin penetration and permeation of chemicals. However, recent discoveries in the immunological and metabolic capabilities of the skin have expanded enormously our appreciation of the functional complexities and biochemical versatilities of this organ. The skin, in addition to being an organ active in the intermediary metabolism of carbohydrates, lipids, proteins, and nucleic acids (Odland, 1983; Rongone, 1983), is also active in the

The authors gratefully acknowledge Heather Morin for her help in preparing the manuscript. The assistance of Liz Graichen in performing literature searches and Ruthann Llewellyn for the graphics is greatly appreciated.

metabolism of a variety of hormones, vitamins, essential nutrients, and xenobiotics. It produces a host of potent factors that regulate growth and differentiation, as well as mediators and inflammatory and immune responses. We are only just beginning to appreciate the functional significance of some of the newly discovered but important physiological and metabolic capabilities of this organ (Milstone and Edelson, 1988).

Since skin contains enzymes capable of metabolizing xenobiotics, any chemicals that are applied to the surface of the skin will, during the course of penetration and translocation through this organ, be exposed to available biotransformation systems that are present in the skin. Consequently, the capacity of the skin to function as an organ of xenobiotic metabolism is of considerable interest. For example: What is the functional significance of skin metabolism in the cutaneous and systemic disposition of chemicals, and can it be an important determinant in the development of local and systemic toxicity? What are the modulating factors that may affect skin metabolism, and consequently disposition of topically applied chemicals? What are the implications of skin metabolism in dermatotoxicity and dermatopharmaceutics? Indeed, will the capacity of the skin to metabolize drugs prove to be a desirable advantage or a confounding factor that complicates the development of novel transcutaneous therapeutic devices? Perhaps more importantly, what conceptual and experimental approaches are readily available to evaluate the functional significance of skin metabolism on the percutaneous fate of topically applied chemicals?

To ascertain the role of skin metabolism in the physiological disposition and fate of chemicals following dermal exposure, it will be necessary to have some knowledge of the metabolic capabilities of the skin. Also, some appreciation of the magnitude of the metabolic process that can act on the chemical during skin permeation will be important. Furthermore, some understanding of the processes that govern the passage of chemicals into and across the skin will be essential. While the diffusional bases governing skin absorption have been defined, and the metabolic capabilities of the skin are relatively well appreciated, experimental evaluations of skin metabolism as it pertains to dermal exposure are still in their infancy. Nevertheless, studies employing various experimental designs to specifically address some of these questions have been reported.

The purpose of this chapter is to review our current knowledge concerning the skin as a drug-metabolizing organ. We will summarize some of the metabolic reactions that have been observed in the skin, describe some of the properties of the enzymes involved, and critically evaluate experimental approaches that have been employed to assess the significance of skin metabolism in the percutaneous fate of topically applied chemicals.

CUTANEOUS METABOLIC REACTIONS

An extensive literature exists to illustrate the capacity of the skin to metabolize chemicals. The supporting evidence is derived primarily from *in vitro* studies in which chemicals were incubated with various skin preparations such as tissue slices, homogenates, isolated cell preparations, and subcellular fractions. A myriad of cutaneous metabolic reactions have been described. As summarized in recent reviews (Bickers, 1983; Bucks, 1984; Noonan and Wester, 1985; Martin et al., 1987), they include Phase I oxidative, reductive, and hydrolytic reactions and Phase II conjugation reactions, and it is clear that a full complement of drug metabolizing enzyme activities is present in the skin. Selected examples of skin-mediated metabolic reactions are presented in Table 1. Although recent investigations have included other chemicals, such as pesticides and model compounds that are routinely used to assess microsomal mixed-function oxidase activities, the steroids and the polycyclic hydrocarbons remain the most heavily studied classes of chemicals in skin metabolism, providing much of the available information concerning the drug metabolizing capabilities of the skin.

The biotransformation of these and other chemicals in the skin can be viewed as being mediated by enzymatic reactions that are either "cofactor-dependent" or "cofactor-independent" reactions. Cofactor-dependent biotransformations are characterized by reactions that require activation, with the utilization of energy from an external source, such as high-energy cofactors. Typically, these reactions are integrated with redox cycles or ATP-generating systems. For example, the O-deethylation of ethoxycoumarin by cutaneous microsomal P-450 utilizes NADPH as an essential cofactor (Fig. 1). Cofactor-independent biotransformation, on the other hand, requires only that the reaction is catalyzed enzymatically. The reactions do not involve an external energy source and do not require activation with high-energy cofactors, for example, the hydrolysis of esters of salicylic acid (Fig. 2). In the following discussion,

TABLE 1. Skin as a Drug-Metabolizing Organ

Phase I reactions Phase II reactions	
Oxidative reactions	Glucuronic acid conjugation
Alcohol oxidation	Sulfate conjugation
Hydroxylation	
Aliphatic	
Alicylic	
Aromatic	
Deamination	Methylation
Dealkylation	
Reductive reactions	Glycine conjugation
Carbonyl reduction	
C = C reduction	
Hydrolytic reactions	Glutathione conjugation
Ester hydrolysis	
Epoxide hydrolysis	

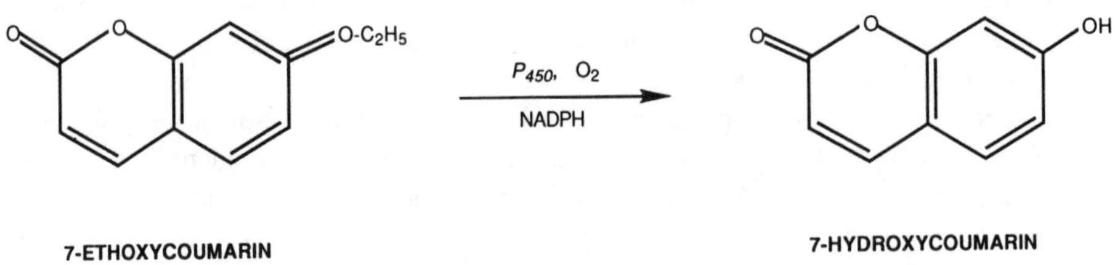

7-ETHOXYCOUMARIN   7-HYDROXYCOUMARIN

FIGURE 1   Cutaneous microsomal *O*-deethylation of 7-ethoxycoumarin.

the characteristics of cutaneous metabolic reactions will be addressed from this perspective.

Cofactor-Dependent Biotransformation

Metabolic reactions.   A range of clinical conditions, such as acne, hirsutism, and testicular feminization syndrome, is thought to be associated with anomalies in the cutaneous metabolism of endogenous steroids (Sansone and Reisner, 1971; Bingham and Shaw, 1973; Hay and Hodgins, 1974; Price, 1975), and topical steroid therapy is a common practice in treating many dermatological disorders; consequently, interest in the steroid-metabolizing capability of the skin has received much recent attention. Skin metabolism of steroids has been reviewed (Kuttenn and Mauvais-Jarvis, 1975; Hsia, 1980; Longcope, 1980; Kuttenn et al., 1980), and the spectrum of metabolites described provides many examples of cofactor-dependent reactions. The cutaneous metabolism of steroids involves primarily two reactions: (1) the interconversion of keto and hydroxyl groups in the steroid molecule, which is mediated by various hydroxysteroid dehydrogenases, and (2) the metabolism of steroid molecules with the 3-keto-Δ-4 structure at the C_5 position to produce the skin-specific 5α-reduced derivatives, mediated by cutaneous 5α-reductases. In the skin, both the hydroxysteroid dehydrogenase and 5α-reductase activities are reported to be associated with the microsomal fraction of skin preparations, and both activities have requirements of pyridine nucleotides as cofactors (Hsia, 1980). Classic examples of cutaneous biotransformations that are catalyzed by

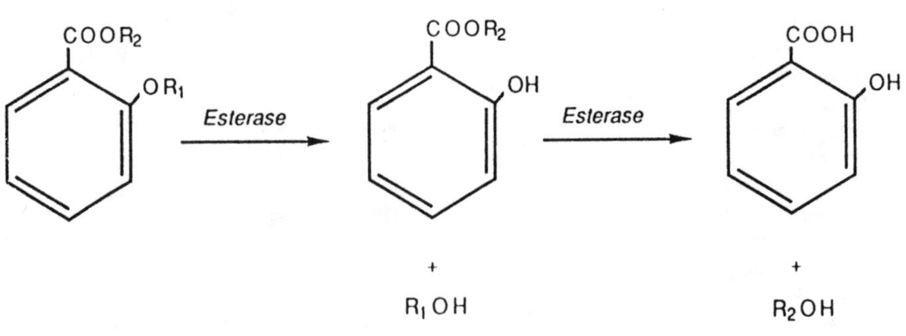

FIGURE 2   Cutaneous hydrolysis of salicylate ester(s).

hydroxysteroid dehydrogenases include the interconversions of estradiol with estrone, cortisone with hydrocortisone (Fig. 3), and testosterone with androstenedione where NAD is the preferred cofactor in these reactions (Hsia, 1980). In contrast, NADPH is utilized by 5α-reductase as the preferred cofactor in the formation of 5α-dihydrotestosterone (Fig. 4) and 5α-pregnane derivatives from testosterone and progesterone, respectively, and they provide examples of typical cutaneous 5α-reduction reactions (Hsia, 1980). Other cutaneous metabolic reactions involving steroids have also been described, and with the observed 7α-hydroxylation of dehydroepiandrosterone in human skin, the possible involvement of cutaneous cytochrome P-450 in the metabolism of steroids was implicated (Faredin et al., 1969).

Evidence for the presence of mixed-function monooxygenase enzymes in the skin was obtained initially from studies dealing with the carcinogenic effects of polycyclic aromatic hydrocarbons on this organ. From these studies, it is generally recognized that, as a prerequisite to inducing skin carcinomas, polycyclic aromatic hydrocarbons must undergo metabolic activation to form reactive intermediates, which can interact with tissue macromolecules, and this interaction is ultimately responsible for the induction of tumors (Harvey, 1982). Studies with model compounds such as benzo[a]pyrene (Fig. 5), dimethylbenz-[a]anthracene, and 3-methylcholanthrene have shown that skin metabolism of polycyclic hydrocarbons produces a variety of metabolites, including phenols, quinones, dihydrodiols, and reactive diol-epoxides (MacNicoll et al., 1980; Weston et al., 1982; Bickers, 1983; Kao et al., 1984). The diol-epoxides are thought to be the ultimate carcinogens, forming covalent adducts with the target macromolecules (Koreeda et al., 1978; Baer-Dubowska and Alexandrov, 1981; Ashurst and Cohen, 1981). Studies based on measurements of aryl hydrocarbon hydroxylase activities in various skin preparations from rats and mice have demonstrated that the properties of the skin enzymes responsible for activating these carcinogens, both basal and induced, are similar to those forms of the hepatic microsomal cytochrome P-450 that are induced by polycyclic hydrocarbons such as 3-methylcholanthrene (Bucks, 1984).

Using model hepatic mixed-function monooxygenase substrates, other cytochrome P-450-mediated reactions have also been demonstrated in the skin. The NADPH-cytochrome P-450-dependent *O*-dealkylation of ethoxyresorufin, 7-ethoxycoumarin, and other alkylumbelliferone ethers, the hydroxylation of aniline to *p*-aminophenol (Pohl et al., 1976; Moloney et al., 1982b; Rettie et al., 1986b), and the epoxidation of aldrin to dieldrin (Rettie et al., 1986a) (Fig. 6) have been reported in studies with skin microsomes.

Glucuronidation and sulfation are typical Phase II reactions. They require the cofactors UDP-glucuronic acid and phosphoadenosylphosphosulfate (PAPS), respectively, and represent another type of cofactor-dependent metabolic reactions, which take place in the skin. Studies with skin strips and isolated epidermal cells from rats and mice have shown that model xenobiotics such as benzo[a]pyrene and ethoxycoumarin are metabolized, and the resultant phenols are readily conjugated to give water soluble glucuronides (Fig. 7) and

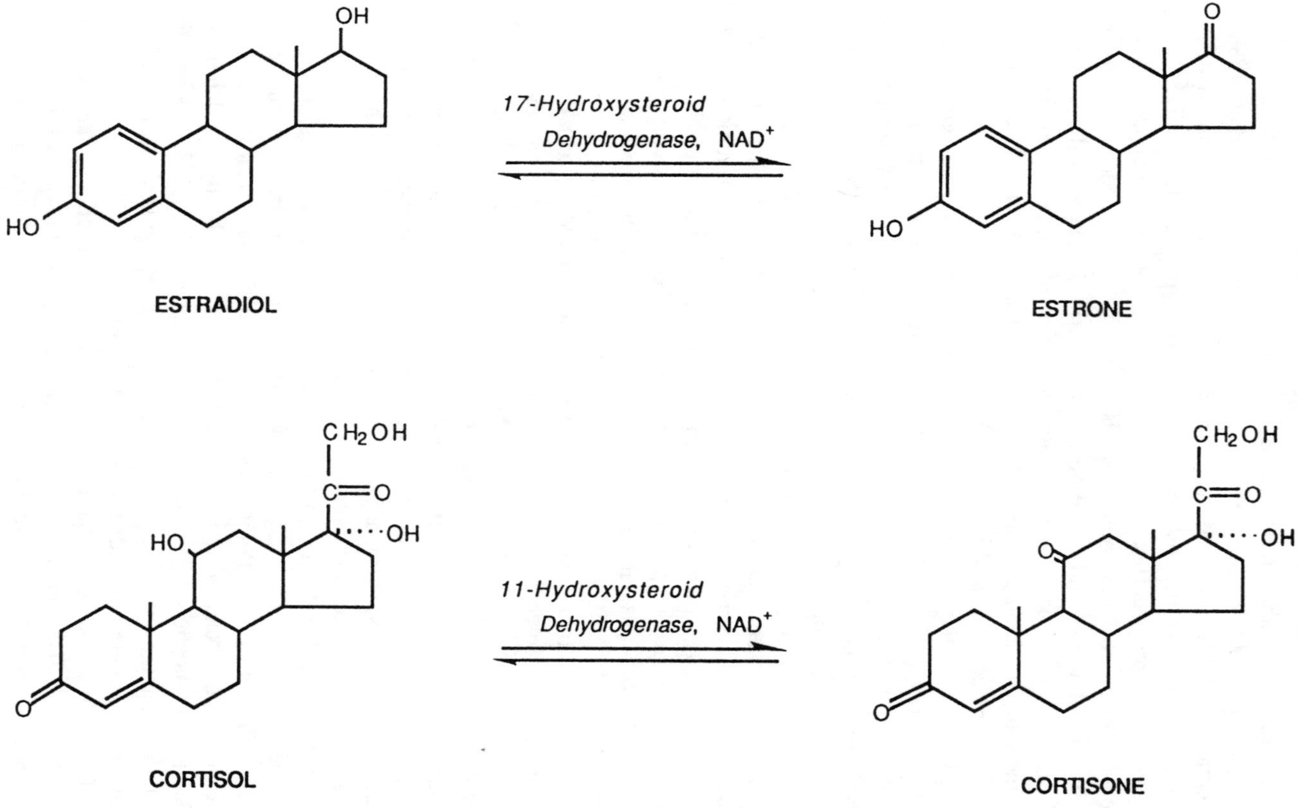

ESTRADIOL ⟶ **ESTRONE**

17-Hydroxysteroid Dehydrogenase, NAD⁺

CORTISOL ⟶ **CORTISONE**

11-Hydroxysteroid Dehydrogenase, NAD⁺

FIGURE 3 Typical hydroxysteroid dehydrogenase reactions in skin.

148

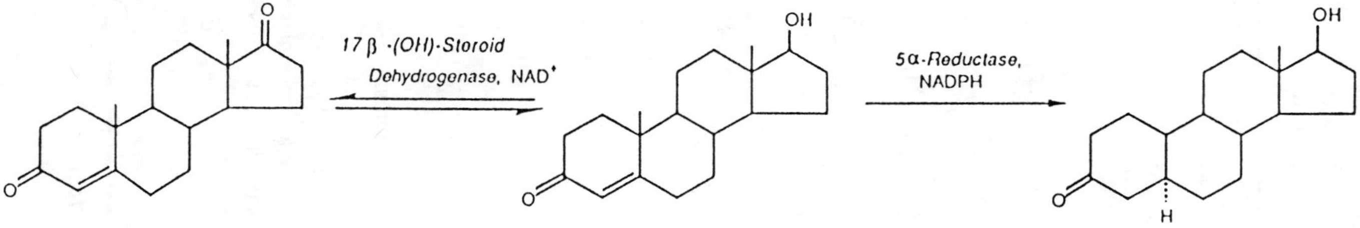

FIGURE 4 Cutaneous metabolic pathways for testosterone.

ANDROSTENEDIONE

17β-(OH)-Steroid Dehydrogenase, NAD⁺

TESTOSTERONE

5α-Reductase, NADPH

5α-DIHYDROTESTOSTERONE

149

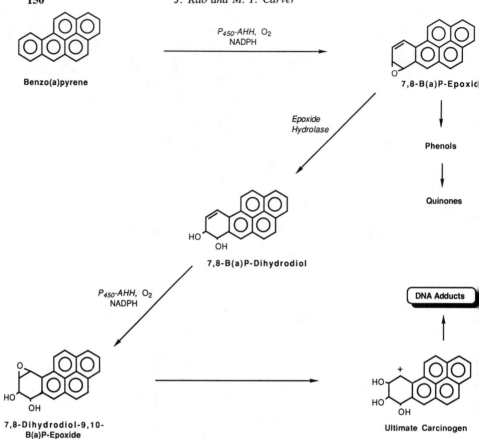

Benzo(a)pyrene

P_{450}-AHH, O_2
NADPH

7,8-B(a)P-Epoxide

Epoxide
Hydrolase

Phenols

Quinones

7,8-B(a)P-Dihydrodiol

P_{450}-AHH, O_2
NADPH

DNA Adducts

**7,8-Dihydrodiol-9,10-
B(a)P-Epoxide**

Ultimate Carcinogen

FIGURE 5   Cutaneous biotransformation of benzo[a]pyrene.

sulfates (Moloney et al., 1982a, 1982c; Finnen, 1987). Other phenols such as naphthol (Harkness et al., 1971; Hemels, 1971, 1972) and aminophenols (Stevenson and Dutton, 1960; Rugstad and Dybing, 1975) are readily conjugated in skin homogenates, and endogenous chemicals such as cholesterol and certain steroids are also substrates of cutaneous UDP-glucuronosyl transferase

ALDRIN

Cytochrome
P_{450}

DIELDRIN

FIGURE 6   Aldrin epoxidation to dieldrin in cutaneous microsomes.

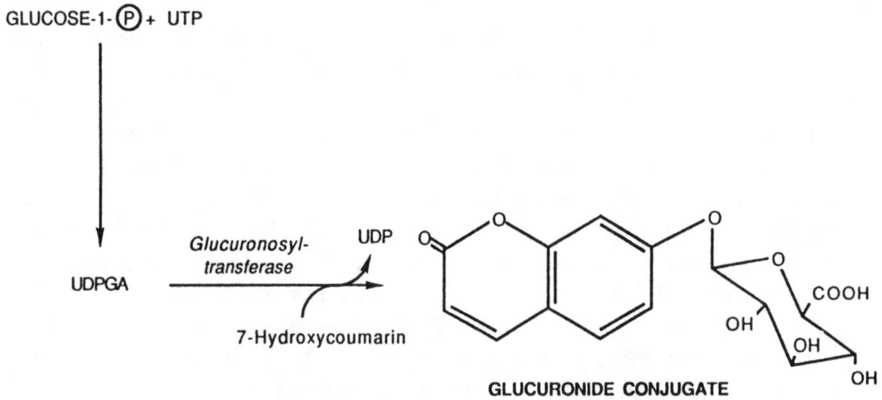

GLUCOSE-1-Ⓟ + UTP

FIGURE 7 Conjugation (phase II metabolism) of 7-hydroxycoumarin in skin.

and sulfotransfase enzymes. Methylation of norepinephrine in skin preparations from rat, mouse, rabbit, and human has also been reported, and catechol-*O*-methyltransferase was implicated in the reaction (Hakanson and Moller, 1963).

Enzymology of cutaneous P-450. Cutaneous microsomal P-450 enzyme activities, in common with similar activities of the liver, are readily modulated by chemical inducers and inhibitors. Indeed, evidence that cytochrome P-450-dependent enzymes are present in the skin was derived primarily from comparative studies of the effects of classical hepatic P-450 inducers and inhibitors on the mixed-function monooxygenase activities in the skin. The hepatic enzymes have been studied extensively, and several forms of the cytochrome P-450 enzyme have been described. These isozymes have different physicochemical and immunological properties, individual substrate specificities, and they differ in their characteristic response to treatment with inducers and inhibitors (Wolf, 1986; Netter, 1987; Gonzalez, 1989). The presence of multiple forms of the mixed-function monooxygenase enzymes in the skin has been suggested in a number of recent studies. In the following sections, evidence for the multiplicity of cutaneous P-450, based on their observed induction and inhibition characteristics, in addition to their differential substrate specificities in the skin will be discussed.

Induction. The inducibility of cutaneous mixed-function monooxygenase activity was first demonstrated in skin homogenates prepared from rats (Schlede and Conney, 1970). A tenfold increase in aryl hydrocarbon hydroxylase activity was observed in the skin homogenates prepared from rats treated, 24 h previously, with a topical application of 3-methylcholanthrene. Subsequently, extensive studies with skin microsomes have demonstrated that various topically applied polycyclic hydrocarbons, coal tar, and petroleum derivatives are effective as inducers of aryl hydrocarbon hydroxylase in mammalian skin, including that of humans (Bickers and Kappas, 1978; Kumar et al., 1982; Mukhtar et al., 1986).

Besides polycyclic hydrocarbons, other chemicals have also been shown to induce P-450-mediated activities in the skin. Indeed, the heme protein cytochrome P-450 itself was first characterized spectrally in the skin using induced cutaneous microsomes prepared from rats and mice pretreated *in vivo* with potent hepatic inducers, such as polychlorinated biphenyls (Arochlor 1254), 1,1,1-trichloro-2,2-bis(*p*-cholorophenyl)ethane (DDT), and 2,3,7,8-tetrachlorodibenzo-*p*-dioxin (TCDD) (Bickers et al., 1974, 1975; Pohl et al., 1976). Topically applied nitropyrenes were also shown to be potent inducers of cutaneous, as well as hepatic, monooxygenase activities (Asokan et al., 1985, 1986). Furthermore, it was reported that topical pretreatment with 5,6-benzoflavone resulted in significant induction of ethoxycoumarin *O*-deethylase activities in microsomes prepared from rat and hairless mouse skin (Bickers et al., 1982; Moloney et al., 1982c).

Topical corticosteroids are often used in treating dermatologic diseases, and studies of the cutaneous microsomal hydroxylation of benzo[a]pyrene and the dealkylation of ethoxycoumarin and ethoxyresorufin have shown that corticoids, such as pregnenolone-16α-carbonitrile and clobetasol propionate, represent another class of agents capable of inducing cutaneous cytochrome P-450 activities (Finnen et al., 1984, 1985). Moreover, it was reported that clobetasol propionate and 3-methylcholanthrene had differential effects on the activities of cutaneous ethoxycoumarin and ethoxyresorufin dealkylase (Damen and Mier, 1982). Consistent with findings in hepatic P-450 systems, this indicated that corticosteroids may induce a form of cutaneous P-450 that is distinct from those induced by the polycyclic hydrocarbons.

The barbiturates are normally recognized as effective inducers of certain hepatic P-450 isozymes (Wolf, 1986). When administered topically, phenobarbital generally had little or no effect on cutaneous aryl hydrocarbon hydroxylase activity. However, induction of ethoxycoumarin *O*-deethylase was observed in mouse skin microsomes following multiple subcutaneous injections of phenobarbital (Damen and Mier, 1982). Furthermore, it was reported that benzo[a]pyrene hydroxylase activities in skin microsomes were induced in the rat following multiple intraperitoneal doses of phenobarbital (Vizethum et al., 1980). While many of the recent investigations of skin metabolism are concerned with the inducibility of cutaneous P-450-mediated activities, it is perhaps worth noting that other skin-metabolizing activities are also inducible. For example, topical exposure to polycyclic hydrocarbons, TCDD, and polychlorinated biphenyls has been reported to induce cutaneous UDP-glucuronosyl transferase and epoxide hydrolase activities (Bucks, 1984).

Inhibition. Because P-450-dependent biotransformation is an important step in the activation of polycyclic hydrocarbons, it has been postulated that inhibiting the enzyme activities could reduce the potential carcinogenicity of these compounds in target tissues such as skin (Bickers et al., 1986). *In vitro* studies with synthetic flavones have demonstrated that both 5,6-benzoflavone and 7,8-benzoflavone inhibited mouse skin aryl hydrocarbon hydroxylase activity (Bowden et al., 1974) and the ethoxycoumarin deethylase activity of skin microsomes from both control and induced rats and hairless mice (Moloney et al., 1982b; Rettie et al., 1986a). Moreover, it was reported that coadministration of 7,8-benzoflavone with dimethylbenzanthracene to mice diminished the binding of the carcinogen to cellular macromolecules and decreased papilloma formation (Bowden et al., 1974). On the other hand, it was also reported that 7,8-benzoflavone did not inhibit benzo[a]pyrene-induced skin tumorigenesis, and actually increased the incidence of skin tumors induced by 1,2,5,6-dibenzanthracene (Kinoshita and Gelboin, 1972a, 1972b). In contrast, pretreatment with 5,6-benzoflavone 3 days prior to topical application of benzo[a]pyrene produced a significant reduction in subsequent skin tumor formation (Bowden et al., 1974). These results demonstrated that the *in vivo* effects of the benzoflavones, which can act as both inducers and inhibitors of mixed-function monooxygenases, are complex, and their influence on polycyclic hydrocarbon-induced skin tumorigenesis will require further investigation.

Although the studies with benzoflavones were somewhat inconclusive, as an approach to the prevention of cutaneous malignancy, the modulation of P-450-mediated activation of carcinogens with chemical inhibitors has stimulated much recent interest. A number of investigations have demonstrated that certain plant phenols have substantial antimutagenic activities with respect to polycyclic hydrocarbons (Bickers et al., 1986). Studies with ellagic acid, a naturally occurring plant polyphenol, demonstrated that this compound was a potent inhibitor of epidermal microsomal aryl hydrocarbon hydroxylase activity, inhibiting both the cutaneous metabolism of benzo[a]pyrene and the enzyme-mediated binding of benzo[a]pyrene to epidermal DNA (Mukhtar et al., 1984a, 1984d; Shugart and Kao, 1984). Furthermore, topical application of ellagic acid to skin of BALB/c mice afforded a substantial delay in skin tumorigenesis due to 3-methylcholanthrene (Mukhtar et al., 1984b). These observations, together with substantiating results from feeding studies (Das et al., 1985), indicate that the anticarcinogenic properties of ellagic acid in murine skin may be related to its capacity to modulate the cutaneous metabolism of carcinogenic polycyclic hydrocarbons. Additional studies with other naturally occurring plant phenols such as tannic acid, quercetin, myricetin, and anthraflavic acid have also demonstrated that these compounds were inhibitory with respect to cutaneous microsomal mixed-function monooxygenase activities, and *in vitro* metabolism of benzo[a]pyrene. These findings suggest the possibility that plant phenols or structurally related compounds may have potential usefulness as antagonists in polycyclic hydrocarbon-induced tumorigenesis in skin (Das et al., 1987a, 1987b, 1989).

The imidazole antifungal agents, such as clotrimazole, are another class of compounds that are widely used in a number of dermatological indications. These drugs have also been shown to be potent inhibitors of microsomal P-450-dependent monooxygenase activities (James and Little, 1983; Kahl et al., 1980). In the skin, clotrimazole was a potent inhibitor of not only epidermal aryl hydrocarbon hydroxylase activity, but also epoxide hydrolase activity. Moreover, it was an inducer of epidermal gluthathione *S*-transferase activity and inhibited, to some extent, the cutaneous metabolism, macromolecular binding, and carcinogenicity of topically applied benzo[a]pyrene (Mukhtar et al., 1984c; Das et al., 1986). These studies suggest that clotrimazole, like ellagic acid, may also be useful in the prevention of polycyclic hydrocarbon skin malignancies, by modulating cutaneous drug metabolizing enzymes.

As we have seen, the focus of many recent studies has been on identifying chemical inhibitors of cutaneous drug metabolizing enzymes as potential candidates for antineoplastic agents in skin. It is worth noting, however, that other, more classical inhibitors of hepatic P-450 are also inhibitors of cutaneous mixed-function monooxygenase activities. The differential effects of these inhibitors, which include compounds such as carbon monoxide, SK&F 525A, metyrapone, and 7,8-benzoflavone, on the metabolism of model compounds may thus assist in demonstrating and characterizing the multiplicity of cytochrome P-450 isozymes in the skin.

Multiplicity of cutaneous P-450.   Traditionally, inducers of hepatic cytochrome P-450 are categorized into different types based on their differential effects on a spectrum of P-450-mediated reactions (Snyder and Remmer, 1982). The basis for differentiating hepatic cytochrome P-450 in this manner is that each type of inducer increases the synthesis of a characteristic range of P-450 isozymes that have distinctive, but not necessarily unique, substrate and reaction specificities (Guengerich et al., 1982b). As summarized above, induction of P-450-mediated activities in the skin was observed with various chemicals that can be categorized as belonging to the aromatic hydrocarbon, the phenobarbital, or the corticosteroid family of inducing agents. Therefore, by inference, multiforms of cytochrome P-450 are thought to be present and are inducible in the skin.

Although significant advances have been made with immunological and recombinant DNA technologies, measuring the metabolism of isozyme-selective substrates remains one of the more practical approaches in identifying and assessing the multiplicity of P-450 isozymes. Unfortunately, many of the "model" P-450 substrates used in the past for assessing microsomal mixed-function monooxygenase activities do not differentiate between individual induced isozymes, nor between constitutive and induced isozymes (Guengerich et al., 1982a; Kaminsky et al., 1983). Furthermore, with cutaneous microsomal P-450-mediated activities the problem is compounded by the extremely low constitutive and induced activities often encountered, and the limited sensitivity of the assays then becomes a challenging technical problem. Consequently, much of our knowledge concerning cutaneous cytochrome P-450 is based on the use of benzo[a]pyrene and, more recently, ethoxycoumarin as model substrates.

The metabolism of a number of alternative substrates for the mixed-function monooxygenase system was studied recently in mouse skin microsomes, and highly sensitive assay techniques were employed. Ethoxyresorufin and aldrin, considered to be "diagnostic" substrates for the P-450 isozymes that are induced by aromatic hydrocarbons (Burke and Mayer, 1974; Burke et al., 1977) and phenobarbital (Wolff et al., 1979, 1980), respectively, were studied along with benzo[a]pyrene, diphenyloxazole coumarin, and a homologous series (C_1–C_4) of 7-alkylcoumarins (Rettie et al., 1986a). Cutaneous microsomal metabolism was evident for all substrates studied. However, depending on the substrate, the metabolic rates in skin microsomes (expressed in terms of microsomal protein content) ranged from 0.5% to 15% of the corresponding rates observed in the liver microsomes. Furthermore, the skin microsomes showed a preference for metabolizing ethoxyresorufin, benzo[a]pyrene, and diphenyloxazole. Also, 7,8-benzoflavone, a selective inhibitor of aromatic hydrocarbon-induced P-450 isozymes, blocked the cutaneous microsomal metabolism of ethoxyresorufin, but had no effects on aldrin metabolism. On the other hand, metyrapone, an inhibitor for phenobarbital-inducible cytochrome P-450, was only partially effective (at high concentrations) in reducing the cutaneous microsomal metabolism of either substrate. Based on these observations, it was concluded that mouse skin contains multiple forms of cytochrome P-450, and the constitutive enzymes are analogous to those rodent hepatic P-450 isozymes induced by polycyclic hydrocarbons (Rettie et al., 1986a). In another study, the *in vitro* metabolism of a number of phenoxazone ethers, homologous with ethoxyresorufin, was examined in mouse skin microsomes. These phenoxazone ethers had clearly differing substrate selectivities for each type of inducible hepatic cytochrome P-450 (Rettie et al., 1986b), and the results were consistent with the presence of constitutive P-450 isozymes in mouse skin that are analogous to those isozymes induced by aromatic hydrocarbons.

Studies using purified hepatic cytochrome P-450 isozymes have shown the hydroxylation of testosterone to be both regiospecific and stereoselective (Wood et al., 1983). Recently, it was reported that testosterone, in the presence of NADPH, was hydroxylated at the 6α, 7α, and 16α positions following incubation with microsomes prepared from neonatal rat skin. Moreover, the formation of these hydroxylated metabolites was inhibited by SK&F 525A and metyrapone. These observations, therefore, provided clear evidence that the biotransformation of steroids in skin is also mediated by cytochrome P-450-associated mixed-function monooxygenases, and the results of this investigation indicated that other P-450 isozymes may also be found in the skin (Mukhtar et al., 1987). In recent studies, the presence of several isoforms of P-450 in skin microsomes was revealed from their cross-immunoreactivity using specific antibodies raised against different purified rat hepatic P-450s (Khan et al., 1989a, 1989b; Pham et al., 1989). The results showed that rat skin microsomes contain mixed-function monooxygenase activities associated with cytochrome P-450IA1 (P-450 induced by 3-methylcholanthrene) and cytochrome P-450IIB1 (P-450 induced by phenobarbital). Furthermore, based on substrate specificities, the results from one of these studies (Pham et al., 1989) indicated that multiple forms of epoxide hydrolase, glutathione S-transferase, and UDP-glucuronosyl transferase were also present in rat skin.

Cofactor-Independent Biotransformation

Hydrolytic reactions, such as the hydrolysis of esters catalyzed by esterases are not dependent upon the presence of cofactors, nor do they require the presence of functional redox cycles or ATP-generating systems in the skin. The skin is known to contain nonspecific enzymes capable of mediating the hydrolysis of esters (Montagna, 1955; Findlay, 1955; Tauber and Rost, 1987), and there are many examples of cutaneous hydrolytic reactions involving compounds with ester linkages. Typical examples were observed in recent efforts toward the development and evaluation of safe and efficacious prodrugs such as corticosteroids (Cheung et al., 1985), p-nitrobenzoate (Pannatier et al., 1981), theophylline (Sloan and Bodor, 1982), antibiotics (Baines et al., 1984), cromolyn (Bodor et al., 1980), and metronidazole (Johansen et al., 1986) for topical delivery.

The major barrier to the topical delivery of drugs is the stratum corneum, but it is also recognized that cutaneous metabolism could influence the bioavailability of topically applied drugs. Therefore, in the prodrug approach to topical therapy, the primary objective is to improve the diffusion of the parent drug by manipulating its physicochemical properties through derivatization. Once increased permeation is achieved, a secondary objective is to exploit the capacity of the skin to regenerate the active drug through metabolism and/or alter the metabolic fate of the absorbed drug, thereby improving bioavailability. Esterification is the method of choice for accomplishing these goals in the design of many prodrugs (Higuchi and Yu, 1987). Therefore, ester derivatives should provide the ideal chemical modification necessary for the synthesis of successful topical prodrugs and, indeed, topical corticosteroid esters are recognized as one of the most important classes of drugs in contemporary dermal therapeutics (Stoughton and Cornell, 1988). Unfortunately, this approach does not yet have universal application, as suggested by a recent study of 16 prodrugs for 6-mercaptopurine. Classical structure-activity relationships predicted that amide group substitution for carboxyesters in α-(acylhetero)alkyl prodrugs would impart greater hydrophilicity and increase dermal delivery; however, only one of 16 candidates tested produced the desired effect and the relative increase obtained was small (Siver and Sloan, 1990).

Other examples of cutaneous metabolic reactions that may be considered to be cofactor-independent include, for example, the hydrolysis of benzoyl peroxide, a compound used in the treatment of acne vulgaris, to benzoic acid (Nacht et al., 1981); the metabolism of topical nitroglycerin, which is used in the treatment for angina (Wester et al., 1983); and the metabolism of T-2 toxins (Kemppainen et al., 1986a, 1986b). Various organophosphates, including paraoxon (Fredriksson et al., 1961; Fredriksson, 1962, 1964), diisopropylfluorophosphate (Loden, 1985), and the chemical warfare agents soman, sarin, and tabun (Blank et al., 1957; Fredriksson, 1958; vanHooidonk, 1979), have also been shown to be hydrolyzed by enzymes found in human and animal skin. The enzymatic hydrolysis of intermediate epoxides from benzo[a]pyrene metabolism, mediated by microsomal epoxide hydrolase (Oesch et al., 1978; Bickers and Kappas, 1980; Del Tito et al., 1984), and the glutathione conjugation of arene oxides have been demonstrated in skin preparations (Mukhtar and Bresnick, 1976; Mukhtar and Bickers, 1982), providing further examples of cofactor-independent cutaneous metabolism.

Distribution of Enzyme Activities

The skin is generally viewed as consisting of two broadly distinguishable, anatomical regions. The outer region, the epidermis, is comprised of a basal layer of actively dividing cells, which undergo progressive terminal differentiation and migration outward, eventually forming the keratinized cell layer known as the stratum corneum. The thicker dermis, underlying the epidermis, is essentially a matrix of connective tissues containing a preponderance of fibroblasts. Blood vessels, nerves, and lymphatics form networks across and within this matrix, and embedded in this tissue are skin appendages such as the pilosebaceous apparatus, eccrine glands, and apocrine glands. Although skin is recognized as an organ capable of metabolizing xenobiotics, the exact anatomical distribution and localization of this metabolic activity within the skin remains uncertain.

Epidermal, dermal, and appendageal metabolism. Histochemical examination of skin has demonstrated that enzymes such as nonspecific esterases and catechol-*O*-methyl transferases in the skin are localized primarily in the epidermis, and there is evidence indicating that these enzyme activities are also present in the skin appendages (Montagna, 1955; Bamshad, 1969; Meyer and Neurand, 1976). Indeed, using a combination of histochemical, freeze-fracture/scraping, and biochemical techniques, a number of hydrolytic enzymes have been localized in the "dead" cell layers comprising the stratum corneum. Thus phospholipases (Elias et al., 1988), sphingomyelinase (Menon et al., 1986), transglutaminase (DeYoung et al., 1984), γ-glutamyl cyclotransferase (Barrett and Scott, 1983), aryl and steroid sulfatases (Baden et al., 1980), glycosidases (Nemanic et al., 1983), and acid phosphatase (Weinstock and Wilgram, 1970) have all been found within this tissue and are believed to play important roles in desquamation processes in health and disease. Their role, if any, in xenobiotic metabolism has not been addressed.

Using both histochemical and autoradiographic methods, initial studies have shown that benzo[a]pyrene hydroxylase activity in mouse skin was located in the dermis, primarily in the vicinity of the sebaceous glands and upper portion of the hair follicles, and it appears that each skin region exhibits a different rate of carcinogen metabolism (Wattenberg and Leong, 1970). Others, using relatively crude tissue separation procedures, also reported that cutaneous aryl hydrocarbon hydroxylase activity was highest in the superficial layers of the dermis (Wiebel et al., 1975). Subsequently, in studies with better-defined procedures for separating dermis and epidermis, a number of investigators have demonstrated that drug metabolizing activities in mammalian skin are localized primarily in the epidermis (Akin and Norred, 1976; Thompson and Slaga, 1976; Bickers, 1980). However, it is worth commenting that the apparent localization of activity in the epidermis is dependent on the units used to express enzyme activity, and in these studies specific activities were compared in terms of microsomal protein content. When compared on the basis of wet tissue weight, it was noted that enzyme activities in the whole skin and the dermis were approximately equal, if somewhat lower than that found using the epidermis alone. However, when enzyme activity was expressed per unit area of skin, it was concluded that the dermis and not the epidermis was the major site of metabolic activity within the skin. This conclusion takes into account the greater mass of the dermis, relative to that of the epidermis, in a given unit area of skin, and it is argued that the dermis will make the larger contribution to the total metabolic activity of skin. Consequently, the authors concluded that the dermis possesses the greater overall capacity to metabolize chemicals (Finnen et al., 1985; Finnen, 1987).

There are a number of problems associated with the measurement of cutaneous drug metabolizing activities. A major hurdle has been the extremely low intrinsic levels of activity found in this tissue, a problem complicated by the difficulties in sample preparation. The skin is extremely resistant to homogenization, and the harsh techniques required to homogenize cutaneous tissue often result in the destruction of enzyme activities (Akin and Norred, 1976; Moloney et al., 1982b). Furthermore, skin contains relatively large amounts of metabolically inert material (i.e., collagen and keratin) and, depending on the preparation procedures and the reference units used to express enzyme activity, variations in the amounts of these nonenzymic contaminants could greatly influence the apparent specific activities measured in this tissue. Consequently, caution must be exercised when interpreting and comparing measurements of cutaneous drug metabolizing activities.

Because of their easy accessibility, hair follicles have been exploited as biopsy specimens for the detection of some genetic diseases (Gartler et al., 1971; deBruyn et al., 1974; Vermorken et al., 1978). They have also been shown to be capable of metabolizing steroids and polycyclic hydrocarbons (Fazekas and Lanthier, 1971; Fazekas and Sandor, 1973; Vermorken et al., 1979a, 1979b); therefore, hair follicles may be a useful test system for examining genetically determined differences in drug metabolism. It has been postulated that the expression of carcinogen-activating enzymes may be an important determinant in individual susceptibility to chemical carcinogenesis, especially those malignancies attributable to aromatic hydrocarbons. Therefore, the possible use of hair follicles as a tool for population studies in humans was introduced recently, and significant interindividual variation has been demonstrated in the metabolite profiles of benzo[a]pyrene in human hair follicles

(Hukkelhoven et al., 1982, 1983; Merk et al., 1987). This approach may prove to be useful in identifying high-risk groups within the general population; however, correlations of enzyme activities and metabolite profile differences with individual susceptibility to chemical carcinogens are not yet adequate to accomplish this broader goal.

Isolated cells and cell culture. Skin slices, whole skin homogenates, and subcellular fractions have been the principle preparations utilized in many of the previous investigations of cutaneous metabolism. However, recent advances in cell isolation, enrichment, and culture techniques make it possible to study metabolism in the various cell populations that comprise and inhabit the integument. The consequences of cutaneous metabolic transformation activity on topical drug therapies and its interaction with the physiological function of skin, both in health and in various disease states, are areas of interest in which studies with isolated cells may have a profound impact.

Benzo[a]pyrene and ethoxycoumarin biotransformations have been the most well-characterized reaction pathways in cultured mouse and human epidermal cells (Chapman et al., 1979; Kuroki et al., 1980, 1982; Coomes et al., 1983; Finnen and Shuster, 1985). Furthermore, it is widely believed that most, if not all, of the reactions that take place in cutaneous tissue homogenates and subcellular fractions also occur in cultured keratinocytes. Although dermal fibroblasts may possess similar metabolic activities in culture, they have not been as extensively investigated in this regard. In a study of the metabolism of benzo[a]pyrene by isolated human and mouse skin cells, variations in metabolism related to cell type (epidermal keratinocytes versus dermal fibroblasts) and species were observed. The activity of aryl hydrocarbon hydroxylase was greater in human keratinocytes than fibroblasts (Kuroki et al., 1980), and this was consistent with previous observations, which showed that this enzyme is localized almost exclusively within the epidermis (Chapman et al., 1979). In contrast, the opposite (i.e., aryl hydrocarbon hydroxylase activity in fibroblasts was greater than that of keratinocytes) was demonstrated in the two cell types of rodent origin (Kuroki et al., 1982).

In addition to putative species differences in the relative activities of different skin layers, the reaction pathways and the extent of metabolism *in vitro* may be dependent on the culture conditions. For example, cultures of newborn rat skin, maintained in a state of terminal differentiation by high Ca^{2+} concentrations in the medium, demonstrated much greater basal and benzanthracene-induced aryl hydrocarbon hydroxylase activities than germinative cells (low Ca^{2+}) (Guo et al., 1990). These findings are consistent with increased metabolism of both benzo[a]pyrene and dimethylbenzanthracene (DMBA), as well as shifts in the release of water-soluble metabolites and decreased formation of DMBA glucuronides, due to calcium-induced differentiation of mouse epidermal cultures (DiGiovanni et al., 1989). As expected, a corresponding increase in DNA adduct formation was found in association with the increased metabolism of these carcinogens (DiGiovanni et al., 1989).

Others have shown that 12-O-tetradecanoyl phorbol 13-acetate induced differentiation of sencar mouse keratinocytes is accompanied by a xanthine dehydrogenase to xanthine oxidase conversion (Reiners and Rupp, 1989) and that minoxidil sulfation is greater in proliferating (low Ca^{2+}) than in differentiated (high Ca^{2+}) rat skin cells in culture (Hamamoto and Mori, 1989). The latter result takes on added significance in light of the recent interest in minoxidil as a topical therapy for male pattern baldness and the belief that sulfation represents a bioactivation step in its metabolism. Retinoids are also currently of interest from a dermatotherapeutic standpoint, and their relationship with epidermal keratinization/differential processes and a number of cutaneous pathologies is intriguing (Vahlquist and Torma, 1988). The cutaneous biotransformation of various vitamin A congeners has been previously shown to occur in human, mouse, and hairless mouse skins (Torma and Vahlquist, 1985, 1987; Torma et al., 1987). Recently, using a combination of cell culture and fractionation techniques, enhanced esterification of vitamin A in terminally differentiating keratinocytes was not attributable to aryl-CoA:retinol acyltransferase (ARAT) concentration differences in the various cell types (Torma and Vahlquist, 1990). Rather, it was hypothesized that the pH near the skin surface more closely matched the pH optimum for the cutaneous enzyme, which was, in turn, found to differ from ARAT isolated from other tissues. However, this did not explain the presence of low ARAT activities in the basal and squamous carcinoma cell types also studied (Torma and Vahlquist, 1990), and the possibility that altered enzyme activities may be a consequence of the differentiation state cannot be ruled out.

By incorporating a density-gradient centrifugation step in the isolation procedures, fractions enriched with epidermal cells at different stages of differentiation and proliferative potentials are readily isolated from the skin of mice. Studies on the capacity of these cell fractions to metabolize exogenous arachidonic acid to prostaglandins and hydroxyeicosatetraenoic acids indicated that fractions containing less dense, more differentiated cells also had greater cyclooxygenase and lipoxygenase enzyme activities (Cameron et al., 1990). Similar studies with the model substrate ethoxycoumarin demonstrated that increased cell size and differentiation was accompanied by increases in drug-metabolizing activities. The sebaceous cells were the most active population, while the basal cell layer possessed the lowest enzyme activities (Pohl et al., 1984; Coomes et al., 1984). These results reemphasized the apparently high relative distribution of drug-metabolizing activities seen in the sebaceous glands by others (Wattenberg and Leong, 1970). Interestingly, the sebaceous glands are also reported to participate extensively in the metabolism of steroid hormones (Bardin et al., 1973; Sansone-Bazzono and Reisner, 1974; Hay and Hodgins, 1978). Indeed, recent studies have demonstrated the presence of 3β-hydroxysteroid dehydrogenase in sebaceous gland cells, in much greater concentrations than those found in keratinocytes (Milewich and Sontheimer, 1989; Milewich et al., 1988). Moreover, the contents of this enzyme were twice as high in the cytosolic fraction of sebaceous gland isolates from bald versus hirsute scalp sites (Sawaya et al., 1988).

Although 5α-reductase activity did not vary much in the study of sebaceous gland isolates (Bardin et al., 1973), certain lactamates and other analogs of testosterone have been shown to inhibit hair loss in primate models of male-pattern baldness (Metcalf et al., 1989). When 5α-reductase activity from cultured beard dermal papillary cells was compared with that of dermal fibroblasts from the same skin sample, a three- to fivefold increase in activity of the beard cells was demonstrated and the major metabolite identified was dihydrotestosterone. In contrast, hairy scalp follicular papilla cells were not enriched in this enzyme (Itami et al., 1990). Steroid 5α-reductase inhibitors have also been shown to block dihydrotestosterone formation in sebaceous gland cells in culture, but did not reduce sebaceous gland size *in vivo* in hamster ear and flank organ models, suggesting that acne and seborrhea are more amenable to androgen antagonist therapy (Schroder et al., 1989).

These and similar studies serve to demonstrate the impact that an understanding of cutaneous metabolism can have on delineating the mechanisms of various skin disorders and in identifying promising therapeutic strategies. As culture techniques for other cell types become commonplace, their affect on the percutaneous fate of topical xenobiotics can then be assessed. An example, albeit negative, of comparative cellular metabolism in the skin is the recent demonstration that melanocytes in culture do not activate benzo[a]pyrene to a significant extent (Grunberger et al., 1983). Is it possible for melanocytes to make a significant contribution to particular metabolic pathways, and what happens when other constituent populations, such as Langerhans' cells, blood infiltrates, or transformed cell types, interact with xenobiotics permeating through the integument? Finally, there has been a great deal of academic and commercial (Naughton et al., 1989; Bell et al., 1989) interest recently in techniques for growing fully competent synthetic skin, particularly that of humans, in culture. Although some progress has been made in reproducing the conditions necessary for terminal differentiation and barrier layer formation in culture (Asselineau et al., 1986; Williams et al., 1988; Ponec et al., 1989), a next logical step in the development of synthetic skin models would be to compare the absorption and disposition of topically applied xenobiotics with other *in vitro* models and with that found *in vivo*.

Microbial metabolism. Microorganisms are ubiquitous residents on and within the skin surface layers, and it is possible that they are capable of metabolizing topically applied substances. For example, during an investigation of the *in vitro* permeation of nandrolone decanoate, metabolism of a small percentage of the applied compound was observed, and it was suggested that skin microorganisms were responsible for this biotransformation (Foreman and Clanachan, 1975). Indeed, the bioconversion of topically applied benzoylperoxide to benzoic acid, observed during skin absorption studies, was assumed to be almost exclusively due to skin microbes (Nacht et al., 1981). Cutaneous microorganisms have also been reported to be capable of metabolizing topically applied drugs such as betamethasone-17-valerate (Brookes et al., 1982) and glyceryl trinitrate (Denyer et al., 1984).

In contrast, during the development of methods for assessing pregraft viability of skin, metabolism of various substrates by cutaneous microorganisms was shown to be negligible (May and DeClement, 1982). Furthermore, in a recent survey of lipase and steroid metabolism by commensal and transient skin isolates, there was no evidence that microbial enzymatic activity approached that of the skin itself, and only clinical isolates (pathogens) were capable of metabolizing betamethasone esters (Denyer and McNabb, 1989). Nevertheless, the significance of cutaneous microorganisms in the fate of topically applied chemicals remains to be established, and the avoidance of treatments which might increase the relative proportion of opportunistic pathogens in the skin is considered to be a prudent course of action when studying the metabolic potential of the skin.

CUTANEOUS METABOLISM AND THE FATE OF TOPICALLY APPLIED SUBSTANCES

Prior to any discussions concerning the functional significance of skin metabolism in the percutaneous fate of topically applied chemicals, it is pertinent to assess the processes considered to be important in percutaneous absorption. Early investigations into the mechanisms of percutaneous absorption can be viewed as an attempt to provide the simplest theoretical framework in which to conceptualize and interpret skin absorption investigations. Despite the relatively crude experimental techniques available prior to the past 10–15 years, a great deal of progress was made. Much of what is now known about skin pharmacology and topical therapeutics can be derived directly from these early experiments, and most concepts are valid and applicable to current methodological and model development efforts.

The historical background and chronology of early events leading to present concepts of diffusion being the principle determinant in barrier function of skin have been extensively reviewed (Scheuplein and Blank, 1971; Scheuplein and Bronaugh, 1983) and will not be discussed here. Moreover, there is also a body of literature concerned both with cutaneous anatomy and with the interaction of skin structure and function, vis-à-vis diffusional pathways of percutaneous absorption. The reader is referred to the excellent reviews of Katz and Poulsen (1971) and Kligman (1964), as well as relevant chapters in this book. In this chapter our discussion will focus primarily on the pharmacokinetics of percutaneous absorption, with particular emphasis on conceptual models that have evolved to describe percutaneous absorption and metabolism. In addition, we will discuss recent developments in experimental methodology, which can be used in conjunction with the conceptual models to provide the framework for testing hypotheses and assessing the functional significance of skin metabolism in the percutaneous fate of topically applied chemicals.

Conceptual Approaches

It has long been known that the first-pass effect after oral administration can produce significantly altered clearance profiles for some xenobiotics. However, when topical and parenteral dispositions and clearance differ, as several recent studies have demonstrated (Andersen et al., 1980; Sanders et al., 1986; Carver and Riviere, 1990), first-pass cutaneous metabolism as a potential determining factor is frequently overlooked (Greaves, 1971). Because of the general inability to distinguish cutaneous from systemic metabolic processes, biotransformation in skin is difficult to assess directly in traditional *in vivo* study designs. Nevertheless, with the proper combination of topical dose, absorption rate, species, drug and metabolites, and assay specificity and sensitivity, a reasonable estimate of first-pass cutaneous biotransformation may be possible. An investigation on the pharmacokinetics and bioavailability of topical and intravenous [14C]nitroglycerin in the rhesus monkeys (Wester et al., 1983) provides a classic example where the extent of cutaneous first-pass metabolism was estimated *in vivo*.

Aldrin epoxidation (Graham et al., 1986) and benzoyl peroxide (Nacht et al., 1981) and paraoxon hydrolysis (Fredriksson, 1962, 1964) are other examples of cutaneous metabolism that have been reported following topical administration *in vivo*. Unfortunately, these *in vivo* data are limited in scope, particularly from the perspective of assessing the contribution of cutaneous metabolism in the overall metabolic fate of the applied compound. Because of the technical difficulties associated with *in vivo* investigation, it is necessary to consider *in vitro* techniques using excised skin for examining the pharmacokinetics of skin absorption and metabolism. *In vitro* studies generally afford the investigator the ability to manipulate and control the experimental conditions, and the approach provides the unique opportunity to monitor the rate and extent of percutaneous absorption in skin tissues that are isolated from the confounding influences of the rest of the body. In addition, *in vitro* methodologies provide the most practical approach currently available for studying cutaneous metabolism concomitant with skin absorption, and the results can be obtained relatively quickly and inexpensively. However, caution must be exercised in extrapolating *in vitro* observations to *in vivo* situations (Kao, 1990a).

Traditionally, diffusion principles are recognized as the only important determinants in skin absorption, and Fick's laws of diffusion provided the mathematical basis for the development of *in vitro* models in percutaneous absorption. Equations derived from Fick's laws form the simplest mathematical framework describing many *in vitro* skin penetration investigations. However, percutaneous absorption is a complex phenomenon, involving a myriad of diffusional and metabolic processes that are proceeding either concurrently or sequentially. Consequently, theoretical models describing the overall process will be approximations and will reflect our current knowledge concerning the most relevant events.

Diffusion models. The thermodynamics of membrane flux and development of more complex models describing diffusion processes within skin have been reviewed elsewhere (Higuchi, 1960; Dugard, 1983; Kubota and Ishizaki, 1985; Flynn, 1985; Zatz, 1985; Hadgraft, 1987; Sato et al., 1988a, 1988b). Similar mathematical principles have been used to describe transdermal drug delivery profiles (Gienger et al., 1986; Yu et al., 1979a, 1979b; Chandrasekaran et al., 1978; Kubota et al., 1990) and such complex phenomena as diffusion through multilaminate transdermal drug delivery systems (Berner, 1985). From these models mathematical expressions have been derived that relate the extent of skin absorption to physiochemical parameters of the penetrants and the biophysical properties of the skin, and have provided the theoretical bases for designing and interpreting *in vitro* studies using excised skin in diffusion chambers.

Appreciation of the possibility that skin metabolism may influence the percutaneous fate of topically applied chemicals has led to the development of mathematical models, based on Fick's principles, that describe simultaneous diffusion and metabolism in biological membranes (Ando et al., 1977; Fox et al., 1979; Stehle et al., 1989). Unfortunately, complete evaluation of these models often requires a degree of mathematical sophistication and analytical measurement that cannot be matched by current experimental techniques in skin absorption.

The methodology for *in vitro* skin absorption studies including diffusion chamber designs, methods for assessing the diffusional integrity of the excised tissue, and techniques for controlling important variables such as skin temperature, hydration state, and donor/receptor solution mixing have been extensively reviewed (Tojo, 1987; Huang, 1987; Kao, 1990b). There is no doubt that steady-state diffusion experiments have made substantial contributions to our current knowledge concerning the diffusional aspects of skin absorption; however, there are limitations to their usefulness, particularly for developing predictive models for assessing skin absorption and metabolism. A recent study of the kinetics of skin absorption and metabolism of several salicylate esters demonstrated that the esterase activity was overestimated *in vitro* compared to *in vivo*, except when sink conditions were employed to simulate clearance properties of the vascular system *in vivo* (Guzek et al., 1989; Potts et al., 1989). Results obtained after addition of an esterase inhibitor suggested that drug distribution in the outer layers (i.e., initial stages of absorption) was more sensitive to altered enzyme activity, while vascular clearance primarily affects drug disposition in the deeper regions (Potts et al., 1989). An important concept that can be derived from such studies is the applicability of tissue concentration gradient data toward more accurate pharmacokinetic models of percutaneous drug absorption with concurrent metabolism.

The underlying assumptions inherent in the validity of using excised skin for diffusion experiments are that (1) living processes have little or no effect on percutaneous absorption mechanism or kinetics, (2) penetration through dermis is not rate-limiting, (3) skin condition, particularly that of the stratum corneum, is comparable to that found *in situ* (Wester and Maibach, 1977), and (4) recovery of the applied substances in the receptor fluid provides a true reflection of the rates and extent of percutaneous absorption, such that tissue binding and partitioning into the receptor fluid are not confounding factors. All of these premises are becoming increasingly difficult to justify in light of what we now know about metabolism of drugs within the skin, binding to cutaneous macromolecules, and the influence of cutaneous blood flow on the clearance of drugs and their metabolites from the skin.

Linear compartmental models. From a kinetic perspective the relevant events that are important in skin absorption may be characterized as the partitioning of the compound from the delivery vehicle to the stratum corneum, transport through the stratum corneum, partitioning from the lipophilic stratum corneum into the more aqueous viable epidermis, transport across the epidermis/dermis with uptake by the cutaneous microvasculature, and subsequent systemic distribution and elimination. As has been discussed in detail in previous sections of this chapter, at any stage during this process cutaneous metabolism of the applied compound may occur.

Conceptual models of percutaneous absorption that are rigidly adherent to general solutions of Fick's equation are not always readily adaptable to *in vivo* conditions, primarily because such models are not physiologically relevant. Linear kinetic models describing percutaneous absorption in terms of mathematical compartments that have approximate physical or anatomical correlates have been proposed (Hadgraft, 1979; Guy and Hadgraft, 1984b). In these models, the various relevant events, including cutaneous metabolism, considered to be important in the overall process of skin absorption are characterized by first-order rate constants (Fig. 8) (Guy and Hadgraft, 1984b). The rate constants associated with diffusional events in the skin are assumed to be proportional to mass transfer parameters and may be estimated by *in vitro* diffusion experiments. Other rate constants such as those related to metabolism may be estimated based on *in vitro* experiments, and constants associated with the systemic distribution and elimination are estimated from pharmacokinetic parameters derived from plasma concentration-time profiles obtained following intravenous administration of the penetrant.

These linear kinetic models and diffusion models of skin absorption kinetics have a number of features in common, they are subject to similar constraints, and they have a similar theoretical basis. The compartmental models, however, are more versatile and are potentially powerful predictive tools used to simulate various aspects of percutaneous absorption (Hadgraft, 1987; Guy et al., 1987b). Techniques for simulating multiple-dose behavior (Guy et al., 1983); evaporation, cutaneous metabolism, microbial degradation, and other surface loss processes (Guy and Hadgraft, 1984a; Denyer et al., 1985); dermal

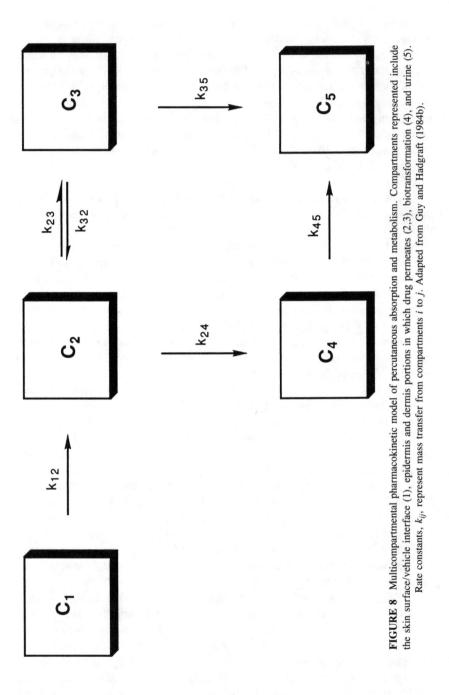

FIGURE 8 Multicompartmental pharmacokinetic model of percutaneous absorption and metabolism. Compartments represented include the skin surface/vehicle interface (1), epidermis and dermis portions in which drug permeates (2,3), biotransformation (4), and urine (5). Rate constants, k_{ij}, represent mass transfer from compartments i to j. Adapted from Guy and Hadgraft (1984b).

risk assessment (Guy and Maibach, 1984); transdermal drug delivery (Guy and Hadgraft, 1985a, 1985b, 1986; Guy et al., 1987a, 1987b); and vehicle effects (Guy and Hadgraft, 1987) have all been described. However, these simulations are only theoretical, and in some cases the predictions compare favorably with the experimental observations, but in others, such as those dealing with varying degrees of cutaneous metabolism, experimental confirmation will require a better understanding of skin as a drug-metabolizing organ.

As was the case for diffusional kinetic models, deficiencies of current experimental and analytical methods limit our ability to appreciate and fully utilize these compartmental models. The model parameters (i.e., rate constants) are usually based on assumed partitioning phenomena or kinetic behavior, assumptions that are necessitated by the paucity of kinetic information provided by current experimental methods. For example, little is known about how volatility affects absorption of the applied dose (Spencer et al., 1979; Reifenrath and Robinson, 1982; Reifenrath and Spencer, 1985), and the concept of mass-balance studies following topical doses has only recently been addressed (Guy et al., 1987b; Bucks et al., 1988). Moreover, the influence of cutaneous metabolism on the evaluation of percutaneous absorption pharmacokinetics using deconvolution techniques (Fisher et al., 1985; Sato et al., 1988a, 1988b) has not yet been investigated.

Physiologically relevant models. A more recent trend in pharmacokinetic modeling is reflected in the development of physiologically based pharmacokinetic (PBPK) models, which are reviewed elsewhere (Rowland, 1984; Gerlowski and Jain, 1983). Skin and other poorly perfused tissues are generally treated together in PBPK models as a single entity (i.e., poorly perfused or slowly equilibrating compartments), whenever the route of administration is parenteral or by inhalation exposure. However, there has been at least one such model published that simulated, to some extent, dihalomethane dispositions after exposure of the skin to these lipophilic vapors (McDougal et al., 1986). Since it is recognized that for certain penetrants skin absorption and metabolism are functions of cutaneous blood flow, pharmacokinetic models have recently been described that incorporate flow components into the traditional compartmental models (Williams et al., 1990; Williams and Riviere, 1989a, 1989b). Although these physiologic pharmacokinetic models are not PBPK models in the classical sense, they represent a hybrid approach that seems particularly suited for extrapolating from isolated organ experiments to the whole animal (Williams and Riviere, 1989a). In addition, one such pharmacokinetic model has been reported that also accounted for metabolite profiles of a topically applied drug (Fig. 9) (Nakashima et al., 1987). These models provide the conceptual framework from which experiments may be designed to simultaneously assess the role of the cutaneous vasculature and cutaneous metabolism in percutaneous absorption.

Because the modeling efforts have advanced in complexity far beyond the capabilities of prevailing experimental techniques used to assess their validity,

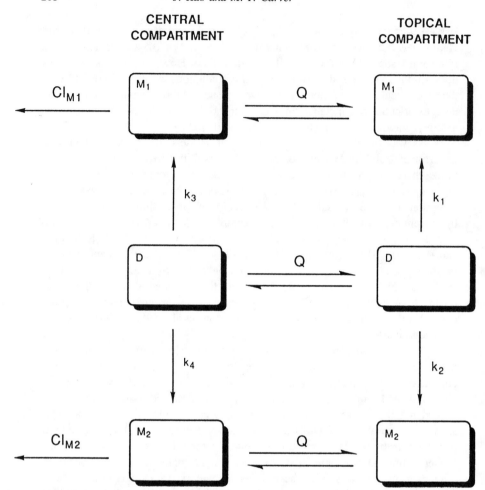

FIGURE 9   Physiologic pharmacokinetic model of nitroglycerin percutaneous absorption and metabolism. The rate constants (k_1-k_4) represent metabolic clearance of the parent nitroglycerin to its two dinitrate metabolites and Q is the reversible, cutaneous blood flow-dependent transfer of drug and metabolites to plasma. Cl_{M1} and Cl_{M2} represent plasma clearance of metabolites into urine (Cl_D = 0). Adapted from Nakashima et al. (1987).

particulary when the skin is considered in terms of a drug-metabolizing organ, parameters described in these models (i.e., rate constants) are not necessarily "identifiable" as measurable entities (Godfrey et al., 1980; Jacquez, 1985; Venot et al., 1987). Nevertheless, the models themselves occasionally appear to simulate *in vivo* results and do serve as a framework for developing new hypotheses, thus satisfying important validity criteria for mathematical constructs (Zierler, 1981; Rescigno and Beck, 1987). It is obvious that newer *in vitro* systems are needed to generate the appropriate data that can be used to properly evaluate these physiologically relevant models. It will be the focus of the remainder of this review to describe recent development of such methodologies and demonstrate their relevance in understanding the relationship between skin absorption and biotransformation processes.

Experimental Approaches

Mammalian skin organ cultures. A major assumption in using excised skin or inert stratum corneum membranes to examine dermal penetration is that living processes do not affect the rates or mechanisms of percutaneous absorption. However, a strong relationship between permeability of the skin to topically applied compounds and both viability and metabolic status of the tissue has been demonstrated in a series of experiments using freshly excised skin preparations maintained in short-term organ culture (Kao, 1988, 1989, 1990b). In these studies, full-thickness mammalian skin preparations were maintained as short-term raised organ cultures. The techniques described were relatively simple. Basically, the skin preparations were supported over the culture medium, which also served as the receptor fluid, so that their epidermal surfaces were exposed and above the air-culture medium interface. Compounds of interest could be applied topically in a manner similar to exposure *in vivo*; the compounds reach the epidermal cells by diffusion through the various matrices of the skin where they may be metabolized. The recovery of both metabolites and parent compound in the tissue layers and culture media then provides a measure of skin absorption and extent of cutaneous first-pass metabolism. In this *in vitro* system, the percutaneous fate of topically applied [^{14}C]benzo[a]pyrene in skin preparations from humans and five laboratory animals exhibited marked species differences (Kao et al., 1985). *In vitro* permeation, as determined by the recovery of radioactivity in the receptor fluid, was accompanied by varying degrees of cutaneous first-pass metabolism. A full spectrum of metabolites was found in both the skin and the receptor fluid following topical application (Fig. 10), and the metabolite profiles showed substantial species differences (Kao et al., 1985).

Skin permeation *in vitro* appears to be directly dependent on metabolic viability of the skin samples. For example, if potassium cyanide (a metabolic inhibitor) is added to the culture medium, or if frozen nonviable skin samples were used, a dramatic reduction in benzo[a]pyrene permeation and metabolism *in vitro* was observed. Also, *in vitro* permeation of benzo[a]pyrene in cultured mouse skin preparations that have been subjected to frozen storage, transient freeze-thawing on dry ice, exposure to high temperatures, or sodium azide in the culture medium was shown to be decreased in all cases (Smith and Holland, 1981; Kao et al., 1983; Holland et al., 1984). Moreover, carbon monoxide, which inhibited the activities of cytochrome P-450 in cultured skin preparations from TCDD-induced C3H or tape-stripped hairless (HRS) mice, also decreased *in vitro* permeation of topical benzo[a]pyrene (Kao, 1989).

The results of studies using skin preparations from metabolically induced

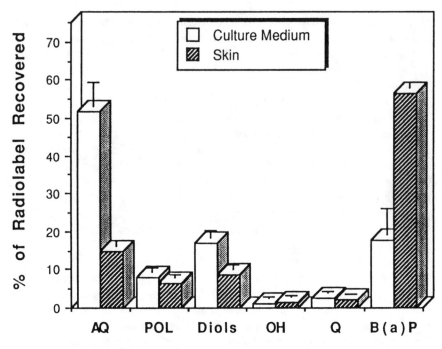

FIGURE 10   Metabolite profile of [^{14}C]benzo[a]pyrene 24 h after *in vitro* topical application to human skin in organ culture. Abbreviations used are B(a)P, benzo[a]pyrene; AQ, aqueous residue (unextracted radioactivity); POL, organic solvent-extractable polar metabolites; Diol, B(a)P dihydrodiols; OH, B(a)P phenols; Q, B(a)P quinones. Results are expressed as percent of radiolabel recovered in skin and culture medium, mean ± SE for four skin samples. Adapted from Kao et al. (1985).

mice were as expected. Induction by topical or systemic pretreatment with TCDD increased the *in vitro* permeation of benzo[a]pyrene in mouse skin, and this was accompanied by a shift in the profile of metabolites found in the receptor fluid (Table 2; Fig. 11). In addition, 3-methylcholanthrene induction *in vivo* increased benzo[a]pyrene permeation in skin from the "inducible" C57BL6 mice, but not for "noninducible" DBA2 mouse skin (Holland et al.,

TABLE 2. Influence of TCDD Induction on the Distribution of Radioactivity 24 Hours after Topical Application of [^{14}C]Benzo(a)pyrene to Mouse Skin in Raised Organ Culture

Group	Skin	Receptor fluid	Recovery
Controls	70.7 ± 1.2	24.3 ± 0.9	95.0 ± 1.7
Induced	53.5 ± 1.4	38.3 ± 2.9	91.9 ± 2.5

Note. Results are expressed as percent of the dose applied (5 μg/5 cm^2), mean ± SE from four individual skin preparations. Skin was induced by *in vivo* topical administration of TCDD (2 μg/200 μl acetone/animal), 48 h before each *in vitro* experiment. Data are adapted from Kao et al. (1984).

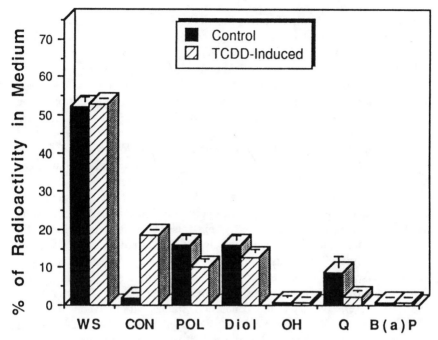

FIGURE 11 Metabolite profile of [^{14}C]benzo[a]pyrene 24 h after *in vitro* topical application to mouse skin in organ culture. Abbreviations are those used in Fig. 10, with the addition of CON = B(a)P conjugates. Results are expressed as percent of radiolabel recovered in the culture medium, mean ± SE for four skin samples. Adapted from Kao et al. (1985).

1984; Kao et al., 1985). These findings, in combination with the above results, provided strong evidence to support the concept that cutaneous metabolism may have an important role in skin absorption and percutaneous fate of some topically applied chemicals.

It has been reported that relatively high xenobiotic metabolizing activities are localized in the differentiated cells of the skin appendages (Coomes et al., 1983; Hukkelhoven et al., 1983; Pohl et al., 1984). In studies with skin preparations from various haired, "fuzzy" haired, and hairless mouse strains it was demonstrated that the rate and extent of *in vitro* skin permeation of benzo[a]pyrene may be correlated with the presence or absence of normal hair follicles, and, in general, permeation in haired mice was higher than in hairless mice (Kao, 1989). These studies support the possibility that the transfollicular pathway may play an important role in the percutaneous absorption of this compound (Scheuplein, 1967; Foreman et al., 1979; Holland et al., 1979); these results also provided further evidence to indicate that cutaneous metabolism may facilitate percutaneous absorption of highly lipophilic compounds.

In contrast to benzo[a]pyrene, *in vitro* permeation of topically applied testosterone was somewhat higher in nonviable tissues as compared to viable tissues (Table 3). However, compared to viable tissue where there was substantial first-pass metabolism, in nonviable tissues testosterone diffused through the skin unchanged, and essentially only the parent compound was found in the receptor fluid and the skin preparation (Fig. 12). Furthermore, in studies using viable skin preparations it was evident that when the topically applied dose of testosterone was increased, the relative extent of permeation was decreased. This decrease was accompanied by a decrease in the relative extent of cutaneous first-pass metabolism (Kao and Hall, 1987), indicating the potential saturability of the cutaneous drug metabolizing enzymes.

In contrast with these findings, Marzulli et al. (1969) reported that less than 5% of radiolabeled testosterone penetrated isolated human stratum corneum as testosterone, when tested in a diffusion cell system.

Because skin penetration is assumed to be essentially a diffusional process, the relative ease by which steroids permeate skin can be deduced mathematically in terms of their permeability constants (Scheuplein et al., 1969). For three structurally related estrogens, namely, estrone, estradiol, and estriol, their respective permeability constants, obtained from in vitro diffusion studies with human cadaver skin, indicated that permeation of estrone was 100 times higher than estradiol, which in turn was 100 times that of estriol (Schaefer et al., 1982). However, contrary to this conclusion, studies with metabolically viable mouse skin maintained in organ culture have shown that at an equivalent topical dose, the percutaneous permeation of estradiol was greater than that of estrone, which in turn was significantly greater than that of estriol (Kao and Hall, 1987). It has been demonstrated that skin metabolism may play a major role in the redistribution of endogenous steroid hormones and their metabolites (Gomez and Hsia, 1968); this metabolic capability may also affect disposition of exogenously administered steroids. The metabolic reactions involving steroid hormones are often found to be reversible. For example, estradiol is reversibly metabolized to estrone in human skin. The equilibrium for the reaction in vitro

TABLE 3. Species Differences and the Influence of Tissue Viability on the In Vitro Permeation of Topical [^{14}C]Testosterone

	Permeation (%)[a]	
Species	Fresh, viable skin	Frozen, nonviable skin
Mouse	70.33 ± 2.37	74.29 ± 4.11
Rat	25.20 ± 5.21	38.47 ± 2.74
Rabbit	47.22 ± 0.08	50.39 ± 7.66
Guinea pig	16.61 ± 0.81	27.75 ± 3.16
Marmoset	16.62 ± 4.77	not determined
Human	46.45 ± 1.09	62.30 ± 4.02

[a]Permeation is determined as the recovery of radioactivity in the culture fluid and supporting filter paper 24 h after topical application of [^{14}C]testosterone (10 μg/5 cm^2) to skin preparations maintained in the static culture system. Data are expressed as mean ± SE of four skin samples. Adapted from Kao et al. (1985).

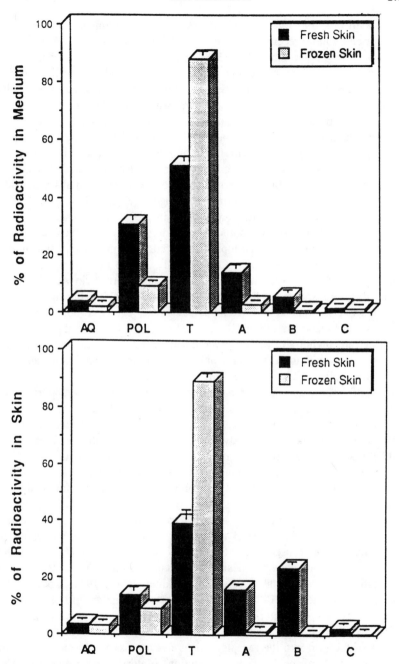

FIGURE 12 Metabolite profile of [^{14}C]testosterone 24 h after *in vitro* topical application to human skin in organ culture. Abbreviations AQ and POL are those used in Fig. 10; T, testosterone; A, 4-androstene-3,17-dione; B, 5α-dihydrotestosterone; and C, 5α-androsten-3,17-dione. Results are expressed as percent of radiolabel recovered in the skin and culture medium, mean ± SE for four skin samples. Adapted from Kao et al. (1985).

is in favor of ketone formation (Frost et al., 1966), and this hypothesis has been supported by more recent studies of the metabolism of estrogens incubated with various skin preparations (Hsia, 1980; Longcope, 1980). However, in mouse skin maintained in organ culture permeation of topically applied estrone was accompanied by extensive first-pass metabolism to estradiol and water soluble metabolites. In contrast, only limited first-pass metabolism of estradiol to estrone was reported (Fig. 13). Cutaneous first-pass metabolism of estriol was also essentially negligible (Kao and Hall, 1987). Whether these incongruent findings represent true species effects or merely differences in experimental methodology has not been resolved; however, studies using viable human breast skin and guinea pig skin have shown that there were substantial species differences in the percutaneous fate of these estrogens (Kao, 1989).

More recently, various compounds, including various toxins and azo dyes, have also been shown to undergo varying degrees of cutaneous first-pass metabolism following *in vitro* topical application to mammalian skin in organ culture (Bronaugh et al., 1989; Collier et al., 1989). For example, trichothecenes, such as T2 toxin, diacetoxyscirpenol, and verrucarin A, administered topically were shown to be metabolized to some effect during penetration through excised human skin (Kemppainen et al., 1986a, 1986b, 1987). Similarly, some metabolism of topically applied butylated hydroxytoluene and acetyl ethyl tetramethyltetralin was observed during *in vitro* penetration through fuzzy rat skin. However, under the same *in vitro* conditions, cutaneous metabolism of topically applied DDT, salicylic acid, and caffeine was not observed (Collier et al., 1989). These and the aforementioned studies all serve to support the view that both diffusional and metabolic processes are involved in the percutaneous fate of topically applied chemicals. They also serve to illustrate the utility of this experimental model for studying percutaneous absorption and metabolism, which must be considered intimately related for certain compounds.

Techniques for maintaining viable skin and presumably fully competent synthetic skin *in vitro*, capable of accommodating both static (Kao et al., 1984) and flow-through diffusion-cell studies (Holland et al., 1984), have been described to provide a simple and versatile experimental model system. However, a limitation of this experimental approach is the lack of normal vascular uptake mechanisms. One consequence of this inadequacy has been a large effort aimed at better diffusion-chamber designs, particularly through the use of flow-through devices (Holland et al., 1984; Akhter et al., 1984; Cooper, 1984; Bronaugh and Stewart, 1985). Another important limitation of this approach is that the recovery of material in the receptor fluid, which provides an overall measure of *in vitro* permeation (i.e., the net penetration through the various layers of the skin into the receptor), does not necessarily produce an accurate measure of overall percutaneous absorption. Materials that penetrate the skin but remain in the tissue have undergone absorption, but would not be accounted for when only receptor fluid is assessed. Furthermore, various tissue slicing techniques (Middleton and Hasmall, 1977; Schaefer et al., 1978; Zesch et al.,

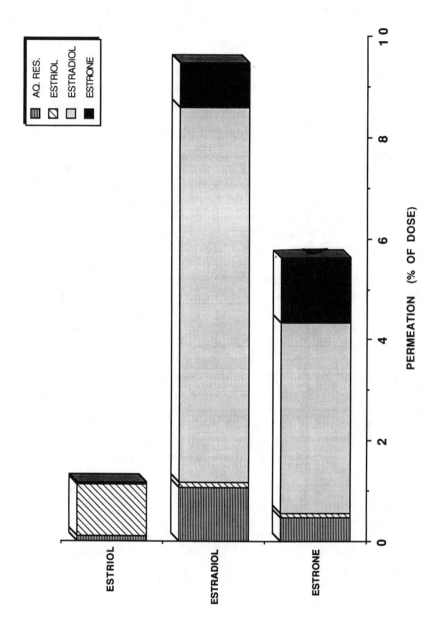

FIGURE 13 *In vitro* permeation and metabolite profile of [³H]estrogens 8 h after *in vitro* topical application to mouse skin in organ culture. Abbreviation (AQ) is the same as that used in Fig. 10. Results are expressed as percent of dose (5 μg/cm²) recovered in the receptor medium. Mean of five skin samples. Adapted from Kao and Hall (1987).

1979; Bronaugh and Stewart, 1986) or apparatus design considerations (Bronaugh and Stewart, 1984; Hawkins and Reifenrath, 1984; Reifenrath et al., 1984a, 1984b) have failed to totally resolve the possibility that the thick dermis may represent an artificial and selective barrier limiting the permeation of lipophilic penetrants *in vitro*. Indeed, a recent comparison of the *in vivo* and *in vitro* dispositions of topical salicylate esters provided ample evidence that this "dermal reservoir" may have a dramatic impact on the interpretation of both penetration and metabolism data obtained from *in vitro* studies (Guzek et al., 1989; Potts et al., 1989). Therefore, the compound may accumulate and the longer residence time in the skin tissue may provide the viable epidermis and dermis a greater opportunity to convert the water-insoluble compound to water-soluble metabolites that are capable of partitioning freely into the receptor. The recovery of significant amounts of metabolites in the receptor may be artifactual, and the influence of skin metabolism overestimated.

Metabolites found in the receptor are often assumed to be the product of cutaneous metabolism, formed during permeation through the skin. However, it has been suggested that these metabolites may result from transformation in the receptor fluid after skin permeation. The inherent instability of the parent compound in the receptor could be a possible reason for these chemical transformations, for example, hydrolysis. Alternatively, these transformations may be mediated by enzymes (i.e., skin esterases) that have leaked into the receptor from the excised tissue (Yu et al., 1979b; Bundgaard et al., 1983). In assessing the relevance of cutaneous metabolism in skin absorption *in vitro*, it will be important to determine the origin of the metabolites found in the receptor. Moreover, the influence of culture medium or receptor fluid composition on both metabolism and skin penetration remains to be clearly defined. There is no consensus on what constitutes an ideal receptor fluid. The selection of a suitable receptor fluid for a particular compound of interest is frequently empirical and often reflects the biases of the investigator. Therefore, caution should be exercised and *in vitro* observations should not always be considered true and accurate representations of the *in vivo* situation, with respect to cutaneous absorption and metabolism.

Skin flaps and perfused skin preparations. Given the obvious physiological limitations of the above organ culture and diffusion-cell approaches, perfused skin preparations, with an intact and functional cutaneous microcirculation, appear to represent an ideal experimental methodology for investigating the pharmacokinetics and mechanisms of percutaneous absorption and metabolism. However, following the development of the perfused rabbit ear model in the early 1900s and the subsequent demonstration of its potential as a tool for studying skin absorption (Nyiri and Jannitti, 1932), surprisingly little progress was made over the next half century. Reports of perfused feline and canine skin flaps, both *in situ* and *in vitro*, appeared sporadically in the literature (reviewed in Riviere and Carver, 1990), and these models have provided useful information in studies of skin physiology and the basic pathways of cutaneous respiration and energy production. However, with the possible exception of a recent study of methylsalicylate absorption and metabolism in perfused rabbit ears (Behrendt and Kampffmeyer, 1989), they have not been used to study percutaneous absorption and cutaneous biotransformation.

Recently, techniques for creating and maintaining isolated arterial sandwich skin flaps, *in situ*, in rats have been reviewed (Pershing and Krueger, 1987). This rat skin flap (RSF) is created on athymic nude rats by surgically raising a small area of skin, perfused by the superficial epigastric artery, and grafting a split-thickness skin sample from syngenetic rats onto the underneath side. Cutaneous blood flow in the RSF has been well characterized using both fluorescent dyes and laser Doppler velocimetry (Wojciechowski et al., 1987), and recent studies involving the percutaneous absorption of both benzoic acid and caffeine have shown that better *in vitro* estimates of percutaneous absorption are obtained when cutaneous blood flow is measured rather than assumed constant (Pershing et al., 1989a). The effects of temperature- and vasoconstrictor- (phenylephrine) induced alterations in skin perfusion on absorption have also been examined (Pershing et al., 1986; Krueger et al., 1985; Wojciechowski et al., 1985). In addition, the kinetics of vidarabine (ara-A) deamination to 9-β-D-arabinofuranosylhypoxanthine (ara-H) have also been studied in this skin preparation (Krueger et al., 1985; Burton et al., 1985). Although athymic rats reject foreign skin grafts at a relatively high rate (up to 90%), some success has been achieved in creating and maintaining a hybrid rat-human sandwich flap (RHSF) on this animal by repeated low-dose cyclosporine therapy (Biren et al., 1986). It has been proposed that the RHSF might be useful for studying percutaneous absorption in human skin if it can be shown that the absorption mechanisms are unaffected by the surgical manipulations and cyclosporine treatments (Wojciechowski et al., 1987; Pershing et al., 1988, 1989b). The experimental advantages afforded by such human-grafted skin flaps, in addition to the fact that they are reusable, are intuitive. Unfortunately, the complicated surgical procedures, costly animals and husbandry requirements, and expensive cyclosporine therapy, with its confounding effects on skin absorption (Pershing et al., 1988, 1989b), coupled with the apparently high variability in xenobiotic flux through the xenografts, place severe limitations on the utility of RSF and RHSF as experimental models for studying cutaneous metabolism and skin absorption.

Given the known anatomical and physiological similarities in skin obtained from certain pale-skinned porcine species and humans, it is not surprising that various pig skin flaps have been pursued. The biochemistry and utility of pig buttock flaps, created surgically in several different patterns, for dermatological purposes have been extensively investigated (Daniel and Kerrigan, 1982; Harmon et al., 1986). Proposed advantages for using pig skin flaps include the availability of large surface areas, similar vasculature and anatomic structure, and the ease and similarity in the types of clinical observations that can be made. Perhaps the most promising perfused skin preparation is the isolated perfused porcine skin flap (IPPSF), which has been developed recently and provides a novel *in vitro* approach for examining percutaneous absorption processes in intact, living skin (Riviere et al., 1986a, 1986b). The biochemistry and morphology of the IPPSF have been examined in great detail and appear to be consistent with that found in porcine integument *in vivo* (Monteiro-Riviere, 1986; Riviere et al., 1986a, 1986b; Monteiro-Riviere et al., 1987). Moreover, patterns of cutaneous glucose metabolism/respiration found in the IPPSF are strikingly similar to those observed in humans (Freinkel, 1983). Furthermore, in assessing the potential advantage of the IPPSF as an experimental model in skin absorption and metabolism, the close correspondence between other anatomical (Forbes, 1967; Meyer et al., 1978) and biochemical features (Meyer and Neurand, 1976; Gray et al., 1978; Klain et al., 1986) of human and porcine skin should not be overlooked.

Although early attempts to develop human skin perfusion models have been documented (Winkelmann, 1966) and, more recently, an isolated perfused human groin flap was reported (Hiernickel, 1985), progress has been slow. For example, despite the presence of inducible, P-450-dependent arylhydrocarbon hydroxylase activity in the human groin flap (Hiernickel, 1985; Hiernickel et al., 1986; Merk and Hiernickel, 1986), the viability of this preparation and the methodology for using it in *in vitro* studies of percutaneous absorption and metabolism remain to be optimized (Riviere et al., 1987a). On the other hand, the absorption of a wide variety of topically applied xenobiotics has already been demonstrated using the IPPSF, including such diverse chemicals as organic acids and bases, organophosphate insecticides, steroid hormones (Riviere et al., 1987b; Carver et al., 1989), and organochlorines (Chang et al., 1990). In addition, the effects of applied surface concentration and coadministration of vasoactive drugs (tolazoline, norepinephrine) on lidocaine iontophoresis have been examined using the IPPSF, demonstrating its potential for testing novel transdermal drug delivery systems (Riviere et al., 1989/1990).

Cutaneous biotransformation of xenobiotics during percutaneous absorption has been demonstrated using the IPPSF with the chlorinated hydrocarbon, chlorbenzilate (J. E. Riviere and R. A. Rogers, unpublished observations), and with the insecticides carbaryl (Chang et al., 1990) and parathion (Carver et al., 1990). Parathion bioconversion to paraoxon and *p*-nitrophenol occurred following topical administration (Fig. 14), and the extent of *in vitro* permeation was dependent on cutaneous metabolism (Fig. 15). Occlusion and inhibition of P-450-dependent drug metabolizing activities in the skin resulted in decreases in skin absorption and alteration of the metabolite profile of parathion. The results obtained using 1-aminobenzotriazole (ABT), a suicide substrate inhibitor of cytochrome P-450 that has no other known physiologic or toxicologic effects *in vivo* (Ortiz de Montellano and Correia, 1983; Ortiz de Montellano, 1988), serve as an excellent example to reemphasize the concept that metabolism can have a dramatic impact on the absorption and systemic exposure profiles of drugs and environmental agents, without necessarily affecting the diffusional

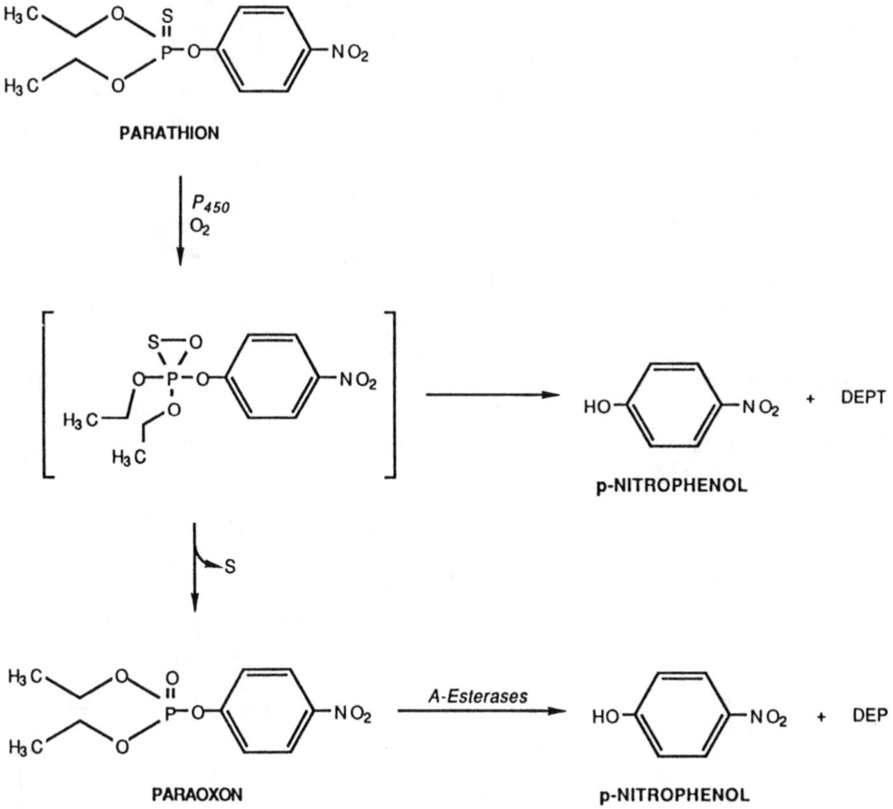

FIGURE 14 Putative parathion biotransformation pathways in porcine skin. Reactions shown include both cofactor-dependent and cofactor-independent steps.

resistance of stratum corneum. The occlusion results also suggest the possibility that competing cutaneous biotransformation pathways may be present, perhaps involving multiple P-450 isozymes (Levi et al., 1988), since occlusion inhibited parathion penetration in the IPPSF and altered the ratio of phenol to *p*-oxon products formed. More recent experiments have shown that the extent of first-pass metabolism may be better estimated in a single-pass (nonrecirculating) perfusion system (Chang et al., 1990). Furthermore, enzyme immunohisto-chemical techniques have demonstrated the presence of flaxin-containing mono-oxygenases in pig skin (Levi et al., 1990), suggesting that the IPPSF may be a useful tool for exploring other cutaneous enzyme systems as well. These types of experiments represent important steps in understanding the mechanisms of cutaneous biotransformation reactions, which have not been fully explored, and for developing empirical models of the rates and extent of first-pass cutaneous metabolism.

Preliminary studies using the IPPSF have shown that compounds such as the cancer chemotherapeutic agents cisplatin and carboplatin and the antibiotics tetracycline and doxycycline readily distribute into the skin following intravascular administration (Riviere and Williams, 1988; Williams and Riviere, 1989a). Also, compounds such as parathion, ABT, and 25-hydroxyvitamin D are bioactivated in the skin following intravascular administration in the IPPSF (Bikle et al., 1989; Carver et al., 1990). The vitamin D results may be important in light of recent interest in topical vitamin D and its analogues as a new therapeutic strategy for treating psoriasis (Kragballe et al., 1988; Holick, 1989; Kragballe, 1989). Therefore, these studies suggest a role for the IPPSF as an ideal experimental model for studying skin metabolism of xenobiotics that are distributed to skin from the systemic circulation. Interest in the so-called outward transdermal migration or reverse penetration concept, namely, that skin may function as a clearance organ following delivery of systemically administered substances via the cutaneous vasculature, has been stimulated by the development of non-invasive techniques for measuring and analyzing the pharmacokinetics of the distribution of substances to skin *in vivo* (Peck et al., 1981, 1987, 1988). Metabolites isolated in the transcutaneous collection system cannot be distinguished from those produced in the liver or other internal organs

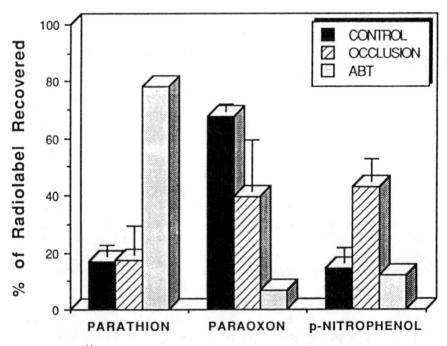

FIGURE 15 [^{14}C]Parathion metabolite profiles during percutaneous absorption in perfused porcine skin. ABT, pretreatment by intravascular administration of 1-aminobenzotriazole (50 μg/g). Results are expressed as percent of radiolabel recovered in the perfusion medium 8 h after topical application. Mean of $n = 4$ (control, occluded) or $n = 2$ (ABT) separate skin flap experiments. Adapted from Carver et al. (1990).

using the experimental methods described by Peck and co-workers (Peck et al., 1987, 1988). However, the absence of these confounding, extracutaneous metabolizing organs is a distinct advantage in IPPSF investigations of this reverse penetration phenomenon.

Given the relatively lengthy viability period of approximately 12–18 h, the IPPSF offers a very attractive approach for studying mechanisms of percutaneous absorption and metabolism, particularly the role of the cutaneous microvasculature. In addition to the presence of an intact and functional circulatory system, a principal advantage in using the IPPSF is the greater sensitivity afforded in determining model parameters necessary to describe percutaneous absorption mathematically. Pharmacokinetic models currently under evaluation have been shown to accurately simulate *in vitro* flux profiles, while also providing meaningful extrapolations to the longer time frames of *in vivo* experiments (Carver et al., 1989; Carver and Riviere, 1990). Absorption rate-time profiles obtained from the IPPSF have been used to derive and test both multicompartment and physiologic pharmacokinetic models of skin absorption (Williams et al., 1989; Carver et al., 1989; Williams and Riviere, 1989, 1990). The latter, or physiologically relevant, model (Fig. 16) incorporates cutaneous blood or perfusate flow information in a manner adaptable to transcutaneous permeation in either direction (Williams and Riviere, 1989a; Williams et al., 1990). The proposed pharmacokinetic models are physiologically consistent with those discussed earlier in this review and, in conjunction with the experimental techniques now available, provide a framework in which to test new hypotheses regarding the mechanisms of skin penetration and metabolism, as well as uptake by the cutaneous microcirculation.

CONCLUSIONS

It is self-evident that the skin is not just an inert protective barrier surrounding the body. It is a dynamic, living tissue involved in a variety of important physiological and metabolic functions. The skin possesses the metabolic capability to biotransform a variety of endogenous and exogenous chemicals. Furthermore, results from a host of *in vitro* studies strongly indicate that the cutaneous drug metabolizing enzymes may have an important role in the barrier functions of the skin. Percutaneous absorption can be regarded as the translocation of surface-applied chemicals through the various strata of the epidermis and dermis to a location where the penetrating substances may enter systemic circulation via the dermal vasculature and lymphatics, or remain in the deeper layers of skin. This is a dynamic process, involving both diffusional and metabolic events, and the percutaneous fate of topically applied substances is the net result of the penetration, outward migration, cutaneous metabolism, binding, and permeation into and through the various strata of the skin.

There are many fundamental questions concerning skin absorption and metabolism that remain to be addressed. The potential role of the dermal vascu-

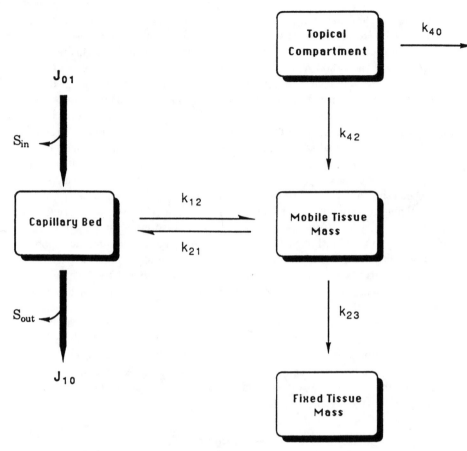

FIGURE 16 Physiologic pharmacokinetic model of drug disposition in the isolated perfused porcine skin flap. J_{01} and J_{10} represent arterial drug influx and venous effluent, respectively, while rate constants (k_{ij}) describe mass transfer from compartments i to j. Fixed tissue mass represents drug irreversibly sequestered within cutaneous tissues during a 10 to 12 h (typically) experiment. S_{in} and S_{out} indicate sampling ports on the perfusion apparatus. Adapted from Williams and Riviere (1989a) and Williams et al. (1990).

lature, the contribution of skin appendages such as hair follicles and sebaceous glands, and the influence of skin condition, age, disease state, and anatomic sites are just a few examples of questions that need to be resolved. When topical exposure results in local effects, pathological changes in the skin may be expected to affect its barrier functions. These changes may involve alteration of the physical barrier as well as the biochemical properties, such as the metabolic status of the skin. Such local changes may have important implications on the outcome of dermal absorption and fate of topically applied xenobiotics. The experimental techniques necessary to address these questions are available, and productive research in these areas will provide means whereby species differences in skin absorption and metabolism may be investigated. These studies should provide not only a better understanding of the mechanisms important in the percutaneous fate of topically applied chemicals, but also a rational basis for cross-species extrapolation and, therefore, more predictive estimates for skin absorption and metabolism in humans.

In this review we have described, albeit briefly, the xenobiotic metabolizing capabilities of the skin, and some of the conceptual models and *in vitro* methodologies that may be used to examine skin metabolism and its functional significance in the percutaneous fate of topically applied xenobiotics. Research in this area is in its infancy, and it is anticipated that as our knowledge accumulates, experimental techniques will continue to evolve and conceptual models will be revised to reflect the most recent trends. However, the future development of this area requires an appreciation of the fact that the skin, in addition to being a drug-metabolizing organ and a portal of entry for a variety of topically applied agents, is also a target organ for local toxicity. Understanding the interrelationships of these skin functions is important and will provide valuable insight into the processes that can influence the percutaneous fate of surface-applied xenobiotics.

REFERENCES

Akhter, S. A., Bennett, S. L., Waller, I. L. and Barry, B. W. 1984. An automated diffusion apparatus for studying skin penetration. *Int. J. Pharm.* 21:17–26.

Akin, F. J. and Norred, W. P. 1976. Factors affecting measurement of aryl hydrocarbon hydroxylase activity in mouse skin. *J. Invest. Dermatol.* 67:709–712.

Andersen, K. E., Maibach, H. I. and Anjo, M. D. 1980. The guinea-pig: An animal model for human skin absorption of hydrocortisone, testosterone and benzoic acid? *Br. J. Dermatol.* 102:447–453.

Ando, H. Y., Ho, N. F. H. and Higuchi, W. I. 1977. Skin as an active metabolizing barrier I: Theoretical analysis of topical bioavailability. *J. Pharm. Sci.* 66:1525–1528.

Ashurst, S. W. and Cohen, G. M. 1981. *In vivo* formation of benzo(a)pyrene diol epoxide-deoxyadenosine adducts in the skin of mice susceptible to benzo(a)pyrene-induced carcinogenesis. *Int. J. Cancer* 27:357–364.

Asokan, P., Das, M., Bik, D. P., Howard, P. C., McCoy, G. D., Rosenkranz, H. S., Bickers, D. R. and Mukhtar, H. 1986. Comparative effects of topically applied nitrated arenes and their nonnitrated parent arenes on cutaneous and hepatic drug and carcinogen metabolism in neonatal rats. *Toxicol. Appl. Pharmacol.* 86:33–43.

Asokan, P., Das, M., Rosenkranz, H. S., Bickers, D. R. and Mukhtar, H. 1985. Topically applied nitropyrenes are potent inducers of cutaneous and hepatic monooxygenases. *Biochem. Biophys. Res. Commun.* 129:134–140.

Asselineau, D., Bernard, B. A., Bailly, C., Darmon, M. and Pruieras, M. 1986. Human epidermis reconstructed by culture: Is it "normal"? *J. Invest. Dermatol.* 86:181–186.

Baden, H. F., Hooker, P. A., Kubilus, J. and Tarascio, A. 1980. Sulfatase activity in X-linked ichithyosis. *Pediatr. Res.* 14:1347–1348.

Baer-Dubowska, W. and Alexandrov, K. 1981. The binding of benzo[a]pyrene to mouse and rat skin DNA. *Cancer Lett.* 13:47–52.

Baines, P. J., Jackson, D., Mellows, G., Swaisland, A. J. and Tasker, T. C. G. 1984. Mupirocin: Its chemistry and metabolism. In *Mupirocin: A Novel Topical Antibiotic*, eds. D. S. Wilkinson and J. D. Price, pp. 13–22. London: Royal Society of Medicine.

Bamshad, J. 1969. Catechol-*O*-methyl transferase in epidermis, dermis and whole skin. *J. Invest. Dermatol.* 52:351–352.

Bardin, C. W., Bullock, L. P., Sherins, R. J., Mowszowicz, I. and Blackburn, W. R. 1973. Part II. Androgen metabolism and mechanism of action in male pseudohermaphroditism: A study of testicular feminization. *Recent Prog. Horm. Res.* 29:65–109.

Barrett, J. G. and Scott, I. R. 1983. Pyrrolidone carboxylic acid synthesis in guinea pig epidermis. *J. Invest. Dermatol.* 81:122–124.

Behrendt, H. and Kampffmeyer, H. G. 1989. Absorption and ester cleavage of methyl salicylate by skin of single-pass perfused rabbit ears. *Xenobiotica* 19:131–141.

Bell, E., Gay, R., Swiderek, M., Class, T., Kemp, P., Green, G., Haimes, H. and Bilbo, P. 1989. Use of fabricated living tissue and organ equivalents as defined higher order systems for the study of pharmacologic responses to test substances. *Proc. NATO Advanced Research Workshop: Pharmaceutical Application of Cell and Tissue Culture to Drug Transport*, Bandol, France.

Berner, B. 1985. Pharmacokinetics of transdermal drug delivery. *J. Pharm. Sci.* 74:718–721.

Bickers, D. R. 1980. The skin as a site of drug and chemical metabolism. In *Current Concepts in Cutaneous Toxicity*, eds. V. A. Drill and P. Lazar, pp. 95–126. New York: Academic Press.

Bickers, D. R. 1983. Drug, carcinogen, and steroid hormone metabolism in the skin. In *Biochemistry and Physiology of the Skin*, vol. II, ed. L. A. Goldsmith, pp. 1169–1186. New York: Oxford University Press.

Bickers, D. R. and Kappas, A. 1978. Human skin aryl hydrocarbon hydroxylase. Induction by coal tar. *J. Clin. Invest.* 62:1061–1068.

Bickers, D. R. and Kappas, A. 1980. In *Extrahepatic Metabolism of Drugs and Foreign Compounds*, ed. T. E. Grams, pp. 295–310. New York: Spectrum.

Bickers, D. R., Das, M. and Mukhtar, H. 1986. Pharmacological modification of epidermal detoxification systems. *Br. J. Dermatol.* 115(Suppl. 31):9–16.

Bickers, D. R., Dutta-Choudhury, T. and Mukhtar, H. 1982. Epidermis: Site of drug metabolism in neonatal rat skin. Studies on cytochrome P-450 content and mixed-function oxidase and epoxide hydrolase activity. *Mol. Pharmacol.* 21:239–247.

Bickers, D. R., Eiseman, J., Kappas, A. and Alvares, A. P. 1975. Microscope immersion oils: Effects of skin application on cutaneous and hepatic drug-metabolizing enzymes. *Biochem. Pharmacol.* 24:779–783.

Bickers, D. R., Kappas, A. and Alvares, A. P. 1974. Differences in inducibility of cutaneous and hepatic drug metabolizing enzymes and cytochrome P-450 by polychlorinated biphenyls and 1,1,1-trichloro-2,2,-bis(p-chlorophenyl)ethane (DDT). *J. Pharmacol. Exp. Ther.* 188:300–309.

Bikle, D. D., Gee, E., Halloran, B. P. and Riviere, J. E. 1989. Production of 1,25-dihydroxyvitamin D by pig skin in situ. *J. Invest. Dermatol.* 92:404.

Bingham, K. D. and Shaw, D. A. 1973. Male pattern baldness and the metabolism of androgens by human scalp skin. *J. Soc. Cosmet. Chem.* 24:523–536.

Biren, C. A., Barr, R. J., McCullough, J. L., Black, K. S. and Hewitt, C. W. 1986. Prolonged viability of human skin xenografts in rats by cyclosporine. *J. Invest. Dermatol.* 86:611–614.

Blank, I. H., Griesemer, R. D. and Gould, E. 1957. The penetration of an anticholinesterase agent (sarin) into skin. I. Rate of penetration into excised human skin. *J. Invest. Dermatol.* 29:299–309.

Bodor, N., Zupan, J. and Selk, S. 1980. Improved delivery through biological membranes. VII. Dermal delivery of chromoglycic acid (cromolyn) via its prodrugs. *Int. J. Pharm.* 7:63–75.

Bowden, G. T., Slaga, T. J., Shapas, B. G. and Boutwell, R. K. 1974. The role of aryl hydrocarbon hydroxylase in skin tumor initiation by 7,12-dimethylbenz[a]anthracene and 1,2,5,6-dibenzanthracene using DNA binding and thymidine-^{3}H incorporation into DNA as criteria. *Cancer Res.* 34:2634–2642.

Bronaugh, R. L. and Stewart, R. F. 1984. Methods for *in vitro* percutaneous absorption studies III: Hydrophobic compounds. *J. Pharm. Sci.* 73:1255–1258.

Bronaugh, R. L. and Stewart, R. F. 1985. Methods for *in vitro* percutaneous absorption studies IV: The flow-through diffusion cell. *J. Pharm. Sci.* 74:64–67.

Bronaugh, R. L. and Stewart, R. F. 1986. Methods for *in vitro* percutaneous absorption studies VI: Preparation of the barrier layer. *J. Pharm. Sci.* 75:487–491.

Bronaugh, R. L., Stewart, R. F. and Storm, J. E. 1989. Extent of cutaneous metabolism during percutaneous absorption of xenobiotics. *Toxicol. Appl. Pharmacol.* 99:534–543.

Brookes, F. L., Hugo, W. B. and Denyer, S. P. 1982. Transformation of betamethasone 17-valerate by skin microflora. *J. Pharm. Pharmacol.* 34:61P.

Bucks, D. A. W. 1984. Skin structure and metabolism: Relevance to the design of cutaneous therapeutics. *Pharm. Res.* 1:148–153.

Bucks, D. A. W., Maibach, H. I. and Guy, R. H. 1988. Mass balance and dose accountability in percutaneous absorption studies: Development of a nonocclusive application system. *Pharm. Res.* 5:313–315.

Bundgaard, H., Hoelgaard, A. and Mollgaard, B. 1983. Leaching of hydrolytic enzymes from human skin in cutaneous permeation studies as determined by metronidazole and 5-fluorouracil pro-drugs. *Int. J. Pharm.* 15:285–292.

Burke, M. D. and Mayer, R. T. 1974. Ethoxyresorufin: Direct fluorimetric assay of a microsomal *O*-dealkylation which is preferentially inducible by 3-methylcholanthrene. *Drug Metab. Dispos.* 2:583–588.

Burke, M. D., Prough, R. A. and Mayer, R. T. 1977. Characteristics of a microsomal cytochrome P-448-mediated reaction. Ethoxyresorufin O-de-ethylation. *Drug Metab. Dispos.* 5:1–8.

Burton, S. A., Wojciechowski, Z. J., Rohr, U., Krueger, G. G. and Higuchi, W. I. 1985. Comparison of *in vivo* and *in vitro* transdermal drug absorption and dermal drug metabolism of vidarabine using a unique isolated skin flap model. *Clin. Res.* 33:628A.

Cameron, G. S., Baldwin, J. K., Jasheway, D. W., Patrick, K. E. and Fischer, S. M. 1990. Arachidonic acid metabolism varies with the state of differentiation in density gradient-separated mouse epidermal cells. *J. Invest. Dermatol.* 94:292–296.

Carver, M. P. and Riviere, J. E. 1990. Percutaneous absorption and excretion of xenobiotics after topical and intravenous administration to pigs. *Fundam. Appl. Toxicol.* 13:714–722.

Carver, M. P., Levi, P. E. and Riviere, J. E. 1990. Parathion metabolism during percutaneous absorption in perfused porcine skin. *Pestic. Biochem. Physiol.* 38:245–254.

Carver, M. P., Williams, P. L. and Riviere, J. E. 1989. The isolated perfused porcine skin flap (IPPSF). III. Percutaneous absorption pharmacokinetics of organophosphates, steroids, benzoic acid, and caffeine. *Toxicol. Appl. Pharmacol.* 97:324–337.

Chandrasekaran, S. K., Bayne, W. and Shaw, J. E. 1978. Pharmacokinetics of drug permeation through human skin. *J. Pharm. Sci.* 67:1370–1374.

Chang, S. K., Williams, P. L. and Riviere, J. E. 1990. Percutaneous absorption of parathion, malathion, carbaryl and lindane in the isolated perfused porcine skin flap (IPPSF). *Toxicologist* 10:257.

Chapman, P. H., Rawlins, M. D. and Shuster, S. 1979. The activity of aryl hydrocarbon hydroxylase in adult human skin. *Br. J. Clin. Pharmacol.* 7:499–503.

Cheung, Y. W., Po, A. L. W. and Irwin, W. J. 1985. Cutaneous biotransformation as a parameter in the modulation of the activity of topical corticosteroids. *Int. J. Pharm.* 26:175–189.

Collier, S. W., Storm, J. E. and Bronaugh, R. L. 1989. Structure-related differences in the metabolic fate of aniline during azo color metabolism in Sencar mouse skin. *Toxicologist* 9:164.

Coomes, M. W., Norling, A. H., Pohl, R. J., Muller, D. and Fouts, J. R. 1983. Foreign compound metabolism by isolated skin cells from the hairless mouse. *J. Pharmacol. Exp. Ther.* 225:770–777.

Coomes, M. W., Sparks, R. W. and Fouts, J. R. 1984. Oxidation of 7-ethoxycoumarin and conjugation of umbelliferone by intact, viable epidermal cells from the hairless mouse. *J. Invest. Dermatol.* 82:598–601.

Cooper, E. R. 1984. Increased skin permeability for lipophilic molecules. *J. Pharm. Sci.* 73:1153–1156.

Damen, F. M. J. and Mier, P. D. 1982. Cytochrome P-450-dependent *O*-dealkylase activity in mammalian skin. *Br. J. Pharmacol.* 75:123–127.

Daniel, R. K. and Kerrigan, C. L. 1982. The omnipotential pig buttock flap. *Plast. Reconstr. Surg.* 70:11–15.

Das, M., Bickers, D. R. and Mukhtar, H. 1985. Effect of ellagic acid on hepatic and pulmonary xenobiotic metabolism in mice: Studies on the mechanism of its anticarcinogenic action. *Carcinogenesis* 6:1409–1413.

Das, M., Bickers, D. R. and Mukhtar, H. 1989. Protection against chemically induced skin tumorigenesis in SENCAR mice by tannic acid. *Int. J. Cancer* 43:468–470.

Das, M., Khan, W. A., Asokan, P., Bickers, D. R. and Mukhtar, H. 1987a. Inhibition of polycyclic aromatic hydrocarbon-DNA adduct formation in epidermis and lungs of SENCAR mice by naturally occurring plant phenols. *Cancer Res.* 47:767–773.

Das, M., Mukhtar, H., Bik, D. P. and Bickers, D. R. 1987b. Inhibition of epidermal xenobiotic metabolism in SENCAR mice by naturally occurring plant phenols. *Cancer Res.* 47:760–766.

Das, M., Mukhtar, H., Del Tito Jr., B. J., Marcelo, C. L. and Bickers, D. R. 1986. Clotrimazole, an inhibitor of benzo[a]pyrene metabolism and its subsequent glucuronidation, sulfation, and macromolecular binding in BALB/c mouse cultured keratinocytes. *J. Invest. Dermatol.* 87:4–10.

deBruyn, C. H. M. M., Oei, T. L. and terHaar, B. G. A. 1974. Studies on hair roots for carrier detection in hypoxanthine-guanine phosphoribosyl transferase deficiency. *Clin. Genet.* 5:449–456.

Del Tito Jr., B. J., Mukhtar, H. and Bickers, D. R. 1984. *In vivo* metabolism of topically applied benzo[a]pyrene-4,5-oxide in neonatal rat skin. *J. Invest. Dermatol.* 82:378–380.

Denyer, S. P. and McNabb, C. 1989. Microbial metabolism of topically applied drugs. In *Transdermal Drug Delivery: Developmental Issues and Research Initiatives,* eds. J. Hadgraft and R. H. Guy, pp. 113–134. New York: Marcel Dekker.

Denyer, S. P., Guy, R. H., Hadgraft, J. and Hugo, W. B. 1985. The microbial degradation of topically applied drugs. *Int. J. Pharm.* 26:89–97.

Denyer, S. P., Hugo, W. B. and O'Brien, M. 1984. Metabolism of glyceryl trinitrate by skin staphylococci. *J. Pharm. Pharmacol.* 36:61P.

DeYoung, L., Ballaron, S. and Epstein, W. 1984. Transglutaminase activity in human and rabbit ear comedogenesis: A histochemical study. *J. Invest. Dermatol.* 82:275–279.

DiGiovanni, J., Gill, R. D., Nettikumara, A. N., Colby, A. B. and Reiners, J. J. 1989. Effect of extracellular calcium concentration on the metabolism of polycyclic aromatic hydrocarbons by cultured mouse keratinocytes. *Cancer Res.* 49:5567–5574.

Dugard, P. H. 1983. Skin permeability theory in relation to measurements of percutaneous absorption in toxicology. In *Dermatotoxicology*, 2nd ed., eds. F. N. Marzulli and H. I. Maibach, pp. 91–116. Washington, D.C.: Hemisphere.

Elias, P. M., Menon, G. K., Grayson, S. and Brown, B. E. 1988. Membrane structural alterations in murine stratum corneum: Relationship to the localization of polar lipids and phospholipases. *J. Invest. Dermatol.* 91:3–10.

Faredin, I., Fazekas, A. G., Toth, I., Kokai, K. and Julesz, M. 1969. Transformation *in vitro* of [4-^{14}C]-dehydroepiandrosterone into 7-oxygenated derivatives by normal human male and female skin tissue. *J. Invest. Dermatol.* 53:357–361.

Fazekas, A. G. and Lanthier, A. 1971. Metabolism of androgens by isolated human hair follicles. *Steroids* 18:367–379.

Fazekas, A. G. and Sandor, T. 1973. The metabolism of dehydroepiandrosterone by human scalp hair follicles. *J. Clin. Endocrinol. Metab.* 36:582–586.

Findlay, G. H. 1955. The simple esterases of human skin. *Br. J. Dermatol.* 67:83–91.

Finnen, M. J. 1987. Skin metabolism by oxidation and conjugation. In *Pharmacology and the Skin: Skin Pharmacokinetics,* eds. B. Shroot and H. Schaefer, pp. 163–169. Basel: Karger.

Finnen, M. J. and Shuster, S. 1985. Phase 1 and Phase 2 drug metabolism in isolated epidermal cells from adult hairless mice and in whole human hair follicles. *Biochem. Pharmacol.* 34:3571–3575.

Finnen, M. J., Herdman, M. L. and Shuster, S. 1984. Induction of drug metabolizing enzymes in the skin by topical steroids. *J. Steroid Biochem.* 20:1169–1173.

Finnen, M. J., Herdman, M. L. and Shuster, S. 1985. Distribution and sub-cellular localization of drug metabolizing enzymes in the skin. *Br. J. Dermatol.* 113:713–721.

Fisher, H. L., Most, B. and Hall, L. L. 1985. Dermal absorption of pesticides calculated by deconvolution. *J. Appl. Toxicol.* 5:163–177.

Flynn, G. L. 1985. Mechanism of percutaneous absorption from physicochemical evidence. In *Percutaneous Absorption: Mechanisms—Methodology—Drug Delivery,* eds. R. L. Bronaugh and H. I. Maibach, pp. 17–42. New York: Marcel Dekker.

Forbes, P. D. 1967. Vasuclar supply of the skin and hair in swine. In *Advances in Biology of Skin,* eds. W. Montagna and R. Dobson, pp. 419–432. New York: Pergamon Press.

Foreman, M. I. and Clanachan, I. 1975. The percutaneous penetration of nandrolone decanoate. *Br. J. Dermatol.* 93:47–52.

Foreman, M. I., Picton, W., Lukowiecki, G. A. and Clark, C. 1979. The effect of topical crude coal tar treatment on unstimulated hairless hamster skin. *Br. J. Dermatol.* 100:707–715.

Fox, J. L., Yu, C.-D., Higuchi, W. I. and Ho, N. F. H. 1979. General physical model for simultaneous diffusion and metabolism in biological membranes. The computational approach for the steady-state case. *Int. J. Pharm.* 2:41–57.

Fredriksson, T. 1958. Studies on the percutaneous absorption of sarin and two allied organophosphorus cholinesterase inhibitors. *Acta Dermato-Venereol.* 38(suppl. 41):1–83.

Fredriksson, T. 1962. Studies on the percutaneous absorption of parathion and para-oxon. V. Rate of absorption of paraoxon. *J. Invest. Dermatol.* 38:233–236.

Fredriksson, T. 1964. Studies on the percutaneous absorption of parathion and para-oxon. VI. *In vivo* decomposition of paraoxon during the epidermal passage. *J. Invest. Dermatol.* 42:37–40.

Fredriksson, T., Farrior, W. L. and Witter, R. F. 1961. Studies on the percutaneous absorption of parathion and paraoxon. I. Hydrolysis and metabolism within the skin. *Acta Dermato-Venereol.* 41:335–343.

Freinkel, R. K. 1983. Carbohydrate metabolism of epidermis. In *Biochemistry and Physiology of the Skin,* vol. I, ed. L. A. Goldsmith, pp. 328–337. New York: Oxford University Press.

Frost, P., Weinstein, G. D. and Hsia, S. L. 1966. Metabolism of estradiol-17β and estrone in human skin. *J. Invest. Dermatol.* 46:584–585.

Gartler, S. M., Scott, R. C., Goldstein, J. L., Campbell, B. and Sparkes, R. 1971. Lesch-Nyhan syndrome: Rapid detection of heterozygotes by use of hair follicles. *Science* 172:572–574.

Gerlowski, L. E. and Jain, R. K. 1983. Physiologically based pharmacokinetic modeling: Principles and applications. *J. Pharm. Sci.* 72:1103–1127.

Gienger, G., Knoch, A. and Merkle, H. P. 1986. Modeling and numerical computation of drug transport in laminates: Model case evaluation of transdermal delivery system. *J. Pharm. Sci.* 75:9–15.

Godfrey, K. R., Jones, R. F. and Brown, R. F. 1980. Identifiable pharmacokinetic models: The role of extra inputs and measurements. *J. Pharmacokin. Biopharm.* 8:633–648.

Gomez, E. C. and Hsia, S. L. 1968. *In vitro* metabolism of testosterone-4-^{14}C and Δ^4-androstene-3,17-dione-4-^{14}C in human skin. *Biochemistry* 7:24–32.

Gonzalez, F. J. 1989. The molecular biology of cytochrome P450s. *Pharmacol. Rev.* 40:243–288.

Graham, M. J., Williams, F. M. and Rawlins, M. D. 1986. Aldrin epoxidation by rat skin during percutaneous absorption *in vivo*. *Br. J. Clin. Pharmacol.* 21:111P.

Gray, G. M., White, R. J. and Majer, J. R. 1978. 1-(3'-O-Acyl)-β-glucosyl-*N*-dihydroxypentatriacontadienoylsphingosine, a major component of the gluco-sylceramides of pig and human epidermis. *Biochim. Biophys. Acta* 528:127–137.

Greaves, M. S. 1971. The *in vitro* catabolism of cortisol by human skin. *J. Invest. Dermatol.* 57:100–107.

Grunberger, D., Theall, G. and Eisinger, M. 1983. Metabolism and DNA binding of carcinogens in cultured human epidermal cells. In *Human Carcinogenesis,* eds. C. C. Harris and H. N. Autrup, pp. 195–216. New York: Academic Press.

Guengerich, F. P., Dannan, G. A., Wright, S. T., Martin, M. V. and Kaminsky, L. S. 1982a. Purification and characterization of liver microsomal cytochromes P-450: Electrophoretic, spectral, catalytic, and immunochemical properties and inducibility of eight isozymes from rats treated with phenobarbital or β-naphthoflavone. *Biochemistry* 21:6019–6030.

Guengerich, F. P., Dannan, G. A., Wright, S. T., Martin, M. V. and Kaminsky, L. S. 1982b. Purification and characterization of microsomal cytochrome P-450s. *Xenobiotica* 12:701–716.

Guo, J. F., Brown, R., Rothwell, C. E. and Bernstein, I. A. 1990. Levels of cyto-chrome P-450-mediated aryl hydrocarbon hydroxylases (AHH) are higher in differentiated than in germinative keratinocytes. *J. Invest. Dermatol.* 94:86–93.

Guy, R. H. and Hadgraft, J. 1984a. Percutaneous absorption kinetics of topically applied agents liable to surface loss. *J. Soc. Cosmet. Chem.* 35:103–113.

Guy, R. H. and Hadgraft, J. 1984b. Pharmacokinetics of percutaneous absorption with concurrent metabolism. *Int. J. Pharm.* 20:43–51.

Guy, R. H. and Hadgraft J. 1985a. Kinetic analysis of transdermal nitroglycerin delivery. *Pharm. Res.* 2:206–211.

Guy, R. H. and Hadgraft, J. 1985b. Pharmacokinetic interpretation of the plasma levels of clonidine following transdermal delivery. *J. Pharm. Sci.* 74:1016–1018.

Guy, R. H. and Hadgraft, J. 1986. Interpretation and prediction of the kinetics of transdermal drug delivery: Oestradiol, hyoscine and timolol. *Int. J. Pharm.* 32:159–163.

Guy, R. H. and Hadgraft, J. 1987. The effect of penetration enhancers on the kinetics of percutaneous absorption. *J. Controlled Release* 5:43–51.

Guy, R. H. and Maibach, H. I. 1984. Correction factors for determining body exposure from forearm percutaneous absorption data. *J. Appl. Toxicol.* 4:26–28.

Guy, R. H., Hadgraft, J. and Bucks, D. A. W. 1987a. Transdermal drug delivery and cutaneous metabolism. *Xenobiotica* 17:325–343.

Guy, R. H., Hadgraft, J. and Maibach, H. I. 1983. Percutaneous absorption: Multidose pharmacokinetics. *Int. J. Pharm.* 17:23–28.

Guy, R. H., Hadgraft, J., Hinz, R. S., Roskos, K. V. and Bucks, D. A. W. 1987b. *In vivo* evaluations of transdermal drug delivery. In *Drugs and the Pharmaceutical Sciences—Transdermal Controlled Systemic Medications,* ed. Y. W. Chien, pp. 179–224. New York: Marcel Dekker.

Guzek, D. B., Kennedy, A. H., McNeill, S. C., Washkull, E. and Potts, R. O. 1989. Transdermal drug transport and metabolism: I. Comparison of *in vitro* and *in vivo* results. *Pharm. Res.* 6:33–39.

Hadgraft, J. 1979. The epidermal reservoir: A theoretical approach. *Int. J. Pharm.* 2:265–274.

Hadgraft, J. 1987. Variables associated with a kinetic analysis of skin penetration. In *Pharmacology and the Skin: Skin Pharmacokinetics,* eds. B. Shroot and H. Schaefer, pp. 154–162. Basel: Karger.

Hakanson, R. and Moller, H. 1963. On metabolism of noradrenaline in the skin: Activity of catechol-*O*-methyl transferase and monoamine oxidase. *Acta Dermato-Venereol.* 43:552–555.

Hamamoto, T. and Mori, Y. 1989. Sulfation of minoxidil in keratinocytes and hair follicles. *Res. Commun. Chem. Pathol. Pharmacol.* 66:33–44.

Harkness, R. A., Beveridge, G. W. and Davidson, D. W. 1971. Percutaneous absorption of 1-naphthol-(^{14}C) in man. *Br. J. Dermatol.* 85:30–34.

Harmon, C. S., Phil, D., Masser, M. R. and Phizackerly, P. J. R. 1986. Effect of ischemia and reperfusion of pig skin flaps on epidermal glycogen metabolism. *J. Invest. Dermatol.* 86:69–73.

Harvey, R. G. 1982. Polycyclic hydrocarbons and cancer. *Am. Sci.* 70:386–393.

Hawkins, G. S. and Reifenrath, W. G. 1984. Development of an *in vitro* model for determining the fate of chemicals applied to skin. *Fundam. Appl. Toxicol.* 4(suppl.):S133–S144.

Hay, J. B. and Hodgins, M. B. 1974. Metabolism of androgens by human skin in acne. *Br. J. Dermatol.* 91:123–133.

Hay, J. D. and Hodgins, M. B. 1978. Distribution of androgen metabolizing enzymes in isolated tissues of human forehead and axillary skin. *J. Endocrinol.* 79:29–39.

Hemels, H. G. W. M. 1971. Percutaneous absorption of 1-naphthol in man. *Br. J. Dermatol.* 85:494–495.

Hemels, H. G. W. M. 1972. Percutaneous absorption and distribution of 2-naphthol in man. *Br. J. Dermatol.* 87:614–622.

Hiernickel, H. 1985. An improved method for *in vitro* perfusion of human skin. *Br. J. Dermatol.* 112:299–305.

Hiernickel, H., Merk, H. and Steigleder, G. K. 1986. *In vitro* perfusion of preputial flaps. *Clin. Exp. Dermatol.* 11:316.

Higuchi, T. 1960. Physical chemical analysis of percutaneous absorption process from creams and ointments. *J. Soc. Cosmet. Chem.* 11:85–97.

Higuchi, W. I. and Yu, C.-D. 1987. Prodrugs in transdermal delivery. In *Transdermal Delivery of Drugs,* vol. III, eds. A. F. Kydonieus and B. Berner, pp. 43–83. Boca Raton, Fla.: CRC Press.

Holick, M. F. 1989. Will 1,25-dihydroxyvitamin D_3, MC903, and their analogues herald a new pharmacologic era for the treatment of psoriasis? *Arch. Dermatol.* 125:1692–1697.

Holland, J. M., Kao, J. Y. and Whitaker, M. J. 1984. A multisample apparatus for kinetic evaluation of skin penetration *in vitro*: The influence of viability and metabolic status of the skin. *Toxicol. Appl. Pharmacol.* 72:272–280.

Holland, J. M., Whitaker, M. S. and Wesley, J. W. 1979. Correlation of fluorescence intensity and carcinogenic potency of synthetic and natural petroleums in mouse skin. *Am. Ind. Hyg. Assoc. J.* 40:496–503.

Hsia, S. L. 1980. Metabolism of steroids in human skin. In *Percutaneous Absorption of Steroids,* eds. P. Mauvais-Jarvis, C. F. H. Vickers and J. Wepierre, pp. 81–88. New York: Academic Press.

Huang, Y.-C. 1987. *In vitro* evaluations of transdermal drug delivery. In *Drugs and the Pharmaceutical Sciences—Transdermal Controlled Systemic Medications,* ed. Y. W. Chien, pp. 159–178. New York: Marcel Dekker.

Hukkelhoven, M. W. A. C., Dijkstra, A. C. and Vermorken, A. J. M. 1983. Human hair follicles and cultured hair follicle keratinocytes as indicators for individual differences in carcinogen metabolism. *Arch. Toxicol.* 53:265–274.

Hukkelhoven, M. W. A. C., Vermorken, A. J. M., Vromans, E. and Bloemendal, H. 1982. Human hair follicles, a convenient tissue for genetic studies on carcinogen metabolism. *Clin. Genet.* 21:53–58.

Itami, S., Kurota, S. and Takayasu, S. 1990. 5α-reductase activity in cultured human dermal pailla cells from beard compared with reticular dermal fibroblasts. *J. Invest. Dermatol.* 94:150–152.

Jacquez, J. A. 1985. *Compartmental Analysis in Biology and Medicine,* 2nd ed., pp. 277–310. Ann Arbor, Mich.: University of Michigan Press.

James, M. O. and Little, P. J. 1983. Modification of benzo(a)pyrene metabolism in hepatic microsomes from untreated and induced rats by imidazole derivatives which inhibit monooxygenase activity and enhance epoxide hydrolase activity. *Drug Metab. Dispos.* 11:350–354.

Johansen, M., Mollgaard, B., Wotton, P. W., Larsen, C. and Hoelgaard, A. 1986. *In vitro* evaluation of dermal prodrug delivery—Transport and bioconversion of a series of aliphatic esters of metronidazole. *Int. J. Pharm.* 32:199–206.

Kahl, R., Friederici, D. E., Kahl, G. F., Ritter, W. and Krebs, R. 1980. Clotrimazole as an inhibitor of benzo[a]pyrene metabolite-DNA adduct formation *in vitro* and of microsomal mono-oxygenase activity. *Drug Metab. Dispos.* 8:191–196.

Kaminsky, L. S., Guengerich, F. P., Dannan, G. A. and Aust, S. D. 1983. Comparisons of warfarin metabolism by liver microsomes of rats treated with a series of poly-brominated biphenyl cogeners and by the component-purified cytochrome P-450 isozymes. *Arch. Biochem. Biophys.* 225:398–404.

Kao, J. 1988. Estimating the contribution by skin to systemic metabolism. *Ann. NY Acad. Sci.* 548:90–96.

Kao, J. 1989. The influence of metabolism on percutaneous absorption. In *Percutaneous*

Absorption: Mechanisms—Methodology—Drug Delivery, 2nd ed., eds. R. L. Bronaugh and H. I. Maibach, pp. 259–281. New York: Marcel Dekker.

Kao, J. 1990a. Validity of skin absorption and metabolism studies. In *CRC Handbook: Methods in Percutaneous Absorption,* eds. B. W. Kemppainen and W. G. Reifenrath. Boca Raton, Fla.: CRC Press.

Kao, J. 1990b. *In vitro* assessment of dermal absorption. In *Fundamentals and Methods of Dermal and Ocular Toxicology,* ed. D. W. Hobson. Caldwell, N.J.: Telford Press.

Kao, J. and Hall, J. 1987. Skin absorption and cutaneous first pass metabolism of topical steroids: *In vitro* studies with mouse skin in organ culture. *J. Pharmacol. Exp. Ther.* 241:482–487.

Kao, J., Hall, J. and Holland, J. M. 1983. Quantitation of cutaneous toxicity: An *in vitro* approach using skin in organ culture. *Toxicol. Appl. Pharmacol.* 68:206–217.

Kao, J., Hall, J., Shugart, L. R. and Holland, J. M. 1984. An *in vitro* approach to studying cutaneous metabolism and disposition of topically applied xenobiotics. *Toxicol. Appl. Pharmacol.* 75:289–298.

Kao, J., Patterson, F. K. and Hall, J. 1985. Skin penetration and metabolism of topically applied chemicals in six mammalian species, including man: An *in vitro* study with benzo[a]pyrene and testosterone. *Toxicol. Appl. Pharmacol.* 81:502–516.

Katz, M. and Poulsen, B. J. 1971. Absorption of drugs through the skin. In *Handbook of Experimental Pharmacology,* eds. B. Brodie and J. Gillette, pp. 103–174. New York: Springer-Verlag.

Kemppainen, B. W., Riley, R. T. and Biles-Thurlow, S. 1987. Comparison of penetration and metabolism of [³H]diacetoxyscirpenol, [³H]verrucarin A and [³H]T-2 toxin in skin. *Food Chem. Toxicol.* 25:379–386.

Kemppainen, B. W., Riley, R. T., Pace, J. G. and Hoerr, F. J. 1986a. Effects of skin storage condition and concentration of applied dose on [³H]T-2 toxin penetration through excised human and monkey skin. *Food Chem. Toxicol.* 24:221–227.

Kemppainen, B. W., Riley, R. T., Pace, J. G., Hoerr, F. J. and Joyave, J. 1986b. Evaluation of monkey skin as a model for *in vitro* percutaneous penetration and metabolism of [³H]T-2 toxin in human skin. *Fundam. Appl. Toxicol.* 7:367–375.

Khan, W. A., Park, S. S., Gelboin, H. V., Bickers, D. R. and Mukhtar, H. 1989a. Epidermal cytochrome P-450: Immunochemical characterization of isoform induced by topical application of 3-methylcholanthrene to neonatal rat. *J. Pharmacol. Exp. Ther.* 249:921–927.

Khan, W. A., Park, S. S., Gelboin, H. V., Bickers, D. R. and Mukhtar, H. 1989b. Monoclonal antibodies directed characterization of epidermal and hepatic cytochrome P-450 isozymes induced by skin application of therapeutic crude coal tar. *J. Invest. Dermatol.* 93:40–45.

Kinoshita, N. and Gelboin, H. V. 1972a. Aryl hydrocarbon hydroxylase and polycyclic hydrocarbon tumorigenesis: Effect of the enzyme inhibitor 7,8-benzoflavone on tumorigenesis and macromolecule binding. *Proc. Nat. Acad. Sci. USA* 69:824–828.

Kinoshita, N. and Gelboin, H. V. 1972b. The role of aryl hydrocarbon hydroxylase in 7,12-dimethylbenz(a)anthracene skin tumorigenesis: On the mechanism of 7,8-benzoflavone inhibition of tumorigenesis. *Cancer Res.* 32:1329–1339.

Klain, G. J., Bonner, S. J. and Bell, W. G. 1986. The distribution of selected metabolic processes in the pig and human skin. In *Swine in Biomedical Research,* ed. M. E. Tumbleson, pp. 667–671. New York: Plenum Press.

Kligman, A. M. 1964. The biology of the stratum corneum. In *The Epidermis,* eds. W. Montagna and W. C. Lobitz, pp. 387–433. New York: Academic Press.

Koreeda, M., Moore, P. D., Wislocki, P. G., Levin, W., Conney, A. H., Haruhiko, Y. and Jerina, D. M. 1978. Binding of benzo[a]pyrene 7,8-diol-9,10-epoxides to DNA, RNA, and protein of mouse skin occurs with high stereoselectivity. *Science* 199:778–781.

Kragballe, K., Beck, H. I. and Sogaard, H. 1988. Improvement of psoriasis by a topical vitamin D_3 analogue (MC903) in a double-blind study. *Br. J. Dermatol.* 119:223–230.

Kragballe, K. 1989. Treatment psoriasis by the topical application of the novel cholecalciferol analogue cacipotriol (MC903). *Arch. Dermatol.* 125:1647–1652.

Krueger, G. G., Wojciechowski, Z. J., Burton, S. A., Gilhar, A., Huether, S. E., Leonard, L. G., Rohr, U. D., Petelenz, T. J., Higuchi, W. I. and Pershing, L. K. 1985. The development of a rat/human skin flap served by a defined and accessible vasculature on a congenitally athymic (nude) rat. *Fundam. Appl. Toxicol.* 5(suppl.):S112–S121.

Kubota, K. and Ishizaki, T. 1985. A theoretical consideration of percutaneous drug absorption. *J. Pharmacokin. Biopharm.* 13:55–72.

Kubota, K., Tamada, T., Ogura, A. and Ishizaki, T. 1990. A novel differentiation method of vehicle models for topically applied drugs: Application to a therapeutic timolol patch. *J. Pharm. Sci.* 79:179–184.

Kumar, S., Antony, M. and Mehrota, N. K. 1982. Induction of benzo[a]pyrene hydroxylase in skin and liver by cutaneous application of jute batching oil. *Toxicology* 23:347–352.

Kuroki, T., Hosomi, J., Munakata, K., Onizuka, T., Terauchi, M. and Nemoto, N. 1982. Metabolism of benzo(a)pyrene in epidermal keratinocytes and dermal fibroblasts of humans and mice with reference to variation among species, individuals, and cell types. *Cancer Res.* 42:1859–1865.

Kuroki, T., Nemoto, N. and Kitano, Y. 1980. Metabolism of benzo[a]pyrene in human epidermal keratinocytes in culture. *Carcinogenesis* 1:559–565.

Kuttenn, F. and Mauvais-Jarvis, P. 1975. Testosterone 5α-reduction in the skin of normal subjects and of patients with abnormal sex development. *Acta Endocrinol.* 79:164–176.

Kuttenn, F., Mowszowicz, I. and Mauvais-Jarvis, P. 1980. Androgen metabolism in human skin. In *Percutaneous Absorption of Steroids,* eds. P. Mauvais-Jarvis, C. F. H. Vickers and J. Wepierre, pp. 99–121. New York: Academic Press.

Levi, P. E., Hollingworth, R. M. and Hodgson, E. 1988. Differences in oxidative dearylation and desulfuration of fenitrothion by cytochrome P-450 isozymes and in the subsequent inhibition of monooxygenase activity. *Pestic. Biochem. Physiol.* 32:224–231.

Levi, P. E., Inman, A., Venkatesh, K., Misra, R., Hodgson, E. and Monteiro-Riviere, J. E. 1990. Immunohistochemical and enzymatic studies of the flavin-containing monooxygenase (FMO) in mouse and pig skin. *Toxicologist* 10:186.

Loden, M. 1985. The *in vitro* hydrolysis of diisopropyl fluorophosphate during penetration through human full-thickness skin and isolated epidermis. *J. Invest. Dermatol.* 85:335–339.

Longcope, C. 1980. The metabolism of oestrogens by human skin. In *Percutaneous Absorption of Steroids,* eds. P. Mauvais-Jarvis, C. F. H. Vickers and J. Wepierre, pp. 89–98. New York: Academic Press.

MacNicoll, A. D., Grover, P. L. and Sims, P. 1980. The metabolism of a series of polycyclic hydrocarbons by mouse skin maintained in short-term organ culture. *Chem.-Biol. Interact.* 29:169–188.

Martin, R. J., Denyer, S. P. and Hadgraft, J. 1987. Skin metabolism of topically applied compounds. *Int. J. Pharm.* 39:23–32.

Marzulli, F., Brown, W. C. and Maibach, H. 1969. Techniques for studying skin penetration. *Toxicol. Appl. Pharmacol. Suppl.* 3:76–83.

May, S. R. and DeClement, F. A. 1982. Development of radiometric metabolic viability testing method for human and porcine skin. *Cryobiology* 19:362–371.

McDougal, J. N., Jepsen, G. W., Clewell, H. J., MacNaughton, M. G. and Andersen, M. E. 1986. A physiological pharmacokinetic model for dermal absorption of vapors in the rat. *Toxicol. Appl. Pharmacol.* 85:286–294.

Menon, G. K., Grayson, S. and Elias, P. M. 1986. Cytochemical and biochemical localization of lipase and sphingomyelinase activity in mammalian epidermis. *J. Invest. Dermatol.* 86:591–597.

Merk, H. and Hiernickel, H. 1986. New method: *In vitro* perfusion of human skin grafts. *Clin. Exp. Dermatol.* 11:316–317.

Merk, H. F., Mukhtar, H., Kaufmann, I., Das, M. and Bickers, D. R. 1987. Human hair follicle benzo[a]pyrene and benzo[a]pyrene-7,8-diol metabolism: Effect of exposure to a coal tar-containing shampoo. *J. Invest. Dermatol.* 88:71–76.

Metcalf, B. W., Levy, M. A. and Holt, D. A. 1989. Inhibitors of steroid 5α-reductase in benign prostatic hyperplasia, male pattern baldness and acne. *Trends Pharmacol. Sci.* 10:491–495.

Meyer, W. and Neurand, K. 1976. The distribution of enzymes in the skin of the domestic pig. *Lab. Anim.* 10:237–247.

Meyer, W., Schwarz, R. and Neurand, K. 1978. The skin of domestic mammals as a model for human skin, with special reference to domestic pig. *Curr. Prob. Dermatol.* 7:39–52.

Middleton, M. C. and Hasmall, R. 1977. A rapid method for preparing epidermal slices of reproducible thickness from excised rat skin. *J. Invest. Dermatol.* 68:108–110.

Milewich, L. and Sontheimer, R. D. 1989. Steroid hormone metabolism by human epidermal keratinocytes. *J. Invest. Dermatol.* 92:292.

Milewich, L., Shaw, C. B. and Sontheimer, R. D. 1988. Steroid metabolism by epidermal keratinocytes. *Proc. NY Acad. Sci.* 548:66–89.

Milstone, L. M. and Edelson, R. L. 1988. Endocrine, metabolic and immunologic functions of keratinocytes. *Ann. NY Acad. Sci.* 548:1–366..

Moloney, S. J., Bridges, J. W. and Fromson, J. M. 1982a. UDP-glucuronosyltransferase activity in rat- and hairless mouse-skin microsomes. *Xenobiotica* 12:481–487.

Moloney, S. J., Fromson, J. M. and Bridges, J. W. 1982b. Cytochrome P-450 dependent deethylase activity in rat and hairless mouse skin microsomes. *Biochem. Pharmacol.* 31:4011–4018.

Moloney, S. J., Fromson, J. M. and Bridges, J. W. 1982c. The metabolism of 7-ethoxycoumarin and 7-hydroxycoumarin by rat and hairless mouse skin strips. *Biochem. Pharmacol.* 31:4005–4009.

Montagna, W. 1955. Histology and cytochemistry of human skin. IX. The distribution of non-specific esterases. *J. Biophys. Biochem. Cytol.* 1:13–16.

Monteiro-Riviere, N. A. 1986. Ultrastructural evaluation of the porcine integument. In *Swine in Biomedical Research,* ed. M. E. Tumbleson, pp. 641–655. New York: Plenum Press.

Monteiro-Riviere, N. A., Bowman, K. F., Scheidt, V. J. and Riviere, J. E. 1987. The isolated perfused porcine skin flap (IPPSF). II. Ultrastructural and histological characterization of epidermal viability. *In Vitro Toxicol.* 1:241–252.

Mukhtar, H. and Bickers, D. R. 1982. Evidence that coal tar is a mixed inducer of microsomal drug-metabolizing enzymes. *Toxicol. Lett.* 11:221–227.

Mukhtar, H. and Bresnick, E. 1976. Glutathione-S-epoxide transferase in mouse skin and human foreskin. *J. Invest. Dermatol.* 66:161–164.

Mukhtar, H., Athar, M. and Bickers, D. R. 1987. Cytochrome P-450 dependent metabolism of testosterone in rat skin. *Biochem. Biophys. Res. Commun.* 145:749–753.

Mukhtar, H., Das, M. and Bickers, D. R. 1986. Skin tumor initiating activity of therapeutic crude coal tar as compared to other polycyclic aromatic hydrocarbons in SENCAR mice. *Cancer Lett.* 31:147–151.

Mukhtar, H., Das, M., Del Tito Jr., B. J. and Bickers, D. R. 1984a. Epidermal benzo[a]pyrene metabolism and DNA-binding in BALB/c mice: Inhibition by ellagic acid. *Xenobiotica* 14:527–531.

Mukhtar, H., Das, M., Del Tito Jr., B. J. and Bickers, D. R. 1984b. Protection against 3-methylcholanthrene induced skin tumorigenesis in BALB/c mice by ellagic acid. *Biochem. Biophys. Res. Commun.* 119:751–757.

Mukhtar, H., Del Tito Jr., B. J., Das, M., Cherniack, E. P., Cherniack, A. and Bickers, D. R. 1984c. Clotrimazole, an inhibitor of epidermal benzo[a]pyrene metabolism and DNA binding and carcinogenicity of the hydrocarbon. *Cancer Res.* 44:4233–4240.

Mukhtar, H., Del Tito Jr., B. J., Marcelo, L. C., Das, M. and Bickers, D. R. 1984d. Ellagic acid: A potent naturally occuring inhibitor of benzo[a]pyrene metabolism and its subsequent glucuronidation, sulfation and covalent binding to DNA in cultured BALB/c mouse keratinocytes. *Carcinogenesis* 5:1565–1571.

Nacht, S., Yeung, D., Beasley Jr., J. N., Ango, M. D. and Maibach, H. I. 1981. Benzoyl peroxide: Percutaneous penetration and metabolic disposition. *J. Am. Acad. Dermatol.* 4:31–37.

Nakashima, E., Noonan, P. K. and Benet, L. Z. 1987. Transdermal bioavailability and first-pass skin metabolism: A preliminary evaluation with nitroglycerin. *J. Pharmacokin. Biopharm.* 15:423–437.

Naughton, G. K., Jacob, L. and Naughton, B. A. 1989. A physiological skin model for *in vitro* toxicity studies. In *Alternative Methods in Toxicology*, vol. 7, ed. A. M. Goldberg, pp. 183–189. New York: Mary Ann Liebert.

Nemanic, M. K., Whitehead, J. S. and Elias, P. M. 1983. Alterations in membrane sugars during epidermal differentiation: visualization with lectins and role of glycosidases. *J. Histochem. Cytochem.* 31:887–897.

Netter, K. J. 1987. Mechanisms of monooxygenase induction and inhibition. *Pharmacol. Ther.* 33:1–9.

Noonan, P. K. and Wester, R. C. 1985. Cutaneous metabolism of xenobiotics. In *Percutaneous Absorption: Mechanisms—Methodology—Drug Delivery*, 2nd ed., eds. R. L. Bronaugh and H. I. Maibach, pp. 65–85. New York: Marcel Dekker.

Nyiri, W. and Jannitti, M. 1932. About the fate of free iodine upon application to the unbroken animal skin in an experimental study. *J. Pharmacol. Exp. Ther.* 45:85–107.

Odland, G. F. 1983. Structure of the skin. In *Biochemistry and Physiology of the Skin*, vol. I, ed. L. A. Goldsmith, pp. 3–63. New York: Oxford University Press.

Oesch, F., Schmassmann, H. and Bentley, P. 1978. Specific activity of human, rat and mouse skin epoxide hydratase towards K-region epoxides of polycyclic hydrocarbons. *Biochem. Pharmacol.* 27:17–20.

Ortiz de Montellano, P. R. 1988. Suicide substrates for drug metabolizing enzymes: Mechanisms and biological consequences. In *Progress in Drug Metabolism*, vol. 11, ed. G. G. Gibson, pp. 99–148. New York: Taylor & Francis.

Ortiz de Montellano, P. R. and Correia, M. A. 1983. Suicidal destruction of cytochrome P-450 during oxidative drug metabolism. *Annu. Rev. Pharmacol. Toxicol.* 23:481–503.

Pannatier, A., Testa, B. and Etter, J.-C. 1981. Enzymatic hydrolysis by mouse skin homogenates: Structure-metabolism relationships of para-nitrobenzoate esters. *Int. J. Pharm.* 8:167–174.

Peck, C. C., Conner, D. P., Bolden, B. J., Almirez, R. G., Kingsley, T. E., Mell, L. D., Murphy, M. G., Hill, V. E., Rowland, L. M., Ezra, D., Kwiatkowski, T. E., Bradley, C. R. and Abdel-Rahim, M. 1988. Outward transcutaneous chemical migration: Implications for diagnostics and dosimetry. *Skin Pharmacol.* 1:14–23.

Peck, C. C., Conner, D. P., Bolden, B. J., Almirez, R. G., Rowland, L. M., Kwiatkowski, T. E., McKelvin, B. A. and Bradley, C. R. 1987. Outward transdermal migration of theophylline. In *Pharmacology and the Skin: Skin Pharmacokinetics*, eds. B. Shroot and H. Schaefer, pp. 201–208. Basel: Karger.

Peck, C. C., Lee, K. and Becker, C. E. 1981. Continuous transepidermal drug collection: Basis for use in assessing drug intake and pharmacokinetics. *J. Pharmacokin. Biopharm.* 9:41–58.

Pershing, L. K. and Krueger, G. G. 1987. New animal models for bioavailability studies. In *Pharmacology and the Skin: Skin Pharmacokinetics*, eds. B. Shroot and H. Schaefer. Basel: Karger.

Pershing, L. K., Conklin, R. L. and Krueger, G. G. 1986. Effects of reduced body temperature on blood flow and percutaneous absorption of ^{14}C benzoic acid across grafted nude rat skin. *Clin. Res.* 34:418A.

Pershing, L. K., Huether, S., Conklin, R. L. and Krueger, G. G. 1989a. Cutaneous blood flow and percutaneous absorption: A quantitative analysis using a laser Doppler velocimeter and a blood flow meter. *J. Invest. Dermatol.* 92:355–359.

Pershing, L. K., Jederberg, W. J., Conklin, R. L. and Krueger, G. G. 1988. Mechanisms of cyclosporine enhanced absorption in the skin sandwich flap model. *J. Invest. Dermatol.* 90:597.

Pershing, L. K., Lambert, L. D. and Krueger, G. G. 1989b. Oral cyclosporine A increases the diffusivity of skin *in vivo* thereby enhancing percutaneous absorption. *J. Invest. Dermatol.* 92:500.

Pham, M.-A., Magdalou, J., Totis, M., Fournel-Gigleux, S., Siest, G. and Hammock, B. D. 1989. Characterization of distinct forms of cytochrome P-450, epoxide metabolizing enzymes and UDP-glucuronosyltransferase in rat skin. *Biochem. Pharmacol.* 38:2187–2194.

Pohl, R. J., Coomes, M. W., Sparks, R. W. and Fouts, J. R. 1984. 7-Ethoxycoumarin O-deethylation activity in viable basal and differentiated keratinocytes isolated from the skin of the hairless mouse. *Drug Metab. Dispos.* 12:25–34.

Pohl, R. J., Philpot, R. M. and Fouts, J. R. 1976. Cytochrome P-450 content and mixed-function oxidase activity in microsomes isolated from mouse skin. *Drug Metab. Dispos.* 4:442–450.

Ponec, M., Weerheim, A., Kempenaar, J., Elias, P. M. and Williams, M. L. 1989. Differentiation of cultured human keratinocytes: Effect of culture conditions on lipid composition of normal versus malignant cells. *In Vitro Cell. Dev. Biol.* 25:689–696.

Potts, R. O., Mcneill, S. C., Desbonnet, C. and Washkull, E. 1989. Transdermal drug transport and metabolism: II. The role of competing kinetic events. *Pharm. Res.* 6:119–124.

Price, V. H. 1975. Testosterone metabolism in the skin. A review of its function in androgenetic alopecia, acne vulgaris, and idiopathic hirsutism including recent studies with antiandrogens. *Arch. Dermatol.* 11:1496–1502.

Reifenrath, W. G. and Robinson, P. B. 1982. *In vitro* skin evaporation and penetration characteristics of mosquito repellents. *J. Pharm. Sci.* 71:1014–1018.

Reifenrath, W. G. and Spencer, T. S. 1985. Evaporation and penetration from skin. In

Percutaneous Absorption: Mechanisms—Methodology—Drug Delivery, eds. R. L. Bronaugh and H. I. Maibach, pp. 305–325. New York: Marcel Dekker.

Reifenrath, W. G., Chellquist, E. M., Shipwash, E. A. and Jederberg, W. W. 1984a. Evaluation of animal models for predicting skin penetration in man. *Fundam. Appl. Toxicol.* 4(suppl.):S224–S230.

Reifenrath, W. G., Chellquist, E. M., Shipwash, E. A., Jederberg, W. W. and Krueger, G. G. 1984b. Percutaneous penetration in the hairless dog, weanling pig, and grafted athymic nude mouse: Evaluation of models for predicting skin penetration in man. *Br. J. Dermatol.* 111(suppl. 27):123–135.

Reiners, J. J. and Rupp, T. 1989. Conversion of xanthine dehydrogenase to xanthine oxidase during keratinocyte differentiation: Modulation by 12-*O*-tetradecanolyphorbol-13-acetate. *J. Invest. Dermatol.* 93:132–135.

Rescigno, A. and Beck, J. S. 1987. The use and abuse of models. *J. Pharmacokin. Biopharm.* 15:327–340.

Rettie, A. E., Williams, F. M. and Rawlins, M. D. 1986a. Substrate specificity of the mouse skin mixed-function oxidase system. *Xenobiotica* 16:205–211.

Rettie, A. E., Williams, F. M., Rawlins, M. D., Mayer, R. T. and Burke, D. M. 1986b. Major differences between lung, skin and liver in the microsomal metabolism of homologous series of resorufin and coumarin ethers. *Biochem. Pharmacol.* 35:3495–3500.

Riviere, J. E. and Carver, M. P. 1990. Isolated perfused skin flap and skin grafting techniques. In *Fundamentals and Methods of Dermal and Ocular Toxicology,* ed. D. W. Hobson. Caldwell, N.J.: Telford Press.

Riviere, J. E. and Williams, P. L. 1988. Interaction of regional hyperthermia with antineoplastic agent delivery pharmacokinetics: Studies in an isolated perfused skin flap system. *Proc. Radiol. Res. Soc.* 36A:16.

Riviere, J. E., Bowman, K. F. and Monteiro-Riviere, N. A. 1986a. The isolated perfused porcines skin flap: A novel animal model for cutaneous toxicologic research. In *Swine in Biomedical Research,* ed. M. E. Tumbleson, pp. 657–666. New York: Plenum Press.

Riviere, J. E., Bowman, K. F. and Monteiro-Riviere, N. A. 1987a. On the definition of viability in isolated perfused skin preparations. *Br. J. Dermatol.* 116:739–741.

Riviere, J. E., Bowman, K. F., Monteiro-Riviere, N. A., Dix, L. P. and Carver, M. P. 1986b. The isolated perfused porcine skin flap (IPPSF). I. A novel *in vitro* model for percutaneous absorption and cutaneous toxicology studies. *Fundam. Appl. Toxicol.* 7:444–453.

Riviere, J. E., Carver, M. P., Monteiro, N. A. and Bowman, K. F. 1987b. Percutaneous absorption of organophosphates, steroids, caffeine, and benzoic acid *in vivo* and *in vitro* using the isolated perfused porcine skin flap (IPPSF). In *Proc. Sixth Medical Chemical Defense Bioscience Review,* pp. 763–766. Columbia, Md.: Johns Hopkins Applied Physics Laboratory.

Riviere, J. E., Sage, B. H. and Monteiro-Riviere, N. A. 1989/1990. Transdermal lidocaine iontophoresis in isolated perfused porcine skin. *J. Toxicol.-Cutan. Ocul. Toxicol.* 8:493–504.

Rongone, E. L. 1983. Skin structure, function, and biochemistry. In *Dermatotoxicology,* 2nd ed., eds. F. N. Marzulli and H. I. Maibach, pp. 1–70. New York: Hemisphere.

Rowland, M. 1984. Physiological pharmacokinetic models: Relevance, experience, and future trends. *Drug Metab. Rev.* 15:55–74.

Rugstad, H. E. and Dybing, E. 1975. Glucuronidation in cultures of human skin epithelial cells. *Eur. J. Clin. Invest.* 5:133–137.

Sanders, C. L., Skinner, C. and Gelman, R. A. 1986. Percutaneous absorption of 7,10

^{14}C-benzo[a]pyrene and 7,12 ^{14}C-dimethylbenz[a]anthracene in mice. *J. Environ. Pathol. Toxicol. Oncol.* 7:25–34.

Sansone, G. and Reisner, R. M. 1971. Differential rates of conversion of testosterone to dihydrotestosterone in acne and in normal human skin—A possible pathogenic factor in acne. *J. Invest. Dermatol.* 56:366–372.

Sansone-Bazzono, G. and Reisner, R. M. 1974. Steroid pathways in sebaceous glands. *J. Invest. Dermatol.* 62:211–216.

Sato, K., Oda, T., Sugibayaski, K. and Morimoto, Y. 1988a. Estimation of blood concentration of drugs after topical application from *in vitro* skin permeation data. I. Prediction by convolution and confirmation by deconvolution. *Chem. Pharm. Bull. (Tokyo)* 36:2232–2238.

Sato, K., Oda, T., Sugibayashi, K. and Morimoto, Y. 1988b. Estimation of blood concentration of drugs after topical application from *in vitro* skin permeation data. II. Approach by using diffusion model and compartmental model. *Chem. Pharm. Bull. (Tokyo)* 36:2624–2632.

Sawaya, M. E., Honig, L. S., Garland, L. D. and Hsia, S. L. 1988. Δ^5-3β-Hydroxysteroid dehydrogenase activity in sebaceous glands of scalp in male-pattern baldness. *J. Invest. Dermatol.* 91:101–105.

Schaefer, H., Stuttgen, G., Zesch, A., Schalla, W. and Gazith, J. 1978. Quantitative determination of percutaneous absorption of radiolabelled drugs *in vitro* and *in vivo* by human skin. *Curr. Prob. Dermatol.* 7:80–94.

Schaefer, H., Zesch, A. and Stuttgen, G. 1982. *Skin Permeability*. New York: Springer-Verlag.

Scheuplein, R. J. 1967. Mechanism of percutaneous absorption. II. Transient diffusion and the relative importance of various routes of skin penetration. *J. Invest. Dermatol.* 48:79–88.

Scheuplein, R. J. and Blank, I. H. 1971. Permeability of the skin. *Physiol. Rev.* 51:702–747.

Scheuplein, R. J. and Bronaugh, R. L. 1983. Percutaneous absorption. In *Biochemistry and Physiology of the Skin*, vol. II, ed. L. A. Goldsmith, pp. 1255–1295. New York: Oxford University Press.

Scheuplein, R. J., Blank, I. H., Brauner, G. J. and MacFarlane, D. J. 1969. Percutaneous absorption of steroids. *J. Invest. Dermatol.* 52:63–70.

Schlede, E. and Conney, A. H. 1970. Induction of benzo[α]pyrene hydroxylase activity in rat skin. *Life Sci.* 9(part II):1295–1303.

Schroder, H. G., Ziegler, M., Nichisch, K., Kaufmann, J. and Fathy El Etreby, M. 1989. Effects of topically applied antiandrogenic compounds on sebaceous glands of hamster ears and flank organs. *J. Invest. Dermatol.* 92:769–773.

Shugart, L. R. and Kao, J. 1984. Effect of ellagic and caffeic acids on covalent binding of benzo[a]pyrene to epidermal DNA of mouse skin in organ culture. *Int. J. Biochem.* 16:571–573.

Siver, K. G. and Sloan, K. B. 1990. Alkylation of 6-mercaptopurine (6-MP) with *N*-alkyl-*N*-alkoxycarbonylaminomethyl chlorides: S^6-(*N*-Alkyl-*N*-alkoxycarbonyl)-aminomethyl-6-MP prodrug structure effect on the dermal delivery of 6-MP. *J. Pharm. Sci.* 79:66–73.

Sloan, K. B. and Bodor, N. 1982. Hydroxymethyl and acyloxymethyl prodrugs of theophylline: Enhanced delivery of polar drugs through skin. *Int. J. Pharm.* 12:299–313.

Smith, L. H. and Holland, J. M. 1981. Interaction between benzo[a]pyrene and mouse skin in organ culture. *Toxicology* 21:47–57.

Snyder, R. and Remmer, H. 1982. Classes of Hepatic Microsomal Mixed Function

Oxidase Inducers. In *Hepatic Cytochrome P_{450} Monooxygenase Systems*, eds. J. B. Schenkman and D. Kupfer, pp. 227–268. New York: Pergamon Press.

Spencer, T. S., Hill, J. A., Feldmann, R. J. and Maibach, H. I. 1979. Evaporation of diethyltoluamide from human skin *in vivo* and *in vitro*. *J. Invest. Dermatol.* 72:317–319.

Stehle, R. G., Ho, N. F. H., Barsuhn, C. L. and Stefanski, K. J. 1989. Local topical delivery of drugs: A model incorporating simultaneous diffusion and metabolic interconversion between drug and a single metabolite in the skin. *J. Theor. Biol.* 138:1–15.

Stevenson, I. H. and Dutton, G. J. 1960. Mechanism of glucuronide synthesis in skin. *Biochem. J.* 77:19P.

Stoughton, R. B. and Cornell, R. C. 1988. In *Topical Corticosteroid Therapy: A Novel Approach to Safer Drugs*, eds. E. Christophers, E. Schopf, A. M. Kligman and R. B. Stoughton, pp. 1–12. New York: Raven Press.

Tauber, U. and Rost, K. L. 1987. Esterase activity of the skin including species variations. In *Pharmacology and the Skin: Skin Pharmacokinetics*, eds. B. Shroot and H. Schaefer, pp. 170–182. Basel: Karger.

Thompson, S. and Slaga, T. J. 1976. Mouse epidermal aryl hydrocarbon hydroxylase. *J. Invest. Dermatol.* 66:108–111.

Tojo, K. 1987. Design and calibration of *in vitro* permeation apparatus. In *Drugs and the Pharmaceutical Sciences—Transdermal Controlled Systemic Medications*, ed. Y. W. Chien, pp. 127–158. New York: Marcel Dekker.

Torma, H. and Vahlquist, A. 1985. Biosynthesis of 3-dehydroretinol (vitamin A_2) from all-*trans*-retinol (vitamin A_1) in human epidermis. *J. Invest. Dermatol.* 85:498–500.

Torma, H. and Vahlquist, A. 1987. Retinol esterification by mouse epidermal microsomes: Evidence for acyl-CoA:retinol acyltransferase activity. *J. Invest. Dermatol.* 88:398–402.

Torma, H. and Vahlquist, A. 1990. Vitamin A esterification in human epidermis: A relation to keratinocyte differentiation. *J. Invest. Dermatol.* 94:132–138.

Torma, H., Brunnberg, L. and Vahlquist, A. 1987. Age-related variations in acyl-CoA:retinol acyltransferase activity and vitamin A concentration in the liver and epidermis of hairless mice. *Biochim. Biophys. Acta* 921:254–258.

Vahlquist, A. and Torma, H. 1988. Retinoids and keratinization: Current concepts. *Int. J. Dermatol.* 27:81–95.

vanHooidonk, C. 1979. Percutaneous absorption of toxic agents. II. The nerve gases and some other toxic organophosphates. A survey of the literature. Defense Technical Information Center Technical Report USAMIIA-K-9739.

Venot, A., Walter, E., Lecourtier, Y., Raksanyi, A. and Chauvelot-Moachon, L. 1987. Structural indentifiablity of "first-pass" models. *J. Pharmacokin. Biopharm.* 15:179–189.

Vermorken, A. J. M., Goos, C. M. A. A., Henderson, P. T. and Bloemendal, H. 1979a. Hydroxylation of dehydroepiandrosterone in human scalp hair follicles. *Br. J. Dermatol.* 100:693–698.

Vermorken, A. J. M., Goos, C. M. A. A., Roelofs, H. M. J., Henderson, P. T. and Bloemendal, H. 1979b. Metabolism of benzo[a]pyrene in isolated scalp hair follicles. *Toxicology* 14:109–116.

Vermorken, A. J. M., Weterings, P. J. J. M., Spierenburg, G. T., van Bennekom, C. A., Wirtz, P., deBruyn, C. H. M. M. and Oei, T. L. 1978. Fabry's disease: Biochemical and histochemical studies on hair roots for carrier detection. *Br. J. Dermatol.* 98:191–196.

Vizethum, W., Ruzicka, T. and Goerz, G. 1980. Inducibility of drug-metabolism enzymes in rat skin. *Chem.-Biol. Interact.* 31:215–219.

Wattenberg, L. W. and Leong, J. L. 1970. Benzpyrene hydroxylase activity in mouse skin. *Proc. Am. Assoc. Cancer Res.* 11:81.

Weinstock, M. and Wilgram, G. F. 1970. Fine-structural observations on the formation and enzymatic activity of keratinosomes in mouse tongue filiform papillae. *J. Ultrastruct. Res.* 30:262–274.

Wester, R. C. and Maibach, H. I. 1977. Percutaneous absorption in man and animal: A perspective. In *Cutaneous Toxicity,* eds. V. A. Drill and P. Lazar, pp. 111–126. New York: Academic Press.

Wester, R. C., Noonan, P. K., Smeach, S. and Kosobud, L. 1983. Pharmacokinetics and bioavailability of intravenous and topical nitroglycerin in the rhesus monkey: Estimate of percutaneous first-pass metabolism. *J. Pharm. Sci.* 72:745–748.

Weston, A., Grover, P. L. and Sims, P. 1982. Metabolism and activation of benzo[a]pyrene by mouse and rat skin in short-term organ culture and *in vivo. Chem.-Biol. Interact.* 31:233–250.

Wiebel, F. J., Leutz, J. C. and Gelboin, H. V. 1975. Aryl hydrocarbon (benzo[a]pyrene) hydroxylase: A mixed-function oxygenase in mouse skin. *J. Invest. Dermatol.* 64:184–189.

Williams, M. L., Brown, B. E., Monger, D. J., Grayson, S. and Elias, P. M. 1988. Lipid content and metabolism of human keratinocyte cultures grown at the air-medium interface. *J. Cell. Physiol.* 136:103–110.

Williams, P. L. and Riviere, J. E. 1989a. Definition of a physiologic pharmacokinetic model of cutaneous drug distribution using the isolated perfused porcine skin flap (IPPSF). *J. Pharm. Sci.* 78:550–555.

Williams, P. L. and Riviere, J. E. 1989b. Estimation of physiological volumes in the isolated perfused porcine skin flap. *Res. Commun. Chem. Pathol. Pharmacol.* 66:145–158.

Williams, P. L., Carver, M. P. and Riviere, J. E. 1990. A physiologically relevant pharmacokinetic model of xenobiotic percutaneous absorption utilizing the isolated perfused porcine skin flap (IPPSF). *J. Pharm. Sci.* 79:305–311.

Winkelmann, R. K. 1966. Technique of dermal perfusion. *J. Invest. Dermatol.* 46:220–223.

Wojciechowski, Z. J., Burton, S. A., Petelenz, T. J. and Krueger, G. G. 1985. Role of microcirculation in percutaneous absorption. *Clin. Res.* 33:696A.

Wojciechowski, Z., Pershing, L. K., Huether, S., Leonard, L., Burton, S. A., Higuchi, W. I. and Krueger, G. G. 1987. An experimental skin sandwich flap on an independent vascular supply for the study of percutaneous absorption. *J. Invest. Dermatol.* 88:439–446.

Wolf, C. R. 1986. Cytochrome P-450s: Polymorphic multigene familes involved in carcinogen activation. *Trends Genetics* Aug.:209–214.

Wolff, T., Deml, E. and Wanders, H. 1979. Aldrin epoxidation, a highly sensitive indicator specific for cytochrome P-450-dependent mono-oxygenase activities. *Drug Metab. Dispos.* 7:301–305.

Wolff, T., Greim, H., Huang, M.-T., Miwa, G. T. and Lu, A. Y. H. 1980. Aldrin epoxidation catalyzed by purified rat-liver cytochromes P-450 and P-448. High selectivity for cytochrome P-450. *Eur. J. Biochem.* 111:545–551.

Wood, A. W., Ryan, D. E., Thomas, P. E. and Levin, W. 1983. Regio- and stereoselective metabolism of two C_{19} steroids by five highly purified and reconstituted rat hepatic cytochrome P-450 isozymes. *J. Biol. Chem.* 258:8839–8847.

Yu, C.-D., Fox, J. L., Ho, N. F. H. and Higuchi, W. I. 1979a. Physical model evaluation of topical prodrug delivery—Simultaneous transport and bioconversion of vidarabine-5'-valerate I: Physical model development. *J. Pharm. Sci.* 68:1341–1346.

Yu, C.-D., Fox, J. L., Ho, N. F. H. and Higuchi, W. I. 1979b. Physical model evaluation of topical prodrug delivery—Simultaneous transport and bioconversion of vidarabine-5'-valerate II: Parameter determinations. *J. Pharm. Sci.* 68:1347–1357.

Zatz, J. L. 1985. Percutaneous absorption. Computer simulation using multicompartmented membrane models. In *Percutaneous Absorption: Mechanisms—Methodology—Drug Delivery,* eds. R. L. Bronaugh and H. I. Maibach, pp. 165–181. New York: Marcel Dekker.

Zesch, A., Schaefer, H. and Stuttgen, G. 1979. The quantitative distribution of percutaneously applied caffeine in the human skin. *Arch. Dermatol. Res.* 266:277–283.

Zierler, K. 1981. A critique of compartmental analysis. *Annu. Rev. Biophys. Bioeng.* 10:531–562.

10

predictive skin irritation tests in animals and humans

■ **Esther Patrick** ■ **Howard I. Maibach** ■

Many authors have defined skin irritation by exclusion: chemically induced skin inflammation not produced by activated T lymphocytes or antibodies. This definition does not reflect the range of skin damage and change in function that have been categorized as skin irritation. Indeed, defining irritation reactions is similar to the proverbial blind men and the elephant. The definition depends on which aspect of skin change you are considering! While the blind men dealt with walls, tree trunks, or ropes, the skin toxicologist deals with tissue destruction, erythema and edema, changes in surface characteristics, and occasionally changes in anatomy and physiology. Like the elephant the true form(s) of skin irritation remains elusive although many aspects have been studied. In attempting to describe how to conduct predictive tests for skin irritation one must always define which aspect of irritation is under consideration.

Irritation tests are conducted for a variety of reasons. A single contact with some chemicals may result in acute inflammation and in some cases skin necrosis at the application site. Chemicals producing necrosis are termed corrosive. Animal tests mandated by regulatory agencies are routinely used to screen materials for their capability to produce acute irritation and corrosion. Since only a small area of skin need be tested, acute irritation assays can also be performed in humans provided systemic toxicity (from absorption through the skin) is low and informed consent is obtained. One should approach testing in humans cautiously; new materials and those of unknown or unfamiliar composition should be tested on animal skin first to determine if application to humans is warranted [National Academy of Science, (NAS), 1977] and testing should be conducted in stepwise fashion, with short exposure period and open application tests being conducted first.

Chemicals that do not produce acute irritation from a single irritation may produce inflammation following repeated application to the skin. This type of response is often described as cumulative irritation. Many consumer product companies and others interested in predictive testing have developed animal assays for ranking materials within selected product classes. However, cumulative irritation is most often evaluated in humans. The patch test is often thought of as the test for irritation; however, investigators have employed a variety of exaggerated exposure tests in animals and in humans. A few have also used human usage tests in small populations to detect differences in irritancy potential of materials under conditions similar to normal use.

Assays evaluating the capacity of chemicals to produce acute irritation and corrosion differ extensively from those used to predict cumulative irritation. A few of the published procedures are described here. For ease of organization, animal assays are presented first followed by human assays. Tests for acute irritation (and corrosion in animals) are presented first in sections on animal and human assays. The final section deals with factors affecting skin irritation potential that may be manipulated to develop more sensitive assays.

ANIMAL TESTS FOR PREDICTING IRRITATION

Primary irritation and corrosion are usually evaluated by modifications of the method described by John Draize and his colleagues (1944). Although the test was widely used in the late 1940s and 1950s it was not mandated by regulatory agencies until enactment of the Federal Hazardous Substance Act (FHSA).

In the test described under the FHSA, materials to be tested are applied to two 1-in square sites of skin on the back of albino rabbits. The test is usually performed on six animals. One site is abraded prior to applying the test material and one is tested intact. Abrasion of the site is accomplished in such a way that while the stratum corneum is opened, no bleeding is produced. Typically, abrasions are produced by drawing a hypodermic needle across the skin repeatedly or an instrument such as the Berkely Scarifier or Maryland Plastics skin abrader (Haley and Hunziger, 1974) is used. Liquids are tested undiluted by applying 0.5 ml to each test area. For solids 0.5 g of material is applied to moistened skin or an equal volume of solvent is applied to moisten the material. Each test site is covered with two layers of 1-in square surgical gauze secured in place with tape. The entire trunk of the animal is then wrapped with rubberized cloth or other occlusive impervious material to retard evaporation of the material and protect the patches from the animal. Twenty-four hours after application the wrappings are removed and the test sites are evaluated for erythema and edema using the scale described in Table 1. Evaluations for intact and abraded sites are recorded separately. Test sites are evaluated again 48 h later. If severe reactions

TABLE 1. Grading Scale Typically Used in Performing Draize Type Tests in Albino Rabbits[a]

Description	Score assigned
Erythema and eschar formation	
No erythema	0
Very slight erythema (barely perceptible)	1
Well-defined erythema	2
Moderate to severe erythema	3
Severe erythema (beet redness) to slight eschar formations (injuries in depth)	4
Edema formation	
No edema	0
Very slight edema (barely perceptible)	1
Slight edema (edges of area well defined by definite raising)	2
Moderate edema (raised approximately 1 mm)	3
Severe edema (raised more than 1 mm and extending beyond the area of exposure)	4

[a]The scale as defined by Draize and adopted by various regulatory agencies.
Note: The PII (primary irritation index) is calculated by averaging the erythema values and averaging the edema values then combining the averages (maximum PII = 8).

were noted, delayed observations are also made, usually on day 7 or 14. Additional observations through 35 days may be made in order to determine if scarring develops. Some investigators have supplemented visual evaluations of skin damage with histologic evaluation of the tissue (Mezei et al., 1966; Landsdown, 1972; Ingram and Grasso, 1975; Murphy et al., 1979). Use of biochemical techniques or radiolabeled tracers to monitor healing has been reported (Mezei et al., 1966; Mezei, 1970), but on an experimental basis, not as components of routine tests.

Results of the tests are usually presented in tabular form showing the erythema and edema responses for each animal, and the Primary Irritation Index (PII) is calculated. The PII values are calculated by averaging values for erythema from all sites (abraded and nonabraded), averaging the values for edema from all sites, and adding the average values. Agents producing PII of < 2 are considered only mildly irritating, 2–5 moderately irritating, and > 5 severely irritating. Materials that produce a PII of greater than 5 require precautionary labeling.

This test varies somewhat from the original method described by Draize. In the original assay four materials were evaluated on six animals with three intact and three abraded sites exposed to each material. Other variations of this method are currently required by the Department of Transportation [Code of Federal Regulations (CFR), 1989b], Environmental Protection Agency (CFR, 1989a), and the Consumer Product Safety Committee by administration of the FHSA (CFR, 1989c). The basic exposure has been further modified by the

Organization for Economic Cooperation and Development to test for corrosion alone (OECD, 1981). Under a directive of the European Economic Community (1983), a 3-min exposure was added in which the sites were not wrapped. The United Nations recommendations for the Transport of Dangerous Goods is based on exposure times of 4 h, 1 h and 2 min; the 1-h assay is usually performed first. Evaluations are made 1 h after application and again at 24, 48, and 72 h and 7 days after dosing. The variations on the method differ principally in the number of animals tested, the length of exposure, and whether some sites are abraded. Recently one group of investigators developed a composite test protocol that incorporated several tests required by different agencies (Cruzan et al., 1986). The differences in tests required by some agencies are summarized in Table 2. The method of applying materials and evaluation of the responses are similar for all Draize type procedures.

The reproducibility of the FHSA procedure (Weil and Scala, 1971) and the relevance of test results to human experience (Edwards, 1972; Nixon et al., 1975; MacMillan et al., 1975; Guillot et al., 1962) have been questioned, and numerous modifications to the procedure have been proposed to improve its prediction of human experience. Modifications that have been proposed include changing the preferred species, reduction of the exposure period, use of fewer animals, and testing on intact skin only (Edwards, 1972; Nixon et al., 1975; Griffith and Buehler, 1976; Motoyoshi et al., 1979). It should be noted that the method has generally erred on the side of safety in that it overpredicts the severity of skin damage produced by chemicals, thus providing a safety factor for those exposed. One criticism that is often repeated is that the test is not sensitive enough to separate mild from moderate irritants. In fairness to the developer one should remember that the purpose was to identify chemicals that posed a severe hazard to the public, not to compare products. Criticisms of the Draize test have been embraced by groups supporting abolition of animal testing as demonstrating that use of the method is unwarranted. *This overlooks the tremendous value of the test in warning consumers, workers, and manufacturers of potential dangers associated with specific chemicals so that appropriate precautions could be taken.* While Draize-type tests may be replaced by *in vitro* assays at some time in the future, they are currently recommended by regulatory agencies and have served society well for over 40 years. We have no validated *in vitro* substitute at present.

In order to distinguish between mild and moderate irritants in an acute exposure test, Finkelstein and his colleagues (1963, 1965) used pretreatment of test sites with an irritant and enhanced visualization of the response by injection of trypan blue in order to increase test sensitivity. The technique was performed in anesthetized rabbits, rats, or guinea pigs. A circular area of the shaved abdomen was painted with a 20% solution of formaldehyde that was allowed to dry for 5 min. This was repeated three times and then 1-in cotton flannel pads were saturated with test material and applied to each site. A control substance of known irritancy was tested in each study. Pads were secured in place and the

TABLE 2. Comparison of Skin Irritation Tests Based on Draize Method

	Draize	DOT	FHSA	OECD
Abrasion	Intact/abraded	Intact	Intact/abraded	Intact
Occlusion	Rubberized cloth	Yes	Impervious material	Semiocclusive
Exposure period	24 h	4 h	24 h	4 h
Examined at	24 and 72 h	4 and 48 h	24 and 72 h	0.5, 1, 24, 48, 72 h
Labeling criteria	—	Corrosion	PII $\geq$ 5	Narrative/corrosion

entire trunk was wrapped in polyethylene. A solution of trypan blue was injected into subcutaneous tissue away from the dosages sites. The dye was absorbed and served as a marker for plasma leakage because it spontaneously binds to albumin. After 16 h, patches were removed and the degree of bluing at each site was evaluated on a 0–100% scale. In light of more recent work comparing the reactivity of dorsal and abdominal animal skin (Vinegar, 1979), one wonders if the enhanced sensitivity was due in part to choice of test site.

A few tests in which material is not applied topically have been developed claiming to evaluate the intrinsic irritancy of test materials. The persistence of edema in the skin of depilated juvenile white mice following intracutaneous injection of solutions has been used to assess local irritation (Bucher et al., 1981; Walz, 1985). The number of wrinkles observed on reefing the skin with thin pinchers is counted before and at selected time points through 6 h after injection of 0.01 ml test solution. Although the number of test animals has varied between 8 and 25, the developers considered 20–25 to be optimal. An obvious limitation of this method is that materials must be administered as isosmotic solutions, which requires substantial pretest formulation. Although the developers claim this procedure has good predictive power for eye, skin, and mucosal irritation, it has not been adopted extensively.

Justice et al. (1961) described a repeat animal patch (RAP) test for comparing irritation potential of surfactants. Solutions were applied to the clipped back of immobilized albino mice with a saturated cotton-tipped applicator. The test site was covered with rubber dam to prevent evaporation. This process was repeated seven times at 10-min intervals. The skins were evaluated microscopically for epidermal erosion.

Brown (1971) used both open and closed exposures to rank surfactants for skin irritation potential. Tests ranged from 6 h patch exposures each day for 3 consecutive days in rabbits to daily open application to the skin of rabbits, guinea pigs, or hairless mice for up to 4 1/2 weeks. Good agreement among the test methods was not obtained and none of the methods gained wide acceptance, although they are similar to techniques developed by others later.

Repeat application patch tests in which diluted materials are applied to the same site each day for 15–21 days have been used to rank products for their irritant potential. While use of several species was investigated, the guinea pig and rabbit are used most often (Phillips et al., 1972; Steinberg et al., 1975). Patches used vary considerably, with Draize-type gauze dressings and Duhring metal chambers being the extremes. Since the degree of occlusion is an important determinant of percutaneous penetration, the choice of covering material may influence the sensitivity of a given test. A reference material of similar use or which produces a known effect in humans is usually included in the test. The cumulative irritancy assay in rabbits (Marzulli and Maibach, 1975) utilizes open applications and control reference compounds. The degrees of inflammation produced by the materials are compared by visual inspection and measurement of swelling with a skinfold thickness caliper. Test sites may be evaluated using either the scales for erythema and edema used for Draize-type tests or more descriptive scales developed by the investigator.

A 5-day dermal irritation test in rabbits was used to compare consumer products of various types (MacMillan et al., 1975). After shaving the animals' backs 0.5 ml of test materials was spread over a 5 by 4.5 cm area of skin. The test sites were protected from grooming by placing the animal in a leather harness or Elizabethan collar. After 4 h, sites were cleaned and graded using the Draize scoring system. This procedure was repeated each day for 5 days. The authors showed good agreement between this assay and 21-day human patch tests of liquid detergents, afterbath colognes, and hair preparations. The technique was less satisfactory for other types of materials.

The guinea pig immersion assay was developed to evaluate the irritancy of aqueous detergent solutions and other surfactant-based products (Opdyke and Burnett, 1965; Calandra, 1971; Opdyke, 1971; MacMillan et al., 1975). Ten guinea pigs are placed in restraining devices and immersed in a 40°C test solution for 4 h. The apparatus is designed to maintain the guinea pig's head above the solution. Immersion is repeated daily for 3 days. Concentration of test material is usually below 10% to limit systemic toxicity. Only materials of limited toxic potential are suitable for this assay because systemic absorption of a lethal dose is possible. A second group of animals is usually tested with a reference material for comparison to the material of interest. Twenty-four hours after the final immersion, the flank is shaved and the skin is evaluated for erythema, edema, and fissures using the scale presented as Table 3. A photographic grading scale for this assay was presented in MacMillan et al. (1975).

An open application procedure in guinea pigs uses microscopic examination of skin biopsies of sites treated with weak irritants to rank materials. (Anderson et al., 1986). Biopsies are taken after three daily applications of 10% solvent or 5% aqueous test solutions to 1-cm^2 areas of the shaved flank. Sites were evaluated visually for erythema and edema, and microscopically, three histologic sections were stained with May-Grunward-Giemsa under oil immersion, for epidermal thickness and dermal infiltration. A composite score reflecting the macroscopic evaluation, the number of applications before development of visible response, the epidermal thickness, and the cellular response was used to rank chemicals. While this method provides information on pathogenesis of the response to each chemical, the extensive processing may limit its application to special studies.

Uttley and Van Abbe (1973) developed a mouse ear test in which undiluted shampoos were applied to one ear of mice daily for 4 days. The degree of inflammation was evaluated visually and the degree of inflammation produced by materials of interest was compared to that produced by reference materials tested on other groups of mice. One confounding factor with this assay may be the use of anesthetics, which may alter development of inflammation, to facilitate performance of the procedure.

TABLE 3. Grading Scale for the Guinea Pig Immersion Test

Number	Indication
10	Normal skin
9	First signs of scattered scaling
8	Moderate scaling
7	Scurfing over entire abdomen, capillaries not visible, slight loss in elasticity
6	Flank skin drawn, severe scurfing
5	Flank skin drawn, severe scurfing with cracking and fissuring
4	Dehydration evident, animal constricted
3	Dehydration evident, bleeding evident
2	Eschar formation(s)
1	Death

Source: Opdyke and Burnett, 1965.

We have used an assay in which dilute solutions of surfactants and other chemicals are applied to one ear of 5 or 6 mice each day for 4 days (Patrick and Maibach, 1987). Ear thickness was measured at various time points after each treatment to quantify the degree of inflammation. Multiple groups (at least four) were compared using different doses of test material that produced a 50% maximum response following a single treatment. The slope of the dose-response lines was also used to compare chemicals. Pretreating the ear with croton oil or 12-*O*-tetradecanoylphorbol 13-acetate 72 h before application of the material of interest increased the sensitivity of the assay. While the procedure was useful for most surfactant-based products, it was not suitable for oily and highly perfumed materials since animals attempt to remove the materials by grooming. Moloney and Teal (1988) also used ear thickness to quantify inflammatory changes produced by *n*-alkanes applied to ears of mice. They dosed animals twice per day for 4 days in order to produce inflammation.

The principles of general toxicology should be remembered when one designs and interprets any animal (and human) assay for skin irritation. One should consider dose-response relationships. Draize scores require careful interpretation; they are best interpreted by comparison to related compounds or formulations with a history of human exposure. Knowledge of intended human use (and foreseeable uses) permits more rational interpretation. With occlusive application techniques, one should remember that occlusion increases the permeability of some but not all moieties. Although there is a consistent, reasonably good correlation between responses in rabbits and humans, occasional inconsistencies have occurred. Wise investigators conduct carefully planned and executed tests in humans when rabbit tests indicate materials may be irritants. One should follow the guidelines of the NAS committee (1977) when this course of action is followed.

HUMAN TESTS FOR PREDICTING IRRITATION

Draize et al. (1944) suggested that after screening materials in animals the irritant potential of materials should be evaluated in humans. They outlined a procedure for a human 24-h patch test. Many variations of single application patch tests have been developed. The procedure outlined by an advisory committee of the National Academy of Sciences (NAS, 1977) is summarized here. Because of the risk of human injury, tests in humans should be performed under the supervision of individuals who have extensive experience in human skin testing, and informed consent must be obtained. Tests are conducted on normal, nondiseased skin. Test site is either the intrascapular region of the back or the dorsal surface of the upper arm(s). Multiple materials can be tested simultaneously, up to 10 on the back or four on each arm. Because of the variability in human responses each test usually includes one reference material. In order to minimize risk to the subjects, it is desirable to first test new materials and volatiles using short exposure periods, 30 min to 1 h, with no covering being applied ("open" patch).

For routine use a 4-h exposure was suggested by the NAS panel. Although materials may be tested as described for the Draize-type test, it may be desirable to test dilutions of new materials and unknowns. If the test is intended to supplement Draize-type animal studies, 1-inch gauze squares can be used with the same amount of material applied as in the animal study. Commercial patches, chambers, gauze squares, or cotton bandage material such as Webril may be used. If commercial patches/devices are used, the volume of test material may need to be adjusted. Pads of these devices should be saturated with liquid, and a sufficient amount of solid/slurry should be used to cover the surface of the pad. Because of variations in patch size, it is helpful to express the dose in the form of mg/cm^2 and to report both the area of exposure and amount of material applied. Patches are secured in place with surgical tape without wrapping the trunk or arm. The degree of occlusion of the patch/device and of the surgical tape will affect the degree of irritation that develops. Increasing the degree of occlusion by use of Duhring or Hilltop Chambers or occlusive tapes such as Blenderm will generally increase the severity of the response. When volatiles are tested under patch conditions (after screening in an open application test), a relatively nonocclusive tape should be used.

After the desired period of exposure, test patches/devices are removed and the area is rinsed with water to remove any residue. Because some tapes may produce skin damage that could be falsely attributed to the test material, test sites are marked to facilitate locating treatment sites for evaluation. Evaluation of the response is usually deferred for 30 min to 1 h after patch removal to allow hydration and pressure effects of the patch to subside. Test sites are reevaluated 24 h after patch removal. The dual scale used to evaluate Draize-type animal tests (Table 1) can also be used for grading human skin responses. Since this scale does not include papular, vesicular, or bullous responses, integrated scales ranging from four to 16 points have been proposed. An example of such scales is presented in Table 4. Typically, scores from all subjects are averaged for each material, and intensities of responses to test materials are compared to a reference material. Although a few investigators have used abrasion in acute irritation tests involving humans (Nixon et al., 1975), it is not recommended as a routine procedure with undiluted materials. There is a possibility of scarring, and the human data base is limited so that extrapolation to use situations is difficult.

Single-application patch tests are also used to rank materials for their irritation potential, especially dilute solutions of commercial products. While many investigators have adopted 24-h exposures, others have customized the length of exposure, concentration tested, and evaluation schedule for tests on specific classes of products. These modifications may increase the capacity of

TABLE 4. Human Patch Test Grading Scales

Number	Indication
	Detailed
0	No apparent cutaneous involvement
1/2	Faint, barely perceptible erythema or slight dryness (glazed appearance)
1	Faint but definite erythema, no eruptions or broken skin, OR no erythema but definite dryness; may have epidermal fissuring
1 1/2	Well-defined erythema or faint erythema with definite dryness; may have epidermal fissuring
2	Moderate erythema, may have a few papules or deep fissures, moderate to severe erythema in the cracks
2 1/2	Moderate erythema with barely perceptible edema OR severe erythema not involving a significant portion of the patch (halo effect around the edges), may have a few papules OR moderate to severe erythema
3	Severe erythema (beet redness), may have generalized papules OR moderate to severe erythema with slight edema (edges well defined by raising)
3 1/2	Moderate to severe erythema with moderate edema (confined to patch area) OR moderate to severe erythema with isolated eschar formations or vesicles
4	Generalized vesicles or eschar formations OR moderate to severe erythema and/or edema extending beyond the area of the patch
	Simple
0	Negative, normal skin
±	Questionable erythema not covering entire area
1	Definite erythema
2	Erythema and induration
3	Vesiculation
4	Bullous reaction

the assay to detect differences in the irritancy potential of milder products. Wooding and Opdyke (1967) investigated the effects of modifying some test parameters on intensity of response. Intensity of inflammation has been shown to increase after patch removal in some cases (Dahl and Trancik, 1977; Rietschell, 1982). Kooyman and Snyder (1942) used a 6-h exposure to 8% solutions of bar soaps and evaluated test sites 24-h after patch application. Griffith et al. (1969) reported using single application patch tests with exposures of less than 24 h to evaluate laundry detergents containing enzymes. Justice et al. (1961) varied exposure time between 18 and 24 h to test bar soaps, liquid detergents, and laundry detergents. Others have suggested that a 48-h patch exposure is more suitable for some products (Rostenberg, 1961).

Patch test responses generally heal rapidly, within a week or so. More severe reactions should be evaluated periodically over a longer period to determine how the inflammatory response is resolved. Some subjects may develop changes in pigmentation level at the test site following severe responses.

Shelanski (1951) observed that during the induction phase of sensitization tests some chemicals produced inflammation, although no response to the initial patch and challenge patches was observed. He coined the phrase "skin fatigue," but secondary irritation and cumulative irritation also refer to the same phenomenon. Because of the conditions of the original observation most repeat application patch tests were patterned after human sensitization studies using 24-h exposures, with or without a rest period between patches. Kligman and Wooding (1967) proposed that statistical analyses be applied to repeated application patch tests. They applied the Litchfield and Wilcoxon probit analysis and calculated IT50 (time to produce irritation in 50% of the subjects) and ID50 (dose required to produce irritation in 50% of the subjects after a 24-hour exposure). Their early work formed the basis for the 21-day cumulative irritation assay that is widely used.

The cumulative irritation assay as described by Lanman and his co-workers (1968) was developed to identify components of products producing adverse reactions in consumers. The test was developed to screen new formulas prior to marketing. In the original assay a 1-in square of Webril was saturated with liquid test material or the surface was covered with viscous substances. After application to the upper back, patches were sealed in place with occlusive tape. After a 24-h exposure period patches were removed, the test sites were evaluated, and a fresh set of patches was applied. Although their work was patterned after tests described by Kligman and Wooding (1967), they increased the number of applications from 10 to 21 and the number of subjects to 24. These modifications were needed because of the low level of response normally produced by antiperspirants/deodorants and bath oils. The number of applications required to produce inflammation was estimated using the IT50 method of Kligman and Wooding. Some investigators have also varied the interval between application of fresh patches (Rapaport et al., 1978) and other data evaluation schemes have been proposed (Rapaport et al., 1978; Berger and Bowman,

1982; Carabello, 1985). The assay described by Lanman et al. (1968) came to be known as the 21-day cumulative irritation assay, though in fact they varied the number of applications depending on the type of materials being tested, 21 applications being the maximum number used for antiperspirants and bath oils. Other investigators have recently reconfirmed that fewer applications are sufficient for surfactant-based products (Bowman and Berger, 1982; Carabello, 1985).

Numerous other repeated application patching schedules have been used successfully for comparing commercial products. Finkelstein et al. (1963, 1965) described tests utilizing one of two patching schedules, a 5–6 or a 17–18 h exposure each day for 4 days. Test sites were evaluated 1-h after patch removal. Modifications of this procedure have also been used to evaluate shaving creams and toilet soaps (Smiles and Pollack, 1977).

After observing that conventional repeated application patch tests failed to predict adverse reactions to many consumer products, Frosch and Kligman (1979) reasoned that there were intrinsic differences in reactivity of normal skin, damaged skin, and sensitive skin. The chamber scarification test was developed to evaluate materials that would normally be applied to damaged tissue. Because of the clinical observation that certain individuals were more sensitive than others, subjects were prescreened to identify sensitive individuals. Light-skinned Caucasians who developed severe erythema with edema and vesicles following a 24-h exposure to 5% sodium lauryl sulfate applied via Duhring chambers to the inner forearm were selected as test subjects. Six to eight 10-mm^2 areas on the volar forearm were scarified with eight criss-cross scratches made with a 30-gauge needle. In scarifying the tissue, the bevel of the needle is held to the side and the needle is drawn across the skin with enough pressure to scratch the epidermis without drawing blood. Four scratches are parallel, with another four at right angles. After scarification, Duhring chambers containing the test material, 0.1 g of ointments, creams, or powders, or a fitted pad saturated with 0.1 ml of liquid are placed over the scarified area. In some cases identical sets of test materials are applied to intact skin as well as to abraded areas. Chambers are held in place by wrapping the forearm with non-occlusive tape. Chambers containing fresh solutions of test materials are applied to the same sites each day for 3 days. Thirty minutes after removal of the last set of chambers test sites are evaluated using the scale described in Table 5. The grades are averaged and irritation potential of materials producing average responses of 0–0.4 is considered low, responses of 0.5–1.4 are considered as slight, 1.5–2.4 moderate, and 2.5 severe. If both normal and scarified skin has been tested, results can also be expressed as the scarification index, the scores of scarified sites divided by scores from intact skin. The scarification index is used to estimate the relative risk for damaged and normal tissue. Published results using this assay have been limited. The appropriateness of extrapolation to predicting responses during routine use has not been established.

Although bar soaps produce erythema when tested by conventional patch

TABLE 5. Grading Scale for the Chamber Scarification Test

Number	Indication
0	Scratch marks barely perceptible
1	Erythema confined to scratches
2	Broader bands of erythema with or without rows of vesicles, pustules, or erosions
3	Severe erythema with partial confluency with or without other lesions
4	Confluent, severe erythema sometimes with edema, necrosis, or bulla

Source: Frosch and Kligman, 1976. "The chamber scarification test for irritancy." *Contact Dermatitis* 2:314–324. Reproduced by permission. Copyright Munksgaard International Publishers.

test techniques, the typical clinical response is dryness and flaking, sometimes with erythema and fissuring. Frosch and Kligman (1979) developed the soap chamber test to compare the "chapping" potential of bar soaps. Sensitive subjects were preselected as described for the chamber scarification test or by ammonium hydroxide blistering time (Frosch and Kligman, 1982). Duhring chambers fitted with Webril pads are used to apply 0.1 ml of an 8% solution of soap to the forearm. Chambers are secured in place by encircling the arm with porous tape. Patch contact time is 24 h for day 1 (Monday) and 6 h each day for the next 4 days (Tuesday through Friday). Test sites are monitored each day before application of fresh solutions. If severe erythema is noted, dosing is discontinued. Unless treatment was discontinued before the fifth exposure, skin reactions are evaluated on day 8 (Monday) using the scales listed in Table 6. This test showed good agreement with skin washing procedures but overpredicted irritant responses to some materials (Frosch, 1982).

While patch tests have been useful in detecting differences in the irritation potential of some materials, they have overpredicted differences in some cases, that is, differences that were predicted were not apparent when the materials were used by consumers. Various exaggerated exposure tests have been developed to bridge the gap between responses occurring during product use and patch tests. Perhaps the oldest nonpatch irritancy test still in use is the arm immersion technique (Kooyman and Snyder, 1942), in which the relative irritancy of two soap or detergent products is compared. As originally described, soap solutions of up to 3% were prepared in troughs. Temperature was maintained at 105 °F while subjects immersed one hand and arm to just above the elbow in one test solution and the other arm in a solution containing a second product. The period of exposure varied between 10 and 15 min three times each day for 5 days or until observable irritation was produced on both arms. In most persons the first sign of irritation was erythema of the anticubital surface of the arm (Kooyman and Snyder, 1942; Justice et al., 1961). Later the hands developed dryness and cracking. These observations led to the development of separate assays on the anticubital area and the hands.

Numerous versions of the anticubital washing test, also known as flex

TABLE 6. Grading Scale for the Soap Chamber Test[a]

	Erythema
1	Slight, spotty, or diffuse
2	Moderate, uniform redness
3	Intense
4	Firey red with edema or epidermal defect (vesicles or necrosis)
	Scaling
1	"Shiny" dryness
2	Fine scales
3	Moderate
4	Severe with large flakes
	Fissures
1	Fine cracks
2	Single or multiple broader fissures
3	Wide cracks with hemorrhage

[a]Exposure is discontinued when grade 4 erythema is reached. Maximal scores for each parameter are assigned for the final evaluation if treatment was discontinued.
    Source: Frosch and Kligman, 1979. "The soap chamber test. A new method for assessing the irritancy of soaps." *J. American Acad. Dermatol.* 1:35–41. Adapted by permission.

washing tests and elbow crease washing tests, have been used. Published methods compare two products; however, dosing regimes differ somewhat. Investigators have used two (Frosch, 1982) or three (Griffith et al., 1969) washing procedures per day, and some specify that lather is allowed to remain on the skin for a brief period. Erythema and edema are evaluated as end points in all studies. Frosch (1982) used a similar procedure on the cheeks to evaluate toilet soaps. Simple 1–4 (i.e., slight, moderate, severe, and very severe) grading scores are used to evaluate the severity of the response. Products can be compared in terms of the average grades or the number of washes required to produce an effect. Some investigators have tested up to four samples per forearm by washing in glass cylinders, then rinsing the area (Imokowa et al., 1975).

At least two types of hand immersion procedures have been used. On a small scale (i.e., 10 subjects), relatively concentrated solutions, up to 2%, of two materials are tested. Up to four hand dishwashing products have been compared at near use concentration in studies on 64 subjects using a Latin square dosing pattern (E. A. Bannan, personal communication, 1975). Exposure conditions have varied from two or three 10–15 min immersions each day (Griffith et al., 1969) to a single 30-min exposure each day (E. A. Bannan, personal communication, 1975). Grading scales for this type of assay focus on scaling and cracking as well as erythema.

Evaluation of skin condition before and after use in the home has also been used to compare the irritation potential of various products. These tests represent skin tolerance studies, since either irritation or allergy could be detected. The clinical method published by Johnson et al. (1953) has been varied to include tests of bar soaps, laundry soaps and detergents, and dishwashing detergents. Essentially the method is a double-blind crossover study with 2-week usage periods (Carter and Griffith, 1965). Skin condition is evaluated by a dermatologist before the study and after use of each product. Magnification of the area is used to facilitate grading using a 0–10 scale. Tests are conducted using large panels, >300 housewives per product, and up to eight materials can be evaluated simultaneously using a Latin square design. The principles in conducting this type of large scale usage study have been applied to laundry presoaks for diapers and bar soaps used in infants (Griffith et al., 1969; Ellickson and Jungermann, 1967) and to fabric softeners in adult populations (Weaver, 1976).

Irritant response to chemicals may include changes in transepidermal water loss (TEWL), changes in electrical impedance of the skin, changes in carbon dioxide emission, and changes in electrolyte flux through the skin. Measurements of these biophysical parameters of skin function have been proposed as adjuncts to visual evaluations of the inflammatory response (Malten and Thiele, 1973a, 1973b; Thiele and Malten, 1973a, 1973b; Wilhelm et al., 1989). Changes in TWEL and electrical resistance have been detected before inflammatory changes are apparent. These techniques compare the irritancy potential of soaps tested at near use levels (Hassing et al., 1982). One unique way of evaluating irritancy uses *in vivo* measurements of the water-binding capacity of the stratum corneum after occlusion (Berardesca and Maibach, 1989). In most cases investigators constructed their own instruments to perform these measurements. As availability of commercial instruments increases, assessment of the biophysical changes in skin is expected to be an important component of predictive irritation testing.

FACTORS INFLUENCING THE DEVELOPMENT
OF SKIN IRRITATION

Many factors have been shown to be related to the development of skin irritation. These factors have been classified as extrinsic or intrinsic (Mathias, 1987; Mathias and Maibach, 1978). Extrinsic factors were defined as factors that influence the capacity of the chemical to penetrate the skin, generally conditions of exposure, while intrinsic factors are those constitutional factors that determine individual (human or animal) susceptibility to the irritant. Some of the factors shown experimentally to be important in predictive testing for skin irritation are shown in Table 7. These factors were recognized by early investigators developing predictive tests (Kooyman and Snyder, 1942). Many extrinsic factors that enhance the development of irritation were manipulated in developing the predictive assays described above. A few investigators also considered intrinsic variables in their study design.

The type of appliance, patch or chamber, and tape used to secure patches in place has been shown to influence the intensity of irritant responses (Magnusson and Hersh, 1965a, 1965b; Kooyman and Snyder, 1942). More

TABLE 7. Factors Influencing Irritation Test Sensitivity

Variables	Examples/references
Extrinsic	
Degree of occlusion	Magnusson and Hersle (1965a, 1965c)
Choice of vehicle	Patrick et al. (1985)
Frequency of dosing	Kligman and Wooding (1967)
	Frosch and Kligman (1979)
Duration of exposure	Wooding and Opdyke (1967)
Dose (concentration)	Patrick et al. (1985)
	Kligman and Wooding (1967)
Temperature	Rothenberg et al. (1977)
Environmental conditions	Hannuksela et al. (1975)
	Carter and Griffith (1965)
Altered barrier function	
Abrasion	Draize-Type Tests
	Frosch and Kligman (1976)
Chemical damage	Finkelstein et al. (1963, 1965)
	Patrick and Maibach (1987)
Tape stripping	Kligman (1969)
Intrinsic	
Anatomical site	Magnusson and Hersh (1965b, 1965c)
Concomitant disease	Skög (1960); Bjornberg (1974)
Species differences	Davies et al. (1972)
Age	Rockl et al. (1966)
Sex (effect disputed)	Wagner and Purschel (1962)
	Bjornberg (1975)
Race	Frosch and Kligman (1977)
	Weigand et al. (1974)
	Weigand and Gaylor (1976)

intense inflammatory responses are produced as the degree of occlusion is increased. The search for good techniques of occlusion ultimately led to the development of the Pirila (Finn), Duhring, and Hilltop Chambers now routinely used in patch testing.

Increases in occlusion are usually accompanied by local increases in surface temperature and increased temperature is thought to predispose to irritation. The temperature of solutions used in immersion assays is usually around 105 °F (Opdyke and Burnett, 1965; Justice et al., 1961; Griffith et al., 1969). Although systematic studies demonstrating that those temperatures were necessary were not presented, increased temperature has been shown to be necessary to reproduce irritant dermatitis in some instances (Rothenberg et al., 1977).

The influence of vehicle in diagnostic patch testing for allergy is well recognized. Similar effects are seen when irritation is studied. These effects are demonstrated most convincingly in open systems because patch occlusivity and interactions between vehicles and adhesives used in patch systems also influence the intensity of response; for example, a dose of croton oil that produces no measurable edema in the mouse ear when applied in olive oil produces the maximum response when applied in acetone (Patrick et al., 1985). In most predictive irritation tests the choice of solvent is related to use conditions and water is the solvent often used.

Dosing schedules have been developed that maximize the development of the response of interest. In general, the longer the duration of contact, the greater the intensity of the response. Multiple exposures at frequent intervals are the basis for most cumulative irritation assays, although there is some disagreement on the optimal time between exposures. In developing the soap chamber test, Frosch and Kligman (1979) varied both the frequency and duration of exposure in order to produce a more sensitive test.

Like other toxic responses, skin irritation is related to dose. If the duration of contact and the dosing procedure is held constant, intensity of response increases as concentration of the solution increases. Under patch test conditions Wooding and Opdyke (1967) showed that the rate of increase decreases as the concentration increases.

The seasonal variability in human response to normal exposure to irritants is well documented (Hannuksela et al., 1975). Conducting usage studies in late fall and winter increases the tests discriminating ability (Carter and Griffith, 1965). Some investigators have demonstrated similar effects using patch test procedures (Wooding and Opdyke, 1967; Kligman, 1969) and small-scale exaggerated exposure tests (Justice et al., 1961). While the basis for this variability is not well understood, it is thought to be due in part to changes in the barrier properties of the skin.

Many investigators have experimentally altered the barrier properties of skin in order to develop more sensitive assays. Alteration varies from the abrasion of Draize-type tests (Draize et al., 1944) and the chamber scarification test (Frosch and Kligman, 1976) to tape stripping to remove the outer surface of the epidermis (Kligman, 1969). Pretreating the test sites with damaging agents has been shown to increase the skin's reactivity to other chemicals (Finkelstein et al., 1963, 1965; Patrick and Maibach, 1987). While these procedures are extrinsic factors modifying barrier function, intrinsic factors governing barrier properties are also important. Barrier function would be expected to contribute to responses observed in screening tests used to identify sensitive subjects (Frosch and Kligman, 1976, 1979, 1982).

The demonstration that persons with some skin diseases develop more intense response to irritants (Bjornberg, 1974) was not unexpected. Susceptibility to develop irritant responses is thought to be under genetic control. The prevalence of irritant responses in atopic individuals supports this theory.

The variable response to identical patches applied to different skin sites (Magnusson and Hersle, 1965b, 1965c) is convincing evidence that there is regional variation in susceptibility to irritants. The reactivity of the various sites appears to correlate with the capacity of chemicals to penetrate the skin in that area (see skin penetration chapter). As discussed in the section on animal testing regional differences in skin response are not limited to humans!

Susceptibility to irritation is thought to vary with age, sex, and race. Children have been shown to develop inflammatory responses to lower levels of a variety of chemicals than adults (Rockl et al., 1966). Some investigators have suggested that the skin of women is more sensitive to irritants than that of men (Wagner and Purschel, 1962). However, sex differences in reactivity were not confirmed by other investigators (Bjornberg, 1975). Investigators have reported that higher doses of irritants are required to produce inflammation of the skin of blacks (Weigand and Gaylor, 1976; Weigand et al., 1976; Frosch and Kligman, 1976, 1982). This difference in reactivity disappeared when black skin was tape stripped, leading some investigators to the hypothesis that black skin contains a more efficient barrier. Berardesca recently questioned whether these differences are real (Berardesca and Maibach, 1989a).

SUMMARY

Many predictive tests have been developed to evaluate the potential of materials to damage the skin and to rank materials for their irritation potential so that less irritating products can be developed. Although some tests for irritation and corrosion are mandated by government regulation, the choice of other test designs is determined by the investigator. We have provided an overview of published methods for predicting skin irritation; nevertheless it does not summarize all the methods that have been successful. Various factors that influence the response to irritants and their application to predictive testing have been discussed. Ultimately it is up to the individual investigator to consider the purpose in performing a study and apply principles and techniques that others have used successfully. Only in this way can one successfully evaluate new materials! The area is sufficiently complex to favor the well-trained, experienced, and innovative scientist over those performing studies in cookbook fashion.

REFERENCES

Anderson, C., Sundberg, K. and Groth, O. 1986. Animal model for assessment of skin irritancy. *Contact Dermatitis* 15:143–151.

Berger, R. S. and Bowman, J. P. 1982. A reappraisal of the 21-day cumulative irritation test in man. *J. Toxicol. Cutaneous Ocular Toxicol.* 1:109–115.

Berardesca, E. and Maibach, H. I. 1989a. Physical anthropology of skin. In *Models in Dermatology*, vol. 4, eds. H. I. Maibach and N. J. Lowe, pp. 202–208. New York: Karger.

Berardesca, E. and Maibach, H. I. 1989b. Effect of nonvisible damage on the water-holding capacity of the stratum corneum, utilizing the plastic occlusion stress test (POST). In *Current Topics in Contact Dermatitis,* eds. P. J. Frosch, A. Dooms-Goossens, J.-M. Lachapelle, R. J. G. Rycroft and R. J. Scheper, pp. 554–559. New York: Springer-Verlag.

Bjornberg, A. 1974. Skin reactions to primary irritants and predisposition to eczema. *Br. J. Dermatol.* 91:425.

Bjornberg, A. 1975. Skin reactions to primary irritants in men and women. *Acta Dermatol. Venereol. (Stockh.)* 55:191.

Brown, V. K. H. 1971. A comparison of predictive irritation tests with surfactants on human and animal skin. *J. Soc. Cosmet. Chem.* 22:411–420.

Bucher, K., Bucher, K. E. and Walz, D. 1981. The topically irritant substance: Essentials-bio-tests-predictions. *Agents Actions* 11:515–519.

Calandra, J. 1971. Comments on the guinea pig immersion test. *CTFA Cosmet. J.* 3(3):47.

Carabello, F. B. 1985. The design and interpretation of human skin irritation studies. *J. Toxicol. Cutaneous Ocular Toxicol.* 4:61–71.

Carter, R. O. and Griffith, J. F. 1965. Experimental basis for the realistic assessment of the safety of topical agents. *Toxicol. Appl. Pharmacol.* 7:60–73.

Code of Federal Regulations. 1989a. Office of the Federal Registrar, National Archives of Records Service. General Services Administration Title 40, part 162.10, 163.31, 771.

Code of Federal Regulations. 1989b. Office of the Federal Registrar, National Archives of Records Service. General Services Administration Title 49, part 173.240.

Code of Federal Regulations. 1989c. Office of the Federal Registrar, National Archives of Records Service. General Services Administration Title 16, part 1500.40, part 1500.41, part 1500.42.

Cruzan, G., Dalbey, W. E., D'Aleo, C. J. and Singer, E. J. 1986. A composite model for multiple assays of skin irritation. *Toxicol. Ind. Health* 2:309–320.

Dahl, M. V. and Trancik, R. J. 1977. Sodium lauryl sulfate irritant patch test: Degree of inflammation at various times. *Contact Dermatitis* 3:263–266.

Davies, R. E., Harper, K. H. and Kymoch, S. R. 1972. Interspecies variation in dermal reactivity. *J. Soc. Cosmet. Chem.* 23:371–381.

Draize, J. H., Woodard, G. and Calvery, H. O. 1944. Methods for the study of irritation and toxicity of substances applied topically to the skin and mucous membrane. *J. Pharmacol. Exp. Ther.* 82:377–390.

Edwards, C. C. 1972. Hazardous substances. Proposed revision of test for primary skin irritants. *Fed. Reg.* 37:27, 635-27, 636.

Ellickson, B. E. and Jungermann, E. 1967. Comparative soap mildness test on infants. *Current Ther. Res.* 9:441–446.

European Economic Community. 1983. Sixth amendment to the council directive on the classification and labelling of dangerous substances, Annex VI. *Offic. J. Eur. Communities* L257:13–33.

Finkelstein, P., Laden, K. and Meichowski, W. 1963. New methods for evaluating cosmetic irritancy. *J. Invest. Dermatol.* 40:11–14.

Finkelstein, P., Laden, K. and Miechowski, W. 1965. Laboratory methods for evaluating skin irritancy. *Toxicol. Appl. Pharmacol.* 7:74–78.

Frosch, P. J. 1982. Irritancy of soap and detergent bars. In *Principles of Cosmetics for the Dermatologist,* eds. P. Frost and S. N. Howitz, pp. 5–12. St. Louis: C. V. Mosby.

Frosch, P. J. and Kligman, A. M. 1976. The chamber scarification test for irritancy. *Contact Dermatitis* 2:314–324.

Frosch, P. J. and Kligman, A. M. 1979. The soap chamber test. A new method for assessing the irritancy of soaps. *J. Am. Acad. Dermatol.* 1:35–41.

Frosch, P. J. and Kligman, A. M. 1982. Recognition of chemically vulnerable and delicate skin. In *Principles of Cosmetics for the Dermatologist,* eds. P. Frost and S. N. Horwith, pp. 287–296. St. Louis: C. V. Mosby.

Gilman, M. R., Evans, R. A. and DeSalva, S. J. 1978. The influence of concentration, exposure duration, and patch occlusivity upon rabbit primary dermal irritation indices. *Drug Chem. Toxicol.* 1(4):391–400.

Griffith, J. F., Weaver, J. E., Whitehouse, H. S., Poole, R. L., Newman, E. A. and Nixon, C. A. 1969. Safety evaluation of enzyme detergents. Oral and cutaneous toxicity, irritancy and skin sensitization studies. *Food Cosmet. Toxicol.* 7:581–593.

Griffith, J. F. and Buehler, E. 1976. Prediction of skin irritancy and sensitization potential by testing with animals and man. In *Cutaneous Toxicity*, eds. V. Drill and P. Lazer. New York: Academic Press.

Guillot, J. P., Gonnet, J. F., Clement, C., Caillard, L. and Truhaut, R. 1982. Evaluation of the cutaneous-irritation potential of 56 compounds. *Food Chem. Toxicol.* 20:563–572.

Haley, T. and Hunziger, J. 1974. Instrument for producing standardized skin abrasions. *J. Pharm. Sci.* 63:106.

Hannuksela, M., Prilia, V. and Salo, O. P. 1975. Skin reactions to propylene glycol. *Contact Dermatitis* 1:112.

Hassing, J. H., Nater, J. P. and Bleumink, E. 1982. Irritancy of low concentrations of soap and synthetic detergents as measured by skin water loss. *Dermatologica* 164:312–314.

Imokowa, G., Sumura, K. and Katsumi, M. Study on skin roughness caused by surfactants: I. A new method *in vivo* for evaluation of skin roughness. *J. Am. Oil Chem. Soc.* 52:479–483.

Ingram, A. J. and Grasso, A. 1975. Patch testing in the rabbit using a modified human patch test method. Application of histological and visual assessment. *Br. J. Dermatol.* 92:131–142.

Johnson, S. A. M., Kile, R. L., Kooyman, D. J., Whitehouse, H. S. and Brod, J. S. 1953. Comparison of effects of soaps and detergents on the hands of housewives. *Arch. Dermatol. Syphilol.* 68:643–650.

Justice, J. D., Travers, J. J. and Vinson, L. J. 1961. The correlation between animal tests and human tests in assessing product mildness. *Proc. Scientific Section of the Toilet Goods Association* 35:12–17.

Kligman, A. 1969. Evaluation of cosmetics for irritancy. *Toxicol. Appl. Pharmacol. Suppl.* 3:30–44.

Kligman, A. M. and Wooding, W. M. 1967. A method for the measurement and evaluation of irritants on human skin. *J. Invest. Dermatol.* 49:78–94.

Kooyman, D. J. and Snyder, F. H. 1942. Tests for the mildness of soaps. *Arch. Dermatol. Syphilol.* 46:846–855.

Lanman, B. M., Elvers, W. B. and Howard, C. S. 1968. The role of human patch testing in a product development program. In *Proc. Joint Conference on Cosmetic Sciences*, pp. 135–145. Washington, D.C.: Toilet Goods Association.

Landsdown, A. B. G. 1972. An appraisal of methods for detecting primary skin irritants. *J. Soc. Cosmet. Chem.* 23:739–772.

MacMillan, F. S. K., Rafft, R. R. and Elvers, W. B. 1975. A comparison of the skin irritation produced by cosmetic ingredients and formulations in the rabbit, guinea pig, beagle dog to that observed in the human. In *Animal Models in Dermatology*, ed. H. I. Maibach, pp. 12–22. Edinburgh: Churchill-Livingstone.

Magnusson, B. and Hersle, K. 1965a. Patch test methods I. A comparative study of six different types of patch tests. *Acta Dermatol.* 45:123–128.

Magnusson, B. and Hersle, K. 1965b. Patch test methods II. Regional variations of patch test responses. *Acta Dermatol.* 45:257–261.

Magnusson, B. and Hersle, K. 1966c. Patch test methods III. Influence of adhesive tape on test response. *Acta Dermatol.* 46:275–278.

Malten, K. E. and Thiele, F. A. J. 1973a. Some theoretical aspects of orthoergic (= irritant) dermatitis. *Arch. Belges Dermatol.* 28:9–22.

Malten, K. E. and Thiele, F. A. J. 1973b. Evaluation of skin damage. II. Water loss and carbon dioxide release measurements related to skin resistance measurements. *Br. J. Dermatol.* 89:565:569.

Marzulli, F. N. and Maibach, H. I. 1975. The rabbit as a model for evaluating skin irritants: A comparison of results obtained on animals and man using repeated skin exposure. *Food Cosmet. Toxicol.* 13:533–540.

Mathias, C. G. T. 1987. Clinical and experimental aspects of cutaneous irritation. In *Dermatotoxicology*, 3rd ed., eds. H. I. Maibach and F. N. Marzulli, pp. 173–190. Washington, D.C.: Hemisphere.

Mathias, C. G. T. and Maibach, H. I. 1978. Dermatoxicology monographs. I. Cutaneous irritation: Factors influencing the response to irritants. *Clin. Toxicol.* 13:333–346.

Mezei, M. 1970. Dermatitic effect of nonionic surfactants. V. The effect of nonionic surfactants on rabbit skin as evaluated by radioactive tracer techniques in vivo. *J. Invest. Dermatol.* 54:510–516.

Mezei, M., Sager, R. W., Stewart, W. D. and DeRuyter, A. L. 1966. Dermatitic effect on nonionic surfactants I. Gross, microscopic, and metabolic changes in rabbit skin treated with nonionic surface-active agents. *J. Pharm. Sci.* 55:584–590.

Moloney, S. J. and Teal, J. J. 1988. Alkane-induce edema formation and cutaneous barrier dysfunction. *Arch. Dermatol. Res.* 280:375–379.

Motoyoshi, K., Toyoshima, Y., Sato, M. and Yoshimura, M. 1979. Comparative studies on the irritancy of oils and synthetic perfumes to the skin of rabbit, guinea pig, rat, miniature swine, and man. *Cosmet. Toiletries* 94:41–42.

Murphy, J. C., Watson, E. S., Wirth, P. W., Skierkowski, P., Folk, R. M. and Peck, G. 1979. Cutaneous irritation in the topical application of 30 antineoplastic agents to New Zealand white rabbits. *Toxicology* 14:117–130.

National Academy of Sciences, Committee for the Revision of NAS Publication 1138. 1977. *Principles and Procedures for Evaluating the Toxicity of Household Substances*, pp. 23–59. Washington, D.C.: National Academy of Sciences.

Nixon, G. A., Tyson, C. A. and Wertz, W. C. 1975. Interspecies comparisons of skin irritancy. *Toxicol. Appl. Pharmacol.* 31:481–490.

Opdyke, D. 1971. The guinea pig immersion test—A 20 year appraisal. *CTFA Cosmet. J.* 3(3)46–47.

Opdyke, D. L. and Burnett, C. M. 1965. Practical problems in the evaluation of the safety of cosmetics. *Proc. Scientific Section, Toilet Goods Association* 44:3–4.

Organization for Economic Cooperation and Development. 1981. *OECD Guidelines for Testing of Chemicals*, Section 404, 1–6. Paris: OECD.

Patrick, E., Maibach, H. I. and Burkhalter, A. 1985. Mechanisms of chemically induced skin irritation I. Studies of time course, dose response, and components of inflammation in the laboratory mouse. *Toxicol. Appl. Pharmacol.* 81:476–490.

Patrick, E. and Maibach, H. I. 1987. A novel predictive irritation assay in mice. *Toxicologist* 7:84.

Phillips, L., Steinberg, M., Maibach, H. I. and Akers, W. A. 1972. A comparison of rabbit and human skin responses to certain irritants. *Toxicol. Appl. Pharmacol.* 21:369–382.

Rapaport, M., Anderson, D. and Pierce, U. 1978. Performance of the 21 day patch test in civilian populations. *J. Toxicol. Cutaneous Ocular Toxicol.* 1:109–115.

Rietschell, R. L. 1982. Advances and pitfalls in irritant and allergen testing. *J. Soc. Cosmet. Chem.* 33:309–313.

Rockl, H., Muller, E. and Haltermann, W. 1966. Zum aussagewert positiver epicutantest bei sauglingen and kindern. *Arch. Klin. Exp. Dermatol.* 226:407.

Rostenberg, A. 1961. Methods for the appraisal of the safety of cosmetics. *Drug Cosmet. Ind.* 88:592.

Rothenberg, H. W., Menne, T. and Sjolin, K. E. 1977. Temperature dependent primary irritant dermatitis from lemon perfume. *Contact Dermatitis* 3:37.

Shelanski, H. A. 1951. Experience with and considerations of the human patch test method. *J. Soc. Cosmet. Chem.* 2:324–331.

Skög, E. 1960. Primary irritant and allergic eczematous reactions in patients with different dermatoses. *Acta Derm. Venereol.* 40:307–312.

Smiles, K. A. and Pollack, M. E. 1977. A quanative human patch testing procedure for low level skin irritants. *J. Soc. Cosmet. Chem.* 28:755–764.

Steinberg, M., Akers, W. A., Weeks, M., McCreesh, A. H. and Maibach, H. I. 1975. I. A comparison of test techniques based on rabbit and human skin responses to irritants with recommendations regarding the evaluation of mildly or moderately irritating compounds. In *Animal Models in Dermatology,* ed. H. I. Maibach, pp. 1–11. Edinburgh: Churchill-Livingstone.

Thiele, F. A. J. and Malten, K. E. 1973a. Some measuring methods for the evaluation of orthoergic contact dermatitis. *Arch. Belges Dermatol.* 28:23–46.

Thiele, F. A. J. and Malten, K. E. 1973b. Evaluation of skin damage. I. Skin resistance measurements with alternating current (impedance measurements). *Br. J. Dermatol.* 89:373–382.

Uttley, M. and Van Abbe, N. J. 1973. Primary irritation of the skin: mouse ear test and human patch test procedures. *J. Soc. Cosmet. Chem.* 24:217–227.

Vinegar, M. B. 1979. Regional variation in primary skin irritation and corrosivity potentials in rabbits. *Toxicol. Appl. Pharmacol.* 49:63–69.

Wagner, G. and Purschel, W. 1962. Klinisch-analytische studie zum neurodermitisproblem. *Dermatologica* 125:1.

Walz, D. 1985. Quantitative assessment of irritation in the mouse skin test. *Food Chem. Toxicol.* 23:199–203.

Weaver, J. E. 1976. Dermatologic testing of household laundry products: A novel fabric softener. *Int. J. Dermatol.* 15:297–300.

Weigand, D. A. and Gaylor, J. R. 1976. Irritant reaction in Negro and Caucasian skin. *South Med. J.* 67:548–551.

Weigand, D. A., Haygood, C. and Gaylor, J. R. 1974. Cell layer and density of Negro and Caucasian stratum corneum. *J. Invest. Dermatol.* 62:563–568.

Weil, C. S. and Scala, R. A. 1971. Study of intra- and inter-laboratory variability in the results of rabbit eye and skin irritation tests. *Toxicol. Appl. Pharmacol.* 19:276–360.

Wilhelm, K. P., Surber, C. and Maibach, H. I. 1989. Quantification of sodium lauryl sulfate irritant dermatitis in man: Comparison of four techniques: skin color reflectance, transepidermal water loss, laser doppler flow measurement and visual scores. *Arch. Dermatol. Res.* 281:293–295.

Wooding, W. H. and Opdyke, D. L. 1967. A statistical approach to the evaluation of cutaneous responses to irritants. *J. Soc. Cosmet. Chem.* 18:809–829.

11

irritant dermatitis
(irritation)

■ Margaret Bason ■ K. Lammintausta ■
■ Howard I. Maibach ■

CLINICAL ASPECTS

Irritation, or irritant dermatitis, previously considered a monomorphous process, is now understood to be a complex biologic syndrome, with a diverse pathophysiology, natural history, and clinical appearance. Thus, the clinical appearance of irritant contact dermatitis varies depending on multiple external and internal factors. The actual types, with reference to major characteristics in the clinical appearance, are listed in Table 1.

Acute Irritant Dermatitis (Primary Irritation)

When exposure is sufficient and the offending agent is potent, classic symptoms of acute skin irritation are seen. Contact with a strong primary irritant is often accidental, and an acute irritant dermatitis is elicited in almost anyone independent of constitutional susceptibility. This classic, acutely developing dermatitis usually heals soon after exposure. In unusual cases the dermatitis may persist for months after exposure, followed by complete resolution.

The availability of the material Safety Data Sheet and data from the single-application Draize rabbit test combined with activities of industrial hygienists and other informed personnel greatly decreased the frequency of such dermatitis in industry. Further educational efforts and appropriate industrial engineering should make this form of irritation a rarity.

Adapted from "Contact dermatitis due to irritation" (Lammintausta and Maibach, 1990).

M. Bason et al.

TABLE 1. Types of Irritation

Irritation	Onset	Prognosis
Acute irritant dermatitis	Acute—often single exposure	Good
Irritant reaction	Acute—often multiple exposure	Good
Delayed acute irritant dermatitis	Delayed—12–24 h or longer	Good
Cumulative irritant contact dermatitis	Slowly developing (weeks to years)	Variable
Traumatic irritant dermatitis	Slowly developing after preceding trauma	Variable
Pustular and acneiform dermatitis	Moderately slowly developing (weeks to months)	Variable
Nonerythematous irritation	Slowly developing	Variable

Irritant Reaction

Individuals who are extensively exposed to various irritants often develop erythematous, chapped skin in the first months of exposure. This irritant reaction (Fregert, 1981; Griffiths and Wilkinson, 1985; Hjorth and Avnstorp, 1986) may be considered a pre-eczematous expression of acute skin irritation. It is frequently seen in hairdressers and variable wet work-performing employees who are repeatedly exposed. Repeated irritant reactions sometimes lead to contact dermatitis, with good prognosis, although chronic contact dermatitis may also develop. We do not understand what separates the pathophysiology of the low-grade irritant reaction from that of cumulative irritant dermatitis (see below). Once this information becomes available, we may be able to develop interventions to prevent the latter.

Delayed, Acute Irritant Contact Dermatitis

Some chemicals produce acute irritation in a delayed manner so that inflammation is not seen until 8–24 h or more after exposure (Malten et al., 1979; Lovell et al., 1985) (Table 2). Except for the delayed onset, the clinical appearance and course resemble those of acute irritant contact dermatitis. The delayed

TABLE 2. Effect of Duration of Occlusion on Percutaneous Absorption of Malathion in Humans

Duration (h)	Absorption (%)
0^a	9.6
0.5	7.3
1	12.7
2	16.6
4	24.2
8	38.8
24	62.8

[a]Immediate wash with soap and water. From Feldmann and Maibach (1974).

acute irritant dermatitis, because of its delayed onset, is often confused with allergic contact dermatitis; appropriately performed diagnostic patch tests easily separate the two.

Cumulative Irritant Dermatitis

When exposure inducing an acute irritant dermatitis is repeated, the dermatitis tends to last longer, and becomes chronic. In cumulative cutaneous irritation, the frequency of exposure is too high in relation to the skin recovery time. Acute irritant skin reaction is not seen in the majority of patients, but mild or moderate invisible skin changes. Repeated skin exposures and minor reactions lead to a manifest dermatitis when the irritant load exceeds the threshold for visible effects. The development of a cumulative irritant dermatitis was carefully documented by Malten and den Arend (1978) and Malten et al. (1979). Cumulative irritant dermatitis was called "traumiterative dermatitis" in the older German literature ("traumiterative" = traumas repeating) (von Hagerman, 1957; Agrup, 1969). Classic signs are erythema and increasing dryness, followed by hyperkeratosis with frequent cracking and occasional erythema.

Cumulative irritant dermatitis is the most common type of irritant contact dermatitis. This syndrome may develop after days, weeks, or years of subtle exposure to chemical substances. Variation in individual susceptibility increases the multiplicity of clinical findings. Delayed onset and variable attack lead to confusion with allergic contact dermatitis. To rule out allergic etiology, appropriate diagnostic patch testing is indicated.

Traumatic Irritant Dermatitis

Traumatic irritant dermatitis develops after acute skin trauma. The skin does not heal, but erythema, vesicles and/or vesicopapules, and scaling appear. The clinical course later resembles nummular (coin-shaped) dermatitis. This may occur after burns or lacerations and after acute irritant dermatitis. It may be compounded by a concurrent allergen exposure. The healing period is generally prolonged.

Often these patients are considered to have a factitial dermatitis because of a healing phase followed by exacerbation. Although factitial (unnatural) aspects may occur in some patients, this peculiar form of irritation appears to be a disease *sui generis*. Its chronicity and recalcitrance to therapy provides a challenge to both patient and physician. We have no information explaining why the occasional patient develops this phenomenon, and how this patient differs from the general population.

Pustular and Acneiform Irritant Dermatitis

Pustular and acneiform irritant dermatitis may develop from exposure to metals, oils and greases, tar, asphalt, chlorinated naphthalenes, and polyhalogenated naphthalenes. Certain substances have a capacity to elicit these reactions (Wahlberg and Maibach, 1981, 1982; Dooms-Goossens et al., 1986), and even allergic reactions may sometimes be pustular or follicular (Fischer and Rystedt, 1985). In occupational exposure, only a minority of subjects develop pustular or acneiform dermatitis. Thus, the development of this type of irritant contact dermatitis appears to be dependent on both constitutional and chemical factors.

Nonerythematous Irritation

In the early stages of skin irritation, subtle skin damage may occur without visible inflammation. As a correlate of nonvisible irritation, objectively registered alterations in the damaged epidermis have been reported (Berardesca and Maibach, 1988; van der Valk et al., 1985; Lammintausta et al., 1988b). It is customary in Japan to screen new chemicals, cosmetics, and textiles for subtle signs of stratum corneum damage, employing replicas of stratum corneum (the Kawai method). Consumer dissatisfaction with many chemicals may result from exposure to this low-grade irritation; thus the patient feels more than the physician observes.

Subjective Irritation

Subjective irritation is experienced by some individuals ("stingers") in contact with certain chemicals (Frosch and Kligman, 1982; Lammintausta et al., 1988b). Itching, stinging, or tingling is experienced, for example, from skin contact with lactic acid, which is a model for nonvisible cutaneous irritation. The threshold for this reaction varies between subjects, independent of susceptibility to other irritation types. The quality as well as the concentration of the exposing agent is also important, and neural pathways may be contributory, but the pathomechanism is unknown. Some sensory irritation may be subclinical contact urticaria. Screening raw ingredients and final formulations in the guinea pig ear swelling test (Lahti and Maibach, 1985) or the human forehead assay allows us to minimize the amount of subclinical contact urticaria.

Although subjective irritation may have a neural component, recent studies by Lammintausta et al. (1988b) suggest that the blood vessel may be more responsive in "stingers" than nonstingers. At least 10% of women complain of stinging with certain facial products; thus, further work is needed to develop a strategy to overcome this type of discomfort.

Localization of Irritant Contact Dermatitis

In irritant contact dermatitis the exposed sites are first affected. The dorsal and lateral aspects of the hands and fingers have the greatest contact with chemical irritants. Thick stratum corneum provides better protection for palms in most occupations. Other unidentified factors may also protect the palms and soles. The degree of protection may be greater than what might be expected from decreases in skin penetration. Some compounds are almost as permeable through the palm as the forearm (Feldmann and Maibach, 1967). Dermatitis on the anterior thighs, upper back, axillary areas, and feet may be due to an irritant in clothing. When dermatitis is observed on the face, under the collar or belt, or in the flexures, airborne irritants (e.g., dust) may be involved.

EXTERNAL FACTORS

Irritants

Many chemicals qualify as irritant when the exposing dose is high (Kligman and Wooding, 1967). Molecular size, ionization, polarization, fat solubility, and other factors that are important in skin penetration are also important in cutaneous irritation. The threshold of strength and quality of irritation depends on the physicochemical properties of the substance. Temperature may be important, with warm temperatures generally more damaging than cool (Rothenborg et al., 1977). Warm citral perfume produced more irritation than citral at lower temperature.

Exposure

The absorbed dose may vary when the substance is suspended in different vehicles (Cooper, 1985; Gummer, 1985). The solubility of the irritant in the vehicle and the inherent irritancy of the vehicle have an impact on each reaction (Flannigan and Tucker, 1985). The effective tissue dose depends on concentration, volume, application time, and duration on and in the skin. Long exposure time and large volume increase penetration. Thus, greater response may be expected. If exposure is repeated, the recovery from previous exposure(s) affects the subsequent response. Sometimes a shorter, repeated exposure leads to a lengthened recovery period (Malten and den Arend, 1978). This was demonstrated in experimental studies with dimethyl sulfoxide (DMSO). Intermittent application leads to a different response as compared with one lengthened application (Lammintausta et al., 1988a). These experimental observations are consistent with the multiple clinical appearances of cumulative irritant dermatitis.

Multiple Simultaneous Exposure

Simultaneous or subsequent exposure may lead to an additive effect and increased reaction, although each chemical alone would elicit only a minor reaction, or none. On the other hand, subsequent exposure may lead to a decreased response. For instance, exposure to a detergent and then to a soap led to a response less than exposure to a detergent alone. The detergent was washed away by the subsequent soap exposure (Malten, 1981).

The outcome of multiple, subsequent, or simultaneous exposures is sometimes unexpected (Lammintausta et al., 1987a) and rules must be sought (Pittz et al., 1985).

Other Irritation Sources

Physical trauma from friction often facilitates the harmful effects of a chemical irritant. Repeated microtrauma and friction typically lead to dry, hyperkeratotic and abraded skin (Susten, 1985). Although physical irritation alone may produce irritant dermatitis, the additive effect with chemical exposure may lead to irritant contact dermatitis. Corresponding impact is seen with other physical irritants.

Quantification of physical trauma from friction and differences in individual susceptibility to friction are expected to lead to appropriate interventions to decrease such damage.

Environmental Factors

Low environmental humidity enhances irritability: skin tests with irritants produce more and stronger reactions in winter when the weather is cool, windy, and dry (Hannuksela et al., 1975). It also produces variable irritation symptoms: itching and erythema associated with whealing or erythema and scaling (Rycroft, 1981).

Occlusion often enhances penetration and increases acute irritation (Table 2). Thus, skin reactions frequently become stronger when the chemical is applied under occlusion, providing a humid environment that minimizes evaporation and makes the stratum corneum more permeable. Gloves and clothing increase the susceptibility for irritant dermatitis. Frequent changes of these articles is important, to minimize the humid and occlusive environment.

Airborne Irritation

Airborne irritation dermatitis is located most commonly in exposed skin areas, such as the face, hands, and arms (Lachapelle, 1986). Volatile chemicals and dusts are common sources of exposure, but even sharp particles in dust may induce lesions (Table 3). Airborne irritation is a type of exposure in which physical sources of irritation frequently exacerbate the response with an additive influence. For instance, sunlight, wind, and cold air are additive to chemical exposure. Depending on the occupational situation, multiple environmental and occupational irritants may induce airborne irritation (Dooms-Goossens et al., 1986).

PREDISPOSING FACTORS

Methodological Aspects

Although irritant contact dermatitis accounts for most occupational skin diseases, and many nonoccupational eczemas are exclusively or partially in-

TABLE 3. Common Airborne Irritants

Volatile substances
Acids and alkalis, ammonia
Cleaning products
Formaldehyde
Industrial solvents
Noncarbon required (NCR) paper
Epoxy resins
Foams, e.g., insulation foams in urea-formaldehyde process
Powders
Aluminum
Anhydrous calcium silicate
Cement
Cleaning products
Metallic oxides
Particles
Tree-sawing particles
Wool
Plastics, dry
Particles from plants
Stone particles in mining

duced by irritation, in-depth investigation of irritant contact dermatitis is rare. Epidemiologic studies have identified many important irritants, and some information is available about subjects who appear vulnerable to irritant dermatitis in occupational circumstances that induce dermatitis. Detergents and soaps are considered principal causes of occupational irritant dermatitis. However, in controlled experimental trials, this implied harmful effect of soap has not been documented (Jambor, 1955; Bettley, 1960; Suskind et al., 1963; Stoughton et al., 1969; White et al., 1987). Correspondingly, with evaluation of patch test reactions to detergents by direct visualization, individual differences in irritant reactivity was not documented in healthy skin. Only those subjects with a concurrent eczema reacted more strongly (Bjornberg, 1968; Lammintausta et al., 1988b). Bioengineering methods now make it possible to quantitate minor differences in cutaneous reactivity; it is expected that the development of methods is still proceeding.

Nonvisible cutaneous changes are measurable with various methods in which different aspects of skin function are quantitated. Table 4 lists the available and most useful instrumentation with reference to the measured physicochemical parameters. Documented are alterations in skin impedance (Thiele and Malten, 1973), in the amount of transepidermal water loss (TEWL), in dielectric characteristics (Maibach et al., 1984), and in conductance and resistance (Tagami et al., 1980), and alterations in blood flow velocity (Guy et al., 1985b) and skin thickness (Maibach et al., 1971). Skin pH (Grice et al., 1973) and O_2 resistance and CO_2 effusion rate (Frame et al., 1972; Grice et al., 1975)

TABLE 4. Bioengineering Techniques Used in the Evaluation of Cutaneous Irritation

Technique	Measured skin function	Advantages	Disadvantages
Laser Doppler velocimetry	Velocity of the moving erythrocytes with the blood flow	Slight, preerythema	Does not measure nonerythematous irritation
Evaporimeter	Transepidermal water exchange evaluated	Epidermal damage evaluated Easy to use	Visible erythema Inflammation contributes but does not directly correlate Standardized environmental circumstances important
Ultrasound	Skin thickness	Edematous inflammation measured	Minimal correlation with visible erythema or epidermal damage
Impedance, conductance, and capacitance	Skin hydration	Correlation with epidermal damage	
Colorimeter	Skin colors	Correlation with erythema, inflammation	Correlates with the amount of pigment, too Minimal correlation with epidermal damage and other nonerythematous inflammation

are further measurable skin changes in skin irritation. Measurements of these variables often show poor correlation with each other, probably because these methods give information about different aspects of cutaneous irritation and skin function.

In addition to patch testing with irritants accompanied by visual scoring, alkali resistance and alkali neutralization capacity have been evaluated in some European countries by using ammonium hydroxide applications. Their capacity to reflect individual susceptibility appears to be limited or minimal (Ummenhofer, 1980) and their value is questioned.

Recently K. Wilhelm (unpublished data) utilized sodium hydroxide to produce transepidermal water loss as a measure of skin damage. This assay shows a high correlation between subjects developing increased water loss after application of sodium hydroxide and a propensity for sodium lauryl sulfate damage. This simple approach may provide a first step toward a preemployment test for irritant dermatitis potential.

Individual susceptibility to chemicals has been studied by documenting skin reactivity to model irritants. The intensity of the wheal created by DMSO, the time required to raise a blister (MBT) after cutaneous application of aluminum hydroxide solution, and reactivity to sodium lauryl sulfate (SLS) are examples of objective methods that have been used (Frosch, 1985). Stinging occurs with certain test substances (e.g., lactic acid), and clinical experiments provide some information about individual susceptibility (Frosch and Kligman, 1982).

Despite important steps taken in the investigation of the pathogenesis of irritant contact dermatitis, no experimental design has proved entirely successful for the clinical evaluation of individual susceptibility. Hopefully, the Wilhelm studies will lead to an objective test.

Regional Anatomic Differences

Anatomic differences in the exposure site are important. Because skin permeability is variable in different skin sites, being generally greatest in thin-skin areas (Cronin and Stoughton, 1962; Feldmann and Maibach, 1967; Wester and Maibach, 1985, 1989b; Tur et al., 1985), corresponding association between permeability, skin thickness, and skin irritation is expected, but direct correlation is lacking (Fig. 1). Regional variation has been studied comparing the whealing response—a variation of immediate irritation—to DMSO and measuring differences in minimal blistering time (MBT) after topical ammonium hydroxide application in different skin sites (Frosch and Kligman, 1982). Both

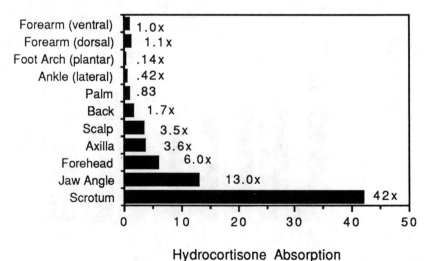

Hydrocortisone Absorption

FIGURE 1 Anatomic regional variation of percutaneous absorption in humans. *Source:* Wester and Maibach, 1989. Reprinted by permission of Marcel Dekker.

tests showed the mandibular area to be most reactive, followed by the upper back, forearm, lower leg, and palm. With DMSO whealing, the forehead was more sensitive than the back, the antecubital area reaction preceded that of the rest of the upper extremity, and the wrist was more sensitive than the leg.

In patch testing, the irritant benzalkonium chloride and several allergens produced maximal reactivity in the upper back (Magnusson and Hersle, 1965), an observation recently extended to the middle scapula (Flannigan et al., 1984). The greater reactivity may be related to pressure in this area when sleeping (von Hornstein and Kienlein-Kletschka, 1982; Gollhausen and Kligman, 1985). Certain "inherent" differences between different skin sites in irritation reactivity may also exist. Vulvar skin is much more sensitive than forearm skin (Britz and Maibach, 1979; Oriba et al., 1989) (Fig. 2). On the other hand, it is often noted in clinical occupational dermatology that male genitalia are affected in occupational irritant dermatitis.

Age

The threshold for skin irritation is decreased in babies, who develop dermatitis from irritation that does not occur in adult skin (Jordan and Blaney, 1982). Except for structural and functional immaturity of infant's skin, other factors (intestinal *Candida albicans*, completed breast feeding, low frequency of diaper changes) are contributory (Seymour et al., 1987). Children below the age of 8 years are generally considered more susceptible to skin irritation (Mobly and Mansman, 1974; Epstein, 1971; Fisher, 1975). Irritation susceptibility gradually decreases after this age. Maibach and Boisits (1982) define this data base; unfortunately, despite extensive chemical exposure of infants and

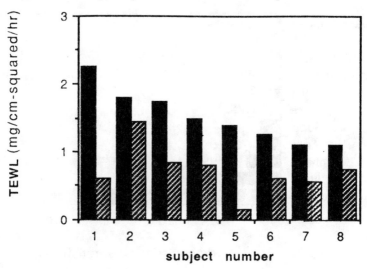

FIGURE 2 Transepidermal water loss from vulva and forearm. ■ vulva ▨ forearm. *Source:* Oriba et al., 1989. Rerpinted by permission of W. B. Saunders.

TABLE 5. Laser Doppler Velocimetry (LDV) Values in Blacks and Whites

LDV (mV)	Preoccluded	
	0.5%[a]	2.0%
Whites	73.6 ± 34	179 ± 128
	p < .01	
Blacks	58 ± 25	234 ± 194
	p < .01	

Note. p Values refer to the comparison between 0.5% and 2% sodium lauryl sulfate (SLS) concentration.
[a]*p* ≤ .04 for Blacks versus Whites.

children, our experimental evidence is lacking because of methodologic problems and limited data.

Skin problems commonly occur in the elderly (Beauregaard and Gilchrest, 1987), who do not routinely seek help from physicians. In a majority of cutaneous symptoms, cutaneous irritation is contributory. Elderly subjects may develop reactions to skin irritants less sharply and more slowly than younger individuals (Lejman et al., 1984; Grove et al., 1981). A corresponding alteration occurs with regard to cutaneous reactivity to allergens. With ammonium hydroxide skin tests, older subjects had a shorter reaction time (MBT, minimal blistering time), whereas the time needed to develop a tense blister was longer (Frosch and Kligman, 1977a), and a longer time was needed for the resorption of a wheal elicited by saline injection (Kligman, 1976).

Age-associated alterations in skin reactivity may be related to altered cutaneous permeation, although contradictory results have been reported (Christophers and Kligman, 1965; Tagami, 1971; DeSalva and Thompson, 1965; Guy et al., 1985a). Alterations in structural lipids (Elias, 1981) and in cell composition (Gilchrest et al., 1982) and renewal (Roberts and Marks, 1980; Baker and Blair, 1968) are reported in association with structural alteration (Montaga and Carlisle, 1979; Holzle et al., 1986). Thus, age-associated alterations in cutaneous reactivity are expected; however, the subject requires more investigation.

Race

It is difficult to compare irritant reactions in white and black skin, although black skin less frequently seems (to the naked eye) to develop irritation from chemicals eliciting irritant reactions in white skin (Weigand and Gaylor, 1974; Anderson and Maibach, 1979). When blood flow velocity is altered in an irritant reaction, the reaction is measurable with laser Doppler velocimetry (LDV). Observations in experimental studies using LDV support *increased* reactivity to a detergent in black subjects (Berardesca and Maibach, 1988) (Table 5).

Black skin has higher electrical resistance than does caucasoid skin (Johnson and Corah, 1960). Owing to this characteristic it may have increased resistance to irritants that themselves often lower electrical skin resistance. Structural differences are reported, too, such as difference in skin reactivity to irritants when minimal perceptible erythema was registered (Weigand and Gaylor, 1974). Black skin, however, needs more stripping for the removal of stratum corneum (Weigand et al., 1974). With methacholine-induced erythema and flare response, blacks appear to be less reactive than whites (Buckley et al., 1982).

Clinical experiments suggest that black skin has differences in the modulation of irritation reactivity as compared with white skin (Berardesca and Maibach, 1988). It may be reflected in certain aspects of the multifactoral development of skin irritation, which is, however, still poorly understood. Cutaneous erythema induced by methacholine injections was compared in Warain Indians, Tibetans, and Caucasians. Caucasians reacted to the greatest degree (Buckley et al., 1985), and associations between skin irritation and cholinergic reactivity may exist (Berardesca and Maibach, 1988).

Gender

The incidence of irritant contact dermatitis—most often located in the hands—is higher in females than in males (Agrup, 1969; Rystedt, 1985; Lantinga et al., 1984). Because of this clinical observation, susceptibility to skin irritation has been related to female skin, which also seems to elicit more tape irritation (Wagner and Porshel, 1962; Magnusson and Hillgren, 1962). Skin tests with surfactants, however, have not experimentally documented a difference (Bjornberg, 1975; Lammintausta et al., 1987b). The increased occurrence of irritant contact dermatitis may be related to the more extensive exposure to irritants and wet work. A minimal relationship between gender and constitutional skin irritability is supported by the fact that the female preponderance in the irritant contact dermatitis populations does not hold true for all geographic areas (Olumide, 1987). Socioeconomic factors may be responsible.

Genetics

Interindividual variation based on genetic constitutional differences has been demonstrated (Bjornberg, 1968; Frosch, 1985). When patch-test reactivity to common irritants was compared between monozygotic and dizygotic twins with control subjects, the highest degree of concordance was demonstrated for the monozygotic twin pairs (Holst and Moller, 1975).

Susceptibility to sunlight has been associated with vulnerability to chemical irritants. Sun-sensitive skin and low minimal erythema dose (MED) seem to be correlated with high cutaneous irritability (Frosch and Wissing, 1982; Maurice and Greaves, 1983). Marked interindividual variation in skin reactivity has been demonstrated with the alkali resistance test, although the relevance to clinical irritant reactivity is minor (Ummenhofer, 1980).

In a large series, individual skin irritability varied for different chemical irritants when reactions were evaluated with visual scoring (Bjornberg, 1968). These results were confirmed by Cerwinska-Ditram and Rudzki (1981). Both sets of data support the simultaneous influence of the quality of irritant, individual susceptibility, and multiple environmental factors. For experimental studies, certain model irritants are needed; however, the results may not be generalizable.

A test battery consisting of DMSO reactivity, blistering susceptibility to ammonium hydroxide, and SLS reactivity was found to be useful (Frosch, 1985). Unfortunately, it is too complicated to be used in clinical practice for preemployment testing.

Newer bioengineering test methods show great interindividual variation. For example, TEWL, which is easy to measure, reflects important components of detergent-induced irritation. In the evaluation of individual irritant reactivity, however, repeated follow-up measurements are needed, because baseline values do not necessarily reflect the reactivity when irritation is produced.

Previous and Preexisting Skin Diseases

Subjects with a previous or present atopic dermatitis have an increased susceptibility to develop irritant dermatitis (Rystedt, 1985; Hanifin and Rajka, 1980). Ichthyosis vulgaris is sometimes seen in association with atopic dermatitis; in ichthyosis vulgaris, patients' irritant reactivity has been shown to be increased to alkali irritants (Ziierz et al., 1960). The increased general cutaneous irritability related to atopic dermatitis (Hanifin and Lobitz, 1977) could not be demonstrated with regular patch tests when skin irritants were used (Skog, 1960; Rajka, 1975).

Reduced capacity to bind water has been related to atopic skin (Werner et al., 1982), which in noneczematous sites demonstrates greater transepidermal water loss than does nonatopic skin. Stratum corneum water content may even be increased (Finlay et al., 1980; Al Jaber and Marks, 1984; Gloor et al., 1981). An increased water loss was induced with detergent patch tests in atopic skin (van der Valk et al., 1985). Itchy and dry atopic skin has been connected with an increased risk for developing hand dermatitis (Lammintausta and Kalimo, 1981; Rystedt, 1985). However, certain atopic subjects with rhinitis or asthma have normal, nonirritable skin, and an itchy and dryness-prone skin may be seen in some nonatopic subjects. Accurate objective tools are not available to evaluate the atopic cutaneous characteristics or atopic skin diathesis.

Seborrheic skin has not been shown to possess increased susceptibility to skin irritants; reports and interpretations are contradictory (Vickers, 1962; Holland, 1958; von Hornstein et al., 1986). Clinical experience suggests that some increased irritability is associated with a seborrheic constitution in certain subjects. This may be true in certain geographic areas, where environmental humidity is low in the winter in relation to the cold temperatures.

Different methods have been used in studies on skin irritability in psoriatic individuals. Those studies revealed decreased and increased irritant reactivity (Kingston and Marks, 1983; Maurice and Greaves, 1983; Lawrence et al., 1984; MacDonalds and Marks, 1986) when anthralin (dithranol) irritancy was the main interest. Psoriatic skin is particularly irritable in certain individuals (Epstein and Maibach, 1985), and the development of psoriatic lesions in irritation sites (Koebner phenomenon) is often seen.

In the presence of eczema, the threshold for skin irritation is decreased (Bjornberg, 1968; Mitchell, 1981; Bruynzeel et al., 1983; Bruynzeel and Maibach, 1986). A whole-body examination of employees sometimes reveals nummular lesions or other constitutional eczema symptoms. Such a clinical finding may suggest an increased skin irritability in different locations. Pompholyx (dyshidrosis) type dermatitis is harmful. As a constitutional eczema, it probably increases skin irritability in general. These patients often have difficulty wearing gloves, since phompholyx is made worse by occlusion.

A history of contact dermatitis may be important when susceptibility to irritant contact dermatitis is evaluated (Nilsson et al., 1985; Lammintausta et al., 1988a). Although increased irritability has been hard to demonstrate (Bjornberg, 1968; Lammintausta et al., 1988a), further improvement of methodological equipment in the bioengineering industry should make this possible.

Systemic Skin Disease

Atopic Dermatitis. On the basis of dermatologic clinical experience, atopic dermatitis patients have irritable skin manifested by reactivity to all types of irritants (Hanifin and Rajka, 1980). Since facial dermatitis and hand dermatitis are common in atopic dermatitis, it appears that irritation is an important factor. In wet work, for example, in which exposure to water, detergents, or other chemicals is frequent or continuous, the subjects with a history of atopic dermatitis develop hand dermatitis more often than those without a history of atopic symptoms (Lammintausta and Kalimo, 1981; Nilsson et al., 1985; van der Valk et al., 1985). The studies also suggest that atopic subjects with dry, itchy skin have skin problems more often than nonatopic subjects in environments where exposure to irritants is extensive, although they would not have histories of manifest skin effects (Lammintausta and Kalimo, 1981). In these subjects, the threshold level for cutaneous irritation from repeated irritant attacks appears intermediate between those with atopic dermatitis and those with a non-atopic constitution.

Cutaneous irritability in atopic subjects shows considerable clinical variation. The degree is dependent on the number of characteristics in the skin that make the skin particularly prone to develop cutaneous irritation. The scale is wide. Simultaneously, many atopic subjects—some 30–40% of those with only mucosal symptoms—have normal skin without any demonstrable susceptibilities. The importance of motivated protection and self care for vulnerable groups appears evident. Although many atopic subjects learn to handle difficulties, despite some skin effects appearing intermittently, problems may arise in occupations with repeated irritation exposure. A subject with a history of severe atopic dermatitis, with atopic hand problems as a child, or with relapsing atopic skin effects in adulthood should not start work in conditions where irritation exposure is extensive until both the individual and the employer have been apprised of the risk.

STUDIES IN IRRITANT DERMATITIS SYNDROME

Experimental Irritant Dermatitis

Irritant dermatitis is induced with patch-test technique and read on the basis of visual scoring of elicited irritant reactions of variable degree. The strength of one reaction does not usually predict reactivity to other irritants (Bjornberg, 1968). The alkali resistance test as a predictive test for irritability has not proven reliable (Ummenhofer, 1980).

In human experiments, visible reactions to different irritants—whealing from dimethyl sulfoxide contact, blister formation from ammonium hydroxide, and eczematous reactions after contact with sodium lauryl sulfate, alkyldimethyl benzyl ammonium chloride, croton oil, or kerosene—have suggested that some part of individual variation in cutaneous irritant reactivity may be predictable (Frosch, 1985). Hyper- and hyporeacting groups may be recognizable to some extent.

Investigators have worked on methodologic improvements in irritant dermatitis studies, because visual assessment measures mainly erythema and edema and is subjective.

Besides the limitations in qualitative aspects, the reliability of observed and visually quantitated results may be limited. Tools employed in clinical experiments are the laser Doppler flowmeter, evaporimeter, micrometers, and ultrasonography. Skin impedance and water content have been measured and replica systems developed to qualify and quantify reactions (Maibach et al., 1984). In experimental irritant dermatitis studies, certain model irritants, usually detergents, were used. Sodium lauryl sulfate is the model surfactant that has been used most frequently. It induces epidermal damage as well as visible erythematous irritation and thus is a useful model irritant for such experiments.

The laser Doppler flowmeter gives information about cutaneous circulatory changes associated with erythematous irritation. Results obtained with laser Doppler generally correlate with visible changes (Guy et al., 1985b; van der Valk et al., 1984). This method appears slightly more sensitive than the naked eye in evaluating erythema, which is often correlated with the amount of epidermal damage (Lammintausta et al., 1988a, 1988b).

Edema may sometimes interfere with measurements, and thus reactions with associated edema yield lower flowmeter values, although irritation-induced reaction in skin vasculature is apparent (Lammintausta et al., 1988b). Nonerythematous irritation cannot be detected with this method.

The evaporimeter is a practical tool for the measurement of transepidermal loss. Cumulative irritation leads to increased transepidermal water loss (Lammintausta et al., 1988a). Increased irritation from more concentrated irritants leads to greater increase in transepidermal water loss, although no erythema is seen. These alterations can be demonstrated before visible changes appear. Transepidermal water loss often increases in association with erythematous irritation (Blanker et al., 1986; Lammintausta et al., 1988a), which makes this method useful in studies of more acute irritant responses. The recovery of epidermis after irritant attacks has been demonstrated with gradually normalizing transepidermal water loss values. Evaporimeter measurements are quick: measurement can be registered in minutes. But the resting time needed before individual values can be evaluated has to be 20–30 min, since nonsweating baseline values must first be obtained. Environmental circumstances (temperature and humidity) must be standardized. For evaluations of individual reactivity, repeated values have to be followed up, since individual baseline values are different. On the other hand, baseline values for an individual subject show day-to-day variation. Transepidermal water loss measurements still need standardization and improvement before this tool is useful for routine clinical purposes.

The measurement of skin electrical impedance and water content provides further means of studying cutaneous hydration (Maibach et al., 1984; Tagami et al., 1980; Thiele and Malten, 1973). Impedance measurement is based on the facilitated current conduction in stratum corneum related to the ionic movements of hydrates. Stratum corneum water content is assessed by means of a microwave dielectric probe.

Future efforts will be directed to developing these methods for practical purposes. Studies of the mechanisms of irritant contact dermatitis on the cellular and biochemical level will reveal new aspects to this syndrome. Increasing knowledge about mediators (Csato and Czarnetzki, 1988; Rosenbach et al., 1988) and cell interactions (Frosch and Czarnetzki, 1987; Gawkrodger et al., 1987) will also help us to understand this multifactorial clinical problem.

Concomitant Disease

Generalized wasting and debilitation in patients with advanced carcinoma have been associated with decreased skin reactivity to croton oil and DNCB (Johnson et al., 1971). Decreased reactivity to croton oil (Weidenfeld, 1912) and increased susceptibility to alkali (Ziierz et al., 1960) were reported in patients with ichthyosis vulgaris. Other investigators noted increased reactivity to phenol (Schultz, 1912) but decreased reactivity to croton oil (Halter, 1941) on the depigmented skin in patients with vitiligo. The literature on patch-test reactions to irritants in the presence of eczema is conflicting. This subject has been partly clarified by Bjornberg (1968), who showed that an increased susceptibility to irritants may be demonstrated in eczematous patients with some but *not all* irritants. Susceptibility to irritation has also been correlated with the extent of the eczema. Patients with *localized* hand eczema had increased reactivity to sodium lauryl sulfate; patients with *generalized* eczema had increased reactivity to four additional irritants (croton oil, trichloroacetic acid, mercury bichloride, and sapo kalinus). Bjornberg (1974) further demonstrated that patients with healed hand eczema have no greater susceptibility to irritants than noneczematous controls. The type of eczema may also influence the response to irritants. Skog (1960) showed an increased incidence of primary irritant reactions to pentadecylcatechol in patients with preexisting allergic contact eczema but not in patients with preexisting irritant eczema or atopic dermatitis. Although clinical observations have suggested that individuals with atopic dermatitis or atopic diathesis are more susceptible to skin irritation, experimental proof is lacking.

Neurologic Influence

Neurologic factors may influence cutaneous reactivity. Biberstein (1940) reported an increased inflammatory response to mustard oil on sympathectomized ears in rabbits, compared with nonsympathectomized contralateral control ears. Others reported decreased reactivity to phenol in areas of peripheral paralysis but increased reactivity to phenol in areas of central paralysis (Schaefer, 1921), decreased reactivity to tincture of iodine in areas of peripheral anesthesia (Kaufman and Winkel, 1922), and a generalized increase in reactivity in areas of peripheral neuritis (Halter, 1941).

The nervous system is obviously involved in the subjective response to irritants. A specific somatosensory receptor, selectively stimulated by certain irritants (e.g., lacrimators), has been identified in cat skin (Foster and Ramaze, 1976).

Medication

Corticosteroids in sufficient dose administered either topically or systemically may suppress subsequent irritant responses to croton oil (Nilzen and Wikstrom, 1955), but not to turpentine or cantharidin (Goldman et al., 1952). In general, there appears to be a limiting dose of systemically administered corticosteroid below which the inflammatory response is not inhibited. Although there is not universal agreement, the limiting dose appears to be in the range of 15 mg of prednisone or equivalent (Feuerman and Levy, 1972). Antihistamines in any dose probably do not impair responses to irritants. No data exist on the cutaneous response to irritants in patients with Addison's or Cushing's disease.

PREDICTIVE IRRITANCY TESTING

Predictive irritancy testing involves specific tests for the irritant potential of individual chemicals as well as tests for individual susceptibility to irritation.

Predictive Testing for Chemical Irritant Potential

Predictive testing is widely performed to determine the irritant potential of various chemicals. The most popular methods are bioassays with human or animal subjects. Most procedures employ a single application of a test substance, with evaluation of the response in 24–48 h. The oldest of these assays is the Draize rabbit test, in which test substances are applied for 24 h under occlusion to abraded and nonabraded skin. While this procedure detects severe irritants for human skin, it is unsatisfactory for mild to moderate irritants (Phillips et al., 1972). Numerous modifications adaptable to special situations have been developed. The reader is referred to the National Research Council (1977) special publication that discusses the principles and practices involved.

Because of species variability, correlation of irritancy studies of animal skin with human skin has not been entirely satisfactory. A rabbit cumulative irritancy test has been described that compares favorably with a cumulative human irritancy assay (Marzulli and Maibach, 1975; Steinberg et al., 1975).

Bioassays involving human subjects are patterned after those involving animal models. Frosch and Kligman (1977b) introduced a chamber-scarification test, which enhances the capacity to detect mild irritants. The forearm is scarified in a crisscross pattern; the suspected irritant is applied to this area in a large aluminum chamber once daily for 3 days.

To date, bioassays have utilized visible degrees of erythema and edema as indices of irritancy; this method is simple and convenient. The development of physical techniques for measuring subtle degrees of noninflammatory skin damage has improved our understanding of this area. Skin permeability to water vapor (transepidermal water loss) was the first physical measurement to be used for this purpose. Early investigations clearly established that chemicals that provoked inflammation increased transepidermal water loss (Rollins, 1978; Spruit, 1970, 1971). Malten and Thiele (1973) subsequently showed that increases in transepidermal water loss occurred *before* visible inflammation when ionic, polar, water-soluble substances (e.g., sodium hydroxide, soaps, detergents) were used as irritants. Malten and den Arend (1978) showed that an unionized, polar irritant (dimethyl sulfoxide) did not provoke increased water vapor loss until visible inflammation had already occurred. Similarly, two unionized nonpolar (water-insoluble) irritants, hexanediol diacrylate and butanediol diacrylate, did not provoke increased skin water vapor loss until visible inflammation occurred (Malten et al., 1979). Thus, transepidermal water loss measurements may detect the irritant capacity of certain chemicals in the absence of visible inflammation, but possibly only for ionizable, polar, water-soluble substances.

Measurements of the electrical impedance (resistance) of human skin also detect subtle degrees of skin damage before skin inflammation occurs (Thiele and Malten, 1973). This method has the advantage over water loss measurements that it is capable of detecting subtle changes produced by unionizable or nonpolar substances as well as ionizable, polar ones (Malten et al., 1979). Measurements of carbon dioxide emission from human skin have been developed (Malten and Thiele, 1973). Rates of carbon dioxide emission from irritated skin increase roughly in proportion to the degree of irritation (Thiele, 1974).

Electrolyte flux through the skin barrier may be measured with the aid of ion-specific skin electrodes (Grice et al., 1975; Anjo et al., 1978). Measurements of chloride ion flux through psoriatic or eczematous skin indicate that, despite the dramatic increases in permeability to water vapor, the electrolyte barrier remains relatively intact (Grice et al., 1975). Chloride ion flux may provide another noninflammatory index of cutaneous irritation. A potassium ion electron has been of value in quantifying potassium flux postdamage (Lo et al., 1990).

Predictive Testing for Susceptibility to Irritation

The ability to predict which individuals are more prone to irritant skin reactions has practical significance as a preemployment screening test. The ability of the skin to neutralize solutions of sodium hydroxide was first proposed as a screening test for susceptibility to irritation by Gross et al. (1954). Bjornberg (1968) reviewed previous attempts to predict general susceptibility by determining irritant responses to selected irritants. He was unable to corroborate early claims that inability to neutralize alkaline solutions, decreased resistance to alkaline irritation, or that increased susceptibility to common experimental irritants could be used to predict susceptibility to irritations in a preemployment setting.

Frosch and Kligman (1977a) used the length of time to slight blister formation after experimental exposure to ammonium hydroxide as a predictive index. They found that short times were highly correlated with the intensity of inflammation produced by irritating concentrations of sodium lauryl sulfate. They also found that patients with atopic dermatitis (who were presumably more susceptible to irritation) had shorter times to blister formation than controls (Frosch, 1978).

HISTOLOGY, HISTOPATHOLOGY, AND PATHOLOGY

Contact dermatitis, eczema, and eczematous lesions are imprecise terms in dermatologic histology. Irritant contact dermatitis cannot be characterized on the basis of histologic findings. The histology is different in acute and chronic contact dermatitis. The degree and severity of the dermatitis and the interval between the onset and the actual time of biopsy influence the histological findings.

If the acute irritant or toxic skin reaction is strong, vesicles may be seen. In the vesicle, a mixture of neutrophils and lymphocytes is seen. In initial acute irritant contact dermatitis, dermal changes may be absent or minimal. Dermal infiltrates appear and increase during the first day of the developing dermatitis. The cell infiltrates in irritant and allergic contact dermatitis are not significantly or diagnostically different. In chronic irritant contact dermatitis, scaling, hyperkeratosis, and lichenification are apparent in older skin lesions, often resembling neurodermatitis.

In immunohistologic studies, identical composition of peripheral T lymphocytes, associated with peripheral HLA-DR (histocompatibility locus A) positive macrophages and Langerhans cells, is seen in irritant and allergic contact dermatitis (Scheynius et al., 1984; Ferguson et al., 1985). In the lymphocyte population, helper/inducer lymphocytes exceed the number of T-suppression/cytotoxic cells (Scheynius et al., 1984; Avnstorp et al., 1987). In irritant contact dermatitis, keratinocytes have been demonstrated to express major histocompatibility complex (MHC) class II antigens concerned with the antigen presentation and the elicitation of the T-lymphocyte-dependent immune response (Gawkrodger et al., 1987). These antigens were expressed by the keratinocytes in both allergic and irritant contact dermatitis.

The inflammatory cell response has also been characterized in guinea pigs treated with toxic croton oil application or repeated sodium lauryl sulfate (SLS) applications. In both reactions monocyte counts were increased, even as compared with an allergic reaction. The heterogeneous monocyte group, however, consisted of lymphocytes, fibroblasts, and monocytes. Only a minority of basophils was seen, less than in allergic contact reactions. Mast cells were also slightly increased, suggesting some association between nonimmunologic contact urticaria and an acute irritant contact reaction (Anderson et al., 1988).

Irritants, such as surfactants, removed skin lipids and keratins. The mechanisms of inflammation in the development of irritant contact dermatitis are still poorly understood. In laboratory animals, the importance of the function and inflammation mediators of different cell types is appreciated, and certain preliminary observations have been reported in constructed experimental designs. For example, SLS and alkyl dimethyl benzammonium chloride (ADBC) were shown to enhance the migration of polymorphonuclear leukocytes. A corresponding inhibition was induced by leukotriene B4; that is, SLS and ADBC also induced the secretion of preformed mediators, such as histamine and lysozymal enzyme beta-G from the cells (Frosch and Czarnetzki, 1987). Wide variation in the inhibitory response was documented for cutaneous inflammation elicited by different irritants, whether induction was by histamine antagonists, prostaglandin and kinin synthesis inhibitors, or neutropenia-inducing agents (Patrick et al., 1987).

The importance of leukotrienes in irritant contact dermatitis appears evident (Rosenbach et al., 1988), and a peptidoleukotriene antagonist and an antagonist of platelet-activating factor (PAF) were documented to be less effective in irritant contact dermatitis than in the allergic type, suggesting that cytotoxic effects predominate in irritant contact dermatitis (Csato and Czarnetzki, 1988).

A corresponding interpretation was made based on the observation that lipoxy-genesis pathway is enhanced in irritant contact dermatitis, being inhibited in allergic contact dermatitis (Ruzicka and Printz, 1982).

Ulcerations

Ulcerative lesions can develop from skin contact with strong acids or strong alkalies. Calcium oxide and calcium hydroxide, sodium hydroxide, sodium metasilicate and sodium silicate, potassium cyanide, and trisodium phosphate may induce strong cutaneous irritation with ulcerations. Chrome ulcers are the most common type of cutaneous ulcers induced by irritation of dichromates. Compounds of beryllium, arsenic, or cadmium are also capable of inducing strong irritation and ulcers.

Solvents such as acrylonitrile and carbon bisulfide as well as gaseous ethylene oxide are examples of contactants that may induce ulceration in certain occupations. Cutaneous ulcerations develop from the direct corrosive and necrotizing effect of the chemical on the living tissue. Exposed areas, where both friction and chemical irritation are associated, are most susceptible for ulcers; minor preceding trauma in the exposed skin increases the risk. The ulcerations tend to be deeper, with an undermined thickened border, and the exudate under the covering crusts predisposes to infection. The treatment for ulcers is usually conservative, with dressings, powders, and different coverings according to the phase of healing. In some cases, such as beryllium ulcerations, excision has been recommended.

Granulomas

Cutaneous granulomas are considered a variant of irritant contact dermatitis when caused by a biologically inactive substance inoculated into the skin. A granuloma appears as a focal, tumid lesion persisting chronically in its primary site. It is subjectively symptomless. Macrophages respond with phagocytosis to the foreign body inoculation, and even giant cells may be seen (Epstein, 1983).

In clinical occupational dermatitis, the development is generally due to an accidental foreign body inoculation of hard and sharp plant parts, hairs, or different hard keratin animal parts into the skin of the employee. Powders, lead, and metals such as metallic mercury, beryllium, and silica are examples of substances that elicit toxic skin granulomas (Kresbach et al., 1971). Infectious granulomas may be caused by deep fungi, bacteria, or parasites. In these cases, inflammation and macrophage response, with phagocytic secretory and mixed-function macrophages, are seen.

The examining occupational dermatologist should keep the possibility of irritation granuloma in mind when studying and performing biopsy on this type of lesion; he should remind the histopathologist to utilize the special maneuvers needed to demonstrate possible foreign bodies. Special stains, electron microscopy, and the use of polarized light are often useful (Andreas et al., 1981).

TABLE 6. Clinical Features That May Suggest the Etiology of Irritant Contact Dermatitis

Ulcerations
  Strong acids, especially chromic, hydrofluoric, nitric, hydrochloric, sulfuric
  Strong alkalis, especially calcium oxide, sodium hydroxide, potassium hydroxide, ammonium
    hydroxide, calcium hydroxide, sodium metasilicate, sodium silicate, potassium cyanide,
    trisodium phosphate
  Salts, especially arsenic trioxide, dichromates
  Solvents, especially acrylonitrile, carbon bisulfide
  Gases, especially ethylene oxide, acrylonitrile
Folliculitis and acneiform
  Arsenic trioxide
  Glass fibers
  Oils and greases
  Tar
  Asphalt
  Chlorinated naphthalenes
  Polyhalogenated biphenyls and others
Miliaria
  Occlusive clothing and dressing
  Adhesive tape
  Ultraviolet
  Infrared
  Aluminum chloride
Pigmentary alterations
  Hyperpigmentation
    Any irritant or allergen, especially phototoxic agents such as psoralens, tar, asphalt,
      phototoxic plants, others
    Metals, such as inorganic arsenic (systemically), silver, gold, bismuth, mercury
    Radiation: ultraviolet, infrared, microwave, ionizing
  Hypopigmentation
    p-tert-Amylphenol
    p-tert-Butylphenol
    Hydroquinone
    Monobenzyl ethyl hydroquinone
    Monomethyl hydroquinone ether
    p-tert-Catechol
    p-Cresol
    3-Hydroxyanisole
    Butylated hydroxyanisole
    1-*tert*-Butyl-3,4-catechol
    1-Isopropyl-3,4,catechol
    4-Hydroxypropriophenone
Alopecia
  Borax
  Chloroprene dimers
Urticaria
  Numerous chemicals, cosmetics, animal products, foods, plants, textile, woods
Granulomas
  Keratin
  Silica
  Beryllium
  Talc
  Cotton fibers
  Bacteria
  Fungi
  Parasites and parasite parts

TABLE 7. Major Industrial Uses for Fibrous Glass

Insulation
Weatherproofing
Plastic reinforcement: laminates with polyesters, epoxy, polyurethanes, and other resins
Filtration media
Structural materials
Textiles

Hardening

Extensive and repeated exposure often produces an increased resistance to further irritation in the course of weeks or months. The importance of interindividual variation in the development of hardening may be even greater than the threshold level for cutaneous irritation, since the individual capacity to recover from previous attacks is a factor. The developed resistance or hardening is specific to the substance inducing it. It is restricted to the affected skin area; certain subjects appear to be unable to develop hardening. Relatively short periods away from work decrease the resistance, again increasing the vulnerability for irritant contact dermatitis after holidays. The "hardened" skin appears coarse, thickened, and somewhat lichenified. Increased skin thickness may play a role in the development of hardening. Skin thickening was evident in the experimental "hardening" state in guinea pigs (McOsker and Beck, 1967). Unfortunately, the main biologic mechanisms are unknown.

Repeated UV exposures also increase the capacity to resist irritation in the skin. This effect appears to be nonspecific (Thorvaldsen and Volden, 1980). Repeated UV exposures are therapeutic, followed by a period of "hardening" in the treatment of subacute or chronic irritant contact dermatitis. When the acute phase of an irritant contact dermatitis is over and relapses are expected, repeated UV exposures may elicit nonspecific "desensitization" in the skin, increasing the capacity to avoid relapses. Alterations at the cellular level, in cell surface proteins, and in the releasability of inflammatory mediators probably are important in the therapeutic benefit achieved by UV therapies of irritant contact dermatitis.

SUMMARY OF CLINICAL ASPECTS

The clinical appearance of irritant contact dermatitis is dependent on multiple factors. Some clinical features that may suggest the etiology are listed in Table 6. Fibrous glass is one of the most common causes of occupational contact dermatitis, and dermatitis elicited by fibrous glass appears variable depending on individual characteristics, exposure, and mechanisms. Table 7 showed the major industrial uses for fibrous glass.

The diagnosis of irritant contact dermatitis is always clinical, and patch testing is done to exclude allergic contact dermatitis. Hardening against certain irritants may sometimes develop.

REFERENCES

Agrup, G. 1969. Hand eczema and other dermatoses in South Sweden. (Thesis.) *Acta Dermatol. Venereol. [Suppl.] (Stockh.)* 49:61.

Al Jaber, H. and Marks, R. 1984. Studies of the clinically uninvolved skin in patients with dermatitis. *Br. J. Dermatol.* 111:437–443.

Andersen, K. E. and Maibach, H. I. 1979. Black and white human skin differences. *J. Am. Acad. Dermatol.* 1:276–228.

Anderson, K. E., Sjolin, K. E. and Soelgaard, P. 1988. Acute irritant contact folliculitis in a galvanizer. European Symposium on Contact Dermatitis, Heidelberg, May 27–29, p. 62.

Andreas, T. L., Vallyathan, N. V. and Madison, J. F. 1981. Electron probe microanalysis: Aid in the study of skin granulomas. *Arch. Dermatol.* 116:1272–1276.

Anjo, D. M., Cunico, R. L. and Maibach, H. I. 1978. Transepidermal chloride diffusion in man. *Clin. Res.* 26:208A.

Avnstorp, C., Ralfkiaer, E., Jorgensen, J. et al. 1987. Sequential immunophenotypic study of lymphoid infiltrate in allergic and irritant reactions. *Contact Dermatitis* 16:239–245.

Baker, H. and Blair, C. P. 1968. Cell replacement in the human stratum corneum in old age. *Br. J. Dermatol.* 80:367–372.

Beauregaard, S. and Gilchrest, B. A. 1987. A survey of skin problems and skin care regimens in the elderly. *Arch. Dermatol.* 123:1638–1643.

Berardesca, E. and Maibach, H. I. 1988. Racial differences in sodium lauryl sulphate-induced cutaneous irritation: Black and white. *Contact Dermatitis* 18:65–70.

Bettley, F. R. 1960. Some effects of soap on the skin. *Br. Med. J.* 1:1675–1679.

Biberstein, H. 1940. The effects of unilateral cervical sympathectomy on reactions of the skin. *J. Invest. Dermatol.* 3:201.

Bjornberg, A. 1968. Skin reactions to primary irritants in patients with hand eczema. (Thesis.) Gothenburg, Sweden: Oscar Isacsons Tryckeri AB.

Bjornberg, A. 1974. Skin reactions to primary irritations and predisposition to eczema. *Br. J. Dermatol.* 91:425.

Bjornberg, A. 1975. Skin reactions to primary irritants in men and women. *Acta. Derm. Venereol. (Stockh.)* 55:191–194.

Blanker, R., van der Valk, P. G. M. and Nater, J. P. 1986. Laser Doppler flowmetry in the investigation of irritant compounds on human skin. *Dermatosen* 34:5.

Britz, M. B. and Maibach, H. I. 1979. Human cutaneous vulvar reactivity to irritants. *Contact Dermatitis* 5:375–377.

Bruynzeel, D. P. and Maibach, H. I. 1986. Excited skin syndrome (angry back). *Arch. Dermatol.* 12:323–328.

Bruynzeel, D. P., van Ketel, W. G. and Scheper, R. J. 1983. Angry back of the excited skin syndrome: A prospective study. *J. Am. Acad. Dermatol.* 8:392–397.

Buckley, C. E. III, Larrick, J. W. and Kaplan, J. E. 1985. Population differences in cutaneous metacholine reactivity and circulating IgE concentrations. *J. Allergy Clin. Immunol.* 76:847–854.

Buckley, C. E. III, Lee, K. L. and Burdick, D. S. 1982. Metacholine-induced cutaneous flare response: Bivariate analysis of responsiveness and sensitivity. *J. Allergy Clin. Immunol.* 69:25–64.

Cerwinska-Ditram, I. and Rudzki, E. 1986. Skin reactions to primary irritants. *Contact Dermatitis* 7:315–319.

Christophers, E. and Kligman, A. M. 1965. Percutaneous absorption in aged skin. In *Advances in the Biology of the Skin*, ed. E. Montagna, pp. 160–179. Oxford: Pergamon Press.

Cooper, E. R. 1985. Vehicle effects on skin penetration. In *Percutaneous Absorption*, eds. H. I. Maibach and R. L. Bronaugh, pp. 525–530. New York: Marcel Dekker.

Cronin, E. and Stoughton, R. B. L. 1962. Percutaneous absorption: regional variations and the effect of hydration and epidermal stripping. *Br. J. Dermatol.* 74:7265–7272.

Csato, M. and Czarnetzki, B. M. 1988. Effect of BN 52021, a platelet activating factor antagonist on experimental murine contact dermatitis. *Br. J. Dermatol.* 118:475–480.

DeSalva, S. J. and Thompson, G. 1965. Na^{22}Cl skin clearance in humans and its relation to skin age. *J. Invest. Dermatol.* 45:315–318.

Dooms-Goossens, E., Delusschene, K. M., Gevers, D. M., et al. 1986. Contact dermatitis caused by airborne irritant. *J. Am. Acad. Dermatol.* 15:1–10.

Elias, P. M. 1981. Lipids and the epidermal permeability barrier. *Arch. Dermatol. Res.* 270:95–117.

Epstein, E. and Maibach, H. I. 1985. Eczematous psoriasis: what is it? In *Psoriasis*, eds. H. H. Roenigk, Jr. and H. I. Maibach, pp. 9–14. New York: Marcel Dekker.

Epstein, E. 1971. Contact dermatitis in children. *Pediatr. Clin. North Am.* 18:839–852.

Epstein, W. L. 1983. Cutaneous granulomas as a toxicologic problem. In *Dermatoxicology*, 2nd ed., eds. F. M. Marzulli and H. I. Maibach, pp. 533–545. New York: Hemisphere.

Feldmann, R. and Maibach, H. I. 1967. Regional variation in percutaneous penetration. *Int. J. Dermatol.* 48:1813–1819.

Feldmann, R. J. and Maibach, H. I. 1967. Regional variations in percutaneous absorption of C-cortisol in man. *J. Invest. Dermatol.* 48:181–183.

Feldmann, R. J. and Maibach, H. I. 1974. Systemic absorption of pesticides through the skin of man. Occupational Exposure to Pesticides: Report to the Federal Working Group on Pest Management from the Task Group on Occupational Exposure to Pesticides, Appendix B, pp. 120–127.

Ferguson, J., Gibbs, J. H. and Swanson Beck, J. 1985. Lymphocyte subsets and Langerhans cells in allergic and irritant patch test reactions: Histometric studies. *Contact Dermatitis* 13:166–174.

Feuerman, E. and Levy, A. 1972. A study of the effect of prednisone and an antihistamine on patch test reactions. *Br. J. Dermatol.* 86:68.

Finlay, A. Y., Nocholls, S., King, C. S., et al. 1980. The "dry" non-eczematous skin associated with atopic eczema. *Br. J. Dermatol.* 102:249–256.

Fischer, T. and Rystedt, I. 1985. False positive, follicular and irritants patch test reactions to metal salts. *Contact Dermatitis* 12:93–98.

Fisher, A. A. 1975. Childhood allergic contact dermatitis. *Cutis* 15:635–645.

Flannigan, S. A., Smith, R. E. and McGovern, J. P. 1984. Intraregional variation between contact irritant patch test sites. *Contact Dermatitis* 10:123–124.

Flannigan, S. A. and Tucker, S. B. 1985. Influence of the vehicle on irritant contact dermatitis. *Contact Dermatitis* 12:177–178.

Foster, R. W. and Ramaze, A. G. 1976. Evidence for a specific somatosensory receptor in the cat skin that responds to irritant chemicals. *Br. J. Pharmacol.* 57:436.

Frame, G. W., Strauss, W. G. and Maibach, H. I. 1972. Carbon dioxide emission of the human arm and hand. *J. Invest. Dermatol.* 59:155–158.

Fregert, S. F. 1981. Irritant contact dermatitis. In *Manual of Contact Dermatitis*, 2nd ed., ed. S. F. Fregert, pp. 55–62. Copenhagen: Munksgaard.

Frosch, P. J. and Czarnetzki, B. M. 1987. Surfactants cause in vitro chemotaxis and chemokinesis of human neutrophils. *J. Invest. Dermatol.* 88:525–555.

Frosch, P. J. and Kligman, A. M. 1977a. Rapid blister formation in human skin with ammonium hydroxide. *Br. J. Dermatol.* 96:461–473.

Frosch, P. J. and Kligman, A. M. 1982. Recognition of chemically vulnerable and delicate skin. In *Principles of Cosmetics for Dermatologists*, pp. 287–296. St. Louis: C. V. Mosby.

Frosch, P. J. and Wissing, C. 1982. Cutaneous sensitivity to ultraviolet light and chemical irritants. *Arch. Dermatol. Res.* 272:269–278.

Frosch, P. J. 1985. Hautirritation und empfindliche Haut (Thesis), pp. 1–118. Grosse Scripta 7, Berlin: Grosse Verlag.

Frosch, P. J. and Kligman, A. M. 1977b. The chamber scarification test for assessing irritancy of topically applied substances. In *Cutaneous Toxicity*, eds. V. A. Drill and P. Lazar, p. 150. New York: Academic Press.

Frosch, P. J. 1978. Rapid blister formation in human skin with ammonium hydroxide. Presented before the Society of Investigative Dermatology, San Francisco.

Gawkrodger, D. J., Carr, M. M., McVittie, E., et al. 1987. Keratinocyte expression of MCH class III antigens in allergic sensitization and challenge reactions and in irritant contact dermatitis. *J. Invest. Dermatol.* 88:11–20.

Gilchrest, B. A., Murphy, G. F. and Sotter, N. A. 1982. Effects of chronologic aging and ultraviolet irradiation on Langerhans cells in human skin. *J. Invest. Dermatol.* 79:85–88.

Gloor, M., Heyman, B. and Stuhlert, T. 1981. Infrared spectrocopic determination of water content of the horny layer in healthy subjects and in patients suffering from atopic dermatitis. *Arch. Dermatol. Res.* 271:429–458.

Goldman, L., Preston, R. and Rockwell, E. 1952. The local effect of 17-hydroxycorticosterone-21-acetate (compound F) on the diagnostic patch test reaction. *J. Invest. Dermatol.* 18:89.

Gollhausen, R. and Kligman, A. M. 1985. Effects of pressure on contact dermatitis. *Am. J. Ind. Med.* 8:223–328.

Grice, K., Sattar, H., Casey, T. and Baker, H. 1975. An evaluation of Na^+, Cl^-, and pH ion-specific electrodes in the study of the electrolyte contents of epidermal transudate and sweat. *Br. J. Dermatol.* 92:511–518.

Grice, K., Sattar, H. and Baker, H. 1973. The cutaneous barrier to salts and water in psoriasis and in normal skin. *Br. J. Dermatol.* 88:459–463.

Griffiths, W. A. D. and Wilkinson, D. S. 1985. Primary irritants and solvents. In *Essentials of Industrial Dermatology*, eds. W. D. Griffiths and D. S. Wilkinson, pp. 58–72. Oxford: Blackwell Scientific.

Gross, P., Blade, M. O., Chester, J. and Sloane, M. B. 1954. Dermatitis of housewives as a variation of nummular eczema. A study of pH of the skin and alkali neutralization by the Burckhart technique. Further advances in therapy and prophylaxis. *Arch. Dermatol.* 70:94.

Grove, G. L., Lavker, R. M., Hoelzle, E., et al. 1981. Use of nonintrusive tests to monitor age-associated changes in human skin. *J. Soc. Cosmet. Chem.* 32:15–26.

Gummer, C. L. 1985. Vehicles as penetration enhancers. In *Percutaneous Absorption*, eds. H. I. Maibach and R. L. Bronaugh, pp. 561–570. New York: Marcel Dekker.

Guy, R. H., Tur, E., Bjerke, S., et al. 1985a. Are there age and racial differences in methyl nicotinate-induced vasodilatation in human skin? *J. Am. Acad. Dermatol.* 12:1001–1006.

Guy, R. H., Tur, E. and Maibach, H. I. 1985b. Optical techniques for monitoring cutaneous microcirculation. *Int. J. Dermatol.* 2:88–94.

Halter, K. 1941. Zur pathogenese des ekzems. (Cited in Bjornberg [1968], p. 21.) *Arch. Dermatol. Syph.* 181:593.

Hanifin, J. M. and Lobitz, W. C. 1977. Newer concepts of atopic dermatitis. *Arch. Dermatol.* 113:663–670.

Hanifin, J. M. and Rajka, G. 1980. Diagnostic features of atopic dermatitis. *Acta Derm. Venereol. [Suppl.] (Stockh.)* 92:44–47.

Hannuksela, M., Pirila, V. and Salo, O. P. 1975. Skin reactions to propylene glycol. *Contact Dermatitis* 1:112–116.

Hjorth, N. and Avnstorp, C. 1986. Rehabilitation in hand eczema. *Derm. Beruf. Umwelt* 34:74–76.

Holland, B. D. 1958. Occupational dermatoses—Predisposing and direct causes. *JAMA* 167:2203–2205.

Holst, R. and Moller, H. 1975. One hundred twin pairs tested with primary irritants. *Br. J. Dermatol.* 93:145–149.

Holzle, E., Plewig, G. and Ledolter, A. 1986. Corneocyte exfoliative cytology: A model to study normal and diseased stratum corneum. In *Skin Models,* eds. R. Marks and G. Plewig, pp. 183–193. New York: Springer Verlag.

Jambor, J. J. 1955. Etiologic appraisal of hand dermatitis. *J. Invest. Dermatol.* 24:387–392.

Johnson, L. C. and Corah, N. L. 1960. Racial skin differences in skin resistance. *Science* 139:766–767.

Johnson, M. A., Maibach, H. I. and Salmon, S. E. 1971. Skin reactivity in patients with cancer-impaired delayed hypersensitivity of faulty inflammatory response. *N. Engl. J. Med.* 284:1255.

Jordan, W. E. and Blaney, T. L. 1982. Factors influencing infant diaper dermatitis. In *Neonatal Skin,* eds. H. I. Maibach and E. K. Boisits, pp. 205–221. New York: Marcel Dekker.

Kaufman, A. M. and Winkel, M. 1922. Entzundung und nervensystem. *Klin. Wochenschr.* 1:12.

Kingston, T. and Marks, R. 1983. Irritant reactions to dithranol in normal subjects and in psoriatic patients. *Br. J. Dermatol.* 108:307–313.

Kligman, A. M. and Wooding, W. A. 1967. A method for the measurement and evaluation of irritants on human skin. *J. Invest. Dermatol.* 49:78–94.

Kligman, A. M. 1976. Perspectives and problems in cutaneous gerontology. *J. Invest. Dermatol.* 73:39–46.

Kresbach, H., Karl, H. and Wawschink, O. 1971. Cutaneous mercury granuloma. *Berufsdermatoisen* 18:173–186.

Lachapelle, J. M. 1986. Industrial airborne irritant or allergic contact dermatitis. *Contact Dermatitis* 14:137–145.

Lahti, A. and Maibach, H. I. 1985. Guinea pig ear swelling test as an animal model for nonimmunologic contact urticaria. In *Models in Dermatology,* vol. II, eds. H. I. Maibach and N. I. Lowe, pp. 356–359. New York.

Lammintausta, K. and Maibach, H. I. 1990. Contact dermatitis due to irritation. In *Occupational Skin Disease,* ed. R. M Adams, pp. 1–15. Philadelphia: W. B. Saunders.

Lammintausta, K. and Kalimo, K. 1981. Atopy and hand dermatitis in hospital wet work. *Contact Dermatitis* 7:301–308.

Lammintausta, K., Maibach, H. I. and Wilson, D. 1987a. Human cutaneous irritation: induced hyperreactivity. *Contact Dermatitis* 17:193–198.

Lammintausta, K., Maibach, H. I. and Wilson, D. 1987b. Irritant reactivity in males and females. *Contact Dermatitis* 17:276–280.

Lammintausta, K., Maibach, H. I. and Wilson, D. 1988a. Susceptibility to cumulative and acute irritant dermatitis. An experimental approach in human volunteers. *Contact Dermatitis* 19:84–90.

Lammintausta, K., Maibach, H. I. and Wilson, D. 1988b. Mechanisms of subjective (sensory) irritation propensity to nonimmunologic contact urticaria and objective irritation in stingers. *Derm. Beruf. Umwelt* 36:45–49.

Lantinga, H., Nater, J. P. and Coenraads, P. J. 1984. Prevalence, incidence and course of eczema on the hand and forearm in a sample of the general population. *Contact Dermatitis* 10:135–139.

Lawrence, C. M., Howel, C. and Schester, S. 1984. The inflammatory response to anthralin. *Clin. Exp. Dermatol.* 9:336.

Lejman, E., Stoudemayer, T., Grove, G., et al. 1984. Age differences in poison ivy dermatitis. *Contact Dermatitis* 11:163–167.

Lo, J. S., Oriba, H. A., Maibach, H. I. and Bailin, P. L. 1990. Transepidermal potassium ion, chloride ion, and water flux across delipidized and cellophane tape-stripped skin. *Dermatologica* 180:66–68.

Lovell, C. R., Rycroft, R. C. G., Williams, D. M. J., et al. 1985. Contact dermatitis from the irritancy (immediate and delayed) and allergenicity of hydroxy acrylate. *Contact Dermatitis* 12:117–118.

MacDonalds, K. J. S. and Marks, J. 1986. Short contact anthralin in the treatment of psoriasis: A study of different contact times. *Br. J. Dermatol.* 114:235–239.

Magnusson, B. and Hersle, K. 1965. Patch test methods: II. Regional variation of patch test responses. *Acta Derm. Venereol. (Stockh.)* 45:226–257.

Magnusson, B. and Hillgren, L. 1962. Skin irritating and adhesive characteristics of some different adhesive tapes. *Acta Derm. Venereol. (Stockh.)* 42:463–472.

Maibach, H. I. and Boisits, E. K., eds. 1982. *Neonatal Skin: Structure and Function.* New York: Marcell Dekker.

Maibach, H. I., Bronaugh, R., Guy, R., et al. 1984. Noninvasive techniques for determining skin function. In *Cutaneous Toxicity,* eds. V. A. Drill and P. Lazar, pp. 63–97. New York: Raven Press.

Maibach, H. I., Feldmann, R. J., Millby, T. H., et al. 1971. Regional variation in percutaneous penetration in man. Pesticides. *Arch. Environ. Health* 23:208–294.

Malten, K. E., den Arend, J. and Wiggers, R. E. 1979. Delayed irritation: hexanediol diacrylate and butanediol diacrylate. *Contact Dermatitis* 5:178–184.

Malten, K. E. and den Arend, J. 1978. Topical toxicity of various concentrations of DMSO recorded with impedance measurements and water vapour loss measurements. *Contact Dermatitis* 4:80–92.

Malten, K. E. and Thiele, F. A. J. 1973. Evaluation of skin damage. II. Water loss and carbon dioxide release measurements related to skin resistance measurements. *Br. J. Derm.* 89:565.

Malten, K. E. 1981. Thoughts on irritant contact dermatitis. *Contact Dermatitis* 7:238–247.

Marzulli, F. N. and Maibach, H. I. 1975. The rabbit as a model for evaluating skin irritants: A comparison of results in animals and man using repeated skin exposures. *Food Cosmet. Toxicol.* 13:533.

Maurice, P. D. L. and Greaves, M. W. 1983. Relationship between skin type and erythema response to anthralin. *Br. J. Dermatol.* 109:337–341.

McOsker, D. E. and Beck, L. W. 1967. Characteristics of accommodated (hardened) skin. *J. Invest. Dermatol.* 48:372–383.

Mitchell, J. C. 1981. Angry back syndrome. *Contact Dermatitis* 7:359–360.

Mobly, S. L. and Mansmann, H. C. 1974. Current status of skin testing in children with contact dermatitis. *Cutis* 13:995–1000.

Montaga, W. and Carlisle, K. 1979. Structural changes in aging human skin. *J. Invest. Dermatol.* 73:47–53.

National Research Council. 1977. *Principles and Procedures for Evaluating the Toxicity of Household Substances.* Washington, DC: National Academy of Sciences.

Nilsson, E., Mikaelsson, B. and Andersson, S. 1985. Atopy, occupation and domestic work as risk factors for hand eczema in hospital workers. *Contact Dermatitis* 13:216–223.

Nilzen, A. and Wikstrom, K. 1955. Factors influencing the skin reaction in guinea pigs sensitized with 2,4-dinitrochlorobenzene. *Acta Derm. Venereol. (Stockh.)* 35:415.

Olumide, G. 1987. Contact dermatitis in Nigeria. II. Hand dermatitis in men. *Contact Dermatitis* 17:136–138.

Oriba, H. A., Elsner, P. and Maibach, H. I. 1989. Vulvar physiology. *Semin. Dermatol.* 8:2–6.

Patrick, E., Burkhalter, A. and Maibach, H. I. 1987. Recent investigations of mechanisms of chemically induced skin irritation in laboratory mice. *J. Invest. Dermatol.* 88:245–315.

Phillips, L., Steinberg, M., Maibach, H. I. and Akers, W. A. 1972. A comparison of rabbit and human skin responses to certain irritants. *Toxicol. Appl. Pharmacol.* 21:369.

Pittz, E. P., Smorbeck, R. V. and Rieger, M. M. 1985. An animal test procedure for the simultaneous assessment of irritancy and efficacy of skin care products. In *Models in Dermatology,* eds. H. I. Maibach and N. J. Lowe, vol. II, pp. 209–224. New York: S. Karger.

Rajka, G. 1975. The aetiology of atopic dermatitis. In *Atopic Dermatitis,* ed. G. Rajka, pp. 46–104. Philadelphia: W. B. Saunders.

Roberts, D. and Marks, R. 1980. The determination of regional and age variations in the rate of desquamation: A comparison of four techniques. *J. Invest. Dermatol.* 74:13–16.

Rollins, T. G. 1978. From xerosis to nummular dermatitis: The dehydration dermatosis. *J. Am. Med. Assoc.* 206:637.

Rosenbach, T., Csato, M. and Czarnetzki, B. M. 1988. Studies on the role of leukotrienes in murine allergic and irritant contact dermatitis. *Br. J. Dermatol.* 18:1–6.

Rothenborg, H. W., Menne, T. and Sjolin, K. E. 1977. Temperature dependent primary irritant dermatitis from lemon perfume. *Contact Dermatitis* 1:37–48.

Ruzicka, T. and Printz, M. P. 1982. Arachidonic acid metabolism in skin: Experimental contact dermatitis in guinea pigs. *Int. Arch. Allergy Appl. Immunol.* 69:347–353.

Rycroft, R. J. G. 1981. Occupational dermatoses from warm dry air. *Br. J. Dermatol.* 105(Suppl.)(21):29–34.

Rystedt, I. 1985. Factors influencing the occurrence of hand eczema in adults with a history of atopic dermatitis in childhood. *Contact Dermatitis* 12:247–254.

Schaefer, W. 1921. Beitrage zum klinischen Studium und der quantatitiven Prufung der Hautreaktion auf chemische Reize. II. Uberdie chemische Hautreaktion bei Peripheren und zentralen Lahmungen. *Arch. Dermatol. Syph.* 132:87. Cited in Bjornberg (1968).

Scheynius, A., Fischer, T., Forsum, U., et al. 1984. Phenotypic characterization in situ of inflammatory cells in allergic and irritant contact dermatitis in man. *Clin. Exp. Immunol.* 55:81–90.

Schultz, I. H. 1912. Beitrage zum klinischen Studium und der quantatitiven Prufung der

Hautreaktion auf chemische Reize. I. Mitteilung: Uber das verhalten normaler und leukopathischer lautstellen hautranker und Hautreaktion bei peripheren und zentralen Lahmungen. *Arch. Dermatol. Syph.* 13:987. Cited in Bjornberg (1968, p. 21).

Seymour, J. L., Keswich, B. H., Hanifin, J. M., et al. 1987. Clinical effects of diaper types on the skin of normal infants and infants with atopic dermatitis. *J. Am. Acad. Dermatol.* 17:988–997.

Skog, E. 1960. Primary irritant and allergic eczematous reactions in patients with different dermatoses. *Acta Derm. Venereol. (Stockh.)* 40:307.

Spruit, D. 1970. Evaluation of skin function by the alkali application technique. *Curr. Probl. Dermatol.* 3:148.

Spruit, D. 1971. Interference of some substances with water vapor loss of human skin. *Am. Perfum. Cosmet.* 8:27.

Steinberg, M., Akers, W. A., Weeks, M., McCreesh, A. H. and Maibach, H. I. 1975. A comparison of test techniques based on rabbit and human skin responses to irritants with recommendations regarding the evaluation of mildly or moderately irritating compounds. In *Animal Models in Dermatology,* ed. H. I. Maibach, pp. 1–11. New York: Churchill Livingstone.

Stoughton, R. B., Potts, L. W., Clendenning, W., et al. 1969. Management of patients with eczematous diseases: use of soap vs. no soap. *JAMA* 175:1196–1198.

Suskind, R. R., Meister, M. M., Scheen, S. R., et al. 1963. Cutaneous effects of household synthetic detergents and soaps. *Arch. Dermatol.* 88:117–124.

Susten, A. S. 1985. The chronic effects of mechanical trauma to the skin: A review of the literature. *Am. J. Intern. Med.* 18:281–288.

Tagami, H., Masatoshi, O., Iwatsuki, K., et al. 1980. Evaluation of the skin surface hydration in vivo by electrical measurements. *J. Invest. Dermatol.* 75:500–507.

Tagami, H. 1971. Functional characteristics of aged skin. *Acta Derm. Venereol. (Stockh.)* 66:19–21.

Thiele, F. A. J. and Malten, K. E. 1973. Evaluation of skin damage I. Skin resistance measurements with alternative current impedance measurements. *Br. J. Dermatol.* 89:373–382.

Thiele, F. A. J. 1974. *Measurements on the Surface of the Skin,* p. 81, Nijmegen, Netherlands: Drukkeij van Mammeren BV.

Thorvaldsen, J. and Volden, G. 1980. PUVA-induced diminution of contact allergic and irritant skin reactions. *Clin. Exp. Dermatol.* 5:43–46.

Tur, E., Maibach, H. I. and Guy, R. H. 1985. Spatial variability of vasodilatation in human forearm skin. *Br. J. Dermatol.* 113:197–303.

Ummenhofer, B. 1980. Zum Methodik der Alkaliresistenzprufung. *Dermatosen Beruf Umwelt* 28:104.

van der Valk, P. G. M., Nater, J. P. and Bleumink, E. 1984. Skin irritancy of surfactants as assessed by water vapour loss measurements. *J. Invest. Dermatol.* 89:291.

van der Valk, P. G. M., Nater, J. P. K. and Bleumink, E. 1985. Vulnerability of the skin to surfactants in different groups of eczema patients and controls as measured by water vapour loss. *Clin. Exp. Dermatol.* 101:98.

Vickers, H. R. 1962. The influence of age on the onset of dermatitis in industry. Prague, Symposium Dermatologorum de Morbis Cutaneis, pp. 145–148.

von Hagerman, G. 1957. Uber das "traumiterative" (toxische) Ekzem. *Dermatologica* 115:525–529.

von Hornstein, O. P., Baurle, G. and Kienlein-Kletschka, B. M. 1986. Prospktiv-Studie zur bedeutung konstitutioneller Parameter fur die Ekzemgenese im Friseur und Baugewerbe. *Derm. Beruf. Umwell* 33:43–498.

von Hornstein, O. P. and Kienlein-Kletschka, B. M. 1982. Improvement of patch test allergen exposure by short-term local pressure. *Dermatologica* 165:607–611.

Wagner, G. and Porschel, W. 1962. Klinisch-analytische studie zum neuroder-matitisproblem. *Dermatologica* 125:1–32.

Wahlberg, J. E. and Maibach, H. I. 1986. Sterile cutaneous pustules: A manifestation of contact pustulogens. *J. Invest. Dermatol.* 76:381–383.

Wahlberg, J. E. and Maibach, H. I. 1982. Identification of contact pustulogens. In *Dermatotoxicology,* 2nd ed., eds. F. N. Marzulli and H. I. Maibach, pp. 627–635. New York: Hemisphere.

Weidenfeld, S. 1912. Beitrage zur Pathogenese des Ekzems. *Arch. Dermatol. Syph.* 111:891. Cited in Bjornberg (1968, p. 21).

Weigand, D. A. and Gaylor, J. R. 1974. Irritant reaction in Negro and Caucasian skin. *South. Med. J.* 67:548–551.

Weigand, D. A., Haygood, C. and Gaglor, J. R. 1974. Cell layers and density in Negro and Caucasian stratum corneum. *J. Invest. Dermatol.* 62:563–568.

Werner, Y., Lindberg, M. and Forslind, B. 1982. The water binding capacity of stratum corneum in dry non-eczematous skin of atopic eczema. *Acta Derm. Venereol. (Stockh.)* 62:334–336.

Wester, R. C. and Maibach, H. I. 1989a. Dermal decontamination and percutaneous absorption. In *Percutaneous Absorption,* eds. R. L. Bronaugh and H. I. Maibach, pp. 335–342. New York: Marcel Dekker.

Wester, R. C. and Maibach, H. I. 1985. Dermatopharmocokinetics. In *Clinical Dermatology in Percutaneous Absorption,* eds. H. I. Maibach and R. L. Bronaugh, pp. 525–530. New York: Marcel Dekker.

Wester, R. C. and Maibach, H. I. 1989b. Regional variation in percutaneous absorption. In *Percutaneous Absorption,* eds. R. L. Bronaugh and H. I. Maibach, pp. 111–119. New York: Marcel Dekker.

White, M. I., Jenkinson, D. M. and Lloyd, D H. 1987. The effect of washing on the thickness of the stratum corneum in normal and atopic individuals. *Br. J. Dermatol.* 116:525–530.

Ziierz, P., Kiessling, W. and Berg, A. 1960. Experimentelle Prufung der Hautfunktion bei Ichthyosis Vulgaris. *Arch. Klin. Exp. Dermatol.* 209:592.

12

advances in mechanisms of allergic contact dermatitis: *in vitro* and *in vivo* research

■ **B. M. E. von Blomberg** ■ **D. P. Bruynzeel** ■
■ **R. J. Scheper** ■

OPTIONS

The skin is notorious as a sensitive monitor for diseases developing within the internal organs. In particular, systemic immune function is sharply reflected by skin reactivity. Allergic contact dermatitis (ACD) is a prototype skin manifestation of systemic immune reactivity, mediated by circulating, specifically sensitized T lymphocytes (Polak, 1980) (Fig. 1).

Interestingly, typical contact allergens are small, chemically reactive molecules that may bind to skin constituents and thus modify "self" to "nonself," bringing the immune system into alert. It has been recognized for long that the sensitization process triggered by simple epicutaneous application of such contact allergens could provide valuable information on mechanisms determining systemic T-cell-dependent immune function. T-cell-mediated reactions became known to play a central role in various "modified-self"-related immune diseases, including transplantation reactions and autoimmunity, as well as in tumor rejection. Experimental contact sensitivity has thus been widely used as a model for cell-mediated immune diseases.

The convenience, however, of ACD models primarily applies to *in vivo* studies. This became clear when *in vitro* studies on T-cell immunity in ACD were designed, initially to elucidate the different elements involved in contact allergic reactions. Since—in the early 1970s—*in vitro* tests were also considered extremely desirable from a clinical point of view, that is, for diagnosing ACD, research in this field was intensified. The initial progress was promising: contact sensitivity reactions could be successfully elicited *in vitro* by stimulating

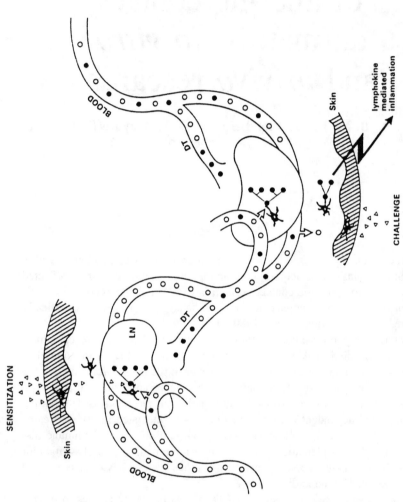

FIGURE 1 Pathogenesis of allergic contact dermatitis: sensitization and challenge. Upon sensitization, allergen-specific T lymphocytes proliferate in the draining lymph nodes (LN) and reach the blood through the thoracic duct (DT). Subsequent challenge of the skin with allergen results in a local lymphokine-mediated inflammation and may further increase the frequency of allergen-specific cells in the circulation. △, Allergen; ⋆, allergen-presenting cell; ●, allergen-specific T

lymphocytes with allergen. Introduction of *in vitro* tests for diagnosing ACD in clinical settings then became within reach.

In a review on *in vitro* tests for ACD, Scheper and Oort (1973) speculated on the potential use of these tests in diagnostic procedures. Replacement of traditional skin tests by *in vitro* tests was considered to "depend on the progress in filling up the large gaps in theoretical knowledge on cellular immunity." Now, almost 20 years later, many gaps have been filled and the time has come to reconsider the value of *in vitro* tests in clinical ACD as compared to the perennial patch tests.

The aim, therefore, of the present review is:

1. To delineate the progress in fundamental knowledge in ACD
2. To evaluate the impact of this extended knowledge on *in vivo* and *in vitro* testing in ACD, and
3. To evaluate the current clinical applicability of *in vitro* tests in ACD.

THE MECHANISM OF T-CELL ACTIVATION IN ACD

Introduction

Although in established allergic contact dermatitis (ACD) humoral antibody-mediated reactions can participate, ACD depends primarily on the activation of specifically sensitized T cells. Upon local allergen triggering, these cells initiate an inflammatory cascade leading to overt skin disease. Contact sensitivity can thus be regarded as an example of delayed-type hypersensitivity (DTH). Although the term DTH has been used in the past for all skin reactions taking more than 24 h to develop after antigenic challenge, it now refers to a state of hypersensitivity associated with systemically increased numbers of antigen-specific T lymphocytes (Turk, 1975). In contrast to the classical, tuberculin-type DTH reaction, which is induced by intradermal injection of protein antigens, ACD is generally elicited by epicutaneous contact with allergens and affects in particular superficial skin layers. Although partly different mechanisms are involved in the development of these two delayed-type reactions, at the level of T-cell activation they are essentially similar. This chapter will focus on how T-cell activation takes place *in vivo* upon sensitization and challenge, since this provides the clues for understanding *in vitro* assays in ACD.

Although distinct differences can be noted in macroscopic appearance, time course, and histopathology of contact allergic reactions in mice, guinea pigs, and humans, mechanisms of T-cell activation in these species share many features. Most cell surface molecules involved in T-cell activation have been detected and characterized on human as well as on murine leukocyte membranes (Horejsi and Bazil, 1988; Holmes and Morse, 1988). These and other leukocyte surface molecules have been grouped into clusters of differentiation (CD). A selection of human CD designations relevant for ACD has been listed in Table 1. This list includes molecules of the human major histocompatibility complex (MHC), the human leukocyte antigens (HLA). Other basic elements involved in triggering, amplification, and regulation of allergic reactions, such as intercellular adhesion molecules, lymphokines, and vasoactive amines, are also found in mice, guinea pigs, and humans. Their relative contribution to skin reactivity may, however, vary, leading to subtle differences in the manifestations of ACD. As both mouse and guinea pig models have strongly contributed to our present knowledge of ACD, in this review data from animal studies have been taken together with results obtained from studies on T-cell-mediated reactions in humans.

Depending on the site of primary allergen contact, sensitization or tolerance may result. From animal studies it is clear that upon allergen application onto or into the skin both hypersensitivity and tolerance-inducing mechanisms are triggered, the balance, however, being tipped in favor of sensitization. In contrast, oral or intravenous administration of allergen in animals rather induces tolerance (Van Hoogstraten et al., 1989; Vreeburg et al., 1990). Unfortunately, still little is known about the cells and restriction elements determining the induction of tolerance in humans. As to the sensitization process, however, much progress has been made in identifying the cells and molecular structures involved. This chapter will concentrate on sensitization and highlight the unique environment the skin provides in this process.

All constituents essential for sensitization, that is, allergen-specific T cells, antigen-presenting cells (APC), and mediators facilitating lymphocyte activation (Kupper, 1989), can be found in the skin. Thus, a highly elaborate defensive mechanism is provided, completing the physicomechanical barrier function of the skin. Keratinocytes, Langerhans cells (LC), epidermotropic T lymphocytes, and peripheral lymph nodes have been described as an integrated system of "skin-associated lymphoid tissue" (SALT; Streilein, 1983) mediating cutaneous immunosurveillance. To stress the immunologically autonomous role of the epidermis and the complexity of the cell system it harbors, another term, now excluding peripheral lymph nodes, was introduced by Bos and Kapsenberg (1986): the "skin immune system" (SIS).

With the acceptance of the epidermis as an immunological organ in its own right, the long-disputed question of peripheral versus central sensitization (Polak, 1980) became less compelling. Theoretically, sensitization as well as elicitation could take place all along the route of allergen-bearing APC, from the skin to the lymph nodes. The actual site of T-cell triggering is determined by the local frequency of specific T cells and by their activational state. The more specific T cells abound, the sooner an allergen-bearing APC will by chance meet one. As memory T lymphocytes show high migratory capacity and are, in addition, readily triggered by skin LC, the process of elicitation, that is, T-cell activation in hypersensitive individuals, generally takes place within the

TABLE 1. Cell Surface Molecules in ACD, Selected Cluster of Differentiation (CD) Designations

Cluster	mAbs[b]	Name	MW[a] (kD)	Ligand/ function	Leukocyte distribution
D1a	OKT6, leu6		49		Langerhans cells
D2	OKT11, leu5	LFA-2	50	LFA-3, SRBC	T cells
D3	OKT3, leu4	T3 complex	27, 20, 20 (16, 16)	Transducer TCR signal	T cells
D4	OKT4, leu3		55	MHC-class II	T subset (help)
D8	OKT8, leu2		32	MHC-class I	T subset (sup/cyt)
D11a/CD18	CLB-LFA1 2/1	LFA-1 a/β	(180, 95)	ICAM-1	Leukocytes
D16	leu11	Fc-gamma R	50–60	Low affinity for Fc gamma	Granulocytes, NK cells
D25	OKT26a (Tac)	IL-2 R	55	Low affinity for IL-2	Activated lymphocytes
D27	OKT18		(55, 55) 32		T cells activated T cells
D28		Tp44 antigen	44		T cells, plasma cells
D29	4B4	VLA β-chain	130		T subset (help inducer), myeloid cells
D45		Leukocyte Common antigen LCA, T200	180, 190, 205,220		Leukocytes
D45RA	2H4, WR16	Restricted LCA	205, 220		T subset Suppressor inducer/naive B lymphocytes, monocytes
D45R0	UCHL1	Restricted LCA	180		T subset (help/memory)
D4g	VLA-1	VLA-1	(210, 130)		Activated cells
	VLA-4	VLA-4	(150, 130)	VCAM-1	Lymphocytes, monocytes Myeloid cells
D54		ICAM-1	90	LFA-1	Lymphocytes, myeloid cells
D58		LFA-3	40–70	CD2	Broad
D71	OKT9	Transferrin R	(90, 90)	transferrin	Activated cells
	WT31	TCR α/β	(44, 40)	antigen + MHC	
	W6/32	MHC-class I HLA-A, B, C	45	CD8	Nucleated cells
	OKDr	MHC-class II HLA-DR, DQ, DP	(34, 29)	CD4	B cells, monocytes Activated T cells

[a]Molecular weights of the different chains are given between brackets if they are covalently linked. rom Bierer and Burakoff (1988), Hemler (1990), Horejsi and Bazil (1988), Knapp et al. (1989), and Van ongen et al. (1988).
[b]Monoclonal antibodies.

skin. Sensitization, on the other hand, is rather localized in the draining lymph nodes, where large numbers of T cells can be contacted by the now fully active allergen-bearing APC (Romani et al., 1989; see also next subsection).

The guiding principle in selecting data for the present review is given by their value for designing and interpreting *in vivo* and *in vitro* tests in human ACD. We will deal with allergen presentation (next subsection), T-cell activation and T-cell products, T-lymphocyte traffic and compartmentalization, and T cells mediating ACD.

Allergen Presentation and Sensitization

Most contact allergens are small, chemically reactive molecules. Upon penetration through the epidermis they readily bind to skin components forming "hapten-carrier" complexes. The ability to associate with carrier molecules, either covalently or through weak interaction bonds, is a prerequisite for contact sensitization. Whereas most allergens bind spontaneously, some need enzyme- or UV-induced activation before binding can take place.

In the skin not only soluble amino acids or macromolecules but also cell membrane-bound structures may serve as carriers. Nevertheless, only those allergen molecules eventually associated with MHC-class II molecules present on allergen-presenting cells (APC) will stimulate specific T cells. That is, the T-cell receptor for antigen (TCR) recognizes allergens only in MHC-class II context. The density of class II molecules [collectively termed "Ia" (immune response associated) molecules] on the cell membrane of APCs may vary considerably and roughly correlates with the capacity to stimulate T lymphocytes (Janeway et al., 1984; Nunez et al., 1987). Up-regulation of the Ia density on the APC membrane can be induced *in vitro* by cytokines like interferon-gamma (IFN-gamma) but, interestingly, also by incubation with contact allergens (Picut et al., 1987).

In humans the HLA-D region of the MHC encodes three types of Ia molecules: HLA-DP, DQ, and DR. Although the three MHC-class II genes can be independently expressed, stimulatory agents like IFN-gamma generally induce surface expression of all three HLA-D region products (Collins et al., 1984; Nunez et al., 1987). Correspondingly, all three Ia molecules can contribute to T-cell activation. Nevertheless, DR-restricted allergen-specific T-helper clones apparently are most frequently found (Ottenhof et al., 1985; Botham et al., 1989). When in mice strong support was obtained for a determining role of defined Ia molecules ("I-J") in the activation of suppressor pathways (Grantstein, 1985) a human analogue has been looked for. HLA-DQ was put forward as a promising candidate in a study on schistosomal antigens (Hirayama et al., 1987). Nevertheless, a clear suppressor function for DQ molecules or any other particular Ia antigen has up to now not been convincingly demonstrated.

In ACD, sensitization is most likely to occur through allergen directly bound to MHC-class II molecules or to the peptides associated with them at the peptide binding sites or "grooves" (Grey and Chesnut, 1985; Cresswell, 1987; Claverie et al., 1989).

In addition, degradation and processing of haptenated proteins or cell membrane constituents, followed by class II-associated exposition on the cell membrane may contribute to the actual sensitization of T lymphocytes.

It would appear that the immune response in ACD is directed to a large variety of hapten-carrier determinants, involving at least three different Ia molecules (DP, DQ, and DR), whereas in addition, binding may be to various reactive molecular groups, such as the nucleophilic groups $-NH_2$ and $-SH$ (Parker et al., 1985). The obstinate search for one putative "true" sensitizing carrier in contact sensitization has considerably hampered the development of *in vitro* diagnostic assays in ACD.

In healthy skin, the epidermal dendritic Langerhans cell (LC), bearing high numbers of Ia molecules on its cell membrane, is the primary antigen-presenting cell (Fig. 2) (Stingl et al., 1978; Wolff and Stingl, 1983; Breathnach, 1988). LC stem from the bone marrow (Tamaki and Katz, 1980), but their

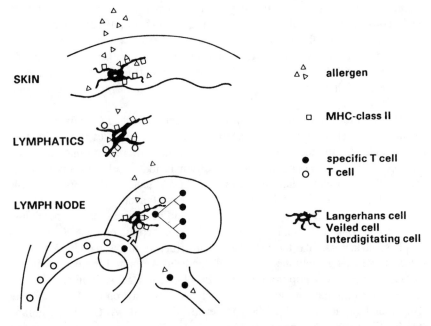

FIGURE 2   Allergen presentation in ACD. Upon penetration through the skin allergen molecules are carried to the lymph nodes by Langerhans cells/veiled cells. These APC readily interact with T cells ("clustering") and will eventually present the allergen to a specific T lymphocyte. In nonsensitized individuals this encounter usually takes place in the lymph nodes (above), and in sensitized individuals within the skin. Only those allergen molecules that associate with MHC-class II structures on the APC membrane will cause T-lymphocyte triggering. △, Allergen; □, MHC-class II molecule; ⚡, allergen-presenting cell; ●, allergen-specific T lymphocyte; ○, T lymphocyte of irrelevant specificity.

continuous presence in the epidermis is at least partly maintained by local LC proliferation (Czernielewsky and Demarchez, 1987; Parent et al., 1989). In mice the sensitization rate was found to be determined by the density of LC at the site of allergen application (Rheins and Nordlund, 1986; Bigby et al., 1987). Moreover, absence or functional inactivation of LC rather was associated with tolerance induction (Toews et al., 1980; Halliday and Muller, 1986; Kanagawa et al., 1983).

If allergen-specific memory T cells are encountered in the skin, as is likely to occur in hypersensitive individuals, allergen-bearing LC may trigger these cells immediately, thus giving rise to an overt inflammatory reaction of the skin. Since skin LC should be considered as still relatively immature APC (Schuler and Steinman, 1985; Streilein and Grammer, 1989; Romani et al., 1989; Teunissen et al., 1989), only previously activated, memory T cells, expressing sufficient cellular adhesion molecules on their surface, will be triggered locally. Upon subsequent lymphokine release, during the course of the ACD reaction, several cell types (endothelial cells, keratinocytes) may become Ia positive. Although all Ia-positive cells should be considered as potential stimulators of memory T lymphocytes, their actual contribution to allergen presentation *in vivo* is still speculative (Burger and Vetto, 1982; Hirschberg et al., 1982; Pober et al., 1983; Nickoloff et al., 1986; Nishioka et al., 1987). Interestingly, Ia expression of keratinocytes is associated rather with suppressor T cell—than with helper T cell—infiltration (Nickoloff et al., 1988; Smolle et al., 1988), which might suggest a down-regulating role of Ia-positive keratinocytes.

In nonsensitized individuals, the allergen-bearing LC will travel as "veiled cells" (Drexhage et al., 1980) through the lymphatics to the draining lymph nodes. In the meantime the LC may further differentiate into fully mature APC. In the paracortical area of the lymph nodes, cell contacts between these APC, now called "interdigitating cells" (Veldman, 1970; Veerman, 1974; Hoefsmit et al., 1982), and lymphocytes are sufficiently close to allow for triggering naive, allergen-specific cells. It should be realized that the formation of these cell contacts depends not just simply on Ia expression by APC, but also on physical factors, like the intricate tissue structure of the paracortical area, the characteristic membrane ruffling of dendritic APC, and the electrical cell surface charge. More importantly, the APC–T-cell contact is facilitated by sets of specialized interaction molecules, which are expressed on the T lymphocyte (Bierer and Burakoff, 1988; Makgoba et al., 1989) and APC cell membrane (De Panfilis, 1989), as shown in Fig. 3a.

T-cell triggering in the lymph nodes is followed by abundant proliferation of specific T lymphocytes (Fig. 1) (Oort and Turk, 1965; Polak, 1980). Notably, this obligatory proliferative response of draining lymph node cells upon contact sensitization has provided the basis for new "*ex vivo*" parameters for evaluation of the sensitizing potential of chemicals (Kimber et al., 1986). The process of sensitization is now completed by the subsequent release of specific

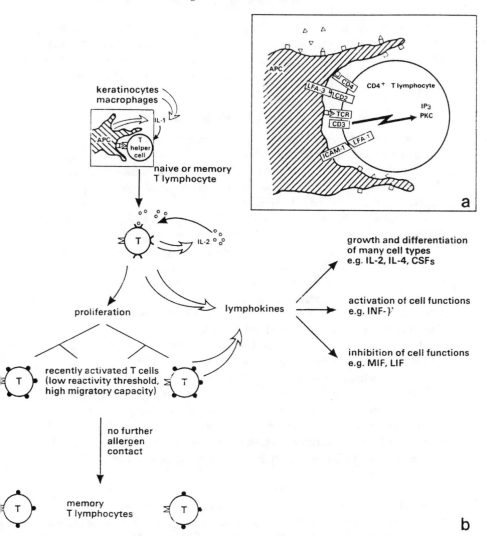

FIGURE 3 T-Cell activation. (a) Specific T lymphocytes are triggered by allergen associated with MHC-class II molecules on the APC membrane. IL-1, produced by APC, macrophages, or keratinocytes, provides a growth signal for T lymphocytes essential in this phase. A close lymphocyte-APC contact is maintained by several sets of molecules. The actual function of these molecules is, however, not yet clear. (b) Upon triggering, T lymphocytes produce their own growth factor (IL-2) and start to proliferate. The activated T lymphocytes now start to express increased numbers of cell surface molecules, such as transferrin receptors, adhesion molecules, and MHC-class II molecules. Activated T cells have a low reactivity threshold and a high migratory capacity. At the same time they produce an array of lymphokines with various biological activities. In the absence of further allergen contact, activated T lymphocytes gradually lose their "activation markers" and become memory cells. These memory cells, however, will continue to express higher levels of several surface glycoproteins as compared to naive T lymphocytes. △, Allergen; □, MHC-class II molecule; ⥲, TCR; ⟨, IL-2R; °°, IL-2; ⟨, different cell-surface glycoproteins associated with activation (see Fig. 4).

cells into the circulation. This can be monitored by evaluation of the "flare-up" of the sensitization site, where generally sufficient MHC class-II associated allergen molecules are retained to allow for a local ACD reaction. Such flare-up reactivity can be observed in humans at about 10 days after DNCB application (Skog, 1966).

T-Lymphocyte Activation

In recent years the T-cell receptor for antigen (TCR) has been identified and characterized (Dembic et al., 1986; Royer and Reinherz, 1987; Claverie et al., 1989). It consists of two linked polypeptide chains, each containing a variable and a constant domain. These domains are encoded in different gene segments, which are rearranged during T-cell ontogeny within the thymus. Interestingly, CD4$^+$ ("helper") T cells and CD8$^+$ ("cytotoxic/suppressor") T cells (Table 1) share the same set of TCRs. Upon exposition on the cell surface, the T-cell receptor associates with three nonvariable peptide chains bearing the CD3 determinant that is widely used as a T-cell marker. It is now assumed that, in addition to a TCR-mediated signal, T-cell activation requires an interleukin-mediated signal (presumably given by interleukin-1, IL-1; Fig. 3) (Mizel, 1987). In the skin IL-1 (or: epidermal cell-derived thymocyte activating factor: ETAF) can be produced by both Langerhans cells and keratinocytes (Sauder et al., 1984; Oppenheim et al., 1986; Lisby et al., 1987) and may be available in the epidermis as a preformed pool (Didierjean et al., 1989).

The biochemical pathways involved in T-cell stimulation are essentially the same as commonly observed in mammalian cell types upon hormone stimulation. In brief, membrane-bound phospholipids are converted into inositol 1,4,5-triphosphate (IP3), which mobilizes intracellular calcium, and diacylglycerol, which activates protein kinase c (Isakov et al., 1986). These signals initiate cellular proliferation, production of interleukin-2 (IL-2), and IL-2 receptor components.

Allergen-driven T-cell stimulation is terminated by a transient disappearance (probably by internalization) of the TCR. The process of T-cell activation then enters a second, allergen-independent phase, in which T-cell expansion is primarily mediated by growth factors such as IL-2, now abundantly released by the activated T cells. Low-affinity receptors for IL-2 (carrying the CD25 or "Tac" antigen), appear on the cell membrane early (within 48 h) after activation (Isakov and Altman, 1986). They combine with other IL-2-binding proteins to form high-affinity receptors for IL-2 (Smith, 1988). Internalization of the occupied receptors then further supports T-cell proliferation (Kumar et al., 1987). Additional receptors for growth factors including the transferrin receptor also appear on the cell membrane in this period (Holter et al., 1985). Allergen-activated T cells become morphologically "transformed" into blastoid cells, and subsequently differentiate into effector cells, producing, in addition to IL-2, a vast number of biologically active mediators, collectively known as lymphokines. In addition to the IL-2 and transferrin receptors, several other surface molecules have been detected with monoclonal antibodies on activated T cells (Fig. 4) (Holter et al., 1985; Horejsi and Bazil, 1988). Most of these molecules are still ill defined and are currently only being used as markers for T-cell activation in immunological studies. Interestingly, the "late" T-cell activation markers (expressed from about 4 days after stimulation) include the MHC-class II molecules. Different HLA-D region products may be expressed, depending on their (allo)antigen specificity (Schendel and Johnson, 1985). These molecules are actively synthesized by T cells (Holter et al., 1980). One may speculate that Ia molecules present on T cells contribute to down-regulation of T-cell immune responses by presenting the T-cell receptor (idiotype) to other T cells, thereby evoking an anti-idiotypic (suppressive) immune response.

T-Lymphocyte Products: Lymphokines

Introduction. Lymphokines (LK) comprise a fascinating group of primarily locally active peptide regulatory factors (PRF) (Green, 1989) whose biological significance is only beginning to be recognized (Dinarello and Mier, 1987). As outlined in the previous section, LK can be released by T cells as a metabolic consequence of signals provided by allergen-modified Ia molecules and IL-1. LK play an essential role in immune responses, not only as effector molecules but also as participants in immune regulation (Cohen, 1982). LK act antigen-nonspecifically and exert various effects on virtually all nucleated cells. To date at least 100 different biological activities have been ascribed to lymphokines. Although it is well established that different lymphokines may be produced by one T-cell subset, it is not yet clear how many different lymphocyte subsets produce how many different lymphokines. Research in this field has been complicated by the requirement of heterogeneous cell populations for optimal LK production, and the fact that LK may in turn induce the release of various mediators from macrophages and vasoamine-containing cells. Moreover, both antagonistic and synergistic lymphokines may be present in the same culture supernatants, and LK assessments strongly depend on bioassays that are at best semiquantitative. When, however, cell clones became available for production of LK and as targets in bioassays, LK research leapt forward. Simultaneously, progress was made with the generation of monoclonal antibodies to several individual LK, as well as with the introduction of molecular cloning techniques, resulting in recombinant lymphokines such as rIL-2 and rIFN-gamma (Hamblin, 1985). We now have learned that T-cell subsets may release characteristic sets of lymphokines upon appropriate stimulation. "Lymphokine-profiles" may thus be used to discriminate between functionally different subsets of T-helper cells. Notably, IL-2, IFN-gamma and MIF production have been associated with the ability of T-helper cells to mediate DTH in mice (Moorhead et al., 1982; Cher and Mosmann, 1987).

Evidence for LK participation in DTH reactions accumulated ever since Bennet and Bloom (1968) reported that upon injection of supernatants from

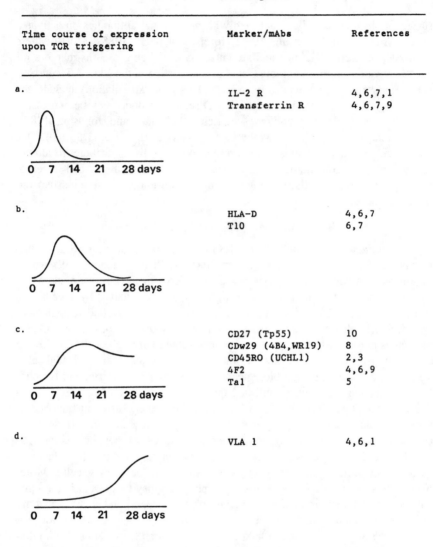

Time course of expression upon TCR triggering	Marker/mAbs	References
a.	IL-2 R Transferrin R	4,6,7,1 4,6,7,9
0 7 14 21 28 days		
b.	HLA-D T10	4,6,7 6,7
0 7 14 21 28 days		
c.	CD27 (Tp55) CDw29 (4B4,WR19) CD45RO (UCHL1) 4F2 Ta1	10 8 2,3 4,6,9 5
0 7 14 21 28 days		
d.	VLA 1	4,6,1
0 7 14 21 28 days		

FIGURE 4 Cell surface glycoproteins associated with T-cell activation. Surface glycoproteins expressed in increased densities on the T-cell membrane upon TCR triggering can be divided into four groups: Transient expression (a,b) with early (a) or delayed (b) appearance, and persistent expression (c,d) with early (c) and delayed or very late (d) appearance. Examples of each type are given as (mAbs detecting) the antigen. References: (1) ACT-T-SET[TM] TLiSA1 (T Cell Sciences); (2) Beverley (1987, 1988); (3) Byrne et al. (1988); (4) Furue and Katz (1988); (5) Hafler et al. (1986); (6) Hemler (1990); (7) Holter et al. (1985); (8) Moore and Nesbitt (1987); (9) Suomalainen et al. (1986); (10) Van Lier et al. (1988).

antigen-stimulated lymphocyte cultures into the skin, a DTH-like reaction developed within 3–5 h. This biologic activity was attributed to the putative "skin reactive factor" (SRF), at present considered to represent a number of different LK working in concert. Importantly, LK could be extracted from DTH lesions, and antilymphokine antibodies were reported to inhibit delayed skin reactions when administered locally or systemically (Geczy, 1984). The lymphokines actually initiating a local inflammatory reaction include LK acting on the cutaneous vessels, either directly (SRF) or indirectly, for instance by causing vasoamine-containing cells (basophils, mast cells) to release their mediators. Further development of the DTH reaction was found to be facilitated by LK activating the coagulation cascade, by LK attracting leukocytes to the site of inflammation, and by migration-inhibitory lymphokines (Geczy, 1984). The following paragraphs will focus on lymphokines involved in allergic contact dermatitis and considered of potential relevance for diagnostic *in vitro* tests in ACD (Table 2).

Interleukin-2 (IL-2). IL-2, formerly known as T-cell growth factor, is an early product of activated T lymphocytes. Maximum IL-2 concentrations in culture supernatants are usually reached within 24 h after T-cell stimulation. IL-2 promotes the proliferation of all IL-2 receptor-bearing cells, thus amplifying T-cell immune responses as soon as one or more T cells are stimulated by allergen contact. In recent years IL-2 research has successfully concentrated on isolation, purification, sequencing, and cloning. Recombinant IL-2 (rIL-2) produced in *Escherichia coli* proved to be as effective as the glycosylated "natural" IL-2, produced by activated lymphocytes. Availability of rIL-2 not only allowed for large-scale tumor therapeutical studies, but also contributed substantially to our insight in mechanisms of T-cell activation, by facilitating *in vitro* T-cell cloning and by enabling detailed analyses of the IL-2 receptor moieties. Both high- and low-affinity receptors have been demonstrated on activated helper T cells. High-affinity receptors, required for IL-2 induced T-cell proliferation, are expressed upon occupation of the TCR by antigen. They consist of two cooperating, non-covalently bound IL-2 binding proteins, each with a low affinity for IL-2 (Smith, 1988). One of these proteins, bearing the Tac epitope (CD25), is abundantly expressed on T cells upon IL-2 stimulation and is widely used as an activation marker. Obviously, growth factors promoting expression of their own receptors on target cells need strict control. Down-regulation is achieved by endocytosis of the high-affinity IL-2 receptor upon occupation by IL-2 (Isakov and Altman, 1986) or by release of the IL-2 receptor molecules. Soluble, IL-2 binding, Tac-positive proteins are indeed detectable in lymphocyte culture supernatants as well as in serum of patients with inflammatory disease (Rubin et al., 1986). Negative feedback control is also mediated by activated monocytes releasing prostaglandins (PGE_2) known to interfere with both production of and response to IL-2 (Tilden and Balch, 1982).

Although direct IL-2 measurements have not yet received much attention for *in vitro* monitoring of DTH reactivity, the most widely employed *in vitro*

TABLE 2. Some Important Lymphokines Produced by Allergen-Activated Helper T Cells

Lymphokine	Acronym	Function
Interleukin-2	IL-2	Growth/activation factor for T cells, NK cells
Interleukin-4	IL-4	Growth factor for activated B cells, resting T cells, mast cells
		Induces DR-expression on B cells
		Enhances T cell cytotoxicity
Colony-stimulating factors	IL-3	Bone marrow growth factors
		Multilineage stem cells
	GM-CSF	Granulocyte and macrophage stem cells
	G-CSF	Granulocyte stem cells
	M-CSF	Macrophage stem cells
Interferon-gamma	IFN-gamma	Induces class I and II expression, activates
(macrophage	(MAF)	macrophages, endothelial cells, killer cells
activating factor)		Exerts antiviral activity
Tumor necrosis	TNF β	Cytotoxic for tumor cells
factor β		Activates macrophages, endothelial cells
(= lymphotoxin)		Induces acute-phase response
Chemotactic factors	LCF	Lymphocyte chemotactic factor
	IL-8	Chemotactic for T cells and neutrophils
Migration inhibition	MIF	Inhibits macrophage migration
factors	LIF	Inhibits granulocyte migration
	TIF	Inhibits T cell migration
Macrophage	MPIF	Activates monocytes to produce procoagulant
procoagulant inducing		
factor		

assay, the lymphocyte transformation test (LTT), actually strongly depends on IL-2-mediated lymphocyte proliferation.

Immune interferon (IFN-gamma). IFN-gamma also plays a key role in the cascade of lymphokines produced during an immune response. Functional studies with T-lymphocyte clones revealed that both cytotoxic T cells and helper T cells are capable of producing IFN-gamma if appropriately stimulated, in particular in the presence of IL-2 (Trinchieri and Perussia, 1985). Interestingly, previously activated memory T lymphocytes produce much more IFN-gamma than unprimed, naive T cells do (Dohlsten et al., 1988). This already points toward an important role of IFN-gamma in the efferent immune response.

Two active species of IFN-gamma have initially been identified, with molecular weights of 20 and 25 kD reflecting different degrees of glycosylation. Homogeneous (nonglycosylated) human recombinant IFN-gamma is available now, and as this material is as active as the natural product(s), much progress has been made in studying IFN-gamma biology (Trinchieri and Perussia, 1985).

The capacity of IFN-gamma to up-regulate membrane expression of various cellular interaction molecules is of paramount importance for the development of the DTH reaction. Expression of both class I and class II (Ia) molecules is induced or enhanced by IFN-gamma in a large number of cell types (Rosa and Fellous, 1984), including vascular endothelial cells (Collins et al., 1984), keratinocytes (Nickoloff et al., 1986), monocytes (Gonwa et al., 1986), and Langerhans cells (Berman et al., 1985). Surprisingly, B and T lymphocytes are not susceptible to this effect of IFN-gamma (Gonwa et al., 1986; Gerrard et al., 1988). MHC class II expression by vascular endothelium may contribute to DTH reactivity by facilitating circulating $CD4^+$ lymphocytes to locally adhere and to enter the skin (Masuyama et al., 1986). Moreover, IFN-gamma has been found to increase vascular permeability (Martin et al., 1988). In skin cells increased Ia expression endows an enhanced capacity to present allergens, resulting in further local activation of specific T lymphocytes.

Besides enhancement of Ia expression, IFN-gamma has a plethora of effects on inflammatory cells recruited into DTH skin sites. At this point macrophage activation deserves mentioning, as can be detected by the increase of phagocytosis, O_2 metabolism, cytotoxic capacity, or by the induction of high-affinity Fc-receptors. These activities have earlier been ascribed to the macrophage-activating factor (MAF), now assumed to be identical to IFN-gamma (Talmadge et al., 1987).

From the biological activities of IFN-gamma the antiviral activity in particular has offered the opportunity to quantitatively measure IFN-gamma production in a bioassay (Trinchieri and Perussia, 1985).

Although direct IFN-gamma measurements have not become popular in DTH studies, indirect assays such as detecting Ia expression can provide important information on *in situ* or *in vitro* T-cell activation.

Migration-enhancing lymphokines. Local generation of chemotactic lymphokines in the skin further enables the development of DTH reactions, as these mediators cause inflammatory cells to migrate along concentration gradients to the actual site of allergen–T-cell contact. Upon arrival, however, another group of lymphokines, the so-called migration inhibitory factors (see below), supposedly maintain the cellular infiltrate *in situ*. The fact that stimulated lymphocytes release apparently counteracting mediators simultaneously or sequentially within only a short time interval has strongly complicated studies on these various lymphokines.

Several different chemotactic lymphokines have been described, attracting either or both eosinophils, macrophages, basophils, and lymphocytes (Geczy, 1984). Lymphocyte chemotactic factors (LCF) have most thoroughly been studied. The role of LCFs in delayed hypersensitivity was stressed by the group of Hayashi, who were able to demonstrate that out of four different LCF species isolated from guinea pig DTH reactions, at least two were T-cell derived (Hayashi et al., 1984; Shimokawa et al., 1984). In humans, LCFs distinct from IL-1 and IL-2 have also been isolated from DTH and ACD blister fluids (Ternowitz and Thestrup-Pedersen, 1986; Elmets et al., 1987). Human epidermal LCFs are, however, still poorly characterized, and no certainty exists as to their cellular source. Human LCF preparations were shown to attract preferentially CD4⁺ lymphocytes (Zachariae, 1988; Berman et al., 1985). Surprisingly, CD8⁺ cells, rather than CD4⁺ cells, may produce these factors upon *in vitro* stimulation (Potter and Van Eps, 1986). In addition, IL-8, a well characterized chemotactic for both T cells and neutrophils, may be produced by activated T lymphocytes (Nickoloff et al., 1990; Shall et al., 1990).

Since so much uncertainty still exists about the cells producing or responding to LCF, and about the biochemical nature of LCFs, employment of LCF production as a parameter of T-cell activation is not to be expected in the near future.

Migration-inhibitory lymphokines. Local production of migration inhibitory lymphokines by activated lymphocytes contributes to the retention of inflammatory cells in the area of allergen contact, thus enabling the DTH reaction to fully develop.

Migration inhibition factor (MIF) was the first lymphokine described and defined by its inhibitory effect on the migration of macrophages from capillary tubes (Bloom and Bennet, 1966). Its release by cultured mononuclear cells upon antigenic challenge has long been taken as the key molecular event in DTH reactivity.

The important role of MIF in the development of DTH reactions was shown by experiments in guinea pigs, in which DTH reactions could be suppressed by local or systemic administration of polyclonal anti-MIF antibodies (Geczy et al., 1976; Sorg and Geczy, 1976). In accordance with these results DTH reactions could also be suppressed by administration of alpha-L-fucose, which competes for MIF with the MIF receptor on the macrophage cell membrane (Hasegawa et al., 1980).

Biochemical characterization of both guinea pig MIF (Remold and Mednis, 1977) and human MIF (Weiser et al., 1981; David et al., 1983) revealed that the inhibitory activity is associated with a heterogeneous group of glycoproteins (Table 3). Following *in vitro* lymphocyte stimulation the biochemical MIF characteristics shift within a few days: the isoelectric point decreases (pH 5 to 3), the molecular weight increases (8–70 kD), and the MIF protein becomes more glycosylated. Structural homology of the different MIF molecules is confirmed by considerable cross reactivity observed with monoclonal anti-MIF antibodies (Table 3).

It has been widely accepted that cells capable of producing MIF upon antigenic stimulation reside in the helper T-cell population. Recent studies, however, by Malorny et al. (1988) unsettled the idea that human lymphocytes are MIF producers at all. Using monoclonal anti-MIF no positive lymphocytes could be detected *in situ* in either ACD reactions or activated lymph nodes, whereas both endothelial cells and macrophages were MIF-positive. It was suggested that lymphocytes upon stimulation cause macrophages to release their MIF. Since commonly heterogeneous cell suspensions, containing both macrophages (as APC) and lymphocytes, are used for MIF production, this hypothesis is hard to

TABLE 3. Properties of Human MIFs and Anti-Human MIF mAbs

	Early ("first day") MIF		Late ("second day") MIF	
MW	8/14 kD	23 kD	23–40 kD	65 kD
Isoelectric point	5	4.3–5.2	4.3–5.6	2.4–3.3
Neuraminidase-sensitive	nt	No	Yes	Yes
Trypsin-sensitive	nt	Yes	No	No
Chymotrypsin-sensitive	nt	nt	Yes	Yes
Anti-MIF D11[a]	Inactivation		Inactivation	
Anti-MIF E7[b]	Inactivation		Inactivation	
Anti-MIF 1C5[c]	Binding only		nt	nt

[a]Weiser et al. (1985): mAbs were raised against a 68-kD MIF preparation, pI 5, obtained from mitogen-stimulated T-cell hybridomas.
[b]Kawaguchi et al. (1986): mAbs were raised against 55–90 kD MIF, pI 5, obtained from a mitogen-stimulated T-cell line.
[c]Burmeister et al. (1986): mAbs were raised against 14-kD MIF, pI 5, obtained from mitogen-stimulated PBL.
Note: nt = not tested.

reject. Certainly more experimental data are needed to disprove the lymphokine nature of MIF. In this review MIF is still taken as a T-cell product.

MIF production is not inhibited by blocking lymphocyte proliferation (Rocklin, 1973). In mice, MIF-producing cells were enriched in those cell suspensions containing DTH effector cells (Tamura et al., 1982; Moorhead et al., 1982). In humans, support for MIF being produced by T-helper (CD4$^+$) lymphocytes came from various *in vitro* studies using virus-immortalized T cells (Szigeti et al., 1986), T-cell hybridomas, (Kobayashi et al., 1982) or peripheral blood-derived T-cell clones (Vyakarnam and Lachmann, 1984). More importantly, studies on fresh peripheral blood lymphocytes (PBL) showed that, upon stimulation, CD4$^+$ lymphocytes produced MIF (Kowalczyk et al., 1986; MacSween et al., 1986), whereas CD8$^+$ lymphocytes generally produced migration stimulatory factors instead of MIF (MacSween et al., 1986). It should be noted that in these experiments the potential role of monocytes or macrophages as MIF producers has not rigidly been excluded.

MIF acts on macrophages through a glycolipid receptor containing both fucose and sialic acid residues. Elegant proof for the existence of such receptors was given by Liu et al. (1985). Glycolipids could be isolated from MIF-sensitive macrophages and inserted into cell membranes of nonsensitive macrophages, thus rendering these cells sensitive to MIF.

The primary effect of MIF on macrophages, that is, inhibition of random migration, provided the basis for several *in vitro* bioassays for monitoring DTH reactivity. This inhibition is probably due to activation of the coagulation cascade, resulting in cross-linking of macrophage surface-bound fibrinogen, leading to impairment of the migratory capacity of the cells (Geczy, 1983). The same process actually is also mediated by another lymphokine, called the macrophage procoagulant inducing factor (MPIF). Interestingly, MPIF is produced by activated lymphocytes and induces the release of procoagulant from macrophages, analogous to the recently suggested pathway of lymphokine-induced release of MIF from macrophages (Malorny et al., 1988). The relationship between MPIF and MIF remains to be elucidated. Monoclonal MIF-binding antibodies are now available, and could be used to verify the homology suggested by Geczy (1983, 1984) between the two lymphokines. MPIF production, which can be readily measured in lymphocyte cultures upon antigenic stimulation, is also considered to be a close *in vitro* correlate of DTH (Geczy and Meijer, 1982; Geczy, 1984; Aldridge et al., 1985).

Not only macrophages, but also polymorphonuclear leukocytes (PMN) and lymphocytes are retained at sites of DTH-reactivity by locally released lymphokines. LIF (leukocyte migration inhibition factor) has been studied extensively, particularly in humans, with buffycoats providing an easy supply of target cells. Like MIF production, LIF production has also repeatedly been propagated as a relevant *in vitro* correlate of DTH.

From biochemical and functional studies it is clear that MIF and LIF are distinct molecules, but they may be produced simultaneously by the same helper T lymphocytes upon antigenic stimulation (Szigeti et al., 1986). Unlike MIF, LIF was found to display esterase activity, and the amount of hydrolytic activity present in a given supernatant could be correlated to its effect on PMN-migration (Rocklin and Urbano, 1978).

Using a highly purified LIF preparation [molecular weight (MW) 58,000] Borish et al. (1986b) found that LIF, apart from inhibiting random migration of PMN, induces neutrophil degranulation and an increased expression of receptors on the PMN-cell membrane for the chemoattractant f-Met-Leu-Phe.

The T-cell migration inhibition factor (TIF) is a novel and still ill-defined lymphokine, distinct from all other migration inhibitory factors (Kowalczyk et al., 1986; Berman et al., 1985). It is noteworthy that $CD8^+$ cells in particular are able to produce this TIF, whereas both $CD4^+$ and $CD8^+$ lymphocyte migration can be inhibited (Kowalczyk et al., 1986). Mediators like TIF and LCF, produced by and acting on distinct lymphocyte subsets, are likely to play an important role in the formation of characteristic cell infiltrates in ACD.

Evaluation of both MIF and LIF production by lymphocytes upon stimulation with contact allergens has so far provided valuable *in vitro* correlates of ACD in humans. Gene technology will undoubtedly in the near future allow for better characterization of these and many other lymphokines. A plethora of peptide regulatory factors still waits for identification before their potential value for diagnostic or therapeutic application can even be envisaged.

T-Lymphocyte Traffic

T-Cell-mediated allergic reactions are characterized by lymphocytic infiltrates at the site of allergen contact. The migration of T lymphocytes between the blood, skin, and lymphoid tissue compartments and the factors determining this traffic are visualized in Table 4.

The process of lymphocyte extravasation has been studied extensively in the lymph nodes, where T lymphocytes leave the bloodstream to populate the paracortical areas. To enter the lymphoid tissue, lymphocytes adhere to the postcapillary high endothelial venules (HEV), a process that now can be mimicked *in vitro* with frozen lymph node sections. Adhesion of lymphocytes to HEV is not a random event but achieved by receptor-ligand type of interactions, facilitating extravasation of those lymphocytes that express proper ligands on their surface (Kraal et al., 1987). The existence of tissue-specific ligands explains why some lymphocytes migrate preferentially to mucosa-associated lymph nodes, while another subpopulation rather enters peripheral lymph nodes (Cavender, 1989; Pals et al., 1986, 1988, 1989; Duyvestein et al., 1988, 1989; Picker et al., 1990).

In normal skin no specialized endothelium for lymphocyte extravasation has yet been found, but receptor-ligand interactions resembling those observed in the lymph nodes, may play a role in the preferential migration of T cells toward this organ. Several adhesion molecules have now been identified on lymphoid cells, such as H-cam(CD44), VLA-4(CD2g/CD4g^d) and LFA-1 (lymphocyte function-associated antigen), a structure present on the surface of most of the peripheral leukocytes. One of the major counter structures of LFA-1 is called ICAM-1 (intercellular adhesion molecule 1), which is not only expressed on different dendritic cell populations and macrophages, but also on endothelial cells (Dustin et al., 1986) and keratinocytes upon lymphokine activation (Griffiths et al., 1989). Intense staining with an anti-ICAM-1 monoclonal antibody (mAb) was found on endothelial cells in the T-cell areas of activated lymph nodes and, interestingly, also in DTH reactions in the skin (Dustin et al., 1986). In ACD reactions keratinocytes also express ICAM-1 (Wantzin et al., 1988). Strong support for involvement of LFA-1 in the adhesion of T lymphocytes to skin vascular endothelium was provided by Haskard et al. (1987), who demonstrated that monoclonal antibodies to LFA-1 could substantially reduce the binding of T-lymphocytes to cultured human dermal endothelial cells. Notably, T-cell binding to dermal endothelium could be potentiated, both by preincubation of the endothelial cells with IFN-gamma, IL-1, or bacterial lipopolysaccharides and by preactivation of the T lymphocytes with phorbol esters (Haskard et al., 1987). The latter finding fits with earlier reports on the predominant extravasation of lymphoblasts or their immediate descendants to sites of inflammation (Asherson et al., 1973; Van Dinther-Janssen et al., 1983; Jungi and McGregor, 1978).

Binding of lymphocytes bearing receptors for MHC class II (the CD4 determinants) to vessel walls may additionally be facilitated by the expression of class II molecules on endothelial cells (Masuyama et al., 1986). The Ia-positive endothelium is a characteristic feature of strong DTH reactions (Wood et al., 1986) or skin inflammatory reactions induced by IFN-gamma (Pober et

TABLE 4. Factors Determining T-Lymphocyte Traffic through the Skin and Draining Lymph Nodes

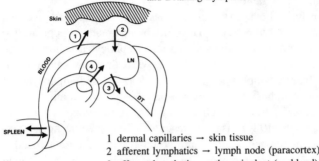

1 dermal capillaries → skin tissue
2 afferent lymphatics → lymph node (paracortex)
3 efferent lymphatics → thoracic duct (→ blood)
4 postcapillary HEV → lymph node (paracortex)

Migratory step	(Potential) determining factor (ref.)[a]	Effect on migration
1	T cell:	
	Activational stage (4, 12)	+
	Expression of adhesion/homing molecules (11, 15)	+
	Endothelial cells:	
	Expression of homing ligands (2, 3)	+
	Expression of antigen and/or class II molecules (9)	+
	Skin:	
	Release of vasoactive amines (1)	+
	Production of LCF, IL-1 (10)	+
	Production of IFN-gamma (6)	+
2	Skin:	
	Release of migration inhibitory cytokines	−
	Presence of allergen (13)	−
	Langerhans cells in the skin (14)	−
	ICAM-1 expressing keratinocytes? (8, 16)	−
3	Lymph node:	
	Release of migration inhibitory cytokines/sinusal blocking (7)	−
	IFN-alpha-2a (5)	−
4	T cells: Expression of adhesion/homing molecules (2, 11)	+
	HEV:	
	Expression of homing ligands (2, 11)	+
	Expression of antigen and/or class II molecules	+

[a]References: (1) Askenase and Van Loveren (1983); (2) Cavender (1989); (3) Dustin et al. (1986); (4) Haskard et al. (1987); (5) Hein et al. (1988); (6) Issekutz et al. (1988); (7) Kelly et al. (1972); (8) Lewis et al. (1989); (8) Masuyama et al. (1986); (10) Miossec et al. (1988); (11) Pals et al. (1989); (12) Pitzalis et al. (1988); (13) Scheper et al. (1983); (14) Shiohara et al. (1988); (15) Stoolman (1989); (16) Wantzin et al. (1988).

al., 1983; Collins et al., 1984). When allergen is present and associates with Ia-bearing endothelial cells, preferential adhesion and extravasation of antigen-specific helper T cells may occur. A lymphocyte homing receptor that may convey preferential adhesion to cutaneous, in contrast to mucosal, vessels has recently been described: the cutaneous lymphocyte associated antigen (CLA-a.g.), defined by the mAb HECA 452 (Picker et al., 1990).

The actual extravasation of lymphocytes following the binding to endothelial cells is obviously facilitated by locally released chemotactic factors. Such factors could be isolated from the epidermis overlying a tuberculin DTH reaction (Ternowitz and Thestrup-Pedersen, 1986; Zachariae et al., 1988). Locally acting lymphocyte chemotactic factors are assumed to include IL-1/ETAF (epidermal cell-derived thymocyte activating factor) and leukotriene B4, activated serum components, and chemotactic lymphokines like IL-2, LCF, and IL-8. Interestingly, IL-1 may be present in the epidermis as a preformed pool, allowing for early action (Didierjean et al., 1989). During an ongoing DTH reaction the increased production of lymphocyte chemotactic factors by activated T cells further contributes to lymphocyte infiltration. Notably, these chemotactic lymphokines mainly act on T cells, particularly CD4-positive T cells (Zachariae, 1988; Nickoloff et al., 1990; Sauder, 1990; Schall et al., 1990).

It has been reported that the massive infiltration of T lymphocytes early in DTH reactions is facilitated by the local release of vasoactive amines from mast cells (Askenase and Van Loveren, 1983). Serotonin is known to induce contraction of endothelial cells, thus forming "gaps" in the endothelial lining of the microvessel wall. The mechanism of early mast-cell activation in DTH reactions has been elucidated in the mouse, in which circulating antigen-specific T cell factors were found to be able to sensitize peripheral mast cells to secrete serotonin upon allergen contact. Such IgE-like T cell factors, however, have not yet been identified in other species.

A few days after allergenic challenge, most of the infiltrated T cells emigrate from the skin to the lymph nodes and may eventually join the recirculating pool of lymphocytes. For a long period of time, however (up to several months; Scheper et al., 1983), significant numbers of T cells are retained at former sites of allergen challenge. Generally, the frequency of allergen-specific cells in residual infiltrates will be markedly increased. Retained specific cells may give rise to local "flare-up" reactions upon renewed supply of allergen from the circulation or to enhanced skin reactivity upon subsequent epicutaneous allergen contact ("retest" reaction). Retention of antigen-reactive cells may be further enhanced by persistent antigen display, for instance, in draining lymph nodes in tuberculosis (Rook et al., 1976) or in the synovia (in reactive arthritis; Ford et al., 1985). In ACD, flare-up reactions are often observed at sites of (previous) eczema.

Since both *in vivo* and *in vitro* tests for T-cell immunity bear upon the circulating pool of allergen-specific lymphocytes, insight into the local traffic of lymphocytes (compartmentalization) upon allergen stimulation is of paramount importance for the design and interpretation of such tests. Remarkably few solid data are, however, available on compartmentalization in human ACD.

T Cells Mediating ACD

The nature of the cells that mediate contact sensitivity has been intriguing researchers for decades and has led to much speculation. Earliest relevant information was obtained in experimental studies by transferring immune cell subpopulations to naive recipients. Both in guinea pigs and mice contact sensitivity could be transferred with T lymphocytes (see Polak, 1980a). When appropriate reagents became available, T cells mediating DTH (T_{DTH}) could be further characterized in mouse models. Dennert and Hatlen (1975) postulated that specific cell-mediated cytotoxicity and contact sensitivity are mediated by different T-cell populations. In another model, however, contact sensitivity [to the 4-hydroxy-3-nitrophenyl (NP) hapten] could be transferred with both MHC-class I and MHC-class II restricted T-cell clones, assumed to display cytotoxic and helper functions, respectively (Minami et al., 1982). Possible involvement of cytotoxic T-cell-mediated skin damage in ACD was supported by data of Tamaki et al. (1981) and Shimada and Katz (1985), who observed that proliferating cytotoxic T lymphocytes, obtained from mice after contact sensitization, were able to kill hapten-coated epidermal cells *in vitro*. Nevertheless, most experimental data support the view that T_{DTH} and T_{ACD} primarily belong to the helper subclass (see below).

Phenotypic characterization of subsets of helper T cells mediating DTH in mice proved to be a difficult task. Nevertheless, functionally different subsets of murine helper T cells could be distinguished. T Cells able to mediate DTH reactions rather than providing B-cell help were found to be Ia negative, nonadherent to nylon wool, nonproliferating, and MIF producing (Moorehead et al., 1978, 1982; Tamura et al., 1982). On the other hand it was strongly suggested that the same T cell can mediate DTH and provide B-cell help depending on its environment (Milon et al., 1983). More recently, it has been found that individual spleen-derived helper T cells show dissimilar responses upon stimulation: some T cells produced IL-2 without providing detectable help for Ig synthesis; others led to Ig production but did not produce IL-2, or showed both functions (Powers and Miller, 1987). A similar subdivision of T-helper clones was described independently by Mosmann et al. (1986). The ability to mount DTH reactions upon local transfer resided in the T-helper subset "T_H1" or "inflammatory" subset, able to produce IL-2, IFN-gamma, and lymphotoxin. Help for specific antibody production, on the other hand, as well as IL-4 release was restricted to the "T_H2" or "helper" subset (Cher and Mosmann, 1987; Bottomly, 1988).

In humans a direct causal relationship between distinct T-cell subsets and DTH obviously can not be tested by passive cell transfer experiments. Identification of T cells mediating clinical contact hypersensitivity must, therefore, be based on analysis of skin infiltrates or on *in vitro* analysis of circulating allergen-specific T lymphocytes in contact allergic patients. A major role of $CD4^+$ cells in mediating human contact sensitivity was supported by the finding of a predominant early $CD4^+$ infiltrate in ACD reactions (Scheynius et al., 1984), as well as in other delayed-type skin reactions (Platt et al., 1983), and the finding that all nickel-specific clones isolated not only from peripheral blood from allergic patients but also from patch-test reaction sites showed the $CD4^+$ phenotype (Sinigaglia et al., 1985; Kapsenberg, 1987). Interestingly, isolation of urushiol-specific T-cell clones from PBL several months after rhus dermatitis resulted in only $CD8^+$ clones (Kalish and Morimoto, 1989). The authors suggest a role of these $CD8^+$ cells in down-regulating the DTH response.

Several mouse mAbs have been developed recently that allow for phenotypic subdivisions of human $CD4^+$ cells in various different subsets (Table 5) (Beverley, 1987). Most of these monoclonal antibodies are directed to one of the four polypeptides of the CD45 complex, a ubiquitous leukocyte antigen of unknown function (Beverley et al., 1988). Functional analyses of these subsets focussed on capacities for help or suppression in B-cell Ig production assays. A clear dissociation of $CD4^+$ cells in "helper-inducer" and "suppressor-inducer" subsets could be demonstrated with different mAbs (Moore and Nesbitt, 1987). Nevertheless, attempts to group human helper T-cell clones, in analogy to the mouse T_H1 and T_H2 subsets, into different nonoverlapping subsets related to either IL-2 and IFN-gamma or IL-4 production have failed so far (Paliard et al., 1988; Maggi et al., 1988). However, considering the kinetics of IL-2 release, distinct differences were found between $CD45RA^-$ helper T cells as early (within 24 h) producers of IL-2 and $CD45RA^+$ cells as late producers of IL-2. Also, higher amounts of IFN-gamma were produced by the former T-helper subset (Dohlsten et al., 1988).

In line with these results, an attractive view was recently presented by Sanders et al. (1988a), who regard the $CD45RA^+$ subset and the $CD29^+$ countersubset as different stages of differentiation: namely, as naive and memory (previously activated) T cells, respectively. This would also fit with the observation that upon PHA stimulation normal human $CD4^+$ cells change their $WR16^+$ phenotype into a $WR19^+$ phenotype (Moore and Nesbitt, 1987) and start to express the UCHL1 antigen (Terry et al., 1987). The UCHL1 epitope is located on the smallest CD45 peptide chain (CD45RO), whereas the CD45RA (naive) antigens are located on the longer chains of this complex (Smith et al., 1986; Beverley et al., 1988). UCHL1 as well as 4B4 mAbs have been shown to bind to $CD45RA^-$ helper T cells; they may now be considered as markers for previously activated, memory T lymphocytes. It is of particular interest that such memory T lymphocytes express increased numbers of cell adhesion molecules, thus facilitating effective allergen presentation by APCs (Table 5). Accordingly, $CD29^+$ helper T cells respond vigorously *in vitro* to antigen stimulation, whereas CD45RA-high-density cells fail to do so (Table 5) (Sanders et al., 1988).

TABLE 5. Characteristics of Human CD4$^+$ Subpopulation[a]

Subpopulation	Naive CD45RA-high		Memory CD29-high
Phenotype (mAb)	(relative expression)		
CD 3	1	:	1
CD45RA (2H4)	10	:	1
CD45RO (UCHL1)	1	:	30
CD29 (4B4)	1	:	4
LFA-3	1	:	>8
CD 2	1	:	3
LFA-1	1	:	3
Function			
Proliferation:			
Recall antigen	±		+ + + +
Mitogen	+ + + +		+ +
Lymphokine production:			
IL-2	+ + + +		+ + + +
	(late production)		(early production)
IL-3	+		+ + + +
IFN-gamma	±		+ + + +
BCGF	+ + + +		+ + + +
Modulation of B response:			
Help Ig production	±		+ + + +
Suppression of			
Polyclonal Ig production	+ + + +		±
Specific Ig production	±		+ + + +
Cell-mediated cytotoxicity	±		+ + + +
Binding to endothelial cells	+		+ + + +
Clustering with dendritic cells	+ +		+ + +

[a]Some characteristics of human CD4$^+$ T cell subsets phenotypically dissociated into 40–50% naive/suppressor-inducer and 50–60% memory/helper-inducer T cells. References: Byrne et al. (1988); Dohlsten et al. (1988); Pitzalis et al. (1988); Sanders et al. (1988); Vakkila (1989).

Notably, in normal human skin CD29 expression predominates in the CD4-positive lymphocytes (> 95% of CD4$^+$ cells) (Bos et al., 1987). These apparently activated (HLA-DR$^+$, IL-2 receptor$^+$) cells are situated perivascularly in the skin and are obviously ready to proliferate upon exogenous antigen stimulation. If a phenotypically distinct T$_{DTH}$ subset of helper T cells exists in humans, CD4$^+$, CD29$^+$ memory lymphocytes are likely candidates. An additional selective factor may be given by their expression of cutaneous lymphocyte-associated antigen (CLA-a.g.) as detected by mAb HECA 452 (Picker et al., 1990).

In conclusion, although human CD4$^+$ cells can now phenotypically be divided into several distinct subsets, and in mouse models relevant functional properties of T$_{DTH}$ have been further defined, T$_{DTH}$ still cannot be viewed as a well confined subset of helper T cells in either species. For the time being, it would appear prudent, therefore, to consider essentially all CD4$^+$ lymphocytes capable of contributing to ACD upon allergen-specific stimulation.

Conclusions

This section has focused on the process of specific T-cell activation representing the primordial event in allergic contact dermatitis. As to the site of T-cell activation, upon recognition of the epidermis as a distinct immunological organ in its own right (SIS), the long-disputed question of peripheral versus central sensitization lost much of its vigor. Frequency and activational stage of allergen-specific T cells entering insulted skin should be considered as the major factors determining the site of T-cell activation: within the draining lymph nodes (usually upon primary allergen contact) or peripherally in the skin (usually upon allergen challenge).

The central role of MHC class II (Ia) bearing allergen-presenting cells (APC), in particular Langerhans cells in the skin, is now well established. Contact sensitization occurs exclusively upon presentation of the allergen in context with one of the Ia molecules DR, DP, or DQ. Although a variety of carrier molecules may additionally be involved, hapten-modified Ia molecules should be considered to provide the major sensitizing determinants.

Our knowledge on mechanisms of T-cell activation has also rapidly grown: the T-cell receptor for antigen has been identified and its molecular structure characterized, and important interaction molecules and mediators were discovered.

Triggering of specific T cells by allergen-modified Ia on one hand leads to clonal expansion and on the other hand to the production of lymphokines, which mediate recruitment of other leukocytes. Many important lymphokines have now been fully characterized and their individual effects on the immune system could be extensively studied, especially since pure, recombinant lymphokines became available.

Upon activation, T lymphocytes express on their cell membranes increasing numbers of various glycoproteins (Fig. 5), which can be readily detected by monoclonal antibodies. Simultaneously, other surface structures may be lost. Phenotypically defined T cell subsets, such as CD45RA-positive and CD29-positive cells, were thus found to represent different stages of activation, namely, naive and memory T cells, respectively. The increased numbers of adhesion molecules, expressed on recently activated T cells and now known to be required for good migratory capacity and rapid triggering, gradually decrease in the absence of stimulating allergen. Interestingly, a distinctly increased level of adhesion molecules apparently persists on the cell membrane of previously activated memory T cells, keeping these cells distinguishable from naive T cells. Although final answers are not yet obtained, it does seem likely that in humans primarily CD29$^+$ helper T cells account for contact sensitivity reactions. However, so far little evidence has been obtained to support the

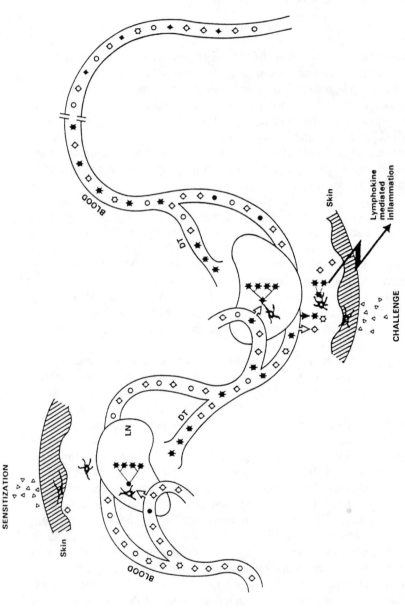

FIGURE 5 Activation of T lymphocytes upon sensitization and challenge. Once activated by allergen, T lymphocytes express increased numbers of adhesion molecules on their surface. These facilitate migration into the skin and cluster formation with allergen-presenting cells (see also Fig. 12). After a period of allergen restraint the activated lymphocytes lose many of their activation-associated cell surface glycoproteins and become memory cells. △ , Allergen; ⅄ , allergen-presenting cell; ● , allergen-specific T lymphocyte, naive; ★ , allergen-specific T lymphocyte, recently activated; ◆ , allergen-specific T lymphocyte, memory; ○ , T cell of irrelevant specificity, naive; ⬡ , T cell of irrelevant specificity, recently activated; ⬡ , T cell

existence of an a priori distinct subset of T cells (T_{DTH}) mediating allergic contact dermatitis.

IN VIVO TESTS IN ACD

Introduction

Patients presenting with the clinical picture of contact dermatitis are currently skin tested to verify whether the dermatitis is of allergic origin. If allergic, it is important to identify the allergen involved. Since allergic contact dermatitis (ACD) reflects systemic immune function, challenging uninvolved areas of the body with suspected allergens allows for answering these questions. Skin testing provides a sensitive methodology for diagnosing hypersensitivity, and its value for detecting causative agents in contact allergy is beyond dispute. In this chapter the capacity of skin testing to enlighten underlying immunological mechanism(s) will be evaluated.

In ACD epicutaneous skin tests are usually preferred to intracutaneous tests, as epicutaneous application most directly relates to pathogenesis. Upon epicutaneous application, allergen readily binds to epidermal Langerhans cells as required for T-cell triggering, while allergen overflow into the circulation may be kept at a low level. Occlusion of skin test sites with patches (Fig. 6) favors skin penetration without disrupting the Langerhans cell "curtain" in the epidermis, thus allowing for a very sensitive test procedure (Jadassohn, 1896; Adams, 1981; Calnan, 1982). Patch testing has thus gained an important place in dermatological practice, even more since patches are easy to apply and not really inconvenient for the patients. Moreover, prolonged allergen exposure may intensify and protract reactivity, thereby reducing the risk of missing weak reactions.

Ever since the introduction of patch testing by Jadassohn in 1896, much effort has been put in reducing test variables. Extensive research on chemical and toxicological aspects of allergens, and on suitable vehicles, skin penetration, and patch test materials all contributed to optimal and standardized patch test techniques allowing for interlaboratory comparison of test results (Fregert and Bandmann, 1975; Fischer, 1989). Further developments are still underway (Andersen et al., 1987; Fischer, 1989); new allergens related to new industrial or cosmetic products are regularly added to the test batteries, whereas others can be left out. "Ready-to-use" patch test devices containing standardized quantities of allergen in optimal vehicles have recently been developed (TRUE TEST, Pharmacia, Sweden; Fischer and Maibach, 1985, 1989; Lachapelle et al., 1988; EPIQUICK, Hermal Kurt Herrmann, West Germany) (Fig. 7). Knowledge about different potential allergens processed in food, cosmetics, synthetic materials, etc. is growing and, more importantly, this data has become accessible for individual dermatologists through computer-assisted monitoring systems as developed by Benezra et al. (1985) and Dooms-Goossens (1986).

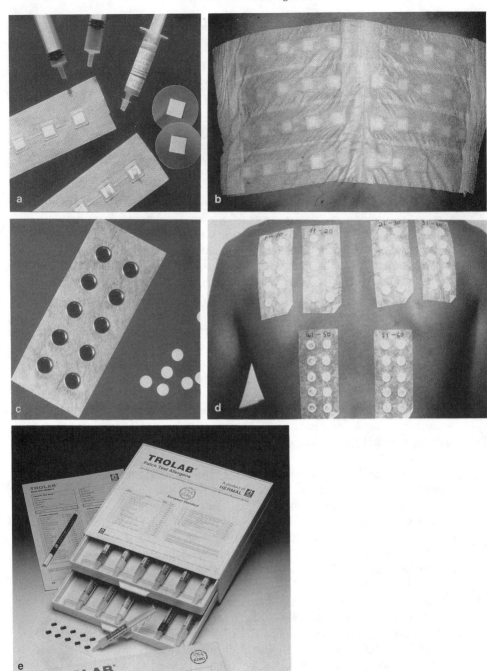

FIGURE 6 Patch test systems currently used in clinical practice; (a,b) Square chambers and silver patches (Van der Bend BV, The Netherlands). (c,d) Finn Chambers on Scanpor (Epitest Ltd., Bipharma BV, The Netherlands). (e) Trolab patch test allergens (Hermal Kurt Herrmann, West Germany).

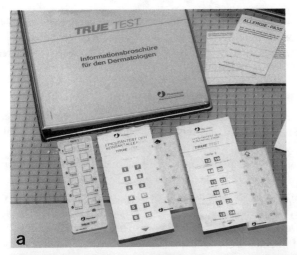

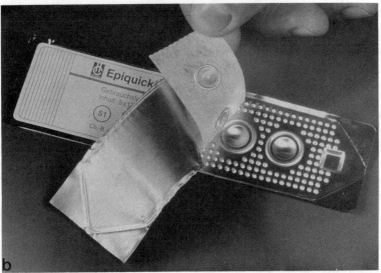

FIGURE 7 Recently developed ready-to-use patch test systems. (a) TRUE TEST (Pharmacia AB, Sweden). (b) EPIQUICK (Hermal Kurt Herrmann, West Germany).

This section will focus on the skin test reaction as an *in vivo* parameter for T-cell-mediated allergy, thereby leaving aside all aspects concerning clinical indications, optimization of patch test ingredients, and allergen chemistry. Data from both experimental and clinical ACD research have been integrated to better understand the mechanisms of contact sensitivity reactions. Different methods to evaluate skin test reactions will be discussed as to their value for classifying underlying immunological mechanisms. In addition, conditions will be described favoring positive skin test reactions in the absence of circulating sensitized T cells, or lack of reactivity in sensitized individuals. The legitimacy of the term "false positive" and "false negative" for such reactions will be discussed. Finally, attention will be paid to possible interference of skin tests with the immune status of an individual.

Evaluation of Skin Test Kinetics

From the time course of macroscopical features, hypersensitivity reactions in the skin have been classified as type I (reaching maximum skin reactivity within 30 min), type III (at 4–6 h) and type IV reactions (at 24–72 h), representing IgE-, immune complex-, and T-cell-mediated immune reactivity respectively (Fig. 8). In practice, these reaction types are seldomly observed as pure entities. Even after a single application of DNCB in guinea pigs, T-cell sensitization is invariably accompanied by low titres of circulating hapten-specific antibodies (De Hurtado and Osler, 1975). These antibodies, however, have no detectable influence on the expression of contact hypersensitivity (Boerrigter et al., 1988).

Chronic exposure to contact allergens may induce high levels of hapten-specific antibodies (Oort et al., 1974; Boerrigter et al., 1988). In clinical ACD, therefore, a distinct role of humoral antibodies in the primarily T-cell-mediated reaction can not be excluded. Conversely, T-cell reactivity may play a role in the chronicity of IgE-mediated atopic dermatitis. Here, T cells may be triggered by allergen, bound to Langerhans cells by specific IgE (Bruynzeel-Koomen, 1986; Barker et al., 1988a).

Analysis of the nature of skin-test reactions is important, not only for a better understanding of the pathogenesis of eczematous skin diseases, but also for guiding therapy. It is helpful in this respect that, in contrast to type IV reactivity, type I reactivity is typically elicited by relatively large protein allergens, which are generally unable to penetrate the epidermis (Hjorth and Roed-Petersen, 1976). Incidentally, however, typical contact allergens may also induce type I reactions upon epicutaneous application (immunologic or nonimmunologic contact urticaria) (Maucher, 1972; Andersen et al., 1987).

As shown in Fig. 8, type I and type IV reactions are generally well differentiated by their characteristic time courses. Reaction kinetics can, however, be misleading. A delayed time course is not always the result of type IV hypersensitivity. In humans, "late phase" reactions following immediate type wheal and flares may be encountered after 48 hours (Deshazo et al., 1983). Biphasic responses to typical type I allergens, with peaks at 15 min and at 24–48 h, have been ascribed to IgE, particularly since comparable reactions could be evoked in mice passively sensitized with hapten-specific IgE antibodies (Ray et al., 1983). Late-phase reactions, showing distinct basophilic infiltration and erythema in the absence of strong induration resemble the so-called "Jones Mote" reactions, which have been described in both humans and experimental animals (Jones and Mote, 1934; Dvorak et al., 1970; Mahapatro and Mahapatro, 1984). Jones Mote reactions are readily induced by protein allergens; they

Reaction type	Mechanism	Time course

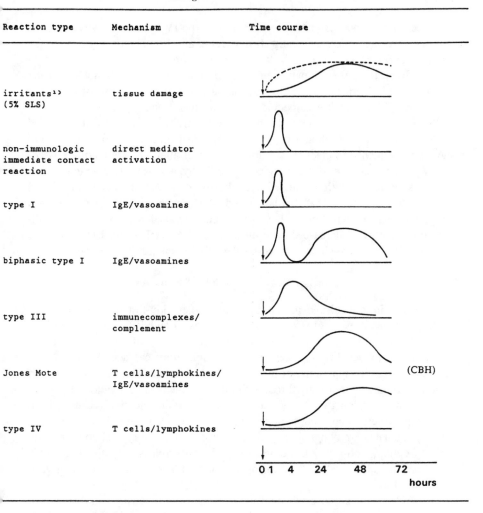

irritants[1] (5% SLS) — tissue damage

non-immunologic immediate contact reaction — direct mediator activation

type I — IgE/vasoamines

biphasic type I — IgE/vasoamines

type III — immunecomplexes/ complement

Jones Mote — T cells/lymphokines/ IgE/vasoamines — (CBH)

type IV — T cells/lymphokines

0 1 4   24   48   72
hours

FIGURE 8 Skin-test reactions may display different time courses depending on the reaction type. [1] Variable time courses depending on agent, concentration, etc.

can be characterized as delayed erythematous reactions with numerous infiltrating basophils. For this reason they have also been referred to as cutaneous basophil hypersensitivity (CBH) (Mahapatro and Mahapatro, 1984). Both IgE and sensitized T cells are likely to play a role in these reactions (Mitchell et al., 1984). Degranulation of antibody-loaded basophils recruited from the circulation upon allergen exposure would account for the delayed onset of this reaction.

To further confuse matters, nonallergic, irritant skin reactions may also show a delayed time course ("delayed irritancy;" Malten et al., 1979). Sodium lauryl sulfate (SLS), an irritant widely used to monitor skin hyperirritability, induces skin responses that closely resemble type IV hypersensitivity reactions both macro- and microscopically (Bruynzeel et al., 1982). Differences between irritant and type IV reactions will be discussed further.

Given the complex nature of delayed skin reactions, it is not surprising that in clinical practice little attention is paid to the time course of patch-test reactions. Most patch-test methods just aim at screening potentially relevant allergens and revealing delayed-type hypersensitivity. Occlusion of the applied allergen for 24–48 h obviously obscures the exact time course of the reaction. As a consequence immediate reactions to contact allergens are readily missed. However, the chance of detecting any type IV hypersensitivity reaction is high when skin test sites are evaluated both shortly after patch removal (day 2) and again after another 24–48 h (day 3 and 4) (Rietschel et al., 1988). Such a regimen enables detection of both accelerated delayed reactions (e.g., facilitated by DMSO to increase skin permeability) (Van Ketel, 1979, 1981) and very delayed reactions, such as induced by the slowly penetrating drug neomycin.

Macroscopical Evaluation of Skin Tests

Both in clinical and in experimental studies skin-test reactions are routinely evaluated by macroscopical scoring (Figs. 9 and 10). Skin-test parameters are based on erythema, induration, and vesiculation of the reaction. These parameters reflect different steps in the inflammatory cascade. In ACD, erythema represents hyperemia of the skin due to direct action of lymphokines on the vasculature or indirectly through lymphokine-mediated activation of vasoactive amine-containing cells. Induration relates to fluid retention (edema), local fibrin polymerization, and cellular infiltration, which is also directly or indirectly mediated by lymphokine activity. Vesiculation is a typical epidermal lesion, regularly observed in human ACD. Locally released lymphokines may induce intercellular edema also in superficial skin layers, thereby causing vesicle formation.

In the guinea pig, erythema-related parameters (intensity and diameter of erythema) and induration (measured as increase in skin fold thickness) may vary independently when intracutaneous skin tests are performed with proteins under different experimental conditions (Scheper et al., 1977). In contact sensitivity a dissociation between erythema and induration can also be observed. Here, induration seems to be more readily suppressed than erythema, for instance, by leukopenia (Polak and Rufli, 1981), antibody transfer (Boerrigter et al., 1988), or iv-induced desensitization (Van Hoogstraten, personal communication). Generally, however, in guinea pig ACD the intensity of erythema correlates well with the increase in skin fold thickness. Regardless whether T-cell hypersensitivity was accompanied by circulating allergen-specific antibodies or not, both erythema and induration measurements closely reflected the number of inflammatory cells (Przybilla et al., 1984; Boerrigter et al., 1988). In mice, on the other hand, induration is the predominating feature of contact allergic

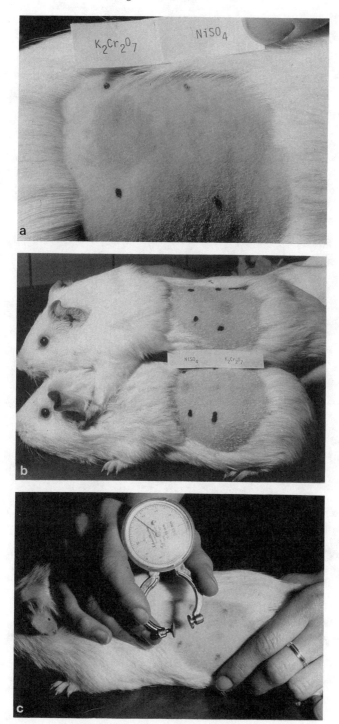

FIGURE 9 Contact skin-test reactions in the guinea pig: (a) open epicutaneous skin-test reaction to chromium; (b) intracutaneous skin-test reactions to chromium and nickel, respectively; (c) induration measurement using mechanical calipers.

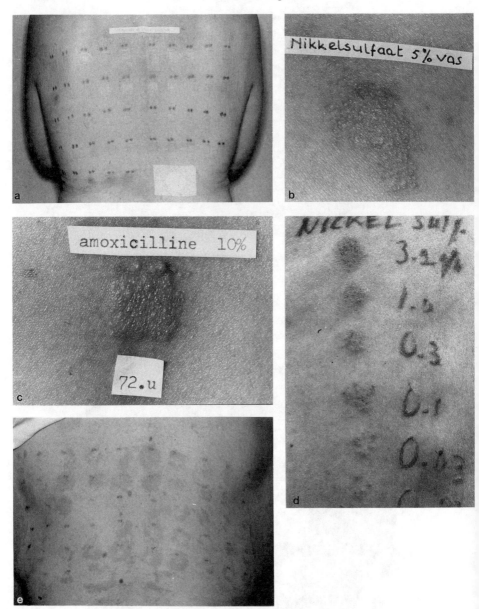

FIGURE 10 Contact skin-test reactions in humans: (a) a few positive patch test reactions appear upon patch removal. (b,c) Examples of typical patch test reactions. (d) Dose-response test with nickel sulfate. (e) Multiple positive patch test reactions ("angry back").

reactions, and rather than erythema provides a valuable parameter for quantitative assessment (see below).

In human ACD vesicles and papules are often seen in addition to erythema and induration. To standardize clinical patch-test reading, guidelines (IC-DRG: Fregert and Bandmann, 1975) have been internationally accepted. According to these guidelines the grading of contact skin test reactions is based on an integrated visual score of erythema, induration, papules, and vesicles. In contrast to intradermal tuberculin-type DTH reactions, which are readily evaluated by measuring the diameter of induration (Van de Plassche-Boers et al., 1985), ACD reactions are relatively hard to quantitate. The need for quantitation of the different parameters has, nevertheless, always been strongly felt. Even more so since the most obvious quantitative approach, that is, by dose-response studies (Kligman, 1958; Bleumink et al., 1974; Burrows, 1983; Friedman et al., 1983) is not feasible for a whole battery of test allergens.

The erythematous reaction upon intracutaneous skin tests can be quantitatively evaluated by measuring the area or diameter of erythema. In contact allergy, however, this method is very dependent on the way of allergen application and was found to be insufficient for patch-test evaluations (Przybilla et al., 1984). The introduction of laser Doppler flowmetry (LDF) has provided a more sophisticated way of quantitating erythematous reactions and has also been applied in humans. LDF enables, to some extent, registration of changes of the microvascular flow in the skin, which—under strict conditions—is related to the intensity of erythema. Promising results have been reported on the use of LDF in ACD (Andersen and Staberg, 1985), although the method does not discriminate allergic from irritant reactions (Staberg and Serup, 1988). Application of LDF for routine assessment of either human or animal contact allergic reactions is, however, not to be expected in the near future, mainly because the method is time consuming and, in addition, highly susceptible to irrelevant fluctuations in the microvascular blood flow (Berardesca and Maibach, 1988; Willis et al., 1988). Nevertheless, in carefully controlled settings LDF may still successfully be used, for example, for assessing skin irritancy (Guy et al., 1985; De Boer et al., 1989; Wahlberg, 1989). Another promising technique for erythema quantitation is provided by the chromometer (Minolta, Japan), which reproducibly measures the color of the skin at the skin test site (Berardesca and Maibach, 1988).

It would appear that the most practicable and reliable method for erythema measurement still is by visual scoring of the intensity of erythema at the reaction sites (by two persons independently).

With respect to quantitation of the induration parameter, vast experience has been obtained in experimental animals, particularly mice, in which induration is the most prominent feature of ACD. Using pressure-controlled calipers (Fig. 9), skin induration can be accurately measured, not only in mice (footpad swelling; Kerckhaert et al., 1974; ear swelling; Van Loveren et al., 1984), but also in guinea pigs (Przybilla et al., 1984; Boerrigter et al., 1988) and humans

(Friedman et al., 1983). Possibly, high-frequency pulsed ultrasound measurements could also contribute to sensitivity register increases in skin fold thickness (Serup et al., 1984).

However, the ease, accuracy, and low costs of using small mechanical or electronic calipers for induration measurements would prevent broad application of more sophisticated methods.

Microscopical Evaluation of Skin Tests

Microscopical evaluation of skin-test reactions provides insight into the composition and localization of infiltrating cells, as well as in structural changes of the skin (Dvorak et al., 1976). The motive for taking biopsies from skin test reactions resides in the fact that macroscopic evaluation does not classify the underlying (immunological) mechanism of the reaction.

Conventional histological methods admittedly allow for localization and quantitative evaluation of cellular infiltrates, as well as for differentiation of the major types of white cells. Classical DTH reactions characterized by mononuclear cell infiltrates (Fig. 11) can thus be distinguished from Arthus reactions. Appropriate staining procedures (Giemsa staining of semithin sections; Boerrigter et al., 1988) may also give information on the number of infiltrating basophils. Although basophil infiltration initially was considered to feature a separate form of hypersensitivity (CBH), basophil infiltration actually is a common phenomenon in contact allergic reactions in humans. In virtually all patch test reactions basophils are found in the infiltrates (Dvorak et al., 1974). The mechanism of their recruitment and activation has not yet completely been clarified. Both T-cell-derived factors and IgE, but also additional undefined serum factors, seem to be involved in human CBH (Mahapatro and Mahapatro, 1984; Mitchell et al., 1984).

Further refinement of histological methods by introducing enzyme histochemical staining techniques enabled detection of Langerhans cells (ATPase) and T lymphocytes (ANAE spots) in skin-test reactions. Using these techniques DTH, including ACD reactions in humans, have been extensively studied. Surprisingly, no essential differences between irritant and allergic reactions could be detected, neither at 5 h, nor at 24, 48, or 72 h after patch appliance (Hartman et al., 1976; Reitamo et al., 1981).

Electron-microscopic studies on subcellular aspects of skin reactions also failed to reveal essential differences between irritant and allergic reactions. Numbers of Langerhans cells (LC) or the frequency of LC-mononuclear cell contacts were similar in allergic and irritant reactions (Forslind and Wahlberg, 1978; Ranki et al., 1983), but cellular infiltrates and intercellular edema tended to be more pronounced in allergic reactions (Lindberg, 1982; Kanerva et al., 1984). A target role of LC for sensitized T cells in ACD, based on the observation of damaged LC (Silberberg, 1976), was not confirmed by others (Forslind and Wahlberg, 1977; Gianotti et al., 1986; Hunter, 1986).

A new incentive for skin-test histology came from the introduction of

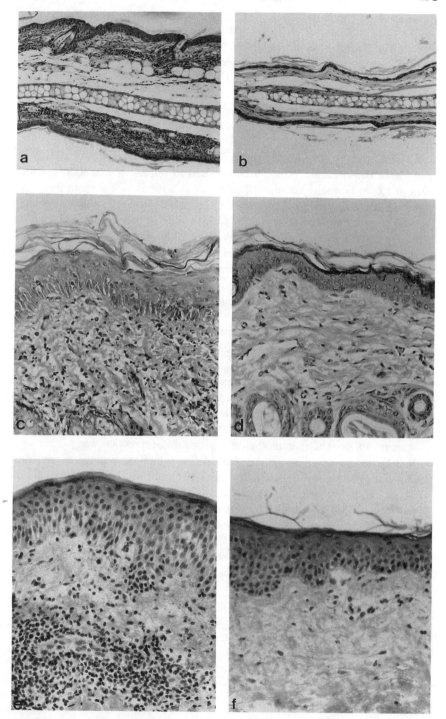

FIGURE 11 Microscopic evaluation of skin test infiltrates: (a,b) ACD reaction to chromium and control skin of mouse ear (Vreeburg et al., 1989). (c,d) ACD reaction to chromium and control skin of guinea pig flank. (e,f) ACD reaction to nickel and control skin of human back.

monoclonal antibodies (mAbs) to leukocyte differentiation antigens. Almost all inflammatory cells in both irritant and allergic patch test reactions were found to be T lymphocytes, the majority showing CD4 (T helper), the minority CD8 (T suppressor/cytotoxic) determinants (Table 6). T4:T8 ratios varied considerably, ranging from 1 to 5 in both perivascular foci and diffuse intervening infiltrates and, more importantly, again revealed no differences between irritant and allergic patch test reactions (Bruynzeel et al., 1983a; Ralfkiaer and Wantzin, 1984; Scheynius et al., 1984; Ferguson et al., 1985).

The availability of mAbs, particularly those directed to class II (HLA-D) and CD1a determinants, strongly contributed to reliable quantitation of numbers of LC in normal epidermis (De Jong et al., 1986) and in patch test reactions (Table 6). A clear picture now emerges from careful time-response studies in which epidermal and dermal LCs were evaluated separately. Whereas the numbers of LCs in the epidermis may be slightly elevated during the first 2 days after either allergen or irritant skin contact, they dramatically decrease thereafter, leading to increased numbers of dermal LCs. In irritant reactions to SLS, these dermal LCs rapidly disappear, whereas in allergic reactions LCs remain detectable in the dermis for at least several days. How far this finding represents a general feature of irritant contact dermatitis remains to be established. After 14–21 days both epidermal and dermal LC numbers return to control values in both allergic and irritant reactions (Marks et al., 1987).

In further search for histochemical differences between allergic and irritant contact dermatitis (ICD), Scheynius and Fischer (1986) reported that as a late (after 4 days) sequel of allergic reactions, but not of irritant reactions, class II molecules are expressed on human keratinocytes, confirming earlier findings in rats (Suitters and Lampert, 1982), mice (Roberts et al., 1985), and humans (Lampert, 1984). The immunological basis of this expression was further supported by *in vitro* studies, which showed that lymphokine preparations from nickel-sensitive patients (Tjernlund et al., 1987) and in particular IFN-gamma (Wikner et al., 1986) could induce HLA-DR expression in cultured human keratinocytes. More recently, however, further analysis of Ia molecules on ~ keratinocytes in different dermatoses including irritant and allergic contact dermatitis, revealed that HLA-DR expression is relatively common, accompanying helper T-cell infiltration. All class II antigens, with the exception of DP, were found to be expressed on keratinocytes in both ACD and ICD (Gawkrodger et al., 1987a; Barker et al., 1988b).

In conclusion, although antibody and T-cell-mediated skin reactions can be often differentiated by microscopic evaluation, so far surprisingly little differences have been observed between allergic and irritant contact dermatitis reactions.

Further studies are therefore warranted on the value of other potentially relevant features:

TABLE 6. Immunohistochemical Evaluation of Human Contact Skin Test Reactions

Characteristic features of ACD reaction	References[a]
Histology	
Epidermal edema, vesiculation	1, 4, 12
Dermal edema	1, 4, 12
Mononuclear cell infiltrate	1, 4, 12, 23
Comparison ACD ↔ ICD: no essential differences, but:	12, 23
More epidermal necrosis in ICD	1
More dermal edema in ACD	1
Denser cell infiltrates in ACD	5, 24, 25
Langerhans cells	
Epidermal LC number (day 0–2) normal or increased,	2, 3, 6, 13, 24, 28, 29
(day 2–7) decreased	3, 14, 18
Dermal LC numbers (day 2–14) increased	3, 14, 17, 18, 23, 29
LC damage and LC-lymphocyte apposition still disputed	3, 10, 22, 28
CD4 expression on LC	11, 28
Comparison ACD ↔ ICD: no essential differences, but:	2, 13, 22, 24, 28
Dermal LC increase in ICD only till day 2	18
Loss of epidermal LC in ICD at day 2	5, 6
Keratinocytes	
HLA-DP, DQ, DR positive (day 1–20)	7, 20, 25, 29
ICAM-1 expression (day 2)	17, 26, 27
Comparison ACD ↔ ICD: no essential differences, but:	19
No DR$^+$ keratinocytes in ICD	25
No DP$^+$ keratinocytes in ICD	7
No ICAM-1$^+$ keratinocytes in ICD	27
Cellular infiltrate	
Few or no B cells, NK cells	13, 18, 20, 21, 29
Few or no macrophages (0–4%)	4, 8, 21
Marked basiphilic infiltration (5–10%)	4
Relative increase in CD8$^+$ lymphocytes with time	14, 15, 17, 28
CD4$^+$ >> CD8$^+$, both perivascularly and in diffuse infiltrated (day 0–20)	2, 5, 6, 13, 18, 20, 21, 24, 25, 29
Around epidermal vesicles mainly CD8$^+$ lymphocytes	2
T cells activated (OKT9, HLA-DR, IL2R or Ki-67 positive)	8, 14, 16, 21, 24, 29
Comparison ACD ↔ ICD: no essential differences, but:	2, 5, 13, 24, 25, 28
IL2R expression higher in ACD	16

[a]References: (1) Avnstorp et al. (1989); (2) Bruynzeel et al. (1983a); (3) Carr et al. (1984); (4) Dvorak et al. (1976); (5) Ferguson et al. (1985); (6) Gawkrodger et al. (1986); (7) Gawkrodger et al. (1987a); (8) Gawkrodger et al. (1987b); (9) Gawkrodger et al. (1988); (10) Gianotti et al. (1986); (11) Groh et al. (1986); (12) Hartman et al. (1976); (13) Kanerva et al. (1984); (14) Kanerva et al. (1987); (15) Kanerva et al. (1988); (16) Klareskog et al. (1986); (17) Lewis et al. (1989); (18) Marks et al. (1987); (19) McKenna et al. (1989); (20) McMillan et al. (1985); (21) Ralfkiaer and Wantzin, (1984); (22) Ranki et al. (1983); (23) Reitamo et al. (1981); (24) Scheynius et al. (1984); (25) Scheynius and Fischer (1986); (26) Singer et al. (1989); (27) Wantzin et al. (1988); (28) Willis et al. (1986); (29) Wood et al. (1986).

Expression of T-cell activation markers (IL-2 receptor or Tac antigen, transferrin receptor, etc.) and proliferation-associated antigens has been observed in both tuberculin and ACD reactions (Table 6). Significantly more Tac-positive cells were found in ACD and tuberculin reactions than at irritant reaction sites, the difference being most pronounced at 24 h (Klareskog et al., 1986).

Histological staining for local lymphokine production has now also become feasible. Fullmer et al. (1987) reported on the presence of IL-2 producing cells in the dermal infiltrate of tuberculin reactions. Using monoclonal anti-MIF in a conventional immunoperoxidase staining, Neumann et al. demonstrated MIF-producing lymphocytes infiltrating the skin at contact reaction sites (1987). More recent results of this group, however, provided conflicting data, namely, on MIF production by non-lymphoid cells (endothelium, macrophages) early in irritant and allergic inflammation (Malorny et al., 1988). Further research on lymphokine-producing cells *in situ,* including the use of *in situ* hybridization techniques, is required to evaluate in how far MIF or IL-2 production is an exclusive characteristic of T-cell-mediated reactions.

Future studies should also focus on the expression of leukocyte adhesion molecules by endothelial cells and keratinocytes at contact reaction sites. An interesting finding in this context is the fact that in allergic contact dermatitis, particularly at sites of massive infiltration keratinocytes start to express ICAM-1, an adhesion molecule present also on the membrane of antigen presenting cells. In contrast, ICAM-1 is only seldom found on keratinocytes at irritant skin reaction sites (Wantzin et al., 1988). The regulatory role of keratinocytes in the homing of lymphocyte subpopulations certainly warrants further investigation (Nickoloff et al., 1988).

Functional Analysis of Skin Test Infiltrates

In diagnosing ACD it would be attractive if both the underlying mechanism and the causative agent could be identified by evaluating skin biopsies. Obviously this would require specificity measurements on the infiltrating lymphocytes. The wish to assess the specificity of infiltrating lymphocytes has been felt for a long time, in particular in inflammatory diseases, where lymphocytes of unknown specificity accumulate locally and apparently are involved in the pathogenesis.

Direct antigen-specific staining of T cells is not feasible since antigens are only recognized in association with proper class II molecules, and TCR-mediated antigen binding may be weak. Also, *in situ* hybridization with T-cell-receptor idiotype-related RNA/DNA probes cannot be expected to soon provide a satisfactory technique for detection of allergen-reactive T cells in inflammatory infiltrates. So as yet allergen specificity of infiltrating cells can only be revealed by indirect functional analysis. In the last decade much progress has been made in functional infiltrate analysis, following three different routes:

1. Experimentally, Cr^{51}-labeled allergen-specific T cells (*in vitro* selected T cell lines or clones) have been injected into the circulation, followed by assessment of accumulating radioactivity at skin test reaction sites (Scheper et al., 1985).

2. Clinically, lymphocytes have been isolated from skin biopsies, after which further expansion and cloning allowed for *in vitro* testing (Kapsenberg et al., 1987).

3. Retained allergen-specific cells in (former) skin reaction sites have been revealed *in situ* by evoking "flare-up" or "retest" reactions in guinea pigs (Scheper et al., 1983, 1987b).

Concordant data were obtained by these different methods, showing that considerable allergen-specific T cell accumulation occurs at contact reaction sites during the inflammatory process. Cloning and testing of lymphocytes derived from human 72-h $NiSo_4$ skin test reactions revealed as many as 7–15% nickel-specific T cells in the infiltrate (Kapsenberg et al., 1987).

This high frequency may be due to several factors. Infiltration of allergen-specific cells into contact skin reactions is primarily determined by their frequency in the circulation and their activational stage. Every allergen contact may induce transient peaks in this frequency and will, in addition, preferentially activate specific T lymphocytes. The fact that recently activated T lymphocytes exhibit an exceptionally high migratory capacity contributes to a preferential influx of such allergen-specific cells to (all) inflammatory sites (Fig. 12a).

Specific accumulation of hapten-reactive T lymphocytes at contact reaction sites may be further enhanced at the skin level by preferential binding of these cells to hapten-presenting endothelial cells, as well as by local proliferation and retention of specific T lymphocytes (Fig. 12b). For these mechanisms the amount of hapten locally present is of major importance, rather than the intensity of the allergic reaction.

Accordingly, despite a fall in absolute numbers of T lymphocytes, the frequency of allergen-specific T cells at contact reaction sites will gradually increase, particularly during the first week following the peak reaction (Fig. 12c) (Scheper et al., 1984, 1987a). Up to months after the reaction has disappeared, locally persisting specific T cells may cause allergen-specific hyperreactivity at these sites, as can be measured in the so-called "retest" reaction (Scheper et al., 1983).

False and True Skin Test Reactions

The definition of false positive and false negative reactions strongly depends on the viewer's aims. Obviously, clinical interest is not restricted to type

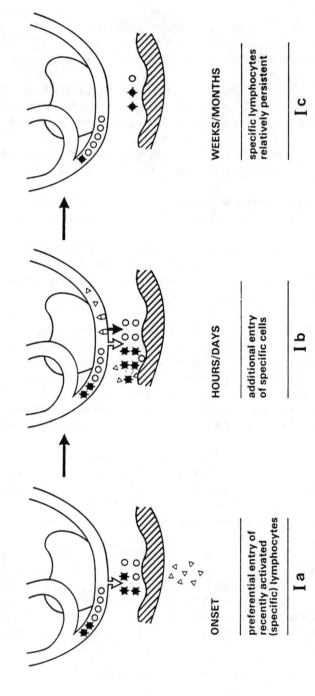

FIGURE 12 T-lymphocyte infiltration at ACD reaction sites, (I) in allergic patients shortly after sensitization or boosting and (II) after a period of allergen restraint. (a) During the onset of ACD reactions, infiltration is determined by allergen-independent extravasation of lymphocytes (Ia, IIa, ⇗). As recently activated lymphocytes enter the skin more readily than memory lymphocytes, preferential infiltration of specific T cells at the skin test site can be expected when individuals have been sensitized or boosted with the challenging allergen shortly beforehand (Ia).

ONSET

preferential entry of
recently activated
(specific) lymphocytes

I a

HOURS/DAYS

additional entry
of specific cells

I b

WEEKS/MONTHS

specific lymphocytes
relatively persistent

I c

296

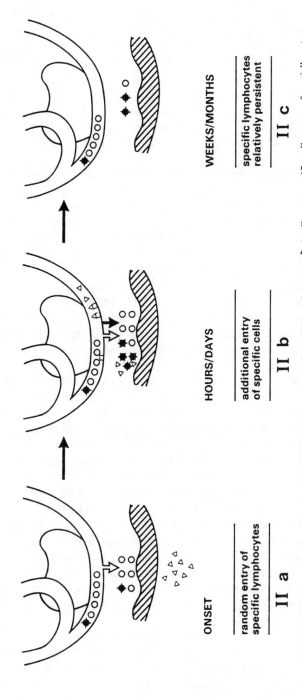

ONSET

random entry of
specific lymphocytes

II a

HOURS/DAYS

additional entry
of specific cells

II b

WEEKS/MONTHS

specific lymphocytes
relatively persistent

II c

FIGURE 12 (*Continued*). (b) After the initial allergen-independent influx of T lymphocytes (⇨), allergen-specific cells may preferentially enter the skin (IIb, IIb, ➤) upon binding to the endothelial cells exposing MHC-class II molecules associated with allergen. *In situ* proliferation, as well as local retention of allergen-specific cells, may further contribute to an increased frequency of specific T cells at "old" ACD reaction sites (Ic, IIc). △, Allergen; □, MHC-class II molecules; ●, allergen-specific T lymphocyte, naive; ✦, allergen-specific T lymphocyte, recently activated; ◆, allergen-specific T lymphocyte, memory; ○, T cell of other specificity, naive.

297

IV hypersensitivity. Detection of late-phase IgE-mediated reactions therefore may be positively appreciated, whereas missed contact urticarial reactions subsided at the time of reading may be considered as false negatives (Calnan, 1982). Even nonimmunological contact urticaria reactions, involving direct mediator activation without immune recognition (Lahti and Maibach, 1987), may reveal a disease related agent and therefore be considered as a true reaction. The term "relevant" in contrast to "irrelevant" would thus be more appropriate. In the present review skin testing is, however, evaluated as a method for measuring T-cell-mediated ACD and false reactions will be considered accordingly.

False positive reactions, that is, positive skin tests in the absence of sensitization, are readily observed with an inappropriate test technique or with too high allergen concentrations (Table 7). The maximum nonerythematous dose varies not only interindividually (Frosch, 1989) but also intraindividually from time to time and from site to site. Clinical conditions, like concomitant dermatitis or chronic inflammation remote from the site of skin testing, may lower the irritancy threshold of the skin (Björnberg, 1968; Maibach, 1981; Bruynzeel and Maibach, 1986). Whether strongly positive skin test reactions may have such an effect is still a matter of controversy (Mitchell, 1977; Bruynzeel et al., 1983a; Kligman and Gollhausen, 1986). Recently, however, support has been presented for activation of the whole skin during patch testing: the amount of epidermal IL-1 and epidermal LCF in normal-looking skin appeared to be elevated during a positive patch test reaction at a remote site (Larsen et al., 1988). Hyperirritable skin, described as the "angry back" or "excited skin syndrome (ESS)" may account for 8% to over 40% of weakly positive reactions (Mitchell, 1977; Bandmann and Agathos, 1981; Maibach et al., 1982; Bruynzeel et al., 1983b; Kligman and Gollhausen, 1986). Mechanisms playing a role in ESS have been studied in experimental models: in guinea pigs ESS could be induced by mere injection of Freund's complete adjuvant (FCA) (Bruynzeel et al., 1983c) as well as by irritant or allergen-induced acute dermatitis (Roper and Jones, 1985). In (nude) mice a model for studying ESS was created by epicutaneous phenol application (Van der Lugt and Veninga, 1981). In humans application of Trafuril cream induced skin hyperirritability (Sonnex and Ryan, 1987), but the value of this hyperreactivity as a model for ESS has been disputed (Bruynzeel, 1987). Although hard data are still lacking, it may be concluded from these studies that release of inflammatory mediators, such as prostaglandins, primarily accounts for skin hyperirritability, whereas, in addition, bone marrow activation, resulting in increased numbers of peripheral blood leukocytes, may play an additional role (Bruynzeel et al., 1983c).

Attempts to develop reliable methods to quantitate the degree of nonspecific skin excitation failed. Although sodium lauryl sulfate (SLS) skin reactions were generally elevated in patients with eczema, and in particular at skin sites in the vicinity of strong skin test reactions, SLS hyperreactivity did not predict false positive, presumably ESS related reactions (Bruynzeel et al., 1983b). A

TABLE 7. Some Important Causes of False Positive and False Negative Skin Test Reactions

Reactions	Cause
False positive	
Allergen restricted	Test concentration too high
	Inappropriate vehicle
	Local hyperreactivity due to previous allergic reaction at the test site
Non-allergen restricted	ESS, e.g., due to inflammatory reaction elsewhere
False negative	
Allergen restricted	Test concentration too low
	Inappropriate vehicle
	Slow penetration
	Present or recent allergic reaction to the same allergen
	Systemic presence of allergen
Non-allergen restricted	Local or systemic UV effect
	Suppressing factors (e.g., tumor or virus derived)
	Medication (e.g., corticosteroids)

practical strategy for dealing with ESS is therefore still based on retesting with the allergens that have elicited dubious positive reactions (Bruynzeel and Maibach, 1986).

As discussed in the preceding subsection, allergen-specific hyperreactivity of distinct skin areas can also be caused by local persistence of allergen-reactive cells at previously involved skin reaction sites. Although positive reactions in such areas should be considered as true reactions, reflecting sensitization of the patient, they are not representative for overall immune reactivity, since insufficient allergen-specific cells may be left in the circulation to mount allergic reactions at distant skin sites.

As to the frequency of false negative reactions in humans ("the silent back syndrome"; Kligman and Gollhausen, 1986), few hard data exist. This is despite several reports concerning possible underlying mechanisms of false negative reactions. Apart from technical shortcomings in skin testing, various immunological factors may cause transient or local hyporesponsiveness (Table 7). A hyporesponsive state may easily lead to false negative reactions in routine assays, when only one single concentration per test allergen is used, or when patch tests are only read at 48 and 72 h (Bruynzeel, 1986).

A major cause of local allergen-specific hyporesponsiveness is a transient lack of circulating antigen-specific cells. This may occur when allergic reactions elsewhere in the body withdraw specific cells from the circulation. Such allergen-specific suppression can be readily demonstrated in experimental animals: contact hypersensitivity reactions are significantly suppressed by repeated allergen application at distant sites (Boerrigter and Scheper, 1987) or even by one strong skin-test reaction elicited simultaneously by the same allergen at the contralateral flank of the guinea pig (Thestrup-Pedersen, 1975; Von Blomberg et al., 1978). Similar hyporeactive states have been observed in humans during acute poison ivy dermatitis (Kligman, 1958). It would appear that for sequestration of allergen-reactive cells into an inflammatory site the local amount of hapten is of primary importance rather than the degree of inflammation (Scheper and Polak, 1984).

Large systemic amounts of hapten, induced by intravenous injection or orally taken allergen (Van Hoogstraten et al., to be published), may also cause transient hyporesponsiveness (desensitization), presumably by transient blockage of T-cell receptors (Polak, 1980d). On this basis therapeutical protocols involving allergen ingestion have been developed (poison ivy: Shelmire, 1941; penicillin: Wendel et al., 1985). To our knowledge these oral desensitization protocols are only of transient benefit to the patients.

Nonspecific hyporesponsiveness of the skin can result from UV light exposure or sunburning (O'Dell et al., 1980; Hersey et al., 1983). Such reduced skin reactivity does not necessarily apply to irritant reactions and may be related to UV damage of Langerhans cells (Maurer, 1983; Koulou and Jansén, 1988). Apart from its effects on Langerhans cells, UVB has systemic immune-suppressive effects (Morison et al., 1984). In mice this suppression was shown to be mediated by T-suppressor cells that were activated by irradiation-converted urocanic acid, a normal component of epidermis (Harriot-Smith and Halliday, 1988).

Another immunosuppressive factor, resembling the retroviral envelope protein P15E, may be released from tumors, and probably accounts for low skin-test reactions in cancer patients (Tan et al., 1986; Chanh et al., 1988).

Surprisingly, the presence of an inflammatory reaction elsewhere in the body instead of enhancing skin reactivity (ESS), may also suppress skin-test reactions (Bruynzeel et al., 1983c). DTH to microbial antigens was thus found to be suppressed in guinea pigs with oil-induced peritonitis (McGuire and Fox, 1979), irritant dermatitis or ACD (Uehara and Ofuji, 1977), and in humans suffering from atopic eczema (McGeady and Buckley, 1975). This anergy is probably due to general depletion of monocytes (McGuire and Fox, 1979) and T lymphocytes (McGeady and Buckley, 1975) from the blood. Contact skin reactions, however, appeared to be much less susceptible to shortage of circulating monocytes than the tuberculin type IV reaction (McGuire and Fox, 1979; Polak and Rufli, 1981).

Methods to retrospectively analyze possibly false negative reactions, for instance to nickel, may consist of retesting with higher concentrations in the same vehicle (Dooms-Goossens et al., 1980), or retesting with the allergen dissolved in DMSO (Van Ketel, 1978), intracutaneous testing (Meneghini and Angelini, 1979; Möller, H., 1989), or oral provocation (Veien et al., 1983).

Immunological Effects of Skin Testing

An unavoidable consequence of *in vivo* skin testing is interference with the patient's immune system. Not only the presence of allergen in the skin under most immunogenic conditions, as required for optimal skin testing, but also the allergic reaction itself inevitably influences immune status.

Three different aspects of immune modulation by skin testing deserve to be considered: sensitization to new allergens or boosting of existing immune reactivity, "flare-ups" of clinically healed allergic reactions, and mobilization or retention of allergen-reactive cells (compartmentalization).

Sensitization and boosting. Although in experimental studies low dosages (within the skin test concentration range) of potent contact allergens may induce contact allergy, primary sensitization in current human skin testing seems to be rare (Meneghini and Angelini, 1977). Nevertheless, particularly when testing new substances, sensitization by skin testing cannot be excluded (Kanerva et al., 1988). Boosting of previous sensitization is also occasionally seen when contact allergens are tested repeatedly (penicillin: Bruynzeel and Van Ketel, 1981). For comparison, booster effects are commonly seen after repeated intracutaneous injections with microbial antigens, particularly with *Candida albicans* antigens (Keystone et al., 1980; Christou et al., 1983).

Flare-up phenomena. In mice topical provocation with contact allergens may readily induce sufficiently high levels of allergen in the circulation to cause a flare-up of previous reaction sites (Möller, 1984). In humans, however, the risk of flare-ups upon patch testing is relatively small, since the amount of allergen leaking from patch-test sites is usually too small to reactivate T cells persisting at previous eczematous areas. Nevertheless, flare-ups of old eczema sites upon patch testing may be observed (e.g., for poison ivy; Kligman, 1958).

Although such flares are diagnostically important as they support the relevance of positive patch tests, they are clinically undesirable: they are usually inconvenient for the patients and may in addition boost the patient's hypersensitivity. Obviously, with intracutaneous testing one should be even more aware of the potential consequences of circulating allergen molecules.

Compartmentalization of specific T cells. When skin-test reactions subside, part of the locally activated T cells will in turn leave the skin, enter the draining lymph nodes, and eventually (re-)join the circulating pool of lymphocytes (Fig. 5). Persistence of immunogenically bound allergen in the skin and in the lymph nodes may, however, delay or protract this process for several days or even weeks. Therefore, early after skin testing—that is, before allergen-reactive T cells are released from the lymph nodes—a decreased frequency of allergen-specific T cells may be found in the circulation, whereas shortly thereafter this frequency may become increased. Although changes in the circulating pool of specific T cells would affect both *in vivo* and *in vitro* measurements of contact sensitivity, these immune-modulating effects of skin testing have been analyzed mainly by probing peripheral blood lymphocyte reactivity *in vitro*.

Levis and co-workers systematically studied the proliferative responsiveness of blood lymphocytes to DNCB-antigen upon DNCB-sensitization (Miller and Levis, 1973) and subsequent challenge (Powell et al., 1975) in humans. DNCB-specific lymphocyte transformation of peripheral blood cells reached a peak at 14–21 days after sensitization and showed a rapid decline afterward, despite persisting positive skin reactivity to DNCB. Rechallenge with DNCB, some months after sensitization, boosted the proliferative response of blood lymphocytes with a delay of 10 days.

In patients suffering from ACD, however, it is usually more difficult to keep track of circulating allergen-reactive cells. This is because frequent oral and skin contacts may take place with ubiquitous allergens such as nickel and also because multiple sites of previous or current dermatitis may be involved in compartmentalization of allergen-specific cells. Not surprisingly, therefore, Svejgaard et al. (1978) could detect nickel-specific *in vitro* respones in patients' blood lymphocytes regardless of the period after skin testing (4 days to 2.5 years).

Taking together data from literature and our own experience we conclude that for most allergens, particularly those that are not ubiquitous, local or oral challenges will transiently raise the numbers of antigen-reactive cells in the circulation within 10–20 days (Veien et al., 1979).

Conclusions

Epicutaneous skin testing provides a sensitive and convenient method for diagnosing hypersensitivity to unlimited numbers of chemicals. Its value for detecting the causative agent in ACD is beyond question. In this chapter we commented on the capacity of skin testing to reveal underlying immunological mechanism(s). For this purpose the different evaluable parameters of skin test reactions have been discussed.

Skin test kinetics may shed some light on the underlying mechanism after either intracutaneous or open epicutaneous application of the allergen, provided that skin penetration is not a limiting factor. Occlusion of skin test sites, however, as is common practice in human ACD testing, obscures time courses of hypersensitivity reactions. Since irritant and IgE-mediated reactions may also show a delayed appearance, generally the time course of the skin test reaction does not provide important information in evaluating human T-cell-mediated hypersensitivity.

Macroscopical evaluation of human skin test reactions should comprise assessment of erythema, induration, papules, and vesicles, since all these parameters are primary, and partly independent, features of contact sensitivity reactions in humans. This also holds true for guinea pigs, although vesiculation is quite exceptional in this species. In mice, induration is a predominant feature of ACD. Generally, indurated reactions in the absence of erythema may indicate a lack of basophil/mastcell involvement.

Skin test biopsies have been microscopically evaluated in many studies, using various techniques, primarily in attempts to characterize the underlying immunological mechanism. Although clear-cut Arthus type reactivity, CBH and DTH may be distinguished histologically, so far no obvious differences have been observed between irritant and allergic contact sensitivity skin reactions. Actually, this stresses the extent of the "nonspecific" components of the inflammatory reaction, shared by both irritant and allergic reactions. Apparently, allergic skin reactions only differ from irritant reactions in the initiating event, that is, the activation of allergen-specific T lymphocytes. Future research on expression of T-cell activation markers and adhesion molecules, as well as on local lymphokine production (e.g., using mAbs or RNA probes), might reveal distinct features of T-cell-mediated reactions.

The recently developed technology of T-cell cloning and expansion facilitated progress in evaluating numbers of allergen-specific cells in contact allergic reactions. Relatively high (10%) proportions of allergen-specific lymphocytes could be detected in ACD reactions, but obviously such techniques are not feasible in a routine setting. Future research should concentrate on *in situ* detection of allergen-specific cells.

Conditions resulting in hypo- and hyperreactivity of the skin, *in extremo* perceived by the dermatologist as either false negative or false positive reactions, have been summarized in Table 7. An important factor mediating allergen-specific hypo- and hyperresponsiveness is compartmentalization of allergen-specific T cells. More insight into the migratory patterns of these cells upon allergen contact (e.g., after skin testing) is, however, required to fully understand changes in skin test and *in vitro* test reactivity in ACD.

In conclusion, skin patch testing is an easy technique, relatively cheap and very sensitive. It provides an adequate method for detecting causative agents in ACD, and often reveals underlying immunological mechanisms (type I versus type IV). Skin test reactions may, however, be easily misinterpreted, such as when allergen-specific cells are transiently sequestered from the circulation by a remote inflammatory reaction, or when the skin displays general hyperreactivity (excited skin syndrome). Finally, a substantial drawback of skin testing is the fact that any allergenic contact is bound to interfere with the immune status of an individual. In this respect availability of reliable *in vitro* assays measuring sensitized T cells in the blood would be of great advantage.

IN VITRO STUDIES IN ACD

Introduction

Cellular transfer studies were initiated by Landsteiner and Chase (1942), and in the years to follow it became clear that lymphocytes could mediate ACD (see Bloom and Chase, 1967; Polak, 1980a). The mechanisms involved, however, still had to wait for elucidation. Aiming at a suitable model for studying delayed hypersensitivity (DTH), George and Vaughan (1962) reported on an *in vitro* correlate of DTH in the guinea pig. Macrophage migration inhibition could be detected when peritoneal exudate cells from mycobacteria-sensitized animals were cultured with tuberculin. At that time the authors did not yet associate this *in vitro* phenomenon with lymphocyte function. It took another few years before sensitized lymphocytes were identified as the source of macrophage migration inhibitory factor (MIF) (David et al., 1964). At that time lymphocytic blast transformation and proliferation were also observed in lymph nodes draining sites of allergen contact (Oort and Turk, 1965), and subsequently provided new *in vitro* parameters for DTH (Oppenheim, 1968; Polak, 1980c). Basic mechanisms of DTH could now be studied at the cellular level, and results from these studies contributed to our present knowledge of T-cell activation.

Most of this basic *in vitro* research on DTH was initially performed in animal models. Clinical *in vitro* studies on cell-mediated immunity did not get well underway until suitable procedures had been developed for isolation of lymphocytes from the peripheral blood. Böyum (1968) introduced density-gradient centrifugation with Ficoll-Hypaque, thus providing a most successful method, still in vogue. In recent years basic immunological research has shifted strongly toward the human system. Major developments that facilitated this rapid shift are the progress in cell culture technology, allowing for expansion and long-term culture of human cell lines and clones, the development of broad panels of mAbs identifying human cell surface antigens, the large-scale production of human recombinant lymphokines, and the growing reward of clinically applied research.

In contact allergy studies the need for reliable *in vitro* assays to directly measure sensitized lymphocytes in the circulation has always been strongly felt, and even more so when the limitations of *in vivo* skin testing became clear. Thus, ever since the first successful *in vitro* lymphocyte stimulation studies, unceasing attempts have been made to optimally design lymphocyte cultures with contact allergens.

This chapter will focus on those issues of particular importance for understanding the scope and limitations of diagnostic *in vitro* assays in human ACD. We will deal with potential *in vitro* parameters for DTH, with the source, sampling, and type of responder cells, and with molecular and cellular requirements for allergen presentation *in vitro*. In addition, a literature survey will be presented of diagnostic *in vitro* assays performed in human ACD. Currently available results will be analyzed and future perspectives will be discussed of *in vitro* diagnostic procedures in contact allergy.

In Vitro Parameters for ACD

Direct identification of allergen-specific cells.   Basically, the frequency of circulating allergen-specific cells determines the degree of contact sensitivity.

Thus, the ultimate goal of *in vitro* testing in ACD is to establish the presence and the frequency of specific T lymphocytes in the circulation. Unfortunately, direct identification of allergen-specific T lymphocytes by incubation with labeled allergen, a method successfully used for antigen-specific staining of B lymphocytes (Van Dinther-Janssen et al., 1986), has not yet been possible. Antigen binding to the T-cell receptor alone is relatively weak, and many different allergen-MHC class II complexes would be needed for such staining. This would also apply to methods to identify specific T cells by allergen-specific rosette or cluster formation. Alternatively, allergen-specific staining of T lymphocytes might be achieved with anticlonotypic antibodies, that is, antibodies directed toward the variable part of the T-cell receptor. Such antibodies could be raised against allergen-specific T-cell clones, but to our knowledge have not yet been described in ACD. It remains, however, unlikely that the large numbers of allergen-specific T-cell receptors including different MHC class II restriction patterns could be stained by one or a limited pool of monoclonal antibodies. The same would apply for RNA/DNA probes to be used for *in situ* hybrization procedures, or the detection of RNA, coding for T-cell receptor idiotypes, such as after polymerase chain reaction (PCR) amplification (Saiki et al., 1988).

As direct staining of allergen-specific cells is not expected to reach routine status in the near future, assessment of the presence of allergen-reactive cells still requires functional assays.

In vitro *stimulation of T lymphocytes.* To determine the presence of allergen-reactive T cells in a cell preparation lymphocytes can be challenged with allergen *in vitro,* and either cellular changes, related to T-cell activation and proliferation, or the amount of lymphokines produced is assessed as parameters for T-cell activation. For accurate determination of the frequency of allergen-specific cells, limiting-dilution analyses of the cultured lymphocytes are required (Van Oers et al., 1978; Lefkovits and Waldmann, 1984).

Essential ingredients for such lymphocyte cultures are T lymphocytes, allergen-presenting cells, and allergen. Extensive studies on the culture conditions required for optimal lymphocyte stimulation by antigens showed that strict control of the following test conditions is of paramount importance (Schellekens and Eijsvoogel, 1968; Knight, 1982):

Numbers of lymphocytes per culture: Obviously, the frequency of allergen-specific cells determines the minimum number of lymphoid cells to be cultured. "Macro" cultures containing 10^6 cells per well or tube should therefore be preferred when few circulating specific cells are to be detected. Routinely, however, microcultures containing around 10^5 cells can be used. To provide optimal intercellular contacts, U- or V-bottomed microtitre plates are recommended. When aiming at the production of high lymphokine concentrations to be tested in a secondary assay, higher cell concentrations can be used, as only relatively short culture periods (1–3 days) are required.

Numbers of allergen-presenting cells in the cultures: Nonlymphoid cells are primarily needed for allergen presentation to T lymphocytes. The number of APC required per culture depends on their efficiency and varies from 1% of the lymphocyte number for human dendritic cells to about 10% for monocytes. Usually the proportion of monocytes in Ficoll-Hypaque isolated mononuclear cell suspensions suffices. Monocytes (up to maximally 10–15%) also favor culture conditions by keeping the cultures clean due to their phagocytic activity. Higher numbers of monocytes often suppress lymphocyte proliferation by prostaglandin production. Such suppression is particularly pronounced in animal studies with activated peritoneal inflammatory macrophages, but may be readily prevented by adding indomethacin (3.10^{-6} M) to the culture media (Mullink and Von Blomberg, 1980).

Concentration of allergens in the cultures: Since complex interrelationships exist in lymphocyte cultures between numbers of cells, culture periods, and allergen concentrations, at least one of these variables should be varied. By testing serial dilutions of allergen, the test limitations that result from fixing the cell number and culture period are largely abolished. For example, low allergen concentrations may allow 6 days of culture for detection of strong proliferative responses, which would have subsided at that time with higher allergen concentrations.

Nutrients in the cultures: Although the type or brand of culture medium does not seem to be very critical, RPMI 1640, buffered with both HEPES and sodium bicarbonate, has proven to be a reliable lymphocyte culture medium and is now widely used for this purpose. The medium can be supplemented with 10% fetal calf serum (FCS) for short culture periods (1–4 days). When human lymphocytes are cultured for 6 days with allergen, FCS may considerably increase base-line proliferation. A human serum supplement is then to be preferred (10–20% pooled, inactivated, human serum). The use of autologous serum should be avoided, since erratic lymphotoxic effects of individual sera are regularly observed.

Culture periods: Optimal culture periods may vary depending on the parameters chosen for evaluating T-cell stimulation. Allergen-specific lymphocyte proliferation can be detected between day 4 and day 7. As stated above, by testing with serial dilutions of allergen, a culture period of around 6 days generally suffices. When using lymphokine production as a parameter for T-cell stimulation, culture periods are commonly fixed at 24 h for IL-2 and LIF evaluation and at 24–72 h for MIF-production.

Evaluation of* in vitro *stimulated T cells.   Classical evaluation of T-cell activation is by counting the numbers of lymphoblasts in cell smears of the cultures (lymphocyte transformation test, LTT). In allergen stimulated cultures up to 15% of the lymphocytes may be transformed into blastoid cells versus less than 1% in control cultures. For comparison, mitogens such as concanavalin A (ConA) or phytohemagglutinin (PHA) may induce transformation in up to 80% of the lymphocytes. Quantitation of the blastogenic response is, however, time consuming, and although morphological evaluation still should be considered as a valuable parameter, lymphocyte transformation is most reliably measured by [^{3}H]thymidine incorporation (Fig. 13) (Maluish and Strong, 1986). The lymphocyte transformation assay using [^{3}H]thymidine incorporation thus is by far the most frequently performed *in vitro* assay in ACD.

In the LTT allergen-specific responses can be expressed by the proportional increase (stimulation index, SI) or by the absolute increase (delta cpm) in thymidine uptake in allergen containing cultures as compared to appropriate control cultures. Whatever parameter being chosen, base-line proliferation should always be presented, since it may provide information on previous *in vivo* activation, for instance, by ongoing hypersensitivity reactions (Gill, 1967; Lachapelle et al., 1980; Tosca et al., 1981).

In ACD the LTT primarily provides information on CD4$^+$ lymphocyte activation, since this subset accounts for IL-2 production in the cultures. Furthermore, proliferating cells in nickel ACD appeared to be CD4$^+$ lymphocytes in several studies (Silvennoinen-Kassinen et al., 1986; Sinigaglia et al., 1985).

Although the [^{3}H]thymidine assay is very sensitive, it is time consuming, expensive, and entails the drawbacks of radioactive work. Effort has therefore been put in finding alternatives for T-cell activation measurements. Besides blast formation and increased DNA synthesis, upon stimulation various other cytoplasmic and membrane-associated events take place in T cells. It is still expected that one of these events may provide such an alternative.

Within few hours after stimulation biochemical reactions can be recorded in the lymphocytes, as detected by different fluorescent probes and flow cytometry (Nairn and Rolland, 1980). Despite promising results, however, with mitogen-stimulated lymphocytes, so far no reports on the use of such probes for measuring antigenic stimulation have appeared. Another parameter for T-cell activation is based on the conversion of MTT [3-(4,5-dimethylthiazol-2-yl)-2,5-diphenyl-tetrazolium bromide] into a colorimetrically measurable blue formazan. This conversion is associated with mitochondrial activation, and correlates well with cell growth in IL-2 or mitogen-stimulated cultures (Mosmann, 1983; Denizot and Lang, 1986). None of these methods, however, seems to be sensitive enough to detect antigenic T-cell stimulation, let alone the usually weak stimulation observed with contact allergens. More sensitive alternatives have been provided by Dotsika and Sanderson (1987), who developed a fluorometric cell growth assay, and by Magaud et al. (1988), who reported on an ELISA-like procedure for measurement of bromodeoxyuridine uptake, both closely correlating with thymidine uptake. The value of these promising techniques in routine evaluation of lymphocyte stimulation in ACD still has to be investigated.

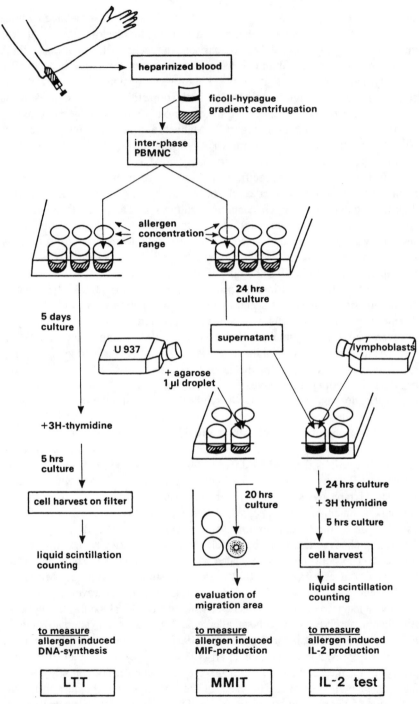

FIGURE 13 *In vitro* assays for T-cell immunity in ACD: methodology. (a) The lymphocyte transformation test (LTT). (b) The macrophage migration inhibition test (MMIT). (c) The IL-2 test.

The appearance of "activation markers" such as Ia molecules, IL-2 receptors (Tac, CD25), transferrin receptors (CD71), and the nuclear Ki-67-antigen (associated with cell proliferation in general) is widely used for monitoring T-cell-mediated processes *in situ*. Principally they might as well be applied to assess *in vitro* T-cell activation. Palutke et al. (1987) showed that the increase in Ki-67 positivity in mixed lymphocyte cultures correlated nicely with both [³H]thymidine uptake and blast transformation. However, quantitation of lymphocyte surface determinants requires flow cytometry. Since access to the apparatus still may be restricted, and in clinical testing hundreds of samples would have to be run, routine use of this method is not to be expected soon.

In conclusion, the method most commonly used for evaluating T-cell activation *in vitro,* measurement of [³H]thymidine uptake, is relatively convenient and very sensitive. Alternatives for the use of radioisotopes should nevertheless be explored because of the long-lasting environmental pollution caused by tritiated molecules.

Evaluation of T-cell products. Lymphokines that received much attention in studies on diagnostic *in vitro* tests for T-cell immunity are MIF, LIF, and to a lesser extent IL-2. Upon antigenic stimulation these lymphokines are primarily produced by helper T lymphocytes.

Both human and guinea pig MIF have originally been assayed with guinea pig peritoneal exudate macrophages as target cells in the macrophage migration inhibition test (MMIT) (Marsman et al., 1972; Von Blomberg et al., 1976; MacSween et al., 1982). Erratic variations in MIF sensitivity of individual macrophage suspensions, however, regularly led to inconsistent results. The development of MIF-sensitive macrophage tumor cell lines (McSween, 1982) strongly facilitated reproducible MIF bioassays. Both human and guinea pig MIF are now successfully detected with the human monocytoid cell line U937 as target (Fig. 14) (Van de Plassche-Boers et al., 1986; Von Blomberg et al., 1984, 1987). The mouse cell line Wehi3 provides a sensitive target for the detection of mouse and rat MIF (Limpens et al., 1989).

Several systems have been developed for the assessment of cell migration (Borish et al., 1986a). In our hands the micro-agarose-droplet assay as originally developed by Harrington and Stastny (1973) and Thurman et al. (1983) provides a most convenient and reproducible assay with both U937 and Wehi3 cells as targets.

In various clinical studies LIF measurement has been assessed as a parameter for T-cell sensitization (Fritz and Sandhofer, 1979). The LMIT (leukocyte migration inhibition test) is most conveniently performed in a direct assay in which production of LIF and response to LIF are measured simultaneously over a 24-h period. Human buffycoats are used containing both lymphocytes as producers and granulocytes as targets of LIF. Unlike macrophages, polymorphonuclear (PMN) leukocytes readily migrate underneath an agarose layer in petri dishes. As alternative for the original capillary tube technique (Søborg and Bendixen, 1967) an agarose LMIT was developed allowing for routine assess-

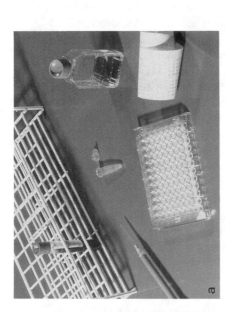

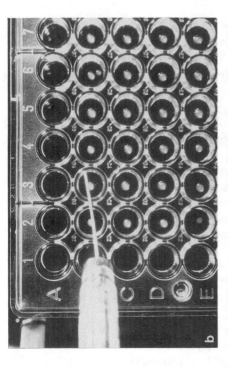

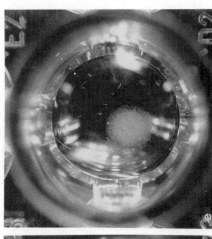

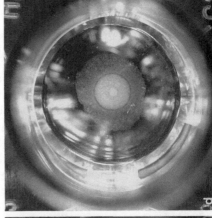

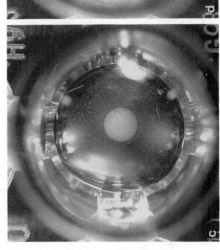

FIGURE 14 Macrophage migration inhibition test (MMIT). (a) Evaluation of MIF production by peripheral blood lymphocytes upon antigenic stimulation. (b) One-microliter droplets of a macrophage (U937 cells) suspension in agarose are being placed in flat-bottomed microtitre plates and overlaid with test culture supernatants. (c–e) Depending on the amount of MIF, macrophage migration is strongly (e) or moderately (d) inhibited as compared to

310

ment of LIF (Clausen, 1971). As the patient's leukocytes may not always provide reliable indicator cells, LIF can also be measured in lymphocyte culture supernatants by using healthy donor leukocytes as target cells. However, in this LIF-2-phase system also, individual differences in LIF sensitivity of the target granulocytes limit reproducibility.

Allergen-induced IL-2 production can be assayed by monitoring the growth of IL-2-dependent lymphoblasts in the presence of lymphocyte culture supernatants (Fig. 13). With IL-2 lacking substantial species restriction, mouse CTL lines are commonly used as a source for IL-2-dependent lymphoblasts (Gillis et al., 1978). Since culturing these cells requires considerable attention, the IL-2 bioassay has not yet become widely in use for evaluating cell mediated immunity *in vitro*. A less demanding alternative, which is both sensitive (down to 0.5 U IL-2/ml) and reproducible, is provided by the use of Con-A-stimulated mouse spleen cells as indicator cells (Weigent et al., 1986; Oostendorp et al., 1989). Recently, radioimmunoassays (RIAs) have also been developed with sensitivities comparable to this bioassay (Cardenas et al., 1986). Both methods for IL-2 measurement are promising, and evaluation of T-cell-mediated immunity by detection of IL-2 release is now within reach.

In conclusion, lymphokine-based assays for T-cell sensitization are subject to considerable biological and technical variation, as can be expected when two bioassays (i.e., for LK production and for LK assessment) are to be used in sequence. The development of sensitive enzyme-linked immunoassays (ELISAs) and RIAs for LK detection may partly solve these problems.

Responder Cells *In Vitro*

Introduction. Whereas in experimental animals lymphocytes can be readily obtained from lymph nodes draining the site of sensitization, or the spleen, human peripheral blood is the main source of responder cells. The following paragraphs, therefore, will concentrate on *in vitro* responses of peripheral blood lymphocytes (PBL).

Before evaluating *in vitro* responsiveness of PBL to contact allergens, one important point should be stressed: When sampling the peripheral blood compartment for *in vitro* lymphocyte stimulation, it should be realized how limited the sample is in terms of both volume and time. Whereas *in vivo* skin test reactions may recruit all circulating lymphocytes passing by for the period of testing (i.e., at least 24–48 h), *in vitro* cultures just bear upon the lymphocytes circulating at the time and site of venipuncture, and present in only a few milliliters of blood (Table 8).

Since the numbers of circulating antigen-specific lymphocytes may fluctuate, depending on various factors, it is of vital importance to carefully choose the time of blood sampling and to register all parameters that could affect *in vitro* responsiveness.

In the next paragraphs some important factors influencing allergen responsiveness of peripheral blood lymphocytes in ACD will be discussed.

TABLE 8. Quantitative Aspects of Blood Lymphocyte Sampling[a]

In vitro	
Total lymphocyte sample (routinely 10 ml of blood, assuming at least 2×10^6 lymphocytes/ml)	2×10^7 lymphocytes
Lymphocytes per test (culture/well)	2×10^5 lymphocytes
In vivo	
Assuming that the average normal skin blood flow is around 250 ml/min/m^2, one skin test (1 cm^2) bears upon 7.10^7 lymphocytes (36 ml of blood) per day, that is, in 48 h	14×10^7 lymphocytes
Some reference data:	
Total blood lymphocytes (5 liter $\times 2 \times 10^6$)	1×10^{10} lymphocytes
Average duration of lymphocyte stay in the circulation	30 min
Total pool of recirculating lymphocytes	25×10^{10} lymphocytes
Total body lymphocytes	50×10^{10} lymphocytes

[a]References: Guyton (1976); Pabst (1988): Schick et al. (1975); Trepel (1975).

Factors affecting blood lymphocyte responsiveness. Total numbers and differential cell counts of peripheral white blood cells depend on several nonimmunological factors (Table 9). Some of these factors may in addition interfere with lymphocyte responsiveness, as measured by mitogenic or antigenic stimulation *in vitro*. As skin test reactions recruit inflammatory cells from the circulation, such suppressive factors will generally also affect skin test reactivity (Pownall et al., 1979). However, as stated above, blood samples for *in vitro*

TABLE 9. Some Factors Affecting Blood Lymphocyte Responsiveness

Factor	T-Lymphocyte responsiveness	References
Circadian rhythm	Increased/decreased	Lévi et al. (1985, 1988) Indiveri et al. (1985) Eskola et al. (1975)
Stress	Decreased	Calabrese et al. (1987) Khansari et al. (1990) Biondi and Pancheri (1987)
Corticosteroid medication	Decreased	Yu (1978); Lomnitzer et al. (1983); Pinkston et al. (1987)
Extensive inflammation	Increased background responses	Gill (1967)
Viral infection	Decreased	Rouse and Horohov (1986)
Recent surgery	Decreased	Berenbaum (1973)
Retroviral or tumor-derived proteins	Decreased	Cianciolo et al. (1980) Chanh et al. (1988)

tests are small as compared to the volume of blood "filtered" by a delayed skin reaction. *In vitro* tests therefore are more susceptible to shortlasting fluctuations in blood lymphocyte numbers.

The most pronounced fluctuations in blood lymphocyte numbers are those related to the circadian rhythm (Abo et al., 1981; Lévi et al., 1985, 1988). Although lymphocyte numbers as well as PBL responsiveness tend to inversely correlate with plasma cortisol levels (Abo et al., 1981; Eskola et al., 1976) the role of the adrenal cortex in regulating the circadian rhythm of lymphocyte counts is still disputed (Lévi et al., 1988). As not only spontaneous proliferation but also antigen responsiveness, as well as the composition of lymphocyte subpopulations, show partly independent circadian rhythms (Eskola et al., 1976; Lévi et al., 1985, 1988) the overall picture is blurred.

It is advisable, therefore, to collect blood samples for *in vitro* studies at a fixed time of the day.

Compartmentalization of allergen-specific lymphocytes. Any renewed skin contact with an allergen in contact hypersensitive individuals will reactivate specific T lymphocytes and cause sequestration of specific T lymphocytes into the resulting inflammatory reaction site. Subsequently a new generation of specific cells may be released from the draining lymph nodes into the circulation. Thus, after allergen contact the numbers of specific T cells might be transiently decreased in the peripheral blood.

In different studies, *in vitro* allergen responsiveness of peripheral blood lymphocytes has been evaluated at various periods after skin testing (Powell et al., 1975; Hamilton et al., 1976; Svejgaard et al., 1978; Byers et al., 1979; Veien et al., 1979; Al-Tawil et al., 1985b). Surprisingly, only little attention has been paid to lymphocyte responsiveness during the first days after skin testing. In clinical practice these days are most convenient for blood sampling, when skin test results become available and the patient is still around. A possible dip in frequency of allergen-specific cells in the blood during a positive skin-test reaction was not observed by Al-Tawil et al. (1985b), as nickel-specific lymphocyte transformation was unaffected 2 days after skin testing. This suggests that early lymphocyte sequestration may hardly be detectable at the systemic level. However, when studying the effects of skin testing in guinea pigs, Tosca et al. (1981) showed that even small dosages of ic antigen reduced the *in vitro* responsiveness of PBL, presumably by means of circulating lymphokines. Interestingly, increased allergen-specific lymphocyte transformation was often observed when testing patients at 2–3 weeks after challenge (Powell et al., 1975; Byers et al., 1979; Al-Tawil et al., 1985b), particularly after oral challenge (Veien et al., 1979). Such a "booster" effect of skin testing was most pronounced when the initial degree of lymphocyte stimulation was very low, for instance, several months after sensitization with a nonubiquitous allergen like DNCB (Powell et al., 1975; Hamilton et al., 1976). It is important to note that skin reactivity was still detectable at that time (Powell et al., 1975). Apparently allergen-specific memory cells in the circulation may at a certain point require reactivation to become fully responsive *in vitro,* whereas the capacity to mount an ACD reaction is still intact. Such a "discrepancy" may be explained by the low numbers of cellular adhesion molecules on memory cells preventing their triggering by allergen-presenting blood monocytes. As discussed earlier, such memory cells still can be readily triggered by skin Langerhans cells.

The effect of active (widespread) contact dermatitis on *in vitro* PBL responsiveness to related allergens has been poorly studied. In drug hypersensitivity it has been found that *in vitro* assays with blood lymphocytes may remain negative up to 6 months after an exacerbation (Houwerzijl, 1977a, 1977b). In this context it should be mentioned that sequestration of antigen-reactive cells, resulting in negative PBL responses to antigen, has also been observed in tuberculosis and rheumatoid arthritis. Antigen-reactive cells were found to be retained in lymph nodes or synovia respectively (Rook et al., 1976; Ford et al., 1985).

In conclusion, when designing *in vitro* assays in ACD one should be aware of the possibility that specific cells have been transiently sequestered from the circulation into sites of (persistent) allergen contact. Optimal *in vitro* test results are to be expected when blood samples are collected in the absence of clinical eczema at 2–3 weeks after challenge.

Interference of circulating suppressor cells. When responder cells are isolated from peripheral blood using Ficoll-Hypaque gradient centrifugation, the resulting mononuclear cell suspensions consist of 5–20% monocytes, 5–15% B lymphocytes, 20–30% $CD8^+$ cells, and 40–60% $CD4^+$ cells. In lymphocyte cultures of allergic donors T helper cells rather than B cells or $CD8^+$ cells proliferate upon antigenic stimulation (Sinigaglia et al., 1985; Silvennoinen-Kassinen et al., 1986; Löfström and Wigzell, 1986). IL-2 and MIF also are primarily produced by $CD4^+$ lymphocytes.

When immune responsiveness to contact allergens has been actively down-regulated, as in individuals with intravenously or orally induced tolerance (Polak, 1980c; Van Hoogstraten et al., 1989) and possibly also in other nonallergic individuals, one might theoretically expect circulating allergen-specific suppressor cells to be present, potentially interfering with *in vitro* parameters for T-cell-mediated immunity. Clinically, however, definite proof of the existence of such suppressor cells has never been obtained. A search for nickel-specific suppressor cells in nonallergic siblings was carried out by Silvennoinen-Kassinen (1981a, 1981b, 1986). Either histamine-receptor-positive (Silvennoinen-Kassinen, 1981a) or CD8-positive (Silvennoinen-Kassinen, 1981b, 1986), putative suppressor cell preparations from healthy siblings were added to proliferating helper cell cultures from HLA-identical nickel-allergic siblings. These experiments did not provide any support for an active role of efferently acting, T suppressor cells in the maintenance of unresponsiveness to nickel in nonallergic individuals. An important role of afferently acting suppressor cells, as has been described in tolerized guinea pigs (Polak, 1980d), cannot be excluded. As animal data supporting the existence of such suppressor cells are rather convincing, this issue certainly warrants further investigation.

In conclusion, it is highly unlikely that the presence of circulating suppressor cells will affect *in vitro* responsiveness of blood lymphocytes in ACD.

Allergen Presentation *In Vitro*

Historical views on allergen presentation. In 1935 Landsteiner and Jacobs, when studying the relationship between immunogenicity and chemical structure of allergens, showed that the immunogenicity of small, chemically reactive allergens like picryl chloride depends on conjugation with macromolecular carriers. Since then scientists have been questioning which carrier in the skin would render an allergen molecule fully recognizable by T lymphocytes. Search for the "true" sensitizing carrier was strongly expanded in the early 1970s, when it was felt necessary to develop effective, nontoxic allergen preparations for *in vitro* assays in contact sensitivity studies.

Initially effectivity of hapten-carrier complexes was studied *in vivo* by sensitizing animals with the conjugates, followed by epicutaneous testing with the free hapten. Despite some successful studies with homologous guinea pig serum proteins (Parker et al., 1970), haptenated serum protein generally failed to induce (Salvin and Smith, 1961; Baumgarten and Geczy, 1970; Chase and Kawata, 1971) or elicit (Geczy and Baumgarten, 1970; Nakagawa and Tanioku, 1972) contact sensitivity in guinea pigs. So the belief in soluble proteins as "true" carriers dwindled away. Research then focused on fractionation of allergen-treated skin, and microsomal fractions were found to display distinct activity as allergen carriers, *in vivo* as well as *in vitro* (Nishioka et al., 1971; Nakagawa and Tanioku, 1972; Nishioka and Amos, 1973; Von Blomberg et al., 1976; Nishioka, 1976; Polak, 1980). Whole cells also received attention as potential allergen carriers in this period. Positive reports by Levis et al. (1974, 1975) using haptenated erythrocytes in clinical *in vitro* lymphocyte transformation studies remained isolated. On the other hand, nucleated cells, in particular mononuclear cells, preferably syngeneic and alive, were effective in inducing contact sensitivity in experimental animals (Baumgarten and Geczy, 1970; MacFarlin and Balfour, 1973; Polak and Macher, 1974; Jones and Amos, 1975). Haptenated mononuclear cells could also be used for *in vitro* stimulation of lymphocytes obtained from contact-sensitized guinea pigs (Geczy and Baumgarten, 1970), rabbits (Hinrichs and Gibbins, 1975), and humans (Miller and Levis, 1973).

Up to 1977 macrophages were employed *in vitro* for degradation and processing of protein antigens. Their relevance as allergen-presenting cells was first demonstrated by Thomas et al. (1977) in guinea pigs and by Greene et al. in mice (1978). From that time macrophages were generally used as allergen-bearing cells both *in vivo* (Von Blomberg et al., 1984) and *in vitro* (Scheper and Polak, 1981; Polak and Scheper, 1981; Von Blomberg et al., 1982). The process of allergen presentation was, however, not appreciated until the discovery of the central role of MHC-class II antigens in macrophage-T cell interactions. In the last decade research on allergen presentation focused on antigen-presenting cells (APC), and ideas about relevant carriers other than MHC-class II molecules subsided. Birth was given to the concept of the dendritic cell family, in which different antigen presenting cells, such as Langerhans cells, veiled cells, interdigitating cells, and other dendritic cells are brought together (Austyn, 1987).

MHC-class II (Ia) molecules.   The presence of Ia molecules on APC apparently is a prerequisite for effective allergen presentation. As outlined earlier, in humans the HLA-DR, DP, and DQ molecules are suitable carriers for allergens to be recognized by the TCR. *In vivo,* reactive chemicals may bind to any skin protein, including cell-surface-bound Ia molecules. ACD most likely results from sensitization to either or both hapten-modified Ia molecules and haptenated protein fragments (peptides) associated with Ia molecules. Serum proteins probably play a minor role as carrier in ACD, since both homologous and heterologous haptenated serum proteins regularly failed to stimulate lymphocytes from contact-sensitized animals (Geczy and Baumgarten, 1970; Hinrichs and Gibbins, 1975; Von Blomberg et al., 1976). In contrast, culturing with chemically reactive haptens, or APC preincubated with free hapten, was generally successful in this respect (Polak, 1980b). The relevance of direct "coating" of APC with allergen was stressed by experiments with nickel salts in human ACD (Kapsenberg, 1988): *in vitro* T-cell responses to nickel sulfate remained high when culturing in serum-free medium or in the presence of chloroquine, which prevents potential macrophage processing by inhibiting lysosomal catabolism. It would appear that the stimulatory capacity of haptenated APC is primarily due to direct binding of haptens with MHC class II and class II associated peptides.

The crucial role of Ia molecules in allergen presentation was underlined by the finding that non-APC such as fibroblasts may present antigens upon treatment with interferon-gamma to induce Ia expression (Maurer et al., 1987) or upon transfection with class II molecules (Norcross et al., 1984). Even allergen-containing liposomes were found to specifically stimulate sensitized T lymphocytes, provided additional Ia molecules had been incorporated (Nishioka et al., 1987). It should be kept in mind, however, that autopresentation by APC contaminating the responder lymphocyte preparations, or by activated T lymphocytes themselves, is hard to exclude in such experiments.

A minimal density of Ia molecules on APC membranes is required to endow cells with full capacity to present allergen (Janeway et al., 1984; Bjercke et al., 1985; Nunez et al., 1987). Further increasing the number of Ia molecules on, for instance, peritoneal macrophages (Von Blomberg, 1982) or liposomes (Nishioka et al., 1987) did not further heighten the T-cell response to contact allergens.

In most of these experiments T-cell clones or recently activated T cells have been used as responder cells. Antigenic stimulation of resting T cells (Umetsu,

1986) and memory T cells (Inaba and Steinman, 1984), as well as of some T-cell clones (Maurer et al., 1987; Kapsenberg, 1987), is now thought to require more than just MHC-class II expression. Apparently, additional cellular interaction molecules determine effective allergen presentation to resting T cells.

Antigen processing by APC. The capacity of APC to process antigen is of particular importance for the induction of T-cell responses to internal epitopes of protein antigens. Proteolytically digested antigen fragments may, however, directly associate with Ia molecules on the APC membrane and stimulate T cells, that is, without being internalized or processed (Cresswell, 1987; Claverie et al., 1989). Also, for contact allergens, processing is not required, since such allergens bind spontaneously to cell membrane components of the APC.

Processing of hapten-carrier complexes may nevertheless occur, particularly when monocytes or macrophages are being used as APC *in vitro*. Cell-bound allergens may also be processed by macrophages. This explains the observation that Ia-incompatible macrophages may present contact allergens both *in vivo* (Baker et al., 1987) and *in vitro* (Von Blomberg et al., 1980; Chang et al., 1987).

Clustering of APC and lymphocytes. An absolute requirement for *in vitro* stimulation of T lymphocytes by APC is a close, immediate cell contact between the two cell types (Austyn et al., 1988). Experimentally this can be observed as "cell clustering." Two types of clustering have been described: antigen-independent and antigen-dependent clustering (Inaba and Steinman, 1986).

Antigen-independent clustering is exclusively observed when dendritic cells are used as APC. This type of clustering, characterized by frequent, short-lasting cell contacts, may be teleologically regarded as reflecting the search of APC for the right (allergen-specific) T cell to stimulate. Antigen-independent cluster formation is temperature dependent (only at 37 °C), and MHC-class II molecules do not participate in the binding (Inaba and Steinman, 1987). Besides the adhesion molecules ICAM-1 on APC and LFA-1 on lymphocytes, other physical properties of the APC cell membrane, like reduction of the negative cell surface charge and the formation of "veils," are likely to play a role in this antigen-independent cell clustering (Austyn and Morris, 1988; King and Katz, 1990).

The initial binding between APC and T cell is further stabilized when allergen-modified Ia molecules interact with the TCR. Several pairs of adhesion molecules, including CD2 and LFA-1 on T cells, and LFA-3 and ICAM-related molecules on APC (Fig. 3), participate in stabilization of the cluster (Breitmeyer, 1987; Inaba and Steinman, 1987). Interestingly, this process of antigen-dependent clustering may *in vitro* already take place at 4 °C and is, in contrast to the initial clustering, not limited to dendritic cells as APC (Inaba and Steinman, 1984). Within these clusters antigenic stimulation of specific cells may occur through the TCR complex.

The electrical surface charges of the APC and lymphocyte are important for both types of cluster formation. Neuraminidase treatment (reducing the negative charge of the cell surface) of either allergen-bearing cells or responder lymphocytes enhanced monocyte-T lymphocyte clustering (Kapsenberg, 1989). This parallels similar enhancement by neuraminidase of B/T-cell contacts. Cell clustering could also be facilitated by adding 2% polyethylene glycol to the cultures (Krieger et al., 1988).

It is not only the APC that determines the rate of cluster formation. The activation stage of the T cell is another important factor in this process. The fact that memory T cells and particularly recently activated cells, as compared to naive T lymphocytes, are less fastidious as to the type of APC probably relates to increased expression of adhesion molecules on previously activated lymphocyte cell membranes (Inaba and Steinman, 1984; Sanders, 1988) (see Table 5).

This obviously has important implications for performing *in vitro* tests in ACD. Since these tests aim at stimulating previously activated, and often recently activated, T lymphocytes, allergen presentation need not be restricted to "dendritic" allergen-presenting cells.

IL-1 production by APC.   It has been well established that antigenic stimulation of T lymphocytes through the TCR requires an additional signal from interleukin-1 (IL-1) (Weaver and Unanue, 1990). Macrophages as well as dendritic APC can produce this mediator. The degree of IL-1 production in human peritoneal macrophages was shown to directly correlate with the ability of the cells to induce antigen specific T-cell proliferation (Becker et al., 1986). During an immune response, macrophages are stimulated to synthesize and to release IL-1 by direct contact with T cells (Breitmeyer, 1987) and T-cell products (CSF) or by complement-fixing antigen-antibody complexes (Weaver and Unanue, 1986; Oppenheim et al., 1986). Other cell types (including keratinocytes, endothelial cells, B cells, and neutrophils) can also be induced to release IL-1 (Oppenheim et al., 1986). It has been noted that for signal delivery IL-1 does not need to be in the fluid phase. Using fixed APCs for T-cell stimulation, membrane-bound IL-1 on macrophages (Weaver and Unanue, 1986; Unanue and Allen, 1986) and dendritic cells (Nagelkerken and Van Breda Vriesman, 1986) was found to provide the appropriate signal. Surprisingly, in some studies, dendritic cells are regarded as target rather than as producer cells of IL-1. Koide et al. (1987) reported on activation of dendritic cells by IL-1 (optimal at a dose of 5 U/ml and 18 h of exposure) becoming manifest by an enhanced capacity to cluster with helper T cells. In line with these findings are the results of Heufler et al. (1988), who activated Langerhans cells *in vitro* with keratinocyte-derived IL-1 and GM-CSF, rendering the Langerhans cells more potent in stimulating resting T cells. It would appear that, like IL-2, IL-1 represents a mediator with considerable autoendocrine function.

As to *in vitro* activation of T cells by allergen, it is apparently of paramount importance that an IL-1-related signal is provided in the cultures. Since recombinant IL-1 is now available, routine addition of this mediator to the cultures may improve the conditions for *in vitro* contact sensitivity tests.

The dendritic cell family.   The dendritic cell (DC) family has been considered as a distinct lineage of cells, specialized in antigen presentation (Steinman and Nussenzweig, 1980; Knight et al., 1986; Austyn, 1987). Others still consider them as members of the mononuclear phagocyte family (Drexhage et al., 1980; Kraal et al., 1986; Kabel et al., 1989). Consensus exists, however, with respect to their role in the immune response (King and Katz, 1990). The most important role of DC is in primary immune responses, which explains their location in skin and peripheral lymph nodes. The DC family has been studied extensively *in situ,* in particular the Langerhans cells, veiled cells, and interdigitating cells, as well as *in vitro* using lymphoid DC, isolated from spleen, lymph nodes, or blood. Although Langerhans cells, interdigitating cells, and lymphoid DC all originate from bone marrow precursors (Austyn, 1987), little is still known about their interrelationships, sites of maturation, and phenotypes of blood precursors. Depending on the organ sources, as well as on *in vitro* culture periods, DC show morphologic and phenotypic differences (Austyn, 1987). Remarkably, because of the considerable intrafamily variation, no hard criteria are available to distinguish DC from mononuclear phagocytes (Table 10). Some important members of this family of APC will be described below.

Langerhans cells. Langerhans cells (LC), isolated from suction blister roofs by trypsinization, acquire DC characteristics when cultured *in vitro* (Schuler and Steinman, 1985): they lose their Birbeck granules, express increased numbers of class II molecules and gain in potency to stimulate immune responses (Austyn, 1987; Shimada et al., 1987; Schuler and Steinman, 1985; Streilein and Grammer, 1989; Romani et al., 1989; Teunissen et al., 1989). Interestingly, the capacity of LC to stimulate T cells can also be enhanced by *in vitro* exposure to contact allergens (Picut et al., 1987) or to keratinocyte-derived GM-CSF and IL-1 (Heufler et al., 1988; Gaspari et al., 1989). Even without preculture, however, LC appeared to be effective *in vitro* stimulators of memory lymphocytes with contact allergens (Braathen and Thorsby, 1980, 1983; Res et al., 1987), tuberculin (Bjercke et al., 1985), and viral antigens (Bagot et al., 1985). The efficacy of LC to present antigens to sensitized T lymphocytes equals that of blood-derived DC, but differences in technical conditions and (im)purities of cell preparations allow only for rough comparisons. A functional dichotomy between LC and blood-derived DC was nevertheless suggested by Kapsenberg (1987), since some nickel-specific T cell clones could recognize nickel only when presented by LC (Kapsenberg et al., 1987). However, differences in the activation stages of the T cell clones could also lead to such discrepancies.

Despite their excellent capacity to present contact allergens *in vitro,* LC are of little importance for routine diagnostic procedures in human ACD, since suction blistering would be required in every patient to be tested.

Dendritic cells. DC derived from mouse spleens have been used extensively for studying DC/T-cell interactions (Inaba and Steinman, 1984, 1986, 1987). Utilizing some DC features (low buoyant density, transient glass adherence, absence of Fc receptors), these cells can be isolated also from other organs, as well as from peripheral blood (Van Voorhis et al., 1983; Bjercke et al., 1985; Nau and Peters, 1986; Knight, 1986). Blood-derived dendritic cells

TABLE 10. Characteristics Favoring APC Function *In Vitro*

	Contact allergens presented to		Protein antigens presented to	
APC characteristics	Naive T cells	Memory T cells	Naive T cells	Memory T cells
MHC-class II expression	+	+	+	+
Antigen processing	−	−	+	+
Antigen-independent clustering	+	−	+	−
Antigen-dependent clustering	+	+	+	+
IL-1 production	+	+	+	+

are extremely efficient in antigen presentation as compared to blood monocytes (10–100 times; Van Voorhis et al., 1983; Bjercke et al., 1985). Although Ia expression of DC, as well as their ability to cluster with T cells, is beyond dispute, DC are relatively deficient in antigen processing and IL-1 production (Table 10). The simultaneous presence of monocytes or macrophages in the cultures may therefore further enhance the stimulatory capacity of DC, in particular for protein antigens (Guidos et al., 1987).

The importance of dendritic cells *in vivo* for triggering T lymphocytes in contact allergy was revealed from studies in mice. Allergen-specific T cells could be strongly stimulated with DC isolated from the draining lymph nodes 1 day after allergen application on the skin (Knight et al., 1985). Although few studies have yet been made on DC as allergen-presenting cells in human contact sensitivity, the *in vitro* effectiveness of peripheral blood-derived dendritic cells as APC was clear in nickel allergy (Res et al., 1987).

For those interested in clinical *in vitro* testing, it is a relief that DC are among the mononuclear cells isolated from human blood by routine Ficoll-

TABLE 11. Capacity of Various Allergen Presenting Cells to Display Characteristics Favoring APC Function[a]

	Cell type			
APC characteristics	LC	DC blood	Monocytes	B cells
HLA-DR expression	+ + +	+ + +	+ +	+ +
HLA-DP expression	+ + +	+ + +	+	+ +
HLA-DQ expression	+ + +	+ + +	+	+ +
Antigen processing	±	±	+ +	+
Antigen-independent clustering	+ +	+ + +	±	−
Antigen-dependent clustering	+ +	+ + +	+ +	+ +
IL-1 production	+	±	+ +	±

[a]References: Gonwa et al. (1986); Brooks and Moore (1988).

Hypaque centrifugation procedures. Considering that only very few DC are required to activate large numbers of responder T cells, efficient allergen presentation would be guaranteed, even without further purification of the mononuclear cells.

Monocytes and macrophages (MØ). In experimental animals the most readily available cell type for antigen processing and presentation is the peritoneal exudate macrophage, as obtained after ip injection of mineral oil or thioglycollate. Peritoneal exudates contain up to 80% macrophages, and can be obtained in large quantities (3×10^8 peritoneal exudate cells per guinea pig; 10^7 per mouse). These macrophages meet all requirements for allergen presentation (Tables 10 and 11), except for the ability to form antigen-independent clusters (Inaba and Steinman, 1986).

In studies on experimental contact allergy, MØ have been employed successfully *in vitro* as antigen-presenting cells for stimulating memory lymphocytes with the allergens dinitrochlorobenzene (DNCB), picrylchloride, and oxazolone (Thomas et al., 1977; Greene et al., 1978; Von Blomberg et al., 1980; Polak and Scheper, 1981; Von Blomberg et al., 1982). In these studies optimal results were obtained by preincubating MØ with high, marginally toxic doses of free hapten to avoid toxic effects in the lymphocyte cultures. Inhibitory effects of PGE_2, produced by activated peritoneal exudate macrophages, could be reduced with indomethacin (Mullink and Von Blomberg, 1980). For some allergens, like picryl chloride, but not for DNCB, peritoneal macrophages could also be used for *in vitro* stimulation of unprimed lymphocytes (L. Polak, personal communication). The success of peritoneal macrophages as APC *in vitro* may be due to their intrinsic capacity to present allergen, or to DC, which may also be present in peritoneal exudate preparations. Experimentally, other sources of MØ have been less well documented, as isolation and purification procedures usually are more complicated. Adherent spleen cells as well as alveolar macrophages were successfully used as APC in mice and guinea pigs. Alveolar macrophages, however, induced relatively high background lymphocyte responses (Von Blomberg et al., 1982; Lipscomb et al., 1981).

Very few animal studies have been devoted to the allergen-presenting capacity of peripheral blood monocytes. As the blood is the primary source of APC for experimental and routine diagnostic *in vitro* assays in humans, knowledge about this type of APC mainly stems from clinical studies. Peripheral blood monocytes are quite heterogeneous both in terms of physical properties and functional capacities. As discussed above, it is still far from clear whether different cell lineages or different maturation stadia account for this heterogeneity. Evaluation of the capacity of monocyte subpopulations to present (microbial) antigens, revealed a slight but consistent increase of antigen presenting capacity with decreasing monocyte density. Subdivision of the total monocyte population in MØ-like monocytes (FcR-positive cells, Bjercke et al., 1985; 24-h adherent cells, Mittal and Nath, 1987) and dendritic cells (FcR-negative, Bjercke et al., 1985; transiently adherent cells, Mittal and Nath, 1987) revealed a relative deficiency in antigen presentation of the MØ-like monocytes. However, despite much effort, a distinct dendritic cell precursor within the monocyte population could not be demonstrated. In contrast, upon *in vitro* culturing under nonadhering conditions and in the presence of stimulatory agents as metrizamide, up to 40% of the monocytes acquire a dendritic appearance as well as the capacity for antigen-independent clustering (Kabel et al., 1989). This finding confirms earlier observations of Peters et al. (1987), who isolated DC from *in vitro* blood monocyte cultures.

From these studies it may be concluded that monocytes should be regarded as a very suitable source of APC for *in vitro* tests, since they seem to harbor high numbers of immature DC, which "mature" upon culturing.

B lymphocytes as APC. The capacity of B cells to serve as APC for stimulating helper (CD4⁺) T cells has become firmly established. All B cells express high levels of HLA-DP, DQ, and DR molecules, even in the absence of IFN-gamma (Table 12). Whereas B cells are poor IL-1 producers and do not show antigen-independent clustering, they are quite able to pinocytose, to process protein antigens, and to reexpress antigen fragments on their cell membrane (Lanzavecchia, 1985). The presence of antigen-specific immunoglobulins on the B cells considerably enhances their ability to capture and to process these antigens. The immunoglobulin receptor molecules are not themselves involved in the actual antigen presentation (Lanzavecchia, 1985; Howard, 1985). Interestingly, as a consequence of TCR triggering by B-cell-bound antigen, T cells produce B-cell activating lymphokines, thus in turn stimulating the B cells to secrete antibodies (Liano and Abbas, 1987). This may explain the frequent occurrence of hapten-specific antibodies in allergic contact dermatitis. The functional relevance of such antibodies seems, however, to be low (Boerrigter et al., 1988).

In contact allergy studies, HLA-compatible Epstein-Barr virus-transformed B cells, which are easily kept in long-term cultures, offer satisfactory APC function, particularly when used to stimulate specific T-cell clones (Sinigaglia et al., 1985). Routine clinical application of such cells for diagnostic T-cell stimulation is, however, not to be expected because sets of EBV-B cells would be required, expressing all known MHC-class II antigens.

Other cells or artifacts. Theoretically, all Ia-bearing cells or particles can function as APC to specifically stimulate memory T cells. Indeed, data from various groups indicate that recently activated T lymphocytes or T-cell clones can be stimulated by any cell or particle bearing antigen and proper Ia determinant(s) under appropriate culture conditions. Thus, activated, Ia⁺ T lymphocytes appeared to be capable of autopresentation (Brown et al., 1984), whereas functional antigen presentation was also found for Ia-positive fibroblasts (Maurer et al., 1987), endothelial cells (Hirschberg et al., 1982), neutrophils (Okuda et al., 1980), and keratinocytes (Morikawa et al., 1989). Keratinocytes are, however, less efficient accessory cells, as they may produce mediators in the cultures that inhibit lymphocyte proliferation (Nickoloff et al.,

TABLE 12. Studies on Diagnostic *In Vitro* Tests in ACD[a]

Author	Year	Allergen	LTT bl	LTT thy	LMIT	MMIT	Other	Sens[b]	Spec[c]	Sign[d]	Conclusion as to clinical use[e]
pegren	1962	Nickel	*					+ + +	−	−	−
rdquist	1967	Neomycin		*				+ + +	+ + +	+	+
nifin	1970	Beryllium		*				+ + +	+ + +	+	
höpf	1970	Gold	*					+ + +	+ + +	nt	
cLeod	1970	Nickel		*				+ + +	+ + +	+	
ppas	1970	Nickel	*	*				+ + +	−	−	−
nz	1971	Chromium	*					+ + +	nt	nt	+ +
nz	1971	Cobalt	*					+ + +	nt	nt	+ +
nz	1971	Formalin	*					+ + +	nt	nt	+ +
nz	1971	Mercury	*					+ + +	nt	nt	+ +
nz	1971	Nickel	*					+ + +	nt	nt	+ +
nz	1971	PPDA	*					+ + +	nt	nt	+ +
nz	1971	Procaine	*					+ + +	nt	nt	+ +
chka	1971	Chromium	*					+	+ + +	+	−
lágyi	1971	Tuliposide		*				+ + +	+ + +	+	+ +
rman	1972	Nickel				*		+	+ + +	nt	±
rman	1972	Nickel	*	*				+ + +	+	+	±
nderson	1972	Beryllium				*		+ + +	+ + +	nt	+ +
tchinson	1972	Nickel		*				+ +	+ + +	+	
vene	1972	DNCB		*				+	+ + +	nt	
ulin	1972	Chromium#			*			+ + +	+ + +	+	+
mada	1972	Chromium	*					+ +	+ +	+	−
mada	1972	Cobalt	*					+ + +	+ + +	nt	±
mada	1972	Formalin	*					−	nt	nt	−
mada	1972	Iodine	*					+ + +	+	nt	−
mada	1972	Mercury	*					+ + +	−	−	−
mada	1972	PPDA	*					+ + +	+	−	−
mada	1972	Urushiol	*					+ +	−	nt	−
ler	1973	DNCB #		*				+ + +	+ + +	+	+
likan	1973	Nickel		*				+ + +	+ + +	+	+
lner	1974	DNCB #		*				+ + +	+ +	+	±
menez	1975	Nickel		*				+ + +	+ + +	+	
vis	1975	DNCB #		*				+ + +	nt	nt	
vis	1975	DNCB #					1	+	nt	nt	
rza	1975	Nickel			*			+	+ + +	−	−
rza	1975	Nickel #			*			+ + +	+ +	+	+
milton	1976	DNCB #			*			nt	nt	+	+
dan	1976	Nickel			*			+ + +	+ + +	+	+
n	1976	Nickel		*				+ + +	+ + +	+	±
vis	1976	DNCB		*				+ + +	+ + +	+	
cLeod	1976a	Nickel					2	+ +	+ + +	+	
cLeod	1976b	Nickel			*			nt	nt	−	−
hioka	1976	DNCB #				*		+ + +	+ + +	+	±

(Table continues on next page)

TABLE 12. Studies on Diagnostic *In Vitro* Tests in ACD[a] (*Continued*)

Author	Year	Allergen	LTT bl	LTT thy	LMIT	MMIT	Other	Sens[b]	Spec[c]	Sign[d]	Conclusion as to clinical use
Soeberg	1976	DNCB #	*					nt	+ + +	+	
Soeberg	1976	NDMA #	*					nt	nt	+	
Tio	1976	Chromium #			*			+ + +	+ + +	+	+ +
Thulin	1976	Nickel			*			+	+	−	−
Thulin	1976	Nickel #			*			+ +	+ +	+	−
Goering	1977	Diverse	*					+ +	+ + +	+	
Goering	1977	DNCB	*					+ + +	nt	+	
Goering	1977	NDMA	*					+ + +	nt	nt	
Swoboda	1977	Nickel			*			+ + +	+ + +	+	+
Houwerzijl	1977b	CBZ	*					+ + +	+ + +	+	+
Svejgaard	1978	Nickel	*					+ + +	+ + +	+	+
Adam	1979	Chloramphenicol	*					+ + +	nt	nt	+
Byers	1979	Urushiol #	*					+ +	+ + +	nt	
Dupuis	1979	Urushiol #	*					+ +	+ +	+	±
Veien	1979	Nickel	*					+ + +	+ +	+	
Silvennoinen	1980	Nickel	*					+ + +	+ +	+	+
Al-Tawil	1981	Nickel	*					+ + +	+ +	+	+ +
Nakano	1981	DNFB			*			+ +	+ + +	nt	
Oehling	1981	Chromium	*					−	+ + +	−	−
Oehling	1981	Nickel	*					−	+ + +	−	−
MacLeod	1982	Nickel					1	+ +	+ +	−	
MacLeod	1982	Nickel			*			+ +	+ +	−	
Rytter	1982	Chromium			*			+ + +	+ + +	+	+ +
Williams	1982a	Beryllium	*					+ + +	nt	nt	+
Williams	1982b	Beryllium				*		+ +	+ + +	+	−
Williams	1982b	Beryllium			*			+ + +	+ + +	+	+ +
Al-Tawil	1983	Chromium	*					+ + +	+ + +	+	+ +
Nordlind	1983	Chromium			*			+ +	+ + +	+	±
Nordlind	1983	Nickel			*			−	+ + +	−	−
Al-Tawil	1984	Cobalt	*					+ +	+ + +	+	+ +
Camarasa	1984	Mercury	*					+ + +	+ + +	+	
Nordlind	1984a	Nickel	*					+ + +	+	+	±
Nordlind	1984b	Nickel	*					+ + +	+ +	+	±
Silvennoinen	1984	Gold	*					+ + +	nt	nt	+ +
Aldridge	1985	Nickel					3	+ +	+ + +	+	+ +
Al-Tawil	1985	Nickel	*					+ + +	+ +	+	±
Bruynzeel	1985	Penicillin g	*					+ +	nt	nt	
Stejskal	1986	Alprenolol	*	*				+ + +	+ + +	+	+
Stejskal	1986	Bacampicillin	*	*				+ + +	+ + +	+	+
Stejskal	1986	Quinidine	*	*				+ + +	+ + +	+	+
Tjernlund	1987	Nickel					4	+ +	+ + +	nt	
V. Blomberg	1987	Nickel				*		+ +	+ + +	+	±
V. Blomberg	1987	Nickel			*			+ + +	+ +	+	±

TABLE 12. Studies on Diagnostic *In Vitro* Tests in ACD[a] (*Continued*)

Author	Year	Allergen	LTT bl	thy	LMIT	MMIT	Other	Sens[b]	Spec[c]	Sign[d]	Conclusion as to clinical use[e]
ham	1988	Nickel	*					+ + +	+ + +	+	+
ns	1988	Nickel	*					+ + +	+ + +	+	+
rttunen	1988	Nickel					5	nt	nt	+	
rttunen	1988	Nickel					6	nt	nt	−	

[a]Key: #, allergen preconjugated to cells or proteins; in all other experiments allergens were added to the ‹ure as reactive chemicals or metal salts; NDMA, para-*N*-dimethylnitrosaniline; CBZ, carbamazepine; LTT bl, phocyte transformation test evaluated by counting the percentages of blastoid cells; LTT thy, LTT evaluated by asuring thymidine uptake; LMIT, leukocyte migration inhibition test (one-phase system: production and effect lymphokine measured simultaneously); MMIT, macrophage migration inhibition test (two-phase system: ‹duction and effect of lymphokine measured separately); 1, assay for blastogenic factor production; 2, leukocyte ‹regation assay; 3, assay for procoagulant production; 4, supernatants are assayed for their potential to induce ‹C-class II expression in keratinocytes in cultured skin biopsies; 5, assay for IL-2 production; 6, assay for ‹-gamma production; nt, not tested, not explicitly mentioned, or not evaluable because too few people were ‹mined.

[b]Sens, sensitivity of tests defined as the percentage of patch-test positive, allergic patients showing a ‹sitive *in vitro* response. *In vitro* responses were considered positive when stimulation indices exceeded 2 (in T) or migration inhibition exceeded 20% (LMIT and MMIT).

[c]Spec, specificity of tests defined as the percentage of negative *in vitro* tests in healthy controls. Both ‹sitivity and specificity were graded as <20%, −; 20–50%, +; 50–80%, + +; and >80%, + + +.

[d]Sign, the difference between patch test positive patients and negative controls was recorded as − if not ‹nificant, and as + if *p* < .05 (significance only tested when more than four patients per group).

[e]Clinical use, the authors' conclusion as to clinical use of the test was graded as not applicable −; dubious ‹licability ±; restricted applicability +; and applicability stressed + +.

1986). Artificially constructed liposomes, containing both antigen and class II molecules, could also be used for antigen presentation (Nishioka et al., 1984). Although such conditioned liposomes, kept in stock, might be promising for diagnostic assays in ACD, general application would be limited by the many different allergen–MHC-class II combinations needed in clinical practice.

Conclusions. In diagnostic procedures in human ACD, (recently) activated lymphocytes, rather than resting memory cells, are being addressed. This implies that antigen-independent clustering is not required for effective allergen presentation. Therefore, monocytes as present in typical Ficoll-Hypaque peripheral blood mononuclear cell suspensions will sufficiently support allergen presentation. Moreover, dendritic cells are among those mononuclear cells and their numbers may even increase upon culturing.

Finally, culture media may be supplemented to guarantee optimal antigen presentation and accessory function in the system: biological response modifiers (BRM) like IL-1 stimulate APC-clustering and T-cell activation, whereas other substances like neuraminidase or polyethylene glycol may facilitate contacts between APC and T cells.

Diagnostic Relevance of *In Vitro* Tests in ACD

Introduction.   The aim of this section is to evaluate the impact of two decades of *in vitro* studies in contact allergy on the clinical applicability of *in vitro* tests. For this purpose at first an inventory was made of published reports on *in vitro* tests in ACD. The literature data were used to study the diagnostic value of these tests in relation to a number of variables, like lymphocyte sampling, allergen presentation, and culture techniques, as discussed in the preceding paragraphs.

In addition, the literature data were supplemented with results from a small inquiry, held during the first European Contact Dermatitis Society meeting (Heidelberg, 1988) to record current dermatologists' opinion as to the clinical applicability of *in vitro* assays in diagnosing ACD (Von Blomberg et al., 1989).

Literature review.   In Table 12, diagnostic *in vitro* tests in ACD have been listed chronologically. All studies aiming at *in vitro* testing as a diagnostic tool and providing sufficient data to allow for a comparison between patch test results and *in vitro* tests have been included. Thus, those reports on *in vitro* tests lacking skin test data had to be omitted. Diagnostic use was evaluated by scoring both sensitivity and specificity of the *in vitro* test for detecting positive patch-test reactivity, using fixed criteria for positivity of the assays. In addition, the capacity of an *in vitro* test to differentiate between groups of patch-test positive patients and negative controls, as well as the authors' opinion as to the clinical applicability of the test, has been given (for details see Table 12).

From the table it is clear that positive reports have been published consistently since 1967. Notably, neither the absolute number of published tests nor the percentage of successful tests has substantially changed during this period.

Peripheral blood cells served as responder cells in all these studies. In most reports little or no information is given on the time of blood sampling, neither in relation to the diurnal rhythm nor in relation to recent allergen contacts. The importance of sampling peripheral blood for *in vitro* testing well after disappearance of clinical symptoms of drug hypersensitivity was nevertheless stressed by Houwerzijl et al. (1977). Data on other relevant conditions known to affect lymphocyte responsiveness (Table 9) are also rarely provided. Occasionally, however, corticosteroid treatment (Millikan et al., 1973; Williams and Williams, 1982a, 1982b) or the presence of an active eczema (Lischka, 1971; Gimenez-Camarasa et al., 1975) has explicitly been mentioned. Active dermatitis was found to coincide with high "background" proliferation of PBL, thereby possibly reducing the sensitivity of allergen-specific testing (e.g., for chromium; Lischka, 1971). In other studies, however, nickel-specific lymphocyte proliferation was readily detectable at a time of clinically active dermatitis (Gimenez-Camarasa et al., 1975). Interestingly, systemic steroid treatment of the patients did not prevent allergen-specific proliferation to either nickel or beryllium (Millikan et al., 1973; Williams and Williams, 1982a, 1982b).

Although diagnostically successful tests have been recorded for a broad range of water-soluble and insoluble allergens, about 50% of the published tests concern nickel and DNCB (Table 13). For comparison the allergens most frequently causing positive patch tests have been listed in Table 14. As regards the presentation of contact allergens *in vitro*, a clear pattern emerges from Table 12. Initially, allergens were added to *in vitro* cultures just as they were applied onto the skin for patch testing, that is, as free haptens. Later, in the period 1972–1978, haptens were often conjugated to cells or soluble proteins before being added to the cultures, reflecting the extensive studies on the "true" carrier in ACD in these years. Since 1979, however, contact allergens were again regularly added as free haptens to the lymphocyte cultures. Apparently the diagnostic value does not really require adding preformed allergen-conjugate preparations. Nevertheless, highly toxic allergens (urushiol, DNCB) might still be more effective when preconjugated either to cells (Miller and Levis, 1973; Levis et al., 1975; Byers et al., 1979) or to soluble proteins (Dupuis, 1979). In the leukocyte migration inhibition test also relatively nontoxic allergens, like nickel and chromium, had to be used as conjugates (Mirza et al., 1975; Thulin, 1976; Tio, 1976).

Regarding the techniques used for diagnostic *in vitro* testing through the years, the lymphocyte transformation test (LTT) remains the favorite: until 1972 evaluation was done by scoring percentages of blastoid cells, and thereafter by measuring thymidine uptake. Data obtained with both methods of evaluating lymphocyte transformation generally correlate well, and have therefore been combined for diagnostic value scoring in Table 12. Lymphokine production was evaluated most often with the leukocyte migration inhibition test (LMIT), that is, by simultaneous assessment of both the production of LIF by, and the effect on, buffycoat cells. When lymphocyte transformation and lymphokine production were assessed in parallel, the LTT was usually more sensitive, whereas the lymphokine assays showed greater specificity (Forman and Alexander, 1972; Levis et al., 1975; Williams and Williams, 1982b; Von Blomberg et al., 1987). Both LTT and lymphokine assays regularly show high diagnostic scores for sensitivity, specificity, and clinical applicability of the tests.

Inquiry results. In order to challenge our literature-based findings, this survey was completed with an inquiry, held among about 250 participants of the clinically oriented Heidelberg meeting on ACD in 1988 (Von Blomberg et al., 1989). Most of the 74 inquiry responders had no experience with *in vitro* testing, because they were insufficiently acquainted with the techniques involved (41%) or considered these tests too laborious (32%), not yet reliable (7%), or unnecessary (25%). Dermatologists with *in vitro* test experience applied the tests mainly for research purposes. The LTT was the most frequently used assay, and metals and drugs were the most frequently tested allergens. It became furthermore clear that no consensus existed in the group of experienced inquiry responders with respect to clinical applicability of *in vitro* tests. Remarkably, only a minority of the experienced inquiry responders (33%) consid-

TABLE 13. Contact Allergens Used for *In Vitro* Testing
in the Period 1962–1987 (Extracted from Table 12)

Contact allergen	Number of published reports on *in vitro* tests
Nickel	30
DNP	10
Chromium	9
Beryllium	4
Urushiol	3
Cobalt	3
Mercury	3
Formalin	2
p-Phenylene diamine	2
Gold	2
NDMA	2
Alprenolol	1
Bacampicillin	1
Chloramphenicol	1
Iodine	1
Neomycin	1
Penicillin g	1
Carbamazepine	1
Procaine	1
Quinidine	1
Tuliposide	1

ered *in vitro* tests not clinically applicable. The opinion on clinical applicability of the tests was not clearly related to the allergens tested.

Conclusions. Clinical application of *in vitro* tests in ACD has been promoted consistently since 1967. In the early 1970s it was generally expected that increase in fundamental knowledge of T-cell activation would facilitate the introduction of diagnostic *in vitro* assays (Scheper and Oort, 1973). As shown in previous paragraphs, the increase in knowledge has been tremendous, particularly as to the molecular requirements for allergen presentation and T-cell activation. However, this has not led to a widespread use of *in vitro* tests for ACD in clinical practice. As has been discussed in the preceding chapters, with increasing knowledge about the mechanisms involved, awareness has also grown as to the great number of factors that inevitably restrict wide clinical applicability. The inquiry revealed some additional reasons for the fact that, despite a consistent number of positive reports appearing yearly, still so little use is being made of *in vitro* tests in ACD. Most dermatologists are poorly informed about *in vitro* technologies, whereas the "insiders" often consider the tests too laborious as compared to *in vivo* tests, and are deterred by the frequent erratic results inherent to bioassays.

As most literature data provide little information on the time of blood sampling in relation to recent allergen contacts, the actual limiting effects of compartmentalization on diagnostic *in vitro* testing remain unclear. Even in the presence of a clinically active dermatitis, nickel-specific *in vitro* responses remained detectable in the peripheral blood (Gimenez-Camarasa et al., 1975). Nevertheless, active dermatitis may reduce the overall sensitivity of *in vitro* testing by increasing "background" proliferation of blood lymphocytes (Gill, 1967; Lischka, 1971).

In vitro tests have been performed with a wide variety of allergens. However, only a minority of the allergens most frequently causing positive patch tests were tested *in vitro*. Moreover, the majority of reports concern the allergens nickel and DNCB, thus indicating that models for evaluating optimal *in vitro* conditions were studied, rather than diagnostic tools. Nickel salts apparently are exceptionally convenient for *in vitro* stimulation of T cells, probably because these are water soluble and, in contrast to, for instance, mercury salts, can be used in high concentrations without showing cytotoxicity. Interestingly, the inquiry showed that apart from these model allergens, drugs have been frequently tested *in vitro*. This stresses the need for *in vitro* tests in this field. However, both *in vitro* and *in vivo* establishment of drug allergies meet with considerable difficulties: some drugs, particularly upon systemic administra-

TABLE 14. Top 10 Contact Allergens in Canada, Germany, and Holland

	Percent of positive patch tests		
Contact allergens	Canada 1967–1981	Germany 1977–1983	Holland 1985–1988
Nickel sulfate	14.7%	9.2%	16.0%
Balsam of Peru	10.8%	6.3%	4.0%
Potassium dichromate	10.6%	4.3%	3.2%
Caine mix	7.4%	4.2%	
p-Phenylene diamine	7.3%	4.1%	
Neomycin	6.6%	3.2%	1.8%
Carba mix	6.1%		1.5%
Thiuram mix	5.4%		
Formaldehyde	5.2%	3.5%	2.6%
Thiomersal	5.0%		
Fragrance mix		8.9%	5.7%
Cobalt chloride		4.7%	7.3%
Lanolin alcohols		4.3%	
Colophony			3.0%
Kathon CG			4.1%

Note. The prevalence of the ten most frequently encountered contact allergens has been calculated from different patient groups, all consisting of about 65% females and 35% males: 4190 patients tested in Canada in the period 1967–1981 (Lynde et al., 1982); 12,026 patients tested in Germany in the period 1977–1983 (Enders et al., 1988); and 1855 patients tested in Holland in the period 1985–1988 (A.Z.V.U. Bruynzeel, Amsterdam personal communication).

tion, are metabolized in the liver, resulting in ill-defined sensitizing determinants; others may exert unwanted pharmacological activities in the test system (e.g., clonidine; Goeptar et al., 1988).

The progress made in understanding the molecular and cellular requirements for allergen presentation actually had few consequences for *in vitro* testing in contact allergy. Whereas initially, unhampered by too much fundamental knowledge on allergen presentation, free, chemically reactive haptens were used *in vitro,* free haptens are now applied deliberately, to allow for association with Ia molecules on the cell membranes. Only with very toxic allergens does preconjugation seem advisable, preferably to autologous APC. However, if autologous APC are not available, protein conjugates may be stimulatory as well, provided that sufficient monocytes are available for processing. Apparently, peripheral blood as a source of responder cells provides sufficient allergen-presenting capacity. Whether monocytes, eventually upon *in vitro* activation, or dendritic cells present in the blood samples account for the actual allergen presentation still remains to be elucidated.

As to the assays used, both literature data and inquiry results identify the LTT as the most popular test, even despite its relatively low specificity in comparison with migration inhibition tests. As LTT and LK production do regularly provide discordant data, it remains likely that different (activational stages of) memory T cells are being addressed in the assays. Multiparameter analysis, by combination of both assays, therefore can be recommended (Von Blomberg et al., 1987). Since the basic principles of these test systems remained essentially unchanged during the last two decades, the methodologies only underwent minor technical improvements in this period, such as the use of microculture equipment instead of tubes, and cell lines (U937) instead of guinea pig macrophages as target cells for MIF. Importantly, convenient alternatives for measuring lymphocyte growth *in vitro* are now being developed (Dotsika and Sanderson, 1987; Potter et al., 1987), possibly enabling a more routine use of the LTT in the near future.

Since thorough optimization is required for each allergen and for each assay, the performance of *in vitro* tests for ACD will long be restricted to expert centers. These tests are very unlikely ever to become part of common routine diagnostic procedures. In qualified laboratories, however, *in vitro* tests provide valuable diagnostic tools for special cases where *in vitro* tests fail to be conclusive, for example, when dealing with generalized eczema, hyperreactive skin, or drug hypersensitivity. Moreover, *in vitro* tests are invaluable for investigations on pathogenetic mechanisms of ACD and related diseases, as well as for studies on potential effects of pharmacological agents, including BRM, on inflammatory disease.

In conclusion, two decades of *in vitro* studies in ACD have taught us to appreciate *in vitro* testing as a delicacy rather than as daily food.

SUMMARY AND CONCLUSIONS

Recent Advances in ACD Research

In the last 20 years the molecular and cellular mechanisms leading to ACD have been largely unravelled. The skin was disclosed as an immunological organ in its own right, providing all elements required for allergen-specific T-cell activation. The actual site of T-cell activation by allergen was found to primarily depend on the local frequency of specific cells and on their activational stage. Since memory T lymphocytes show high migratory capacity and are, in addition, easy to trigger, it is conceivable that in hypersensitive individuals T-cell activation, mediator release, and overt inflammation will take place within the skin. The process of sensitization, on the other hand, will take place in the lymph nodes, where fully mature APC find optimal conditions to encounter and trigger naive allergen-specific T lymphocytes.

Refinement of cell isolation procedures and cell culture technology, as well as the production of monoclonal antibodies and recombinant lymphokines, provided the tools needed for studying T-cell activation processes in detail. Important recent studies have been devoted to identification of the allergen-specific T-cell receptor and the most commonly recognized determinants, allergen-modified MHC-class II molecules. Much progress has also been made in unravelling the minimal requirements for efficient allergen presentation. Adhesion molecules like LFA-1 were discovered, as well as the biochemical mechanisms behind receptor expression and cytokine production upon T-cell triggering. Thus, functionally different T-cell subsets could be characterized by the use of monoclonal antibodies directed toward different lymphocyte membrane determinants (Table 5).

It now would appear that within the helper T-cell population particularly those cells account for contact sensitivity reactions, which upon allergenic stimulation readily produce high amounts of IL-2 and IFN-gamma, and which express high levels of adhesion molecules, as required for extravasation and subsequent interaction with APC. In humans these cells can be phenotypically characterized as $CD3^+$, 4^+, 8^-, 29^+, $45RA^-$, $45RO^+$ lymphocytes.

The Impact of Compartmentalization on *In Vivo* and *In Vitro* Testing

Clearly our fundamental knowledge on ACD has substantially increased at the level of molecules, cells, and tissues. At the level of the organism, however, much is still left to be explored. Awareness has grown that organisms cannot be simply regarded as large culture bags. In atopy it is known that assessment of systemic immunoglobulin E (IgE) often does not provide relevant information as to local atopic reactivity: IgE molecules do not freely exchange between tissue and blood. Similarly, T lymphocytes are not homogeneously distributed over the body. Although we are now well aware of the fact that blood, skin, and lymphoid tissues represent distinct immunological compartments, laws determining cell traffic between these compartments have only recently begun to be understood (Table 4).

Factors causing lymphocyte sequestration from the blood include the presence of organ-specific homing receptors for T lymphocytes on vascular endothelia, the local presence of allergen-modified MHC class II molecules, and the local release of mediators facilitating lymphocyte extravasation. Little is still known about factors determining the subsequent release of specific cells from the skin to the lymph nodes and from the lymph nodes back into the circulation. The latter factors undoubtedly strongly affect compartmentalization of allergen-specific cells. Also, the roles of various nonimmunological factors (e.g., neuroendocrinological factors, biorhythms) in T-cell activation and compartmentalization are still far from understood. Adequate compartmentalization studies would require methodology for reliable, quantitative evaluation of frequencies of allergen-specific T cells, even in small lymphocyte samples. Since functional assays now available for this purpose require at least millions of cells, frequencies of allergen-specific lymphocytes in small samples can only be assessed after clonal expansion. Such analyses are, however, not attractive for studying frequencies far below 1 in 100, as expected to occur in most compartments, including the peripheral blood.

It would appear therefore that compartmentalization of allergen-specific T cells will for some time remain poorly defined, and will thus continue to complicate interpretation of diagnostic assays. Clinical in vitro tests are based on relatively small blood samples, 0.01% of the total recirculating pool of lymphocytes. In contrast, in vivo skin tests bear upon all recirculating specific T lymphocytes passing the skin-test area over a period of 24–48 hours (in normal skin, approximately 14×10^7; Table 8).

Thus, long-lasting (days, weeks) compartmentalization of allergen-specific cells may similarly affect in vivo and in vitro testing, whereas short-lasting fluctuations in frequencies of circulating specific cells would mainly affect in vitro tests.

The Value of *In Vivo* Tests in Human ACD

The impact of our extended fundamental knowledge about ACD on *in vivo* testing has been very limited. Skin test technology was developed empirically, and considered convenient and diagnostically quite satisfactory, long before immunological research on ACD had even started. Skin testing has now become even more convenient by the introduction of "prefab" patch tests, which removed even the last tedium.

As the nature of a skin test reaction is seldom clear from the macroscopic appearance, and in particular irritant and allergic reactions are often hard to differentiate, a huge effort has been put into immunohistological evaluation of skin test reactions. So far, however, this has not yet led to the development of methodology suitable for routine identification of the (immunological) mechanism underlying skin test reactivity. Amplification mechanisms shared by various types of inflammatory reactions occurring in the skin apparently obscure the initial event of T-cell activation in ACD. We may conclude therefore that although the diagnostic value of current skin testing remains high, its value for revealing pathogenetic mechanisms is very limited. If required, therefore, *in vitro* assays remain to evaluate the nature of specific immunity in contact allergic patients.

The Value of *In Vitro* Tests in ACD

The increased knowledge of the molecular events causing T-cell activation in ACD certainly affected views about *in vitro* testing with contact allergens, although the actual methods underwent only minor technical improvements. Lymphocyte transformation testing still provides the most sensitive information on T-cell sensitization, whereas assays based on *in vitro* lymphokine production can provide more specific data predicting skin reactivity. Although these *in vitro* parameters may show marked independent variation, both types of assays often correlate well with *in vivo* skin reactivity.

Recently acquired insights into the requirements for allergen presentation justify the routine use of Ficoll-Hypaque purified peripheral blood mononuclear cell suspensions. When aiming at the detection of memory T lymphocytes, monocytes represent efficient APCs. Moreover, monocytes may rapidly differentiate within the cultures into fully active allergen-presenting cells even capable of presenting allergen to naive T lymphocytes. Allergen presentation requirements, therefore, do not seriously limit the clinical use of *in vitro* tests in ACD.

Owing to the successful studies on establishing contact sensitivity *in vitro* and culturing allergen-specific T cell clones from blood and ACD-skin infiltrates, we now are able to fill the remaining gaps in our understanding of the basic mechanisms in ACD. Quantitative analyses of the frequencies of allergen-specific T-cell subsets in different compartments will help us to gain further insight in the phenomenon of compartmentalization of allergen-specific cells. Cross-reactivity between potential allergens can now be studied at the clonal level. Cells mediating unresponsiveness to allergens, for instance after oral induction of tolerance, should be identified by *in vitro* studies. *In vitro* tests also offer the opportunity to analyze effects of antiinflammatory drugs on different steps of the contact allergic reaction. Moreover, *in vitro* tests akin to these should contribute to large-scale allergenicity testing, for which unacceptably high numbers of experimental animals are still required.

On the other hand, despite all successful studies on evaluating contact sensitivity *in vitro,* diagnostic use of *in vitro* tests in ACD is unlikely to reach routine status, because blood samples are by nature small in terms of both volume and time, and even the most perfect *in vitro* technique would not compensate that; *in vitro* tests aiming at measurements of frequencies of sensitized cells require bioassays that are time consuming and hard to control in a clinical setting; many allergens are cytotoxic or mitogenic as such, or require metabolization to become allergenic; and skin-test methodologies are unbeatably convenient and cheap compared to any *in vitro* manipulation.

It should be realized that identification of the causative agent is often clinically more important than revealing the underlying immunological mechanisms. Nevertheless, in clinical practice *in vitro* assays may also be extremely useful whenever *in vivo* tests provide equivocal results; whenever support is sought for a potentially immunological pathogenesis of clinical symptoms; or whenever interference with the immune system induced by a renewed allergen contact has to be avoided.

The last options highlight the major advantages of *in vitro* testing (Table 15), that is, in providing unequivocal information about the presence of sensitized T cells in the circulation without disturbing the patient's immune status.

TABLE 15. Major Advantages and Disadvantages of *In Vivo* and *In Vitro* Tests in ACD

Advantages	Disadvantages
In vivo testing	
Overall picture of immune mechanism	Information on immune mechanism limited
Causative agent usually detected	Interference with immune status unavoidable
No special facilities required/cheap	False positives, due to "angry back" and allergen toxicity
Recruitment of lymphocytes over a 48-h period	False negatives, due to compartmentalization
	Interpretation only by experts
In vitro testing	
Information on immune mechanism	"Snapshot" of circulating lymphocytes
No interference with immune status	Tissue culture facilities required/expensive
Different elements of allergic reaction can be studied separately	Fluctuating background response, e.g., due to extensive inflammation
	False negatives, due to allergen toxicity and compartmentalization of specific lymphocytes
	Interpretation only by experts

REFERENCES

Abo, T., Kawate, T., Itoh, K. and Kumagai, K. 1981. Studies on the bioperiodicity of the immune response. I. Circadian rhythms of human T, B and K cell traffic in the peripheral blood. *J. Immunol.* 126:1360–1363.

Adam, H. 1979. Zum Nachweis der chloramphenicol-Sensibilisierung mit Hilfe des auf morphologischen Auswertungskriterien basierenden Lymphozyten-Transformations-Tests. *Dermatol. Mschr.* 165:270–273.

Adams, R. A. 1981. Continuing medical education. Patch testing—A recapitulation. *J. Am. Acad. Dermatol.* 5:629–646.

Aldridge, R. D., Milton, J. I. and Thomson, A. W. 1985. Leukocyte procoagulant activity as an in vitro index of nickel contact hypersensitivity. *Int. Arch. Allergy Appl. Immunol.* 76:350–353.

Al-Tawil, N. G., Marcusson, J. A. and Möller, E. 1981. Lymphocyte transformation tests in patients with nickel sensitivity: An aid to diagnosis. *Acta Dermatol. Venereol. (Stockh.)* 61:511–515.

Al-Tawil, N. G., Marcusson, J. A. and Möller, E. 1983. Lymphocyte stimulation by trivalent and hexavalent chromium compounds in patients with chromium sensitivity. *Acta Dermatol. Venereol. (Stockh.)* 63:296–303.

Al-Tawil, N. G., Marcusson, J. A. and Möller, E. 1984. In vitro testing for cobalt sensitivity: An aid to diagnosis. *Acta Dermatol. Venereol. (Stockh.)* 64:203–208.

Al-Tawil, N. G., Berggren, G., Emtestam, L., Fransson, J., Jernselius, R. and Marcusson, J. A. 1985a. Correlation between quantitative in vivo and in vitro responses in nickel-allergic patients. *Acta Dermatol. Venereol. (Stockh.)* 65:385–389.

Al-Tawil, N. G., Marcusson, J. A. and Möller, E. 1985b. T and B lymphocytes in patients with nickel sensitivity. *Scand. J. Immunol.* 22:495–502.

Andersen, K. E. and Staberg, B. 1985. Quantitation of contact allergy in guinea pigs by measuring changes in skin blood flow and skin fold thickness. *Acta Dermatol. Venereol. (Stockh.)* 65:37–42.

Andersen, K. E., Benezra, C., Burrows, D., et al. (The European Environmental and Contact Dermatitis Research Group). 1987. Contact dermatitis. A review. *Contact Dermatitis* 16:55–78.

Asherson, G. L., Allwood, G. G. and Mayhew, B. 1973. Contact sensitivity in the mouse. XI. Movement of T blasts in the draining lymph nodes to sites of inflammation. *Immunology* 25:485–494.

Askenase, P. W. and Van Loveren, H. 1983. Delayed-type hypersensitivity: Activation of mast cells by antigen-specific T cell factors initiates the cascade of cellular interactions. *Immunol. Today* 4:259–264.

Aspegren, N. and Rorsman, H. 1962. Short term culture of leucocytes in nickel hypersensitivity. *Acta Dermatol. Venereol.* 42:412–417.

Austyn, J. M. 1987. Lymphoid dendritic cells. Review. *Immunology* 62:161–170.

Austyn, J. M. and Morris, P. J. 1988. T cell activation by dendritic cells: CD-18 dependent clustering is not sufficient for mitogenesis. *Immunology* 63:537–543.

Austyn, J. M., Weinstein, D. E. and Steinman, R. M. 1988. Clustering with dendritic cells precedes and is essential for T cell proliferation in a mitogenesis model. *Immunology* 63:691–696.

Avnstorp, C., Balslev, E. and Thomsen, H. K. 1989. The occurrence of different morphological parameters in allergic and irritant patch test reactions. In *Current Topics in Contact Dermatitis*, eds. P. J. Frosch, A. Dooms-Goossens, J. M. Lachapelle, R. J. G. Rycroft and R. J. Scheper, pp. 38–41. Heidelberg: Springer-Verlag.

Bagot, M., Heslan, M., Roujeau, J.-C., Lebon, P. and Levy, J.-P. 1985. Human epidermal cells are more potent than peripheral blood mononuclear cells for the detection of weak allogeneic or virus-specific primary responses in vitro. *Cell. Immunol.* 94:215–224.

Baker, D., Parker, D., Healey, D. G. and Turk, J. L. 1987. Induction of sensitization and tolerance in contact sensitivity with haptenated epidermal cells in the guinea pig. *Immunology* 62:659–664.

Bandmann, H. J. and Agathos, M. 1981. New results and some remarks to the angry back syndrome. *Contact Dermatitis* 7:23–26.

Barker, J. N. W. N., Alegre, V. A. and Macdonald, D. M. 1988a. Surface-bound immunoglobulin E on antigen-presenting cells in cutaneous tissue of atopic dermatitis. *J. Invest. Dermatol.* 90:117–121.

Barker, J. N. W. N., Ophir, J. and Macdonald, D. M. 1988b. Products of class II major histocompatibility complex gene subregions are differentially expressed on keratinocytes in cutaneous diseases. *J. Am. Acad. Dermatol.* 19:667–672.

Baumgarten, A. and Geczy, A. F. 1970. Induction of delayed hypersensitivity by dinitrophenylated lymphocytes. *Immunology* 19:205–217.

Becker, S., Johnson, C., Halme, J. and Haskill, S. 1986. Interleukin-1 production and antigen presentation by normal human peritoneal macrophages. *Cell. Immunol.* 98:467–476.

Benezra, C., Sigman, C. C., Perry, L. R., Helmes, C. T. and Maibach, H. I. 1985. A systematic search for structure-activity relationships of skin contact sensitizers: Methodology. *J. Invest. Dermatol.* 85:351–356.

Bennett, B. and Bloom, B. R. 1968. Reactions in vivo and in vitro produced by a soluble substance associated with delayed-type hypersensitivity. *Proc. Natl. Acad. Sci. USA* 59:756–762.

Berardesca, E. and Maibach, H. I. 1988. Bioengineering and the patch test. Review article. *Contact Dermatitis* 18:3–9.

Berenbaum, M. C., Fluck, P. A. and Hurst, N. P. 1973. Depression of lymphocyte responses after surgical trauma. *Br. J. Exp. Pathol.* 54:597–607.

Bergstresser, P. R., Tigelaar, R. E., Dees, J. H. and Streilein, J. W. 1983. Thy-1 antigen bearing dendritic cells populate murine epidermis. *J. Invest. Dermatol.* 81:286–288.

Berman, B., Duncan, M. R., Smith, B., Ziboh, V. A. and Palladino, M. 1985. Interferon enhancement of HLA-DR antigen expression on epidermal Langerhans cells. *J. Invest. Dermatol.* 84:54–58.

Berman, J. G., Cruikshank, W. W., Center, D. M., Theodore, A. C. and Beer, D. J. 1985. Chemoattractant lymphokines specific for the helper/inducer T-lymphocyte subset. *Cell. Immunol.* 95:105–112.

Beverley, P. C. L. 1987. Human T cell subsets. Minireview. *Immunol. Lett.* 14:263–267.

Beverley, P. C. L., Merkenschlager, M. and Terry, L. 1988. Phenotypic diversity of the CD45 antigen and its relationship to function. *Immunology* (Suppl.) 1:3–5.

Bierer, B. E. and Burakoff, S. J. 1988. T cell adhesion molecules. *FASEB J.* 2:2584–2590.

Bigby, M., Kwan, T. and Sy, M. S. 1987. Ratio of Langerhans cells to Th-1[+] dendritic epidermal cells in murine epidermis influence the intensity of contact hypersensitivity. *J. Invest. Dermatol.* 89:495–499.

Biondi, M. and Pancheri, P. 1987. Mind and immunity. *Adv. Psychosom. Med.* 17:234–251.

Bjercke, S., Braathen, L., Gaudernack, G. and Thorsby, E. 1985. Relative efficiency of human Langerhans cells and blood derived dendritic cells as antigen-presenting cells. *Acta Dermatol. Venereol. (Stockh.)* 65:374–378.

Björnberg, A. 1968. Skin reactions to primary irritants in patients with hand eczema. An investigation with matched controls. Göteborg: Oscar Isacsons Tryckeri.

Bleumink, E., Nater, J. P., Koops, S., and The, T. H. 1974. A standard method for DNCB sensitization testing in patients with neoplasms. *Cancer* 33:911–915.

Bloom, B. R. and Bennett, B. 1966. Mechanism of a reaction in vitro associated with delayed hypersensitivity. *Science* 153:80–82.

Bloom, B. R. and Chase, M. W. 1967. Transfer of delayed-type hypersensitivity. A critical review and experimental study in the guinea pig. *Progr. Allergy* 10:151–255.

Boerrigter, G. H. and Scheper, R. J. 1987. Local and systemic desensitization induced by repeated epicutaneous hapten application. *J. Invest. Dermatol.* 88:3–7.

Boerrigter, G. H., Bril, H. and Scheper, R. J. 1988. Hapten-specific antibodies in allergic contact dermatitis in the guinea pig. *Int. Arch. Allergy Appl. Immunol.* 85:385–391.

Borish, L., Liu, D. Y., Remold, H. and Rocklin, R. E. 1986a. Production and assay of Macrophage Migration Inhibitory Factor, Leukocyte Migration Inhibitory Factor, and Leukocyte Adherence Inhibitory Factor. In *Manual of Clinical Laboratory Immunology*, eds. N. R. Rose, H. Friedman and J. L. Fahey, pp. 282–289. Washington, D.C.: American Society for Microbiology.

Borish, L., O'Reilly, D., Klempner, M. S. and Rocklin, R. E. 1986b. Leukocyte inhibitory factor (LIF) potentiates neutrophil responses to formyl-methionyl-leucyl-phenylalanine. *J. Immunol.* 137:1897–1903.

Bos, J. D. and Kapsenberg, M. L. 1986. The skin immune system. Its cellular constituents and their interactions. *Immunol. Today* 7:235–239.

Bos, J. D., Zonneveld, I., Das, P. K., Krieg, S. R., Van der Loos, C. M. and Kapsenberg, M. L. 1987. The skin immune system (SIS): Distribution and immunophenotype of lymphocyte subpopulations in normal human skin. *J. Invest. Dermatol.* 88:569–573.

Bottomly, K. 1988. A functional dichotomy in CD4$^+$ T lymphocytes. *Immunol. Today* 9:268–274.

Böyum, A. 1968. Isolation of mononuclear cells and granulocytes from human blood: Isolation of mononuclear cells by one centrifugation and of granulocytes by combining centrifugation and sedimentation at 1 g. *Scand. J. Lab. Invest.* 21 (Suppl. 97):77–89.

Braathen, L. R. 1980. Studies on human epidermal Langerhans cells. III. Induction of T lymphocyte response to nickel sulfate in sensitized individuals. *Br. J. Dermatol.* 103:517–526.

Braathen, L. R. and Thorsby, E. 1983. Human epidermal Langerhans cells are more potent than blood monocytes in inducing some antigen-specific T-cell responses. *Br. J. Dermatol.* 108:139–146.

Breathnach, S. M. 1988. The Langerhans cell. Centenary review. *Br. J. Dermatol.* 119:463–469.

Breitmeyer, J. B. 1987. Lymphocyte activation. How T cells communicate. *Nature (Lond.)* 329:760–761.

Brooks, C. F. and Moore, M. 1988. Differential MHC class II expression on human peripheral blood monocytes and dendritic cells. *Immunology* 63:303–311.

Brown, M. F., Cook, R. G. and Rich, R. R. 1984. Cloned human T cells synthesize Ia molecules and can function as antigen presenting cells. *Hum. Immunol.* 11:219–228.

Bruynzeel, D. P. and Van Ketel, W. G. 1981. Repeated patch testing in penicillin allergy. *Br. J. Dermatol.* 104:157–159.

Bruynzeel, D. P., Van Ketel, W. G., Scheper, R. J. and Von Blomberg, B. M. E. 1982. Delayed time course of irritation by sodium lauryl sulfate: Observations on threshold reactions. *Contact Dermatitis* 8:236–239.

Bruynzeel, D. P., Nieboer, C., Boorsma, D. M., Scheper, R. J. and Van Ketel, W. G. 1983a. Allergic reactions, "spillover" reactions, and T cell subsets. *Arch. Dermatol. Res.* 275:80–85.

Bruynzeel, D. P., Van Ketel, W. G., Von Blomberg-Van der Flier, M. and Scheper, R. J.

338   *B. M. E. von Blomberg et al.*

1983b. Angry back or the excited skin syndrome. A prospective study. *J. Am. Acad. Dermatol.* 8:392–397.

Bruynzeel, D. P., Von Blomberg-Van der Flier, B. M. E., Van Ketel, W. G. and Scheper, R. J. 1983c. Depression or enhancement of skin reactivity by inflammatory processes in the guinea pig. *Int. Arch. Allergy Appl. Immunol.* 72:67–70.

Bruynzeel, D. P., Von Blomberg-Van der Flier, B. M. E., Scheper, R. J., Van Ketel, G. and de Haan, P. 1985. Penicillin allergy and the relevance of epicutaneous tests. *Dermatologica* 171:429–434.

Bruynzeel, D. P. 1986. Contact allergy to benzydamine. *Contact Dermatitis* 14:313–314.

Bruynzeel, D. P. and Maibach, H. I. 1986. Excited skin syndrome (angry back). Review. *Arch. Dermatol.* 122:323–328.

Bruynzeel, D. P. 1987. The angry back syndrome and Trafuril. *Br. J. Dermatol.* 117:670–671.

Bruynzeel-Koomen, C. 1986. IgE on Langerhans cells: New insights into the pathogenesis of atopic dermatitis. *Dermatologica* 172:181–183.

Burger, D. R. and Vetto, R. M. 1982. Vascular endothelium as a major participant in T-lymphocyte immunity. *Cell. Immunol.* 70:357–361.

Burmeister, G., Tarcsay, L. and Sorg, C. 1986. Generation and characterization of a monoclonal antibody (1C5) to human migration inhibitory factor (MIF). *Immunobiology* 171:461–474.

Burrows, D. 1983. Adverse chromate reactions on the skin. In *Chromium: Metabolism and Toxicity,* ed. D. Burrows, pp. 141–143. Boca Raton, Fla.: CRC Press.

Byers, V. S., Epstein, W. L., Castagnoli, N. and Baer, H. 1979. In vitro studies of poison oak immunity. I. In vitro reaction of human lymphocytes to urushiol. *J. Clin. Invest.* 64:1437–1448.

Byrne, J. A., Butler, J. L. and Cooper, M. D. 1988. Differential activation requirements for virgin and memory T cells. *J. Immunol.* 141:3249–3257.

Calabrese, J. R., Kling, M. A. and Gold, P. W. 1987. Alterations in immunocompetence during stress, bereavement, and depression: Focus on neuroendocrine regulation. *Am. J. Psychiatr.* 144:1123–1134.

Calnan, C. D. 1982. The use and abuse of patch tests. In *Occupational and Industrial Dermatology,* eds. H. I. Maibach and G. A. Gellin, pp. 35–37. Chicago: Yearbook Medical Publishing.

Camarasa, J. G. and Calderon, P. G. 1984. Lymphocyte transformation test in allergic contact dermatitis by mercury. In *Immunodermatology,* ed. D. M. MacDonald, pp. 37–39. Kent: Butterworths.

Cardenas, J. M., Marshall, P., Henderson, B. and Altman, A. 1986. Human interleukin 2. Quantitation by a sensitive radioimmunoassay. *J. Immunol. Methods* 89:181–189.

Carr, M. M., Botham, P. A., Gawkrodger, D. J., McVittie, E., Ross, J. A., Stewart, I. C. and Hunter, J. A. A. 1984. Early cellular reactions induced by dinitrochlorobenzene in sensitized human skin. *Br. J. Dermatol.* 110:637–641.

Cavender, D. E. 1989. Lymphocyte adhesion to endothelial cells in vitro: Models for the study of normal lymphocyte recirculation and lymphocyte emigration into chronic inflammatory lesions. *J. Invest. Dermatol.* 93:88S–95S.

Chang, J. C. C., Ishioka, G. I. and Moorhead, J. W. 1987. Re-presentation of the hapten dinitrophenol (DNP) to a DNP-specific T cell line. *Cell. Immunol.* 106:1–11.

Chanh, T. C., Kennedy, R. C. and Kanda, P. 1988. Synthetic peptides homologous to HIV transmembrane glycoprotein suppress normal human lymphocyte blastogenic response. *Cell. Immunol.* 111:77–86.

Chase, M. W. and Kawata, H. 1971. Induction of contact sensitivity by hapten-epithelium conjugates. *Clin. Res.* 19:578–585.

Cher, D. J. and Mosmann, T. R. 1987. Two types of murine helper T cell clone. II. Delayed-type hypersensitivity is mediated by T$_H$1 clones. *J. Immunol.* 138:3688–3694.

Christou, N. V., Pietsch, J. B. and Meakins, J. L. 1983. Effect of repeated delayed hypersensitivity skin tests on skin-test responses. *Can. J. Surg.* 26:139–142.

Cianciolo, G. J., Copelan, T. D., Oroszian, S. and Snyderman, R. 1985. Inhibition of lymphocyte proliferation by a synthetic peptide homologous to retroviral envelope proteins. *Science* 230:453–455.

Clausen, J. E. 1971. Tuberculin-induced migration inhibition of human peripheral leukocytes in agarose medium. *Acta Allergol.* 26:56–80.

Claverie, J. M., Prochnicka-Chalufour, A. and Bougueleret, L. 1989. Implications of a Fab-like structure for the T cell receptor. *Immunol. Today* 10:10–14.

Cohen, S. P. 1982. Lymphokines and immune regulation. I. *Fed. Proc.* 41:2478–2479.

Collins, T., Korman, A. J., Wake, C. T., et al. 1984. Immune interferon activates multiple class II major histocompatibility complex genes and the associated invariant chain gene in human endothelial cells and dermal fibroblasts. *Proc. Natl. Acad. Sci. USA* 81:4917–4921.

Cresswell, P. 1987. Antigen recognition by T lymphocytes. *Immunol. Today* 8:67–69.

Czernielewski, J. M. and Demarchez, M. 1987. Further evidence for the self-reproducing capacity of Langerhans cells in human skin. *J. Invest. Dermatol.* 88:17–20.

David, J. R., Al-Askari, S., Lawrence, H. S. and Thomas, L. 1964. Delayed hypersensitivity in vitro. I. The specificity of inhibition of cell migration by antigens. *J. Immunol.* 93:264–273.

David, J. R., Remold, H. G., Liu, H. Y., Weiser, W. Y. and David, R. A. 1983. Lymphokines and macrophages. *Cell. Immunol.* 82:75–81.

De Boer, E. M., Bezemer, P. D. and Bruynzeel, D. P. 1989. A standard method for repeated recording of skin blood flow using laser Doppler flowmetry. *Dermatosen* 37:58–62.

De Jong, M. C. J. M., Blanken, R., Nanninga, J., Van Voorst Vader, P. C. and Poppema, S. 1986. Defined in situ enumeration of T6 and HLA-DR expressing epidermal Langerhans cells: Morphologic and methodologic aspects. *J. Invest. Dermatol.* 87:698–702.

De Hurtado, I. and Osler, A. G. 1975. Serum antibody production—An invariable consequence of sensitization with dinitrochlorobenzene. *Proc. Soc. Exp. Biol. Med.* 149:628–632.

Dembic, Z., Von Boehmer, H. and Steinmetz, M. 1986. The role of T-cell receptor alfa and betha genes in MHC-restricted antigen recognition. *Immunol. Today* 7:308–311.

Denizot, F. and Lang, R. 1986. Rapid colorimetric assay for cell growth and survival. Modifications to the tetrazolium dye procedure giving improved sensitivity and reliability. *J. Immunol. Methods* 89:271–277.

Dennert, G. and Hatlen, L. E. 1975. Are contact hypersensitivity cells cytotoxic? *Nature (Lond.)* 257:486–488.

De Panfilis, G., Soligo, D., Manara, G. C., Ferrari, C. and Torresani, C. 1989. Adhesion molecules on the plasma membrane of epidermal cells. I. Human resting Langerhans cells express two members of the adherence promoting CD11/CD18 family, namely H-Mac-1 (CD11b/CD18) and gp 150,95 (CD11c/CD18). *J. Invest. Dermatol.* 93:60–69.

Deshazo, R. D., Levinson, A. I. and Dvorak, H. F. 1983. The late phase skin reaction: Paradigma or epiphenomenon. *Ann. Allergy* 51:166–172.

Didierjean, L., Salomon, D., Merot, Y., Siegenthaler, G., Shaw, A., Dayer, J.-M. and Saurat, J.-H. 1989. Localization and characterization of the interleukin-1 immunoreactive pool (IL-1 alpha and beta forms) in normal human epidermis. *J. Invest. Dermatol.* 92:809–816.

Dinarello, C. A. and Mier, J. W. 1987. Lymphokines. *N. Engl. J. Med.* 317:940–945.

Dohlsten, M., Hedlund, G., Sjögren, H. and Carlsson, R. 1988. Two subsets of human CD4$^+$ helper cells differing in kinetics and capacities to produce interleukin 2 and interferon-gamma can be defined by the leu 18 and UCHL1 monoclonal antibodies. *Eur. J. Immunol.* 18:1173–1178.

Dooms-Goossens, A., Naert, C., Chrispeels, M. T. and Degreef, H. 1980. Is a 5% nickel sulfate patch test concentration adequate? *Contact Dermatitis* 6:232–234.

Dooms-Goossens, A. 1986. A computerized retrieval system of contact allergenic substances. *Sem. Dermatol.* 5:249–254.

Dotsika, E. N. and Sanderson, C. J. 1987. A fluorometric assay determining cell growth in lymphocyte proliferation and lymphokine assays. *J. Immunol. Methods* 105:55–62.

Drexhage, H. A., Lens, J. W., Kamperdijk, E. W. A., Mullink, H. and Balfour, B. M. 1980. Veiled cells resembling Langerhans cells. In *Mononuclear Phagocytes, Functional Aspects,* vol. 1, ed. R. Van Furth, p. 235. The Hague: Martinus Nijhoff.

Duijvestijn, A. M., Horst, E., Pals, S. T., Rouse, B. T., Steere, A. C., Picker, L. J., Meijer, C. J. L. M. and Butcher, E. C. 1988. High endothelial differentiation in human lymphoid and inflammatory tissues defined by monoclonal antibody HECA-452. *Am. J. Pathol.* 130:147–155.

Duijvestijn, A. and Hamann, A. 1989. Mechanisms and regulation of lymphocyte migration. *Immunol. Today* 10:23–28.

Dupuis, G. 1979. Studies on poison ivy. In vitro lymphocyte transformation by urushiolprotein conjugates. *Br. J. Dermatol.* 101:617–624.

Dustin, M. L., Rothlein, R., Bhan, A. K., Dinarello, C. A. and Springer, T. A. 1986. Induction by IL-2 and IFN-gamma: Tissue distribution, biochemistry and function of a natural adherence molecule (ICAM-1). *J. Immunol.* 137:245–254.

Dvorak, H. F., Mihm, M. C., Dvorak, A. M., Johnson, R. A., Manseau, E. J., Morgan, E. and Colvin, R. B. 1974. Morphology of delayed type hypersensitivity reactions in man. *Lab. Invest.* 31:111–130.

Dvorak, H. F., Mihm, M. C. and Dvorak, A. M. 1976. Morphology of delayed type hypersensitivity reactions in man. *J. Invest. Dermatol.* 67:391–401.

Elmets, C. A., Lederman, M. M. and Czinn, S. 1987. In vivo production of a T lymphocyte chemotactic cytokine in the skin at sites of contact dermatitis. *J. Invest. Dermatol.* 88:487 (abstr).

Enders, F., Przybilla, B., Ring, J., Burg, G. and Braun-Falco, O. 1988. Epikutantestung mit einer Standardreihe. *Hautarzt* 39:79–786.

Eskola, J., Frey, H., Molnar, G. and Soppi, E. 1976. Biological rhythm of cell mediated immunity in man. *Clin. Exp. Immunol.* 26:253–257.

Everness, K. M., Botham, P. A., Gawkrodger, D. J. and Hunter, J. A. A. 1989. The role of MHC class II antigens in mediating accessory cell function in vitro in nickel induced contact sensitivity. In *Current Topics in Contact Dermatitis,* eds. P. J. Frosch, A. Dooms-Goossens, J. M. Lachapelle, R. J. G. Rycroft and R. J. Scheper, pp. 584–591. Heidelberg: Springer-Verlag.

Ferguson, J., Gibbs, J. H. and Beck, J. S. 1985. Lymphocyte subsets and Langerhans cells in allergic and irritant patch test reactions: Histometric studies. *Contact Dermatitis* 23:166–174.

Fischer, T. 1989. The patch test standardization. In *Current Topics in Contact Dermatitis*, eds. P. J. Frosch, A. Dooms-Goossens, J. M. Lachapelle, R. J. G. Rycroft and R. J. Scheper, pp. 514–517. Heidelberg: Springer-Verlag.

Fischer, T. and Maibach, H. I. 1985. The thin layer rapid use epicutaneous test (TRUE-test), a new patch test method with high accuracy. *Br. J. Dermatol.* 112:63–68.

Fischer, T. and Maibach, H. I. 1989. Easier patch testing with TRUE test. *J. Am. Acad. Dermatol.* 20:447–453.

Ford, D. K., Da Roza, D. M. and Schulzer, M. 1985. Lymphocytes from the site of disease but not blood lymphocytes indicate the cause of arthritis. *Ann. Rheum. Dis.* 44:701–710.

Forman, L. and Alexander, S. 1972. Nickel antibodies. *Br. J. Dermatol.* 87:320–326.

Forslind, B. and Wahlberg, J. E. 1978. The morphology of chromium allergic skin reactions at electric microscopic resolution: Studies in man and guinea pig. *Acta. Derm. Venereol. (Stockh.) Suppl* 79:43–51.

Fregert, S. and Bandmann, H. J. 1975. *Patch testing.* Published on behalf of ICDRG. Berlin: Springer-Verlag.

Friedmann, P. S., Moss, C., Shuster, S. and Simpson, J. M. 1983. Quantitative relationships between sensitizing dose of DNCB and reactivity in normal subjects. *Clin. Exp. Immunol.* 53:709–715.

Fritz, J. and Sandhofer, M. 1979. Der Leukozyten-migrations-inhibitionstest in der dermatologie. Eine Zwischenbilanz aufgrund der Literatur und eigener erfahrungen. *Z. Hautkr.* 54:487–500.

Frosch, P. J. 1989. Irritant contact dermatitis. In *Current Topics in Contact Dermatitis*, eds. P. J. Frosch, A. Dooms-Goossens, J. M. Lachapelle, R. J. G. Rycroft and R. J. Scheper, pp. 385–398. Heidelberg: Springer-Verlag.

Fullmer, M. A., Shen, J. Y., Modlin, R. L. and Rea, T. H. 1987. Immunohistological evidence of lymphokine production and lymphocyte activation antigens in tuberculin reactions. *Clin. Exp. Immunol.* 67:383–390.

Furue, M. and Katz, S. I. 1988. Molecules on activated human T cells. *Am. J. Dermatopathol.* 10:349–355.

Gaspari, A., Furue, M., Aiba, S. and Katz, S. I. 1989. Human epidermal Langerhans cells, when cultured, exhibit increased class II MHC expression and become potent immunostimulatory cells. Abstr. *J. Invest. Dermatol.* 92:433.

Gawkrodger, D. J., McVittie, E., Ross, J. A. and Hunter, J. A. A. 1986. Phenotypic characterization of the early cellular responses in allergic and irritant contact dermatitis. *Clin. Exp. Immunol.* 66:590–598.

Gawkrodger, D. J., Carr, M. M., McVittie, E., Guy, K. and Hunter, J. A. A. 1987a. Keratinocyte expression of MHC class II antigens in allergic sensitization and challenge reactions and in irritant contact dermatitis. *J. Invest. Dermatol.* 88:11–16.

Gawkrodger, D. J., McVittie, E. and Hunter, J. A. A. 1987b. Immunophenotyping of the eczematous flare-up reaction in nickel-sensitive subjects. *Dermatologica* 175:171–177.

Geczy, A. F. and Baumgarten, A. 1970. Lymphocyte transformation in contact sensitivity. *Immunology* 19:189–203.

Geczy, C. L., Geczy, A. F. and De Weck, A. L. 1976. Antibodies to guinea pig lymphokines. II. Suppression of delayed hypersensitivity reactions by second generation goat antibody against guinea pig lymphokines. *J. Immunol.* 117:66–72.

Geczy, C. L. and Meyer, P. A. 1982. Leukocyte procoagulant activity in man: An in vitro correlate of delayed type hypersensitivity. *J. Immunol.* 128:331–336.

Geczy, C. L. 1983. The role of clotting processes in the action of lymphokines on macrophages. *Lymphokines* 8:201–247.

Geczy, C. L. 1984. The role of lymphokines in delayed type hypersensitivity reactions. Review. *Springer Sem. Immunopathol.* 7:321–346.

George, M. and Vaughan, J. H. 1962. In vitro cell migration as a model for delayed hypersensitivity. *Proc. Soc. Exp. Biol. Med.* 111:514–521.

Gerrard, T. L., Dyer, D. R., Zoon, K. C., Zur Nedden, D. and Siegel, J. P. 1988. Modulation of class I and class II histocompatibility antigens on human T cell lines by IFN-gamma. *J. Immunol.* 140:3450–3455.

Gianotti, B., De Panfilis, G., Manara, G. C., Cappugi, P. and Ferrari, C. 1986. Langerhans cells are not damaged in contact allergic reactions in humans. *Am. J. Dermatopathol.* 8:220–226.

Gill, F. A. 1967. The association of increased spontaneous lymphocyte transformation in vitro with clinical manifestations of drug hypersensitivity. *J. Immunol.* 98:778–785.

Gillis, S., Ferm, M. M., Ou, W. and Smith, K. A. 1978. T cell growth factor: Parameters of production and a quantitative microassay for activity. *J. Immunol.* 120:2027–2032.

Gimenez-Camarasa, J. M., Garcia-Calderon, P., Asensio, J. and De Moragas, J. M. 1975. Lymphocyte transformation test in allergic contact nickel dermatitis. *Br. J. Dermatol.* 92:9–15.

Goeptar, A. R., De Groot, J., Lang, M., Van Tol, R. G. L. and Scheper, R. J. 1988. Suppressive effects of transdermal clonidine administration on contact hypersensitivity reactions in guinea pigs. *Int. J. Immunopharm.* 10:27–282.

Gonwa, T. A., Frost, J. P. and Karr, R. W. 1986. All human monocytes have the capability of expressing HLA-DQ and HLA-DP molecules upon stimulation with interferon-gamma. *J. Immunol.* 137:519–526.

Göring, H. D., Schwalm, I., Agatha, G. and Schubert, H. 1977. Die Antigen-Testung mit gefrierkonservierten Lymphozyten im LTT und LMHT. *Dermatol. Mschr.* 163:217–219.

Grantstein, R. D. 1985. Epidermal I-J bearing cells are responsible for transferable suppressor cell generation after immunization of mice with ultra violet radiation-treated epidermal cells. *J. Invest. Dermatol.* 84:206–209.

Greene, M. I., Sugimoto, M. and Benacerraf, B. 1978. Mechanisms of regulation of cell-mediated immune responses. I. Effect of the route of immunization with TNP-coupled syngeneic cells on the induction and suppression of contact sensitivity to picryl chloride. *J. Immunol.* 120:1604–1611.

Grey, H. M. and Chesnut, R. 1985. Antigen processing and presentation to T cells. *Immunol. Today* 6:101–106.

Griffiths, C. E. M., Voorhees, J. J. and Nickoloff, B. J. 1989. Gamma interferon induces different keratinocyte cellular patterns of expression of HLA-DR and DQ and intercellular adhesion molecule-1 (ICAM-1) antigens. *Br. J. Dermatol.* 120:1–7.

Groh, V., Tani, M., Harrer, A., Wolff, K. and Stingl, G. 1986. Leu-3/T4 expression on epidermal Langerhans cells in normal and diseased skin. *J. Invest. Dermatol.* 86:115–120.

Guidos, C., Sinha, A. A. and Lee, K. C. 1987. Functional differences and complementation between dendritic cells and macrophages in T cell activation. *Immunology* 61:269–276.

Guy, R. H., Tur, E. and Maibach, H. I. 1985. Optical techniques for monitoring cutaneous microcirculation. Review. *Int. J. Dermatol.* 24:88–94.

Guyton, A. C. 1976. Circulation in the skin. In *Textbook of Medical Physiology,* vol. V: *The Circulation,* 5th ed., p. 379. Philadelphia: Saunders.

Hafler, D. A., Fox, D. A., Benjamin, D. and Weiner, H. L. 1986. Antigen reactive memory T cells are defined by Tal. *J. Immunol.* 137:414–418.

Halliday, G. M. and Muller, H. K. 1986. Induction of tolerance via skin depleted of Langerhans cells by a chemical carcinogen. *Cell. Immunol.* 99:220–227.

Hamblin, A. 1985. Molecular cloning lends credence to lymphokine research. *Immunol. Today* 6:38–39.

Hamilton, D. N. H., Ledger, V. and Diamandopoulos, A. 1976. In vitro monitoring of cell mediated immunity to dinitrochlorobenzene. *Lancet* ii:1170–1171.

Hanifin, J. M., Epstein, W. L. and Cline, M. J. 1970. In vitro studies of granulomatous hypersensitivity to beryllium. *J. Invest. Dermatol.* 55:284–288.

Harrington, J. T. and Stastny, P. 1973. Macrophage migration from an agarose droplet: Development of a micromethod for assay of delayed hypersensitivity. *J. Immunol.* 110:752–759.

Harriot-Smith, T. G. and Halliday, W. J. 1988. Suppression of contact hypersensitivity by short term ultraviolet irradiation: II. The role of urocanic acid. *Immunology* 64:174–177.

Hartman, A., Hoedemaker, P. J. and Nater, J. P. 1976. Histological aspects of DNCB sensitization and challenge tests. *Br. J. Dermatol.* 94:407–416.

Hasegawa, S., Baba, T. and Hori, Y. 1980. Suppression of allergic contact dermatitis by alpha-L-fucose. *J. Invest. Dermatol.* 75:284–287.

Haskard, D. O., Cavender, D., Fleck, R. M., Sontheimer, R. and Ziff, M. 1987. Human dermal vascular endothelial cells behave like umbelical vein endothelial cells in T-cell adhesion studies. *J. Invest. Dermatol.* 88:340–344.

Hayashi, H., Honda, M., Shimokawa, Y. and Hirashima, M. 1984. Chemotactic factors associated with leukocyte emigration in immune tissue injury: Their separation, characterization and functional specificity. *Int. Rev. Cytol.* 89:179–250.

Hein, W. R. and Supersaxo, A. 1988. Effect of interferon-alpha-2a on the output of recirculating lymphocytes from single lymph nodes. *Immunology* 64:469–474.

Hemler, M. E. 1990. VLA proteins in the integrin family: Structures, functions, and their role on leukocytes. *Annu. Rev. Immunol.* 8:365–400.

Henderson, W. R., Fukuyama, K., Epstein, W. L. and Spitler, L. E. 1972. In vitro demonstration of delayed hypersensitivity in patients with berylliosis. *J. Invest. Dermatol.* 58:5–8.

Hersey, P., Hasic, E., Edwards, A., Bradley, M., Haran, G. and McCarthy, W. H. 1983. Immunological effects of solarium exposure. *Lancet* i:545–548.

Heufler, C., Koch, F. and Schuler, G. 1988. Granulocyte/macrophage colony-stimulating factor and interleukin 1 mediate the maturation of murine epidermal Langerhans cells into potent immunostimulatory dendritic cells. *J. Exp. Med.* 167:700–705.

Hinrichs, D. J. and Gibbins, B. L. 1975. The in vitro detection of antigen sensitivity in contact dermatitis by lymphocyte transformation. *Cell. Immunol.* 18:343–350.

Hirayama, K., Matsushita, S., Kikuchi, I., Iuchi, M., Ohta, N. and Sasazuki, T. 1987. HLA-DQ is epistatic to HLA-DR in controlling the immune response to schistosomal antigen in humans. *Nature (Lond.)* 327:426–430.

Hirschberg, H., Braathen, L. R. and Thorsby, E. 1982. Antigen presentation by vascular endothelial cells and epidermal Langerhans cells: The role of HLA-DR. *Immunol. Rev.* 65:57–77.

Hjorth, N. and Roed-Petersen, J. 1976. Occupational protein contact dermatitis in food handlers. *Contact Dermatitis* 2:28–42.

Hoefsmit, E. C. M., Duijvesteijn, A. M. and Kamperdijk, E. W. A. 1982. Relation between Langerhans cells, veiled cells and interdigitating cells. *Immunobiology* 161:255–265.

Holmes, K. L. and Morse, H. C. III. 1988. Murine hematopoietic cell surface antigen expression. *Immunol. Today* 9:344–350.

Holter, W., Majdic, O., Liszka, K., Stockinger, H. and Knapp, W. 1985. Kinetics of activation antigen expression by in vitro stimulated human T lymphocytes. *Cell. Immunol.* 90:322–330.

Horejsi, V. and Bazil, V. 1988. Surface proteins and glycoproteins of human leucocytes. Review article. *Biochem. J.* 253:1–26.

Houwerzijl, J. and De Gast, G. C. 1977a. Lymphocyte transformation test in drug allergy. *Lancet* i:425–426.

Houwerzijl, J., De Gast, G. C., Nater, J. P, Esselink, M. T. and Nieweg, H. O. 1977b. Lymphocyte stimulation tests and patch tests to carbamazepine hypersensitivity. *Clin. Exp. Immunol.* 29:272–277.

Howard, J. C. 1985. Immunological help at last. *Nature (Lond.)* 314:494–495.

Hunter, J. A. A. 1986. Langerhans cell damage does occur in contact allergic reactions. *Am. J. Dermatopathol.* 8:227–229.

Hutchinson, F., Raffle, E. J. and MacLeod, T. M. 1972. The specificity of lymphocyte transformation in vitro by nickel salts in nickel sensitive subjects. *J. Invest. Dermatol.* 58:362–365.

Inaba, K. and Steinman, R. M. 1984. Resting and sensitized T lymphocytes exhibit distinct stimulatory (antigen-presenting cell) requirements for growth and lymphokine release. *J. Exp. Med.* 160:1717–1735.

Inaba, K. and Steinman, R. M. 1986. Accessory cell-T lymphocyte interactions. Antigen-dependent and -independent clustering. *J. Exp. Med.* 163:247–261.

Inaba, K. and Steinman, R. M. 1987. Monoclonal antibodies to LFA-1 and to CD4 inhibit the mixed leukocyte reaction after the antigen-dependent clustering of dendritic cells and T lymphocytes. *J. Exp. Med.* 165:1403–1417.

Indiveri, F., Pierri, I., Rogna, S., Poggi, A., Montaldo, P., Romano, R., Pende, A., Morgano Abarabino, A. and Ferrone, S. 1985. Circadian variations of autologous mixed lymphocyte reactions and endogenous cortisol. *J. Immunol. Methods* 82:17–24.

Isakov, N. and Altman, A. 1986. Lymphocyte activation and immune regulation. *Immunol. Today* 7:155–157.

Isakov, N., Scholz, W. and Altman, A. 1986. Signal transduction and intracellular events in T-lymphocyte activation. *Immunol. Today* 7:273–277.

Issekutz, T. B., Stoltz, J. M. and Van der Meide, P. 1988. The recruitment of lymphocytes into the skin by T cell lymphokines: The role of gamma-interferon. *Clin. Exp. Immunol.* 73:70–75.

Jadassohn, J. 1896. Zur Kenntnis der medicamentösen Dermatosen. In *Verhandlungen der Deutschen Dermatologischen Gesellschaft,* Fünfter Congress. eds. Jarisch and Neisser, pp. 103–129.

Janeway, C. A., Bottomly, K., Babich, J., Conrad, P., Conzen, S., Jones, B., Kaye, J., Katz, M., McVay, L., Murphy, D. B. and Tite, J. 1984. Quantitative variation in Ia antigen expression plays a central role in immune regulation. *Immunol. Today* 5:99–105.

Jones, J. M. and Amos, H. E. 1975. Antigen formation in metal contact sensitivity. *Nature (Lond.)* 256:499–500.

Jones, T. D. and Mote, J. R. 1934. The phases of foreign protein sensitization in human beings. *N. Engl. J. Med.* 210.

Jordan, W. P. and Dvorak, J. 1976. Leukocyte migration inhibition assay (LIF) in nickel contact dermatitis. *Arch. Dermatol.* 112:1741–1744.

Jungi, T. W. and McGregor, D. D. 1978. Activated lymphocytes trigger lymphoblast extravasation. *Cell. Immunol.* 38:76–83.

Kalish, R. S. and Morimoto, C. 1989. Quantitation and cloning of human urushiol specific peripheral blood T cells. Isolation of urushiol riggered suppressed T cells. *J. Invest. Dermatol.* 92:46–52.

Kabel, P. J., De Haan-Meulman, M., Voorbij, H. A. M., Kleingeld, M., Knol, E. F. and Drexhage, H. A. 1989. Accessory cells with a morphology and marker pattern of dendritic cells can be obtained from elutriator-purified blood monocyte fractions. An enhancing effect of metrizamide in this differentiation. *Immunobiology* 179:395–411.

Kanagawa, H., Kotake, K., Semma, M. and Sagami, S. 1983. Induction of suppressor T cells to dinitrofluorobenzene contact sensitivity by application of sensitizer through Langerhans cell-deficient skin. II. Kinetics of the induction of suppressor T cells. *J. Am. Acad. Dermatol.* 9:680–685.

Kanerva, L., Ranki, A. and Lauharanta, J. 1984. Lymphocytes and Langerhans cells in patch tests. An immunochemical and electronmicroscopic study. *Contact Dermatitis* 11:150–155.

Kanerva, L., Estlander, T. and Ranki, A. 1987. Lymphocytes and Langerhans cells in allergic patch tests. *Dermatosen* 35(1):16–19.

Kanerva, L., Estlander, T. and Jolanki, R. 1988. Sensitization to patch test acrylates. *Contact Dermatitis* 18:10–15.

Kapsenberg, M. L., Res, P., Bos, J., Schootemeijer, A., Teunissen, M. B. M., Van Schooten, W. 1987. Nickel specific T lymphocyte clones derived from allergic nickel-contact dermatitis lesions in man: Heterogeneity based on requirement of dendritic antigen presenting cell subsets. *Eur. J. Immunol.* 17:861–865.

Kapsenberg, M. L., Van der Pouw-Kraan, T., Stiekema, F. E., Schootemeijer, A. and Bos, J. D. 1988. Direct and indirect nickel-specific stimulation of T lymphocytes from patients with allergic contact dermatitis to nickel. *Eur. J. Immunol.* 18:977–982.

Kapsenberg, M. L., Stiekema, F. E., Kallan, L., Bos, J. D. and Roozemond, R. C. 1989. The restrictive role of sialic acid in antigen presentation to a subset of human peripheral CD4$^+$ T lymphocytes, that requires antigen presenting dendritic cells. *Eur. J. Immunol.* 19:1829–1834.

Karttunen, R., Silvennoinen-Kassinen, S., Juutinen, K. and Andersson, G. 1988. Nickel antigen induces IL-2 secretion and IL-2 receptor expression mainly on CD4$^+$ T cells, but no measurable gamma interferon secretion in peripheral blood mononuclear cell cultures in delayed type hypersensitivity to nickel. *Clin. Exp. Immunol.* 74:387–391.

Kawaguchi, T., Mednis, A., Golde, D. W., David, J. R. and Remold, H. R. 1986. A monoclonal antibody against migration inhibitory factor (MIF) obtained by immunization with MIF from the human lymphoblast cell line Mo. *J. Leukocyte Biol.* 39:223–232.

Kelly, R. H., Wolstencroft, R. A., Dumonde, D. C., and Balfour, B. M. 1972. Role of lymphocyte activation products (LAP) in cell mediated immunity. II. Effects of lymphocyte activation products on lymph node architecture and evidence for peripheral release of LAP following antigenic stimulation. *Clin. Exp. Immunol.* 10:49–65.

Kerckhaert, J. A. M., Van den Berg, G. J. and Willers, J. M. N. 1974. Influence of cyclophosphamide on the delayed hypersensitivity in the mouse. *Ann. Immunol.* 1250:415–420.

Keystone, E. C., Demerieux, D., Gladman, D., Poplonski, L., Piper, S. and Buchanan,

R. 1980. Enhanced delayed hypersensitivity skin test reactivity with serial testing in healthy volunteers. *Clin. Exp. Immunol.* 40:202–205.

Khansari, D. N., Murgo, A. J., Faith, R. E. 1990. Effects of stress on the immune system. *Immunol. Today* 11:170–175.

Kim, C. W. and Schopf, E. 1976. A comparative study of nickel hypersensitivity by the lymphocyte transformation test in atopic and non-atopic dermatitis. *Arch. Dermatol. Res.* 257:57–65.

Kimber, I., Mitchell, J. A. and Griffin, A. C. 1986. Development of a murine local lymph node assay for the determination of sensitizing potential. *Food Chem. Toxicol.* 24:585–591.

King, P. D. and Katz, D. R. 1990. Mechanisms of dendritic cell function. *Immunol. Today* 11:206–211.

Klareskog, L., Scheynius, A. and Tjernlund, U. 1986. Distribution of interleukin-2 receptor bearing lymphocytes in the skin. *Acta. Derm. Venereol. (Stockh.)* 66:193–199.

Kligman, A. and Gollhausen, R. 1986. The "angry back": A new concept or old confusion? *Br. J. Dermatol.* 115(suppl. 31):93–100.

Kligman, A. M. 1958. Poison ivy (*Rhus*) dermatitis. An experimental study. *AMA Arch. Dermatol.* 77:149–180.

Knapp, W., Rieber, P., Dörken, B., Schmidt, R. E., Stein, H. and Borne, A. E. G. Kr. 1989. Towards a better definition of human leucocyte surface molecules. *Immunol. Today* 10:253–258.

Knight, S. C. 1982. Control of lymphocyte stimulation in vitro: "Help" and "suppression" in the light of lymphoid population dynamics. *J. Immunol. Methods* 50:R51–R63.

Knight, S. C., Krejci, J., Malkovsky, M., Colizzi, V., Gautam, A. and Asherson, G. L. 1985. The role of dendritic cells in the initiation of immune responses to contact sensitizers. *Cell. Immunol.* 94:427–434.

Knight, S. C., Farrant, J., Bryant, A. J., Edwards, S., Burman, S., Lever, A., Clarke, J. and Webster, A. D. B. 1986. Non-adherent low density cells from human peripheral blood contain dendritic cells and monocytes, both with veiled morphology. *Immunology* 57:595–603.

Knop, J. and Riechmann, R. 1982. Suppression of the elicitation phase of contact allergy by epicutaneous application of alpha-L-fucose. *Arch. Dermatol. Res.* 274:155–158.

Kobayashi, Y., Asada, M., Higuchi, M. and Osawa, T. 1982. Human T cell hybridomas producing lymphokines. Establishment and characterization of human T cell hybridomas producing lymphotoxin and migration inhibitory factor. *J. Immunol.* 128:2714–2718.

Koide, S. L., Inaba, K. and Steinman, R. M. 1987. Interleukin-1 enhances T-dependent immune responses by amplifying the function of dendritic cells. *J. Exp. Med.* 165:515–530.

Koulou, K. and Jansen, C. T. 1988. In vivo PUVA and UVB sensitivity of various human epidermal Langerhans cell markers (ATPase, HLA-DR and T6). Dose-response and time-sequence studies. *Clin. Exp. Dermatol.* 13:173–176.

Kowalczyk, D., Pryjma, J. and Zembala, M. 1986. Human T cell subsets differ in their ability to migrate in vitro and to produce T cell migration inhibitory factor. *Immunol. Lett.* 13:33–38.

Kraal, G., Breel, M., Janse, M. and Bruin, G. 1986. Langerhans' cells, veiled cells and interdigitating cells in the mouse recognized by a monoclonal antibody. *J. Exp. Med.* 163:981–997.

Kraal, G., Duijvestijn, A. M. and Hendriks, H. H. 1987. The endothelium of the high endothelial venule: A specialized endothelium with unique properties. *Exp. Cell Biol.* 55:1–10.

Krieger, J., Jenis, D. M., Chesnut, R. W. and Grey, H. M. 1988. Studies on the capacity of intact cells and purified Ia from different B cell sources to function in antigen presentation to T cells. *J. Immunol.* 140:388–394.

Kumar, A., Moreau, J. L., Gilbert, M. and Theze, J. 1987. Internalization of interleukin 2 (IL-2) by high affinity IL-2 receptors is required for the growth of IL-2 dependent T cell lines. *J. Immunol.* 139:3680–3684.

Kupper, T. S. 1989. Production of cytokines by epithelial tissues. A new model for cutaneous inflammation. *Am. J. Dermatopathol.* 1:69–73.

Lachapelle, J. M., Van Neste, D., De Bruyere, M. and Lebacq, A. M. 1980. Increased "in vivo" lymphocyte blastogenesis in the peripheral blood of patients with atopic dermatitis and allergic contact dermatitis. *Arch. Dermatol. Res.* 268:231–237.

Lachapelle, J. M., Bruynzeel, D. P., Ducombs, G., Hannuksela, M., Ring, J., White, I. R., Wilkinson, J. D., Fischer, T. and Billberg, K. 1988. European multicenter study of the TRUE test™. *Contact Dermatitis* 19:91–97.

Lahti, A. and Maibach, H. I. 1987. Immediate contact reactions: Contact uricaria syndrome. *Sem. Dermatol.* 6:313–320.

Lampert, I. A. 1984. Expression of HLA-DR (Ia like) antigen on epidermal keratinocytes in human dermatoses. *Clin. Exp. Immunol.* 57:93–100.

Landsteiner, K. and Jacobs, E. 1935. Studies on the sensitization of animals with simple chemical compounds. *J. Exp. Med.* 61:643–656.

Landsteiner, K. and Chase, M. W. 1942. Experiments on transfer of cutaneous sensitivity to simple chemicals. *Proc. Soc. Exp. Biol. Med.* 49:688–690.

Lanzavecchia, A. 1985. Antigen-specific interaction between T and B cells. *Nature (Lond.)* 314:537–539.

Larsen, C. G., Ternowitz, T., Larsen, F. G. and Thestrup-Pedersen, K. 1988. Epidermis and lymphocyte interactions during an allergic patch test reaction. Increased activity of ETAF/IL-1, epidermal derived lymphocyte chemotactic factor and mixed skin lymphocyte reactivity in persons with type IV allergy. *J. Invest. Dermatol.* 90:230–233.

Lefkovits, I. and Waldmann, H. 1984. Limiting dilution analysis of the cells of immune system. I. The clonal basis of the immune response. *Immunol. Today* 5:265–298.

Lenz, U. and Witkowski, R. 1971. Der Lymphozytentransformations test als Hilfsmittel des Nachweises einer Kontaktallergie. *Derm. Mschr.* 157:68–72.

Levene, G. M. 1972. Lymphocyte transformation in contact sensitivity. *Trans. St. Johns Hosp. Dermatol. Soc.* 58:147–152.

Levi, F. A., Canon, C., Blum, J.-P., Mechkouri, M., Reinberg, A. and Mathe, G. 1985. Circadian and/or circahemidian rhythms in nine lymphocyte-related variables from peripheral blood of healthy subjects. *J. Immunol.* 134:217–222.

Levi, F. A., Canon, C., Touitou, Y., Sulon, J., Mechkouri, M., Ponsart, E. D., Touboul, J. P., Vannetzel, J. M., Mowzowicz, I., Reinberg, A. and Mathe, G. 1988. Circadian rhythms in circulating T lymphocyte subtypes and plasma testosterone, total and free cortisol in five healthy men. *Clin. Exp. Immunol.* 71:329–335.

Levis, W. R., Whalen, J. J. and Miller, A. E. 1974. Blastogenesis of autologous, allogeneic, and syngeneic (identical twins) lymphocytes in response to lymphokines generated in dinitrochlorobenzene-sensitive human leukocyte cultures. *J. Immunol.* 112:1488–1493.

Levis, W. R., Powell, J. A. and Whalen, J. J. 1975. Carrier specificity vs. hapten specificity in classical cell-mediated contact sensitivity to dinitrochlorobenzene. *J. Immunol.* 115:1170–1173.

Levis, W. R., Whalen, J. J. and Powell, J. A. 1975. Studies on the contact sensitization of man with simple chemicals. III. Quantitative relationships between specific lymphocyte transformation, skin sensitivity and lymphokine activity in response to dinitrochlorobenzene. *J. Invest. Dermatol.* 64:100–104.

Levis, W. R., Whalen, J. J. and Powell, J. A. 1976. Specific blastogenesis and lymphokine production in DNCB-sensitive human leucocyte cultures stimulated with soluble and particulate DNP-containing antigens. *Clin. Exp. Immunol.* 23:481–490.

Lewis, R. E., Buchsbaum, M., Whitaker, D. and Murphy, G. F. 1989. Intercellular adhesion molecule expression in the evolving human cutaneous delayed hypersensitivity reaction. *J. Invest. Dermatol.* 93:672–677.

Liano, D. and Abbas, A. K. 1987. Antigen presentation by hapten-specific B lymphocytes. V. Requirements for activation of antigen presenting B cells. *J. Immunol.* 139:2562–2566.

Limpens, J., Garssen, J., Germeraad, W. T. V. and Scheper, R. J. 1990. Enhancing effects of locally administered cytostatic drugs on T effector cell functions in mice. *Int. J. Immunopharm.* 12:77–88.

Lindberg, M. 1982. Studies on the cellular and subcellular reactions in epidermis at irritant and allergic dermatitis. *Acta Derm. Venereol. (Stockh.) Suppl.* 105.

Lipscomb, M. F., Toews, G. B., Lyons, C. R. and Uhr, J. W. 1981. Antigen presentation by guinea pig alveolar macrophages. *J. Immunol.* 126:286–291.

Lisby, G., Arnstorp, C. and Wantzin, G. L. 1987. Interleukin-1. A new mediator in dermatology. *Int. J. Dermatol.* 26:8–13.

Lischka, G. 1971. Lymphocytentransformationstest bei Chromatallergie. *Arch. Derm. Forsch.* 240:212–218.

Liu, D. Y., Yu, S. F., Remold, H. G. and David, J. R. 1985. Macrophage glycolipid receptors for human migration inhibitory factor (MIF): Differentiated HL-60 cells exhibit MIF responsiveness and express surface glycolipids which both bind MIF and convert non-responsive cells to responsive. *Cell. Immunol.* 90:605–613.

Löfström, A. and Wigzell, H. 1986. Antigen specific human T cell lines specific for cobalt chloride. *Acta Derm. Venereol. (Stockh.)* 66:200–206.

Lomnitzer, R., Phillips, R. and Rabson, A. R. 1983. The effect of hydrocortisone (HC) on sodium periodate and PHA-induced ^{3}H-thymidine incorporation and lymphokine production by human lymphocytes. *Clin. Immunol. Immunopathol.* 27:378–386.

Lynde, C. W., Warshawski, L. and Mitchell, J. C. 1982. Screening patch tests in 4190 eczema patients 1972–81. *Contact Dermatitis* 8:417–421.

Macfarlin, D. E. and Balfour, B. 1973. Contact sensitivity in the pig. *Immunology* 25:995–1009.

MacLeod, T. M., Hutchinson, F. and Raffle, E. J. 1970. The uptake of labelled thymidine by leucocytes of nickel sensitive patients. *Br. J. Dermatol.* 82:487–492.

MacLeod, T. M., Hutchinson, F. and Raffle, E. J. 1976a. Leucocyte aggregation in subjects with nickel dermatitis. *Clin. Exp. Immunol.* 26:528–530.

MacLeod, T. M., Hutchinson, F. and Raffle, E. J. 1976b. The leukocyte migration inhibition test in allergic nickel contact dermatitis. *Br. J. Dermatol.* 94:63–64.

MacLeod, T. M., Hutchinson, F. and Raffle, E. J. 1982. In vitro studies on blastogenic lymphokine activity in nickel allergy. *Acta Derm. Venereol. (Stockh.)* 62:249–250.

MacSween, J. M., Rajaraman, K., Rajaraman, R. and Fox, R. A. 1982. Macrophage migration inhibition factor (MIF). Reducing the variables. *J. Immunol. Methods* 52:127–136.

MacSween, J. M., Rajaraman, K. and Rajaraman, R. 1986. The cellular basis for differential lymphokine responses to mitogen stimulation. *Cell. Immunol.* 101:82–92.

Magaud, J. P., Sargent, I. and Mason, D. Y. 1988. Detection of human white cell proliferative responses by immunoenzymatic measurement of bromodeoxy uridine uptake. *J. Immunol. Methods* 106:95–100.

Maggi, E., Del Prete, G., Macchia, D., Paronchi, P., Tiori, A., Chretien, I., Ricci, M. and Romagnani, S. 1988. Profiles of lymphokine activities and helper function for IgE in human T cell clones. *Eur. J. Immunol.* 18:1045–1050.

Mahapatro, D. and Mahapatro, R. C. 1984. Cutaneous basophil hypersensitivity. Review. *Am. J. Dermatopathol.* 6:483–489.

Maibach, H. I. 1981. The ESS-excited skin syndrome (alias the "angry back"). In *New Trends in Allergy*, eds. J. Ring and G. Burg, pp. 208–221. Berlin: Springer-Verlag.

Maibach, H. I., Fregert, S., Magnusson, B., Pirila, V., Hjorth, N., Wilkinson, D., Malten, K., Meneghini, C. and Lachapelle, J. M. 1982. Quantification of the excited skin syndrome (the "angry back"): Retesting one patch at a time. *Contact Dermatitis* 8:78–84.

Makgoba, M. W., Sanders, M. E. and Shaw, S. 1989. The CD-2-LFA-3 and LFA-1-ICAM pathways: Relevance to T cell recognition. *Immunol. Today* 10:417–422.

Malorny, U., Knop, J. and Sorg, C. 1988. Immunohistochemical demonstration of migration inhibitory factor (MIF) in experimental allergic contact dermatitis. *Clin. Exp. Immunol.* 71:164–170.

Malten, K. E., Den Arend, J. A. C. J. and Wiggers, R. E. 1979. Delayed irritation: Hexanediol diacrylate and butanediol diacrylate. *Contact Dermatitis* 5:178–184.

Maluish, A. E. and Strong, D. M. 1986. Lymphocyte proliferation. In *Manual of Clinical Laboratory Immunology*, eds. N. R. Rose, H. Friedman and J. L. Fahey, pp. 274–281. Washington, DC: American Society for Microbiology.

Marks, J. G., Zaino, R. J., Bressler, M. F. and Williams, J. V. 1987. Changes in lymphocyte and Langerhans cell populations in allergic and irritant contact dermatitis. *Int. J. Dermatol.* 26:354–357.

Marsman, A. J. W., Van Der Hart, M., Walig, C. and Eijsvoogel, V. P. 1972. Migration inhibition experiments with mixtures of human peripheral blood lymphocytes and guinea pig peritoneal exudate cells. *Eur. J. Immunol.* 2:546–550.

Martin, S., Maruta, K., Burkart, V., Gillis, S. and Kolb, H. 1988. IL-1 and IFN-gamma increase vascular permeability. *Immunology* 64:301–305.

Masuyama, J., Minato, N. and Kano, S. 1986. Mechanisms of lymphocyte adhesion of human vascular endothelial cells in culture. *J. Clin. Invest.* 77:1596–1605.

Maucher, O. M. 1972. Anaphylaktische reaktionen beim epicutantest. *Der Hautarzt* 23:139–140.

Maurer, D. H., Hanke, J. H., Mickelseon, E., Rich, R. R. and Pollack, M. S. 1987. Differential presentation of HLA-DR, DQ, and DP restriction elements by interferon-gamma-treated dermal fibroblasts. *J. Immunol.* 139:715–723.

Maurer, T. 1983. *Contact and Photocontact Allergens: A Manual of Predictive Test Methods*, vol. 3, eds. C. D. Calnan and H. I. Maibach, p. 121. New York: Dekker.

McGeady, S. J. and Buckley, R. H. 1975. Depression of cell mediated immunity in atopic eczema. *J. Allergy Clin. Immunol.* 56:393–406.

McGuire, R. L. and Fox, R. A. 1979. Suppression of delayed hypersensitivity by the depletion of circulating monocytes. *Immunology* 38:157–161.

McKenna, K., Burrows, D. and Walsch, M. 1989. A comparison of expression of human lymphocyte class II antigens between patients with allergic, irritant and atopic dermatitis. In *Current Topics in Contact Dermatitis*, eds. P. J. Frosch,

A. Dooms-Goossens, J. M. Lachapelle, R. J. G. Rycroft and R. J. Scheper, pp. 404–411. Heidelberg: Springer-Verlag.

McMillan, E. M., Stoneking, L., Burdick, S., Cowan, I. and Husain-Hamzavi, S. L. 1985. Immunophenotype of lymphoid cells in positive patch tests of allergic contact dermatitis. *J. Invest. Dermatol.* 84:229–233.

Meneghini, C. L. and Angelini, G. 1977. Behavior of contact allergy and new sensitivities on subsequent patch tests. *Contact Dermatitis* 3:138–142.

Meneghini, C. L. and Angelini, G. 1979. Intradermal test in contact allergy to metals. *Acta Derm. Venereol.* 59(suppl. 85):123–124.

Menne, T., Brandrup, F., Thestrup-Pedersen, K., Veien, N. K., Andersen, J. R., Yding, F. and Valeur, G. 1987. Patch test reactivity to nickel alloys. *Contact Dermatitis* 16:255–259.

Miller, A. E. and Levis, W. R. 1973. Studies on the contact sensitization of man with simple chemicals. I. Specific lymphocyte transformation in response to dinitrochlorobenzene sensitization. *J. Invest. Dermatol.* 61:261–269.

Miller, A. E. and Levis, W. R. 1973. Lymphocyte transformation during dinitrochlorobenzene contact sensitization. *J. Clin. Invest.* 52:1925–1930.

Millikan, L. E., Conway, F. and Foote, J. E. 1973. In vitro studies of contact hypersensitivity: Lymphocyte transformation in nickel sensitivity. *J. Invest. Dermatol.* 60:88–90.

Milner, J. E. 1974. In vitro lymphocyte responses in contact hypersensitivity IV. *J. Invest. Dermatol.* 62:591–594.

Milon, G., Marchal, G., Seman, M., Truffa-Bachi, P. and Zilberfarb, V. 1983. Is the delayed type hypersensitivity observed after a low dose of antigen mediated by helper T cells? *J. Immunol.* 130:1103–1108.

Minami, M., Okuda, K., Sunday, M. E. and Dorf, M. E. 1982. H-2K, H-2I- and H-2D-restricted hybridoma contact sensitivity effector cells. *Nature (Lond.)* 297:231–233.

Miossec, P., Cavender, D. and Ziff, M. 1988. Interleukin 1 derived from endothelial cells enhances the binding and chemotactic step of T lymphocyte emigration. *Clin. Exp. Immunol.* 73:250–254.

Mirza, A. M., Perera, M. G., Maccia, C. A., Dziubynski, O. G. and Bernstein, I. L. 1975. Leukocyte migration inhibition in nickel dermatitis. *Int. Arch. Allergy Appl. Immunol.* 49:782–788.

Mitchell, E. B., Crow, J., Rowntree, S., Webster, A. D. B. and Platts-Mills, T. A. E. 1984. Cutaneous basophil hypersensitivity to inhalant allergens in atopic dermatitis patients: Elicitation of delayed responses containing basophils following local transfer of immune serum but not IgE antibody. *J. Invest. Dermatol.* 83:290–295.

Mitchell, J. C. 1977. Multiple concomitant positive patch test reactions. *Contact Dermatitis* 3:315–320.

Mittal, A. and Nath, I. 1987. Human T cell proliferative responses to particulate microbial antigens are supported by populations enriched in dendritic cells. *Clin. Exp. Immunol.* 69:611–617.

Mizel, S. B. 1987. Interleukin 1 and T cell activation. *Immunol. Today* 8:330–332.

Möller, H. 1984. Flare-up of allergic contact dermatitis in the mouse after topical distant provocation. *Acta Derm. Venereol. (Stockh.)* 64:125–128.

Möller, H. 1989. Intracutaneous testing in doubtful cases of contact allergy metals. In *Current Topics in Contact Dermatitis,* eds. P. J. Frosch, A. Dooms-Goossens, J. M. Lachapelle, R. J. G. Rycroft and R. J. Scheper, pp. 169–171. Heidelberg: Springer-Verlag.

Moore, K. and Nesbitt, A. M. 1987. Functional heterogeneity of CD4[+] T lymphocytes:

Two subpopulations with counteracting immunoregulatory functions identified with the monoclonal antibodies WR16 and WR19. *Immunology* 61:159–165.

Moorhead, J. W. 1978. Tolerance and contact sensitivity to DNCB in mice. VIII. Identification of distinct T cell populations that mediate in vivo and in vitro manifestation of delayed hypersensitivity. *J. Immunol.* 120:137–144.

Moorhead, J. W., Murphy, J. W., Harvey, R. P., Hayes, R. L. and Fetterhoff, T. J. 1982. Soluble factors in tolerance and contact sensitivity to 2,4-dinitrofluorobenzene in mice. IV. Characterization of migration inhibition factor-producing lymphocytes and genetic requirements for activation. *Eur. J. Immunol.* 12:431–436.

Morikawa, M., Iseki, R. and Ohashi, M. 1989. Functional role of DR$^+$ keratinocytes from tuberculin reactive skin. Abstr. *J. Invest. Dermatol.* 92:485.

Morison, W. L., Bucana, C. and Kripke, M. L. 1984. Systemic suppression of contact hypersensitivity by UVB radiation is unrelated to the UVB-induced alterations in the morphology and numbers of Langerhans cells. *Immunology* 52:299–306.

Mosmann, T. R., Cherwinski, H., Bond, M. W., Giedlin, M. A. and Coffman, R. L. 1986. Two types of murine helper T cell clone. I. Definition according to profiles of lymphokine activities and secreted proteins. *J. Immunol.* 136:2348–2357.

Mullink, H. and Von Blomberg, B. M. E. 1980. Influence of anti-inflammatory drugs on the interaction of lymphocytes and macrophages. *Agents Actions* 10:512–515.

Nagao, S., Tanaka, A., Onozaki, K. and Hashimoto, T. 1982. Differences between macrophage migration inhibition by lymphokines and muramyl dipeptide (MDP) or lipopolysaccharide (LPS): Migration enhancement by lymphokines. *Cell. Immunol.* 71:1–11.

Nagelkerken, L. M. and Van Breda Vriesman, P. J. C. 1986. Membrane associated IL-1-like activity on rat dendritic cells. *J. Immunol.* 136:2164–2170.

Nairn, R. C. and Rolland, J. M. 1980. Fluorescent probes to detect lymphocyte activation. *Clin. Exp. Immunol.* 39:1–13.

Nakagawa, S. and Tanioku, J. 1972. The induction of delayed hypersensitivity to 2,4-dinitrophenyl conjugates in guinea pigs sensitized with DNCB. *Dermatologica* 144:19–26.

Nakano, Y., Nakano, K. and Hara, I. 1981. Induction of leucocyte migration inhibitory factor (LIF) by stimulation with free hapten and water-insoluble epoxy resin. *Clin. Exp. Immunol.* 45:419–426.

Nau, P. and Peters, J. H. 1986. Human peripheral blood accessory cell: Isolation by hypotonic density gradient, functional, and phenotypical characterization. *Immunobiology* 173:82–97.

Neumann, C., Schlegel, R., Steckel, F. and Sorg, C. 1987. Detection of macrophage migration inhibitory factor by monoclonal antibody in Sézary syndrome. *J. Invest. Dermatol.* 88:670–674.

Nickoloff, B. J., Basham, T. Y., Merigan, T. C., Torseth, J. W. and Morhenn, V. B. 1986. Human keratinocyte-lymphocyte reactions in vitro. *J. Invest. Dermatol.* 87:11–18.

Nickoloff, B. J., Reusch, M. H., Bensch, K. and Karasek, M. A. 1988. Preferential binding of monocytes and leu 2$^+$ T lymphocytes to interferon gamma treated cultured skin endothelial cells and keratinocytes. *Arch. Dermatol. Res.* 280:235–245.

Nickoloff, B. J., Griffiths, C. E. M. and Barker, J. N. W. N. 1990. The role of adhesion molecules, chemotactic factors, and cytokines in inflammatory and neoplastic skin disease—1990 update. *J. Invest. Dermatol.* 94:151S–157S.

Nishioka, K., Aoki, T., Nishioka, K. and Tashiro, M. 1971. Studies on carrier substances of DNCB contact allergy. *Dermatologica* 142:232–240.

Nishioka, K. and Amos, H. E. 1973. Contact sensitivity in vitro. *Immunology* 25:423–432.

Nishioka, K. 1976. Detection of human contact sensitivity to dinitrochlorobenzene by the migration inhibition test. *J. Invest. Dermatol.* 66:351–354.

Nishioka, K., Funai, T., Yokozeki, H. and Katayama, I. 1984. Induction of hapten-specific lymphoid cell proliferation by liposome-carrying molecules from haptenated epidermal cells in contact sensitivity. *J. Invest. Dermatol.* 83:96–100.

Nishioka, K., Katayama, I. and Kobayashi, Y. 1987. Ia antigen expressed by keratinocytes can be the molecule of antigen presentation in contact sensitivity. *J. Invest. Dermatol.* 88:694–698.

Norcross, M. A., Bentley, D. M., Margulies, D. H. and Germain, R. N. 1984. Membrane Ia expression and antigen-presenting accessory cell function of L cells transfected with class II major histocompatibility complex genes. *J. Exp. Med.* 160:1316–1337.

Nordlind, K. and Sandberg, G. 1983. Leukocytes from patients allergic to chromium and nickel examined by the sealed capillary migration technique. *Int. Arch. Allergy Appl. Immunol.* 70:30–33.

Nordlind, K. 1984a. Lymphocyte transformation test in diagnosis of nickel allergy. *Int. Arch. Appl. Immunol.* 73:151–154.

Nordlind, K. 1984b. Further studies on the lymphocyte transformation test in diagnosis of nickel allergy. *Int. Arch. Allergy Appl. Immunol.* 75:333–336.

Nordquist, B. and Rorsman, H. 1967. Leucocyte migration in vitro as an indicator of allergy in eczematous contact dermatitis. *Trans. St. Johns Hosp. Dermatol. Soc.* 53:154–159.

Nunez, G., Ball, E. J. and Stastny, P. 1987. Antigen presentation by adherent cells from peripheral blood. Correlation between T cell activation and expression of HLA-DQ and DR antigens. *Hum. Immunol.* 19:29–39.

O'Dell, B. M., Jessen, R. T., Becker, L. E., Jackson, R. T. and Smith, E. B. 1980. Diminished immune response in sun-damaged skin. *Arch. Dermatol.* 116:559–561.

Oehling, A., Dieguez, I. and Lobera, T. 1981. Clinical aspects and cellular immunity in contact dermatitis due to chrome and nickel. *Allergol. Immunopathol.* 9:233–240.

Okuda, K., Tani, K., Ishigatsubo, Y., Yokota, S. and David, C. S. 1980. Antigen-pulsed neutrophils bearing Ia antigen can induce T lymphocyte proliferative response to the syngeneic or semi-syngeneic antigen-primed T lymphocytes. *Transplantation* 30:368–372.

Oort, J. and Turk, J. L. 1965. A histological and autoradiographic study of lymph nodes during the development of contact sensitivity in the guinea pig. *Br. J. Exp. Pathol.* 46:147–154.

Oort, J., Scheper, R. J. and Veldhuizen, R. W. 1974. The effects of local continuous stimulation with the contact agent DNCB. *Monogr. Allergy* 8:136–145.

Oppenheim, J. J. 1968. Relationship of in vitro lymphocyte transformation to delayed hypersensitivity in guinea pigs and man. *Fed. Proc.* 27:21–28.

Oppenheim, J. J. and Gery, I. 1982. Interleukin 1 is more than an interleukin. *Immunol. Today* 3:113–119.

Oppenheim, J. J., Kovacs, E. J., Matsushima, K. and Durum, S. K. 1986. There is more than one interleukin-1. *Immunol. Today* 7:45–55.

Ottenhoff, T. H. M., Elferink, D. G., Hermans, J. and De Vries, R. R. P. 1985. HLA class II restriction repertoire of antigen-specific T cells. I. The main restriction determinants for antigen presentation are associated with HLA-D/DR and not with DP and DQ. *Hum. Immunol.* 13:105–112.

Pabst, R. 1988. The spleen in lymphocyte migration. *Immunol. Today* 9:43–45.

Paliard, X., De Waal Malefijt, R., Yssel, H., Blanchard, D., Chretien, I., Abrams, J., De Vries, J. and Spits, H. 1988. Simultaneous production of IL-2, IL-4, and IFN-gamma by activated human CD4$^+$ and CD8$^+$ clones. *J. Immunol.* 141:849–855.

Pals, S. T., Kraal, G., Horst, E., De Groot, A., Scheper, R. J. and Meijer, C. J. L. M. 1986. Human lymphocyte high endothelial venule interaction: Organ-selective binding of T and B lymphocyte populations to high endothelium. *J. Immunol.* 137:760–763.

Pals, S. T., Den Otter, A., Miedema, F., Kabel, P., Keizer, G. D., Scheper, R. J. and Meijer, C. J. L. M. 1988. Evidence that leukocyte function-associated antigen-1 is involved in recirculation and homing of human lymphocytes via high endothelial venules. *J. Immunol.* 140:1851–1853.

Pals, S. T., Horst, E., Scheper, R. J. and Meijer, C. J. L. M. 1989. Mechanisms of human lymphocyte migration and their role in the pathogenesis of disease. *Immunol. Rev.* 108:111–133.

Palutke, M., Kukuruga, D. and Tabeczka, P. 1987. A flow cytometric method for measuring lymphocyte proliferation directly from tissue culture plates using Ki-67 and propidium iodide. *J. Immunol. Methods* 105:97–105.

Pappas, A., Orfanos, C. E. and Bertram, R. 1970. Non-specific lymphocyte transformation in vitro by nickel acetate. *J. Invest. Dermatol.* 55:198–200.

Parent, D., Godfrine, S., Dezutter-Dambuyant, C., Staquet, M. J., Heenen, M., Schmidt, D. and Thivolet, J. 1989. In situ identification of cycling Langerhans cells in normal human skin. *Arch. Dermatol. Res.* 281:75–77.

Parker, D., Aoki, T. and Turk, J. L. 1970. Studies on the ability of the soluble proteins from skin, painted in vivo with DNFB, to cause contact sensitivity in the guinea pig. *Int. Arch. Allergy Appl. Immunol.* 38:42–56.

Parker, D., Long, P. V., Bull, J. E. and Turk, J. L. 1985. Epicutaneous induction of tolerance with acrylates and related compounds. *Contact Dermatitis* 12:146–154.

Peters, J. H., Ruhl, S. and Friedrichs, D. 1987. Veiled accessory cells deduced from monocytes. *Immunobiology* 176:154–161.

Picker, L. J., Terstappen, L. W. M. M., Rott, L. S., Streeter, P. R., Stein, H. and Butcher, E. C. 1990. Differential expression of homing-associated adhesion molecules by T cell subsets in man. *J. Immunol.* 145:3247–3255.

Picut, C. A., Lee, C. S. and Lewis, R. M. 1987. Ultrastructural and phenotypic changes in Langerhans cells induced in vitro by contact allergens. *Br. J. Dermatol.* 116:773–784.

Pinkston, P., Saltini, C., Müller-Quernheim, J. and Crystal, R. 1987. Corticosteroid therapy suppresses spontaneous interleukin 2 release and spontaneous proliferation of lung T lymphocytes of patients with active pulmonary sarcoidosis. *J. Immunol.* 139:755–760.

Pitzalis, C., Kingsley, G., Haskard, D. and Panayi, G. 1988. The preferential accumulation of helper-inducer T lymphocytes in inflammatory lesions: Evidence for regulation by selective endothelial and homotypic adhesion. *Eur. J. Immunol.* 18:1397–1404.

Platt, J. L., Grant, B. W., Eddy, A. A. and Michael, A. F. 1983. Immune cell population in cutaneous delayed-type hypersensitivity. *J. Exp. Med.* 158:1227–1242.

Pober, J. S., Collins, T., Gimbrone, M. A. J. R., Cotran, R. S., Gitlin, J. D., Fiers, W., Clayberger, C., Krensky, A. M., Burakoff, S. J. and Reiss, C. S. 1983. Lymphocytes recognize human vascular endothelial and dermal fibroblasts Ia antigens induced by recombinant immune interferon. *Nature (Lond.)* 305:726–729.

Pober, J. S., Gimbrone, M. A., Cotran, R. S., Reiss, C. S., Burakoff, S. J., Fiers, W. and Ault, K. A. 1983. Ia expression by vascular endothelium is inducible by activated T cells and by human interferon. *J. Exp. Med.* 157:1339–1353.

Polak, L. and Macher, E. 1974. In vitro sensitization to dinitrochlorobenzene in guinea pigs. *Nature (Lond.)* 252:748–751.

Polak, L. 1980. Immunological aspects of contact sensitivity. An experimental study. *Monogr. Allergy* 15: (a)1–62, (b)14–16, (c)25–29, (d)63–125.

Polak, L. and Rufli, T. 1981. Vasoactive mediators in contact sensitivity. In *New Trends in Allergy*, eds. J. Ring and G. Burg. Berlin: Springer-Verlag.

Polak, L. and Scheper, R. J. 1981. In vitro DNA-synthesis in lymphocytes from guinea pigs epicutaneously sensitized with DNCB. *J. Invest. Dermatol.* 76:133–136.

Polak, L. 1982. Self molecules in induction of hypersensitivity and tolerance in DNCB contact sensitivity in the guinea pig. *Ann. NY Acad. Sci.* 392:90–106.

Potter, J. W. and Van Epps, D. E. 1986. Human T-lymphocyte chemotactic activity: Nature and production in response to antigen. *Cell. Immunol.* 97:59–66.

Potter, J. W. and Van Epps, D. E. 1987. Separation and purification of lymphocyte chemotactic factor (LCF) and interleukin-2 produced by human peripheral blood mononuclear cells. *Cell. Immunol.* 105:9–22.

Powell, J. A., Whalen, J. J. and Levis, W. R. 1975. Studies on the contact sensitization in man with simple chemicals. IV. Timing of skin reactivity, lymphokine production,and blastogenesis following rechallenge with dinitrochlorobenzene using an automated microassay. *J. Invest. Dermatol.* 64:357–363.

Powers, G. P. and Miller, R. A. 1987. Heterogeneity among T helper cells. Interleukin-2 secretion and help for immunoglobulin secretion. *J. Immunol.* 139:2567–2576.

Pownall, R., Kabler, P. A. and Knapp, M. S. 1979. The time of day of antigen encounter influences the magnitude of the immune response. *Clin. Exp. Immunol.* 36:347–354.

Prens, E. P., Benne, K., Van Joost, T. and Benner, R. 1989. In vitro nickel specific lymphocyte proliferation: Methodological aspects. In *Current Topics in Contact Dermatitis*, eds. P. J. Frosch, A. Dooms-Goossens, J. M. Lachapelle, R. J. G. Rycroft and R. J. Scheper, pp. 578–586. Heidelberg: Springer-Verlag.

Przybilla, B., Ring, J. and Schmid, J. G. 1984. Comparison of methods for the macroscopic assessment of epicutaneous allergic contact reactions in guinea pigs. *Contact Dermatitis* 11:229–235.

Ralfkiaer, E. and Wantzin, G. L. 1984. In situ immunological characterization of the infiltrating cells in positive patch tests. *Br. J. Dermatol.* 111:13–22.

Ranki, A., Kanerva, L., Förström, L., Konttinen, Y. and Mustalallio, K. K. 1983. T and B lymphocytes, macrophages and Langerhans cells during the course of contact allergic and irritant skin reactions in man. *Acta Derm. Venereol. (Stockh.)* 63:376–383.

Ray, M. C., Tharp, M. D., Sullivan, T. J. and Tigelaar, R. E. 1983. Contact hypersensitivity reactions to dinitrofluoro benzene mediated by monoclonal IgE anti-DNP antibodies. *J. Immunol.* 131:1096–1102.

Reitamo, S., Tolvanen, E., Konttinen, Y. T., Kähkö, K., Förström, L. and Salo, O. P. 1981. Allergic and toxic contact dermatitis: Inflammatory cell subtypes in epicutaneous test reactions. *Br. J. Dermatol.* 105:521–527.

Remold, H. G. and Mednis, A. D. 1977. Two migration inhibitory factors with different chromatographic behaviour and isoelectric points. *J. Immunol.* 118:2015–2019.

Res, P., Kapsenberg, M. L., Bos, J. D. and Stiekema, F. 1987. The crucial role of human dendritic antigen presenting cell subsets in nickel-specific T cell proliferation. *J. Invest. Dermatol.* 88:550–554.

Rheins, L. A. and Nordlund, J. J. 1986. Modulation of the population density of identifiable epidermal Langerhans cells associated with enhancement or suppression of cutaneous immune reactivity. *J. Immunol.* 136:867–876.

Rietschel, R. L., Adams, R. M., Maibach, H. I., Storrs, F. J. and Rosenthal, L. E. 1988. The case for patch test readings beyond day 2. *J. Am. Acad. Dermatol.* 18:42–44.

Robb, R. J. 1984. Interleukin-2: The molecule and its function. *Immunol. Today* 5:203–209.

Roberts, L. K., Spangrude, G. J., Daynes, R. A. and Krueger, G. G. 1985. Correlation between keratinocyte expression of Ia and the intensity and duration of contact hypersensitivity responses in mice. *J. Immunol.* 135:2929–2936.

Rocklin, R. E. 1973. Production of migration inhibitory factor by non-dividing lymphocytes. *J. Immunol.* 110:674–678.

Rocklin, R. E. and Urbano, A. M. 1978. Human leukocyte inhibitory factor (LIF): Use of benzoyl L-arginine ethyl ester to detect LIF activity. *J. Immunol.* 120:1409–1414.

Romani, N., Lenz, A., Glassel, H., Stössel, H., Stanzl, U., Majdic, O., Fritsch, P. and Schuler, G. 1989. Cultured human Langerhans cells resemble lymphoid dendritic cells in phenotype and function. *J. Invest. Dermatol.* 93:600–609.

Rook, G. A. W., Carswell, J. W. and Stanford, J. L. 1976. Preliminary evidence for the trapping of antigen-specific lymphocytes in the lymphoid tissue of "anergic" tuberculosis patients. *Clin. Exp. Immunol.* 26:129–132.

Roper, S. S. and Jones, H. E. 1985. An animal model for altering the irritability threshold of normal skin. *Contact Dermatitis* 13:91–97.

Rosa, F. and Fellous, M. 1984. The effect of gamma-interferon on MHC antigens. *Immunol. Today* 5:261–262.

Rouse, B. T. and Horohov, D. W. 1986. Immunosuppression in viral infections. *Rev. Infect. Dis.* 8:850–873.

Royer, H. D. and Reinherz, E. L. 1987. T lymphocytes: Ontogeny, function, and relevance to clinical disorders. *N. Engl. J. Med.* 317:1136–1142.

Rubin, L. A., Jay, G. and Nelson, D. L. 1986. The released interleukin-2 receptor binds interleukin-2 efficiently. *J. Immunol.* 137:3841–3844.

Rytter, M. and Hausten, U.-F. 1982. Hapten conjugation in the leucocyte migration inhibition test in allergic chromate eczema. *Br. J. Dermatol.* 106:161–168.

Saiki, R. K., Gelfand, D. H., Stoffel, S., Scharf, S. J., Higuchi, R., Horn, G. T., Mullis, K. B. and Erlich, H. A. 1988. Primer directed enzymatic amplification of DNA with a thermostable DNA polymerase. *Science* 239:487–494.

Salvin, S. B. and Smith, R. F. 1961. The specificity of allergic reactions. III. Contact hypersensitivity. *J. Exp. Med.* 114:185–194.

Sanders, M. E., Makgoba, M. W. and Shaw, S. 1988. Human naive and memory T cells: Reinterpretation of helper-inducer and suppressor-inducer subsets. *Immunol. Today* 9:195–198.

Sauder, D. N., Dinarello, C. A. and Morhenn, B. 1984. Langerhans cell production of interleukin-1. *J. Invest. Dermatol.* 84:605–607.

Sauder, D. N. 1990. The role of epidermal cytokines in inflammatory skin diseases. *J. Invest. Dermatol.* 95:275–285.

Schall, T. J., Bacon, K., Toy, K. J. and Goeddel, D. V. 1990. Selective attraction of monocytes and T lymphocytes of the memory phenotype by cytokine RANTES. *Nature* 347:669–671.

Schellekens, P. T. A. and Eijsvoogel, V. P. 1968. Lymphocyte transformation in vitro. I. Tissue culture conditions and quantitative measurements. *Clin. Exp. Immunol.* 3:571–584.

Schendel, D. J. and Johnson, J. P. 1985. T cells specific for different antigens express different HLA-D region products. *Eur. J. Immunol.* 15:1239–1243.

Scheper, R. J. and Oort, J. 1973. Some in vitro experimental methods in allergic contact dermatitis. *Arch. Belges Dermatol.* 28:59–71.

Scheper, R. J., Noble, B., Parker, D. and Turk, J. L. 1977. The value of an assessment of erythema and increase in thickness of the skin reaction for a full appreciation of the nature of delayed hypersensitivity in the guinea pig. *Int. Arch. Allergy Appl. Immunol.* 54:58–66.

Scheper, R. J. and Polak, L. 1981. Characterization of lymphocyte subpopulations which exhibit enhanced DNA-synthesis in vitro in DNFB contact sensitive guinea-pigs. *Immunology* 43:563–572.

Scheper, R. J., Von Blomberg, M., Boerrigter, G. H., Bruynzeel, D. P., Van Dinther, A. and Vos, A. 1983. Induction of immunological memory in the skin. Role of local T cell retention. *Clin. Exp. Immunol.* 51:141–148.

Scheper, R. J. and Polak, L. 1984. Four reasons why hapten-specific T cells preferentially accumulate at contact sensitivity lesions. In *Experimental Contact Dermatitis*, eds. C. Benezra, N. Hunziker, T. Maurer, R. J. Scheper and J. L. Turk, pp. 119–123. Basel: Roche.

Scheper, R. J., Van Dinther-Janssen, A. C. H. M. and Polak, L. 1985. Specific accumulation of hapten-reactive T cells in contact sensitivity reaction sites. *J. Immunol.* 134:1333–1336.

Scheper, R. J. and Von Blomberg, B. M. E. 1987. Traffic and trapping of T lymphocytes in the skin. *Proc. 17th Congr. Mundi Dermatol.* Berlin, p. 820.

Scheper, R. J., Von Blomberg, B. M. E., Vreeburg, K. J. J. and Van Hoogstraten, I. M. V. 1989. Recent advances in immunology of nickel sensitization. In *Nickel and the Skin: Immunology and Toxicology*, eds. H. I. Maibach and T. Menne. Boca Raton, Fla.: CRC Press.

Scheper, R. J. and Von Blomberg, B. M. E. 1989. Allergic contact dermatitis: T cell receptors and migration. In *Current Topics in Contact Dermatitis*, eds. P. J. Frosch, A. Dooms-Goossens, J. M. Lachapelle, R. J. G. Rycroft and R. J. Scheper, pp. 12–17. Heidelberg: Springer-Verlag.

Scheynius, A., Fischer, T., Forsum, U. and Klareskog, L. 1984. Phenotypic characterization in situ of inflammatory cells in allergic and irritant contact dermatitis in man. *Clin Exp. Immunol.* 55:81–90.

Scheynius, A. and Fischer, T. 1986. Phenotypic difference between allergic and irritant patch test reactions in man. *Contact Dermatitis* 14:297–302.

Schick, P., Trepel, F., Eder, M., Matzner, M., Benedek, S., Theml, H., Kaboth, W., Begemann, H. and Fliedner, T. M. 1975. Autotransfusion of ^{3}H-cytidin labelled blood lymphocytes in patients with Hodgkin's disease and non-Hodgkin patients. *Acta Haematol.* 53:206–218.

Schöpf, E., Wex, O. and Schulz, K. H. 1970. Allergische Kontaktstomatitis mit spezifischer Lymphocyten-stimulation durch Gold. *Hautarzt* 21:422–425.

Schuler, G. and Steinman, R. M. 1985. Murine epidermal Langerhans cells mature into potent immuno-stimulatory dendritic cells in vitro. *J. Exp. Med.* 161:526–546.

Serup, J., Staberg, B. and Klemp, P. 1984. Quantification of cutaneous oedema in patch test reactions by measurement of skin thickness with high-frequency pulsed ultrasound. *Contact Dermatitis* 10:88–93.

Shelmire, B. S. 1941. Cutaneous and systemic reactions observed during oral poison ivy therapy. *J. Allergy* 12:252.

Shimada, S. and Katz, S. I. 1985. TNP-specific Lyt-2$^+$ cytolytic T cell clones preferentially respond to TNP-conjugated epidermal cells. *J. Immunol.* 135:1558–1563.

Shimada, S., Caughman, S. W., Sharrow, S. O., Stephany, D. and Katz, S. I. 1987. Enhanced antigen-presenting capacity of cultured Langerhans cells is associated with markedly increased expression of Ia antigen. *J. Immunol.* 139:2551–2555.

Shimokawa, Y., Harita, S., Mibu, Y. and Hayashi, H. 1984. Lymphocyte chemotaxis in inflammation. VIII. Demonstration of lymphocyte chemotactic lymphokines in

PPD-induced delayed hypersensitivity skin reaction site in the guinea pig. *Immunology* 51:275-285.

Shiohara, T., Moriya, N., Saizawa, K. M. and Nagashima, M. 1988. Role of Langerhans cells in epidermotropism of T cells. *Arch. Dermatol. Res.* 280:33-38.

Silberberg, I., Baer, R. L. and Rosenthal, S. A. 1976. The role of Langerhans cells in allergic contact hypersensitivity. A review of findings in man and guinea pigs. *J. Invest. Dermatol.* 66:210-217.

Silvennoinen-Kassinen, S. 1980. Lymphocyte transformation in nickel allergy: Amplification of T lymphocyte responses to nickel sulfate by macrophages in vitro. *Scand. J. Immunol.* 12:61-65.

Silvennoinen-Kassinen, S. 1981a. Histamine receptor bearing suppressor cells in nickel sensitivity. *Acta Derm. Venereol. (Stockh.)* 62:251-253.

Silvennoinen-Kassinen, S. 1981b. Inhibition of in vitro nickel sulfate reaction by anti HLA D/DR antisera. Lack of demonstrable suppressor cells in peripheral blood in nickel unresponsiveness in man. *J. Invest. Dermatol.* 77:417-420.

Silvennoinen-Kassinen, S. 1984. Gold sensitivity blast transformation. *Contact Dermatitis* 11:156-158.

Silvennoinen-Kassinen, S., Jakkula, H. and Karvonen, J. 1986. Helper cells carry the specificity of nickel sensitivity reaction in vitro in humans. *J. Invest. Dermatol.* 86:18-20.

Singer, K. H., Tuck, D. T., Sampson, H. A. and Hall, R. P. 1989. Epidermal keratinocytes express the adhesion molecule intercellular adhesion molecule-1 in inflammatory dermatoses. *J. Invest. Dermatol.* 92:746-750.

Sinigaglia, F., Scheidegger, D., Garotta, G., Scheper, R. J., Pletscher, M. and Lanzavecchia, A. 1985. Isolation and characterization of Ni-specific T cell clones from patients with Ni-contact dermatitis. *J. Immunol.* 135:3929-3932.

Skog, E. 1966. Spontaneous flare-up reactions induced by different amounts of 1,3-dinitro-4-chlorobenzene. *Acta Derm. Venereol. (Stockh.)* 46:386-395.

Smith, K. A. 1987. The two chain structure of high affinity IL-2 receptors. *Immunol. Today* 8:11-13.

Smith, K. A. 1988. The bimolecular structure of the IL-2 receptor. *Immunol. Today* 9:36-37.

Smith, S. H., Brown, M. H., Rowe, D., Callard, R. E. and Beverley, P. C. L. 1986. Functional subsets of human helper-inducer cells defined by a new monoclonal antibody UCHL1. *Immunology* 58:63-70.

Smolle, J., Soyer, H. P, Juettner, F. M., Torne, R., Stettner, H. and Kel, H. 1988. HLA-DR-positive keatinocytes are associated with suppressor lymphocyte epidermotropism. A biomathematical study. *Am. J. Dermatopathol.* 10:128-132.

Soeberg, B. and Andersen, V. 1976. Hapten-specific lymphocyte transformation in humans sensitized with NDMA or DNCB. *Clin. Exp. Immunol.* 25:490-492.

Sonnex, T. S. and Ryan, T. J. 1987. An investigation of the angry back syndrome using Trafuril[R]. *Br. J. Dermatol.* 116:361-370.

Sorg, C. and Geczy, C. L. 1976. Antibodies to guinea pig lymphokines. III. Reactions with radio labeled lymphocyte activation products. *Eur. J. Immunol.* 6:688-693.

Søborg, M. and Bendixen, G. 1967. Human lymphocyte migration as a parameter of hypersensitivity. *Acta Med. Scand.* 181:247-256.

Staberg, B. and Seruyp, J. 1988. Allergic and irritant skin reactions evaluated by laser Doppler flowmetry. *Contact Dermatitis* 18:40-45.

Steele, R. W., Crabtree, B. L., Smith, R. and Marmer, D. J. 1986. Immunologic responses following serial skin testing. *J. Immunol. Methods* 86:213-216.

Steinman, R. M. and Cohn, Z. A. 1973. Identification of a novel cell type in peripheral lymphoid organs of mice. I. Morphology, quantitation, tissue distribution. *J. Exp. Med.* 137:1142–1162.

Steinman, R. M. and Nussenzweig, M. C. 1980. Dendritic cells: Features and functions. *Immunol. Rev.* 53:127–147.

Stejskal, V. D. M., Olin, R. G. and Forsbeck, M. 1986. The lymphocyte transformation test for diagnosis of drug-induced occupational allergy. *J. Allergy Clin. Immunol.* 77:411–426.

Stingl, G., Katz, S. I., Clement, L., Green, I. and Shevach, E. M. 1978. Immunological functions of Ia-bearing epidermal Langerhans cells. *J. Immunol.* 121:2005–2013.

Stoolman, L. M. 1989. Adhesion molecules controlling lymphocyte migration. *Cell* 56:907–910.

Streilein, J. W. 1983. Skin associated lymphoid tissue (SALT): Origins and function. *J. Invest. Dermatol.* 80(suppl.):125–165.

Streilein, J. W. and Grammer, S. 1989. Evidence that Langerhans cells can exist in two different states of functional activity with respect to antigen presentation. Abstr. *J. Invest. Dermatol.* 92:523.

Suitters, A. J. and Lampert, I. A. 1982. Expression of Ia antigen on epidermal keratinocytes is a consequence of cellular immunity. *Br. J. Exp. Pathol.* 63:207–213.

Suomalainen, H. A. 1986. The monoclonal antibodies TROP-4 and 4F2 detect the same membrane antigen that is expressed at an early stage of lymphocyte activation and is retained on secondary lymphocytes. *J. Immunol.* 137:422–427.

Svejgaard, E., Morling, N., Svejgaard, A. and Veien, N. K. 1978. Lymphocyte transformation induced by nickel sulfate: An in vitro study of subjects with and without a positive nickel patch test. *Acta Derm. Venereol. (Stockh.)* 58:245–250.

Swoboda, B., Fritz, J. and Ludvan, M. 1977. Nickelallergie und leukozyten-Migrations-Hemmung. *Dermatol. Mschr.* 163:208–212.

Szigeti, R., Kagan-Haion, K., Klein, E. and Ben-Sasson, S. Z. 1986. Radiation leukemia virus-transformed immunocompetent T cells. II. Antigen-induced macrophage migration inhibition factor and leukocyte migration inhibition factor production. *Cell. Immunol.* 102:89–98.

Szilagyi, I., Dobozy, A., Hunyadi, J. and Simon, N. 1971. Lymphozyten-Transformations-Test bei der Untersuchung der durch Tulpen verursachten Überempfindlichkeit. *Berufsdermatosen* 19:14–22.

Talmadge, K. W., Gallati, H., Sinigaglia, F., Walz, A. and Garotta, G. 1986. Identity between human interferon-gamma and "macrophage activating factor" produced by human T lymphocytes. *Eur J. Immunol.* 16:1471–1477.

Tamaki, K. and Katz, S. I. 1980. Ontogeny of Langerhans cells. *J. Invest. Dermatol.* 75:12–13.

Tamaki, K., Fujiwara, H., Levy, R. B., Shearer, G. M. and Katz, S. I. 1981. Hapten specific TNP-reactive cytotoxic effector cells using epidermal cells as targets. *J. Invest. Dermatol.* 77:225–229.

Tamura, S.-I., Tsuru, S., Chiba, J. and Kojima, A. 1982. Production by cultured spleen cells of inflammatory substances and other lymphokines that mediate delayed type hypersensitivity in mice. *Microbiol. Immunol.* 26:1065–1077.

Tan, I. B., Drexhage, H. A., Scheper, R. J., Von Blomberg-Van der Flier, B. M. E., De Haan-Meulman, M., Snow, G. B. and Balm, F. J. M. 1986. Immunosuppressive retroviral p15E-related factors in head and neck carcinomas. *Arch. Otolaryngol. Head Neck Surg.* 112:942–945.

Ternowitz, T. and Thestrup-Pedersen, K. 1986. Epidermis and lymphocyte interactions during a tuberculin skin reaction. II. Epidermis contains specific lymphocyte chemotactic factors. *J. Invest. Dermatol.* 87:613–616.

Teunissen, M. B. M., Wormmeester, J., Krieg, S. R., Petes, P. J., Kapsenberg, M. L. and Bos, J. D. 1989. Maturation of human epidermal Langerhans cells in vitro. *Abstr. J. Invest. Dermatol.* 92:531.

Thestrup-Pedersen, K. 1975. Suppression of tuberculin skin reactivity by prior skin testing. *Immunology* 28:343–348.

Thestrup-Pedersen, K., Jórgensen, B., Kaltoft, K. and Jensen, J. R. 1985. In vivo and in vitro changes in cell mediated immunity following tuberculin skin testing in humans. *Br. J. Dermatol.* 113(suppl. 28):81–85.

Thomas, D. W., Forni, G., Shevach, E. M. and Green, I. 1977. The role of the macrophage as the stimulator cell in contact sensitivity. *J. Immunol.* 118:1677–1681.

Thulin, H. and Zachariae, H. 1972. The leukocyte migration test in chromium sensitivity. *J. Invest. Dermatol.* 58:55–58.

Thulin, H. 1976. The leukocyte migration test in nickel contact dermatitis. *Acta Derm. Venereol. (Stockh.)* 56:377–380.

Thurman, G. B., Stull, H. B., Miller, P. J., Stevenson, H. C. and Oldham, R. K. 1983. Utilization of purified human monocytes in agarose droplet assay for measuring migration inhibitory factors. *J. Immunol. Methods* 65:41–53.

Tilden, A. B. and Balch, C. M. 1982. A comparison of PGE2 effects on human suppressor cell function and on interleukin-2 function. *J. Immunol.* 129:2469–2473.

Tio, D. 1976. A study on the clinical application of a direct leukocyte migration test in chromium contact allergy. *Br. J. Dermatol.* 94:65–70.

Tjernlund, U., Scheynius, A. and Strand, A. 1987. In vitro testing of contact sensitivity. *Acta Derm. Venereol. (Stockh.)* 67:417–421.

Toews, G., Bergstresser, P., Streilein, J., et al. 1980. Epidermal Langerhans cell density determines whether contact hypersensitivity or unresponsiveness follows skin painting with DNFB. *J. Immunol.* 124:445–453.

Tosca, N., Parker, D. and Turk, J. L. 1981. The effect of a delayed hypersensitivity skin reaction on in vitro parameters of cell mediated immunity. *Cell. Immunol.* 62:28–37.

Trepel, F. 1975. Kinetik lymphatischer Zellen. In *Lymphozyt und klinische Immunologie*, eds. H. Theml and H. Begemann, pp. 16–26. Berlin: Springer-Verlag.

Trinchieri, G. and Perussia, B. 1985. Immune interferon: A pleiotropic lymphokine with multiple effects. *Immunol. Today* 6:131–136.

Trowsdale, J. 1988. Molecular genetics of the MHC. *Immunology Suppl.* 1:21–23.

Turk, J. L. 1975. *Delayed hypersensitivity,* 2nd ed. Amsterdam: North-Holland Publishing.

Uehara, M. and Ofuji, S. 1977. Suppressed cell mediated immunity associated with eczematous inflammation. *Acta Derm. Venereol. (Stockh.)* 57:137–139.

Unanue, E. R. 1984. Antigen presenting function of the macrophage. *Annu. Rev. Immunol.* 2:375–428.

Unanue, E. R. and Allen, P. M. 1986. Biochemistry and biology of antigen presentation by macrophages. *Cell. Immunol.* 99:3–6.

Vakkila, J. 1989. Both virgin and memory T cells cluster with dendritic cells during autologous and allogeneic mixed leukocyte reaction. *Eur. J. Immunol.* 19:1003–1008.

Van de Plassche-Boers, E. M., Drexhage, H. A. and Kokje-Kleingeld, M. 1985. The use of somatic antigen of *Haemophilus influenzae* for the monitoring of T cell-mediated skin test reactivity in man. *J. Immunol. Methods* 83:353–361.

Van de Plassche-Boers, E. M., Drexhage, H. A., Kokje-Kleingeld, M. and Leezenberg, J. A. 1986. Parameters for T cell mediated immunity to commensal microorganisms in patients with chronic purulent rhino-sinusitis: A comparison between de-

360   B. M. E. von Blomberg et al.

layed type hypersensitivity, lymphocyte transformation test and macrophage migration inhibition factor assay. *Clin. Exp. Immunol.* 66:516–521.

Van der Lugt, L. and Veninga, T. S. 1981. Nonspecific hypersensitivity of the skin. *Dermatologica* 162:438–443.

Van Dinther-Janssen, A. C. H. M., Van Maarseveen, A. C. M. T., De Groot, J. and Scheper, R. J. 1983. Comparative migration of T and B subpopulations into skin inflammatory sites. *Immunology* 48:519–527.

Van Dinther-Janssen, A. C. H. M., Hofland, L. and Scheper, R. J. 1986. Specific plasma cell accumulation in antigen induced chronic inflammation in the guinea pig peritoneal cavity. *Int. Arch. Allergy Appl. Immunol.* 79:14–18.

Van Dongen, J. J. M., Adriaansen, H. J. and Hooijkaas, H. 1988. Review. Immunophenotyping of leukemias and non-Hodgkin's lymphomas. Immunological markers and their CD codes. *Neth. J. Med.* 33:298–314.

Van Hoogstraten, I. M. W., Kraal, G., Boden, D., Vreeburg, K. J. J., Von Blomberg, B. M. E. and Scheper, R. J. 1989. Persistent immune tolerance induced by oral feeding of metal allergens. Abstr. *J. Invest. Dermatol.* 92:537.

Van Hoogstraten, I. M. W., Andersen, K. E., Von Blomberg, M., Boden, D., Bruynzeel, D. P., Burrows, D., Camarasa, J. M. G., Dooms-Goossens, A., Lahti, A., Menne, T., Rycroft, R., Todd, D., Vreeburg, K. J. J., Wilkinson, J. D. and Scheper, R. J. 1989. Preliminary results of a multicenter study on the incidence of nickel allergy in relationship to previous oral and cutaneous contacts. In *Current Topics in Contact Dermatitis*, eds. P. J. Frosch, A. Dooms-Goossens, J. M. Lachapelle, R. J. G. Rycroft and R. J. Scheper, pp. 178–186. Heidelberg: Springer-Verlag.

Van Ketel, W. G. 1978. Patch testing with nickel sulfate in DMSO. *Contact Dermatitis* 4:167–168.

Van Ketel, W. G. 1979. Patch testing with eye cosmetics. *Contact Dermatitis* 5:402–404.

Van Ketel, W. G. 1981. Petrolatum—A reliable vehicle for metal allergens? *Contact Dermatitis* 7:60–62.

Van Lier, A. W., Oudkerk-Pool, M., Kabel, P., Mouse, S., Terpstra, F., De Rie, M. A., Melief, C. J. M. and Miedema, F. 1988. Anti-CD27 monoclonal antibodies identify two functionally distinct subpopulations within the CD4$^+$ T cell subset. *Eur. J. Immunol.* 18:811–816.

Van Loveren, H., Kato, K., Ratzlaff, R. E., Meade, R., Ptak, W. and Askenase, P. W. 1984. Use of micrometers and calipers to measure various components of delayed-type hypersensitivity ear swelling reactions in mice. *J. Immunol. Methods* 67:311–319.

Van Oers, M. H. J., Pinkster, J. and Zeijlemaker, W. P. 1978. Quantification of antigen reactive cells among human T lymphocytes. *Eur. J. Immunol.* 8:477–484.

Van Voorhis, W. C., Valinsky, J., Hoffman, E., Luban, J., Hair, L. S. and Steinman, R. M. 1983. Relative efficacy of human monocytes and dendritic cells as accessory cells for T cell replication. *J. Exp. Med.* 158:174–191.

Veerman, A. J. P. 1974. On the interdigitating cells in the thymus dependent area of rat spleen. A relation between the mononuclear phagocyte system and T lymphocytes. *Cell Tissue Res.* 148:247.

Veien, N. K., Svejgaard, E. and Menne, T. 1979. In vitro lymphocyte transformation to nickel: A study of nickel sensitive patients before and after epicutaneous and oral challenge with nickel. *Acta Derm. Venereol. (Stockh.)* 59:447–451.

Veien, N. K., Hattel, T., Justesen, O. and Nørholm, A. 1983. Oral challenge with metal salts. (1) Vesicular patch-test-negative hand eczema. *Contact Dermatitis* 9:402–406.

Veldman, J. E. 1970. *Histophysiology and Electron Microscopy of the Immune Response*. Groningen: NV Boekdrukkerij Niemeyer.

Von Blomberg, B. M. E., Rijlaarsdam, U. and Scheper, R. J. 1976. Direct macrophage migration inhibition test in DNCB contact sensitized guinea pigs. *Int. Arch. Allergy Appl. Immunol.* 50:503–512.

Von Blomberg, B. M. E., Boerrigter, G. H. and Scheper, R. J. 1978. Interference of simultaneous skin tests in delayed hypersensitivity. *Immunology* 35:361–367.

Von Blomberg, B. M. E. and Scheper, R. J. 1980. Hapten-cell conjugates in DNCB contact sensitivity. In vitro stimulation with DNP-conjugates optimally inducing contact sensitivity in vivo. *Immunology* 39:291–299.

Von Blomberg, B. M. E., Scheper, R. J., Mullink, H. and Polak, L. 1982. Differential capacity of macrophages from various sources to act as hapten-specific stimulator cells in vitro. *Int. Arch. Allergy Appl. Immunol.* 68:392–396.

Von Blomberg, B. M. E., Scheper, R. J., Boerrigter, G. H. and Polak, L. 1984. Induction of contact sensitivity to a broad variety of allergens with haptenized macrophages. *J. Invest. Dermatol.* 83:91–95.

Von Blomberg, B. M. E., Van der Burg, C. K. H., Pos, O., Van de Plassche-Boers, E. M., Van Ketel, W. G. and Scheper, R. J. 1984. In vitro diagnosis of nickel allergy: The MMIT revisited. In *Experimental Contact Dermatitis,* eds. C. Benezra, N. Hunziker, T. Maurer, R. J. Scheper and J. L. Turk, pp. 37–43. Basel: Roche.

Von Blomberg, B. M. E., Bruynzeel, D. P. and Scheper, R. J. 1986. De waarde van in vitro testen bij geneesmiddel overgevoeligheid. In *Geneesmiddelen-erupties,* eds. D. P. Bruynzeel, T. Van Joost, W. G. Van Ketel, G. Smeenk, R. Willemze and E. Young, pp. 39–43. Nieuwegein: Glaxo bv.

Von Blomberg, B. M. E., Van der Burg, C. K. H., Pos, O., Van de Plassche-Boers, E. M., Bruynzeel, D. P., Garotta, G. and Scheper, R. J. 1987. In vitro studies in nickel allergy: Diagnostic value of a dual parameter analysis. *J. Invest. Dermatol.* 88:362–368.

Von Blomberg, B. M. E., Bruynzeel, D. P. and Scheper, R. J. 1989. The impact of 25 years in vitro testing in acd. In *Current Topics in Contact Dermatitis,* eds. P. J. Frosch, A. Dooms-Goossens, J. M. Lachapelle, R. J. G. Rycroft and R. J. Scheper, pp. 569–577. Heidelberg: Springer-Verlag.

Vreeburg, K. J. J., Van Hoogstraten, I. M. W., Von Blomberg, B. M. E., De Groot, K. and Scheper, R. J. 1990. Oral induction of immunological tolerance to chromium. *J. Dental Res.,* in press.

Vreeburg, K. J. J., De Groot, K., Van Hoogstraten, I. M. W., Von Blomberg, B. M. E. and Scheper, R. J. 1989. Successful induction of allergic contact dermatitis to chromium and mercury in mice.

Vreeburg, K. J. J., Van Hoogstraten, I. M. W., Von Blomberg, B. M. E., De Groot, K. and Scheper, R. J. 1990. Oral induction of immunological tolerance to chromium in the guinea pig. *J. Dental Res.,* in press.

Vyakarnam, A. and Lachmann, P. J. 1984. Migration inhibition factor secreting human T cell lines reactive to PPD: A study of their antigen specificity, MHC restriction and the use of Epstein Barr virus-transformed B cell lines as requirement for antigen presenting cells. *Immunology* 53:601–610.

Wahlberg, J. E. 1989. Assessment of erythema—A comparison between the naked eye and laser Doppler flowmetry. In *Current Topics in Contact Dermatitis,* eds. P. J. Frosch, A. Dooms-Goossens, J. M. Lachapelle, R. J. G. Rycroft and R. J. Scheper, pp. 549–553. Heidelberg: Springer-Verlag.

Wantzin, G. L., Ralfkiaer, E., Lisby, S. and Rothlein, R. 1988. The role of intercellular adhesion molecules in inflammatory skin reactions. *Br. J. Dermatol.* 119:141–145.

Weaver, C. T. and Unanue, E. R. 1986. T cell induction of membrane IL-1 on macrophages. *J. Immunol.* 137:3868–3873.

Weaver, C. T. and Unanue, E. R. 1990. The costimulatory function of antigen-presenting cells. *Immunol. Today* 11:49–55.

Weigent, D. A., Hoeprich, P. D., Bost, K. L., Brunck, T. K., Reiher, W. E. and Blalock, J. E. 1986. The HTLV ii envelope protein contains a hexapeptide homologous to a region of interleukin-2 that binds to the interleukin-2 receptor. *Biochem. Biophys. Res. Commun.* 139:367–374.

Weiser, W. Y., Greineder, D. K., Remold, H. G. and David, J. R. 1981. Studies on human migration inhibitory factor: Characterization of three molecular species. *J. Immunol.* 126:1958–1962.

Weiser, W. Y., Remold, H. G. and David, J. R. 1985. Generation of human hybridomas producing migration inhibitory factor (MIF) and of murine hybridomas secreting monoclonal antibodies to human MIF. *Cell. Immunol.* 90:167–178.

Wendel, G. D., Stark, B. J., Jamison, R. B., Molina, R. D. and Sullivan, T. J. 1985. Penicillin allergy and desensitization in serious infections during pregnancy. *N. Engl. J. Med.* 312:1229–1232.

Wikner, N. E., Huff, J. C., Norris, D. A., Boyce, S. T., Cary, M., Kissinger, M. and Weston, W. L. 1986. Study of HLA-DR synthesis in cultured human keratinocytes. *J. Invest. Dermatol.* 87:559–564.

Williams, W. R. and Williams, W. J. 1982a. Development of beryllium lymphocyte transformation tests in chronic beryllium disease. *Int. Arch. Allergy Appl. Immunol.* 67:175–180.

Williams, W. R. and Williams, W. J. 1982b. Comparison of lymphocyte transformation and macrophage migration inhibition tests in the detection of beryllium sensitivity. *J. Clin. Pathol.* 35:684–687.

Willis, C. M., Stephens, C. J. M. and Wilkinson, J. D. 1988. Assessment of erythema in irritant contact dermatitis. *Contact Dermatitis* 18:138.

Willis, C. M., Young, E., Brandon, D. R. and Wilkinson, J. D. 1986. Immunopathological and ultrastructural findings in human allergic and irritant contact dermatitis. *Br. J. Dermatol.* 115:305–316.

Wolff, K. and Stingl, G. 1983. The Langerhans cell. *J. Invest. Dermatol.* 80:17s–21s.

Wood, G. S., Volterra, A. S., Abel, E. A., Nickoloff, B. J. and Adams, R. M. 1986. Allergic contact dermatitis: Novel immunohistologic features. *J. Invest. Dermatol.* 87:688.

Yamada, M., Niwa, Y., Fujimoto, F. and Yoshinaga, H. 1972. Lymphocyte transformation in allergic contact dermatitis. *Jpn. J. Dermatol.* 82:94–97.

Yu, D. T. Y. 1978. Effect of corticosteroids on human in vitro anamnestic response. *Cell. Immunol.* 40:431.

Zachariae, C., Ternowitz, T. H., Larsen, C. G., Nielsen, V. and Thestrup-Pedersen, K. 1988. Epidermal lymphocyte chemotactic factor specifically attracts OKT4$^+$ lymphocytes. *Arch. Dermatol. Res.* 280:354–357.

13

identification of contact allergens: predictive tests in animals

■ Georg Klecak ■

INTRODUCTION

The objective of this chapter is to describe the experimental animal procedures that are claimed to be appropriate for predictive testing of the allergenic potential of chemicals and finished formulations as well as for calculating the risk of sensitization associated with skin contact with these substances and being in line with FDA (1980), EPA (1980), or OECD (1981) guidelines for testing standards. Before dealing with the experimental strategy of individual test procedures, however, some essential aspects of dermatology and experimental immunology should be recalled.

Human modes of behavior in industrial society essentially determine the conditioning data of exposure to allergens and thus the rise of sensitization risk (Turk, 1966, 1967; Rostenberg, 1957). The skin has, among other functions, that of protecting against all insults to the organism from the environment (Stüttgen, 1972; Stüttgen et al., 1965; Blank and Scheuplein, 1969; Jarrett, 1973). The chemical industry introduces a multiplicity of new substances and products, some of which, in case of accidental or intentional contact with the skin surface, may cause an allergic contact dermatitis (Adams et al., 1987; Andersen et al., 1983; Baer, 1964; Bandman et al., 1972; Calnan, 1962; Calnan et al., 1970; Cruickshank, 1969; Department of Health, Education and Welfare, 1975; Ferguson and Rothman, 1959; Fisher, 1967; Fisher et al., 1971; Fregert et al., 1969a, 1969b; Hjorth, 1959, 1961; Hjorth and Fregert, 1972; Magnusson and Möller, 1979; Miescher, 1962; Rantuccio and Meneghini,

1970; Rostenberg, 1953, 1954; NACDG, 1973a, 1973b). The increasing frequency of allergic dermatitis in occupational diseases (Cronin and Wilkinson,
1973) reflects the effect on humans of chemical pollution in the environment
(Agrup, 1969a, 1969b; Agrup and Cronin, 1969; Andersen and Maibach,
1980; Bruze et al., 1989; Cronin, 1980; Epstein, 1962; Ferguson and Rothman,
1959; Foussereau and Benezra, 1970; Grimm and Gries, 1968; Hjorth, 1980;
Lüders, 1976; Magnusson and Mobacken, 1972; Malten et al., 1964, 1969,
1971; Malten, 1979; Marcussen, 1962; Pililä, 1947, 1962; Rudner et al., 1973;
Rudzki and Kleiniewsak, 1970; Schubert et al., 1973; Schwartz and Peck,
1940; Schwartz et al., 1957).

In addition to the relatively small group of substances that are obligatory
allergens (Paschoud, 1967), there is a large and steadily growing group of
facultative allergenic agents (Baer et al., 1973; Epstein, 1962; Epstein et al.,
1968; Fregert et al., 1969b; Meneghini et al., 1971; Mitchell, 1975; Schwartz
and Peck, 1944). As their allergenic potential is variable, it is necessary to have
a reliable predictive method for determining the risk of contact sensitization to
these substances. Because of their selective skin pathogenicity, only part of the
population is at risk. Whether an individual is affected is related to immune
responsiveness as well as momentary skin condition (Evans, 1963). A dysfunction of the skin barrier, with or without overt skin manifestations, favors contact
sensitization. To comprehend a broad spectrum of potential allergens is thus of
interest not only from a clinical (Coombs and Gell, 1968) but also from an
occupational-medical and industrial-hygienic viewpoint (Malten, 1975). The
complexity of this problem reaches far beyond the purely medical aspects; it
also has economic and sociopolitical dimensions. A number of measures within
the compass of technology and occupational and preventive medicine have been
taken and regulations have been issued (Bär, 1969; Behrbohm, 1975; Federal
Register Amendment, 1964; Hopf, 1971).

"Absolute innocuousness" does not exist. Most products are neither
wholly innocuous nor very dangerous. There are opportunities for injury
through misuse or inadequate exposure (Gleason et al., 1969; Gloxhuber, 1967,
1976; Opdyke, 1975; Rand, 1972). The risk of injury resulting from product
exposure must be kept as low as possible; it should be restricted to such a
degree that no special measures for users' protection are necessary (Anderson,
1975; Bär, 1974; Goldemberg, 1962; Weil, 1972). Practical experience is the
best guide for determining which biological properties are relevant to consumer
safety (Idman, 1976; Siegel and Melther, 1948). For new substances, experimental investigations provide a reliable basis for estimating hazards (Calnan et
al., 1964; Carter and Griffith, 1965; Dohr-Lux and Lietz, 1965; Draize et al.,
1944; Gloxhuber, 1974; Gloxhuber et al., 1974; Rowe and Olson, 1965). However, not every test procedure succeeds in doing this. Laboratory experiments
may be conducted under extreme or unrealistic conditions. When evaluating the
results, one considers how the relevant dermatotoxicologic and allergologic
data should be interpreted for humans and what other factors—such as form of

application and conditions of exposure—must be considered (Rand, 1972; Rostenberg, 1959; Weil, 1972).

Numerous biological test procedures in humans and animals have been devised, both for research related to eczema and to help the physician recognize the etiologic agents involved (Hardy, 1973; Steigleder, 1975). Various test procedures with a predictive character have been described (Calnan et al., 1964; Epstein and Kligman, 1964; Griffith, 1969; Holland et al., 1950; Maibach and Epstein, 1965; Newcomer and Landau, 1964; Rostenberg, 1959). These methods determine mainly allergenic capability, and seldom sensitizing capacity (Gloxhuber, 1976; Idson, 1968; Maibach, 1975; Rowe and Olson, 1965). Their development was motivated by clinical experience (Schwartz, 1951). The patch test of Jadassohn (1896a, 1896b) is still used with many variants for both induction and elicitation of contact sensitization (Magnusson et al., 1962, 1965, 1966; Schwartz and Peck, 1944).

In principle, predictive sensitization studies in humans are of two types: the "prophetic" patch test (Brunner and Smiljanic, 1952; Epstein and Kligman, 1964; Schwartz and Peck, 1944, 1946; Traub et al., 1954) and the "repeated-insult" patch test. The repeated-insult test (Draize, 1955, 1959; Shelanski and Shelanski, 1953) was a modification of the Landsteiner technique (Landsteiner and Jacobs, 1935, 1936; Landsteiner and Chase, 1937, 1941; Landsteiner and Di Somma, 1938) for guinea pigs and was intended to evaluate finished formulations. Simultaneous use of mild irritants such as sodium lauryl sulfate (SLS), allergens, and occlusive application potentiates penetration and enhances sensitization (Kligman and Epstein, 1959).

The "maximization provocative patch test" of Kligman (1966a, 1966b, 1966c, 1966d) is intended to classify substances according to the sensitizing capacity they elicit under arbitrarily defined sets of experimental conditions. This method is justifiable from an experimental point of view (Brunner, 1967; Giovacchini, 1972; Greif, 1967; Kligman and Epstein, 1975; Marzulli and Maibach, 1974). With respect to the risk of injury to persons involved in the test, Kligman's maximization test is controversial and is inadmissible in many countries (Agrup, 1968). The experience of many years suggests that humans as well as guinea pigs are suitable for experimental studies on allergic contact dermatitis (Magnusson and Kligman, 1970; Maguire, 1975; Maibach, 1975; Marzulli et al., 1968; Maurer et al., 1985). The sequence for predictive testing should be: animal first, human afterwards.

After Jadassohn in 1896 differentiated between toxic and allergic reactions in an eczematous patient by means of a patch test, experimental studies of delayed-type allergy flourished. With the successful sensitizing assay of Bloch and Steiner-Wourlisch in humans in 1926 and in guinea pigs in 1930 by means of a *Primula veris* extract, experimental studies of the mechanism of contact allergy in animals gained importance. The systematic studies of Landsteiner and co-workers (1935, 1936, 1937) brought about the most significant understanding of incubation period, sensitization routes, dosage dependence, group specificity, technique of application, and duration of sensitization. The later findings of Landsteiner and Chase (1941, 1942) on the formation of antigens by interaction of simple chemical substances with protein carriers in exposed guinea pig skin were corroborated by Sulzberger and Baer (1938), Simon (1936), and Simon et al. (1934). Chase (1941, 1950, 1953) closely examined genetics in guinea pigs in relation to susceptibility to skin sensitization. Landsteiner and Chase (1941) noted the influence of adjuvants. Frey and Wenk (1956, 1958) verified the role of regional lymph nodes in the mechanism of delayed-type allergy. In reviewing the innumerable experimental studies of contact dermatitis, we see that only the test object (guinea pig or human) and the application of generally strong allergens such as dinitrochlorobenzene (DNCB) and picryl chloride were common features until the middle of the 1950s (Chase, 1950, 1954; Chase and Maguire, 1974). This methodological arbitrariness was tolerable in basic research on immunologic processes. Shelanski and Shelanski (1953), Draize et al. (1944), and Draize (1959) took the first step toward standardizing the test methods in humans and animals for predictive purposes.

The factors that most influence the occurrence of allergic contact dermatitis can be divided into physiological and physicochemical ones (Federal Register Amendment, 1964; Katz and Poulsen, 1971; Kligman, 1966a; La Du, 1965; Meyer and Ziegenmeyer, 1975; Rockwell, 1955; Wagner, 1961; Scheuplein, 1965; Stoughton, 1965). When animal models are used as a substitute for experiments in humans in dermatotoxicology, the differences and similarities between species represent the most important physiological factors. The structural and biochemical differences between human and animal skin (Bartek et al., 1972; Davies et al., 1972; Dvorak et al., 1974; Justice et al., 1961; Oberste-Lehn and Wiemann, 1950; Roudabush et al., 1965) influence penetration. Eczematous sensitization occurs in species other than humans and guinea pigs (Asherson and Ptak, 1968; Crowle and Crowle, 1961; Frey and Geleick, 1959; Nobréus et al., 1974; Rostenberg and Haeberlin, 1950; Roudabush et al., 1965; Strauss, 1937). Guinea pigs have proved especially suitable for experimental sensitization. Handling and economy are decisive factors in their choice for screening procedures (Asherson and Ptak, 1968; Ginsburg et al., 1937; Hood et al., 1965; Hunziker, 1969; Jadassohn et al., 1955; Landsteiner and Chase, 1941; Lane-Petter and Porter, 1963; Maguire, 1974a, 1974b; Maibach and Mitchell, 1975; Malten et al., 1966a, 1966b; Middleton, 1978; Nicholas, 1978; Oberste-Lehn and Wiemann, 1950; Paterson, 1966; Polak et al., 1973; Poole et al., 1970; Rackemann and Simon, 1934; Ritz et al., 1975; Rostenberg, 1947; Sulzberger, 1930; Thorgeirsson et al., 1975; Voss, 1958; Ziegler et al., 1972).

Guinea pigs stem from a strain endowed genetically with the property of homogeneously reacting upon antigenic exposure. Appropriate strains include the Hartley and Pirbright ones; animals of either sex are used. Even among the commonly used strains there are striking differences, which Chase (1941, 1953) and Polak and co-workers (Polak et al., 1968a; Polak and Turk, 1968b) attributed to a Mendelian dominant characteristic. The proclivity to sensitization must be verified from time to time by using "standard" sensitizers. Housing and feeding conditions should correspond to those defined in the Guide for the animal care and use of laboratory animals or in OECD guidelines (1981). Some of the physicochemical factors that are important in sensitization are identical with those enhancing skin penetration. How much of a potential allergen can pass the skin barrier is of paramount theoretical and practical importance (Calvery et al., 1946; Cameron and Short, 1966; Idson, 1971; Jungermann and Silberman, 1972; Katz and Poulsen, 1971; Landsdown and Grasso, 1972; Smeenk and Rijnbeek, 1969; Schaefer et al., 1975; Scheuplein, 1965; Schumacher, 1967; Stoughton, 1965; Stüttgen, 1972; Vinson et al., 1965; Wagner, 1961). The physicochemical properties of the vehicle (Bronaugh et al., 1981; Christensen et al., 1984a; Coldman et al., 1969; Higuchi, 1960; Hjorth and Trolle-Lassen, 1963; Katz and Poulsen, 1972; Katz and Shaikh, 1965; Mikkelsen and Trolle-Lassen, 1969; Ostrenga, 1971; Poulsen et al., 1968; Ritschel, 1969; Schaefer, 1974; Schaefer et al., 1975; Stemann, 1965; Wurster, 1968; Zesch, 1974) and of chemicals (Baer et al., 1967; Bleumink et al., 1976; Chulz, 1962; Johnson et al., 1972; Katz and Shaikh, 1965; Lieu and Tong, 1973; Nilzen and Wikström, 1955; Treherne, 1956; Wolter et al., 1970) and the dose or concentration of test articles (Allenby et al., 1989; Marzulli and Maibach, 1974; Stadler et al., 1985; White et al., 1986), duration of exposure, and condition of the skin surface are determining for the occurrence of contact sensitization (Andersen and Maibach, 1985b; Baker, 1968; Bettley, 1961; Blank, 1952; Brauer, 1974; Katz and Poulsen, 1972; Landsdown and Grasso, 1972; Lippold, 1974; Marzulli, 1962; Rischel, 1969; Scheuplein, 1965; Stemann, 1965; Vinson et al., 1965; Wurster, 1968). The intradermal route passes natural barriers and in no way resembles real conditions of handling and consuming chemicals.

This chapter describes in detail the test procedures most frequently used in guinea pigs, including the Draize test (DT), the optimization test (OT), Freund's complete adjuvant test (FCAT), the guinea pig maximization test (GPMT) of Magnusson and Kligman, Maguire's modified "split adjuvant" technique, the Bühler test, and the open epicutaneous test (OET) (see Fig. 1).

These tests may be classified according to use of complete Freund's adjuvant (CAF) in non-FCA tests (DT, Bühler test, OET) and in FCA tests (FCAT, Maguire test, GPMT, single injection adjuvant test); or they may be divided, depending on the strategy used for administration of the test material for induction, into three groups:

1. Epicutaneous methods (Bühler test, OET, and Maguire split adjuvant technique)
2. Intradermal methods (DT, OT, and FCAT)
3. Methods using both application routes (Maguire split adjuvant technique and GPMT)

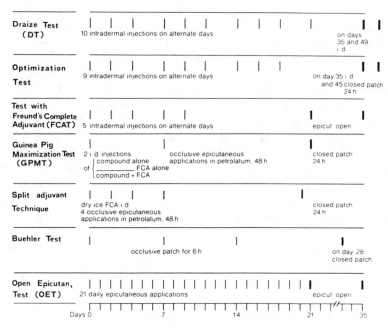

FIGURE 1 Techniques for detecting the capacity of low-molecular-weight compounds to induce contact hypersensitivity in guinea pigs.

To complete the array of guinea pig tests that have proved their predictivity, the following tests should also be mentioned: cumulative contact enhancement test (Tsuchiya et al., 1982, 1985); chamber test (Kero and Hannuksela, 1980); Dossou and Sicard test (Dossou et al., 1985); epicutaneous maximization test (Brulos et al., 1977; Guillot and Gonnet, 1985); modified GPMT (Sato et al., 1981; Sato, 1985); single injection adjuvant test—SIAT—(Goodwin et al., 1981); and TINA test (Ziegler and Süss, 1985).

DRAIZE TEST

In 1944, 1955, and 1959 Draize published the first animal test with a predictive character for determining the allergenicity of new chemical substances. This technique is a variant of the classical Landsteiner and Jacobs technique, which was used in the 1930s for the determination of the allergenicity of simple chemicals in guinea pigs. The Draize test is carried out as follows (see Fig. 2).

Materials and Methods

Animals. One or two groups of albino guinea pigs are used: (1) the experimental group (20 animals) and (2) the control group (facultative; 10 animals).

Materials. The test substance is injected intradermally (id) as a 0.1% solution, suspension, or emulsion in 0.85% NaCl, paraffin oil, or polyethylene glycol.

Induction

Before starting the treatment, an area of the back and the upper anterior flank of the animal are shaved with an electric clipper. Shaving is repeated before each reading and before any further injection. During about 3 wk the animals of the experimental group are given one id injection every second day, a total of 10 injections.

Day 0: Each animal of the experimental group is injected with 0.05 ml of the 0.1% solution, suspension, or emulsion of the test substance.

Day 1: Reading of skin reactions is performed.

Days 2–21: The remaining nine injections are administered as follows: Within an area of 3 × 4 cm on the back and the upper anterior flank, every second day, 0.1 ml of the test material is injected id at different spots; the skin reactions are read 24 h after each id injection.

Challenge

Days 32–35: The challenge is carried out on the contralateral flank of the experimental animal on a skin site that corresponds to the one subjected to the first injection. Control animals, if used, are treated in the same way

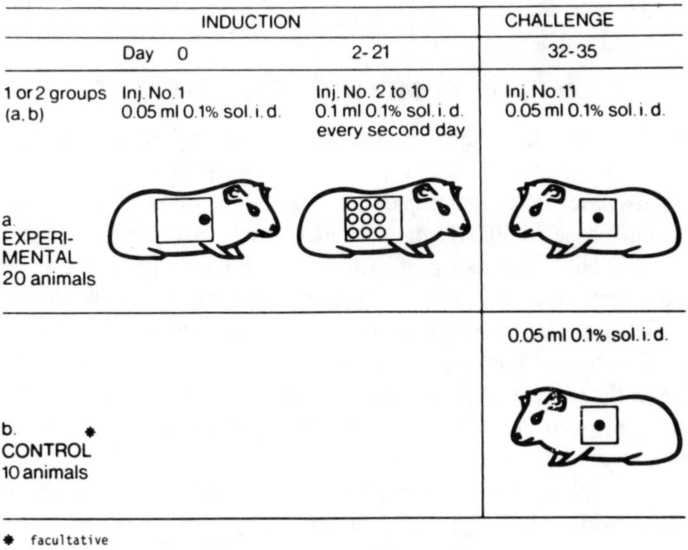

	INDUCTION		CHALLENGE
	Day 0	2- 21	32-35
1 or 2 groups (a, b)	Inj. No.1 0.05 ml 0.1% sol. i. d.	Inj. No. 2 to 10 0.1 ml 0.1% sol. i. d. every second day	Inj. No. 11 0.05 ml 0.1% sol. i. d.
a. EXPERI- MENTAL 20 animals			
			0.05 ml 0.1% sol. i. d.
b. ♦ CONTROL 10 animals			

♦ facultative

FIGURE 2 The Draize test.

and simultaneously, with 0.05 ml of the 0.1% test solution injected id in each animal.

Days 36–37: Animals of both groups are shaved and later are investigated. The intensity of erythema and occurrence and size of edema of the test reaction are evaluated and recorded.

Evaluation

To determine whether a test substance has sensitizing properties, the reactions of all animals after the first id injection (0.05 ml) are compared with the challenge test reactions among themselves and, if negative controls are used, among the control animals. If there are extreme differences between the reactions within a group, the averages of the mean values for the induction and test phases within the group are compared. The same holds for the mean values of the eliciting tests within the experimental and control groups.

Discussion

According to experience, the Draize test fails to identify substances with a weak allergenic potential (Bühler, 1964; Johnson et al., 1985; Klecak et al., 1977; Magnusson and Kligman, 1970; Maguire, 1973a, 1973b, 1980; Marzulli and Maguire, 1982; Maurer, 1974). Besides, it proves merely applicable for chemicals but not for finished preparations. Its modifications (Sharp, 1978) did not improve the predictive value of this testing strategy (Goodwin, 1981). Although recognized by FDA as well as EPA and listed in Japanese guidelines for toxicity studies, the Draize test is not stated in OECD Testing Guidelines (1981) as a predictive test method for assessment of allergenicity of chemical raw materials and final products.

FREUND'S COMPLETE ADJUVANT TEST

Freund's complete adjuvant test was devised by Klecak, Geleick, and Frey (Klecak et al., 1977; Klecak, 1985). This test is a modification of the Landsteiner-Chase (1940) technique that is used in various laboratories. During the induction phase of FCAT, the test material is mixed with FCA, and the mixture is applied id to guinea pigs. The experimental design of FCAT has been continuously optimized with respect to simple performance and high sensitivity. The modification used at present involves 3 id injections within 10 days, while the original technique consisted of 5 id injections on alternate days. The concentration of the test material used for induction was reduced from 50% to 5%, and instead of using the anterior part of the flank skin, the scapula region is used for induction.

The principles for the challenge phase have remained unchanged during the years. A wide range of primary nonirritating concentrations is used, and dose response patterns are established for elicitation concentrations in terms of minimal eliciting and maximal noneliciting ones. This is the most significant difference between the FCAT and other comparable test procedures, like the optimization test, maximization test, single injection adjuvant test, and split adjuvant technique. Intradermal application is preferred for challenging only if substances have to be tested that color the skin and make reading of erythema impossible.

Materials and Methods

Animals. Two groups of 10–20 guinea pigs each are used: (1) the experimental group and (2) the control group. An additional four guinea pigs are needed for the primary skin irritation study.

Materials. For the induction, performed by id injection, oil-soluble test material is incorported in Freund's (FCA) complete adjuvant mixed with an equal amount of twice-distilled water so that the final concentration in the emulsions is usually 5%. This depends on the physicochemical properties and the toxicity of the material to be tested. When incorporated in FCA, water-soluble test material is dissolved in the water phase before emulsification. For the challenge, performed by open epicutaneous application, the test material is diluted, emulsified, or suspended in the most appropriate vehicle (water, acetone, alcohol, petrolatum, polyethylene glycol, and so on). The challenge concentrations vary in steps of three, so that any test substance can be tested epicutaneously undiluted as well as at concentrations of 30, 10, and 3% or less.

Induction

Shortly before the pretreatment, the shoulder region of both test and control animals is shaved.

Days 1, 5, and 9: 0.1 ml of the test material in FCA is injected id in the shoulder region of the animals of the experimental group on an area of 4 × 2 cm. The first injection is at the midline and the remaining two on the left and right sides. Animals of the control group are treated with FCA only (see Fig. 3).

Primary Irritation Study

One day before starting the challenge, a group of four guinea pigs is used to determine the threshold toxic concentration after a single topical application. Four different concentrations (e.g., 100, 30, 10, and 3%) are applied simultaneously to the left flank; 0.025 ml of each test concentration is spread homogeneously on a 2 cm^2 area of the flank skin, which was previously clipped and marked with a circular stamp. The highest concentration of a compound used in this test is limited by its solubility. The application site is left uncovered. It is necessary to rotate the various concentrations of the test substance across the different skin sites to minimize variation in response due to differ-

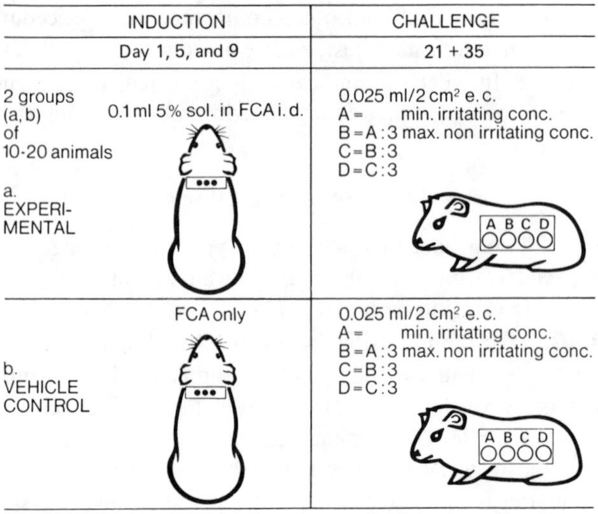

INDUCTION	CHALLENGE
Day 1, 5, and 9	21 + 35
2 groups (a, b) 0.1 ml 5% sol. in FCA i. d. of 10-20 animals a. EXPERI- MENTAL	0.025 ml/2 cm² e. c. A = min. irritating conc. B = A : 3 max. non irritating conc. C = B : 3 D = C : 3 A B C D ○○○○
FCA only b. VEHICLE CONTROL	0.025 ml/2 cm² e. c. A = min. irritating conc. B = A : 3 max. non irritating conc. C = B : 3 D = C : 3 A B C D ○○○○

FIGURE 3   Freund's complete adjuvant test (FCAT).

ent skin areas. Skin reactions are read 24 h after the application of the test substance.

The minimal irritant concentration (A) and maximal nonirritant concentration (B) (threshold concentrations of each substance) are determined by an all-or-none criterion. The minimal irritant concentration is defined as the lowest one causing weak erythema on the test site. The maximal nonirritant concentration is defined as the highest one not causing macroscopic reactions in any of the animals. Estimation of these threshold concentrations is essential for the evaluation of allergic capacity on the basis of end point determination.

Challenge and Rechallenge

Days 21 and 35: To determine whether contact allergy was induced, both groups of animals (experimental and control) are tested on the flank with the same compound at the minimal irritant and some lower (nonirritant) concentrations. Tests are performed by pipetting 0.025 ml of each concentration to skin areas measuring 2 cm². To minimize site-to-site variations in skin reaction, the application of different concentrations of the test material is alternated on the four test sites. For rechallenge on d 35 the contralateral flank can be used.

Days 22–24 and 36–38: The skin sites are always read 24, 48, and 72 h after challenging for erythema, edema, and scaling.

This procedure makes it possible to determine the sensitizing capability of the material tested and the minimal concentration necessary to elicit an allergic reaction. The test material is considered allergenic when animals of the experimental group show positive reactions to nonirritant concentrations used for challenge.

Discussion

This test method is simple to perform and involves low material and operational expenses (Hanau et al., 1983; Klecak, 1985). It is not applicable for testing finished products. Comparative studies show that both FCAT procedures are at least as sensitive as the guinea pig maximization test and the optimization test (Boman et al., 1988; Karlberg et al., 1986, 1988a, 1988b; Klecak et al., 1971; Stampf et al., 1978a, 1978b, 1982b; Stampf and Benezra, 1982a; Van der Walle et al., 1982a, 1982b, 1983).

However, there are some drawbacks, which this technique has in common with all animal models that depend on methods used for induction of sensitization, namely the id injection of the test material incorporated in Freund's complete adjuvant to enhance the immune response in experimental animals. Intradermal application bypasses the penetration-rate-limiting stratum corneum, thus excluding one of the most important variables determining the acquisition of contact sensitization. Like the maximization test and the optimization test, the FCAT procedure provides experimental conditions that represent the very rare situation of skin exposure to a potential allergen. Moreover, the adjuvant may convert chemicals with poor allergenic potential into good sensitizers (See Table 1). Consequently, the FCAT and its modifications can establish the allergenicity of the test material but not the actual risk of contact sensitization under conditions of use (Andersen et al., 1985b; Cheminat et al., 1984; Chung et al., 1977; Hausen et al., 1983, 1986, 1987a, 1987b, 1987c, 1988a, 1988b, 1988c, 1988d; Lepoittevin et al., 1989; Marchand et al., 1982; Schaeffer et al., 1990; Zeller et al., 1985; Zissu et al., 1987).

The foot pad test is another variant of the FCAT. It is used by Polak (1980), and its modification, practiced by Chung et al. (1970; Chung and Giles, 1972; Chung and Carson, 1975), Palazzollo and Di Pasquale (1983), and

TABLE 1. Predictive Value of Human Tests, as Compared to an Animal Test (FCAT)

Number of preparations (268 total)	Human HMT/RIPT	Animal FCAT
136	negative	negative
13	positive	positive
115	negative	positive
4	positive	negative

Parker and Turk (1983). The single injection adjuvant test (SIAT), created and performed by Basketter (1988), Goodwin et al. (1981, 1985a, 1985b), and Johnson et al. (1985) is also a variant of the FCAT. The SIAT procedure is only slightly less sensitive than the GPMT. Maibach and Mitchell (1975) used the SIAT for sensitization of guinea pigs with costus oil.

GUINEA PIG MAXIMIZATION TEST

By determining carefully all factors favoring contact sensitization and combining them in a single procedure, Magnusson and Kligman (1969, 1970, 1975) developed the guinea pig maximization test (GPMT). Assaying known human allergens in the GPMT and the human maximization test, Magnusson and Kligman found a high degree of correlation between the results. Discrepancies were found when the incidences of sensitization by some substances were compared. But agents that sensitized humans invariably sensitized guinea pigs as well. Therefore the GPMT can be considered a reliable procedure for screening of contact allergens and extrapolating the results to humans.

Materials and Methods

Animals.   About equal numbers of male and female guinea pigs are used for (1) the experimental group (10–20 animals), (2) the control or vehicle group (10–20 animals), and (3) the primary irritation group (4 animals).

Materials.   Application is id as well as epicutaneous. For id injections the test material is incorporated into FCA as well as diluted, suspended, or emulsified in NaCl. The concentration of material destined for id injection may elicit neither strong local nor systemic toxic reactions in experimental animals. The concentration is generally between 1 and 5% and seldom, if ever, exceeds 5%. For topical application water-soluble substances are dissolved in water; for oil-soluble ones ethanol or other appropriate vehicles are used. Liquid materials are applied as such or diluted, if necessary. Solids are micronized or reduced to fine powder and then incorporated in a vehicle, usually petrolatum, at a maximum concentration of 25%. If the test agent is an irritant, a concentration is chosen that causes mild to moderate inflammation. If it is not an irritant, the area is pretreated with 10% sodium lauryl sulfate in petrolatum 24 h before the topical induction exposure. The concentrations of test material used for induction are adjusted to the highest one that can be well tolerated systemically.

Induction

Intradermal application.   *Experimental group:*   On d 0 an area of 4 × 6 cm over the shoulder region is clipped short with an electric clipper. Three pairs of id injections are made simultaneously, so that on each side of the midline there are two rows of three injections each. The injection sites are just within the boundaries of the 2 × 4 cm patch, which is applied 1 wk later. Injections are (1) 0.1 ml FCA alone (adjuvant blended with equal amount of water or saline), (2) 0.1 ml test material in saline, and (3) 0.1 ml test material in FCA. Injections 1 and 2 are given close to each other and nearest to the head, injection 3 most caudally (see Fig. 4).

Control group: The animals are given the same injections but without the test agent, that is, FCA and vehicle.

Topical application. Experimental group: on d 7 the same area over the shoulder region is again clipped and shaved with an electric razor. The test agent in petrolatum is spread over a 2 × 4 cm filter paper in an even, rather thick layer or, if liquid, to saturation. The patch is covered by overlapping, impermeable plastic adhesive tape. This, in turn, is firmly secured by an elastic adhesive bandage, which is wound around the torso of the animal. The dressing is left in place for 48 h.

Control group: The animals are exposed to the vehicle without the test agent in the same way as the experimental group. On d 9 the dressings are removed.

The treatment with FCA and occlusive bandage may lower the threshold level for skin irritation. The control group should therefore be exposed to the same maneuvers as the experimental group to exclude any false positive classifications when reading the challenge responses.

Primary Irritation Study

Before the challenge phase is started, the primary irritation study is performed with four fresh animals. Depending on the test material, up to three different concentrations and the vehicle can be applied to the flank skin with a patch, using four aluminum chambers. To minimize site-to-site variations in

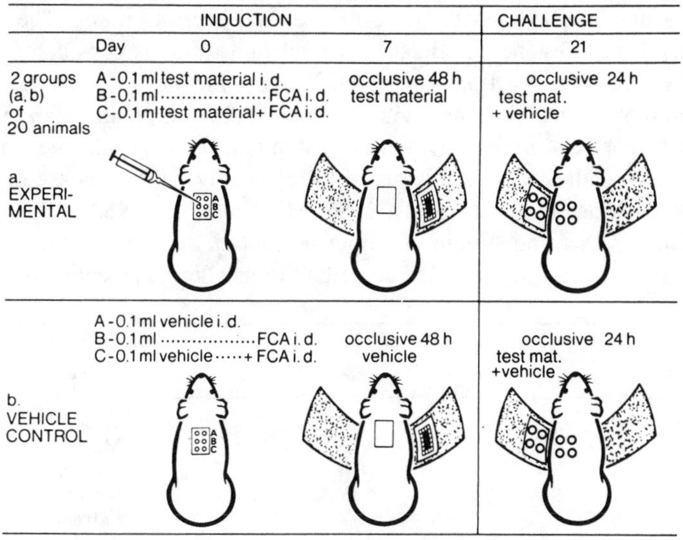

FIGURE 4 Guinea pig maximization test (GPMT).

skin reactivity, the application of different concentrations of test material and vehicle is alternated on the test sites.

Challenge

Day 21: *Patch testing.* In experimental and control animals 5 × 5 cm areas of the flanks are shaved on both sides. Pieces of filter paper measuring 2 × 2 cm are sealed to the flanks for 24 h with the same occlusive bandage as for topical induction: (1) on the left side, a patch with the test agent in the highest nonirritant concentration and the same vehicle as for topical induction, and (2) on the right side, a patch with the vehicle alone. By using smaller ready-made test units, such as aluminum chambers (Finn chambers), challenge with the test agent at different concentrations and the vehicle can be performed on the same flank. If indicated, the contralateral flank can be used for rechallenge.

Days 23 and 24: *Readings.* At 21 h after removing the patches the flank skin is cleaned and shaved, if necessary, and 3 h later the first reading of the reactions is performed. The second reading is made the next day. For evaluation of skin reactions a four-point scale is used:

0 = No reaction
1 = Scattered reactions
2 = Moderate and diffuse reaction
3 = Intense reddening and swelling

Strength and duration of the skin reactions are compared within the experimental group and between the experimental and control groups. The allergic potential of the substance or finished formulation tested is considered proved only when the skin reactions to the challenge with the test material clearly outweigh those to the challenge with the vehicle and are greater than the reactions of the controls. By low frequency of skin reactions to challenge exposure, rechallenge is indicated to confirm any strong positive skin response or invalidate any weak one (Kligman et al., 1986; Mitchell et al., 1982).

Using the scoring system of Kligman (1966c), an individual chemical or finished product may be classified according to its allergic potential as follows:

Sensitization rate (%)	Grade	Class
0–8	I	Weak
9–28	II	Mild
29–64	III	Moderate
65–80	IV	Strong
81–100	V	Extreme

Magnusson and Kligman (1969, 1970) do not regard sensitization of grade I as significant. Material so graded is not considered likely to present a hazard in use. Presumably, this would depend on the type of material, because a final product eliciting a weak reaction would be more hazardous than an individual chemical used as an ingredient in a substantially lower concentration than was tested.

Use of FCA and occlusion may cause some nonspecific effects. Guinea pigs pretreated with FCA have stronger irritant reactions to an occlusive patch of croton oil or other irritant than those not pretreated (B. Magnusson, personal communication). Potential sensitizers, which are also irritants, may show a lower concentration threshold for irritation than for sensitization. To overcome this problem and exclude the nonspecific FCA effect, it is necessary to use a control group pretreated with FCA and vehicle. This is the only way to exclude false positive results. Furthermore, we should point out the influence of the material used for the patch, of the vehicle, and of the tape used (Fernström, 1954, 1955; Magnusson et al., 1962, 1965).

The thickness of the patch is important because it may increase the pressure and therefore the penetration of the sensitizer. For challenging aluminum Finn-chambers (Epitest LDT-Helsinki) or Hilltop plastic chambers are preferred, giving stronger response in sensitized subjects than cellulose or paper disc patches (Pirilä, 1971, 1974; Quisno et al., 1983). Finally, only Elastoplast should be used for the "booster" and challenge occlusive patches. It exerts pressure and holds the patch in position. Pressure is necessary for sensitization and elasticity is necessary for the comfort of the animal.

We have frequently observed strong skin reactions during induction of sensitization by id injection in the neck region, especially when FCA is applied. These sites may ulcerate, bleed, and/or form scales. The animals tolerate the formation of ulcers, which generally heal in a few days.

Discussion

GPMT is an appropriate procedure to determine allergenicity of chemical raw materials, but less adequate to calculate the actual risk of sensitization in man under use conditions, especially for final chemical products. Important criteria are lacking, such as the use of different test concentrations, and the exposure route related to general practice. The modified GPMT (Dossou et al., 1985) partially compensates these handicaps. Evaluation of the challenge reactions may be difficult, particularly when finished products are tested, because even the control animals and placebo sites may show weak to moderate skin reactions. According to Magnusson, "The maximization procedure only establishes the allergenic potentiality or sensitizing capacity of a substance, and not the actual risk of sensitization" (Magnusson, 1975). Other researchers have also noted that the GPMT is considerably more sensitive than the human test (Klecak et al., 1977; Maguire, 1980); Marzulli and Maguire (1982) and Andersen and Hamann (1984) confirmed it.

The GPMT is used in many laboratories in connection with research projections (Andersen et al., 1984a, 1984b, 1984c, 1985a, 1985b, 1985c, 1985d, 1985e, 1985f, 1986; Björkner, 1980, 1981, 1984a, 1984b; Björkner and Niklasson, 1984; Björkner et al., 1984; Bourrinet et al., 1979; Bruze, 1986; Bruze et al., 1985a, 1985b, 1987a, 1987b, 1987c, 1988a, 1988b, 1988c, 1988d, 1988e, 1988f, 1989; Campolmi et al., 1978; Christensen et al., 1984b; Clemmensen, 1985; Fahr et al., 1976; Freeman et al., 1988; Fregert et al., 1984; Goodwin et al., 1981; Guillot et al., 1983; Karlberg et al., 1983; Kero and Hannuksela, 1980; Kojima et al., 1989; Marzulli and Maguire, 1982; Nethercott, 1981; Prince and Prince, 1977; Reller et al., 1985; Sato et al., 1981; Senma et al., 1978; Skog and Wahlberg, 1970; Schubert and Ziegler, 1971; Schubert et al., 1973; Stampf et al., 1978b, 1982a, 1982b; Thorgeirsson, 1978; Thorgeirsson and Fregert, 1977; Thorgeirsson et al., 1975; Tsuchiya et al., 1982; Wahlberg and Boman, 1978, 1979, 1985; Wahlberg and Fregert, 1985; Wahlberg et al., 1985; Van der Walle et al., 1982a, 1983; Warner et al., 1988; Ziegler, 1975, 1977; Ziegler et al., 1972).

The U.S. Food and Drug Administration recommends the GPMT along with the split adjuvant technique (Marzulli and Maibach, 1976) and Bühler test as standard procedures for screening the allergenic capability of new chemicals and finished products.

SPLIT ADJUVANT TECHNIQUE

Maguire and co-workers (1972, 1973b, 1975) utilized an adjuvant technique that enhances the processes leading to sensitization in the guinea pig, so that even weak and moderately weak contact allergens in humans can be identified in small groups of experimental animals (Maguire, 1975). It is derived from the split adjuvant test procedure (Maguire and Chase, 1967, 1972), in which FCA is injected into or near the skin site exposed to the allergen. In his predictive variant of the split adjuvant technique, Maguire used the observations of Bühler (1965) and Magnusson and Kligman (1970) that various adjuvant means can be used to render the guinea pig nonspecifically more susceptible to sensitization. The methodology of the split adjuvant technique is the following (see Fig. 5).

Materials and Methods

Animals. Two groups of 10–20 guinea pigs each are used for the experimental group and the control group, and at least four animals are used for the primary irritation test. The toenails and distal parts of both rear feet are wrapped with adhesive tape to prevent skin injuries.

Materials. Preparations are tested as such or, if necessary, diluted in accordance with use concentrations. Single components of the test material can also be examined in different concentrations by using adequate vehicles (e.g., petrolatum).

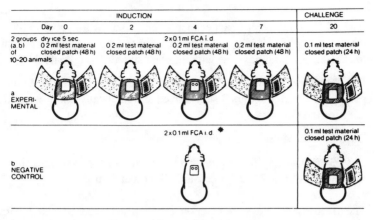

INDUCTION				CHALLENGE
Day 0	2	4	7	20
2 groups dry ice 5 sec (a b) 0 2 ml test material of closed patch (48 h) 10-20 animals	0 2 ml test material closed patch (48 h)	2x0 1 ml FCA i d 0 2 ml test material closed patch (48 h)	0 2 ml test material closed patch (48 h)	0 1 ml test material closed patch (24 h)

a
EXPERI-
MENTAL

2x0 1 ml FCA i d **✻**

0.1 ml test material
closed patch (24 h)

b
NEGATIVE
CONTROL

✻ essential supplement to the original sensitizing schedule

FIGURE 5   Split adjuvant technique.

Induction

Day 0: Before starting the treatment, the skin on the back behind the shoulder girdle of the experimental animals is shaved to remove all the hair and some of the loose keratin. A window dressing is put on the animal, with the window over the shaved area (2 × 2 cm), and fixed in place with adhesive tape. Dry ice is applied for 5 s to this skin site. Then 0.2 ml ointment or 0.1 ml liquid is spread over the sensitization site and covered with Whatman filter paper. Finally, the whole area is covered with an occlusive tape, which is held in place with adhesive tape.

Day 2: The window is opened, the test material reapplied, and the window covered again.

Day 4: The window is opened, 0.1 ml FCA is injected id twice into the sensitization site, the test material is applied epicutaneously, and the window is closed again.

Day 7: Same procedure as on d 2.

Day 9: All wrappings are removed.

Challenge

The challenge is usually performed with a closed-patch test to a new (nonexposed) skin site with various exposure times (maximum, 24 h) and/or with an open test, depending on the toxicity of the test material. The challenge material should not produce substantial irritation in untreated animals. Therefore primary irritation tests must be done before the challenge.

Day 20: In both groups (experimental and control) a 2 × 2 cm area on the dorsal back is closely shaved, and 0.1 ml of the test material is applied to the skin site and covered with an occlusive dressing (patch).

Day 22: After removal of the dressing, the test area is marked with a skin pencil and the whole dorsal skin shaved atraumatically. Skin reactions are read for the first time.

Days 23 and 24: Readings are repeated.

Days 34 and 44: Rechallenging at a different (nonexposed) skin site in the same way as on d 21 may occasionally be performed.

The intensity of the skin reaction is classified according to the rating scale:

0	=	Normal skin
±	=	Very faint, nonconfluent pink
+	=	Faint pink
+ +	=	Pale pink to pink, slight edema
+ + +	=	Pink, moderate edema
+ + + +	=	Pink and thickened
+ + + + +	=	Bright pink, markedly thickened

The estimation of whether a preparation is sensitizing is based on a comparison of the frequency, intensity, and duration of skin reactions in the experimental and control animals.

Discussion

This test method, from a theoretical point of view, has most of the essential features of a predictive procedure. Finished preparations are tested as such and other substances are tested with regard to the use concentration. The mode of application is close to conditions of use. The application of dry ice, FCA, and the occlusive patch makes it possible to detect even weak sensitizers. As in the Bühler test, the closed patch is important, since occlusion enhances penetration and sensitization. Nevertheless, there is a difference between the methods in the duration of exposure, in the number of patches applied during the induction phase, and especially in the utilization of both dry ice and FCA in the split adjuvant technique. Maguire (1980) showed that the Maguire technique is more sensitive and effective in detecting substances and products with weak allergenic potential. To exclude false positive results in the split adjuvant technique it is essential that even the control animals be pretreated with FCA (as discussed in relation to the GPMT). The split adjuvant technique is applicable for screening allergic properties of various chemicals as demonstrated by Chung et al., 1970; Harris et al., 1989; Prince and Prince, 1977; Lachapelle and Tennstedt,

1979; Rao et al., 1981; Maguire, 1980; Marzulli and Maguire, 1982; Maguire, 1985; Maguire and Cipriano, 1985. In the case of finished products, preparation of the same class or range—one with allergenic properties and the other devoid of them—may be included in the screening strategy as additional controls.

A modification of the Maguire procedure that is used in Japan by Tsuchiya et al. (1982, 1985) is called the cumulation contact enhancement test (CCET). The test material is applied by means of an occlusive patch to the same skin site 4–6 times during 2 wk, and just before the third application 0.1 ml FCA is administered id on each side of the patch used for induction. The pretreatment with dry ice is omitted. For challenge, open application of the test material is preferred. If rechallenge is indicated, a closed patch test is recommended. In our experience the sensitivity of this method seems to be equal to that of Maguire's split adjuvant technique and the GPMT. The CCET and the Maguire technique have the same predictive value. They are both much more appropriate than the GPMT for screening of finished preparations that are externally applied to the human skin (toiletries and cosmetics) for their allergenic potential. In our experience, however, the FCA used during induction can convert chemicals with a pure allergenic potential into good sensitizers.

The U.S. Food and Drug Administration recommends the split adjuvant technique (Marzulli and Maibach, 1976) with the Draize test and the GPMT as standard procedures for screening new chemicals and finished products.

BÜHLER TOPICAL CLOSED-PATCH TECHNIQUE

Bühler (1965) and Griffith and Bühler (1969) at Procter & Gamble presented a predictive animal method that resembles the human repeated-insult patch test (RIPT), allows variation of screening conditions to optimize the detection of allergenic chemicals and finished formulations, and avoids unnecessary sensitization of human subjects. They have a number of years of successful experience with this closed-patch technique. Less than 3% of the materials that did not sensitize the guinea pig in the Bühler test were found to sensitize humans in the RIPT. Griffith and Bühler state that the test is sensitive enough to detect a moderate to strong sensitizer and that the probability of false positive results, which might lead to the rejection of an otherwise safe compound or formulation, is very low. The methodology has been modified and adapted several times. At present, experimental skin sensitization in guinea pigs according to Bühler and Griffith (1975) is carried out as follows (see Fig. 6).

Materials and Methods

Animals. About equal numbers of male and female guinea pigs are used for (1) the experimental group (at least 20 animals), (2) the control group(s) (10 animals), and (3) the primary irritation group (4 animals).

Materials. The test substance is diluted, emulsified, or suspended in a

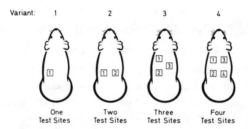

closed patch 6 h 0.4 ml test mat.	INDUCTION		CHALLENGE	
	Week 1+2+3		5	6-7
animal groups:				
EXPERIMENTAL (20 animals)				
VEHICLE • CONTROL (10 animals)				
NEGATIVE CONTROL - primary challenge - (10 animals) - rechallenge - (10 animals)				

• facultative

Various Schedules for Primary Irritation Studies

Variant: 1   2   3   4

One Test Sites	Two Test Sites	Three Test Sites	Four Test Sites

FIGURE 6   Bühler topical closed-patch technique.

suitable vehicle. The concentration used for induction is allowed to provoke only weak skin irritation in the guinea pig and is calculated with respect to the use concentration.

Induction Phase for Primary Sensitization

The animals of the experimental and the vehicle group, if used, are shaved on the left shoulder in an area of about 2 × 2 cm on the day before exposure.

Week 1: Closed patches for the experimental group are prepared as follows: 0.4 ml of freshly prepared test material is applied on a 20 × 20 mm

Webril pad on a 37 × 40 mm Parke-Davis reading bandage. The concentration chosen for induction of sensitization is usually 10 times higher than that calculated for human exposure. If it is found to be too irritating, the concentration may be decreased during the induction phase. After the animal is placed in a special restrainer, the patch is applied to the clipped skin sites as soon as possible. The patch then is occluded with a rubber dental dam pulled tight and fastened to the bottom of the restrainer with binder clips. The restrainer is adjusted to minimize movement of the animal during the 6 h of exposure. Then the dental dam and patch are taken off. The residual material can be washed off with warm water before returning the animals to their cages.

Weeks 2 and 3: The 6-h closed patch with test material or vehicle is repeated (see week 1).

Primary Irritation Study

Before the induction phase is completed, the primary irritation study is performed with four previously unexposed animals. Depending on the test material, up to four different concentrations can be applied by the technique discussed above to various sites on the guinea pig's back. To minimize site-to-site variations in the skin reaction, concentrations of test material are alternated on the various test sites. The 24-h skin response is read and the highest nonirritant concentration determined. The day before challenge one or more virgin skin sites of about 2 × 2 cm are shaved on the backs of animals of the experimental and control groups.

Challenge

Week 5: The challenge test is performed on freshly clipped skin sites in the same way as the 6-h occlusive patch test of the induction phase. The test concentration is chosen such that the guinea pig skin tolerates it without any reaction. Vehicles commonly used for challenging are water and acetone. When other vehicles are chosen, the animals must also be tested with these. Multiple samples may be used to obtain as much data as possible. In principle, the control group is challenged in the same way as the experimental one.

At 18–24 h after application the patches are removed. The area of the challenge is marked and the skin of the whole back is shaved and depilated. At least 2 h after depilation the test site is examined for erythema and edema for the first time. The reaction is graded according to the following scale:

0 = No reaction
0.5 = Very faint erythema, usually confluent
1 = Faint erythema, usually confluent

2 = Moderate erythema

3 = Strong erythema with or without edema

Reading of the skin area is repeated 48 and 72 h after challenge and the skin reactions are graded.

The results of the challenge are expressed in terms of the incidence and severity of the skin response. An incidence index is calculated by dividing the number of animals with responses of grade 1 or more at 24 or 48 h by the number of animals tested. The severity index is the sum of the test grades divided by the number of animals tested. A comparison of the reactions elicited in terms of incidence, severity, and duration between all animal groups is made to determine whether a test substance induces sensitization.

Rechallenge

Sensitized animals can be rechallenged 1 and 2 wk after the primary challenge. For this purpose the animals can be divided into groups of at least 5 each, if more than three components of the sensitizing test material must be tested simultaneously. New control animals must be used for this rechallenge phase.

If the results of primary challenge or rechallenge do not allow clear conclusions and allergenicity of the test material is suspected, a rerun of the test material under aggravated conditions (higher concentrations) is indicated. A special situation occurs if a study with the maximum concentration for both induction and challenge indicates sensitization in animals, but of very low incidence. In this case an additional test is performed involving induction of sensitization by a single id injection of the test material (three concentrations with 10 animals per concentration group) in FCA and a closed-patch test for challenging 14 d later.

Discussion

The authors emphasize the predictive character of their method for determining the allergenic potential of subtances and products (dermatologics, cosmetics, household products, etc.). This animal model allows variations in both the induction and the challenge phase. It mimics the conditions of use in that the epicutaneous mode of application is employed, induction concentrations in most cases correspond to the use concentration, and a solvent or vehicle can be chosen that is identical or similar to the end formulation. Finished preparations are tested as such or, if appropriate, diluted (e.g., shampoos).

The usefulness and limitations of this technique are discussed by Maguire (1980), Marzulli and Maguire (1982), Lamson et al. (1982), Bühler (1982, 1985), and Babiuk et al. (1987). The sensitivity of this method seems to be comparable to that of the RIPT in humans (Poole et al., 1970). Accordingly, a substance tested at a concentration of 10% could not be declared a nonsensitizer because it did not provoke allergic sensitization in guinea pigs or humans, since the possibility exists that the test concentration was below the minimal dose engendering sensitization.

Even an experienced investigator has some difficulty reading and evaluating the challenge test reactions in this procedure. The spots on the controls as well as the experimental animals often show inflammatory reactions, whose strength, duration, and character must be evaluated subjectively. Further, the method requires a relatively large technical and material expenditure. Nevertheless, the technique in many respects satisfies the criteria for a predictive test method. The best recommendation for this technique is that it has been used satisfactorily for more than 15 years by Procter and Gamble for the detection of subtances and products with allergenic capability (Ritz et al., 1980).

OPEN EPICUTANEOUS TEST

Procedures used with guinea pigs to detect sensitizing substances and select compounds that will be tolerated by humans should be simple and reliable, and the results obtained should be valid for humans. Taking into account all the variables that can influence the induction of contact sensitization in humans and guinea pigs, Klecak et al. (1977) developed an animal model, the open epicutaneous test (OET) (see Figs. 7 and 8). With this method one can screen many chemicals and finished formulations under conditions similar to those of human use and obtain quantitative results expressed in terms of a threshold concentration for skin tolerance. In contrast, in current methods compounds are tested at one concentration and the results are expressed in terms of frequency of sensitized animals and grade of intensity of lesions.

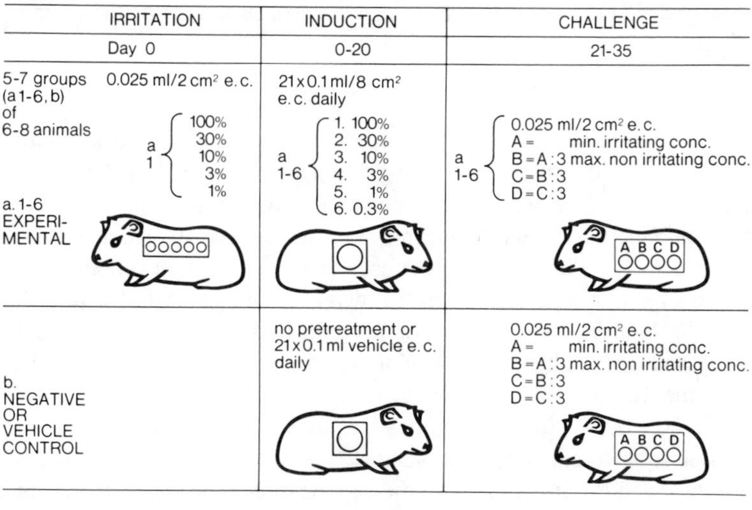

FIGURE 7 Open epicutaneous test.

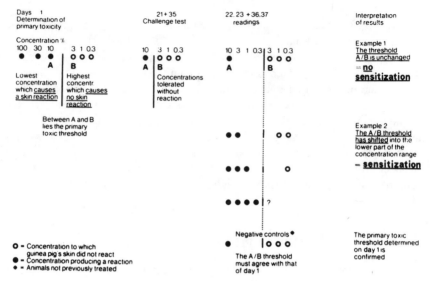

FIGURE 8   Schematic representation of the open epicutaneous test.

Materials and Methods

Animals.   Up to six experimental groups and one control group of 8 guinea pigs are used. One group of 20 animals is used for finished formulations.

Materials.   Substances are applied topically uncovered, undiluted, and, if possible and relevant, dissolved, suspended, or emulsified, in concentrations of 30, 10, 3, and 1% or lower in ethanol, acetone, water, petrolatum, polyethylene glycol, and/or other suitable vehicles. Finished products are tested as such or diluted according to use (shampoos). Constant volumes of each concentration are applied with a pipette or syringe on standard areas of the clipped animal flank.

Skin Irritation

When single chemicals and preparations used in dissolved form for testing are investigated, 1 d before starting the induction procedure the experimental group is used to determine the threshold toxic concentration by simultaneously applying the different concentrations (e.g., 100, 30, 10, and 3%) to the left flank skin. A 0.025-ml portion of each test concentration is homogeneously spread on a 2-cm^2 area of flank skin that was clipped and marked with a circular stamp. The highest concentration of a compound used is determined by its solubility and (for challenge) by its skin irritating capacity. The application site remains uncovered. It is necessary to rotate the various concentrations of test substance across the different application sites to minimize variations in response due to different skin locations.

Skin reactions are read 24 h after application. The minimal irritant concentration (A) and the maximal nonirritant concentration (B) (threshold concentrations) of the test substance are determined by an all-or-none criterion. The minimal irritant concentration is defined as the lowest one causing mild erythema in at least 25% of a group of animals. The maximal nonirritant concentration is the highest one not causing a macroscopic reaction in any animal. Estimation of the threshold concentrations is essential for evaluation of the allergenic capacity of the test material, based on the end point determination.

Induction

Days 0–20: On d 0, a 0.1-ml portion of each undiluted substance (preparation) and/or of its progressive dilutions is applied to an 8-cm^2 area on the clipped flank skin of 20 or 8 guinea pigs per concentration group; one to six such groups are used for each substance. Applications are repeated daily for 3 wk or five times weekly for 4 wk, always on the same skin site. The application site remains uncovered and the reactions, if continuous daily applications are performed, are read 24 h after each application or at the end of each week. The maximal nonirritant and minimal irritant concentrations after repeated applications are determined by the same all-or-none criterion. When strong skin reactions are provoked, the application site is changed.

Challenge

Day 21: To determine whether contact sensitization was induced, all guinea pigs treated for 21 d as described above, as well as 8–10 untreated controls for each substance, are tested on d 21 on the contralateral flank with the same substance at the minimal irritant and some lower concentrations. The minimal irritant concentration is used to confirm the primary irritant capacity determined before starting the induction (d − 1) and to exclude false results due to instability of the test material. These tests are performed by pipetting 0.025 ml of each concentration on skin areas measuring 2 cm^2. It is necessary to rotate the concentrations of test substance across the different application sites to minimize variations in response at different skin locations. Skin reactions are read after 24, 48, and/or 72 h. In sensitized animals this procedure permits determinations of the *minimal sensitizing concentration* necessary for inducing allergic contact hypersensitivity and the *minimal eliciting concentration* necessary to cause a positive reaction. A concentration is considered allergenic when at least one animal in the concentration group shows a positive reaction with nonirritant concentrations.

Day 35: Rechallenge of all experimental animals as well as of old and new controls is performed with the same or lower challenge concentrations to reach the absolute threshold. Readings are made 24, 48, and 72 h after challenging and the results are analyzed. Rechallenge must be performed when finished formulations (shampoos, creams, ointments, etc.) are used for induction and the influence of phenomena such as angry-back syndrome on the results of the first challenge cannot be excluded. False positive results will thereby be avoided.

Discussion

It is important to know how well the OET compares with the tests in use—in other words, how reliably it detects substances with allergenic properties and how accurately it predicts the sensitizing potential of contact allergens. Therefore studies were performed to compare the predictive value of OET results with those of the GPMT, Freund's complete adjuvant test, and the Draize guinea pig test. In addition, the results for the animal models were compared with those of the human maximization test.

Instead of substances with pronounced allergenicity in humans, we chose substances with weak allergenicity for comparative studies with the OET. We selected fragrance materials that are present in most cosmetic, household, and some pharmaceutical products in order to study their biological effects with respect to skin toxicity and/or sensitizing power, determined by clinical investigations and under use conditions (Baer, 1935; Cronin, 1971; Epstein, 1969; Fisher, 1975; Fregert, 1970; Hjorth, 1967; Kahn, 1971; Kastner, 1968; Koch et al., 1971; Larsen, 1975; Mitchell, 1975; Ostbourne, 1956; Rothenborg and Hjorth, 1968; Ziegler et al., 1985).

Initially, we studied 32 fragrance materials that had been described in the literature as allergenic in humans. These compounds were tested concurrently in the four animal tests. The results are summarized in Table 2, which shows a high degree of correlation between clinically verified allergenicity and the results from the OET, GPMT, and FCAT. The Draize test was again found to be less sensitive than the other animal models. The seven substances for which we lacked confirmative data, such as positive history, positive patch test, or reexposure, were negative in all the animal tests. Their allergenicity is questionable or may be due to a cross-sensitizing capacity.

In the next stage, we performed comparative animal tests with 21 concentrated perfume compositions used for commercial products, such as perfumes, toilet waters, colognes, soaps and shampoos, all of which had already passed the test of time—that is, they were found to be harmless in consumer tests. The results are summarized in Table 3, which shows that clinically innocuous substances usually do not sensitize experimental animals by the epicutaneous route. The achievement of sensitization by id procedures may not have clinical relevance and does not correspond to conditions of use.

Both these studies showed a high degree of correlation between clinical innocuousness as well as clinically estimated allergenicity and the results of the OET.

In addition, 268 fragrance materials, which are simple chemical compounds or substances of vegetable origin, were tested with the OET and the

TABLE 2. Number of Compounds Described as Allergenic in Humans and Detected as Allergenic by the Four Animal Tests

Total number of compounds		Epicutaneous OET	Intradermal tests		
			DT	MT	FCAT
Positive					
In OET and id tests	18	18	7	15	17
In OET only	4	4	0	0	0
In id only	3	0	1	3	3
Total positive	25	22	8	18	20
Negative in all tests	7				
Total	32				

results were compared with those of the human maximization test and the repeated-insult patch test (Marzulli and Maibach, 1976; Nakayama et al., 1974; Opdyke, 1974, 1976). For most of these substances there is a high degree of agreement between the test results, as shown in Table 4. The OET results are correlated with those of the HMT and also those of the RIPT (Klecak et al., 1977) when substances of the same origin and the same physical and chemical quality were used (Fisher and Dooms-Goossens, 1976). When these conditions were not fulfilled, differences in skin tolerance and/or allergenic capacity were observed. The OET method was successfully used to sensitize guinea pigs with naturally occurring quinones (Schulz et al., 1977).

The results mentioned above should not be taken to indicate that the OET represents an ideal animal model. Like other techniques, the OET also has some weak points. For instance, it is not suitable for testing substances that color the skin, since this makes reading of skin reactions difficult, if not impossible (Noster and Hausen, 1978). Furthermore, it did not indicate the allergenic potential of epoxy resins, perhaps because these chemicals have a low penetra-

TABLE 3. Allergenicity in Four Animal Tests of 21 Perfume Compositions Harmless in Human Use

Total number of compounds		Epicutaneous OET	Intradermal tests		
			DT	MT	FCAT
Positive					
In all tests	1	1[a]	1	1	1
In OET only	1	1[a]	0	0	0
In id only	11	0	1	5	11
Total positive	13	2	2	6	12
Negative in all tests	8				
Total	21				

[a]Undiluted, positive; at user concentration, negative.

G. Klecak

TABLE 4. Predictive Value of Human Tests, as Compared to an Animal Test (OET)

Number of preparations (268 total)	Human HMT/RIPT	Animal OET
250	negative	negative
12	positive	positive
1	negative	positive
5	positive	negative

tion rate through the intact guinea pig skin. Therefore new chemicals found to be nonallergenic under the test conditions of the OET should also be studied using id application with FCA, such as with Freund's complete adjuvant test. Conclusions concerning their allergenic potential can then be made. Comparative studies involving the OET were done by Andersen et al., 1984b; Cavelier et al., 1988, 1989; Guillot et al., 1985; Hausen et al., 1986, 1988b; Klecak, 1985; Klecak et al., 1977; Lammintausta et al., 1985; Maguire, 1980; Kero and Hannuksela, 1980; Sato et al., 1981; Tsuchiya et al., 1982; Stampf et al., 1982a; and Hausen et al., 1983.

Reasons for recommending OET as a predictive technique for estimating the allergenic potentials of chemicals and finished formulations are as follows:

1. Epicutaneously sensitized guinea pigs appear to be more appropriate models for allergic contact dermatitis in humans than guinea pigs sensitized by other methods. The id routes are likely to produce more heterogeneous forms of sensitization. The question arises whether sensitization induced by nonepicutaneous routes produces an immune response corresponding to that of contact allergy in humans.
2. Mode, frequency, and duration of exposure in the OET are compatible with the texture or consistency of most cosmetic products.
3. The OET allows variations in experimental strategy for the induction and elicitation of contact dermatitis. Moreover, it can be modified by stripping and by ultraviolet (UV-A and UV-B) light exposure.
4. The OET has adequate sensitivity and specificity. When used to test consumer products, there is little likelihood of missing weak sensitizers or misidentifying substances as potent sensitizers when their allergenic potential is weak.
5. The OET results, not only in tests with fragrance materials, agree with those of the HMT, RIPT, and the consumer test.

OPTIMIZATION TEST

In 1974 Maurer published a variant of the Landsteiner-Draize guinea pig test that is highly sensitive (desirable for determining the allergenicity of substances) and easily reproducible. The motivation for developing the optimization test was the failure of the original Draize test (1955, 1959) to detect weak and moderate human sensitizers and the discovery of some drawbacks of the guinea pig maximization test. Moreover, Maurer assumed that humans may be more sensitive than animals to a range of substances with contact allergenic properties. Therefore, to enhance the sensitivity of guinea pig skin, Freund's complete adjuvant is used. In Maurer's opinion, the aim of the animal experiment is not to study the biological effect of a substance when applied by natural means, but to enhance the sensitivity of the animal skin so that substances with a sensitization rate of 1% or less in humans will sensitize a considerably higher percentage of animals in a small experimental group.

Materials and Methods

Animals. Forty guinea pigs of either sex are divided into two groups of 20 animals each (10 females and 10 males) as follows (see Fig. 9): (1) experimental group and (2) vehicle group (negative control).

Test material. In addition to repeated id injections with and without FCA, a single epicutaneous patch is applied. For the id application, solutions, emulsions, or suspensions of the test substance in 0.9% saline and a mixture of FCA and saline containing the test material are prepared. Oil-soluble materials are mixed with FCA before saline is added. The end concentration used is 0.1%. For epicutaneous application (i.e., for the second challenge test), the substance, in subirritant concentrations for guinea pig skin, is dissolved or incorporated in appropriate solvents or vehicles (e.g., water, alcohol, diethyl phthalate, or petrolatum). Test material is always applied to freshly shaved new skin sites.

Induction

Induction is divided into two phases:

Week 1: On d 0 the test material in 0.9% saline is injected id (0.1 ml) into the flank and the dorsal skin sites. On d 2 and d 4 one id injection is made into the dorsal skin toward the region of the neck sites. During the first week, the skin sites are depilated 21 h after application and the 24-h skin reactions are evaluated under standard light conditions. The two largest diameters (in millimeters) of the erythematous reaction in vertical alignment are measured and the skinfold thickness (in millimeters) is determined with a skinfold gauge. Finally, the individual reaction volume (in microliters) is calculated for each reaction for individual animals.

Weeks 2 and 3: On d 7–21 six id injections (0.1 ml each) of the test substance in a 1:1 mixture of FCA and saline are applied every second day in the region of the neck on both sides of the midline. During this period there is no reading of skin reactions.

Challenge

Challenge is performed in two steps, intradermally and epicutaneously.

First challenge step. On d 35 the animals of the experimental and control groups are tested with test material at the same dose and volume used for induction (without adjuvant) at a fresh site on the right shaved flank. On d 36 the test sites and surroundings are shaved and depilated 21 h afer challenging. Readings are made 3 h later to measure the skin reactions (diameter and increase in skinfold thickness) and determine the reaction values.

Assessment: The average extent of the reaction to the first four induction doses (wk 1) and the standard deviation are calculated for each animal. The means and standard deviations are then added up and the sum used as an individual threshold value for each animal. The reactions to the challenge dose and the induction dose are compared in each animal. If the reaction volume on challenge exceeds the corresponding threshold value, the animal is considered sensitized. The number of positive animals in each group is counted and the significance of differences between the treated and control groups is assessed by the exact Fisher test for comparison of the basic probability of two binominal distributions (Sachs, 1971).

Second challenge step. Epicutaneous challenge is performed on d 45. Care must be taken that the test material is applied in nonirritating concentrations. The test substance in vehicle (0.05 ml/cm^2) is fixed during 24 h by means of an occlusive patch, using a 2 × 2 cm filter paper (Whatman 3M) on a shaved area of flank skin. On d 47, about 21 h after removing the patch, the reaction sites are chemically depilated (Butoquick for about 5 min); 3 h later the reactions are evaluated for intensity, size of erythema, and increase in thickness of the skin (edema). A distinctly visible redness within the field of application is considered an allergic reaction. The significance of differences in the number of positive animals between the treated group and the controls is again assessed by the Fisher test.

The number of positively reacting animals in the experimental group is compared with that in the control group, and the test material is classified according to its allergenicity and according to Kligman's system (1966b, 1966c) as shown in the table on p. 377.

Discussion

There is little experience with this technique except that of its authors (Maurer, 1983, 1985; Maurer and Meier, 1984; Maurer et al., 1975, 1978, 1979, 1980a, 1980b, 1985). In principle, this method is a modification of the

Landsteiner-Draize guinea pig technique designed to detect moderate and weak sensitizers. According to Maurer et al. (1975), the optimization test has the following significant advantages: "The measurement of the reaction occurring during the first week of induction, the calculation of the standard deviation and the comparison of induction and challenge in one and the same animal individually makes certain that the effective reaction is objectively measured, the assessment of intradermal reaction by calculation independent of the irritant effect of the substance and the solvent applied."

This seems to be the only appropriate procedure for exact evaluation of results obtained with experimental animals when id application of the test material is used for challenging. The sensitivity and reproducibility of the optimization test were proved in comparative studies with strong, moderate, and weak human sensitizers for which clinical data are available. The results indicate that the optimization test has about the same predictive value as a screening procedure for allergenicity testing as the guinea pig maximization test (Maurer et al., 1975, 1978, 1979; Maurer and Meier, 1984) and Freund's complete adjuvant test (Maurer, personal communication). However, of the three the optimization test seems to be the most complicated and time-consuming.

The crucial points of the optimization test are the following:

1. There is little evidence concerning the correlation between results of the optimization test and those of predictive human tests.
2. The use of id injection limits the applicability of the optimization test to single chemicals and a few formulations. For testing most finished formulations the test seems unsuitable.
3. The natural pathway of the contact allergen and other factors likely to influence the occurrence of contact allergy are not considered.
4. The optimization test (like the GPMT and FCAT) can only establish the allergenic potential or sensitizing capacity of a substance, not the actual risk of sensitization under use conditions.

Nevertheless, this method is a viable alternative to the GPMT or FCAT, particularly for testing synthetic dyes or skin coloring chemicals, since both of them allow no reading of skin reactions with the naked eye during challenge if applied epicutaneously.

CONCLUDING REMARKS

This chapter is meant to give an overview of the predictive animal tests most frequently used for evaluating the allergenic potential of chemicals and finished formulations and to discuss the merits and demerits of these methods. All these tests have been proposed to aid in predicting the probable incidence of adverse effects on the skin caused by contact sensitizers. When critically examined, none of these tests is entirely capable of doing this and none of them is universally applicable to all chemicals and types of formulations. Each substance poses its own unique problems, a fact ignored in recommendations of uniformity in predictive testing.

In practice, experienced dermatologists and toxicologists choose the test that they consider suitable for a specific problem (Andersen and Maibach, 1985a; Bühler, 1982; Guillot et al., 1982; Benezra, 1980; Blomberg et al., 1978; Brulos et al., 1977; Forslind and Wahlberg, 1978; Hunziker, 1969; Ischy et al., 1969; Jadassohn et al., 1955; Lachapelle and Tennstedt, 1979; Meyer et al., 1979; Schäfer et al., 1978; Stampf et al., 1978b). The assumption that a predictive test procedure is reliable is justified when the test technique corresponds to its purpose and the evaluation is sufficiently objective. In this respect, experts must take into account factors related to usage and induction of contact allergy.

The results of animal predictive testing will, of course, serve as guidelines rather than as absolute criteria for safety evaluation of materials and finished formulations before controlled testing on human subjects is indicated. There are some critics who incriminate the use of animal tests. We feel that the *in vitro* studies recommended by them are not suitable alternatives for prediction of safety in use (Goldberg, 1989; Hofmann et al., 1987; Kimber, 1988; Oliver et al., 1986).

REFERENCES

Adams, R. M., Maibach, H. I., Andersen, K. E., Benezra, C., Burrows, D., Camaras, J., Dooms-Goossens, A., Ducombs, G., Frosch, P., Lachapelle, J. M., Lahti, A., Menne, T., Rycroft, R., Scheper, R., White, J. and Wilkinson, J. 1987. Contact dermatitis. A Review. *Contact Dermatitis* 16:55–78.

Agrup, G. 1968. Sensitization induced by patch testing. *Br. J. Dermatol.* 82:631–634.

Agrup, G. 1969a. Hand eczema. *Acta Derm. Venereol. (Stockh.)* 49(Suppl.):40–41.

Agrup, G. 1969b. Hand eczema and other hand dermatoses in south Sweden. *Acta Derm. Venereol. (Stockh.)* 49(Suppl. 61):5–91.

Agrup, G. and Cronin, E. 1969. Contact dermatitis X. *Br. J. Dermatol.* 82:428–433.

Allenby, C. F. and Basketter, D. A. 1989. Minimum eliciting patch test concentrations of cobalt. *Contact Dermatitis* 20:185–190.

Andersen, K. E. and Maibach, H. I. 1980. Cumulative irritancy in the guinea pig from low grade irritant vehicles and the angry skin syndrome. *Contact Dermatitis* 6:430–434.

Anderson, K. E. and Maibach, H. I. 1983. Drugs used topically. In: Allergic reactions to drugs. *Handbook of experimental pharmacology,* eds. A. L. de Weck and H. Bundgaard, Vol. 63. pp. 313–377. Berlin: Springer.

Andersen, K. E., Boman, A., Hamann, K. and Wahlberg, J. E. 1984a. Guinea pig maximization tests with formaldehyde releasers. Results from two laboratories. *Contact Dermatitis* 10:257–266.

Andersen, K. E. and Hamann, K. 1984b. How sensitizing is chloroceresol? Allergy tests in guinea pigs versus the clinical experience. *Contact Dermatitis* 11:11–20.

Andersen, K. E. and Hamann, K. 1984c. The sensitizing potential of metalworking fluid biocides (phenolic and thiazole compounds) in the guinea pig maximization test in relation to patch test reactivity in eczema patients. *Food Chem. Toxicol.* 22:655–660.

Andersen, K. E., Boman, A., Volund, A. A. and Wahlberg, J. E. 1985a. Induction of formaldehyde contact sensitivity: dose-response relationship in the guinea pig maximization test. *Acta Derm. Venereol.* (Stockh.) 65:472–478.

Andersen, K. E., Carlsen, L., Egsgaard, H. and Larsen, E. 1985b. Contact sensitivity and bioavailability of chloroceresol. *Contact Dermatitis* 13:246–251.

Andersen, K. E. and Maibach, H. I. 1985c. Contact allergy predicitive tests in guinea pigs. *Curr. Probl. Derm.* 4:59–61.

Andersen, K. E. and Maibach, H. I. 1985d. Guinea pig sensitization assays an overview. *Curr. Probl. Derm.* 14:263–290.

Andersen, K. E. 1985e. Guinea pig maximization test: effect of type of Freund's complete adjuvant emulsion and of challenge site location. *Derm. Beruf. Umwelt* 33:132–136.

Andersen, K. E. 1985f. Sensitivity and subsequent "down regulation" of sensitivity induced by chlorocresol in guinea pigs. *Arch. Dermatol. Res.* 277:84–87.

Andersen, K. E. 1986. Contact allergy to chlorocresol, formaldehyde and other biocides. Guinea pig tests and clinical studies. *Acta Dermato-Venereologica Supplementum* 125:61.

Anderson, D. W. 1975. Cosmetic safety substantiation. In *5th Annual SCC Seminar, Los Angeles, November 15.* Hollywood, Calif.: Max Factor & Co.

Asherson, G. L. and Ptak, W. 1968. Contact and delayed hypersensitivity in the mouse. I. Active sensitization and passive transfer. *Immunology* 15:405–416.

Babiuk, C., Hastings, K. and Dean, J. H. 1987. Induction of Ethylenediamine Hypersensitivity in the Guinea Pig and the Development of ELISA and lymphocyte Blastogenesis Techniques for its Characterization. *Fundam. Appl. Toxicol.* 9:623–634.

Baer, R. L. 1935. Perfume dermatitis. *J. Am. Med. Assoc.* 104:1926.

Baer, R. L. 1964. Allergic eczematous sensitization in man 1936 and 1964. *J. Invest. Dermatol.* 43:223–229.

Baer, H., Watkins, R. C., Kurtz, A. P., Byck, J. S. and Dawson, C. R. 1967. Delayed contact sensitivity to catechols. III. The relationship of side-chain length to sensitizing potency of catechols of poison ivy. *J. Immunol.* 99:370–375.

Baer, R. L., Ramsey, D. L. and Biondi, E. 1973. The most common contact allergens 1968–1970. *Arch. Dermatol.* 108:74–78.

Bär, F. 1969. Höchstmengen-Verordnung—Pflanzenschutz unter dem Blickpunkt des Gesundheitsschutzes. *Bundesgesundheitsblatt* 2:21–27.

Bär, F. 1974. Die toxikologische Bewertung (Sicherheitsspannen, Höchstmengen) im Rahmen des Lebensmittelgesetzes (Lebensmittel-Zusatzstoffe und Pestizidrückstände). *Arch. Toxikol.* 32:51–62.

Baker, H. 1968. The effects of dimethylsulfoxide, dimethylformamide and dimethylacetamide on the cutaneous barrier to water in human skin. *J. Invest. Dermatol.* 50:282–288.

Bandmann, H. J., Calnan, C. D., Cronin, E., Fregert, S., Hjorth, N., Magnusson, B., Maibach, H., Malten, K. E., Meneghini, C. L., Pirilä, V. and Wilkinson, D. S. 1972. Dermatitis from applied medicaments. *Arch. Dermatol.* 106:335–337.

Bartek, M. J., LaBudde, J. A. and Maibach, H. I. 1972. Skin permeability in vivo: Comparison in rat, rabbit, pig and man. *J. Invest. Dermatol.* 58:114–123.

Basketter, D. A. and Goodwin, B. F. J. 1988. Investigation of the prohapten concept. Cross reactions between 1,4-substituted benzene derivatives in the guinea pig. *Contact Dermatitis* 19:248–253.

Behrbohm, P. 1975. Legislation on prevention of occupational dermatoses. *Contact Dermatitis* 1:207–210.

Benezra, C. 1980. Allergic contact dermatitis to alantolactone: The use of lymphocyte transformation test in experimentally sensitized guinea-pigs. *Abst. 5th Symp. Contact Dermatitis,* Barcelona, p. 76.

Bettley, F. R. 1961. The influence of soap in the permeability of the epidermis. *Br. J. Dermatol.* 73:448–454.

Björkner, B. 1980. Allergenicity of trimethylol propane triacrylate in ultraviolet curing inks in the guinea pig. *Acta Derm. Venerol. (Stockh.)* 60:528–531.

Björkner, B. 1981. Sensitization capacity of acrylated prepolymers in ultraviolet curing inks tested in the guinea pig. *Acta Derm. Venerol. (Stockh.)* 61:7–10.

Björkner, B. 1982. Sensitization capacity of polyester methylcrylate in ultraviolet curing inks tested in the guinea pig. *Acta Derm. Venerol. (Stockh.)* 62:153–182.

Björkner, B. 1984a. Sensitizing potential of urethane (meth)acrylates in the guinea pig. *Contact Dermatitis* 11:115–119.

Björkner, B. 1984b. The sensitizing capacity of multifunctional acrylates in the guinea pig. *Contact Dermatitis* 11:236–246.

Björkner, B. and Niklasson, B. 1984. Influence of the vehicle on elicitation of contact allergic reactions to acrylic compounds in the guinea pig. *Contact Dermatitis* 11:268–278.

Björkner, B., Niklasson, B. and Persson, K. 1984. The sensitizing potential of di-(meth)acrylates based on bisphenol A or epoxy resin in the guinea pig. *Contact Dermatitis* 10:286–304.

Blank, I. H. 1952. Factors which influence the water content of stratum corneum. *J. Invest. Dermatol.* 18:433–439.

Blank, I. H. and Scheuplein, R. J. 1969. Transport into and within the skin. *Br. J. Dermatol.* 81(Suppl. 4):4–10.

Bluemink, E., Mitchell, J. C., Geissman, T. A. and Towers, G. H. N. 1976. Contact hypersensitivity to sesquiterpene lactones in chrysanthemum dermatitis. *Contact Dermatitis* 2:81–88.

Bloch, B. and Steiner-Wourlisch, A. 1926. Die willkürliche Erzeugung der Primelüberempfindlichkeit beim Menschen und ihre Bedeutung für das Idiosynkrasieproblem. *Arch. Dermatol.* 52:283–303.

Bloch, B. and Steiner-Wourlisch, A. 1930. Die Sensibilisierung des Meerschweinchens gegen Primeln. *Arch. Dermatol.* 162:349–378.

Blomberg, M. V., Boerrigter, G. H. and Scheper, R. J. 1978. Interference of simultaneous skin tests in delayed hypersensitivity. *Immunology* 35:361–367.

Boman, A., Karlberg, A. T. and Wahlberg, J. E. 1988. Experiences with Freund's complete adjuvant test (FCAT) when screening for contact allergens in colophony. *Contact Dermatitis* 18:25–29.

Bourrinet, P., Puchault, P., Sarrazin, G. and Bercovic, A. 1979. Etude comparée de quelques substances allergéniques chez l'homme et chez le cobaye. *J. Pharm. Belg.* 34(1):21–26.

Brauer, E. W. 1974. The commission of skin through the medium of the skin patch test. *J. Soc. Cosmet. Chem.* 25:153–158.

Bronaugh, R. L., Congdon, E. R. and Scheuplein, R. J. 1981. The effect of cosmetic vehicles on the penetration of *N*-nitrosodiethanolamine through excised human skin. *J. Invest. Derm.* 76:94–96.

Brulos, M. F., Guillot, J. P., Martini, M. C. and Cotte, J. 1977. The influence of perfumes on the sensitizing potential of cosmetic bases. I. A technique for evaluating sensitizing potential. *J. Soc. Cosmet. Chem.* 28:357–365.

Brunner, M. J. 1967. Pitfalls and problems in predictive testing. *J. Soc. Cosmet. Chem.* 18:323–331.

Brunner, M. J. and Smiljanic, A. 1952. Procedure for evaluation of skin-sensitizing power of new materials. *Arch. Dermatol.* 66:703–705.

Bruze, M. 1985. Contact sensitizers in resins based on phenol and formaldehyde. *Acta Dermato-Venereologica.* Supplementum 119.

Bruze, M., Fregert, S. and Zimerson, E. 1985. Contact allergy to phenol formaldehyde resins. *Contact Dermatitis* 12:81–86.

Bruze, M. 1986. Sensitizing capacity of dihydroxydiphenyl methane(bisphenol F) in the guinea pig. *Contact Dermatitis* 14:228–232.

Bruze, M., Gruvberger, B. and Persson, K. 1987a. Contact allergy to a contaminant in kathon CG in the guinea pig. *Dermatosen* 35:165–168.

Bruze, M., Fregert, S., Gruvberger, B. and Persson, K. 1987b. Contact allergy to the active ingredients of kathon CG in the guinea pig. *Acta Dermato-Venereologica* 67:315–320.

Bruze, M. 1988. Relevance of sensitization studies in guinea pigs. *Acta Dermato-Venereologica* 68: Suppl. 135:21–23.

Bruze, M., Boman, A., Bergqvist-Karlsson, A., Björkner, B., Wahlberg, J. E. and Voog, E. 1988a. Contact allergy to a cyclohexanone resin in humans and guinea pigs. *Contact Dermatitis* 18:46–49.

Bruze, M. and Gruvberger, B. 1988b. Formaldehyde-induced depression of skin reactivity to 5-chloro-2-methyl-4-isothiazolin-3-one in the guinea pig. *Contact Dermatitis:* 19.

Bruze, M., Gruvberger, B. and Agrup, G. 1988c. Sensitization studies in the guinea pig with the active ingredients of Euxyl K 400. *Contact Dermatitis* 18:37–39.

Bruze, M., Dahlquist, I. and Gruvberger, B. 1989. Contact allergy to dichlorinated methylisothiazolinone. *Contact Dermatitis* 20:219–239.

Bühler, E. V. 1964. A new method for detecting potential sensitizers using the guinea pig. *Toxicol. Appl. Pharmacol.* 6:341.

Bühler, E. V. 1965. Delayed contact hypersensitivity in the guinea pig. *Arch. Dermatol.* 91:171–177.

Bühler, E. V. 1982. Comment on guinea pig test methods. *Food Chem. Toxicol.* 20:494–495.

Bühler, E. V. 1985. A rationale for the selection of occlusion to induce and elicit delayed contact hypersensitivity in the guinea pig. A prospective test. *Curr. Probl. Dermatol.* 14:39–58.

Bühler, E. V. and Griffith, F. 1975. Experimental skin sensitization in the guinea pig and man. In *Animal models in dermatology,* ed. H. Maibach, pp. 56–66. Edinburgh: Churchill Livingstone.

Calnan, C. D. 1962. Contact dermatitis from drugs; symposium on drug sensitization. *Proc. R. Soc. Med.* 55:39.

Calnan, C. D., Epstein, W. L. and Kligman, A. M. 1964. Methods of evaluating contact sensitizers. In *Evaluation of therapeutic agents and cosmetics,* eds. T. H. Sternberg and F. C. Newcomer. New York: McGraw-Hill.

Calnan, C. D., Bandmann, H. J., Cronin, E., Fregert, S., Hjorth, N., Magnusson, B., Malten, K., Maneghini, C. L., Pirilä, V. and Wilkinson, D. S. 1970. Hand dermatitis in housewives. *Br. J. Dermatol.* 82:543–548.

Calvery, H. O., Draize, J. H. and Lung, E. P. 1946. The metabolism and permeability of normal skin. *Physiol. Rev.* 26:495–540.

Cameron, G. R. and Short, R. H. D. 1966. Physiology and functional pathology of the skin. In *Modern trends in dermatology,* ed. R. M. B. McKenna. London: Butterworth.

Campolmi, P., Sertoli, A., Fabbri, P. and Panconesi, E. 1978. Alantolactone sensitivity in chrysanthemum contact dermatitis. *Contact Dermatitis* 4:93–102.

Carter, R. O. and Griffith, J. F. 1965. Experimental bases for the realistic assessment of safety of topical agents. *Toxicol. Appl. Pharmacol.* 7(Suppl. 2):60–73.

Cavelier, C., Foussereau, J., Gille, P. and Zissu, D. 1988. Nickel allergy: tolerance to metallic surface-plated samples in nickel sensitive humans and guinea pigs. *Contact Dermatitis* 19:358–361.

Cavelier, C., Foussereau, J., Gille, P. and Zissu, D. 1989. Allergy to nickel or cobalt: tolerance to nickel and cobalt samples in man and in the guinea pig allergic or sensitized to these metals. *Contact Dermatitis* 21:72–78.

Chase, M. W. 1941. Inheritance in guinea pigs of the susceptibility to skin sensitization with simple chemical compounds. *J. Exp. Med.* 73:711–726.

Chase, M. W. 1950. A method for the enhancement of hypersensitivity to a simple chemical substance (picryl chloride). *Fed. Proc.* 9:379.

Chase, M. W. 1953. The inheritance of susceptibility to drug allergy in guinea pigs. *Trans. N.Y. Acad. Sci.* 15:79–82.

Chase, M. W. 1954. Experimental sensitization with particular reference to picryl chloride. *Int. Arch. Allergy* 5:163–191.

Chase, M. W. and Maguire, H. C. 1974. Further studies on sensitization to picric acid. *Monogr. Allergy* 8:1–12.

Cheminat, A., Stampf, J.-L. and Benezra, C. 1984. Allergic contact dermatitis to laurel (*Laurus nobilis* L.): Isolation and identification of haptens. *Arch. Dermatol. Res.* 276:178–181.

Christensen, O. B., Christensen, M. B. and Maibach, H. I. 1984a. Effect of vehicle on elicitation of DNCB contact allergy in guinea pig. *Contact Dermatitis* 10:166–169.

Christensen, O. B., Christensen, M. B. and Maibach, H. I. 1984b. Flare-up reactions and desensitization from oral dosing in chromate-sensitive guinea pigs. *Contact Dermatitis* 10:277–279.

Chulz, K. H. 1962. *Chemische Struktur und allergene Wirkung*, p. 94. Aulendorf, Wurttemberg: Cantor.

Chung, C. W. and Giles, A. L., Jr. 1972. Sensitization of guinea pigs to alpha-chloroacetophenone (CN) and ortho-chloro-benzylidene malanonitrile (CS) tear gas chemicals. *J. Immunol.* 109:284–293.

Chung, C. W. and Carson, Th. R. 1975. Sensitization potential and immunologic specificities of neomycin. *J. Invest. Dermatol.* 64:158–164.

Chung, C. W., Giles, A. L., Jr. and Larson, T. R. 1970. Induction of delayed hypersensitivity in guinea pigs by aflatoxins, other coumarines and furazolium. *J. Invest. Dermatol.* 55:396–403.

Chung, G. W. and Giles, A. L. 1977. Sensitization potentials of methyl, ethyl, and n-buthyl methacrylates and mutual cross-sensitivity in guinea pigs. *J. Invest. Dermatol.* 68:187–90.

Clemmensen, S. 1985. Sensitizing potential of 2-hydroxyethylmethacrylate. *Contact Dermatitis* 12:203–208.

Coldman, M. F., Poulsen, B. J. and Higuchi, T. 1969. Enhancement of percutaneous absorption by the use of volatile-nonvolatile systems as vehicles. *J. Pharm. Sci.* 58:1098–1102.

Coombs, R. R. A. and Gell, P. G. H. 1968. Classification of allergic reactions responsible for clinical hypersensitivity and disease. In *Clinical aspects of immunology*, 2nd ed., pp. 575–596. Oxford: Blackwell.

Cronin, E. 1971. Contact dermatitis from cinnamate. *Contact Dermatitis Newslett.* 9:216.

Cronin, E. 1980. *Contact Dermatitis.* London: Churchill Livingstone.

Cronin, E. and Wilkinson, D. S. 1973. Contact dermatitis. In *Recent advances in dermatology,* ed. A. J. Rook, vol. 3, pp. 134–192. New York: Churchill Livingstone.

Crowle, A. J. and Crowle, C. M. 1961. Contact sensitivity in mice. *J. Allergy* 23:302–320.

Cruickshank, C. N. D. 1969. Contact allergy. *J. Soc. Cosmet. Chem.* 20:479–485.

Davies, R. E., Harper, K. H. and Kynoch, S. R. 1972. Inter-species variation in dermal reactivity. *J. Soc. Cosmet. Chem.* 23:371–381.

Department of Health, Education and Welfare. June 1975. Investigation of consumer's perception of adverse reactions to consumer products. Contracted to Westat, Inc., Rockville, Md., contract 223738052. Rockville, Md.: Consumer Safety Statistic Staff, Office of Planning and Evaluation, Office of the Commissioner, *Food and Drug Administration.*

Dohr-Lux, R. and Lietz, G. 1965. Pharmakologisch-toxikologische und dermatologische Untersuchungsmethoden. *Parfüm. Kosmet.* 46:1:256–259; 2:289–293; 3:232–326.

Dossou, K. G., Sicard, C., Kalopissis, G., Reymond, D. and Schaefer, H. 1985. Guinea pig allergy test adapted to cosmetic ingredients. *Curr. Probl. Dermatol.* 14:248–262.

Draize, J. H. 1955. Dermal toxicity. *Food Drug Cosmet. Law J.* 10:722–732.

Draize, J. H. 1959. Appraisal of the safety of chemicals in foods, drugs and cosmetics. In *Dermal toxicity,* p. 46. Austin, Tex.: Association of Food and Drug Officials of the United States, Texas State Department of Health.

Draize, J. H., Woodgard, G. and Calvery, H. O. 1944. Methods for the study of irritation and toxicity of substances applied topically to the skin and mucous membranes. *J. Pharmacol. Exp. Ther.* 82:377–390.

Dupuis, G., Benezra, C., Schlewer, G. and Stampf, J. L. 1980. Allergic contact dermatitis to alpha-methylene-gamma-butyro-lactones. Preparation of alantonlactone-protein conjugates and induction of contact sensitivity by an alantolactone-skin protein conjugate, in the guinea pig. *Mol. Immunol.* 17:1045–1051.

Dvorak, H. F., Dvorak, A. M. and Mihm, M. C., Jr. 1974. Morphological studies on cellular hypersensitivity in guinea pigs and man. *Monographs in Allergy* 8:54–65.

Epstein, E. 1969. Perfume dermatitis in men. *J. Am. Med. Assoc.* 209:911–913.

Epstein, E., Rees, W. J. and Maibach, H. I. 1968. Recent experience with routine patch test screening. *Arch. Dermatol.* 98:18–22.

Epstein, S. 1962. Newer contact sensitizors in the home. In *Dermatoses due to physical and environmental factors,* ed. C. Rees. Springfield, Ill.: Thomas.

Epstein, W. L. and Kligman, A. M. 1964. Improved methods of prophetic patch testing. In *The evaluation of therapeutic agents and cosmetics,* eds. T. H. Sternberg and V. Newcomer, pp. 160–170. New York: McGraw-Hill.

Evans, D. A. P. 1963. Pharmacogenetics. *Am. J. Med.* 34:639–662.

Fahr, H., Noster, U. and Schulz, K. H. 1976. Comparison of guinea pig sensitization methods. *Contact Dermatitis* 2:335–339.

Federal Register Amendment. 1964. 29 F.R. 13009.

Ferguson, E. H. and Rothman, S. 1959. Synthetic detergents and eczematous hand eruptions. *Arch. Dermatol.* 80:300–310.

Fernström, A. I. B. 1954. Patch-test studies. I. A new patch-test technique. *Acta Derm.-Venereol. (Stockh.)* 34:203–215.

Fernström, A. I. B. 1955. Patch-test studies. II. Details of the pressure test. *Acta Derm.-Venereol. (Stockh.)* 35:420–428.

Fisher, A. A. 1967. *Contact dermatitis.* Philadelphia: Lea & Febiger.

Fisher, A. A. 1975. Patch testing with perfume ingredients. *Contact Dermatitis* 1:166–168.

Fisher, A. A. and Dooms-Goossens, A. 1976. The effect of perfume "ageing" on the allergenicity of individual perfume ingredients. *Contact Dermatitis* 2:155–159.

Fisher, A. A., Pascher, F. and Kanof, N. B. 1971. Allergic contact dermatitis due to ingredients of vehicles. *Arch. Dermatol.* 104:286–290.

Forslind, B. and Wahlberg, J. E. 1978. The morphology of chromium allergic skin reactions at electron microscopic resolution: Studies in man and guinea pig. *Acta Derm.-Venereol. Suppl.* 79:43–51.

Foussereau, J. and Benezra, C. 1970. *Les eczémas allergiques professionnels.* Paris: Masson.

Freeman, J. J., McKee, R. H. and Trimmer, G. W. 1988. Experimental contact sensitization with 3,4,5-trichloropyridazine. *Contact Dermatitis* 18:259–262.

Fregert, S. 1970. Sensitization to phenylacetaldehyde. *Dermatologica* 141:11–14.

Fregert, S. and Hjorth, N. 1969. Results of standard patch tests with substances abandoned. *Contact Dermatitis Newslett.* 5:85–86.

Fregert, S., Hjorth, N., Magnusson, B., Bandmann, H. J., Calnan, D. C., Cronin, E., Malten, K. E., Meneghini, C. L., Pirilä, V. and Wilkinson, D. S. 1969. Epidemiology of contact dermatitis. *Trans. St. John's Hosp. Dermatol. Soc.* 55:17.

Fregert, S., Dahlquist, I. and Trulsson, L. 1984. An attempt to isolate and identify allergens in lanolin. *Contact Dermatitis* 10:16–19.

Frey, J. R. and Geleick, H. 1959. Experimentelles Kontaktekzem durch Dinitrochlorbenzol an Ratten und Kaninchen. *Dermatologica* 119:294–300.

Frey, J. R. and Wenk, P. 1956. Experimentelle Untersuchungen zur Pathogenese des Kontaktekzems. *Dermatologica* 112:265–305.

Frey, J. R. and Wenk, P. 1958. Ueber die Funktion der regionalen Lymphknoten bei der Entstehung des Dinitrochlorbenzol-Kontaktekzems am Meerschweinchen. *Dermatologica* 116:243–259.

Ginsburg, J. E., Becker, F. T. and Becker, S. W. 1937. Sensitization of guinea pigs to poison ivy. *Arch. Dermatol.* 36:1165–1170.

Giovacchini, R. P. 1972. Old and new issues in the safety evaluation of cosmetics and toiletries. *CRC Crit. Rev. Toxicol.* 361–378.

Gleason, M. N., Gosselin, R. E., Hodge, H. C. and Smith, R. P. 1969. *Clinical toxicology of commercial products,* 3rd ed., sect. II, p. 80. Baltimore: Williams & Wilkins.

Gloxhuber, C. 1967. Toxikologische Prüfung von Kosmetika. *J. Soc. Cosmet. Chem.* 18:737–750.

Gloxhuber, C. 1974. Toxikologische und dermatologische Bewertung von chemischen Haushaltprodukten. *Fette Seifen Anstrichm.* 76:504–509.

Gloxhuber, C. 1976. Bewertung der gesundheitlichen Unbedenklichkeit von chemischen Haushaltprodukten und Kosmetika. *Seifen Oele Fette Wachse* 102:173–178.

Gloxhuber, C., Potokan, M., Braig, S., van Raay, H. G. and Schwarz, G. 1974. Untersuchungen über das Vorkommen eines sensibilisierenden Bestandteils in einem technischen Alkyläthersulfat. *Fette Seifen Anstrichm.* 76:126–129.

Goldberg, A. M. Nov. 1989. Alternatives in toxicology. *Cosmetics & Toiletries* 104:53–59.

Goldemberg, R. L. 1962. Cosmetics and the general population: Safety aspects. *Proc. Sci. Sect. Toilet Goods Assoc.* 38:34–39.

Goodwin, B. F. J., Crevel, R. W. R. and Johnson, A. W. 1981. A comparison of three guinea pig sensitization procedures for the detection of 19 reported human contact sensitizers. *Contact Dermatitis* 7:248–258.

Goodwin, B. F. J., Johnson, A. W. and Karge, B. 1985a. Single injection adjuvant test. *Curr. Probl. Derm.* 14:201–207.

Goodwin, B. F. J. and Johnson, A. W. 1985b. Single injection adjuvant test. In *Current problems in dermatology,* eds. K. E. Andersen, and H. I. Maibach, vol. 14. Karger: Basel.

Greif, N. 1967. Cutaneous safety of fragrance material as measured by the maximization-test. *Am. Perfum. Cosmet.* 82:54–57.

Griffith, J. F. 1969. Predictive and diagnostic testing for contact sensitization. *Toxicol. Appl. Pharmacol.* (Suppl. 3):90–102.

Griffith, J. F. and Bühler, E. V. 1969. *Experimental Skin Sensitization in the Guinea Pig and Man.* Cincinnati, Ohio: Procter and Gamble Co. (Presentation at the 26th Annual Meeting, American Academy of Dermatologists, Bar Harbor, Maine.)

Grimm, W. and Gries, H. 1968. Untersuchungen über die Terpentinöl-Allergie. *Berufs-dermatosen* 16:190–203.

Guide for the care and use of laboratory animals. U.S. Department of Health, Education, and Welfare, Public Health Service, National Institutes of Health, *DHEW Publication* no. (NIH) 78-23, Revised 1978.

Guillot, J. P. and Gonnet, J. F. 1985. The epicutaneous maximization test. *Curr. Probl. Dermatol.* 14:220–247.

Guillot, J. P., Martini, M. C., Giauffret, J. Y. and Gonnet, J. F. 1982. Evaluation du pouvoir sensibilisant chez le cobaye de différents échantillons d'alcools de lano-line. *Int. J. Cosmet. Sci.* 4:99–102.

Guillot, J. P., Gonnet, J. F., Clément, C. and Faccini, J. M. 1983. Comparative study of different methods chosen by the 'Association Française de Normalisation' (AF-NOR) for the evaluation of the sensitizing potential in the albino aguinea pig. *Food Chem. Tox.* 21:795–805.

Hanau, D., Grosshan, E., Parbier, P. and Benezra, C. 1983. The influence of Limonene on induced delayed hypersensitivity to Citral in guinea pigs. I. Histological study. *Acta Derm. Venerol. (Stockh.)* 63:1–7.

Hardy, J. 1983. Allergy, hypersensitivity and cosmetics. *J. Soc. Cosmet. Chem.* 24:423–468.

Harris, G. L. and Maibach, H. I. 1989. Allergic contact dermatitis potential of 3 pyri-dostigmine bromide transdermal drug delivery formulations. *Contact Dermatitis* 21:189–193.

Hausen, B. M., Prater, E. and Schubert, H. 1983. The sensitizing capacity of Alstroe-meria cultivars in man and guinea pig. Remarks on the occurrence, quantity and irritant and sensitizing potency of their constituents tuliposide A and tuliplin A (alpha-methylene-gamma-butyrolactone). *Contact Dermatitis* 9:46–54.

Hausen, B. M. and Schmieder, M. 1986. The sensitizing capacity of coumarins (I). *Contact Dermatitis* 15:157–163.

Hausen, B. M., Bröhan, J., König, W. A., Faasch, H., Hahn, H. and Bruhn, G. 1987a. Allergic and irritant contact dermatitis from falcarinol and didehydrofalcarinol in common ivy (Hedera helix L.). *Contact Dermatitis* 17:1–9.

Hausen, B. M., Wollenweber, E., Senff, H. and Post, B. 1987b. Propolis allergy (I). Origin, properties, usage and literature review. *Contact Dermatitis* 17:163–170.

Hausen, B. M., Wollenweber, E., Senff, H. and Post, B. 1987c. Propolis allergy (II). The sensitizing properties of 1,1-dimethylallyl caffeic acid ester. *Contact Derma-titis* 17:171–177.

Hausen, B. M. and Kresken, J. 1988a. The sensitizing capacity of crotamiton. *Contact Dermatitis* 18:298–322.

Hausen, B. M. and Schiedermair, I. 1988b. The sensitizing capacity of chimaphilin, a naturally-occurring quinone. *Contact Dermatitis* 19:180–183.

Hausen, B. M., Devriese, E. G. and Geuns, J. M. 1988c. Sensitizing potency of coleon O in Coleus sp. (Lamiaceae). *Contact Dermatitis* 19:217–238.

Hausen, B. M. and Wollenweber, E. 1988d. Propolis allergy (III). Sensitization studies with minor constituents. *Contact Dermatitis* 19:296–303.

Hausen, B. M. and Sawall, E. M. 1989a. Sensitization experiments with textile dyes in guinea pigs. *Contact Dermatitis* 20:27–31.

Hausen, B. M., Krueger, A., Mohnert, J., Hahn, H. and König, W. A. 1989b. Contact allergy due to colophony (III). Sensitizing potency of resin acids and some related products. *Contact Dermatitis* 20:41–50.

Hausen, B. M. and Spring, O. 1989c. Sunflower allergy on the constituents of the trichomes of Helianthus annuus L. (Compositae). *Contact Dermatitis* 20:326–334.

Hausen, B. M. and Berger, M. 1989d. The sensitizing capacity of coumarins (III). *Contact Dermatitis* 21:141–147.

Higuchi, T. 1960. Physical chemical analysis of percutaneous absorption process from creams and ointments. *J. Soc. Cosmet. Chem.* 11:85–97.

Hjorth, N. 1959. Cosmetic allergy. *J. Soc. Cosmet. Chem.* 10:96–97.

Hjorth, N. 1961. *Eczematous allergy to balsams,* pp. 112–123. Copenhagen: Munksgaard.

Hjorth, N. 1967. Perfume dermatitis. *Contact Dermatitis Newslett.* 1:2–5.

Hjorth, N. 1980. Geschichte der Kontaktdermatitis und ihr Einfluss auf die heutige Arbeitsdermatologie. *Hautarzt* 31:621–626.

Hjorth, N. and Fregert, S. 1972. Contact dermatitis. In *Textbook of Dermatology,* eds. A. Rook, D. S. Wilkinson and F. J. G. Ebling, pp. 305–385. Philadelphia: Davis.

Hjorth, N. and Trolle-Lassen, C. 1963. Skin reactions to ointment bases. *Trans. St. John's Hosp. Dermatol. Soc.* 49:127–140.

Hofmann, T., Diehl, K.-H., Leist, K.-H. and Weigand, W. 1987. The feasibility of sensitization studies using fewer test animals. *Arch. Toxicol.* 60:470–471.

Holland, B. D., Cox, W. C. and Dehne, E. J. 1950. "Prophetic" patch test; report on results of some 14,000 completed tests performed by Army Industrial Hygiene Laboratory. *Arch. Dermatol.* 61:611–618.

Hood, D. B., Neher, R. J., Reinke, R. E. and Zapp, J. A. 1965. Experience with the guinea pig in screening primary irritants and sensitizers. *Toxicol. Appl. Pharmacol.* 7:478.

Hopf, G. 1971. Empfehlungen für Hautverträglichkeitsprüfungen von Körperpflegemitteln (kosmetischen Erzeugnissen). *Fette Seifen Anstrichm.* 73:467–469.

Hunziker, N. 1969. *Experimental studies on guinea pig's eczema.* Berlin: Springer.

Idman, M. 1976. Anticipating the effects of chemicals—an evolving concept. *Ambio* 5:175–179.

Idson, B. 1968. Topical toxicity and testing. *J. Pharm. Sci.* 57:1–11.

Idson, B. 1971. *Percutaneous absorption of topics in medicinal chemistry.* New York: Interscience.

Ischy, R., Hunziker, N., Bujard, E. and Jadassohn, W. 1969. Experimental eczema. 31st communication: Can eczema be provoked in the tongue of the guinea pig? *Dermatologica* 139:413–416.

Jadassohn, J. 1896a. Zur Kenntniss der medicamentösen Dermatosen. *Verhdlg. Deutsch. Derm. Gesellsch. 5. Congress:* 103–129.

Jadassohn, J. 1896b. A contribution to the study of dermatoses produced by drugs. *Verh. Dtsch. Dermatol. Ges.* In *Selected essays and monographs,* transl. L. Elking, 1900:207–229. London: New Sydenham Society.

Jadassohn, W., Bujard, E. and Brun, R. 1955. The experimental eczema of the guinea pig nipple. *J. Invest. Dermatol.* 24:247–253.

Jarrett, A. 1973. *The physiology and pathophysiology of the skin,* Vol. 1. London: Academic Press.

Johnson, A. W. and Goodwin, B. F. J. 1985. The Draize test and modifications. *Curr. Probl. Dermatol.* 14:31–38.

Johnson, R. A., Baer, H., Kirkpatrick, C. H., Dawson, C. R. and Khurana, R. G. 1972. Comparison of the contact allergenicity of the four pentadecyl-catechols derived from poison ivy urushiol in human subjects. *J. Allergy* 49:27–35.

Jungermann, E. and Silberman, H. C. 1972. The absorption and desorption of cosmetic chemicals on skin. *J. Soc. Cosmet. Chem.* 23:139–152.

Justice, J. D., Travers, J. J. and Vinson, L. J. 1961. The correlation between animal tests and human tests in assessing product mildness. *Proc. Sci. Sect. Toilet Goods Assoc.* 35:12.

Kahn, G. 1971. Intensified contact sensitization to benzyl salicylate. *Arch. Dermatol.* 103:497–500.

Karlberg, A. T., Boman, A. and Wahlberg, J. E. 1983. Copper—a rare sensitizer. *Contact Dermatitis* 9:134–139.

Karlberg, A. T., Boman, A., Holmbom, B. and Liden, C. 1986. Contact allergy to acid and neutral fractins of rosins. Sensitization experiments in guinea pigs and patch testing in patients. *Derm. Beruf. Umwelt* 34:31–36.

Karlberg, A. T., Boman, A. and Nilsson, J. L. G. 1988a. Hydrogenation reduces the allergenicity of colophony (rosin). *Contact Dermatitis* 19:22–29.

Karlberg, A. T., Boman, A., Hackseli, Ul., Jacobsson, S. and Nilsson, J. L. G. 1988b. Contact allergy to dehydroabietic acid derivitives isolated from Portugese colophony. *Contact Dermatitis* 19:166–174.

Kastner, E. 1968. Parfüm and Allergie. *J. Soc. Cosmet. Chem.* 19:807–821.

Katz, M. and Poulsen, B. J. 1971. Absorption of drugs through the skin. In *Handbuch der experimentellen Pharmakologie, 28/1,* eds. B. Brodie and J. D. Gilette, pp. 104–174. Berlin: Springer.

Katz, M. and Poulsen, B. J. 1972. Corticoid, vehicle and skin interaction in percutaneous absorption. *J. Soc. Cosmet. Chem.* 23:565–590.

Katz, M. and Shaikh, Z. 1965. Percutaneous corticosteroid absorption correlated to partition coefficient. *J. Pharm. Sci.* 54:591–594.

Kero, M. and Hannuksela, M. 1980. Guinea pig maximization test, open epicutaneous test and chamber test in induction of delayed contact hypersensitivity. *Contact Dermatitis* 6:341–344.

Kimber, I. 1988. Immunotoxicology and allergy: Old problems and new approaches. *Toxic. in Vitro* 2:309–311.

Klecak, G. 1985. The Freund's complete adjuvant test and open epicutaneous test. A complementary test procedure for realistic assessment of allergenic potential. *Curr. Probl. Dermatol.* 14:152–171.

Klecak, G., Geleick, H. and Frey, J. R. 1977. Screening of fragrance materials for allergenicity in the guinea pig. I. Comparison of four testing methods. *J. Soc. Cosmet. Chem.* 28:53–64.

Kligman, A. M. and Epstein, W. 1959. Some factors effecting contact sensitization in man. In *Mechanism of Hypersensitivity,* eds. J. H. Shaffer, G. A. LoGrippo and M. W. Chase, pp. 713–722. Boston, Mass.: Little Brown.

Kligman, A. M. 1966a. The identification of contact allergens by human assay. I. A critique of standard methods. *J. Invest. Dermatol.* 47:369–374.

Kligman, A. M. 1966b. The identification of contact allergens by human assay. II. Factors influencing the induction and measurement of allergic contact dermatitis. *J. Invest. Dermatol.* 47:375–392.

Kligman, A. M. 1966c. The identification of contact allergens by human assay. III. The maximization test. A procedure for screening and rating contact sensitizers. *J. Invest. Dermatol.* 47:393–409.

Kligman, A. M. 1966d. The SLS provocative patch test. *J. Invest. Dermatol.* 46:573–589.

Kligman, A. M. and Epstein, W. 1959. Some factors effecting contact sensitization in man. In *Mechanism of hypersensitivity,* p. 713. Boston: Little, Brown.

Kligman, A. M. and Epstein, W. 1975. Updating the maximization test for identifying contact allergens. *Contact Dermatitis* 1:231–239.

Kligman, A. and Gollhausen, R. 1986. The "angry back": a new concept or old confusion? *Br. J. Dermatol.* 115:Supplement 31:93–100.

Koch, G., Magnusson, B. and Nyquist, G. 1971. Contact allergy to medicaments and materials used in dentistry. II. Sensitivity to eugenol and colophony. *Odontol. Revy* 22:275–289.

Kojima, S. and Momma, J. 1989. Phosgene (2,5-dichlorophenyl)hydrazone, a new strong sensitizer. *Contact Dermatitis* 20:235–236.

Lachapelle, J. M. and Tennstedt, D. 1979. Low allergenicity of triclosan. Predictive testing in guinea pigs and in humans. *Dermatologica* 158:379–383.

La Du, B. N. 1965. Pharmacogenetics. *Toxicol. Appl. Pharmacol.* 7:27–38.

Lammintausta, K., Pitkanen, O. P., Kalimo, K. and Jansen, C. T. 1985. Interrelationship of nickel and cobalt contact sensitization. *Contact Dermatitis* 13:148–152.

Lamson, S. A., Kong, B. M. and de Silva, S. J. 1982. D & C Yellow Nos. 10 and 11: Delayed contact hypersensitivity in the guinea pig. *Contact Dermatitis* 8:200–203.

Landsdown, A. B. G. and Grasso, P. 1972. Physico-chemical factors influencing epidermal damage by surface active damage. *Br. J. Dermatol.* 86:361–373.

Landsteiner, K. and Chase, M. W. 1937. Studies on the sensitization of animals with simple chemical compounds. IV. Anaphylaxis induced by picryl chloride and 2:4 dinitrochlorobenzene. *J. Exp. Med.* 66:337–351.

Landsteiner, K. and Chase, M. W. 1940. Studies on the sensitization of animals with simple chemical compounds. VII. Skin sensitization by intraperitoneal injection. *J. Exp. Med.* 71:237–245.

Landsteiner, K. and Chase, M. W. 1941. Studies on the sensitization of animals with simple chemical compounds. IX. Skin sensitization induced by injection of conjugates. *J. Exp. Med.* 73:431–438.

Landsteiner, K. and Chase, M. W. 1942. Experiments on transfer of cutaneous sensitivity to simple chemical compounds. *Proc. Soc. Exp. Biol. Med.* 49:688.

Landsteiner, K. and DiSomma, A. A. 1938. Studies on the sensitization of animals with simple chemical compounds. V. Sensitization to diazomethane and mustard oil. *J. Exp. Med.* 68:505–512.

Landsteiner, K. and Jacobs, J. 1935. Studies on sensitization of animals with simple chemical compounds. *J. Exp. Med.* 61:643–656.

Landsteiner, K. and Jacobs, J. 1936. Studies on the sensitization of animals with simple chemical compounds, II. *J. Exp. Med.* 64:625–629.

Lane-Petter, W. and Porter, G. 1963. The guinea pig. In *Animals for research,* ed. W. Lane-Petter, pp. 287–321. New York: Academic Press.

Larsen, W. G. 1975. Cosmetic dermatitis due to a perfume. *Contact Dermatitis* 1:142–145.

Lepoittevin, J.-P., Benezra, C. and Asakawa, Y. 1989. Allergic contact dermatitis to Ginkgo biloba L.: relationship with urushiol. *Arch. Dermatol. Res.* 281:227–230.

Liden, C. and Boman, A. 1988. Contact allergy to colour developing agents in the guinea pig. *Contact Dermatitis* 19:290–295.

Lieu, E. J. and Tong, G. L. 1973. Physicochemical properties and percutaneous absorption of drugs. *J. Soc. Cosmet. Chem.* 24:371–384.

Lippold, B. C. 1974. Auswirkungen grenzflächenaktiver Substanzen auf Löslichkeit, chemische Stabilität und Verfügbarkeit cutan applizierter Wirkstoffe. *J. Soc. Cosmet. Chem.* 25:423–435.

Lüders, G. 1976. Reaktionen und Schäden nach äusseren Einwirkungen von Arzneimitteln und Berufsnoxen auf die Haut. *Berufsdermatosen* 24:61–70.

Magnusson, B. 1975. The relevance of results obtained with the guinea pig maximization test. In *Animal models in dermatology,* ed. H. Maibach, pp. 76–83. Edinburgh: Churchill Livingstone.

Magnusson, B. and Hersle, K. 1965. Patch test methods: I. A comparative study of six different types of patch tests. *Acta Derm. Venereol. (Stockh.)* 45:123–128.

Magnusson, B. and Kligman, A. M. 1969. The identification of contact allergens by animal assay. The guinea pig maximization test. *J. Invest. Dermatol.* 52:268–276.

Magnusson, B. and Kligman, A. M. 1970. *Allergic contact dermatitis in the guinea pig. Identification of contact allergens.* Springfield, Ill.: Thomas.

Magnusson, B. and Mobacken, H. 1972. Contact allergy to a self-hardening acrylic sealer for assembling metal parts. *Berufsdermatosen* 20:198–199.

Magnusson, B. and Möller, H. 1979. Contact allergy without skin disease. *Acta Derm.-Venereol. (Stockh.)* 59(Suppl. 85):113–115.

Magnusson, B., Blohm, S. G., Fregert, S., Hjorth, S., Havding, N., Pirilä, V. and Skog, E. 1962. Standardization of routine patch testing. *Acta Derm. Venereol. (Stockh.)* 126–127.

Magnusson, B. et al. 1966. Routine patch testing. II. Proposed basic series of test substances for Scandinavian countries and general remarks on testing technique. *Acta Derm. Venereol. (Stockh.)* 46:153–158. III. Frequency of contact allergy at six Scandinavian clinics. *Acta Derm. Venereol. (Stockh.)* 46:396–400.

Maguire, H. C. 1972. Mechanism of intensification by Freund's complete adjuvant of the acquisition of delayed hypersensitivity in the guinea pig. *Immunol. Commun.* 1:239–246.

Maguire, H. C. 1973. The bioassay of contact allergens in the guinea pig. *J. Soc. Cosmet. Chem.* 24:151–162.

Maguire, H. C. 1974a. Alteration in the acquisition of delayed hypersensitivity with adjuvant in the guinea pig. *Monogr. Allergy* 8:13–26.

Maguire, H. C. 1974b. Induction of delayed hypersensitivity to nitrogen mustard in the guinea pig. *Br. J. Dermatol.* 91:21–26.

Maguire, H. C. 1975. Estimation of the allergenicity of prospective human contact sensitizers in the guinea pig. In *Animal models in dermatology,* ed. H. Maibach, pp. 67–75. Edinburgh: Churchill Livingstone.

Maguire, H. C. 1980. Guinea pig maximization test performs "best overall" of five methods of identifying weak contact allergens, FDA-contracted comparative study finds. *FDS Reports,* Toiletries, Fragrances and Skin Care. "The Rose Sheet" Sept. 8, 3–5.

Maguire, H. C. and Chase, M. W. 1967. Exaggerated delayed-type hypersensitivity to simple chemical allergens in the guinea pig. *J. Invest. Dermatol.* 49:460–468.

Maguire, H. C. and Chase, M. W. 1972. Studies on the sensitization of animals with simple chemical compounds. XIII. Sensitization of guinea pigs with picric acid. *J. Exp. Med.* 135:357–374.

Maguire, H. C., Jr. 1985. Estimation of the allergenicity of prospective human contact sensitizers in the guinea pig. In *Models in Dermatology,* vol. 2, eds. H. Maibach and N. J. Lowe, pp. 234–239. Basel: Karger AG.

Maguire, H. C., Jr. and Cipriano, D. 1984. Allergic contact dermatitis in laboratory animals. In *Cutaneous toxicity,* eds. V. A. Drill and P. Lazar, pp. 55–62. New York: Raven Press.

Maibach, H., ed. 1975. *Animal models in dermatology.* Edinburgh: Churchill Livingstone.

Maibach, H. I. and Epstein, W. L. 1965. Predictive patch testing for allergic sensitization in man. *Toxicol. Appl. Pharmacol.* 7:39–43.

Maibach, H. I. and Mitchell, J. C. 1975. Costus absolute (Saussurea): Predictive assay for allergic contact sensitization in guinea pigs. *Conf. Dermatol.* 1:184.

Malten, K. E. 1975. Cosmetics, the consumer, the factory worker and the occupational physician. *Contact Dermatitis* 1:16–26.

Malten, K. E. 1979. Four bakers showing positive patch-tests to a number of fragrance materials, which can also be used as flavors. *Acta Derm. Venereol. (Stockh.)* 59(Suppl. 85):117–121.

Malten, K. E. and Zielhuis, R. L. 1964. *Industrial toxicology and dermatology in the production and processing of plastic.* New York: Elsevier.

Malten, K. E., Werwilghen, L. M. E. and Seutter, E. 1966a. The sensitization capacity of a simple epoxy resin as demonstrated in the guinea pig nipple test. 1st European Congress on Allergy, Stockholm, 1965. *Acta Derm. Venereol. (Stockh.)* Suppl.

Malten, K. E., Seutter, E., Verwilghen, M. E. and Disse, G. F. 1966b. The sensitization capacity of a simple epoxy resin as demonstrated in the guinea pig nipple test. II *Proc. 15th Int. Congr. Occup. Health, Vienna.*

Malten, K., Meneghini, C. L., Pirilä, V. and Wilkinson, D. S. 1969. Epidemiology of contact dermatitis. *Bull. Johns Hopkins Hosp.* 55:17–35.

Malten, K. E. et al. 1971. Occupational dermatitis in five European dermatological departments. *Berufsdermatosen* 19:1–13.

Marchand, B., Barbier, P., Ducombs, G., Foussereau, J., Martin, P. and Benezra, C. 1982. Allergic contact dermatitis to various salols (phenyl salicylates): A structure-activity relationship study in man and in animal (Guinea Pig). *Arch. Dermatol. Res.* 272:61–66.

Marcussen, P. V. 1962. Eczematous allergy to metals. *Acta Allergol. (Kbh.)* 17:311–333.

Marzulli, F. N. 1962. Barriers to skin penetration. *J. Invest. Dermatol.* 39:387–393.

Marzulli, F. and Maguire, H. C., Jr. 1982. Usefulness and limitations of various guinea pig test methods in detecting human skin sensitizers—validation of guinea pig tests for skin hypersensitivity. *Food Cosmet. Toxicol.* 20:67–74.

Marzulli, F. N. and Maibach, H. I. 1974. The use of graded concentrations in studying skin sensitizers: Experimental contact sensitization in man. *Food Cosmet. Toxicol.* 12:219–227.

Marzulli, F. N. and Maibach, H. I. 1976. Contact allergy: Predictive testing in man. *Contact Dermatitis* 2:1–17.

Marzulli, F. N., Carson, T. R. and Maibach, H. I. 1968. Delayed contact hypersensitivity studies in man and animals. *Proc. Joint Conf. Cosmet. Sci., Washington, D.C.* 107–122.

Marzulli, F. and Maguire, H. C., Jr. 1983. Validation of guinea pig tests for skin hypersensitivity. In *Dermatotoxicology,* eds. F. N. Marzulli and H. I. Maibach, 2nd ed., pp. 237–250. New York: Hemisphere.

Maurer, T. 1974. Tierexperimentelle Methoden zur prädiktiven Erfassung sensibilisierender Eigenschaften von Kontaktallergenen. Inauguraldissertation, Universität Basel.

Maurer, T. 1983. *Contact and photocontact allergens. A manual of predictive test methods.* New York: Becker.

Maurer, T. 1985. The optimization test. *Curr. Probl. Dermatol.* 14:114–151.

Maurer, T. and Meier, F. 1984. Sensitization potential of benzotriazole. *Contact Dermatitis* 10:163–165.

Maurer, T., Thomann, P., Weirich, E. G. and Hess, R. 1975. The optimization test in the guinea pig. A method for the predictive evaluation of the contact allergenicity of chemicals. *Agents Actions* 5:174–179.

Maurer, T., Thomann, P., Weirich, E. G. and Hess, R. 1978. Predictive evaluation in animals of the contact allergenic potential of medically important substances. I. Comparison of different methods of inducing and measuring cutaneous sensitization. *Contact Dermatitis* 4:321–333.

Maurer, T., Thomann, P., Weirich, E. G. and Hess, R. 1979. Predictive evaluation in animals of the contact allergenic potential of medically important substances. II. Comparison of different methods of cutaneous sensitization with "weak" allergens. *Contact Dermatitis* 5:1–10.

Maurer, T., Weirich, E. C. and Hess, R. 1980a. The optimization test in guinea pigs in relation to other prediction sensitization methods. *Toxicology* 15:163–171.

Maurer, T., Weirich, E. G. and Hess, R. 1980b. Predictive animal testing for photocontact allergenicity. *Br. J. Derm.* 63:593–605.

Maurer, T., Hess, R. and Weirich, E. G. 1985. Prädiktive tierexperimentelle Kontaktallergenitätsprüfung. *Dermatosen* 33:6–11.

McKee, R. H. and Maibach, H. J. 1985. The phototoxic and allergenic potential of EDS liquids. *Contact Dermatitis* 13:72–79.

Meneghini, C. L., Rantuccio, R. and Lomuto, M. 1971. Additives, vehicles and active drugs of topical medicaments as causes of delayed-type allergic dermatitis. *Dermatologica* 143:137–147.

Meyer, F. and Ziegenmeyer, J. 1975. Resorptionsmöglichkeiten der Haut. *J. Soc. Cosmet. Chem.* 26:93–104.

Meyer, J. C., Grundmann, H.-P., Weiss, H. and Trachsel, H. 1979. Spättyp-Ueberempfindlichkeit gegenüber Staphylokokkenantigenen bei Meerschweinchen. *Dermatologica* 159:383–385.

Middleton, J. D. 1978. Predictive animal tests for delayed dermal hypersensitivity in man. *Soap Perfum. Cosmet.* 51(5):201–205.

Miescher, G. 1962. Ekzem, Histopathologie, Morphologie, Nosologie. In *Handb. Haut-Geschl. Krankh. Erg.-Werk*, ed. J. Jadassohn, vol. 2, pt. 1, p. 1. Berlin: Springer.

Mikkelsen, T. and Trolle-Lassen, C. 1969. Viscosity of test substances in petrolatum. *Contact Dermatitis Newslett.* 6:128–129.

Mitchell, J. C. 1975. Contact hypersensitivity to some perfume materials. *Contact Dermatitis* 1:196–199.

Mitchell, J. C. and Maibach, H. I. 1982. The angry back syndrome—the excited skin syndrome. *Semin. Dermatol.* 1:9–13.

NACDG (North American Contact Dermatitis Group). 1973a. News and notes. Allergen list. *Arch. Dermatol.* 107–457.

NACDG. 1973b. Epidemiology of contact dermatitis in North America: 1973. *Arch. Dermatol.* 108:537–540.

Nakayama, H. et al. 1974. *Allergen controlled system.* Tokyo: Kamhara Shuppan.

Nethercott, J. R. 1981. Allergic contact dermatitis due to an epoxy acrylate. *Br. J. Dermatol.* 104:697–703.

Newcomer, V. D. and Landau, J. W. 1964. The current role of animals in the development of topically applied preparations. In *The evaluation of therapeutic agents and cosmetics*, eds. T. H. Sternberg and V. D. Newcomer, pp. 102–124. New York: McGraw-Hill.

Nicholas, P. 1978. "Economic" safety evaluation. *Soap Perfum. Cosmet.* 51(5):197-205.

Nilzén, A. and Wikström, K. 1955. The influence of sodium lauryl sulfate on the sensitization of guinea pigs to chrome and nickel. *Acta Derm. Venereol. (Stockh.)* 35:292-299.

Nobréus, N., Magnusson, B., Leander, L. and Attström, R. 1974. Induction of dinitrochlorobenzene contact sensitivity in dogs. Transfer of sensitivity by thoracic duct lymphocytes and suppression of sensitivity by antithymocyte serum. *Monogr. Allergy* 8:100-109.

Noster, U. and Hausen, B. M. 1978. Berufsbedingtes Kontaktekzem durch Chinophthalonfarbstoff (Solvent Yellow 33: C. I. 47000). *Hautarzt* 29:153-157.

Oberste-Lehn, H. and Wiemann, F. W. 1950. Die Meerschweinchenhaut als dermatologisches Testobjeckt. *Arch. Klin. Exp. Dermatol.* 209:539-550.

OECD, Organization for Economic Cooperation and Development, Guidelines for Testing of Chemicals. Director of information, OECD, 2, rue Andre-Pascal, F-75775, Paris Cedex 16, France 1981.

Oliver, G. J. A., Botham, P. A. and Kimber, I. 1986. Models for contact sensitization—novel approaches and future developments. *Br. J. Dermatol.* 115: Supplement 31, 53-62.

Opdyke, D. L. J. 1974. Monographs on fragrance raw materials. *Food Cosmet. Toxicol.* 12:807-1016.

Opdyke, D. L. J. 1975. The safety of fragrance ingredients. *Br. J. Dermatol.* 93:351.

Opdyke, D. L. J. 1976. The safety of fragrances. *Soap Perfum. Cosmet.* 49:237-241.

Ostbourne, R. A. 1956. Dermatological evaluation of perfumes of low sensitizing index. *Proc. Sci. Sect. Toilet Goods Assoc.* 17:80-84.

Ostrenga, J. O. 1971. Significance of vehicle composition. I. Relationship between topical vehicle compositions, skin penetrability, and clinical efficacy. *J. Pharm. Sci.* 60:1175-1179.

Palazzallo, M. J. and DiPasquale, L. C. 1983. The sensitization potential of D & C Yellow No. 11 in guinea pigs. *Contact Dermatitis* 9:367-371.

Parker, D. and Turk, J. L. 1983. Contact sensitivity to acrylate compounds in guinea pigs. *Contact Dermatitis* 9:55-60.

Paschoud, J. M. 1967. Externe Kontaktallergene. Alphabetisch geordnete Uebersicht der Fachliteratur 1960 bis 1965. *Hautarzt* 18:145-149.

Paterson, J. S. 1966. The guinea pig or Cavy. In *The UFAW handbook on the care and management of laboratory animals*, 3rd ed., p. 241. Baltimore: Williams & Wilkins.

Pirilä, V. 1947. On occupational diseases of the skin among paint factory workers and painters in Finland. *Acta Derm. Venereol. (Stockh.)* 27(Suppl. 16).

Pirilä, V. 1962. On the primary irritant and sensitizing effects of organic solvents. *Excerpta Med. Int. Congr. Ser.* 55:463-466.

Pirilä, V. 1971. Patch testing technique. A new modification of the chamber test. *Excerpta Med. Int. Congr. Ser.* 235:50.

Pirilä, V. 1974. Chamber test versus lapptest. *Förh. Nord. Dermatol. Fören.* 20:43.

Polak, L. 1980. Immunological aspects of contact sensitivity. *Monogr. Allergy* 15:1-170.

Polak, L. and Turk, J. L. 1968. Studies on the effect of systemic administration of sensitizers in guinea-pigs with contact sensitivity to inorganic metal compounds. *Clin. Exp. Immunol.* 3:245-254.

Polak, L., Barnes, J. M. and Turk, J. L. 1968. The genetic control of contact sensitization to inorganic metal compounds in guinea-pigs. *Immunology* 14:707-711.

Polak, L., Turk, J. L. and Frey, J. R. 1973. Studies on contact hypersensitivity to chromium compounds. *Progr. Allergy* 17:145–226.

Poole, R. L., Griffith, J. F. and Macmillan, F. S. K. 1970. Experimental contact sensitization with benzoyl peroxide. *Arch. Dermatol.* 102:635–639.

Poulsen, B. J., Young, E., Coquilla, V. and Katz, M. 1968. Effect of topical vehicle composition on the *in vitro* release of fluocinolone acetonide and its acetate ester. *J. Pharm. Sci.* 57:928–933.

Prince, H. N. and Prince, T. G. 1977. Comparative guinea pig assays for contact hypersensitivity. *Cosmet. Toiletr.* 92:53–58.

Quisno, R. A. and Doyle, R. L. January/February 1983. A new occlusive patch test system with a plastic chamber. *J. Soc. Cosmet. Chem.* 34:13–19.

Rackemann, F. H. and Simon, F. A. 1934. The sensitization of guinea pigs to poison ivy. *Science* 79:344.

Rand, M. J. 1972. Toxicological considerations and safety testing of cosmetics and toiletries. *Am. Cosmet. Perfum.* 87:39–48.

Rantuccio, F. and Meneghini, C. L. 1970. Results of patch testing with cosmetic components in consecutive eczematous patients. *Contact Dermatitis Newslett.* 7:156–158.

Rao, K. S., Betso, J. E. and Olson, K. J. 1981. A collection of guinea pig sensitization. Test results grouped by chemical class. *Drug Chem. Toxicol.* 4:331–351.

Reller, H. H. and Bybee, P. M. 1985. Induction in the guinea pig of delayed hypersensitivity to compound 48/80. *Contact Dermatitis* 13:136–139.

Ritschel, W. A. 1969. Sorptionsvermittler in der Biopharmazie. *Angew. Chem.* 81:757–796.

Ritz, H. L., Connor, D. S. and Sauter, E. D. 1975. Contact sensitization of guinea-pigs with unsaturated and halogenated sultones. *Contact Dermatitis* 1:349–358.

Ritz, H. L. and Buehler, E. V. 1980. Planning conduct, and interpretation of guinea pig sensitization patch tests. In *Current Concepts in Cutaneous Toxicity,* eds. V. A. Drill and P. Lazar, pp. 25–40. New York: Academic Press.

Rockwell, E. M. 1955. Study of several factors influencing contact irritation and sensitization. *J. Invest. Dermatol.* 24:35–49.

Rostenberg, A. 1947. Studies on the eczematous sensitization. I. The route by which the sensitization generalizes. *J. Invest. Dermatol.* 8:345–354.

Rostenberg, A. 1953. The allergic dermatoses. *J. Am. Med. Assoc.* 165:1118–1125.

Rostenberg, A. 1954. Concepts of allergic sensitization: Their role in producing occupational dermatoses. *Ind. Med.* 23:1–8.

Rostenberg, A. 1957. Primary irritant and allergic eczematous reactions. *Arch. Dermatol.* 75:547–558.

Rostenberg, A. 1959. A predictive procedure for eczematous hypersensitivity. *Arch. Ind. Health* 20:181–193.

Rostenberg, A. and Haeberlin, J. B. 1950. Studies in eczematous sensitization. III. The development in species other than man or the guinea pig. *J. Invest. Dermatol.* 15:233–247.

Rothenborg, H. W. and Hjorth, N. 1968. Allergy to perfumes from toilet soap and detergents in patients with dermatitis. *Arch. Dermatol.* 97:417–421.

Roudabush, R. L., Terhaar, C. J., Fassett, D. W. and Dzibua, S. P. 1965. Comparative acute effects of some chemicals on the skin of rabbits and guinea pigs. *Toxicol. Appl. Pharmacol.* 7:559–565.

Rowe, V. K. and Olson, K. J. 1965. Prediction of dermal toxicity in humans from studies on animals. *Toxicol. Appl. Pharmacol.* 7:86–92.

Rudner, E. J., Clendenning, W. E., Epstein, E., Fisher, A. A., Jilson, O. F., Jordan, W. P., Kanof, N., Larsen, W., Maibach, H., Mitchell, J. C., O'Quinn, S. E.,

410　　　　　　　　　　　　G. Klecak

Schorr, W. F. and Sulzberger, M. B. 1973. Epidemiology of contact dermatitis in North America. *Arch. Dermatol.* 108:537–540.

Rudzki, E. and Kleiniewsak, D. 1970. The epidemiology of contact dermatitis in Poland. *Br. J. Dermatol.* 83:543–545.

Sachs, L. 1971. *Statistische Auswertungsmethoden.* Stuttgart: Thieme.

Sato, Y. 1985. Modified guinea pig maximization test. *Curr. Probl. Dermatol.* 14:193–200.

Sato, Y., Katsumura, Y., Ichikawa, H., Kobayashi, T., Kozuka, T., Morikawa, F. and Ohta, S. 1981. A modified technique of guinea pig testing to identify delayed hypersensitivity allergens. *Contact Dermatitis* 7:225–237.

Senma, M., Fujuware, N., Sasaki, S., Toxama, M., Sakaguchi, K. and Takaoka, I. 1978. Studies on the cutaneous sensitization reaction of guinea pigs to purified aromatic chemicals. *Acta Derm.-Venereol. (Stockh.)* 58:121–124.

Schaefer, H. 1974. Wechselbeziehungen zwischen Haut, Vehikel und Arzneimittel bei der Penetration in die menschliche Haut. I. Mechanismus der Penetration. *Fette Seifen Anstrichm.* 76:220–222.

Schaefer, H., Zesch, A. and Stüttgen, G. 1975. Penetration von Medikamenten in die Haut. *Hautarzt* 26:449–451.

Schaeffer, M., Talaga, P., Stampf, J. L. and Benezra, C. 1990. Cross-reaction in allergic contact dermatitis from α-methylene-γ-butyrolactones: importance of the cis or trans ring junction. *Contact Dermatitis* 22:32–36.

Schäfer, U., Metz, J., Pevny, I. and Röckl, H. 1978. Sensibilisierungsversuche an Meerschweinchen mit fünf parasubstituierten Benzolderivaten. *Arch. Dermatol. Forsch.* 261:153–161.

Scheuplein, R. J. 1965. Mechanism of percutaneous absorption. I. Routes of penetration and the influence of solubility. *J. Invest. Dermatol.* 45:334–346.

Schlewer, G., Stampf, J. L. and Benezra, C. 1980. Synthesis of alpha-methylene-gamma-butyrolactones; a structure-activity relationship study of their allergenic power. *J. Med. Chem.* 23:1031–1038.

Schubert, H. and Ziegler, V. 1971. Die sensibilisierende Wirkung von flüssigem Polysulfidkautschuk. *Berufsdermatosen* 19:229–239.

Schubert, H., Göring, H. D. and Gans, U. 1973. Untersuchungen zur Sensibilisierungsfähigkeit von Aethoxyquin und p-Pheneditin. *Dermatol. Monatsschr.* 159:791–796.

Schulz, K. H., Garbe, I., Hausen, B. M. and Simatupang, M. H. 1977. The sensitizing capacity of naturally occurring quinones. Experimental studies in guinea pigs. I. Naphthoquinones and related compounds. *Arch. Derm. Res.* 258:41–52.

Schumacher, G. E. 1967. Some properties of dimethyl sulfoxide in man. *Drug. Intell.* 1:188–194.

Schwartz, L. 1951. The skin testing of new cosmetics. *J. Soc. Cosmet. Chem.* 2:321–324.

Schwartz, L. and Peck, S. 1935. The irritants in adhesive plaster. *Public Health Rep.* 50:811–819; cited by L. Schwartz et al. 1940. An outbreak of dermatitis from new resin fabric finishes. *J. Am. Med. Assoc.* 115:906–911.

Schwartz, L. and Peck, S. M. 1944. The patch test in contact dermatitis. *Public Health Rep.* 59:546–557.

Schwartz, L. and Peck, S. M. 1946. *Cosmetics and dermatitis.* New York: Hoeber.

Schwartz, K., Tulipan, L. and Birmingham, D. 1957. *Occupational diseases of the skin.* Philadelphia: Lea & Febiger.

Sharp, D. W. 1978. The sensitization potential of some perfumed ingredients tested using a modified Draize procedure. *Toxicology* 9:261–271.

Shelanski, H. A. and Shelanski, M. V. 1953. A new technique of human patch tests. *Proc. Sci. Sect. Toilet Goods Assoc.* 10:46–49.

Siegel, J. M. and Melther, L. 1948. Patch test versus usage tests with special reference to volatile ingredients. *Arch. Dermatol.* 57:660–663.

Simon, F. A. 1936. Observations on poison ivy hypersensitiveness in guinea pigs. *J. Immunol.* 30:275–286.

Simon, F. A., Simon, M. G., Rackemann, F. M. and Dienes, L. 1934. The sensitization of guinea pigs to poison ivy. *J. Immunol.* 27:113–123.

Skog, E. and Wahlberg, J. E. 1970. Sensitization and testing of guinea pigs with potassium bichromate. *Acta Derm. Venereol. (Stockh.)* 50:103–108.

Smeenk, G. and Rijnbeek, A. M. 1969. The water-binding properties of the water-soluble substances in the horny layer. *Acta Derm. Venereol. (Stockh.)* 49:476–480.

Stadler, J. C. and Karol, M. H. 1985. Use of dose-response data to compare the skin sensitizing abilities of decyclohexylmethane-4,4′-diisocyanate and picryl chloride in two animal species. *Toxicol. Appl. Pharmacol.* 78:445–450.

Stampf, J.-L., Schlewer, G. and Benezra, C. 1978a. Animal and human sensitivity to alpha-methylene-gamma-butyrolactone derivatives. *Contact Dermatitis* 4:306–307.

Stampf, J.-L., Schlewer, G., Ducombs, G., Foussereau, J. and Benezra, C. 1978b. Allergic contact dermatitis due to sesquiterpene lactones. A comparative study of human and animal sensitivity to alpha-methylene-beta-bytyrolactone and derivatives. *Br. J. Dermatol.* 99:163–169.

Stampf, J.-L. and Benezra, C. 1982a. The sensitizing capacity of helenin and of two of its main constituents, the sesquiterpene lactones alantolactone and isoalantolactone: A comparison of epicutaneous and intradermal sensitizing methods and of different strains of guinea pigs. *Contact Dermatitis* 8:16–24.

Stampf, J.-L., Benezra, C. and Asakawa, Y. 1982b. Stereospecificity of allergic contact dermatitis (ACD) to Enantiomers. Part III. Experimentally induced ACD to natural sesquiterpene dialdehyde polygodial in guinea pigs. *Arch. Dermatol. Res.* 274:277–281.

Steigleder, G. K. 1975. Differentialdiagnose des allergisch bedingten Kontaktekzems. *Hautarzt* 26:62–64.

Stemann, G. 1965. Die percutane Penetrationsvermittlung von Rhodamin B durch organische Flüssigkeiten unter besonderer Berücksichtigung ihrer physiko-chemischen Eigenschaften. Dissertation, Hamburg.

Stoughton, R. B. 1965. Percutaneous absorption. *Toxicol. Appl. Pharmacol.* 7(Suppl. 3):1–6.

Strauss, H. W. 1937. Studies in experimental hypersensitiveness in the rhesus monkey. I. Active sensitization with poison ivy. *J. Immunol.* 32:241–246. III. On the manner of development of the hypersensitiveness in contact dermatitis. *J. Immunol.* 33:215–225.

Stüttgen, G. 1965. *Die normale und pathologische Physiologie der Haut.* Stuttgart: Fischer.

Stüttgen, G. 1972. Die Haut als Resorptionsorgan in pharmakokinitischer Sicht. *Arzneim. Forsch.* 22:324–329.

Sulzberger, M. B. 1930. Arsphenamine hypersensitiveness in guinea pigs. *Arch. Dermatol.* 22:839–848.

Sulzberger, M. B. and Baer, R. L. 1938. Sensitization to simple chemicals. III. Relationship between chemical structure and properties, and sensitizing capacities in the production of exzematous sensitivity in man. *J. Invest. Dermatol.* 1:45–58.

Thorgeirsson, A. 1978. Sensitization capacity of epoxy reactive diluents in the guinea pig. *Acta Derm. Venereol. (Stockh.)* 58:329–331.

Thorgeirsson, A. and Fregert, S. 1977. Allergenicity of epoxy resins in the guinea pig. *Acta Derm. Venereol. (Stockh.)* 57:253–256.

Thorgeirsson, A., Fregert, S. and Magnusson, B. 1975. Allergenicity of epoxy reactive diluents in the guinea pig. *Berufsdermatosen* 23:178–193.

Traub, E. F., Tusing, T. W. and Spoor, H. J. 1954. Evaluation of dermal sensitivity. *Arch. Dermatol.* 69:399–409.

Treherne, J. E. 1956. The permeability of skin to some non-electrolytes. *J. Physiol. (Lond.)* 133:171–180.

Tsuchiya, S., Kondo, M., Okamoto, K. and Takase, Y. 1982. Studies on contact hypersensitivity in the guinea pig. The cumulative contact enhancement test. *Contact Dermatitis* 8:246–255.

Tsuchiya, S., Kondo, M., Okamoto, K. and Takase, Y. 1985. The cumulative contact enhancement test. *Curr. Probl. Dermatol.* 14:208–219.

Turk, J. L. 1966. Die Immunreaktion vom verzögerten Typ und ihre Bedeutung in der Medizin. *Triangel* 7:275–280.

Turk, J. L. 1967. *Delayed hypersensitivity.* Amsterdam: North-Holland.

Van der Walle, H. B. and Bensink, T. 1982. Cross reaction pattern of 26 acrylic monomers on guinea pig skin. *Contact Dermatitis* 8:376–382.

Van der Walle, H. B., Klecak, G., Geleick, H. and Bensink, T. 1982a. Sensitizing potentials of 14 mono(meth)acrylates in the guinea pig. *Contact Dermatitis* 8:223–235.

Van der Walle, H. B., Delbressine, L. P. G. and Seutter, E. 1982b. Concomitant sensitizations in the guinea pig to hydroquinone and p-methoxyphenol, inhibitors of acrylic monomers. *Contact Dermatitis* 8:147–154.

Van der Walle, H. B., Waegemaekers, T. and Bensink, T. 1983. Sensitizing potential of 12-di(meth)acrylates in the guinea pig. *Contact Dermatitis* 9:10–20.

Vinson, L. J., Singer, E. J., Koehler, W. R., Lehman, M. D. and Mausrat, T. 1965. The nature of the epidermal barrier and some factors influencing skin permeability. *Toxicol. Appl. Pharmacol.* 7:7–19.

Voss, J. G. 1958. Skin sensitization by mercaptans of low molecular weight. *J. Invest. Dermatol.* 31:273–279.

Waegemaekers, T. H. and Van der Walle, H. B. 1983. The sensitizing potential of 2-ethylhexyl acrylate in the guinea pig. *Contact Dermatitis* 9:372–376.

Wagner, J. G. 1961. Biopharmaceutics: Absorption aspects. *J. Pharm. Sci.* 50:359–387.

Wahlberg, J. E. 1976. Sensitization and testing of guinea pigs with nickel sulphate. *Dermatologica.* 152:321–330.

Wahlberg, J. E. and Boman, A. 1978. Sensitization and testing of guinea pigs with cobalt chloride. *Contact Dermatitis* 4:128–132.

Wahlberg, J. E. and Boman, A. 1979. Guinea pig maximization test method—Cadmium chloride. *Contact Dermatitis* 5:405.

Wahlberg, J. E. and Boman, A. 1985. Guinea pig maximization test. *Curr. Probl. Dermatol.* 14:59–106.

Wahlberg, J. E. and Fregert, S. 1985. Guinea pig maximization test. In *Models in Dermatology,* vol. 2, eds. H. Maibach and N. J. Lowe, pp. 225–233. Basel: Karger AG.

Wang, X. and Suskind, R. R. 1988. Comparative studies of the sensitization potential of morpholine, 2-mercaptobenzothiazole and 2 of their derivatives in guinea pigs. *Contact Dermatitis* 19:11–15.

Warner, R. D., Dorn, C. R., Blakeslee, J. R., Gerken, D. E., Gordon, J. C. and

Angrick, E. J. 1988. Zinc effects on nickel dermatitis in the guinea pig. *Contact Dermatitis* 19:98–108.

White, S. I., Friedmann, P. S., Moss, C. and Simpson, J. M. 1986. The effect of altering area of application and dose per unit area on sensitization by DNCB. *Br. J. Dermatol.* 115:663–668.

Weil, C. S. 1972. Guidelines for experiments to predict the degree of safety of a material for man. *Toxicol. Appl. Pharmacol.* 21:194–199.

Wolter, K., Schaefer, H., Frömming, K. M. and Stüttgen, G. 1970. Partikelgrösse und Penetration. *Fette Seifen Anstrichm.* 72:990–998.

Wurster, D. E. 1968. Factors influencing the design and formulation of dermatological preparations. In *Development of safer and more effective drugs,* ed. S. W. Goldstein, pp. 121–140. Washington, D.C.: American Pharmaceutical Association.

Zeller, W., de Gols, M. and Hausen, B. M. 1985. The sensitizing capacity of compsitae plants VI. Guinea pig sensitization experiments with ornamental plants and weeds using different methods. *Arch. Dermatol. Res.* 277:28–35.

Zesch, A. 1974. Wechselbeziehungen zwischen Haut, Vehikel und Arzneimittel bei der Penetration in die menschliche Haut. II. Vehikel und Penetration. *Fette Seifen Anstrichm.* 76:312–318.

Ziegler, V. 1975. Tierexperimenteller Nachweis stark allergener Eigenschaften von Industrieprodukten. Dissertation zur Promotion B and der Karl-Marx-Universität, Leipzig, DDR.

Ziegler, V. 1977. Der tierexperimentelle Nachweis allergener Eigenschaften von Industrieprodukten. *Dermatol. Monatsschr.* 163:387–391.

Ziegler, V. and Süss, E. 1985. The TINA test. *Curr. Probl. Dermatol.* 14:172–192.

Ziegler, V., Süss, E., Standau, H. and Hasert, K. 1972. Der Meerschweinchen-Maximisationstest zum Nachweis der sensibilisierenden Wirkung wichtiger Industrieprodukte. *Allerg. Immunol.* 18:203–208.

Zissu, D., Cavelier, J. and de Ceaurriz, J. 1987. Experimental sensitization of guinea pigs to nickel and patch testing with metal samples. *Food Chem. Toxicol.* 25:83–85.

14

contact allergy: predictive testing in humans

■ **Francis N. Marzulli** ■ **Howard I. Maibach** ■

INTRODUCTION

Contact dermatitis, an inflammatory skin reaction characterized by redness and vesicles, results from skin contact with either an irritant or with an allergenic substance.

Allergic contact dermatitis (contact allergy), as contrasted with irritant dermatitis, is immunologically mediated, and involves T lymphocytes sensitized to allergens. It is a delayed hyperactivity of skin that follows contact with a specific chemical entity. Clinically, allergic and irritant contact dermatitis may be virtually indistinguishable. Pathophysiologic features of both these dermatoses were reviewed recently (Thestrup-Pedersen et al., 1989). A brief discussion of ultrastructural and vascular changes, mast cell, basophil, leukotriene, interferon, interleukin, tissue antigen and other involvements in these skin reactions is included.

Investigative dermatologists employ basically similar patch test procedures to forecast the allergenic potential of topical skin preparations in subjects without skin disease and to diagnose contact allergy in clinical patients (that is, those who have presented themselves to the physician for treatment).

In diagnostic tests, a preparation is applied to a clinical patient's skin under an occlusive patch for 48 hr and the skin is evaluated for evidence of erythema, edema, or more severe skin changes occurring 24, 48, and 72 hr

The authors thank John Atkinson, Division of Mathematics, Food and Drug Administration, Washington, D.C., for statistical analyses.

after removal of the patch. Allergenic materials are thereby identified by reproducing skin disease on a small scale with offending chemicals. Diagnostic test results obtained in this manner are finding their way into the scientific literature with increasing frequency. There are now three groups of dermatologists, of which the North American Contact Dermatitis Group[1] (NACDG) and the International Contact Dermatitis Research Group (ICDRG) (Fregert et al., 1969), which had its origin in the Northern Dermatologic Society of Scandinavia (Magnusson et al., 1962), have been especially active in this regard. The European Environment Contact Dermatitis Group is the latest such group to be formed.

In this setting, clinical patients from a wide geographic area are tested with a standard screening series tray. Substances, concentrations, and methods are agreed on at the start. Results are centrally reported, analyzed, and evaluated in terms of a sensitization index (percentage of positive skin reactions).

The more recently formed NACDG reported a study of 1,200 clinical patients tested with 16 materials (Rudner et al., 1973). A high incidence of skin reactions was disclosed with nickel sulfate, p-phenylenediamine, potassium dichromate, thimerosal, ethylenediamine, neomycin sulfate, and ammoniated mercury. This suggests the possibility that these, or chemically related substances, might be responsible for skin disease in these patients. A mathematical evaluation of the data of Table 1, reported by the NACDG (Rudner et al., 1973), shows a number of interesting findings. Nickel sulfate, p-phenylenediamine, neomycin sulfate, mercaptothiobenzothiazole, thiram, and paraben show significantly higher sensitization indices (95% confidence) when tested on 1,200 patients by the NACDG than when tested by the ICDRG on 4,825 patients. These results could be interpreted as signifying that climatic or genetic differences might have influenced the outcome or, more likely, greater frequency of exposure of U.S. and Canadian citizens to a wider array of chemicals may be responsible for the higher index in those countries. Marzulli and Maibach (1974b) showed that greater exposure could also occur in the form of a higher concentration of a sensitizing ingredient. This, in turn, could result in elicitation of a higher reaction frequency from chemicals with a proclivity to sensitize.

Two of the six substances that showed a significantly different response rate in tests reported by the NACDG and the ICDRG in 1973 no longer showed this difference in 1983. At this later date, after testing over 20,000 subjects, the ICDRG reported that the rate for nickel sulfate rose from 6.7 to 12.4% and the rate for thiram, from 2 to 3.5%.

The type of patient referred for testing must also be considered in evaluating the significance of the results. For instance, in some clinics (such as that of Fregert et al. in Sweden) many referrals are for alleged occupational exposure;

---

[1]Established in December 1970 by 13 dermatologists. W. G. Larsen, M.D., secretary-treasurer, 2250 N.W. Flanders St., Portland, Oregon 97210.

TABLE 1. Skin Reactions Reported by Two Research Groups
on Clinical Patients Evaluated with a Diagnostic Test Kit[a]

Compound[b]	North American Contact Dermatitis Group			International Contact Dermatitis Research Group			North American vs. International[e]
		Reactors			Reactors		
	Concentration (%)	No. (1,200 tested)[c]	%	Concentration (%)	No. (4,824 tested)[d]	%	
Nickel sulfate	2.5	131	11	5	321	6.7	S
Potassium dichromate	0.5	91	8	5.0	318	6.6	NS
Thimerosal	0.1	91	8				
p-Phenylenediamine	1	98	8	1	237	4.7	S
Ethylenediamine	1	85	7				
Neomycin sulfate	20	71	6	20	176	3.7	S
Benzocaine	5	54	5	5	192	4.0	NS
Ammoniated mercury	1	65	5				
Mercaptobenzothiazole	2	58	5	2	99	2.0	S
Formalin, aqueous	2	43	4	2	169	3.5	NS
Thiram	2	50	4	2	97	2.0	S
Woolwax alcohol	30	37	3	30	127	2.6	NS
Paraben mixture[f]	15	38	3	15	91	1.9	S
Dibucaine HCl	1	32	3				
Cyclomethycaine sulfate	1	23	2				

[a]Data from Rudner et al. (1973).
[b]All prepared in petrolatum, except formalin.
[c]Male and female, black and white subjects.
[d]Male and female, white subjects.
[e]S = significant at 95% level; NS = not significant.
[f]Methyl, ethyl, propyl in equal amounts.

other clinics, because of their location, have few occupationally afflicted patients. Some centers test patients who are referred mainly for intractable eczema, whereas others investigate more acute problems.

A further evaluation of the data of Table 1 is given in Table 2. The table shows that nickel sulfate produces a significantly greater number (95% confidence) of skin reactions in clinical patients than any other material tested by the NACDG. This analysis (Table 2) also suggests that reactions to these 15 compounds can be placed in ten different categories, each of which is significantly different (95% confidence) from the others.

Nickel sulfate, with a reaction rate of 11% the most frequently encountered sensitizer in U.S. and Canadian dermatologic patients, is arbitrarily assigned to category 1. p-Phenylenediamine, potassium dichromate, and thimerosal with an 8% reaction rate and ethylene diamine with a 7% rate represent a

TABLE 2. Reactors Observed by North American Contact Dermatitis Group among 1,200 Patients Tested Diagnostically for Skin Sensitization with 15 Compounds[a]

Compound	No. reactors	1 (131)	2 (98)	3 (91)	4 (91)	5 (85)	6 (71)	7 (65)	8 (58)	9 (54)	10 (50)	11 (43)	12 (38)	13 (37)	14 (32)	15 (23)	Category[b]
1. Nickel sulfate	131		+	+	+	+	+	+	+	+	+	+	+	+	+	+	1
2. p-Phenylenediamine	98			0	0	0	+	+	+	+	+	+	+	+	+	+	2
3. Potassium dichromate	91				0	0	0	+	+	+	+	+	+	+	+	+	2
4. Thimerosal	91					0	0	+	+	+	+	+	+	+	+	+	2
5. Ethylenediamine	85						0	0	+	+	+	+	+	+	+	+	2
6. Neomycin sulfate	71							0	0	0	+	+	+	+	+	+	3
7. Ammoniated mercury	65								0	0	0	+	+	+	+	+	4
8. Mercaptobenzothiazole	58									0	0	0	+	+	+	+	5
9. Benzocaine	54										0	0	0	0	+	+	5
10. Thiram	50											0	0	0	+	+	6
11. Formalin	43												0	0	0	+	7
12. Paraben mixture	38													0	0	0	8
13. Woolwax alcohol	37														0	0	8
14. Dibucaine HCl	32															0	9
15. Cyclomethycaine sulfate	23																10

[a]Items to the right of heavy line are significantly different (95% confidence) from others on that line.
[b]See text.

significantly lower reaction rate and are classified as category 2. Neomycin with a 6% reaction rate represents category 3. Ammoniated mercury with a 5.4% reaction rate is in category 4 and so on to cyclomethycaine, with a reaction rate of 2%, which is category 10.

Background Prior to Human Testing

Human assays (see below) provide useful information; however, they cannot be a substitute for an informed approach to background data on the molecule and related structures.

Structure-function information is invaluable. Numerous scientists have commented on structure-function utilizing human and animal data. Recently Dupuis and Benezra (1983) prepared an extensive summary of the properties of a chemical that suggest a propensity to sensitization. Subsequently, a multidisciplinary team has started to place the literature on allergic contact dermatitis in a main frame computer; their system combines chemical and physical properties of a molecule with biologic data on animals and man (Sigman et al., 1986).

Subsequent to a review of the physical-chemical properties of a molecule and known history of sensitization (see below), appropriate animal testing is often invaluable. A summary of some of the tests available (see chapter 13) gives a starting point for study in this area. Recently, Andersen and Maibach (1985) provided a comprehensive summary of currently available animal techniques. Unfortunately, planning and interpreting such assays requires considerable experience and judgment.

Results of tests performed on clinical patients by the NACDG from July 1, 1981, to June 30, 1982, are shown in Table 3.

The most recently reported results of NACDG diagnostic testing involved 1,199 patients with suspected allergic contact dermatitis during the period Jan. 1984–May 1985 (Storrs et al., 1989). The most common sensitizers identified were nickel, p-phenylenediamine, quaternium-15, neomycin, thimerosol, formaldehyde, cinnamic aldehyde, ethylene diamine, potassium dichomate and thiuram mix. Frequency of positive findings was similar to that reported previously (1973, 1977) except for potassium dichromate, which was somewhat lower (5.2%), and cinnamic aldehyde (5.9%), which was not previously tested as a separate fragrance. The main advance in this publication was attempted documentation of clinical relevance as contrasted to a listing of only patch test positivity. This is a followup of the original study of the ICDRG (Fregert, 1969).

Patch testing of 11,962 patients over a 7 year period (1977–83) in West Germany, using test materials similar to the NACDG and ICDRG, confirmed results obtained by these groups (Gollhausen et al., 1988). In addition, cobalt chloride was identified as a significant allergen (6.3%). Colophony (2.7%), clioquinol (2.6%), eucerin anhydricum (2.6%), mafenide (2.1%), and gentamycin sulphate (1.4%) were also reported.

A five year study (1977–83) involving 13,216 dermatology patients with cosmetic dermatitis was conducted by the NACDG and supported by the FDA. The intent was to find out which cosmetics were responsible for adverse skin effects and to identify the causative ingredients. Products that were most responsible for adverse effects (80%) were skin care products, hair preparations, facial makeup, nail preparations, and fragrance products, in that order. The face, eyes, and forearms were the most frequently involved body sites. Fragrances and preservatives constituted the bulk of the identified reaction-causing components. Among the preservatives, quaternium 15, imidazolidinyl urea, parabens, bronopol, and formaldehyde were the major offenders. Skin sensitization was reported in 81% of the cases and skin irritation in 16%.

PREDICTIVE METHODS

Systematic predictive test procedures (as contrasted with diagnostic) for skin sensitization have evolved over a period of about 30 yr (Draize et al., 1944; Rostenberg and Sulzberger, 1937; Schwartz, 1941, 1951, 1960; Shelanski, 1951). Currently they generally require multiple occlusive patches for induction of sensitization (ten patches, 48 hr each, same site) followed by a 2

TABLE 3. Skin Reactions of Clinical Patients Evaluated
with Standard Screening Tray[a]

	Males		Females	
Compound	Response Fraction	%	Response Fraction	%
Fragrance mix, 16%	94/807	11	166/1220	13
Caine mix, 8%	62/660	9	81/974	8
Potassium dichromate, 0.5%	89/906	9	79/1310	6
Thimerosal, 0.1%	46/591	7	60/880	6
Ethylene diamine, 1%	62/853	7	59/1250	4
Formaldehyde, 2% (A.Q.)	69/937	7	129/1338	9
Formaldehyde, 2% PET.	9/153	5	17/198	8
Nickel sulfate, 25%	47/894	5	192/1345	14
p-Phenylenediamine, 1%	49/904	5	83/1334	6
Neomycin sulfate, 20%	53/890	5	100/1339	7
Carba mix, 1%	34/800	4	41/1167	3
Ammoniated mercury, 1%	26/796	3	53/1215	4
Thiuram mix, 1%	32/833	3	55/1198	4
Quaternium 15-2% (A.Q.)	22/580	3	37/768	4
Mecapto mix, 1%	30/832	3	20/1194	1
MBT, 1%	36/913	3	25/1327	1
Paraben mix, 15%	26/806	3	19/1223	1
Quaternium 15, 12% PET.	371/8	3	21/635	2
Wool alcohols, 30%	20/808	2	25/1188	2
Epoxy resin, 1%	21/887	2	36/1292	2
PCMX, 1%	15/673	2	10/959	1
Imidazolidinyl urea	14/805	1	28/1184	1
PPD mix, 0.6%	12/800	1	15/262	1
Benzoyl peroxide, 1%	2/180	1	5/262	1
p-TERT-Butylphenol, 2%	6/684	1	7/940	1
Lanoline, 100% (hydrous)	7/755	1	11/1081	1

[a]Unpublished data from North American Contact Dermatitis Research Group, 1981–1982.

wk rest period and then challenge (48 hr) with a patch at a new skin site (Marzulli and Maibach, 1973). There are a number of variations in these procedures, including the use of provocative chemical agents such as sodium lauryl sulfate (SLS) (Kligman, 1966b), special skin preparation such as stripping (Spier and Sixt, 1955) or freezing (Epstein et al., 1963), special patches (Magnusson and Hersle, 1965), high concentrations at induction (Marzulli and Maibach, 1974b), and 25–200 test subjects (Draize et al., 1944; Kligman, 1966a). Other background information and references to studies on predictive methods are contained in review papers by Giovacchini (1972) and Hardy (1973). Methods of historic and current interest are summarized in Table 4.

It is apparent from the cited variations in proposed test procedures that methodologies have proliferated. It is not entirely clear, however, how useful these variations are and what limitations obtain under use conditions, as valida-

TABLE 4. Predictive Tests for Skin Sensitization of Humans

Test	No. subjects	Test substance amount or concentration	Vehicle	Skin site	Type patch	Induction — No. patches	Induction — Duration	Induction — Rest	Induction — Challenge	Reference
Schwartz	200	Fabric			Fabric	1	5 days	10 days	48 hr patch; observe 10 days	Schwartz, 1941
Schwartz	200	1 in. fabric liquid or powder		Arm, thigh, or back	Cellophane covered with 2 × 2 in. Elastoplast	1	72 hr	7–10 days	72 hr; same site; observe 3 days	Schwartz, 1960
"Prophetic" Schwartz-Peck	200	1/4 in. square 4-ply gauze, liquid saturated[a]	Petrolatum or corn oil	Arm or back	1 in. square non-waterproof cellophane covered with 2 in. square adhesive plaster	1	24 hr or 3 or 4 days	10–14 days	48 hr; any site especially thin keratin; observe 3 days; compare new and old formulas	Schwartz and Peck, 1944; Schwartz, 1951
"Repeated insult" Shelanski	200	Proportional to area of ultimate use	Mineral oil		Occlusion; follows Schwartz test	10–15	24 hr every other day; same site	2–3 wk	48 hr patch	Shelanski, 1951; Shelanski and Shelanski 1953
"Repeated insult" Draize	100 males 100 females	0.5 ml or 0.5 gram		Arm or back	1 in. square	10	24 hr alternate days	10–14 days	Repeat patch on new site	Draize et al., 1944; Shelanski, 1951; Draize, 1959
Modified Draize	200	0.5 ml or 0.5 gram (high concentration)	Petrolatum	Arm	Square BandAid, no perforations	10	48 hr	2 wk	Patch on new site 72 hr with nonirritant concentration	Marzulli and Maibach, 1973, 1974
"Maximization" Kligman	25	1 ml 5% SLS[b] followed by 1 ml 25% test material	Petrolatum	Forearm or calf	1.5 in. square Webril occluded with Blenderm; held in place with perforated plastic tape	5 (same site)	24 hr SLS followed by 48 hr test material for each of five inducing applications	10 days	1 in. square patch on lower back or forearm; 0.4 ml of 10% SLS for 1 hr followed in 24 hr by 0.4 ml of 10% test material for 48 hr	Kligman, 1966
Modified "maximization"	25	Same as maximization				7	24 hr SLS followed by 48 hr test material for each of seven inducing applications; no patch for 24 hr between each of seven inducing applications	10 days	2% SLS for 1/2 hr followed by 48 hr patch with test material	Kligman and Epstein, 1974

[a] Modified for solids, powders, ointments, and cosmetics. Concentration, amount, area, and site of application are considered important in evaluating results. Authors recommended that cosmetics be tested uncovered. SLS is mixed with test material when compatible. SLS is eliminated when the test material is a strong irritant.

[b] Sodium lauryl sulfate (SLS) pretreatment is used to produce moderate inflammation of the skin.

421

tion has not kept pace with the announcement of each new departure. Furthermore, predictive tests are often performed on a single chemical entity, whereas ultimate use may occur as part of a multicomponent formulation in a marketed product, where the vehicle and associated ingredients may influence the outcome.

If indeed one has an adequate laboratory test for identifying allergenic potential, two important considerations obtain in employing it for successfully marketing a cosmetic or topical drug.

1. The sample size of test subjects must be large enough so that results are valid for the population at large, yet small enough to permit logistic feasibility in the laboratory.
2. The laboratory test must have the capacity to predict likelihood of occurrence under use conditions.

Henderson and Riley (1945) in their classic paper discussed some of the complexities and mathematical considerations involved in extrapolating from a small test population to large numbers of users. Briefly stated, there may be no skin reactions in a test population of 200 random subjects, yet as many as 15 of every 1,000 of the general population may react (95% confidence), and up to 22 of every 1,000 may react (99% confidence). If the test population is reduced to 100 subjects, up to 30 of every 1,000 of the general population may react (95% confidence). Conversely, when 1 of 200 subjects in a test population becomes sensitized, a test population of 10,000 subjects might show from 1 to 275 sensitized, with 95% confidence.

The possibility that the laboratory test may not predict what is likely to happen in the field stems from a large number of variables that may affect the outcome of the test. These include the skin site, climatic conditions, area and frequency of application, and others.

Validation of a laboratory test procedure for predicting skin sensitization in the field can be undertaken in a variety of ways, none of which is completely satisfactory.

One approach is to evaluate the test system by comparing predictive test results with those obtained from other sources, such as:

1. Limited use tests on a final formulation prior to marketing.
2. Industry and Food and Drug Administration (FDA) consumer complaint data.
3. Retrospective epidemiologic data.
4. Monitoring programs such as the Department of Health, Education, and Welfare (HEW)-sponsored investigation of consumer's perceptions of adverse reactions to cosmetic products (HEW, 1975).
5. Diagnostic test results in dermatologic clinics.

All of the above items can be important; however, item 5 represents our major source of precise information at present. When the incidence of sensitization predicted by the prophetic test methods exceeds the incidence observed in the diagnostic clinic, or in other words, when an ingredient is predicted to be a strong sensitizer, yet marketed products containing the ingredient appear to be well tolerated (as evidenced by a lack of sensitized dermatologic patients), it may mean that the concentration used in the marketed product may be exceedingly low or the product may provide limited (time) skin contact (see the section on formaldehyde below). On the other hand, when the sensitization frequency observed in diagnostic tests exceeds that suggested by predictive tests, it may mean that individuals who cannot tolerate a widely used product are being systematically identified by clinical dermatologists (see parabens below). When both diagnostic and predictive tests show a high frequency of sensitization, a substance with strong sensitization potential is suggested (*p*-phenylenediamine), and when both diagnostic and predictive tests show a low frequency of sensitization, it is apparent that the predictive test is accurately forecasting a low allergenic potential and is not revealing false positives.

One can add the art of successful marketing of safe preparations to the aforementioned mathematic and scientific approaches to predicting the safe use of an ingredient. In some cases, despite a careful evaluation of conditions that appear to be of importance, one may not be aware of certain hidden factors that may play a role in the outcome. This aspect is best regulated by comparing a new product with an old one that has stood the test of time in the marketplace. Studies of this kind may occasionally provide a more meaningful interpretation of the likelihood of success (safety) in the marketplace than a carefully obtained sensitization index on a panel of 200 laboratory subjects.

Excited Skin State

Many animal and human studies may be invalid because of a lack of appreciation of hyperirritable skin—the excited skin syndrome. The details of this biologic phenomenon and strategies for handling it in man and animal are discussed by Bruynzeel and Maibach (1986).

EVALUATION OF SOME COMMON CONTACT SENSITIZERS

Kathon

Kathon CG, marketed by Rohm and Haas (Philadelphia), has found increasing use as a cosmetic preservative in Europe and the United States. It consists of two chemicals and a stabilizer; that is, methychlorisothiazolinone (5-chloro-2-methyl-4-isothiazolin-3-one) in 3:1 ratio. $MgCl_2$ and $Mg(NO_3)_2$ are added as stabilizers. De Groot et al. (1988a) reported that Kathon CG was proved responsible for about 2% of contact allergy seen in 150 patients patch tested with aqueous Kathon (100 ppm) for suspected cosmetic allergy. Patients were female clients of beauticians in the Netherlands. In a review article, de Groot (1988b) reported that the risk of adverse skin effects of Kathon CG were related to the use of moisturizing creams on slightly damaged skin. Correlation of concentrations of Kathon in various creams with the risk of sensitization will probably be difficult until Kathon bioavailability data becomes generally available.

Formaldehyde

Formaldehyde (aqueous solution) is a strong sensitizer. In predictive tests conducted on 331 normal subjects with 1-10% formalin (formalin is 37% formaldehyde) at induction, 1% at challenge, 4.5-7.8% of the test population showed evidence of skin sensitization (Marzulli and Maibach, 1974b). Diagnostic tests on clinical patients reported by the NACDG (Rudner et al., 1973) showed a sensitization index of 4%. Earlier reports by other investigators indicate that in earlier times, formaldehyde sensitivity in clinical patients reached as high as 24%. The possibility that some of these reactions were irritant responses (false positives) due to the use of too high a concentration of formaldehyde at challenge has been postulated (Epstein and Maibach, 1966). On the other hand, the general recognition that formaldehyde is a potent sensitizer by both industry and many of those likely to be exposed to it professionally may also have contributed to this decreased incidence in recent years. The Cosmetic Product Registry of the FDA shows that formaldehyde is used in about 5% of 8,000 preparations in the registry (FDA, 1972). Despite this rather extensive use of formaldehyde in cosmetic products, the prediction rate is roughly the same as the incidence seen in diagnostic tests. One explanation for the fact that it has not sensitized a greater number of patients who use cosmetics is that formaldehyde is largely confined to use at low concentrations as a preservative in shampoos. These preparations do not remain in continuous contact with skin, as they are rinsed off. The use of formaldehyde as a nail hardener, on the other hand, is accompanied by a significant number of serious injuries to sensitive nail and adnexal tissues. This type of exposure may contribute substantially to that portion of the 4% sensitization index seen in clinical patients which is cosmetic-related.

Parabens

Methyl and propyl paraben are abundantly used as preservatives in foods, drugs, and cosmetics, providing many opportunities for exposure. Methyl and propyl paraben appear in 36 and 31%, respectively, of cosmetic products registered with the FDA (FDA, 1972). Predictive tests for skin sensitization (Marzulli and Maibach, 1973) show a sensitization index of 0.3% (397 subjects). Diagnostic tests for skin sensitization show a reaction rate of 3% by the NACDG, 1.9% by the ICDRG, and 0.7% when tested in 1968 on 273 chronic dermatitis patients by Schorr (1968) (note correction from 0.8 to 0.7% in the original article). The diagnostic test results show a significantly higher reaction rate in patients than was observed in predictive tests on normal people. This in itself is, of course, not surprising. The fact that each of the diagnostic test results is significantly different from the others is interesting. It may be due to differences in exposure in different geographic areas as well as in different time frames; that is, greater susceptibility as exposure time increases. The widespread use of parabens may account for the tenfold difference between diagnostic and predictive test results obtained with certain test populations. The status of topical parabens with special reference to skin hypersensitivity is discussed in greater detail in a recent review paper (Marzulli and Maibach, 1974a). It was concluded that "allergic contact dermatitis (from parabens) exists. Fortunately, the number of cases is relatively small. The incidence is now so low that it has been removed from the standard series of the NACDG; it is rarely utilized today in the U.S., except in leg ulcer cases. It is hoped that alternatives to the parabens will be carefully studied so that they do not surprise us and prove to be a greater topical or systemic hazard."

p-Phenylenediamine

p-Phenylenediamine (PPDA) is well known as a skin irritant and skin sensitizer. Its principal use in cosmetics is as a hair dye ingredient. In predictive tests at 1% concentration it produced sensitization reactions in 53% of a normal test population (Marzulli and Maibach, 1974b). Other "para" substances are encountered which are immunologically related to *p*-phenylenediamine. These include *p*-aminobenzoic acid, a sunscreen; sulfonamide, an antibacterial agent; procaine, a local anesthetic; and *p*-aminosalicylic acid, an antitubercular agent. In diagnostic tests, 8% of clinical patients showed skin reactions when tested with PPDA (Rudner et al., 1973). An FDA complaint file for 1974 (Cosmetic Injury Reports, 1974) showed that 1.9% of consumer complaints (639) involved oxidative hair dyes containing PPDA or PPDA-like materials. These predictive, diagnostic, and consumer complaint data tend to support the high allergenic potential of PPDA. The fact that a cautionary statement warns the hair dye user to test behind the ear prior to each use may be responsible for reducing the expected reaction rate under use conditions. In addition, hair dyes are applied primarily to the hair, mainly by trained cosmeticians, after admixture with peroxide. These circumstances could also contribute substantially to reducing the reaction rate under use conditions. Nevertheless, PPDA remains in the second highest category (category 2) of diagnostic test reactions seen by investigative clinical dermatologists. Eiermann et al. (1982) recently showed in a prospective cosmetic reaction study that PPDA also remains a leading cause of cosmetic reactions.

Peru Balsam

Peru balsam (or balsam of Peru) is an oleoresin obtained from *Myroxylon pereirae,* a tree that grows mainly in Central America. Peru balsam is a dark brown, viscous liquid which contains 50–60% cinnamein, an ester of cinnamic and benzoic acid, and about 28% resin, styracine, and vanillin. It has had considerable past use in perfumes, flavors, toilet waters, hair lotions, and at one time in topical antiscabic and disinfectant drugs. Peru balsam oil is prepared from Peru balsam by extraction with volatile solvents or by distillation. The oil contains large amounts of benzyl benzoate and benzyl cinnamate. The sensitization potentials of the oil and the parent material are decidedly different (Opdyke, 1974), as are their compositions.

In predictive tests, Shelanski and Shelanski (1953) reported that Peru balsam produced no evidence of skin sensitization when tested at 8% concentration on 50 subjects with a repeated insult method. Failure to elicit sensitization may have resulted from the low concentration of Peru balsam that was used. Hjorth (1961), in a classic and extensive study of Peru balsam, recommended that 25% concentration be used to avoid false negative responses, the same concentration recommended earlier by Bonnevie. Kligman (1966), using a maximization procedure obtained a 28% sensitization rate (Opdyke, 1974) when Peru balsam was tested on 25 human volunteers at 8% concentration. The possibility that the irritant effects of SLS were superimposed on those of Peru balsam cannot be excluded.

In one diagnostic series of tests conducted on 5,558 patients in Scandinavia, a reaction rate of 6.9% to Peru balsam was obtained (Magnusson et al., 1968). In another diagnostic series conducted in 1970 on a selected group of 281 female patients with contact allergy of the hands, 27% of those who reacted to a diagnostic series of allergens showed a reaction to Peru balsam (Calnan et al., 1931). Hjorth (1961) states that 0.4–7% of patients in European clinics react positively to Peru balsam. At the Finsen Institute in Denmark, Hjorth's data, collected from February 1, 1954 to October 31, 1958, show an incidence of 3.2% (239 of 7,500 patients). Records of the NACDG for the period July 1, 1972 to June 30, 1973 show a 4.5% incidence of skin reactions when tested on 177 male and female patients with 25% Peru balsam.

It would appear from the total findings that results for both diagnostic and predictive testing with Peru balsam are complicated as well as variable. On close inspection, some of the factors involved in the variability emerge. Peru balsam is not one substance but several. Benzyl benzoate, benzyl cinnamate, benzoic acid, cinnamic acid, and vanillin are not considered important allergens in Peru balsam (Hjorth, 1961). According to Hjorth (1961), "only resin A (esters of coniferyl alcohol) of which Peru balsam contains 1 to 3% is sensitizing to some patients." The 8% test concentration of Peru balsam used by Shelanski and Shelanski (1953) in predictive tests may therefore be too low. On the other hand, maximization test results of Kligman (1966) may be high if irritant effects of Peru balsam and SLS are additive.

With regard to diagnostic testing, a sensitization rate from about 3.2% (Hjorth, 1961) to 4.5% (NACDG) appears to be representative of the actual reaction rate expected in ordinary clinical patients, whereas higher rates may be observed in selected patients with hand dermatitis of unknown etiology.

Because ingredients of Peru balsam are found in perfumes, spices, and fruits, the allergenic effects of the primary allergen may therefore extend to secondary allergens. Hence, as Hjorth puts it, "sensitization to balsam of Peru results in complicated patterns of multiple sensitivities. The number and kind may vary from subject to subject." In some cases, then, diagnostic reactions are to the primary allergen, in other cases, to related materials (cross-sensitization).

Of interest to the perfume industry is the fact that fractions of Peru balsam that can be eluted with petroleum esters and benzene are rarely allergenic in patients sensitized to Peru balsam (Hjorth, 1961). Thus, highly purified Peru balsam which does not contain resin A, and is available for perfumery, is not expected to be a problem when used in cosmetics. As cosmetic injury reports received by the FDA for the fiscal year 1974 suggest that 3.1% (2.4% for 1970–1973) of the total (639) are due to fragrance preparations, some of which may contain Peru balsam and other potentially allergenic fragrance substances, it would appear that the cosmetic industry may be aware of the requirements for selecting safe perfume ingredients.

Nickel and Chromium

Two metallic substances, nickel and chromium, and compounds containing these metals are responsible for skin irritation, contact dermatitis, and cancer (Sunderman et al., 1973; Baetjer et al., 1974) in industrial workers. They are also among the most frequently encountered contact allergens for the population at large. Nickel offers opportunities for contact in the form of coins, inexpensive jewelry, and metal fastenings on clothing. It is a frequent sensitizer of women, ostensibly because of their greater contact with the metal in the home and in their dress. Sweating skin enhances solubilization of the metal, favoring skin penetration and ultimately sensitization. Hexavalent chromium in the form of dichromate is encountered by contact with tanned leather such as is used for gloves.

A selected population (skewed) of normal human volunteers known to be nonreactive to nickel was exposed experimentally by Vandenberg and Epstein (1963) to a "triple freeze" procedure (irritation, occlusion, freezing, repeated exposure) for inducing sensitization with 25% $NiCl_2$ and 0.1% SLS. On challenge with 5% $NiCl_2$ (nonoccluded), 9% (16 of 172) of the subjects were sensitized. As the latent period in nickel sensitivity appears to be quite long, it was decided to reexpose some of the nonreactors to the triple freeze induction procedure. When the procedure was carried out a second time, 26% (5 of 19) of this group were sensitized. The authors concluded that nickel is slow to sensitize; the rate of sensitization can be raised by prolonged exposure. It is of interest, however, that nickel hypersensitivity induced by this technique did not result in clinical disease in these subjects in skin sites making contact with identification bracelets or watch bands.

Kligman (1966) used his "maximization" procedure to test for the skin sensitization potential of nickel sulfate on healthy subjects, 90% of whom were black. Here, SLS was used both at induction and at challenge, posing greater opportunities for absorption of nickel at the test site. Ten percent nickel sulfate was used at induction and 2.5% at challenge (Kligman, 1966a). Kligman reported that 48% (12 of 25) of the subjects were sensitized, and classified nickel as a "grade 3" sensitizer. (By this technique grade 1 is called a weak sensitizer and is applied to sensitization rates of 0–8%, whereas grade 5 is an extreme sensitizer and is characterized by sensitization rates of 84% or more.)

The results of diagnostic tests (Table 1) show that nickel sulfate is the most frequently encountered sensitizer when tested with tray substances used by the NACDG or the ICDRG on clinical patients. Although the reaction rate is significantly higher in the NACDG subjects (11 vs. 6.7%), the diagnostic test findings of both these groups appear to be more closely related to the original predictive findings of Vandenberg and Epstein (1963), namely, a 9% sensitization rate. Vandenberg and Epstein were able to increase the sensitization rate to 26% by repeating the provocative procedure, and Kligman was able to further increase it to 48% by using SLS at challenge. This fact suggests that although nickel is slow to sensitize, the reaction rate first observed may be increased by further contact with the metal.

It has been reported by several groups that subjects may also lose their hypersensitivity to nickel (probably following a prolonged period of avoidance) (Morgan, 1953; TeLintum and Nater, 1973). In one such study, a persistent positive patch test to nickel sulfate was retained in only 39 of 57 nickel-positive patients after an interval of 2–15 yr (TeLintum and Nater, 1973).

Chromium eczema is one of the most frequently encountered occupational dermatoses; it involves workers in a wide variety of trades. These include industries in which there is frequent contact with chemicals, leather, metal, paint, cement, paper pulp, timber, building materials, and various household articles such as detergents and glue.

A review of our present knowledge of skin hypersensitivity to chromium and its compounds is given in an article by Polak et al. (1973).

Although chromium has been much studied clinically and in basic human and animal experiments, there is little published information regarding its capacity to sensitize normal human subjects. Using the maximization procedure, Kligman (1966a) obtained sensitization rates of 48% (11 of 23) with chromium sulfate and 56% (13 of 23) with chromium trioxide, in predictive tests on healthy subjects. These rates are significantly higher than the 8% incidence of skin reactions reported for clinical patients diagnostically tested by the NACDG (Table 1). These diagnostic findings, as related to the predictive findings, may be at variance with one another for the same reasons as those given for nickel.

Mercury

Mercurials are widely used in inorganic form (mercuric salts and ammoniated mercury) for the topical treatment of skin diseases, disinfection, and a variety of industrial uses. Organic forms of mercurials (phenylmercuric salts and thimerosal, also called Merthiolate, which is sodium ethylmercurithiosalicylate) are used as antiseptics and preservatives.

Many complicating factors may contribute to a proper interpretation of mercury sensitivity. When mercuric chloride is used for elicitation, skin irritation is a strong possibility; when thimerosal is used, the possibility arises that some component (thiosalicylic acid) other than mercury may be responsible (Ellis, 1947; Ellis and Robinson, 1942; Gaul, 1958). Hansson and Moller (1970) suggest that young skin may react differently from old skin to thimerosal; in addition, this compound may have a peculiar predilection to produce false positive responses. Epstein (1974) recommends that in equivocal situations, one must repeat testing, employ various dilutions and usage tests, and use ammoniated mercury for elicitation in order to establish sensitivity to mercury.

Phenylmercuric acetate (PMA) was tested in healthy subjects for skin sensitization potential by Marzulli and Maibach (1973). There was a 2% incidence (1 of 56) of sensitization reactions in a small test panel using 0.125% PMA for induction and 0.01% for challenge (modified Draize test). A 0.01% concentration of PMA was considered to be nonirritating, whereas a 0.05% concentration was irritating to skin.

Anti-infective skin preparations of ammoniated mercury normally do not exceed 5% concentration. In tests by Kligman (1966) using the maximization procedure (25% ammoniated mercury at induction and 10% at challenge) a 59% incidence (44 of 74) of skin reaction was obtained in healthy subjects. By this technique, ammoniated mercury would be characterized as a moderate (grade 3) sensitizer. In diagnostic testing of dermatologic patients, using 1% ammoniated mercury, the NACDG obtained a sensitization index of 5% (Table 1).

Clearly, additional predictive work is needed to provide a more precise interpretation of the sensitization potential of various mercurials in healthy subjects. One cannot overstress the importance of avoiding skin irritation effects with mercurials of any type in such studies.

Neomycin

Neomycin sulfate is a well-known broad-spectrum topical antibiotic of the aminoglycoside family produced from cultures of *Streptomyces fradiae*. It is used for superficial skin infections due to staphylococci and many gram-negative bacteria. When first introduced for these purposes, it produced only rare skin reactions. Widespread, continued use in both prescription and nonprescription ointments in many European communities and the United States resulted in a dramatic rise in the rate of neomycin-related skin reactions (Pirilä and Rouhunkoski, 1959). Sensitivity to neomycin is often accompanied by sensitivity to related compounds (kanamycin, paromomycin, and framycetin) and to unrelated compounds (bacitracin) (Pirilä and Rouhunkoski, 1959, 1962). Whether these are cross-reactions or concomitant sensitization is not entirely clear (Schorr et al., 1973). Neomycin represents a type of substance whose proclivity to sensitize is easily missed. This may be chiefly because it is a poor penetrant of intact skin. Sensitized individuals may show a skin reaction when tested by intradermal injection while at the same time they are patch test negative (Schorr et al., 1973).

Repeated use, especially on broken skin, may be required to produce skin hypersensitivity. Calnan and Sarkany (1958) recognized this early, yet did not recommend the use of SLS and other substances which might enhance absorption for patch testing because of the possibility of producing false positive reactions.

Marzulli et al. (1968) reported provocative patch tests with neomycin on healthy subjects. Results showed a relatively low incidence of skin sensitization (1.6% or 3 of 186) when 5% concentration was used *at both induction and challenge*. No sensitization was induced in similar tests using 0.5% (0 of 54) and 20% (0 of 42) concentrations of neomycin. In further tests, the use of SLS at induction and at challenge increased the incidence of skin reactions. The rates of sensitization appeared to be 5.5% (3 of 54) when tested at 0.5% concentration, 2.6% (5 of 186) at 5% concentration, and 48% (12 of 25) at 20% concentration.

Kligman (1966a) reported a skin reaction incidence of 28% (7 of 25) using the maximization provocative procedure. He used 25% neomycin at induction and 10% at challenge.

The use of SLS in provocative tests with neomycin clearly increases the apparent incidence of skin sensitization reactions. In view of Calnan's warning, however, one must consider the possibility that some of these may have been false positive reactions.

Diagnostic test results on clinical patients evaluated by the NACDG show a 6% incidence of skin reactions to neomycin sulfate (Table 1), using 20% for elicitation.

The overall findings with neomycin suggest that provocative patch tests may fail to detect the proclivity of neomycin to sensitize in some instances and may overstate the incidence when SLS is used.

Thiram

Thiram (tetramethylthiuram disulfide), the methyl analogue of disulfiram, is used as an agricultural fungicide and insecticide for turf and seed treatment. Thiram and disulfiram (tetraethylthiuram disulfide) are also used as accelerators in the rubber industry. Disulfiram has also had limited use as a drug (Antabuse).

Workers in the rubber industry sometimes become sensitized to thiram. In addition, dermatitis has been reported from rubber in wearing apparel and in shoes (Blank and Miller, 1952; Gaul, 1957).

Predictive tests with guinea pigs show that thiram has the capacity to produce skin sensitization in this species (D. Hood, personal communication). Kligman (1966a) found that 16% of a normal test population (4 of 25) became sensitized to thiram when subjected to standard predictive procedures using 25% concentration at induction and 10% at challenge.

Around 1952, thiram was incorporated at about 0.5% concentration in a germicidal soap. Blank (1956) patch-tested six subjects known to be sensitive to thiram with an 8% solution of this soap. As all six reacted to the soap preparation, he notified the manufacturers that persons with rubber-related thiram allergy might develop dermatitis from using this soap. He suggested that the manufacturers monitor this carefully. They did and later reported that consumer complaints from thiram antiseptic soap (1 in 2,000,000 bars sold) were no different in numbers from those received when their more traditional antiseptic soap (cresylic acid) was previously marketed. The manufacturers claimed that they eventually withdrew thiram soap from the market for reasons unrelated to skin sensitization reactions.

These conclusions regarding the lack of adverse effects of thiram when incorporated into soap appear to be somewhat at variance with findings reported by Baer and Rosenthal (1954). These investigators found that 1 in 309 dermatologic patients who used soap containing 1% thiram developed a skin hypersensitivity to the product. Seven other subjects had to discontinue using it because of other adverse effects. The concentration of thiram in these soap studies was higher than that reported above.

Diagnostic tests conducted on dermatologic patients by the NACDG (Rudner et al., 1973), using 2% concentration for elicitation, showed that 4% of the test population reacted to thiram. The rather high incidence of skin reactions to thiram by dermatologic patients in the NACDG test indicates both the ubiquitous nature of this substance and its capacity to produce skin sensitization in significant numbers of persons who come into contact with it.

On the basis of the overall findings, one must conclude that predictive tests accurately foretell the fact that thiram is a contact sensitizer.

Benzocaine

Benzocaine (ethyl aminobenzoate), the ethyl ester of p-aminobenzoic acid, is a procaine-like surface anesthetic with only slight water solubility. It is often used at 2–5% concentration in topical antipruritic dermatologic ointments and creams, for superficial burns, and at 20% concentration for sunburn. Its use for these conditions is questionable in view of the risk of producing dermatitis from this and a host of related materials such as hair dyes with p-phenylenediamine, fabrics treated with azo dyes, sulfonamide-type drugs, and p-aminobenzoic acid-type sunscreens (Wilson, 1966).

In predictive tests on healthy subjects, using the modified Draize procedure, Marzulli and Maibach (1974b) reported that benzocaine produced a 6% incidence (6 of 99), in skin sensitization, using 20% concentration at induction and 10% at challenge. Kligman obtained a 22% incidence (5 of 23) in tests on normal subjects with the SLS maximization procedure. He used 25% at induction and 10% at challenge.

Bandmann et al. (1972) called attention to the possibility of producing iatrogenic allergic contact dermatitis when dermatologists prescribe benzocaine-containing preparations for their patients. In a study of 4,000 eczema patients in five European clinics they concluded that 14% (560 of 4,000) suffered dermatitis from applied medicaments. Benzocaine and neomycin each made up the largest share—4% in each case. Elicitation was accomplished with 5% benzocaine and 20% neomycin sulfate.

Diagnostic tests performed by the NACDG show a reaction rate of 5% (Table 1) when dermatologic patients were patch-tested with benzocaine.

Although benzocaine is known to be a significant skin sensitizer, clinical experience suggests that this potential is not likely to exceed the rate observed in dermatologic test patients.

Ethylenediamine

Ethylenediamine is a strongly alkaline solvent and emulsifier substance. It has been used in an antibiotic anti-inflammatory topical preparation (Mycolog[2]) where, although not an active ingredient, it, like benzocaine, has produced iatrogenic allergic contact dermatitis (Fisher et al., 1971). Cross reactions to chemically related substances used such as topical antihistamines may also occur (Fisher et al., 1971).

Maibach (1975) conducted predictive tests on healthy subjects, using the modified Draize procedure. He obtained a sensitization index of 8% (5 of 61) using 5% ethylenediamine dihydrochloride at induction and 1% at challenge.

Fisher et al. (1971), in a study of 100 patients suspected of allergic contact dermatitis from topical medications, found 18% (18 of 100) sensitive to ethylenediamine dihydrochloride (1%). Six patients who were patch test negative to Mycolog cream containing triamcinolone acetonide, neomycin sulfate, gramicidin nystatin, ethylenediamine hydrochloride, and other minor ingredients showed significant skin reactions when tested with ethylenediamine hydrochloride alone in petrolatum.

In diagnostic tests with dermatologic patients, the NACDG found that 7% of the subjects showed positive reactions. The subjects' responses were elicited with 1% ethylenediamine.

The overall findings with ethylenediamine show that this is a potent sensitizer and suggest that predictive tests by the modified Draize procedure accurately foretell this potential.

Transdermal Systems

Transdermal therapeutic systems employ rate-controlling membranes affixed to skin to deliver medication to the blood stream at a constant rate. The transdermal route of absorption bypasses the gastrointestinal tract and avoids

[2]Nystatin; neomycin sulfate; gramicidintriamcinolone acetonide.

first pass inactivation by the liver. Although the dermal route offers a more direct route to the blood stream and other benefits, as a route of drug administration there are certain disadvantages in some instances. Contact dermatitis, including allergic contact dermatitis, has been reported, when clonidine, nitroglycerin, scopolamine, estradiol, and testosterone were employed as active ingredients. Hogan (1990) summarizes this experience.

Potential Diagnostic Test

From time to time, methods have been proposed to resolve the need for a simple clinical test to distinguish between allergic and irritant skin reactions. Serup and Staberg (1987) have suggested that allergic reactions are characterized by transcutaneous edema, in contrast with irritant reactions, which have more superficial edema. Allergic and irritant skin reactions with similar clinical appearance were reported capable of resolution by noninvasive skin thickness measurements with high frequency ultrasound.

SUMMARY AND CONCLUSION

Essentially three types of tests are needed to evaluate skin sensitization potential. The predictive test is needed to identify allergenic substances; the diagnostic test is used to find out what substances may actually be producing dermatologic problems; and the use test provides information regarding safety of ingredients in a particular combination for a specific use before they enter the marketplace. Inclusion of a known sensitizer or new ingredient in a marketed product will, of course, require more frequent and more careful monitoring than is needed when commonly used substances of known sensitization potential are used.

We have reviewed in some detail skin sensitization predictive and diagnostic data on 11 compounds. These are among the most frequently encountered sensitizers to which large numbers of humans in Western Europe, the United States, and Canada are exposed in normal living. They include drugs (benzocaine and neomycin), cosmetic ingredients (*p*-phenylenediamine and Peru balsam), preservatives (formaldehyde, ethylenediamine, parabens, and mercurials), and ingredients of wearing apparel (nickel, chromium, and thiram).

Eight of these substances have been studied in dermatologic patients by the ICDRG and all 11 have been studied by the NACDG. Use of this type of subject was expected to reveal the (diagnostic) incidence of sensitization in a select population whose skin was seriously enough affected that medical assistance was sought. These individuals would therefore be expected to comprise a dermatologically vulnerable population.

The reported scientific literature contains a paucity of systematic predictive studies of skin sensitization in which a sensitization index is reported on a significant population. For the most part, reported predictive studies have been done by two methodologies, namely, the modified Draize procedure and the maximization procedure. Both methods offer some assistance in forecasting skin sensitization in humans.

The modified Draize procedure showed essentially the same incidence of sensitization potential in predictive tests conducted on a normal test population as was observed by diagnostic tests on clinical patients with four compounds, namely, benzocaine, formaldehyde, ethylenediamine, and paraben. It may have overstated the potential of *p*-phenylenediamine; nevertheless, this is indeed a potent sensitizer. On the other hand, it tended to understate the potential of neomycin.

The maximization procedure is a harsher methodology, whose main usefulness may be in providing a measure of the uppermost limits of sensitization. With a poor skin penetrant such as neomycin, it was useful.

The data for the maximization test must be viewed, like those for all other tests, with judgment. When first promulgated,a high concentration of compound (such as 25% of a single compound) and a high concentration of SLS were suggested (Kligman, 1966). Subsequently the test has frequently been used with final formulations (usually lower concentrations) and lower SLS concentrations instead (Kligman and Epstein, 1975). Data developed with the technique will be required to make an adequate comparison with the more frequently employed modified Draize techniques.

A comparison of results obtained on 21 fragrance ingredients by both the modified Draize and maximization methods was reported recently (Marzulli and Maibach, 1980). The results showed good agreement for 10 of 21 test substances. These included alantroot oil, diethyl malleate, dihydrocoumarin, balsam peru, cinnamon bark oil, ethyl acrylate, and benzilidine acetone, all potent sensitizers by both predictive methods (Table 5). Vetiver acetate appeared intermediate and methyl crotonate a low grade sensitizer by both meth-

TABLE 5. Predictive Test Results with 21 Fragrance Ingredients Tested by Both Draize and Maximization Methods

Both positive	Both negative	Positive maximization only	Positive Draize only
Alantroot oil	Bitter fennel	Dimethyl citraconate	Jasmine
Diethyl maleate			Coumarin
Dihydrocoumarin			Citronellal
Balsam peru			Geraniol
Cinnamon bark oil			Eugenol
Ethyl acrylate			Isoeugenol
Benzilidine acetone			α-amyl cinnamic
Vetiver acetate			alcohol
Methyl crotonate			Hydroxycitronellal
Costus oil			
Cinnamic aldehyde			

ods. Bitter fennel was not considered a skin sensitizer by Draize or by recent maximization tests. Costus oil and cinnamic aldehyde appeared significantly more potent by the maximization test. Dimethyl citraconate was a suspected low grade sensitizer by the maximization method and negative by the Draize procedure. On the other hand, jasmine, coumarin, citronellal, geraniol, eugenol, isoeugenol, α-amyl cinnamic alcohol, and hydroxycitronellal possessed a sensitization potential by the Draize procedure, yet showed no such proclivity by the maximization test. In this series, the vehicle, test concentration, or size of test population may have been responsible for failure of the maximization procedure to detect a sensitization potential seen by the Draize method. The use of sodium lauryl sulfate (SLS) may have been required to elicit a sensitization potential in some of those cases where its absence was accompanied by a negative outcome.

GENERAL COMMENT

Predictive tests in animals are currently under attack by animal rights groups. Related or unrelated to such reviews of animal testing, much remains to be done to understand, perform, and interpret human sensitization assays. Any new assay or modification of the old should be done in context of the expanding depth and quality of worldwide studies of the epidemiology of allergic contact dermatitis.

One approach that merits further attention employs quantitative structure-activity relationships to identify potential sources of contact sensitization, including cross reactants (Benezra et al., 1985, 1989).

REFERENCES

Adams, R. M. and Maibach, H. I., NACDG Group and FDA. 1985. A five-year study of cosmetic reactions. *J. Am. Acad. Dermatol.* 13:1062–1069.

Andersen, K. and Maibach, H. 1985. *Allergic Contact Dermatitis in the Guinea Pig: Principles and Practices.* Basel: Karger.

Baer, R. L. and Rosenthal, S. A. 1954. The germicidal action in human skin of soap containing tetramethylthiuram disulfide. *J. Invest. Dermatol.* 23:193–211.

Baetjer, A. M., Birmingham, D. J., Enterline, P. E., Mertz, W. and Pierce, J. O., II. 1974. *Chromium*, pp. 1–155. Washington, DC: Committee on Biological Effects of Atmospheric Pollutants, National Research Council–National Academy of Sciences.

Bandmann, H. J., Calnan, C. D., Cronin, E., Fregert, S., Hjorth, N., Magnusson, B., Maibach, H., Malten, K. E., Meneghini, C. L., Pirilä, V. and Wilkinson, D. W. 1972. Dermatitis from applied medicaments. *Arch. Dermatol.* 106:335–337.

Benezra, C., Sigman, C. and Maibach, H. 1989. Systematic search for structure-activity relationship of skin contact sensitization: II para-phenylenediamines. *Seminars Derm.* 8:88–93.

Benezra, C., Sigman, C., Penny, L. and Maibach, H. 1985. A systematic search for structure-activity relationships of skin contact sensitization: Methodology. *J. Invest. Derm.* 85:351–356.

Blank, I. H. 1956. Allergic hypersensitivity to an antiseptic soap. *J. Am. Med. Assoc.* 160:1225–1226.

Blank, I. H. and Miller, O. G. 1952. A study of rubber adhesives in shoes as the cause of dermatitis of the feet. *J. Am. Med. Assoc.* 109:1371–1374.

Bruynzeel, D. and Maibach, H. 1986. The excited skin syndrome: A review. *Arch. Dermatol.*, in press.

Calnan, C. D. and Sarkany, I. 1958. Contact dermatitis from neomycin. *Br. J. Dermatol.* 70:435–445.

Calnan, C. D., Bandmann, H. J., Cronin, E., Fregert, S., Hjorth, N., Magnusson, B., Malten, K., Meneghini, C. L., Pirilä, V. and Wilkinson, D. S. 1970. Hand dermatitis in housewives. *Br. J. Dermatol.* 82:543–548.

Cosmetic Injury Reports. FY 1974. Filed in Division of Cosmetics Technology, Bureau of Foods, Food and Drug Administration, Washington, DC.

de Groot, A., Beverdam, E., Tjong Ayong, C., Coenraads, P. and Nater, J. 1988a. The role of contact allergy in the spectrum of adverse effects caused by cosmetics and toiletries. *Contact Derm.* 19:195–201.

de Groot, A. and Weyland, J. 1988b. Kathon CG: A review. *J. Am. Acad. Dermatol.* 18:350–358.

Draize, J. H. 1959. Dermal toxicity. In *Appraisal of the safety of chemicals in foods, drugs and cosmetics.* Austin, Texas: Association of Food and Drug Officials of the United States, Texas State Department of Health.

Draize, J. H., Woodard, G. and Calvery, H. D. 1944. Methods for the study of irritation and toxicity of substances applied topically to the skin and mucous membranes. *J. Pharmacol. Exp. Ther.* 83:377–390.

Dupuis, A. and Benezra, C. 1983. *Allergic Contact Dermatitis to Simple Chemicals: A Molecular Approach.* New York: Dekker.

Eiermann, H. J., Larsen, W., Maibach, H. and Taylor, J. S. 1982. Prospective study of cosmetic reactions: 1977–1981. *J. Am. Acad. Dermatol.* 6(5):909–917.

Ellis, F. A. 1947. The sensitizing factor in merthiolate. *J. Allergy* 18:212–213.

Ellis, F. A. and Robinson, H. M. 1942. Cutaneous sensitivity to merthiolate and other mercurial compounds. *Arch. Dermatol.* 46:425–430.

Epstein, E. 1974. Mercury allergy and patch testing. *Arch. Dermatol.* 109:98–99.

Epstein, E. and Maibach, H. I. 1966. Formaldehyde allergy. *Arch. Dermatol.* 94:186–190.

Epstein, W. L., Kligman, A. M. and Senecal, I. P. 1963. Role of regional lymph nodes in contact sensitization. *Arch. Dermatol.* 88:789–792.

FDA (Food and Drug Administration), Division of Cosmetics Technology/Product Experience Branch, April 11, 1972. Subchapter D-Cosmetics, Part 170, Voluntary registration of cosmetic product establishments, part 171, voluntary filing of cosmetic product ingredients and cosmetic raw material composition statements. *Fed. Regist.* 37(70).

Fisher, A. A., Pascher, F. and Kanof, N. B. 1971. Allergic contact dermatitis due to ingredients of vehicles. *Arch. Dermatol.* 104:186–190.

Fregert, S., Hjorth, N., Magnusson, B., Bandmann, H. J., Calnan, C. D., Cronin, E., Malten, K., Meneghini, C. L., Pirilä, V. and Wilkinson, D. S. 1969. Epidemiology of contact dermatitis. *Trans. St. John's Hosp. Dermatol. Soc.* 55:17–35.

Gaul, L. E. 1957. Results of patch testing with rubber anti-oxidants and accelerators. *J. Invest. Dermatol.* 29:105–110.

Gaul, L. E. 1958. Sensitizing component in thiosalicylic acid. *J. Invest. Dermatol.* 31:91-92.

Giovacchini, R. P. October 1972. Old and new issues in the safety evaluation of cosmetics and toiletries. *CRC Crit. Rev. Toxicol.* 361-378.

Gollhausen, R., Friedemann, E., Przybilla, B., Burg, G. and Ring, J. 1988. Trends in allergic contact sensitization. *Contact Dermatitis* 18:147-154.

Hansson, H. and Moller, H. 1970. Patch test reactions to merthiolate in healthy young subjects. *Br. J. Dermatol.* 83:349-356.

Hardy, J. 1973. Allergy, hypersensitivity and cosmetics. *J. Soc. Cosmet. Chem.* 24:423-468.

Henderson, C. R. and Riley, E. C. 1945. Certain statistical considerations in patch testing. *J. Invest. Dermatol.* 6:227-232.

HEW (Department of Health, Education, and Welfare). June 1975. Investigation of consumer's perceptions of adverse reactions to consumer products. Contracted to Westat, Inc., Rockville, Maryland. Contract No. 223738052. Rockville, Maryland: Consumer Safety Statistics Staff, Office of Planning and Evaluation, Office of the Commissioner, Food and Drug Administration.

Hjorth, N. 1961. Eczematous allergy to balsam, allied perfumes and flavoring agents, with special reference to Balsam of Peru. *Acta Derm. Venereol. (Stockh.)* 41(Suppl. 46):6-216.

Hogan, D. and Maibach, H. 1990. Adverse reactions to transdermal drug delivery systems. *J. Am. Acad. Dermatol.* 22:811-814.

Holdiness, M. R. 1989. A review of contact dermatitis associated with transdermal therapeutic systems. *Contact Dermatitis* 20:3-9.

Jordan, W. 1984. Human studies that determine the sensitizing potential of haptens. *Dermatol. Clinics* 2:533-539.

Kligman, A. M. 1966a. The identification of contact allergens by human assay. III. The maximization test. A procedure for screening and rating contact sensitizers. *J. Invest. Dermatol.* 47:393-409.

Kligman, A. M. 1966b. The SLS provocative patch test in allergic contact sensitization. *J. Invest. Dermatol.* 46:573-585.

Kligman, A. M. and Epstein, W. 1975. Updating the maximization test for identifying contact allergens. *Contact Dermatitis* 1:231-239.

Magnusson, B. and Hersle, K. 1965. Patch test methods. *Acta Derm. Venereol. (Stockh.)* 45:123-128.

Magnusson, B., Blohm, S., Fregert, S., Hjorth, N., Havding, G., Pirilä, V. and Skog, E. 1962. Standardization of routine patch testing. Proceedings of the Northern Dermatologic Society of Gothenburg, *Acta Derm. Venereol. (Stockh.)* 126-127.

Magnusson, B., Blohm, S. G., Fregert, S., Hjorth, N., Havding, G., Pirilä, V. and Skog, E. 1968. Routine patch testing. IV. *Acta Derm. Venereol. (Stockh.)* 48:110-114.

Maibach, H. I. 1975. Report 105 under Contract FDA 223-75-2340. *Skin sensitization.*

Marzulli, F. N. and Maibach, H. I. 1973. Antimicrobials: Experimental contact sensitization in man. *J. Soc. Cosmet. Chem.* 24:399-421.

Marzulli, F. N. and Maibach, H. I. 1974a. Status of topical parabens: Skin hypersensitivity. *Int. J. Dermatol.* 13:397-399.

Marzulli, F. N. and Maibach, H. I. 1974b. The use of graded concentrations in studying skin sensitizers: Experimental contact sensitization in man. *Food Cosmet. Toxicol.* 12:219-227.

Marzulli, F. N. and Maibach, H. I. 1980. Contact allergy: Predictive testing of fragrance ingredients in humans by Draize and maximization methods. *J. Environ. Path. Toxicol.* 3:235–245.

Marzulli, F., Carson, T. and Maibach, H. 1968. Delayed contact hypersensitivity studies in man and animals. *Proceedings of a joint conference on cosmetic sciences.* Washington, DC, April 21–23, pp. 107–122.

Mauer, T. 1983. *Contact and Photocontact Allergens.* New York: Dekker.

Morgan, J. K. 1953. Observations on the persistence of skin sensitivity with reference to nickel eczema. *Br. J. Dermatol.* 65:84–94.

Opdyke, D. L. J. 1974. Monographs on fragrance raw materials. *Food Cosmet. Toxicol.* 12:807–1016.

Pirilä, V. and Rouhunkoski, S. 1959. On sensitivity to neomycin and bacitracin. *Acta Derm. Venereol. (Stockh.)* 39:470–476.

Pirilä, V. and Rouhunkoski, S. 1962. The patterns of cross-sensitivity to neomycin. *Dermatologica* 125:273–278.

Polak, L., Turk, J. L. and Frey, J. R. 1973. Studies on contact hypersensitivity to chromium compounds. *Progr. Allergy* 17:145–226.

Rostenberg, A., Jr. and Sulzberger, M. B. 1937. Some results of patch tests. *Arch. Dermatol. Syphilol.* 35:433–455.

Rudner, E. J., Clendenning, W. E., Epstein, E., Fisher, A. A., Jillson, O. F., Jordan, W. P., Kanof, N., Larsen, W., Maibach, H., Mitchell, J. C., O'Quinn, S. E., Schorr, W. F. and Sulzberger, M. B. 1973. Epidemiology of contact dermatitis in North America. *Arch. Dermatol.* 108:537–540.

Schwartz, L. 1941. Dermatitis from new synthetic resin fabric finishes. *J. Invest. Dermatol.* 4:459–470.

Schwartz, L. 1951. The skin testing of new cosmetics. *J. Soc. Cosmet. Chem.* 2:321–324.

Schwartz, L. 1960. Twenty-two years experience in the performance of 200,000 prophetic-patch tests. *South. Med. J.* 53:478–483.

Schwartz, L. and Peck, S. M. 1944. The patch test in contact dermatitis. *Publ. Health Rep.* 59:546–557.

Serup, J. and Staberg, B. 1987. Ultrasound for assessment of allergic and irritant patch test reactions. *Contact Dermatitis* 17:80–84.

Shelanski, H. A. 1951. Experience with and considerations of the human patch test method. *J. Soc. Cosmet. Chem.* 2:324–331.

Shelanski, H. A. and Shelanski, M. V. 1953. A new technique of human patch tests. *Proc. Sci. Sect. Toilet Goods Assoc.* 19:46–49.

Schorr, W. F. 1968. Paraben allergy: A cause of intractable dermatitis. *J. Am. Med. Assoc.* 204:107–110.

Schorr, W. F., Wenzel, F. J. and Hegedus, S. I. 1973. Cross-sensitivity and aminoglycoside antibiotics. *Arch. Dermatol.* 107:533–539.

Sigman, C., Benezra, C., Helmes, T., and Maibach, H. 1986. *J. Invest. Dermatol.,* in press.

Spier, H. W. and Sixt, I. 1955. Untersuchungen über die Abhängigkeit des Ausfalles der Ekzem Lappchenpraben von der Hornschichtdicke. *Hautarzt* 6:152–159.

Storrs, F., Rosenthal, L., Adams, R., Clendenning, W., Emmett, E., Fisher, A., Larsen, W., Maibach, H., Rietschel, R., Schorr, W. and Taylor, J. 1989. Prevalence and relevance of allergic reactions in patients patch tested in North America— 1984 to 1985. *J. Am. Acad. Dermatol.* 20:1038–1045.

Sunderman, F. W., Jr. 1973. The current status of nickel carcinogenesis. *Ann. Clin. Lab. Sci.* 3:156–180.

TeLintum, J. C. A. and Nater, J. P. 1973. On the persistence of positive patch test reactions to Balsam of Peru, turpentine and nickel. *Br. J. Dermatol.* 89:629–634.

Thestrup-Pedersen, K., Larsen, C. G., and Ronnevig, J. 1989. The immunology of contact dermatology. A review with special reference to the pathophysiology of eczema. *Contact Dermatitis* 20:81–92.

Vandenberg, J. J. and Epstein, W. L. 1963. Experimental nickel contact sensitization in man. *J. Invest. Dermatol.* 41:413–418.

Wilson, H. 1966. Dermatitis from anesthetic ointments. *Practitioner* 197:673–677.

15

diagnostic patch testing

■ Niels Hjorth[†] ■

INTRODUCTION

Although great progress has been made within the field of experimental and clinical immunology, no useful *in vitro* tests have been devised to demonstrate lymphocyte-mediated contact allergy in humans. Instead, the sensitivity must be looked for and proved by a reproduction of the acute lesions after contact with a suspected substance under an occlusive patch.

Like any other clinical or laboratory examination it is subject to sources of error. However, with standardized methods and meticulous attention to detail, patch testing represents a sound and reasonably reliable method for identifying allergens responsible for contact dermatitis.

INDICATIONS FOR PATCH TESTING

Previously, patch testing was performed only if allergic contact dermatitis was suspected. More extensive use of a standard series of diagnostic test substances has, however, revealed that clinical suspicions are most unreliable (Cronin, 1972; Magnusson et al., 1969; Rudner et al., 1975; Wilkinson, 1972) and that, in fact, many cases with nonspecific patterns of dermatitis did suffer from contact dermatitis (Fregert et al., 1969). Recent studies showed that about

[†]Deceased.

40% of patients with contact dermatitis of the hands have one or several contact sensitivities, of which two-thirds are relevant to the dermatitis (Wilkinson et al., 1970a). This justifies a more extensive use of patch testing. Patients with dermatitis of the hands of more than 1 month's duration and all patients with occupational dermatitis causing absence from work must be tested. Possibly the eczema is caused by an allergen that can be avoided—for example, by use of rubber gloves—or whose impact can be diminished by minor changes in the process of work. In chronic dermatitis of the legs, especially stasis dermatitis, the majority of patients are sensitive to one or several medicaments used for topical treatment (Bandmann et al., 1972). Pompholyx or dyshidrotic eczema can develop in sensitive persons after ingestion of traces of their allergens in the daily food, such as nickel (Christensen and Möller, 1975) or chromate (Fisher, 1973).

Any chronic eczema of the anogenital area can be complicated by contact sensitivity.

The observations above justify a more extensive use of patch testing.

PATCH TESTING TECHNIQUE

A standardized procedure for patch testing was developed in the 1960s by a Scandinavian group (Magnusson and Hersle, 1965; Magnusson et al., 1969) and brought into widespread usage by two more recent study groups, the North American Contact Dermatitis Group (Rudner et al., 1975) and the International Contact Dermatitis Research Group (Fregert et al., 1969). Test results can be compared only provided the same techniques are followed.

Basically a patch test implies the application to the skin of a certain amount of the suspected allergen in a suitable concentration and a suitable vehicle. The concentration and the vehicle are usually chosen on the assumption that penetration through the skin is promoted by airtight occlusion.

In practice, the substance is applied to a test unit placed on adhesive tape, which is then fixed onto the skin. The test unit must be left on for at least 24 hr, but because many reactions develop later than that, the units are usually removed after 2 or 3 days.

TEST UNITS

It is common practice to use ready-made test materials. The North American Contact Dermatitis Group at present prefers Al-Test IMECO. This is a unit of circular 10-mm-diameter filter paper disks, welded to polythene foil, which is stiffened by a paper-backed aluminum foil. The Al-Test is supplied in rolls of 1,000 units, convenient for serial patch testing. Aluminum foil affords good occlusion of the centrally placed test material. Many other test units are currently available. One of them, the Finn Chamber Test, is a flat cup of aluminum 10 mm in diameter (Pirilä, 1975). This has the advantage of a stiff brim, which provides sufficient occlusion to allow the use of porous, nonocclusive, less irritant tapes.

Reactions to adhesive tape are common, but most are of a nonallergic nature, and the major concern is interference with the reading of patch test reactions. For that reason many dermatologists prefer Dermicel (Johnson & Johnson), which has, however, less adhesive power than conventional adhesive tape, a drawback of most acrylic tapes. Scanpore (Norgesplaster, Oslo) has better adhesive properties than most other acrylic tapes by virtue of a thicker coat of adhesive and has been recommended for use with the Finn Chamber Test.

VEHICLES

Textiles, leather, and so on can be applied to the skin as they are and covered by adhesive tape. Most chemicals, however, are dissolved in some vehicle in a suitable concentration for testing. Petrolatum is the most suitable, since it does not evaporate, protects against oxidation, and increases the shelf stability of the test substance (Trolle-Lassen and Hjorth, 1966). Petrolatum is therefore used for most diagnostic test substances included in standard series.

Substances brought in by the patients can be diluted in an adequate solvent such as water or alcohol. Irritant solvents such as benzene, chloroform, and kerosene are obviously unsuitable.

CONCENTRATION

The concentration of the test substance is highly important since the choice of too low a concentration causes false negative patch test reactions, and concentrations that are too high cause irritant reactions and a risk of patch test sensitization.

Often a suitable concentration can be found in handbooks on patch testing (Bandmann and Dohn, 1967; Bandmann and Fregert, 1975; Fisher, 1973, 1986; Malten et al., 1976; Rook et al., 1968). The concentrations given in these will usually not cause irritant reactions or sensitizations, but they may, in fact, be too low because they have not been tried out on a sufficient number of sensitive patients. Difficulties arise when patients bring their own materials, such as industrial chemicals, for testing. Open patch tests with various dilutions are advisable for a start. If these give no reactions, occlusive patch tests with lower concentrations can be performed.

It should be realized that the concentration chosen for routine testing will cause false negative reactions in some cases and irritant reactions in others.

Some standard test substances such as formaldehyde, cobalt, and tars cause false positives in children. Presumably the concentrations chosen for routine testing should be selected with regard to the age of the patients tested. No systematic studies of this problem have been performed.

AMOUNT OF TEST MATERIAL

The dose of the test substance applied from a syringe is usually adequate if the string of ointment is 5 mm long. If the test substance is a fluid, the filter paper should be saturated.

Scrapings from solid materials must cover the filter paper and they should be wetted with some solvent.

TEST SITES

Most dermatologists apply the tests on the upper or lower back, but the lateral side of the upper arm can also be chosen. The inner surface of the upper arm, the thighs, and the legs may be unsuitable test sites because of inadequate absorption (Bandmann and Rohrbach, 1964; Bandmann and Fregert, 1975; Magnusson and Hersle, 1965).

TIME OF READING

With most allergens a sufficient amount is usually absorbed within 24 hr to provoke a positive response, which may not develop for one or more further days. Conventionally the tests are left in place for 2 days and then removed. If the patient can come only once, it is advisable to let the patient remove the test 2 days after application and appear for reading the next day. This assumes that all test sites were marked for future identification at the time of application.

Positive reactions usually itch, are red, and are to a varying extent infiltrated and studded with papulovesicles. Such a reaction persists for several days or even weeks.

A positive reaction that develops 6 days or more after the application of a patch test is called a late reaction or a flare-up reaction (Wilkinson et al., 1970b).

Some reactions are of an irritant nature but difficult to distinguish from true allergic responses. But most irritant reactions are sharply demarcated with a brownish eroded or glistening surface. Sometimes they are bullous. Compression of the test site between the fingers may reveal a finely wrinkled surface called a "soap effect." Irritant reactions rarely itch but may burn and be painful.

Sweat retention may develop from patch testing. Such papular nonspecific reactions are particularly common in a hot summer. At all times of the year nonspecific pustular sweat gland reactions can be found in atopic individuals after testing with metal salts.

TEST SUBSTANCES

Common test substances are available from a number of pharmaceutical firms, which supply them in suitable concentrations and in suitable vehicles.[1] The substances available include a standard series of 20–30 substances, known to be the most common allergens (Table 1). There are slight differences between the North American (Rudner et al., 1975) and European (Fregert et al., 1969) recommended series. These substances give a clue to 60–80% of cases of allergic contact dermatitis. The rest are caused by huge numbers of environmental allergens. These derive from several spheres of a patient.

In the personal environment, cosmetics, textiles, and leather are the important allergens. Hair dyes may cause patch test sensitization; permanent wave lotions and mascara and other eye cosmetics may cause irritant reactions. Creams and lipsticks, on the other hand, commonly give false negative reactions.

Textiles should be moistened in water or alcohol in order to wash out the allergen. But even so, up to half of those tested show false negative reactions. Extracts must then be prepared; for example, by means of ether, hot ethanol, or other solvents.

To obtain material from a shoe a mastoid curette must be employed. With proper technique, false positives are rare. In the home and kitchen rubber gloves and indoor plants are reasonably common allergens. It should be noted that not all causes of rubber sensitivity can be revealed by patch testing and that, on the other hand, not all reactions to rubber mixes are indicative of rubber glove sensitivity. Sensitivity to Black Rubber Mix and Naphthyl Mix does not usually coincide with rubber glove sensitivity.

Some plants can be tested as they are, but since the allergen may be largely confined to one organ, several parts of the plant should be employed in the test. Most cases can probably be detected by testing with suitable extracts

---

[1]Patch test substances are supplied by (1) Hollister-Stier Laboratories, Spokane, Washington 94577; (2) Trolab, laboratory for dermatological tests, A. N. Hansensvej 6, DK-2900 Hellerup, Denmark; and (3) Allergopharma, Bahnhofstrasse 4, D-2057 Reinbek, Germany.

TABLE 1. Example of a Patch Test Series Comprising 20 Substances

Substance	Number of tests
Metals (chromium, nickel, cobalt)	3
Mixtures of rubber chemicals	5
Topical medicaments (neomycin, Vioform, local anesthetics, parabens)	5
Balsams (balsam of Peru, rosin, turpentine, wood tars)	4
Miscellaneous agents (formaldehyde, paraphenylenediamine, epoxy resin)	3

and mixtures thereof. Extracts of the Compositae (supplied by Hollister-Stier) are used in the detection of weed allergy in hand eczema and in dermatitis on exposed surfaces, especially in farmers. Primin, the sensitizer in *Primula,* is commercially available for patch testing (supplied by Trolab).

Hobbies involve manifold chemical contacts with substances such as glues, dyes, exotic woods, and so forth, and if they involve amateur gardening, exposures to sensitizing plants—apart from the obvious *Rhus*—are unavoidable.

Industrial allergens are commonly detected by standard testing, which includes nickel, chromate, cobalt, and epoxy resin, but obviously there must be a wealth of different materials not included. They must be selected according to the history of the individual patient. Protective gloves, creams, and cleansers should not be forgotten.

SIGNIFICANCE OF PATCH TEST REACTIONS

A positive reaction to a patch test properly performed indicates that the patient is sensitive to the substance tested and that the allergen may be involved in the causation of dermatitis.

Corroboration of the history determines whether exposure to the substance in question is relevant to the development of dermatitis. Establishment of sensitivity to rubber can explain a nonspecific dermatitis of the leg as being caused by a rubber boot. This is a typical example of an unexpected sensitivity that could only be detected by patch testing and is most easily detected by inclusion of rubber chemicals in a series of standard tests.

Positive reactions can be (1) relevant to the actual dermatitis, (2) of past relevance, (3) of questionable relevance, and (4) of unknown relevance (Wilkinson et al., 1970b).

A reaction of past relevance could be a positive reaction to nickel in the standard series, associated with a history of previous dermatitis from a zip fastener. The finding of a positive reaction to neomycin associated with a clearcut history of dermatitis from an unknown applied medicament would be of questionable relevance.

Some patients are sensitive to substances that are not known to occur in their environment. Such reactions of unknown relevance should challenge the clinician to trace the origin of the sensitization. The positive reaction indicates that the patient has been sensitized by contact either with the test substance or with a chemically related allergen. Reactions of unknown relevance at the time of reading may later prove highly important as a clue to dermatitis. More and more reactions to chromate have proved to be relevant (Table 2). Nonspecific patterns of dermatitis of the body were common in the 1950s in patients sensitive to formaldehyde. These reactions were of unknown relevance until it was established that formaldehyde resins were used as fixatives for textiles. Similarly, reactions to balsam of Peru may indicate a perfume sensitivity. Questionably relevant would apply to a reaction to a common perfume chemical in a patient

TABLE 2. Year of Detection of New
Sources of Chromate Contact

Source	Year
Dichromate	1923
Eau de Javelle (cleansing agent)	1930
Leather	1938
Cement	1950
Matches	1962
Game-table felt	1970
Sodium sulfate	1972

with dermatitis of the hands. The perfume chemical may or may not occur in the toilet soap used, and the reaction is therefore of questionable relevance.

Obviously, the relevance of a positive patch test can only be established provided the clinician has an adequate knowledge of the occurrence of the allergen in the patient's environment. The occurrences of the common allergens are listed in many handbooks (Bandmann and Fregert, 1975; Fisher, 1973, 1986; Malten et al., 1976; Rudner et al., 1975), and at least one should be consulted before a positive reaction is discarded as being of questionable or unknown relevance.

FALSE POSITIVE REACTIONS

False positive reactions are of irritant and of nonimmunological character. Many substances are irritant if applied in a sufficiently high concentration under occlusion on normal skin. Even substances included in the standard patch test series cause irritant reactions in a small number of susceptible individuals.

Materials brought in by the patients pose the greatest problems. Many industrial chemicals are irritant under the condition of a patch test. Some, such as gasoline, kerosene, and detergents, should never be tested. Patients may be sensitive to organic dyes used for motor oils or gasoline, but the vehicle is so irritant that it is impossible to verify the sensitivity by testing with dilutions of the material. Other solvents are also irritant. This applies to benzene and chloroform, which should not be used for testing, even if they are the only solvents suitable for a particular test substance.

Recent dermatitis in the test area, and even an active dermatitis elsewhere, may decrease the threshold for irritant reactions (Björnberg, 1968). If reading of the reaction is performed immediately after removal of the adhesive tape, reactions may be read as positive although the local erythema will disappear after 20–30 min. Rubbing or fingering of the test area will prolong this type of irritant erythema. The adhesive tape employed for fixation of the test units may provoke irritant or allergic reactions or miliaria. Any of these complicates the reading so that nonallergic reactions are read as positives.

Strong positive reactions in the neighborhood of the test site may lower the threshold for both allergic and irritant patch test reactions.

FALSE NEGATIVE REACTIONS

A patch test may give a negative reaction, even if the patient has a clinical (i.e., relevant) sensitivity to the substance tested. Such false negative reactions are generally due to insufficient penetration through the skin.

The most common cause of error is loosening of the adhesive tape. This results in inadequate occlusion and therefore inadequate penetration of test material. Open patch tests require ten times the concentration recommended for occlusive patch tests.

The laboratory technician may apply too little test material to the patch. This is particularly obvious if the filter paper patch is not saturated with a testing solution. An unfortunate choice of vehicle may prevent release and thus penetration of the test substance into the skin. A powdered test substance may be too crude, and for that reason unable to penetrate.

The concentration of the allergen may be too low. Neomycin dermatitis is usually caused by ointment with 0.5% neomycin. However, penetration of neomycin through normal skin is so slow that only half of those who are clinically sensitive will develop a positive patch test reaction to 0.5% neomycin. Testing with an excessive concentration of 20% is required to prove the sensitivity.

If only a small fraction of a composite test mixture is allergenic, the very bulk of inert material may preclude an adequate concentration on normal skin. With eosin in lipstick contact dermatitis could develop when sufficient amounts of an impurity of eosin had accumulated in the skin of the vermilion border. This could not be verified with a 48 hr patch test with the lipstick but only with the excessive concentration of 50% eosin in a lipstick base. Similarly, lanolin sensitivity is best demonstrated by patch testing with wool alcohols, which contain a concentrate of the allergens.

Some irritants must be diluted to avoid irritant reactions, but this may prevent testing in search of allergy to a component of the mixture. Perfumes in toilet soaps and detergents cannot be expected to give positive reactions in persons sensitive to them. To avoid the irritant effect of the alkaline soap or detergent, the product must be diluted to such an extent that testing is no longer meaningful (Sulzberger and Baer, 1945).

Very sensitive individuals react to patch tests applied in nearly all body regions. On average, however, half of the positive reactions obtained by testing on the back will be missed if the tests are applied on the front of the thighs (Magnusson and Hersle, 1965).

Negative reactions may be recorded if only one reading is performed, and this is done after 2 days (Fregert et al., 1969). The time of reaction is commonly longer. Local steroid therapy of the test area can reduce the reactivity of the skin, and so can systemic steroid therapy provided the daily dosage exceeds 20 mg prednisone or equivalent. Exhaustion of the immunological reactivity after a widespread acute dermatitis has been reported but is very rare.

SIDE EFFECTS OF PATCH TESTING

Most patients find it a nuisance to carry strips of adhesive tape on their backs for 2 days, partly because it prevents them from having a bath and partly because some itching is unavoidable, especially in summer. Occlusive tapes may cause miliaria rubra. In a pigmented Caucasian temporary hypopigmentation can follow the removal of the adhesive tape. Some test substances can cause a hypopigmentation from pigment incontinence (Osmundsen, 1970). Sun exposure of the test sites leaves hyperpigmented spots from tar and other photosensitizers. Scarring is very rare.

Positive reactions itch, and if they are strong, they may provoke a flare-up of distant sites of dermatitis, dyshidrotic eruptions and id-like dissemination. Such spread can be stopped by a short course of prednisone (40–60 mg/day).

Patch testing may in some cases sensitize to the substance tested. This is rare with substances included in the standard series, whose concentrations and vehicles have been chosen after mass testing. Materials of unknown composition brought in by the patients bring more problems. Sensitization sometimes becomes apparent as a late reaction develops 7 days or more after testing, but some cases can be established only by repeated testing. For unknown reasons patch test sensitizations are often transient and impossible to verify by repeated testing 1 yr later (White and Baer, 1950).

Contact sensitivity tends to decline with the years, especially with avoidance of contact with the allergen. Repeated patch tests may provoke the sensitivity, and even in such cases a late reaction may develop. The clinical significance of this is probably limited since such a patient will easily be resensitized by clinical contact with the allergen.

New important environmental allergens must be introduced in standard patch test series. A suitable test concentration cannot be predicted. With alantolactone, an allergen in the Compositae plant family, a cautious choice of 1% in petrolatum was found to cause patch test sensitization. Consequently, the concentration was adjusted to a safe 0.1%. Patch test sensitizations may also occur if the test substances undergo chemical changes during storage. This happens with turpentine, whose allergen content initially increases and then declines during storage.

Such phenomena are unpredictable and therefore unavoidable. Systemic symptoms may follow occlusive patch tests with Apresoline (Kligman, 1966). Insecticides and some war gases may similarly cause systemic pharmacological effects after absorption.

Fainting, malaise, and fever have been observed after epicutaneous tests with lauryl ether sulfate containing an allergenic sultone impurity (Magnusson and Gilje, 1973). Such symptoms occurred only in patients with a delayed-type hypersensitivity to the test substance and must have an immunological basis, as does contact urticaria from the insect repellent Deet (Maibach and Johnson, 1975). The general reactions described are rare.

WHY PATCH TEST?

Contact sensitivities are very often missed, even at clinics that are specially focused on contact dermatitis (Agrup et al., 1970; Cronin, 1972). This can have far reaching clinical consequences. If a worker develops occupational hand eczema, contact substances specific for the place of work will be suspected. A change of job may be recommended. This would be unlikely to help if the hand eczema were due to protective rubber gloves. Unless patch tests are performed, rubber gloves may not come into focus, and only patch testing could reveal that sensitivities to specific materials were nonexistent. This worker should change his gloves and not his job.

Several studies have assessed the accuracy of clinical estimates of contact sensitivities. The clinical diagnosis of a primary nickel sensitization is usually obvious, but secondary dyshidrotic eruptions of the hands may not be ascribed to a nickel sensitivity (Agrup et al., 1970; Cronin, 1972; Wilkinson, 1972). Chromate, cobalt and rubber sensitivities are often unexpected findings at standard patch testing (Agrup et al., 1970), and so are sensitivities to individual components of local therapeutics. A bullous streaky dermatitis from a weekend outing is assumed to be diagnostic of *Rhus* dermatitis. Only recently has the phototoxic *Heracleum* dermatitis, which in Europe is the usual cause of streaky plant dermatitis, been recognized in the United States (Camm et al., 1976). Standard patch tests with *Primula obconica* reveal that many cases of dermatitis from it are missed by dermatologists.

Many dermatologists trust their clinical acumen in the diagnosis of allergic contact dermatitis and feel, as a consequence, that the benefits of patch testing do not outweigh the risks of the procedure. Systematic investigation has, however, failed to support this complacency and has, on the contrary, shown that half of all contact sensitivities were relevant and unexpected by the clinician.

REFERENCES

Agrup, G., Dahlquist, J., Fregert, S. and Rorsman, H. 1970. Value of history and testing in suspected contact dermatitis. *Arch. Dermatol.* 101:212–215.

Bandmann, H.-J. and Dohn, W. 1967. *Die Epicutantestung.* Munich: Bergmann.

Bandmann, H.-J. and Fregert, S. 1975. *Patch testing.* New York: Springer Verlag.

Bandmann, H.-J. and Rohrbach, W. 1964. Die epicutane Testreaktion und ihre Abhängigkeit von dem Auflageort der Läppchenprobe. *Arch. Klin. Exp. Dermatol.* 220:155.

Bandmann, H.-J., Calnan, C. D., Cronin, E., Fregert, S., Hjorth, N., Magnusson, B., Maibach, H. J., Malten, K. E., Meneghini, C. P., Pirilä, V. and Wilkinson, D. S. 1972. Dermatitis from applied medicaments. *Arch. Dermatol.* 106:335–337.

Björnberg, A. 1968. *Skin reactions to primary irritants in patients with hand eczema*, p. 117. Göteborg, Sweden: Isacson.

Camm, E., Buck, H. W. L. and Mitchell, J. C. 1976. Phytophotodermatitis from Heracleum mantegazzianum. *Contact Dermatitis* 2:68–72.

Christensen, O. B. and Möller, H. 1975. External and internal exposure of the antigen in the hand eczema of nickel allergy. *Contact Dermatitis* 1:136–141.

Cronin, E. 1972. Clinical prediction of patch test results. *Trans. St. John's Hosp. Dermatol. Soc.* 58:153–162.

Fisher, A. A. 1973. *Contact dermatitis.* Philadelphia: Lea & Febiger.

Fisher, A. A. 1986. *Contact dermatitis* (3rd ed.). Philadelphia: Lea & Febiger.

Fregert, S., Hjorth, N., Magnusson, B., Bandmann, H.-J., Calnan, C. D., Cronin, E., Malten, K., Meneghini, C. L., Pirilä, V. and Wilkinson, D. S. 1969. Epidemiology of contact dermatitis. *Trans. St. John's Hosp. Dermatol. Soc.* 55:17–35.

Kligman, A. M. 1966. The identification of contact allergens by human assay. III. The maximization test: A procedure for screening and rating contact sensitizers. *J. Invest. Dermatol.* 47:393.

Magnusson, B. and Gilje, O. 1973. Allergic contact dermatitis from a dishwashing liquid containing lauryl ether sulphate. *Acta Derm. Venereol. (Stockh.)* 53:136–140.

Magnusson, B. and Hersle, K. 1965. Patch test methods. 2. Regional variations of patch test responses. *Acta Derm. Venereol. (Stockh.)* 45:257.

Magnusson, B., Fregert, S., Hjorth, N., Høvding, G., Pirilä, V. and Skog, E. 1969. Routine patch testing V. *Acta Derm. Venereol. (Stockh.)* 49:556–563.

Maibach, H. J. and Johnson, H. L. 1975. Contact urticaria syndrome. *Arch. Dermatol.* 111:726–730.

Malten, K. E., Nater, J. P. and van Ketel, W. G. 1976. Patch testing guidelines. Nijmegen: Dekker and van de Vegt.

Osmundsen, P. E. 1970. Pigmented contact dermatitis. *Br. J. Dermatol.* 83:296–301.

Pirilä, V. 1975. Chamber test versus patch test for epicutaneous testing. *Contact Dermatitis* 1:48–52.

Rook, A., Wilkinson, D. S. and Elling, F. J. G. 1968. *Textbook of dermatology*, vol. 1. Oxford: Blackwell.

Rudner, E. J., Clendenning, W. E., Epstein, E., Fisher, A. A., Jillson, O. F., Jordan, W. P., Kanoj, N., Larsen, W., Maibach, H. J., Mitchell, J. C., O'Quinn, S. E., Schorr, W. and Sulzberger, M. B. 1975. The frequency of contact sensitivity in North America 1972–1974. *Contact Dermatitis* 1:277–280.

Sulzberger, M. B. and Baer, R. L. 1945. Unusual or abnormal effects of soap on the "abnormal skin." In *Medical uses of soap*, ed. M. Fishbein, pp. 51–59. London: Lippincott.

Trolle-Lassen, C. and Hjorth, N. 1966. Deterioration of substances used for patch testing. *Berufsdermatosen* 14:176–188.

White, W. A. and Baer, R. L. 1950. Failure to prevent experimental sensitization. Observations on the "spontaneous" flare-up phenomenon. *J. Allergy* 21:344–348.

Wilkinson, D. S. 1972. Contact dermatitis of the hands. *Trans. St. John's Hosp. Dermatol. Soc.* 58:163–171.

Wilkinson, D. S., Bandmann, H. J., Calnan, C. D., Cronin, E., Fregert, S., Hjorth, N., Magnusson, B., Maibach, H. J., Malten, K. E., Meneghini, C. L. and Pirilä, V. 1970a. The role of contact allergy in hand eczema. *Trans. St. John's Hosp. Dermatol. Soc.* 56:19–25.

Wilkinson, D. S., Fregert, S., Magnusson, B., Bandmann, H.-J., Calnan, C. D., Cronin, E., Hjorth, N., Maibach, H. J., Malten, K. E., Meneghini, C. L. and Pirilä, V. 1970b. Terminology of contact dermatitis. *Acta Derm. Venereol. (Stockh.)* 50:287–292.

16

systemic contact–type dermatitis

■ **T. Menné** ■ **Howard I. Maibach** ■

INTRODUCTION

Systemic reactions to ingested allergens may occur in patients previously sensitized by percutaneous absorption of an allergen. Until recently, such reactions have mainly been of theoretical interest when they were occasionally observed in patients sensitized to a topically applied medicament who later developed widespread dermatitis when treated with the same medicament systemically.

Contact sensitivity to nickel, chromium, and cobalt is frequent and is often associated with chronic hand eczema (Fregert et al., 1969). As these metals occur in small amounts in our food, it is possible that systemic contact-type dermatitis is a common phenomenon (Veien, 1989).

CLINICAL PICTURE

Pompholyx

Pompholyx, or vesicular hand eczema, is a recurring itching eruption with deep-seated vesicles and some or no erythema localized on the palms, volar aspects, and sides of the fingers. Exacerbations occur at intervals of weeks to months without any obvious external reason (Menné and Hjorth, 1983).

Flare-Ups of Earlier Patch Test and Contact Dermatitis Reactions

This phenomenon has been observed experimentally in provocation studies with nickel and chromium in patients sensitized to these metals and in patients sensitized to medicaments. Periodic flare-up reactions in earlier positive patch tests have not been observed in clinical practice.

The Baboon Syndrome

This entity derives its name from the red, well-demarcated eruption on the buttocks and genital area accompanied by a symmetric eczematous eruption in the elbow flexure, axillae, eyelids, and side of the neck. At the same time, a generalized maculopapular rash may be present (Andersen et al., 1984; Nakayama et al., 1983).

Vasculitis

Circular excoriations on the back, buttocks, and thighs were observed in nickel-sensitive women (Hjorth, 1976; Veien and Krogdahl, 1989). Similar excoriations were noticed in two nickel-sensitive patients treated with a nickel-chelating drug (Kaaber et al., 1979). Histopathology shows superficial allergic vasculitis. Purpuric vasculitis-like eruptions have been observed in a patient with allergic contact dermatitis due to balsam of Peru (Bruynzeel et al., 1984).

Systemic Symptoms

In relation to oral provocation with nickel and medicaments, general symptoms such as headache and malaise may occur in sensitized individuals. In neomycin- and chromate-sensitive patients, oral provocation with the hapten produces nausea, vomiting, and diarrhea (Ekelund and Möller, 1969; Pirilä, 1970; Kaaber and Veien, 1977).

NICKEL

Environmental exposures to nickel and nickel metabolites have been described in detail (National Academy of Sciences, 1975; Underwood, 1977; Brown and Sunderman, 1980; Nriagu, 1980; Sunderman, 1983; Sunderman, 1984; Maibach and Menné, 1989). Daily nickel intake varies from 100 to 800 μg. The highest nickel content is found in vegetables, whole wheat or rye bread, and shellfish. Nickel release from stainless steel cooking utensils during the preparation of food with a low pH value may cause additional exposure (Christensen and Möller, 1978; Brun, 1979). Nickel exposure from drinking water and air pollution is usually negligible, although important exceptions do occur (Fregert, 1971). Intravenous fluids may be contaminated with 100–200 μg/l concentrations of nickel (Sunderman, 1983).

Most ingested nickel remains unabsorbed in the gastrointestinal tract. Only 1–10% is absorbed. The nickel concentration in sweat is high, ranging from 7 to 270 μg/liter. Thus, sweating may be an important route of excretion of nickel from the body.

Oral provocation with 5.6 mg nickel as the sulfate to 12 nickel-sensitive female patients with pompholyx resulted in a flare of the dermatitis, with fresh vesicles in 9 of the patients. The reaction appeared within 2–16 h (Christensen and Möller, 1975). This observation has been confirmed in repeated studies (Table 1). From the table it is evident that there is a marked dose-response relationship. Only a minority of nickel-sensitive patients react to oral doses below 1.25 mg of elementary nickel, although nearly all will react at doses of 5.5 mg. A positive response might be one or more of the following symptoms: flare of vesicular hand eczema, flare of primary dermatitis, or flare of earlier positive nickel patch test.

TABLE 1. Challenge Studies in Nickel Sensitive Patients with an Oral Dose of Nickel Given as the Sulphate

Author	Type of study	Allergen dose (elementary nickel)	Duration of dosing	Response frequency
Christensen and Möller (1975)	Double blind	5.6 mg	Single exposure	9/12
Kaaber et al. (1978)	Double blind	2.5 mg	Single exposure	17/28
Kaaber et al. (1979)	Double blind	0.6 mg	Single exposure	1/11
		1.2 mg	Single exposure	1/11
		2.5 mg	Single exposure	9/11
Veien et al. (1979)	Open	4.0 mg	Single exposure	4/7
Jordan and King (1979)	Double blind	0.5 mg	Two repeated days	1/10
Cronin et al. (1980)	Open	0.6 mg	Single exposure	1/5
		1.25 mg	Single exposure	4/5
		2.50 mg	Single exposure	5/5
Burrows et al. (1981)	Double blind	2.00 mg	Two repeated days	9/22
		4.0 mg	Two repeated days	8/22
Goitre et al. (1981)	Open	4.4 mg	Single exposure	2/2
Pecegueiro and Brandao (1982)	Single blind	2.8 mg 5.6 mg	Repeated dose	34/43
Sertoli et al. (1985)	Open	2.2 mg	Single exposure	13/20
Gawkrodger et al. (1986)	Double blind	0.4 mg	Two repeated days	5/10
		2.5 mg	Two repeated days	5/10
		5.6 mg	Single dose	6/6
Santucci et al. (1988)	Open	2.2 mg	Single exposure	18/25

The clinical significance of these findings is a matter for discussion. The nickel doses used in the provocation studies often exceed the figures given for the normal daily intake of nickel. In experimental studies, we have often observed flare reactions at the site of an earlier nickel patch test. This phenomenon does not appear in clinical practice. After oral provocation with 0.6–5.6 mg nickel, a nonphysiological high urinary nickel value was observed on the following days (20–200 μg/l) (Menné et al., 1978; Veien et al., 1979; Cronin, 1980; Christensen and Lagesson, 1981; Gawkrodger et al., 1986). In two studies involving four patients (Menné and Thorboe, 1976; de Yongh et al., 1978) there was a tendency for higher nickel excretion in the urine to be related to active hand dermatitis, but the urinary nickel level was far from the high concentrations measured on the days after oral nickel provocation.

These observations do not exclude the possibility that systemic exposure to nickel is important for the chronicity of hand eczema related to nickel sensitivity. Undoubtedly, the daily nickel intake will sometimes exceed 0.6 mg, and 2 of 5 patients reacted to this dose in the study of Cronin et al. (1980). A diet with a low nickel content diminished the activity of hand eczema in 9 of 17 patients (Kaaber et al., 1978; Veien, 1989), and after the diet was abandoned, 7 of the 9 experienced a flare of their hand eczema.

A systemic contact dermatitis reaction in nickel-sensitive people can also be provoked by treatment with nickel chelating drugs. The drug of choice in the treatment of nickel carbonyl poisoning is diethyldithiocarbamate (Sunderman, 1979). Tetraethylthiuram disulfide (Antabuse) is metabolized to diethyldithiocarbamate after absorption in the gastrointestinal tract. Treatment with these drugs at a daily dosage of 50–400 mg has been effective in the treatment of nickel hand eczema (Christensen and Kristensen, 1982; Kaaber et al., 1978; Menné, 1980; Spruit et al., 1978). Tetraethylthiuram disulfide treatment of nickel hand eczema was evaluated in a double-blind study (Kaaber et al., 1983a). During the treatment, 5 of 11 in the tetraethylthiuram disulfide group healed completely, compared with 2 of 13 in the placebo-treated group. There was a statistically significant decrease in the number of flare and scaling reactions in the tetraethylthiuram disulfide-treated group. Regarding the other parameters, area of dermatitis, redness, and number of vesicles, the difference between the Antabuse-treated and placebo groups was not statistically significant. In the placebo group, the weekly amount of steroid ointment used was 5.3 g, compared with 1.6 g in the tetraethylthiuram disulfide group. Even with a daily dosage of 50 mg tetraethylthiuram disulfide, some patients had a severe flare of their dermatitis during the first weeks of treatment. This eventual effect of Antabuse on nickel dermatitis is of theoretical interest only, as liver toxicity is a potential problem (Kaaber et al., 1987).

If nickel is given intravenously to nickel-sensitive patients, 1–3 μg may elicit a severe systemic contact dermatitis reaction. This has been observed in patients treated with intravenous infusions through a cannula releasing traces of nickel and by hemodialysis (Olerud et al., 1984; Smeenk and Teunissen, 1977; Stoddart, 1960).

Indomethacin increases absorption of nickel, making adverse reactions possible in nickel-sensitive patients (Spruit, 1979). Nickel associates with a variety of natural occurring proteins and amino acids (Nriagu, 1980). Thus, flare of dermatitis in nickel-sensitive patients may not always be caused by increased oral exposure to nickel, but could be elicited by metabolic and pharmacological reactions.

CHROMIUM

Chromium metabolism and toxicology have been described in detail (Burrows, 1983; National Academy of Sciences, 1974; Underwood, 1977). Chromium intake in the United States varies from 5 to 400 μg/d. Exact figures for absorption are difficult to establish because they depend on the source of chromium. Inorganic chromium compounds are poorly absorbed; among them, hexavalent chromium is more easily absorbed than trivalent chromium, the absorption ranging from 1 to 25% of an oral dose. Most meats are good sources of chromium; fish and most vegetables are poor ones.

Sidi and Melki (1954) suggested that oral intake of dichromate by chromate-sensitive patients might be of importance for the chronicity of the dermatitis. Several studies testing this hypothesis are listed in Table 2. Fregert (1965) challenged 5 patients sensitive to chromium with 0.05 mg potassium dichromate. Within 2 h they developed severe vesiculation of the palms. One of the patients experienced acute exacerbation of a generalized dermatitis. Scheliff (1968) observed a flare in chromate dermatitis in 20 patients challenged with 1–10 mg potassium dichromate contained in a homeopathic drug. Some of the patients also experienced a flare in a previously positive dichromate patch test.

Kaaber and Veien (1977) studied the significance of oral intake of dichromate by chromate-sensitive patients in a double-blind study. Thirty-one patients were challenged orally with either 2.5 mg potassium dichromate or a placebo tablet. Nine of 11 patients with pompholyx hand eczema reacted with a flare of the dermatitis within 1 or 2 d, but did not react to placebo. The patients with another morphology reacted to a lesser degree. A few reacted to placebo. Three patients developed vomiting or abdominal pains and transient diarrhea after the chromate provocation, but not after the challenge with placebo. A systemic contact dermatitis reaction to chromium may also occur after inhalation of chromium contained in welding fumes (Shelley, 1964).

COBALT

Cobalt metabolism has been described by Underwood (1977). Daily intake of cobalt ranges from 0.14 to 1.77 mg in the United States. Among indi-

TABLE 2. Challenge Studies in Chromate-Sensitive Patients with an Oral Dose
of Chromate Given as the Chromate

Author	Type of study	Allergen dose (elementary chromate)	Duration of dosing	Response frequency
Fregert (1965)	Open	0.05	Single exposure	5/5
Schleiff (1968)	Open	1–10 mg	Single exposure	20/20
Kaaber and Veien (1977)	Double blind	7.1 mg	Single exposure	11/31 9/11[a]
Goitre et al. (1982)	Open	7.1–14.2 mg	Repeated exposure	1/1

[a]11 Patients with pompholyx.

vidual types of foods, leafy green vegetables and shellfish have the highest
cobalt contents. Unlike nickel and chromium, cobalt salts are easily absorbed in
the gastrointestinal tract. The absorption in humans ranges from 20 to 95% of
an oral dose. Most of it is excreted in the urine. Cobalt is an essential trace
element, but its function other than as part of the vitamin B_{12} molecule is
unknown.

In nature, cobalt is usually found together with nickel. Cobalt sensitivity
has often been found in association with nickel sensitivity in females and chromate sensitivity in men (Fregert and Rorsman, 1966). Isolated cobalt sensitivity
is rare (Rystedt, 1979). Cronin (1980) found an isolated cobalt reaction relevant
in only 20% of men and 45% of women. Most cases among the women were
due to jewelry dermatitis. The possibility of a systemic contact dermatitis reaction in cobalt-sensitive patients has not been systemically examined. Veien and
Kaaber (1979) challenged patients who had negative standard patch tests and
pompholyx hand eczema with 1 mg cobalt as the chloride. Two of 16 reacted to
the oral dose with a flare in the original dermatitis.

Glendenning (1971) observed a 49-yr-old housewife with persistent eczema of the palms and an isolated cobalt allergy. After the removal of metal
dentures made of a cobalt–chromium alloy (Vitallium), the dermatitis cleared.
The patient had not had any local symptoms in the mouth. After the removal of
the prostheses, she noticed a return of her appetite, the loss of which had been a
definite symptom during the entire period of the dermatitis.

Cobalt dermatitis might also flare in patients treated with tetraethylthiuram disulfide (Menné, 1985).

Because cobalt is so well absorbed, it may play a greater role in systemic
contact dermatitis than nickel or chromium. If this is the case, it could explain
why hand eczema related to combined sensitivity to nickel–cobalt or
chromium–cobalt has a more unfavorable prognosis than that related to isolated

nickel or chromate sensitivity (Christensen and Lagesson, 1981; Förström et al., 1969; Menné et al., 1980).

REACTIONS TO IMPLANTED METAL PROSTHESES

Implantation of metal alloys is performed with increasing frequency in orthopedic reconstructive surgery. The most commonly used alloys are stainless steel (15–20% chromium, 0% cobalt, 10–14% nickel) and Vitallium (27–30% chromium, 60–65% cobalt, 0–4% nickel). Both alloys include molybdenum in small concentrations, and vanadium and copper may be present. As an alternative to these two alloys, titanium 318 can be used.

Often, the implant is a joint replacement with two surfaces articulating against each other. This is either a metal-to-metal or, more commonly, a metal-to-plastic contact. In patients with metal-to-metal prostheses, elevated concentrations of chromium and cobalt have been found in blood and urine (Coleman et al., 1973) and in the tissues adjacent to the joint prostheses (Evans et al., 1974). In patients with metal-to-plastic prostheses, the metal concentrations are normal in blood and urine and only slightly elevated in the tissues (Coleman et al., 1973; Evans et al., 1974).

Nickel is released from stainless steel prostheses by the action of sweat, blood, and physiologic saline solution. In laboratory animals, solubilized nickel is localized in the tissue near the implant (Samitz and Katz, 1975).

The sensitization potential of implanted metal alloys has been evaluated in retrospective and prospective clinical studies. The significance of these studies is difficult to interpret because metal allergy is a common phenomenon in the general population. The prevalence of nickel allergy in women approaches 10% (Menné et al., 1982; Peltonen, 1979; Prystowsky et al., 1979), with the highest value in those 15–30 yr of age. The high prevalence is due to the common use of nickel-plated alloys in direct skin contact, for instance, through ear piercing and costume jewelry. The prevalence of nickel allergy is 0.8–0.9% in men (Peltonen, 1979; Prystowsky et al., 1979).

It is commonly thought that cobalt allergy is often related to nickel allergy. In clinical studies of hospital patients, 53% of the nickel-sensitive women, not including those who were also chromium sensitive, were also sensitive to cobalt (Fregert and Rorsman, 1966). This high figure is probably due to a sampling bias, because most patients referred to hospital departments have had hand eczema and not just a dermatitis related to skin contact with metal. In an investigation of unselected female twins, only 6 of 63 nickel-sensitive twins were also cobalt sensitive. Four of the six had hand eczema (Menné, 1980). Thus, cobalt allergy in the general population is rare compared with nickel allergy, and the prevalence probably does not exceed 1%. Chromium is mainly an industrial sensitizer and is seen in bricklayers, masons, and workers in the metal industries.

In retrospective studies of patients with metal-to-metal prostheses (cobalt, chromium), a high incidence of metal sensitivity was found. In 14 patients with loose prostheses, 9 were sensitive to either cobalt or chromium. In 24 patients with a normally functioning prosthesis, none were sensitive to metal (Evans et al., 1974). Elves et al. (1975) studied 50 patients with metal-to-metal prostheses (cobalt, chromium). Of the 50 patients, 23 had nontraumatic failure of the prostheses. Fifteen of these were sensitive to metals: seven to cobalt, three to cobalt and nickel, two to nickel, two to chromium, and one to both nickel and vanadium. Of the other 27 patients with stable prostheses or with a traumatic failure, only four were metal sensitive. Benson et al. (1975) found an incidence of 28% metal sensitivity in patients with metal-to-metal prostheses. Among 34 patients with pain and loosening of the prostheses, Munro-Ashman and Miller (1976) found 16 with metal sensitivity. Thirteen were sensitive to cobalt, four to nickel, and two to chromium. The results of these studies are similar, and even though the studies are retrospective, they suggest that at least cobalt sensitization occurs as a consequence of systemic exposure to the metal from an implanted metal alloy.

In patients with a metal-to-plastic prosthesis, the number who are metal sensitive does not exceed that in nonoperated control patients (Benson et al., 1975). In prospective studies involving similar patients whose preoperative status was evaluated by patch testing, no evidence was found of sensitization to the implanted metal alloys (Carlsson et al., 1980; Deutman et al., 1977; Nater et al., 1976; Rooker and Wilkinson, 1980; Möller and Carlsson, 1989), when the patients were retested months to years after the operation. In the retrospective part of the study by Carlsson et al. (1980) a statistically significant increase in the number of metal-sensitive patients was found among those with loose prostheses. Among the patients studied prospectively, only a few had complications with pain and loosening of the prostheses. Rooker and Wilkinson (1980) studied 69 patients prospectively. Before the operation, six patients were metal sensitive, but only one remained so afterward. Rooker and Wilkinson suggest that the minimal systemic exposure to the hapten led to immunological tolerance. This finding could not be confirmed by Waterman and Schrik (1985) in a prospective study including 85 patients.

The safety of the metal-to-plastic prostheses with respect to sensitization is in agreement with the small amounts of metal released from this type of prosthesis (Coleman et al., 1973; Evans et al., 1974). Sensitization from metal prostheses has been reported mostly in patients with loosening of the prostheses. This does not prove that the allergy is the cause of the loosening; alternatively, the loosening may cause the allergy. The available evidence supports the latter explanation (Anonymous, 1980a, 1980b). Skin symptoms in patients who have undergone implantation of metal prostheses are rare. They occur in two forms: as a dermatitis localized to the skin that covers the area of the metal prosthesis (Cramers and Locht, 1977; Munro-Ashman and Miller, 1976), or as a generalized dermatitis (Barranco and Solomon, 1973; Deutman et al., 1977; Elves et al., 1975; Foussereau and Laugier, 1966; Kubba et al.,

1981; Oleffe and Wilmet, 1980). One patient first had a localized dermatitis and then developed a generalized dermatitis (Grimalt and Romaguera, 1980).

It is noteworthy that in none of the patients with a dermatitis caused by a metal hip or knee prosthesis was it necessary to remove the prosthesis, as the symptoms were transient (Deutman et al., 1977; Elves et al., 1975; Munro-Ashman and Miller, 1976). Those who develop rashes from osteosynthesis screws have a more persistent disease, and removal of the screws has been followed by rapid clearing of the dermatitis (Barranco and Solomon, 1973; Cramers and Locht, 1977; Grimalt and Romaguera, 1980; Oleffe and Wilmet, 1980).

The limited number of patients with allergic reactions attributable to implanted metal prostheses does not indicate that all patients should be patch-tested preoperatively. Carlsson et al. (1980) recommend that patients with a history of metal allergy should be examined by a dermatologist and patch-tested. If metal allergy is found, stainless steel can be used in patients with an isolated cobalt allergy, and Vitallium in those with isolated nickel allergy. Otherwise, titanium alloys should be used. Only long-term prospective studies can determine whether it is necessary to take any precautions at all (Möller and Carlsson, 1989).

Localized lesions or generalized dermatitis caused by allergic reactions due to metals used in dentistry have not been discussed here. The subject has been reviewed by Fisher (1974), Burrows (1984), and Hensten-Pettersen (1989).

MEDICAMENTS

Systemic contact dermatitis due to medicaments has been reviewed by Cronin (1972), Fisher (1973), and Menné et al. (1989). Usually, sensitization occurs through topical application of the drug and the patient later has a systemic reaction when the drug is taken orally or parenterally. The opposite situation can occur, with a patient first having an exanthema due to an antibiotic and later developing a localized dermatitis when the drug is applied topically (Girard, 1978). Pirilä (1970) termed this phenomenon primary endogenic contact eczema. The most commonly used topical antibiotics are neomycin, bacitracin, and chloramphenicol. Ekelund and Møller (1969) challenged 12 patients with leg ulcers sensitized to neomycin with an oral dose of the hapten. Ten of the 12 had a reaction; 5 developed a flare-up of the original dermatitis, 6 had a flare-up at the site of the earlier positive patch test, 3 developed pompholyx hand eczema, 4 had nausea, and 1 vomited. Pirilä (1970) made a similar study and also observed diarrhea. It is noteworthy that the pompholyx eczema of the hands occurred as a primary event after the systemic administration of the hapten and did not represent a flare-up of the original dermatitis. The gastrointestinal symptoms are signs of a systemic contact allergy reaction.

Systemic contact dermatitis to penicillin has occurred in patients who were sensitized by topical treatment with penicillin and later exposed to very small amounts of penicillin in milk (Vickers et al., 1958). Similarly, nurses contact-sensitized to streptomycin have had systemic reactions during parenteral desensitization with streptomycin (Wilson, 1958).

The pharmacological effectiveness of topically applied antihistamines is questionable. The ethanolamine and ethylenediamine antihistamines are the most common contact-sensitizing antihistamines in the United States (Fisher, 1976). Ethylenediamine-derived antihistamine may elicit reactions in patients sensitized to ethylenediamine from the use of Mycolog Cream (E.R. Squibb & Sons, Princeton, N.J.). In the San Francisco area 0.43% of the general population is sensitized to ethylenediamine (Prystowsky et al., 1979). Aminophylline, containing theophyllamine and ethylenediamine, elicits systemic reactions in ethylenediamine-sensitized patients (Provost and Jillson, 1967). The knowledge in this field rests on anecdotal therapeutic accidents (Sertoli et al., 1985). Based on the common occurrence of ethylenediamine contact sensitivity in the population, systemic contact dermatitis to ethylenediamine must be rare.

During World War II, sulfonamides were the most important antibacterial drugs. Many soldiers were sensitized by topical applications and later developed a local flare-up reaction and a generalized maculopapular rash when the drugs were given orally. Park (1943, 1944) found that the severity of the eruption varied with the sensitivity of the subject and the size of the dose. Sulzberger et al. (1947) frequently found cross-reactions between the different antibacterial sulfonamides.

Sidi and Dobkevitch-Morrill (1951) studied cross-reactions between the *para*-amine compounds. Systemic reactions were seen after oral provocation with procaine in primary sulfonamide-sensitized patients, to p-aminophenylsulfamide in primary procaine-sensitized patients, and to p-aminophenylsulfamide and procaine in primary p-phenylenediamine-sensitized patients. Baer and Leider (1949) challenged 20 p-phenylenediamine-sensitive patients with an oral dose of 15–210 mg azodyes. Seven of the 20 had a flare of their dermatitis. A similar response occurred in 2 of 20 controls. The possible clinical significance of this observation has not been evaluated.

Oral challenge with the sulfonyl urea hypoglycemic drugs to patients sensitive to p-amino compounds (sulfanilamide, paraphenylendiamine, and benzocaine) produced flare reactions in sulfanilamide- but not in p-phenylendiamine- and benzocaine-sensitive patients (Angelini and Meneghini, 1981) (Table 3).

Oral provocation with tartrazine (20 mg) and saccharin (150 mg) to patients sensitive to p-amino compounds and sulfonamide did not produce any flare reactions (Angelini et al., 1982).

Tetraethylthiuram disulfide is used as a rubber chemical, fungicide, and in the treatment of chronic alcoholism. Cross-reactions to other carbamates may occur. In sensitized patients treatment with tetraethylthiuram disulfide can lead

TABLE 3. Oral Challenge with Sulfonyl Urea Hypoglycemic Drugs
to Sulfanilamide-Sensitive Patients

Substance	Allergen dose	Duration dosing	Response
Carbutamide	500 mg	Single exposure	7/25
Tolbutamide	500 mg	Single exposure	3/11
Chlorpropanide	250 mg	Single exposure	1 (1?)/20

Note. From Angelini and Megeghini (1981).

to a systemic contact dermatitis (Pirilä, 1957). Subcutaneous implantation of the drug led to sensitization in two patients (Lachapelle, 1975). Subsequent oral doses of tetraethylthiuram disulfide led to systemic contact dermatitis in one of the patients, while the other tolerated the drug.

Acetylsalicyclic acid (aspirin) is a rare contact sensitizer. One patient sensitized to methyl salicylate developed a systemic contact dermatitis when treated with aspirin. Patch tests were negative with aspirin but positive with sodium salicylate. Hindson (1977) suggested that the common intermediate metabolite was the cause of the systemic reaction.

In a pharmaceutical factory 14 cases of allergic contact dermatitis to the β-adrenergic blocking agent alprenolol (Aptine) occurred. One man developed pruritus and widespread dermatitis after oral provocation with 100 mg of the drug (Ekenvall and Forsbeck, 1978). Following oral provocation with up to 0.2 mg clonidine as a single dose in 29 patients contact sensitized to clonidine from transdermal exposure, only 1 reacted with a localized flare-up at the original site of dermatitis; this arose from an oral dose of 0.05 mg (Maibach, 1987). Merthiolate is a preservative used in sera and vaccines. In the Scandinavian countries, the prevalence of merthiolate sensitivity approaches 7–16% in adolescents (Förström et al., 1980; Hansson and Möller, 1970). Forty-five merthiolate-sensitive patients were tested with 0.5 ml 0.01% merthiolate solution (subcutaneous), a dose equal to that contained in a tetanus toxoid shot; one developed generalized dermatitis and fever (Förström et al., 1980).

Propylene glycol is a vehicle in topical medicaments and cosmetics and is used as a food additive. The Food and Agriculture Organization/World Health Organization has accepted a daily intake of up to 20 mg/kg body weight. Propylene glycol is both a sensitizer and a primary irritant. Hannuksela and Förström (1978) challenged 10 patients with a positive patch test to 2% propylene glycol with 2–15 ml pure propylene glycol. Eight reacted with an exanthema 3–6 h after ingestion; in seven of these the rash disappeared within 24–48 h without treatment. This observation differs from the picture of a systemic contact dermatitis reaction in some respects. Local flare-up of earlier dermatitis and earlier positive patch tests was not seen, and the rapid disappearance of the rash indicates a pharmacological effect rather than an immunologically mediated process.

A positive patch test to a drug usually contraindicates further use of the drug. But based on current knowledge, systemic contact dermatitis reactions rarely occur after a single therapeutic dose.

OTHER CONTACT ALLERGENS

When hyposensitizing persons against rhus dermatitis, Kligman (1958a) observed systemic contact dermatitis reactions. Half of the moderately to severely sensitive patients experienced either pruritus or a rash. Flares at healed contact dermatitis sites occurred with a frequency of 10%. Dyshidrosis of the palms and erythema multiforme were rare. Pruritus ani occurred in 10% of the highly sensitive patients. Sensitization to balsam of Peru often leads to sensitivity to flavors and orange peel. Hjorth (1961) observed two children who were sensitive to balsam of Peru whose dermatitis flared after they ate fruits and ices. Hjorth (1965) also described a doctor having severe hand eczema for 10 yr who, because he reacted to balsam of Peru on patch testing, was told to avoid orange peel. To test the validity of the advice, he ate a jar of orange marmalade. After 12 h he experienced the most severe attack of hand eczema he had ever had. By avoiding perfumes, cola drinks, vermouth, throat lozenges, cinnamon, and similar items, he has since been free of dermatitis.

Veien et al. (1985) challenged 17 patients sensitive to balsam of Peru with 1 g as an oral dose. Ten reacted to balsam of Peru and one to placebo.

Pentadecyl catechols, the sensitizers in poison ivy, cross-react with oil of cashew nuts (Kligman, 1958b). Five patients sensitized to poison ivy had a widespread dermatitis after eating 150–450 g raw cashew nuts purchased in a health food store. The dermatitis involved the palms, medial aspects of the arms, axillae, bathing trunk area, and posterior parts of the legs (Ratner et al., 1974). Tests with commercially available dry-roasted cashew nuts did not produce any symptoms.

The antioxidant butylated hydroxyanisole, which is permitted in both foods and topical preparations, caused systemic contact dermatitis in two patients (Roed-Petersen and Hjorth, 1976). Both patients had a flare of hand eczema after oral intake of 5–10 mg of the agent for 4 d. Other rare sensitizers, vitamin B_1 (Hjorth, 1958) and vitamin C (Metz et al., 1980), have given rise to systemic contact dermatitis.

MECHANISM

The clinical observation of rapid onset (within hours) of the effect of oral exposure to haptens in sensitized individuals suggests that mechanisms other than the allergic type 4 reaction are involved. It is not unusual for a nickel-sensitive patient who is exposed to nickel to develop a systemic rash within hours and a flare of hand dermatitis after 12–48 hours.

Veien et al. (1979a) investigated 14 patients with a positive nickel patch test. All were challenged orally with 2.5 mg nickel. After 6–12 h, 5 developed widespread erythema. In the erythematous area, no clinical dermatitis developed. Three of the five demonstrated precipitating antibodies in their sera against a nickel-albumin complex in a passive immunodiffusion assay. The same phenomenon was observed in chromium-sensitized guinea pigs (Polak and Turk, 1968b). The response began 6–8 h after an injection of chromate. Histologically, at 24 h, there was marked dilatation of the superficial capillaries in the upper dermis but without any obvious perivascular infiltration. As did Veien and Kaaber (1979), Polak and Turk suggested that circulating immune complexes were the triggering mechanism (1968a, 1968b).

Christensen et al. (1981) studied flare-up reactions in 4- to 7-wk-old positive nickel patch tests in 5 patients after oral provocation with 5.6 mg nickel. The histological picture was that of acute dermatitis. Direct immunofluorescence examination for deposits of immunoglobulin G (IgG), IgA, IgM, complement 3, and fibrinogen were negative. The histological picture of flare-up reactions in chromate-sensitive guinea pigs after an intravenous injection of chromate shows a perivascular infiltration with polymorphonuclear leukocytes (Polak and Turk, 1968b).

Veien et al. (1979b) studied lymphocyte stimulation after oral provocation with 4 mg nickel in 8 nickel-sensitive patients. They found a statistically significant increase in the lymphocytic transformation test in those sensitive to nickel compared with controls. The response was independent of the severity of the skin symptoms. There is clinical and experimental evidence that systemic reactions to ingested haptens can be mediated by both a type 3 and a type 4 immunologic reaction. Both types of reactions can be seen in the same patient. The immunologic reactivity, judged from an increase in the lymphocytic transformation test, can be maintained by oral ingestion of a hapten.

DIAGNOSIS

Usually patients with a systemic reaction to ingested haptens have a positive patch test. This is not surprising, because it is a positive patch test that confirms the diagnosis. But patch testing is not always a reliable diagnostic procedure in systemic contact dermatitis.

Veien and Kaaber (1979) investigated 16 patients with pompholyx and negative routine patch tests. An aggravation of hand eczema was seen in 2 after oral provocation with 2.5 mg chromium and in another 2 after provocation with 1.0 mg cobalt. None reacted to placebo.

In an open study, Veien et al. (1983) challenged 202 patients who had pompholyx with a tablet containing 2.5 mg nickel, 1 mg cobalt, and 2.5 mg chromium as salts of the respective metals. Of the 202 patients, 65 reacted to the mixture of salts as well as to one or two of the individual salts. Male patients reacted primarily to chromate and cobalt, while female patients more commonly reacted to nickel and cobalt. Menné (1981) investigated monozygotic twins who both had a history of nickel allergy and a pompholyx hand eczema. One of the twins had a negative patch test to 5% nickel sulfate in petrolatum, repeated twice. In spite of this, oral provocation with 2.5 mg nickel caused a rash in the axillae and the genital area and a recurrence of the hand eczema. The occurrence of a systemic contact dermatitis reaction and a negative patch test was demonstrated experimentally in guinea pigs. Polak et al. (1970) studied dichromate contact-sensitive animals that had been made permanently tolerant with respect to contact sensitivity by intravenous injections of dichromate followed by epicutaneous application of dichromate. When the animals were later given a systemic injection of dichromate, a flare-up at old positive skin test sites followed.

Therefore oral provocation with haptens may be considered as a diagnostic procedure in patients with a negative patch test and a clinical picture of systemic contact dermatitis. In nickel-sensitive patients, we start with a dose of 0.6 mg, progressing after 2 d to 1.25 mg, and after another 2 d to 2.5 mg nickel as the sulfate. If the patient reacts we do not continue with a higher dose. Using this schedule, we have not had any severe reactions. With chromium and cobalt, 2.5 and 1.0 mg as the dichromate and the chloride, respectively, have been used. Studies with lower doses are desirable (Fregert, 1965). Guidelines for challenge with medicaments are difficult to furnish, but to exclude a systemic contact dermatitis reaction it is necessary to challenge with a therapeutic dose. In patients with a history of urticaria or any other anaphylactic reaction, systemic exposure to a hapten may cause a life-threatening reaction, and small amounts must be used for the initial dose.

TOXICOLOGICAL ASSAYS

The many examples of contact-sensitizing chemicals also giving rise to systemic contact dermatitis reactions make it necessary to include the possibility of such reaction when the safety of new chemicals and topical drugs is evaluated. If a chemical is a topical sensitizer in humans or experimental animals, future systemic reactions are a possibility. In evaluating safety it is necessary to include data on the occurrence of the chemicals in foodstuffs or in drugs for systemic use. Data on absorption and metabolism should be considered. A high degree of absorption would suggest the possibility of future systemic reactions. Systemic reactions and local flare-ups after parenteral administration of dichromate to dichromate-sensitized guinea pigs have been observed (Polak and Turk, 1968a, 1968b; Polak et al., 1970; Christensen et al., 1984). This model may be valuable for comparing the capacity of different chemicals to elicit systemic contact dermatitis reactions.

REFERENCES

Andersen, K. E., Hjorth, N. and Menné, T. 1984. The baboon syndrome: Systemically induced allergic contact dermatitis. *Contact Dermatitis* 10:97–101.

Angelini, G. and Meneghini, C. L. 1981. Oral tests in contact allergy to paŕa-amino compounds. *Contact Dermatitis* 7:311–314.

Angelini, G., Vena, G. A. and Meneghini, C. L. 1982. Allergia da contatto e reazioni secondarie ad additivi alimentari. *Giorn. It. Dermatol. Venereol.* 117:195–198.

Anonymous. 1980. Can metal sensitivity loosen joint replacements? *Lancet* ii:1284–1285.

Anonymous. 1980. Metal allergy: A false alarm? *Br. Med. J.* 281:1303–1304.

Baer, R. L. and Leider, M. 1949. The effects of feeding certified food azo dyes in paraphenylenediamine-hypersensitive subjects. *J. Invest. Dermatol.* 13:223–232.

Barranco, V. P. and Solomon, H. 1973. Eczematous dermatitis caused by internal exposure to nickel. *South. Med. J.* 66:447–448.

Benson, M. K., Goodwin, P. G. and Brostoff, J. 1975. Metal sensitivity in patients with joint replacement arthroplastics. *Br. Med. J.* 4:374–375.

Brown, S. S. and Sunderman, F. W., Jr., eds. 1980. *Nickel Toxicology.* New York: Academic Press.

Brun, R. 1979. Nickel in food: The role of stainless-steel utensils. *Contact Dermatitis* 5:43–45.

Bruynzeel, D. P., van Den Hoogenband, H. M. and Koedijk, F. 1984. Purpuric vasculitis-like eruption in a patient sensitive to balsam of Peru. *Contact Dermatitis* 11:207–209.

Burrows, D., Creswell, S. and Merret, J. D. 1981. Nickel, hands and hip prostheses. *Br. J. Dermatol.* 105:437–444.

Burrows, D., ed. 1983. *Chromium: Metabolism and Toxicity.* Boca Raton, Fla.: CRC Press.

Burrows, D. 1984. The effect of systemic and implanted metals on metal dermatitis. *Dermatol. Clin.* 2:603–612.

Carlsson, Å. S., Magnusson, B. and Möller, H. 1980. Metal sensitivity in patients with metal-to-plastic total hip arthroplasties. *Acta Orthop. Scand.* 51:57–62.

Christensen, O. B. and Möller, H. 1975. External and internal exposure to the antigen in the hand eczema of nickel allergy. *Contact Dermatitis* 1:136–141.

Christensen, O. B. and Möller, H. 1978. Release of nickel from cooking utensils. *Contact Dermatitis* 4:343–346.

Christensen, O. B. 1981. Nickel Allergy and Hand Eczema in Females. Thesis, Department of Dermatology, University of Lund, Malmö, Sweden.

Christensen, O. B. and Kristensen, M. 1982. Treatment with disulfiram in chronic nickel hand dermatitis. *Contact Dermatitis* 8:59–63.

Christensen, O. B. and Lagesson, V. 1981. Nickel concentration of blood and urine after oral administration. *Ann. Clin. Lab. Sci.* 8:184–189.

Christensen, O. B., Lindström, G. C., Löfberg, H. and Möller, H. 1981. Micromorphology and specificity of orally induced flare-up reactions in nickel-sensitive patients. *Acta Dermatol. Venereol.* 61:505–510.

Christensen, O. B., Christensen, M. B. and Maibach, H. I. 1984. Flare-up reactions and desensitization from oral dosing in chromate-sensitive guinea pigs. *Contact Dermatitis* 10:277–280.

Coleman, R. F., Harrington, J. and Scales, J. T. 1973. Concentrations of wear products in hair, blood, and urine after total hip replacement. *Br. Med. J.* i:527–529.

Cramers, M. and Locht, U. 1977. Metal sensitivity in patients treated for tibial fractures with plates of stainless steel. *Acta Orthop. Scand.* 48:245–249.

Cronin, E. 1972. Reactions to contact allergens given orally or systematically. *Br. J. Dermatol.* 86:104–107.

Cronin, E. 1980. *Contact Dermatitis.* Edinburgh: Churchill Livingstone.

Cronin, E., DiMichiel, A. D. and Brown, S. S. 1980. Oral challenge in nickel-sensitive women with hand eczema. In *Nickel Toxicology*, eds. S. Brown and F. W. Sunderman, Jr., pp. 149–155. New York: Academic Press.

Deutman, R., Mulder, T. J., Brian, R. and Nater, J. P. 1977. Metal sensitivity before and after total hip arthroplasty. *J. Bone Joint Surg.* 59A:862–865.

deYongh, G. F., Spruit, D., Bongaarts, P. J. M. and Duller, P. 1978. Factors influencing nickel dermatitis. I. *Contact Dermatitis* 4:142–148.

Ekelund, A.-G. and Möller, H. 1969. Oral provocation in eczematous contact allergy to neomycin and hydroxyquinolines. *Acta Dermatol. Venereol.* 49:422–426.

Ekenvall, L. and Forsbeck, M. 1978. Contact eczema produced by a β-adrenergic blocking agent (alprenolol). *Contact Dermatitis* 4:190–194.

Elves, M. W., Wilson, J. N., Scales, J. E. and Kemp, H. B. S. 1975. Incidence of metal sensitivity in patients with total joint replacements. *Br. Med. J.* 4:376–378.

Evans, E. M., Freeman, M. A. R., Miller, A. J. and Vernon-Roberts, B. 1974. Metal sensitivity as a cause of bone necrosis and loosening of the prosthesis in total joint replacement, *J. Bone Joint Surg.* 56B:626–642.

Fisher, A. A. 1973. *Contact Dermatitis*, 2d ed. Philadelphia: Lea & Febiger.

Fisher, A. A. 1974. Allergic reactions due to metals used in dentistry. *Cutis* 14:797–800.

Fisher, A. A. 1976. Antihistamine dermatitis. *Cutis* 18:329–336.

Foussereau, J. and Laugier, P. 1966. Allergic eczema from metallic foreign bodies. *Trans. St. John's Hosp. Dermatol. Soc.* 52:220–225.

Fregert, S. 1965. Sensitization to hexa- and trivalent chromium. In *Pemphigus, Occupational Dermatosis due to Chemical Sensitization*, pp. 50–55. Budapest: Hungarian Dermatological Society.

Fregert, S. 1971. Nickel in tap water. *Contact Dermatitis Newslett.* 9:202.

Fregert, S. and Rorsman, H. 1966. Allergy to chromium, nickel and cobalt. *Acta Dermatol. Venereol.* 46:144–148.

Fregert, S., Hjorth, N., Magnusson, B., Brandmann, H.-J., Calnan, C. D., Cronin, E., Malten, K., Meneghini, C. L., Pirilä, V. and Wilkinson, D. S. 1969. Epidemiology of contact dermatitis. *Trans. St. John's Hosp. Dermatol. Soc.* 55:17–35.

Förström, L., Pirilä, V. and Huju, P. 1969. Rehabilitation of workers with cement eczema due to hypersensitivity to bichromate. *Scand. J. Rehabil. Med.* 1:95–100.

Förström, L., Hannuksela, M., Kausa, M. and Lehmuskallio, E. 1980. Merthiolate hypersensitivity and vaccination. *Contact Dermatitis* 6:241–245.

Gawkrodger, D. J., Cook, S. W., Fell, G. S. and Hunter, J. A. A. 1986. Nickel dermatitis: the reaction to oral nickel challenge. *Br. J. Dermatol.* 115:33–38.

Girard, J. P. 1978. Recurrent angioneurotic oedema and contact dermatitis due to penicillin. *Contact Dermatitis* 4:309.

Glendenning, E. W. 1971. Allergy to cobalt in metal dentures as cause of hand dermatitis. *Contact Dermatitis Newslett.* 10:225–226.

Goitre, M., Bedello, P. G. and Cane, D. 1981. Su due casi di dermatite da nichel. *Giorn. It. Dermatol. Venereol.* 116:43–45.

Goitre, M., Bedello, P. G. and Cane, D. 1982. Chromium dermatitis and oral administration of the metal. *Contact Dermatitis* 8:208–209.

Grimalt, F. and Romaguera, C. 1980. Acute nickel dermatitis from a metal implant. *Contact Dermatitis* 6:441–447.

Hannuksela, M. and Förström, L. 1978. Reactions to peroral propylene glycol. *Contact Dermatitis* 4:41–45.

Hansson, H. and Möller, H. 1970. Patch test reactions to merthiolate in healthy young subjects. *Br. J. Dermatol.* 83:349–356.

Hensten-Pettersen, A. 1989. Nickel allergy and dental treatment procedures. In *Nickel and the Skin: Immunology and Toxicology,* eds. H. I. Maibach and T. Menné, pp. 195–206. Boca Raton, Fla.: CRC Press.

Hindson, C. 1977. Contact eczema from methyl salicylate reproduced by oral aspirin (acetylsalicyclic acid). *Contact Dermatitis* 3:348.

Hjorth, N. 1958. Contact dermatitis for vitamin B_1 (thiamine). *J. Invest. Dermatol.* 30:261–264.

Hjorth, N. 1961. Eczematous Allergy to Balsams. Thesis. Copenhagen: Munksgaard.

Hjorth, N. 1965. Allergy to balsams. *Spectrum Int.* 7:97–101.

Hjorth, N. 1976. Nickel vasculitis. *Contact Dermatitis* 2:356–357.

Jordan, W. P. and King, S. E. 1979. Nickel feeding in nickel-sensitive patients with hand eczema. *J. Am. Acad. Dermatol.* 1:506–508.

Kaaber, K. and Veien, N. K. 1977. The significance of chromate ingestion in patients allergic to chromate. *Acta Dermatol. Venereol.* 57:321–323.

Kaaber, K., Veien, N. K. and Tjell, J. C. 1978. Low nickel diet in the treatment of patients with chronic nickel dermatitis. *Br. J. Dermatol.* 98:197–201.

Kaaber, K., Menné, T., Tjell, J. C. and Veien, N. 1979. Antabuse treatment of nickel dermatitis. Chelation—a new principle in the treatment of nickel dermatitis. *Contact Dermatitis* 5:221–228.

Kaaber, K., Menné, T., Veien, N. and Hougaard, P. 1983a. Treatment of nickel dermatitis with antabuse R: A double blind study. *Contact Dermatitis* 9:297–300.

Kaaber, K., Menné, T., Veien, N. and Baadsgaard, O. 1987. Some adverse effects of disulfiram in the treatment of nickel-allergic patients. *Dermatosen* 35:209–212.

Kligman, A. M. 1958a. Hyposensitization against rhus dermatitis. *Arch. Dermatol.* 78:47–72.

Kligman, A. M. 1958b. Cashew nut shell oil for hyposensitization against rhus dermatitis. *Arch. Dermatol.* 78:359–363.

Kubba, R., Taylor, J. S. and Marks, K. E. 1981. Cutaneous complications of orthopedic implants. A two-year prospective study. *Arch. Dermatol.* 117:554–560.

Lachapelle, J. M. 1975. Allergic "contact" dermatitis from disulfiram implants. *Contact Dermatitis* 1:218–220.

Maibach, H. I. 1987. Oral substitution in patients sensitized by transdermal clonodine treatment. *Contact Dermatitis* 16:1–9.

Maibach, H. I. and Menné, T., eds. 1989. *Nickel and the Skin: Immunology and Toxicology.* Boca Raton, Fla.: CRC Press.

Menné, T. 1980. Relationship between cobalt and nickel sensitization in females. *Contact Dermatitis* 6:337–340.

Menné, T. 1981. Nickel allergy-reliability of patch test. *Dermatosen Beruf Umwelt* 29:156–160.

Menné, T. 1985. Flare-up of cobalt dermatitis from Antabuse R treatment. *Contact Dermatitis* 12:53.

Menné, T. and Hjorth, N. 1983. Pompholyx—Dyshidrotic eczema. *Sem. Dermatol.* 2:75–80.

Menné, T. and Thorboe, A. 1976. Nickel dermatitis-nickel excretion. *Contact Dermatitis* 2:353–354.

Menné, T., Mikkelsen, H. I. and Solgaard, P. 1978. Nickel excretion in urine after oral administration. *Contact Dermatitis* 4:106–108.

Menné, T., Kaaber, K. and Tjell, J. C. 1980. Treatment of nickel dermatitis. *Ann. Clin. Lab. Sci.* 10:160–164.

Menné, T., Borgan, O. and Green, A. 1982. Nickel allergy and hand dermatitis in a stratified sample of the danish female population. An epidemiological study including a statistic appendix. *Acta Dermatol-Venereol.* 62:35–41.

Menné, T., Veien, N. K. and Maibach, H. I. 1989. Systemic contact-type dermatitis due to drugs. *Sem. Dermatol.* 8:144–148.

Metz, J., Hundertmark, U. and Pevny, I. 1980. Vitamin C allergy of the delayed type. *Contact Dermatitis* 6:172–174.

Möller, H. and Carlsson, Å. 1989. Bioimplantation of metals in patients with metal allergy: The late outcome. In *Current Topics in Contact Dermatitis,* eds. P. J. Frosch, A. Dooms-Goossens, M.-M. Lachapnelle, R. M. G. Rycroft, and R. M. Scheper. pp. 199–202. Heidelberg: Springer-Verlag.

Munro-Ashman, D. and Miller, A. J. 1976. Rejection of metal prosthesis and skin sensitivity to cobalt. *Contact Dermatitis* 2:65–67.

Nakayama, H., Niko, F., Shono, M. and Shunroku, H. 1983. Mercury exanthem. *Contact Dermatitis* 9:411–417.

Nater, J. P., Brian, R. G., Deutman, R., and Mulder, T. J. 1976. The development of metal hypersensitivity in patients with metal-to-plastic hip arthroplasties. *Contact Dermatitis* 2:259–261.

National Academy of Sciences. 1974. *Chromium. Medical and Biological Effects of Environmental Pollutants.* Washington, D.C.: National Academy of Sciences.

National Academy of Sciences. 1975. *Nickel. Medical and Biologic Effects of Environmental Pollutants.* Washington, D.C.: National Academy of Sciences.

Nriagu, J. O. 1980. *Nickel in the Environment.* New York: Wiley.

Oleffe, J. and Wilmet, J. 1980. Generalized dermatitis from an osteosynthesis screw. *Contact Dermatitis* 6:365.

Olerud, J. E., Lee, M. Y., Uvelli, D. A., Goble, G. J. and Babb, A. L. (1984). Presumptive nickel dermatitis from hemodialysis. *Arch. Dermatol.* 120:1066–1068.

Park, R. G. 1943. Cutaneous hypersensitivity to sulphonamides. *Br. Med. J.* 2:69–72.

Park, R. G. 1944. Sulphonamide allergy. *Br. Med. J.* 1:781–782.

Pecegueiro, M. and Brandao, M. 1982. Administracao oral de niquel em individuos sensibilizados. *Med. Cut. I.L.A.* 10:295–298.

Peltonen, L. 1979. Nickel sensitivity in the general population. *Contact Dermatitis* 5:27–33.

Pirilä, V. 1957. Dermatitis due to rubber. *Acta Dermatol. Venereol Proc. 11th Int. Congr. Dermatol.* 11:252–255.

Pirilä, V. 1970. Endogenic contact eczema. *Allergy Asthma* 16:15–19.

Polak, L. and Turk, J. L. 1968a. Studies on the effect of systemic administration of sensitizers in guinea-pigs with contact sensitivity to inorganic metal compounds. *Clin. Exp. Immunol.* 3:245–251.

Polak, L. and Turk, J. L. 1968b. Studies on the effects of systemic administration of sensitizers in guinea-pigs with contact sensitivity to inorganic metal compounds. *Clin. Exp. Immunol.* 3:253–262.

Polak, L., Frey, J. R., and Turk, J. L. 1970. Studies on the effect of systemic administration of sensitizers to guinea-pigs with contact sensitivity to inorganic metal compounds. *Clin. Exp. Immunol.* 7:739–744.

Provost, T. T. and Jilson, O. F. 1967. Ethylenediamine contact dermatitis. *Arch. Dermatol.* 96:231–234.

Prystowsky, S. D., Allen, A. M., Smith, R. W., Nonomura, J. H., Odon, R. B. and

Akers, W. A. 1979. Allergic contact hypersensitivity to nickel, neomycin, ethylenediamine and benzocaine. *Arch. Dermatol.* 115:959–962.

Ratner, J. H., Spencer, S. K. and Grainge, J. M. 1974. Cashew nut dermatitis. *Arch. Dermatol.* 110:921–923.

Roed-Petersen, J. and Hjorth, N. 1976. Contact dermatitis from antioxidants. *Br. J. Dermatol.* 94:233–241.

Rooker, G. D. and Wilkinson, J. C. 1980. Metal sensitivity in patients undergoing hip replacement. *J. Bone Joint Surg.* 62B:502–505.

Rystedt, I. 1979. Evaluation and relevance of isolated test reactions to cobalt. *Contact Dermatitis* 5:233–239.

Samitz, M. H. and Katz, S. A. 1975. Nickel dermatitis hazards from prostheses. *Br. J. Dermatol.* 92:287–290.

Santucci, B., Cristaudo, A., Cannistraci, C. and Picardo, M. 1988. Nickel sensitivity—Effects of prolonged oral intake of the element. *Contact Dermatitis* 19:202–205.

Schleiff, P. 1968. Provokation des Chromatekzems zu Testzwechen durch interne Chromzufuhr. *Hautarzt* 19:209–210.

Sertoli, A., Lombardi, P., Francalanci, S., Gola, M., Giorgini, S. and Panconesi, E. 1985. Effetto della somministrazione orale de apteni in soggetti sensibilizzati affetti da eczema allergizo da contatto. *Giorn. It. Dermatol. Venereol.* 120:207–218.

Shelley, W. B. 1964. Chromium in welding fumes as a cause of eczematous hand eruption. *J. Am. Med. Assoc.* 189:772–773.

Sidi, E. and Dobkevitch-Morrill, S. 1951. The injection and ingestion test in cross-sensitization to the para group. *J. Invest. Dermatol.* 16:299–310.

Sidi, E. and Melki, G. R. 1954. Rapport entre dermatitis de cause externe et sensibilisation par voi interne. *Sem. Hop. Paris* 30:1560–1565.

Smeenk, G. and Teunissen, P. C. 1977. Allergische reacties op nikkel uit infusietoedieningssystemen. *Ned. Tijdschr. Geneeskd.* 121:4–9.

Spruit, D. 1979. Increased nickel absorption following indomethacin therapy. *Contact Dermatitis* 5:62.

Spruit, D., Bongaarts, P. J. M. and de Yongh, G. F. 1978. Dithiocarbamate therapy for nickel dermatitis. *Contact Dermatitis* 4:350–358.

Stoddart, J. C. 1960. Nickel sensitivity as a cause of infusion reactions. *Lancet* ii:741–742.

Sulzberger, M. B., Kanof, A., Baer, R. L. and Lowenberg, C. 1947. Sensitization by topical application of sulphonamides. *J. Allergy* 18:92–103.

Sunderman, F. W. 1979. Efficacy of sodium diethyldithiocarbamate (dithiocarb) in acute nickel carbonyl poisoning. *Ann. Clin. Lab. Sci.* 9:1–10.

Sunderman, F. W., Jr. 1983. Potential toxicity from nickel contamination of intravenous fluids. *Ann. Clin. Lab. Sci.* 13:1–4.

Sunderman, F. W., Jr., ed. 1984. *Nickel in the Human Environment.* Lyon: JARC Scientific Publications no. 53.

Underwood, E. J. 1977. *Trace Elements in Human and Animal Nutrition.* New York: Academic Press.

Veien, N. K. 1989. Systemically induced eczema in adults. *Acta Dermatol. Venereol. Suppl.* 147.

Veien, N. K. and Kaaber, K. 1979. Nickel, cobalt and chromium sensitivity in patients with pompholyx (dyshidrotic eczema). *Contact Dermatitis* 5:371–374.

Veien, N. K. and Krogdahl, A. 1989. Is nickel vasculitis a clinical entity. In *Current Topics in Contact Dermatitis,* eds. P. J. Frosch et al., pp. 172–177. Heidelberg: Springer-Verlag.

Veien, N. K., Christiansen, A. H., Svejgaard, E. and Kaaber, K. 1979a. Antibodies against nickel-albumin in rabbits and man. *Contact Dermatitis* 5:378–382.

Veien, N. K., Svejgaard, E. and Menné, T. 1979b. In vitro lymphocyte transformation to nickel: A study of nickel-sensitive patients before and after epicutaneous and oral challenge with nickel. *Acta Dermatol. Venereol.* 59:447–451.

Veien, N. K., Hattel, T., Justensen, O. and Nørholm, A. 1983. Oral challenge with metal salts. (I). Vesicular patch-test-negative hand eczema. *Contact Dermatitis* 9:402–407.

Veien, N. K., Hattel, T., Justesen, O. and Nørholm, N. 1985. Oral challenge with balsam of Peru. *Contact Dermatitis* 12:104–107.

Vickers, H. R., Bagratuni, L. and Alexander, S. 1958. Dermatitis caused by penicillin in milk. *Lancet* i:351–352.

Waterman, A. H. and Schrik, J. J. 1985. Allergy in hip arthroplasty. *Contact Dermatitis* 13:294–301.

Wilson, H. T. H. 1958. Streptomycin dermatitis in nurses. *Br. Med. J.* i:1378–1382.

17

immediate contact reactions: contact urticaria and the contact urticaria syndrome

■ Arto Lahti ■ Howard I. Maibach ■

INTRODUCTION

Immediate contact reactions of the skin comprise a heterogeneous group of inflammatory reactions that appear after contact with the eliciting substance. They include not only wheals and flares but also transient erythematous and eczematous reactions.

The epidemiology of immediate contact reactions is not well known at present. The first such studies were performed in Hawaii (Elpern, 1985a, 1985b, 1986), Poland (Rudzki and Rebandel, 1985), Sweden (Nilsson, 1985), Denmark (Veien et al., 1987), Finland (Turjanmaa, 1987), and Switzerland (Weissenbach et al., 1988). These studies suggested that immediate contact reactions are common in dermatology practice. Some substances cause immediate reactions in almost everyone at the first contact (methyl nicotinate) but others need a period of sensitization (latex rubber).

SYMPTOMS

Immediate contact reactions appear on normal or eczematous skin within minutes to an hour after agents capable of producing this type of reaction have been in contact with the skin. They disappear within 24 h, usually within a few hours. The symptoms can be classified according to morphology and severity: Itching, tingling or burning accompanied by erythema are the weakest type of immediate contact reaction and are often produced by cosmetics (Emmons and Marks, 1985) and fruits and vegetables. Local wheal-and-flare is the prototype reaction of contact urticaria. Generalized urticaria after a local contact is a rare phenomenon but can occur with strong urticant allergens. Tiny vesicles frequently appear on the fingers in protein contact dermatitis. Apart from the skin, effects may also appear in other organs in cases of very strong hypersensitivity, the phenomenon called contact urticaria syndrome. In some cases, immediate contact reactions can be demonstrated only on slightly or previously affected skin, and it can be part of the mechanism responsible for maintenance of chronic eczemas (Hannuksela, 1980; Maibach, 1976; Veien et al., 1987).

There has been confusion in using terms such as contact urticaria, immediate contact reactions, atopic contact dermatitis, and protein contact dermatitis (Table 1). Immediate contact reaction includes both urticarial and other reactions, whereas protein contact dermatitis means allergic or non-allergic eczematous dermatitis caused by proteins or proteinaceous materials. Atopic contact dermatitis is an immediate type (IgE-mediated) of allergic contact reaction in atopic people (Hannuksela, 1980).

ETIOLOGY AND MECHANISMS

The mechanisms underlying contact reactions are divided into two main types, namely, immunologic (IgE-mediated) and nonimmunologic immediate contact reactions (Lahti and Maibach, 1987). However, there are substances causing immediate contact reactions whose mechanism (immunologic or not) may not be known.

Tables 2–4 present agents that have been reported to cause immediate contact reactions. They include chemicals in medications, industrial contactants, components of cosmetic products and of foods and drinks, as well as chemically undefined environmental agents. The pathogenetic classification (nonimmunologic versus immunologic) is also given but in many instances it is

TABLE 1. Terminology of Immediate Contact Reactions

Term	Remarks
Immediate contact reaction	Includes urticarial, eczematous, and other immediate reactions
Contact urticaria	Allergic and nonallergic contact urticaria reactions
Protein contact dermatitis	Allergic or nonallergic eczematous reactions caused by proteins or proteinaceous material
Atopic contact dermatitis	Immediate urticarial or eczematous IgE-mediated immediate contact reaction
Contact urticaria syndrome	Includes both local and systemic immediate reactions precipitated by contact urticaria agents

TABLE 2. Substances That Have Caused Local Reactions
and Anaphylactic Symptoms in Skin Tests

Aminophenazone
Ampicillin
Balsam of Peru
Bacitracin
Chloramphenicol
Diethyltoluamide
Egg
Epoxy resin
Mechlorethamine
Neomycin
Penicillin
Streptomycin

arbitrary, because the mechanisms of various contact reactions are unclear or because a pathogenic evaluation was not performed.

Increasing awareness of immediate contact reactions will expand the list of etiologic agents, and more thorough understanding of pathophysiologic mechanisms will lead to a better and more rational classification of these reactions than at present.

IgE-Mediated Contact Reactions

Immunologic contact urticaria and other immunologic immediate contact reactions are immediate reactions in people who have previously become sensitized to the causative agent. In many cases of immunologic contact reaction, the respiratory and gastrointestinal tracts have been the routes of sensitization. However, natural latex and some foods can sensitize people through the skin.

In skin challenge, the molecules of a contact reactant penetrate the epidermis and react with specific IgE molecules attached to mast cell membranes. Cutaneous symptoms (erythema and edema) are elicited by vasoactive substances, mainly histamine released from mast cells. The role of histamine is important, but other mediators of inflammation, such as prostaglandins, leukotrienes, and kinins, may also influence the intensity of response. However, little is known regarding the dynamics of their interplay in clinical situations.

Not only mast cells and circulating basophils have Fc-receptors for IgE molecules, but also eosinophils (Capron et al., 1981), peripheral B- and T-lymphocytes (Yodoi and Iskizaka, 1979), platelets (Joseph et al., 1983), monocytes (Melewicz and Spiegelberg, 1980), and alveolar macrophages (Joseph et al., 1980) can bind IgE. These findings make the issue of immediate immunologic contact reaction more complicated than was believed earlier.

It has recently been reported that patients with atopic dermatitis, but not other atopics or normal controls, have IgE on their epidermal Langerhans cells (Barker et al., 1988; Bruynzeel-Koomen, 1986; Bruynzeel-Koomen et al.,

TABLE 3. Agents Producing Immunologic Immediate Contact Reactions

Animal products
Amnion fluid
  Blood
  Brucella abortus (Trunnel et al., 1985)
  Cercariae
  Cheyletus malaccensis (Yoshikawa, 1985)
  Chironomidae, Chironomus thummi thummi (Mittelbach, 1983)
  Cockroaches
  Dander (Agrup and Sjöstedt, 1985; Weissenbach et al., 1988)
  Dermestes maculatus Degeer (Lewis-Jones, 1985)
  Gelatine (Wahl and Kleinhans, 1989)
  Gut
  Hair
  Listrophorus gibbus (Burns, 1987)
  Liver
  Locust (Monk, 1988; Tee et al., 1988)
  Mealworm, *Tenibrio molitor* (Bernstein et al., 1983)
  Placenta
  Saliva (Valsecchi and Cainelli, 1989)
  Serum
  Silk
  Spider mite, *Tetranychus urticae* (Reunala et al., 1983)
  Wool
Food
  Dairy
    Cheese
    Egg
    Milk (Boso and Brestel, 1987; Salo et al., 1986)
  Fruits
    Apple (Halmepuro and Löwenstein, 1985; Pigatto et al., 1983)
    Apricot
    Banana
    Kiwi
    Mango
    Orange
    Peach
    Plum
  Grains
    Buckwheat (Valdivieso et al., 1989)
    Maize
    Malt
    Wheat
    Wheat bran
  Honey
  Nuts
    Peanut butter
    Sesame seed
    Sunflower seed
  Meats
    Beef

TABLE 3. Agents Producing Immunologic Immediate Contact Reactions (*Continued*)

Chicken
Lamb
Liver
Turkey
Seafood
  Fish (Kavli and Moseng, 1987; Melino et al., 1987)
  Prawns
  Shrimp (Nagano et al., (1984)
Vegetables
  Beans
  Cabbage
  Carrot (Muñoz et al., 1985)
  Celery (Kremser and Lindemayr, 1983; Wuthrich and Dietschi, 1985)
  Chives
  Cucumber
  Endive
  Lettuce
  Onion
  Parsley
  Parsnip
  Potato (Larkö et al., 1983)
  Rutabaga (swede)
  Tomato
  Soybean
Fragrances and flavorings
  Balsam of Peru
  Menthol
  Vanillin
Medicaments
  Acetylsalicylic acid
  Antibiotics
    Ampicillin
    Bacitracin
    Cephalosporins
    Chloramphenicol (Schewach-Millet and Shpiro, 1985)
    Gentamicin
    Iodochlorhydroxyquin
    Neomycin
    Nifuroxime (Aaronson, 1969)
    Penicillin (Rudzki and Rebandel, 1985)
    Rifamycin (Grob et al., 1987)
    Streptomycin
    Virginiamycin (Baes, 1974)
  Benzocaine (Kleinhans and Zwissler, 1980)
  Benzoylperoxide
  Clobetasol 17-propionate (Gottmann-Lückerath, 1982)
  Dinitrochlorobenzene (Valsecchi et al., 1986; Van Hecke and Santosa, 1985)
  Etophenamate (Pinol and Carapeto, 1984)
  Mechlorethamine
  Phenothiazines
    Chlorpromazine (Lovell et al., 1986)
    Levomepromazine (Johansson, 1988)
    Promethazine

(Table continues on next page)

TABLE 3. Agents Producing Immunologic Immediate Contact Reactions (*Continued*)

Pyrazolones
  Aminophenazone (Lombardi et al., 1983)
  Methamizole
  Propylphenazone
  Tocopherol (Kassen and Mitchell, 1974)
Metals
  Copper (Shelley et al., 1983)
  Nickel (Valsecchi and Cainelli, 1987)
  Platinum
  Rhodium
Plant products (Lahti, 1986b)
  Algae
  Birch
  Camomile
  Castor bean
  Chrysanthemum (Tanaka et al., 1987)
  Cinchona (Dooms-Goossens et al., 1986a)
  Colophony (Rivers and Rycroft, 1987)
  Corn starch (Assalve et al., 1988; Fisher, 1987)
  Cotoneaster
  Emetin
  Fennel (La Rosa et al., 1986)
  Garlic
  Grevillea juniperina (Apted, 1988a)
  Hakea suaveolens (Apted, 1988b)
  Hawthorn, *Crataegus monogyna* (Steinman et al., 1984)
  Henna
  Latex rubber (Axelsson et al., 1987; Frosh et al., 1986; Morales et al., 1989; Spaner et al.,
    1989; van der Meeren and van Erp, 1986; Wrangsjö et al., 1988)
  Lichens
  Lily (Lahti, 1986a)
  Lime (Picardo, 1988)
  Mahogany
  Mustard (Kavli and Moseng, 1987)
  Papain (Santucci et al., 1985)
  Perfumes
  Pickles (Edwards and Edwards, 1984a)
  Rose (Kleinhans, 1985)
  Rouge
  Spices (Niinimäki, 1987)
  Strawberry (Grattan and Harman, 1985)
  Teak
  Tobacco (Tosti et al., 1987)
  Tulip (Lahti, 1986a)
  Winged bean (Lovell and Rycroft, 1984)
Preservatives and disinfectants
  Benzoic acid (Nethercott et al., 1984)
  Benzyl alcohol
  Chlorhexidine (Bergqvist-Karlsson, 1988; Fisher, 1989; Nishioka et al., 1984)
  Chloramine

TABLE 3. Agents Producing Immunologic Immediate Contact Reactions (*Continued*)

Chlorocresol (Goncalo et al., 1987)
1,3-Diiodo-2-hydroxypropane (Löwenfeld, 1928)
Formaldehyde (Andersen and Maibach, 1984; Lindskov, 1982)
Gentian violet (Francois et al., 1970)
Hexantriol (Tachibana et al., 1977)
p-Hydroxybenzoic acid (Böttger et al., 1981)
Parabens (Henry et al., 1979)
Phenylmercuric propionate
ortho-Phenylphenate (Tuer et al., 1986)
Polysorbates
Sodium hypochlorite
Sorbitan monolaurate
Tropicamide (Guill et al., 1979)
Miscellaneous
    Acetyl acetone (Sterry and Schmoll, 1985)
    Acrylic monomer
    Alcohols (amyl, butyl, ethyl, isopropyl) (Rilliet et al., 1980)
    Aliphatic polyamide
    Ammonia
    Ammonium persulfate
    Aminothiazole
    Benzophenone
    Butylated hydroxytoluene
    Carbonless copy paper
    Cu(II)-acetyl acetonate (Sterry and Schmoll, 1985)
    Denatonium benzoate
    Diethyltoluamide
    Epoxy resin (Jolanki et al., 1987)
    Formaldehyde resin
    Lanolin alcohols
    Lindane
    Methyl ethyl ketone (Varigos and Nurse, 1986)
    Monoamylamine
    Naphtha (Goodfield and Saihan, 1988)
    Naphthylacetic acid (Camarasa, 1986)
    Nylon (Dooms-Goossens et al., 1986b; Hatch and Maibach, 1985)
    Oleylamide
    Paraphenylenediamine (Edwards and Edwards, 1984b; Temesvari, 1984)
    Patent blue dye
    Perlon
    Phosphorus sesquisulfide (Payero et al., 1985)
    Plastic
    Polypropylene (Tosti et al., 1986)
    Polyethylene glycol
    Potassium ferricyanide
    Seminal fluid (Blair and Parish, 1985)
    Sodium silicate
    Sodium sulfide
    Sulfur dioxide
    Terpinyl acetate
    Textile finish (De Groot and Gerkens, 1989)
    Vinyl pyridine
    Zinc diethyldithiocarbamate

TABLE 4. Agents Producing Immediate Nonimmunologic Contact Reactions

Animals
  Arthropods
  Caterpillars (Ducombs et al., 1983; Edwards et al., 1986)
  Corals
  Jellyfish
  Moths
  Sea anemones
Foods
  Cayenne pepper
  Fish
  Mustard
  Thyme
Fragrances and flavorings
  Balsam of Peru
  Benzaldehyde
  Cassia (cinnamon oil)
  Cinnamic acid
  Cinnamic aldehyde (Emmons and Marks, 1985; Guin et al., 1984; Larsen, 1985)
Medicaments
  Alcohols (Wilkin and Fortner, 1985)
  Benzocaine
  Camphor
  Cantharides
  Capsaicin
  Chlorophorm
  Dimethyl sulfoxide
  Friar's balsam
  Iodine
  Methyl salicylate
  Methylene green
  Myrrh
  Nicotinic acid esters
  Resorcinol
  Tar extracts
  Tincture of benzoin
  Witch hazel
Metals
  Cobalt
Plants
  Nettles (Kulze and Greaves, 1988)
  Sea weed
Preservatives and disinfectants
  Benzoid acid
  Chlorocresol (Freitas and Brandão, 1986)
  Formaldehyde
  Sodium benzoate
  Sorbic acid (Soschin and Leyden, 1986)
Miscellaneous
  Butyric acid
  Diethyl fumarate (Lahti and Maibach, 1985a; White and Cronin, 1984)
  Histamine
  Pine oil
  Pyridine carboxaldehyde (Archer and Cronin, 1986; Hannuksela et al., 1989)
  Sulfur (Böttger, 1981)
  Turpentine

1986). This finding may provide an explanation for the high frequency of positive patch-test reactions to inhalant allergens, such as house dust mites, birch and grass pollen, and animal danders, in these patients (Adinoff et al., 1988; Leung et al., 1987; Mitchell et al., 1986; Reitamo et al., 1986; Tigalonowa et al., 1988). The most important function of epidermal Langerhans cells is antigen presentation in delayed-type contact allergic reaction, but it can be hypothesized that protein allergens (inhalant, food, etc.) for type I immediate contact reactions bind to specific IgE molecules present on epidermal Langerhans cells, which become apposed to mononuclear cells (Najem and Hull, 1989) and induce a delayed-type hypersensitivity reaction resulting in eczematous skin lesions. This may be the mechanism whereby repeated immediate contact reactions lead to more persistent eczematous skin lesions.

Contact urticaria to rubber latex is a typical example of immediate immunologic contact reaction and is more common than was thought earlier (Estlander et al., 1987; Turjanmaa, 1987; Turjanmaa and Reunala, 1988; Wrangsjö et al., 1986). There have been cases where anaphylactic symptoms and generalized urticaria have occurred after contact with surgical (Axelsson et al., 1988; Carrillo et al., 1986; Spaner et al., 1989; Turjanmaa et al., 1988a) and household rubber gloves (Seifert et al., 1987). These reactions have been shown to be immediate, allergic, and IgE-mediated (Frosch et al., 1986; Seifert et al., 1987; Turjanmaa and Reunala, 1989; Turjanmaa et al., 1989). The allergens are among the proteins that constitute 1–2% of natural latex. Allergy to latex can be established by skin prick tests (Turjanmaa et al., 1988c) and by latex RAST (radioallergosorbent test), which is commercially available (Pharmacia, Sweden) (Turjanmaa et al., 1988b).

Veterinary surgeons can contract contact urticaria on the hand after contact with cows' amnion fluid, but they do not acquire reactions to cows' dander in clinical provocation tests or in skin prick tests with cows' epithelium extracts. RAST investigations have shown that antibodies to cows' amnion fluid and serum, but not to epithelia, can be found in the sera of veterinary surgeons. The allergen causing contact urticaria in these cases is a compound of amnion fluid and serum but not of the epithelium of cows (Kalveram et al., 1986).

Foodstuffs are the most common causes of immediate allergic contact reactions (Table 3). The orolaryngeal area is a site where immediate reactions are provoked by food allergens, frequently among atopic individuals. Of 230 patients allergic to birch pollen, 152 (66%) gave a history of itching, tingling, or edema of the lips and tongue and hoarseness or irritation of the throat when eating raw fruits and vegetables such as apple, potato, carrot, and tomato (Hannuksela and Lahti, 1977). Plum, peach, cherry, kiwi, celery, and parsnip can also elicit immediate contact reactions in birch pollen-allergic people. Positive results ("scratch-chamber" test) with suspected raw fruits and vegetables were noted in 36% of 230 patients. Apple, carrot, parsnip, and potato elicited reactions more often than swede (rutabaga), tomato, onion, celery, and parsley. The clinical relevance of the skin test results with apple, potato, and carrot was 80–

90%. Only 7 of 158 (4%) atopic patients who were not allergic to birch pollen had positive skin test reactions to any of the fruits and vegetables. RAST and RAST-inhibition studies have confirmed the real cross-allergy between birch pollen and fruits and vegetables. All immunological determinants in apple, carrot, and celery tuber appeared to be present also in birch pollen but not vice versa (Halmepuro and Løvenstein, 1986; Halmepuro et al., 1984).

Protein Contact Dermatitis

The term "protein contact dermatitis" was introduced (Hjorth and Roed-Petersen, 1976) for people with hand eczema demonstrating immediate symptoms when the skin was exposed to certain food proteins. Most of these individuals handled job-related food products for a protracted period before the symptoms appeared. Itching, erythema, urticarial swelling, or small vesicles appear on fingers or dorsa of hands within 30 min of contact with fish or shellfish. Baker's dermatitis is another example of immediate contact reaction, caused by wheat flour. Protein contact dermatitis may appear without previous urticarial rashes, but it may also be a result of repeated contact urticaria (Hannuksela, 1986). It is probable that both immunologic and nonimmunologic (irritant) types of protein contact reactions exist. Eczematous reactions are indistinguishable from primary irritant or allergic dermatitis, and careful study of the patient's history and the performance of skin tests ensure correct diagnosis.

Nonimmunologic Immediate Contact Reactions

Nonimmunologic immediate contact reactions occur without previous sensitization and are the most common type of immediate contact reaction. The reaction remains localized and does not spread to become generalized urticaria, nor does it cause systemic symptoms. Typically, the strength of the reaction varies from erythema to an urticarial response, depending on the concentration, the skin area exposed, the mode of exposure, and the substance itself (Lahti, 1980).

The most potent and best studied substances producing nonimmunologic immediate contact reactions (Table 4) are benzoic acid, sorbic acid, cinnamic acid, cinnamic aldehyde, and nicotinic acid esters. Under optimal conditions more than half of the individuals react with local erythema and edema to these substances within 45 min of application if the concentration is high enough. Benzoic acid, sorbic acid, and sodium benzoate, preservatives for cosmetics and other topical preparations, are capable of producing immediate contact reactions at concentrations from 0.1 to 0.2% (Lahti, 1980; Soschin and Leyden, 1986).

Cinnamic aldehyde at a concentration of 0.01% may elicit erythema with a burning or stinging feeling in the skin. Some mouthwashes and chewing gums contain cinnamic aldehyde at concentrations that produce a pleasant tingling or "lively" sensation in the mouth and enhance the sale of the product. Higher concentrations produce lip swelling or contact urticaria.

The face, back skin, and extensor sides of the upper extremities react more readily than other parts of the body; the soles and palms are the least sensitive areas (Gollhausen and Kligman, 1985; Lahti, 1980). Scratching does not enhance the reactivity, nor does occlusion, for benzoic acid.

The mechanism of nonimmunologic immediate contact reactions has not been established, but possible mechanisms are a direct influence upon dermal vessel walls or a non-antibody-mediated release of histamine, prostaglandins, leukotrienes, substance P or other inflammatory mediators (Lahti and Maibach, 1987). No specific antibodies against the causative agent are in the serum.

It was earlier presumed that substances eliciting nonimmunologic immediate contact reactions also result in nonspecific histamine release from mast cells. However, antihistamines, hydroxyzine, and terfenadine did not inhibit reactions to benzoic acid, cinnamic acid, cinnamic aldehyde, methyl nicotinate, or dimethyl sulfoxide but they did inhibit reactions to histamine in the prick test (Lahti, 1980, 1987). The results suggest that histamine is not the main mediator in immediate contact reactions to these model substances.

Effect of nonsteroidal antiinflammatory drugs (NSAIDs). Nonimmunologic contact reactions to benzoic acid, cinnamic acid, cinnamic aldehyde, methyl nicotinate, and diethyl fumarate can be inhibited by peroral acetylsalicylic acid and indomethacin (Lahti et al., 1983, 1987) and by topical application of diclofenac or naproxene gels (Johansson and Lahti, 1988). Inhibition by acetylsalicylic acid can last up to 4 d (Kujala and Lahti, 1989). The mechanism by which NSAIDs inhibit contact reactions in human skin has not been defined but it may be ascribed to a common pharmacological action, that is, inhibition of prostaglandin bioformation.

Role of sensory nerves. Capsaicin (trans-8-methyl-*N*-vanillyl-6-nonenamide), the most abundant of the pungent principles of the red pepper (*Capsicum*), is known to induce vasodilatation and protein extravasation by specific release of bioactive peptides, for example, substance P, from axons of unmyelinated C-fibers of the sensory nerves. Pretreatment with capsaicin inhibits erythema reactions in histamine skin tests (Bernstein et al., 1981; Wallengren and Möller, 1986). However, pretreatment with capsaicin inhibited neither erythema nor edema elicited by benzoic acid or methyl nicotinate (Larmi et al., 1989). The result suggests that pathways sensitive to capsaicin are not substantially involved.

It was also shown that topical anesthesia (lidocaine plus prilocaine) can inhibit erythema and edema reactions to histamine and also to benzoic acid and methyl nicotinate, but it is not known whether the inhibitory effect is due to the influence on the sensory nerves of the skin only, or if the anesthetic affects other cell types or regulatory mechanisms of immediate type skin inflammation (Larmi et al., 1989).

Effect of ultraviolet irradiation. Immediate contact reactions to benzoic acid and methyl nicotinate can also be inhibited by ultraviolet B and A light exposure, an effect that lasts for at least 2 wk (Larmi et al., 1988). An interesting observation was the fact that UV irradiation had systemic effects; it inhibited reactions on nonirradiated skin sites, too (Larmi, 1989). The mechanism of UV inhibition is not known, but it does not seem to be due to thickening of the stratum corneum (Larmi, 1989).

Little is known about the histology of immediate contact reactions. In recent studies with nicotinates, the accumulation of mononuclear cell perivascular infiltrate was seen from 15 min and that of neutrophils from 2 h onward, persisting up to 48 h in normal subjects. Leukocytoclasis was also observed. The cell infiltrate was seen to a lesser degree in 1 of 6 atopic eczema patients but not in normal subjects treated with 600 mg of acetylsalicylic acid before the nicotinate application (Daroczy and Temesvari, 1988; English et al., 1987).

An animal model for nonimmunologic immediate contact reactions. Animal models are needed to identify agents capable of immediate contact reactions and to study mechanisms, but they have not been available until now (Lahti, 1988). Guinea pig body skin reacts with rapidly appearing erythema to cinnamic aldehyde, methyl nicotinate, and dimethyl sulfoxide but not to benzoic acid, sorbic acid, or cinnamic acid. Any of these substances applied to the guinea pig earlobe causes erythema and edema to appear. Quantification of edema by measuring changes in the ear thickness with a micrometer caliper is an accurate, reproducible, and rapid method (Lahti and Maibach, 1984).

Analogous reactions can be elicited in the earlobes of other laboratory animals. Cinnamic aldehyde and dimethyl sulfoxide produce ear swelling in rat and mouse, but benzoic acid, sorbic acid, cinnamic acid, diethyl fumarate, and methyl nicotinate produce no response. This suggests that either several mechanisms are involved in immediate contact reactions from different substances or there are differences in the activation of mediators of inflammation between guinea pig, rat and mouse (Lahti and Maibach, 1985a, 1985b).

The swelling response in the guinea pig earlobe is dependent on the concentrations of the eliciting substance. The maximal response is a roughly 100% increase in ear thickness, which appears within 50 min of application.

Biopsies taken from the guinea pig earlobe 40 min after application of test substances show marked dermal edema and intra- and perivascular infiltrates of heterophilic (neutrophilic in humans) granulocytes, and they appear to be characteristic of nonimmunologic contact urticaria in the guinea pig ear (Anderson, 1988; Lahti and Maibach, 1984; Lahti et al., 1986).

A decrease in response to contact urticants is noticed after reapplication of the test substances to the guinea pig ear on the following day (Lahti and Maibach, 1985c). The tachyphylaxis is not specific to the substance which produces it, and the reactivity to other agents decreases as well. The length of the refractory period varies with the compound used. It is 4 d for methyl nicotinate, 8 d for diethyl fumarate and cinnamic aldehyde, and up to 16 d for benzoic acid, cinnamic acid, and dimethyl sulfoxide.

The reaction of guinea pig earlobe to nonimmunologic contact urticants seems to be similar to that of human skin. The similarities include the morphology, the time course of maximal response, the concentrations of the eliciting substances, the tachyphylaxis phenomenon (Lahti, 1980), and the lack of an inhibitory effect of antihistamines on contact reactions (Lahti, 1987; Lahti et al., 1986).

Specificity of the reaction. Pyridine carboxaldehyde (PCA) is one of the many substances that can produce nonimmunologic immediate contact reactions (Archer and Cronin, 1986). It has three isomers: 2-, 3-, and 4-PCA, according to the position of the aldehyde group on the pyridine ring. In the study on the capacity of these isomers to produce immediate contact reactions it was found that 3-PCA was the strongest and 2-PCA the weakest contact reactant in both the human skin and guinea pig ear swelling test (Hannuksela et al., 1989; Lahti and Maibach, 1984). Only a slight change in the molecular structure of a chemical can greatly alter its capacity to produce nonimmunologic immediate contact reactions.

The mechanism of nonimmunologic immediate contact reactions is not well known. It has, however, been shown that nonsteroidal antiinflammatory drugs (NSAIDs), UV irradiation, and topical anesthesia, but not antihistamine treatment, inhibit these reactions, suggesting that histamine is not substantially involved. Nonimmunologic contact reactions from different agents are probably linked to different mechanisms and combinations of mediators.

DIAGNOSTIC TESTS

The diagnosis of immediate contact reactions is based on a full medical history and on skin tests with suspected substances.

Tests for Both Immunologic and Nonimmunologic Contact Reactions

The simplest test is the rub test. For this test the suspected substance (fish, apple, carrot) is applied and gently rubbed on either normal-looking or slightly affected skin, usually the hand. The test site is observed for 60 min (Hannuksela, 1986). A positive result is seen as an edema and erythema reaction or as tiny intraepidermal spongiotic vesicles typical of acute eczema.

The use test requires the patient to handle the suspected agent precisely as handled when symptoms appeared. Wearing surgical gloves on wet hands to provoke contact urticaria to latex is a typical use test.

In the open test, 0.1 ml of the test substance is spread on a 3 x 3 cm area of the skin of the upper back or on the extensor side of the upper arm. The test should first be performed on nondiseased skin and then, if negative, on previously or currently affected skin (Lahti and Maibach, 1986). Even in immunologic contact urticaria there may be a marked difference between skin sites in their capacity to elicit contact urticaria (Maibach, 1986). This is typical of nonimmunologic contact urticaria. The face has been considered the most sensitive skin area (Gollhausen and Kligman, 1985). Often it is desirable to apply contact urticants to skin sites suggested by the patient's history. The immunologic contact reactions usually appear within 15–20 min and nonimmunologic ones within 45–60 min after application. A positive reaction comprises a wheal-and-flare reaction and sometimes a vesicular eruption indistinguishable from that seen in eczema (Hjorth and Roed-Petersen, 1976).

Occlusive patch and chamber tests on nondiseased or slightly affected skin have been said to be somewhat more sensitive than the open application test in immunologic immediate contact reactions (von Krogh and Maibach, 1982). The occlusion time is 15–20 min, and a positive reaction is usually seen within 45 min after application.

Tests for Immunologic Contact Reactions

Prick testing is often the method of choice for testing patients with suspected allergic contact reactions.

The scratch test is a less standardized method than the prick test but it is useful when nonstandardized allergens must be used (Paul, 1987). The allergen solutions in scratch testing are the same as those used in prick testing. Also, freeze-dried and other powdered allergens moistened with 0.1 N aqueous sodium hydroxide solution and fresh foodstuffs (e.g., potato, apple, carrot) can be used. When testing with poorly standardized or nonstandardized substances, control tests should be made on at least 20 people to avoid false interpretation of the test results.

The chamber scratch test was introduced for testing foodstuffs when commercial allergens with proven efficacy are not available (Hannuksela and Lahti, 1977). Potato, apple, and carrot lose their allergenity when cooked, deep-frozen, or made into juice, and it is therefore best to use them fresh for skin testing.

In the chamber scratch test, the procedure is that of the ordinary scratch test but the scratch and the foodstuff are covered with a small aluminum chamber (Finn Chamber, Epitest Ltd Oy, Hyrylä, Finland) for 15 min. The result is read 5 min after the removal of the chamber according to the criteria of the scratch test. Reactions at least the size of a similarly produced histamine reaction are usually clinically significant. Histamine hydrochloride (10 mg/ml) is the positive reference and aqueous 0.1 N sodium hydroxide the negative reference.

The Prausnitz–Küstner test or passive transfer test has been used in occupational dermatology for detecting immunologic contact urticaria to potato (Tuft and Blumstein, 1942) and to rubber (Köpman and Hannuksela, 1983).

RAST is seldom needed for contact urticaria diagnosis, but RAST inhibition tests are used in investigating cross-allergenity (Halmepuro and Løvenstein, 1985). For this purpose crossed radioimmunoelectrophoresis and its inhibition are also used.

Nonsteroidal antiinflammatory drugs and antihistamines should not be taken by patients during tests for immediate contact reactions because these drugs may inhibit the reactions. Using the same test site repeatedly may result in the tachyphylaxis phenomenon and cause false negative results.

When examining patients with a suspected allergic contact reaction, the prick, scratch, or scratch chamber tests are done first because the test procedures are fast and reliable. The diagnosis should be based on the result of the rub, open application, or use test.

SUMMARY

In clinical practice, patients report immediate contact reactions after applying cosmetics or therapeutic agents and after handling food products. Not only have dermatologists and allergists been uncertain about the nature of these reactions, but manufacturers, their toxicologists, and other involved personnel have had difficulty in understanding this type of reaction and in developing less irritating products.

Studies on the mechanisms of immediate contact reactions from different substances and the standardization of human and animal tests for these reactions are a challenge for future research. Dermatologists, allergists, toxicologists, and medical authorities need to combine their efforts to investigate the capacity of various environmental agents to produce immediate contact reactions, as was done in the past for delayed type skin effects.

REFERENCES

Aaronson, C. M. 1969. Generalized urticaria from sensitivity to nifuroxime. *J. Am. Med. Assoc.* 210:557.

Adinoff, A. D., Tellez, P. and Clark, R. A. 1988. Atopic dermatitis and aeroallergen contact sensitivity. *J. Allergy Clin. Immunol.* 81:736–742.

Agrup, G. and Sjöstedt, L. 1985. Contact urticaria in laboratory technicians working with animals. *Acta Derm. Venereol. (Stockh.)* 65:111–115.

Andersen, K. E. and Maibach, H. I. 1984. Multiple application delayed onset contact urticaria: possible relation to certain unusual formalin and textile reactions. *Contact Dermatitis* 10:227–234.

Andersen, C. 1988. Irritant contact reactions versus non-immunologic contact urticaria. *Acta Derm. Venereol. Suppl. (Stockh.)* 68:45–48.

Apted, J. 1988a. Acute contact urticaria from *Grevillea juniperina*. *Contact Dermatitis* 18:126.

Apted, J. 1988b. Acute contact urticaria from *Hakea suaveolens*. *Contact Dermatitis* 18:126.

Archer, C. B. and Cronin, E. 1986. Contact urticaria induced by pyridine carboxaldehyde. *Contact Dermatitis* 15:308–309.

Assalve, D., Cicioni, P., Perno, P. and Lisi, P. 1988. Contact urticaria and anaphylactoid reaction from cornstarch surgical glove powder. *Contact Dermatitis* 19:61.

Axelsson, J. G. K., Johansson, S. G. O. and Wrangsjö, K. 1987. IgE-mediated anaphylactoid reactions to rubber. *Allergy* 42:46–50.

Axelsson, I. G., Ericksson, M. and Wrangsjö, K. 1989. Anaphylaxis and angioedema due to rubber allergy in children. *Acta Paediatr. Scand.* 77:314–316.

Baes, H. 1974. Allergic contact dermatitis to virginiamycin. *Dermatologica (Basel)* 149:231.

Barker, J. N. W. N., Alegre, V. A. and MacDonald, D. M. 1988. Surface-bound immunoglobulin E on antigenpresenting cells in cutaneous tissue of atopic dermatitis. *J. Invest. Dermatol.* 90:117–121.

Bergqvist-Karlsson, A. 1988. Delayed and immediate-type hypersensitivity to chlorhexidine. *Contact Dermatitis* 18:84–88.

Bernstein, D. I., Gallagher, J. S. and Bernstein, I. L. 1983. Mealworm asthma: Clinical and immunological studies. *J. Allergy Clin. Immunol.* 72:475–480.

Bernstein, J. E., Swift, R. M., Keyoumars, S. and Lorincz, A. L. 1981. Inhibition of axon reflex vasodilatation by topically applied capsaicin. *J. Invest. Dermatol.* 76:394–395.

Blair, H. and Parish, W. E. 1985. Asthma and urticaria induced by seminal plasma in a woman with IgE antibody and T-lymphocyte responsiveness to a seminal plasma antigen. *Clinical Allergy* 15:117–130.

Boso, E. B. and Brestel, E. P. 1987. Contact urticaria to cow milk. *Allergy* 42:151–153.

Böttger, E. M., Mücke, C. and Tronnier, H. 1981. Kontaktdermatitis auf neuere Antikykotika and Kontakturtikaria. *Acta Derm. Venereol. Suppl. (Stockh.)* 7:70.

Bruynzeel-Koomen, C. 1986. IgE on Langerhans cells: New insights into the pathogenesis of atopic dermatitis. *Dermatologica* 172:181–183.

Bruynzeel-Koomen, C., van Wichen, D. F., Toonstra, J., Berrens, J. and Bruynzeel, P. L. B. 1986. The presence of IgE molecules on epidermal Langerhans cells in patients with atopic dermatitis. *Arch. Dermatol. Res.* 278:199–205.

Burns, D. A. 1987. Papular urticaria produced by the mite *Listrophorus gibbus*. *Clin. Exp. Dermatol.* 12:200–201.

Camarasa, J. G. 1986. Contact urticaria to naphthylacetic acid. *Contact Dermatitis* 14:113.

Capron, M., Capron, A., Dessaint, J., Johansson, S. and Prin, L. 1981. Fc-receptors for IgE on human and rat eosinophils. *J. Immunol.* 126:2087–2092.

Carrillo, T., Cuevas, M., Muñoz, T., Hinojosa, M. and Moneo, I. 1986. Contact urticaria and rhinitis from latex surgical gloves. *Contact Dermatitis* 15:69–72.

Daroczy, J. and Temesvari, E. 1988. Light microscopic and electron microscopic (EM) examination of contact urticaria. *Contact Dermatitis* 19:156–158.

De Groot, A. C. and Gerkens, F. 1989. Contact urticaria from a chemical textile finish. *Contact Dermatitis* 20:63–64.

Dooms-Goossens, A., Deveylder, H., Duron, C., Dooms, M. and Degreef, H. 1986a. Airborne contact urticaria due to cinchona. *Contact Dermatitis* 15:258.

Dooms-Goossens, A., Duron, C., Loncke, J. and Degreef, H. 1986b. Contact urticaria due to nylon. *Contact Dermatitis* 14:63.

Ducombs, G., Lamy, M., Michel, M., Pradinaud, R., Jamet, P., Vincendeau, P., Maleville, J. and Texier, L. 1983. La papillonite de Guyane Francaise. Etude clinique et épidémiologique. *Ann. Dermatol. Venereol.* 110:809–816.

Edwards, E. K. and Edwards, E. K. 1984a. Contact urticaria provoked by pickels. *Cutis* 33:230.

Edwards, E. K. and Edwards, E. K. 1984b. Contact urticaria and allergic contact dermatitis caused by paraphenylenediamine. *Cutis* 34:87–88.

Edwards, E. K., Edwards, E. K. and Kowalczyk, A. P. 1986. Contact urticaria and allergic contact dermatitis to saddleback caterpillar with histologic correlation. *Int. J. Dermatol.* 25:467.

Elpern, D. J. 1985a. The syndrome of immediate reactivities (contact urticaria syndrome). An historical study from a dermatology practice. I. Age, sex, race and putative substances. *Hawaii Med. J.* 44:426–439.

Elpern, D. J. 1985b. The syndrome of immediate reactivities (contact urticaria syndrome). An historical study from a dermatology practice. II. The atopic diathesis and drug reactions. *Hawaii Med. J.* 44:466–468.

Elpern, D. J. 1986. The syndrome of immediate reactivities (contact urticaria syndrome). An historical study from a dermatology practice. III. General discussion and conclusions. *Hawaii Med. J.* 45:10–12.

Emmons, W. W. and Marks, J. G. 1985. Immediate and delayed reactions to cosmetic ingredients. *Contact Dermatitis* 13:258–265.

English, J. S. C., Winkelmann, R. K., Louback, J. B., Greaves, M. W. and MacDonald, D. M. 1987. The cellular inflammatory response in nicotinate skin reactions. *Br. J. Dermatol.* 116:341–349.

Estlander, T., Jolanki, R. and Kanerva, L. 1987. Contact urticaria from rubber gloves: a detailed description of four cases. *Acta Derm. Venereol. Suppl. (Stockh.)* 134:98–102.

Fisher, A. A. 1987. Contact urticaria and anaphylactoid reaction due to corn starch surgical glove powder. *Contact Dermatitis* 16:224–225.

Fisher, A. A. 1989. Contact urticaria from chlorhexidine. *Cutis* 43:17–18.

Francois, A., Henin, P., Carli Basset, C. and Ginies, G. 1970. Anaphylactic shock following applications of Milian's solution. *Bull. Soc. Fr. Dermatol. Syphiligr.* 77:834.

Freitas, J. P. and Brandão, F. M. 1986. Contact urticaria to chlorocresol. *Contact Dermatitis* 15:252.

Frosch, P. J., Wahl, R., Bahmer, F. A. and Maasch, H. J. 1986. Contact urticaria to rubber gloves is IgE-mediated. *Contact Dermatitis* 14:241–245.

Gollhausen, R. and Kligman, A. M. 1985. Human assay for identifying substances which induce non-allergic contact urticaria: the NICU-test. *Contact Dermatitis* 13:98–106.

Goncalo, M., Gongalo, S. and Moreno, A. 1987. Immediate and delayed sensitivity to chlorocresol. *Contact Dermatitis* 17:46–47.

Goodfield, M. J. D. and Saihan, E. M. 1988. Contact urticaria to naphtha present in a solvent. *Contact Dermatitis* 18:187.

Gottmann-Lückerath, I. 1982. Kontakturticaria nach Dermoxin[R]. *Soc. Proc. Dermatosen* 30:124.

Grattan, C. E. H. and Harman, R. R. M. 1985. Contact urticaria to strawberry. *Contact Dermatitis* 13:191–192.

Grob, J. J., Pommier, G., Robaglia, A., Collet-Villette, A. M. and Bonerandi, J. J. 1987. Contact urticaria from rifamycin. *Contact Dermatitis* 16:284–285.

Guill, A., Goette, K., Knight, C. G., Peck, C. C. and Lupton, G. P. 1979. Erythema multiforme and urticaria. *Arch. Dermatol.* 115:742.

Guin, J. D., Meyer, B. N., Drake, R. D. and Haffley, P. 1984. The effect of quenching agents on contact urticaria caused by cinnamic aldehyde. *J. Am. Acad. Dermatol.* 10:45–51.

Halmepuro, L. and Løvenstein, H. 1985. Immunological investigation of possible structural similarities between pollen antigens and antigens in apple, carrot and celery tuber. *Allergy* 40:264–272.

Halmepuro, L., Vuontela, K., Kalimo, K. and Björksten, F. 1984. Cross-reactivity of IgE antibodies with allergens in birch pollen, fruits and vegetables. *Int. Arch. Allergy Appl. Immunol.* 74:235–240.

Hannuksela, M. 1980. Atopic contact dermatitis. *Contact Dermatitis* 6:30.

Hannuksela, M. 1986. Contact urticaria from foods. In *Nutrition and the skin*, ed. D. Roe, pp. 153–162. New York: Alan R. Liss.

Hannuksela, M. and Lahti, A. 1977. Immediate reactions to fruits and vegetables. *Contact Dermatitis* 3:79–84.

Hannuksela, A., Lahti, A. and Hannuksela, M. 1989. Nonimmunologic immediate contact reactions to three isomers of pyridine carboxaldehyde. In *Current Topics in*

Contact Dermatitis, eds. P. J. Frosch, A. Dooms-Goossens, J.-M. Lachapelle, R. J. G. Rycroft and R. J. Scheper, pp. 448–452. Berlin: Springer-Verlag.

Hatch, K. L. and Maibach, H. I. 1985. Textile fiber dermatitis. *Contact Dermatitis* 12:1–11.

Henry, J. C., Tschen, E. H. and Becker, L. E. 1979. Contact urticaria to parabens. *Arch. Dermatol.* 115:1231.

Hjorth, N. and Roed-Petersen, J. 1976. Occupational protein contact dermatitis in foodhandlers. *Contact Dermatitis* 2:28–42.

Johansson, G. 1988. Contact urticaria from levomepromazine. *Contact Dermatitis* 19:304.

Johansson, J. and Lahti, A. 1988. Topical non-steroidal anti-inflammatory drugs inhibit non-immunologic immediate contact reactions. *Contact Dermatitis* 19:161–165.

Jolanki, R., Estlander, T. and Kanerva, L. 1987. Occupational contact dermatitis and contact urticaria caused by epoxy resins. *Acta Derm. Venereol. Suppl. (Stockh.)* 134:90–94.

Joseph, M., Tonnel, A., Capron, A. and Voisin, C. 1980. Enzyme release and super oxide anion production by human alveolar macrophages stimulated with immuno-globulin E. *Clin. Exp. Immunol.* 40:416–422.

Joseph, M., Auriault, C., Capron, A., Vorng, H. and Viens, P. 1983. A new function for platelets: IgE-dependent killing of schistosomes. *Nature (Lond.)* 303:810–812.

Kalveram, K.-J., Kästner, H. and Frock, G. 1986. Detection of specific IgE antibodies in veterinarians suffering from contact urticaria. *Z. Hautkr.* 61:75–81.

Kassen, B. and Mitchell, J. C. 1974. Contact urticaria from a vitamin E preparation in two siblings. *Contact Derm. Newslett.* 16:482.

Kavli, G. and Moseng, D. 1987. Contact urticaria from mustard in fish stick produc-tion. *Contact Dermatitis* 17:153–155.

Kleinhans, D. 1985. Kontakt-Urtikaria. *Dermatosen* 33:198–203.

Kleinhans, D. and Zwissler, H. 1980. Anaphylaktischer Schock nach Anwendung einer Benzocainhaltigen Salbe. *Z. Hautkr.* 55:945.

Köpman, A. and Hannuksela, M. 1983. Contact urticaria to rubber. *Duodecim* 99:221–224.

Kremser, M. and Lindemayr, W. 1983. Celery allergy (celery contact urticaria syn-drome) and relation to allergies to other plant antigens. *Wien. Klin. Wochenscher.* 95:838–843.

Kujala, T. and Lahti, A. 1989. Duration of inhibition of non-immunologic immediate contact reactions by acetylsalicylic acid. *Contact Dermatitis* 21:60–61.

Kulze, A. and Greaves, M. 1988. Contact urticaria caused by stinging nettles. *Br. J. Dermatol.* 119:269–270.

Lahti, A. 1980. Non-immunologic contact urticaria. *Acta Derm. Venereol. (Stockh.)* 60 (suppl. 91):1–49.

Lahti, A. 1986a. Contact urticaria and respiratory symptoms from tulips and lilies. *Contact Dermatitis* 14:317–319.

Lahti, A. 1986b. Contact urticaria to plants. *Dermatol. Clin.* 4:127–136.

Lahti, A. 1987. Terfenadine (H_1-antagonist) does not inhibit non-immunologic contact urticaria. *Contact Dermatitis* 16:220–223.

Lahti, A. 1988. Non-immunologic contact urticaria. Animal tests and their relevance. *Acta Derm. Venereol. Suppl. (Stockh.)* 68:43–44.

Lahti, A. and Maibach, H. I. 1984. An animal model for nonimmunologic contact urticaria. *Toxicol. Appl. Pharmacol.* 76:219–224.

Lahti, A. and Maibach, H. I. 1985a. Contact urticaria from diethyl fumarate. *Contact Dermatitis* 12:139–140.

Lahti, A. and Maibach, H. I. 1985b. Species specificity of nonimmunologic contact urticaria: Guinea pig, rat and mouse. *J. Am. Acad. Dermatol.* 13:66–69.

Lahti, A. and Maibach, H. I. 1985c. Long refractory period after one application of nonimmunologic contact urticaria agents to the guinea pig ear. *J. Am. Acad. Dermatol.* 13:585–589.

Lahti, A. and Maibach, H. I. 1986. Immediate contact reactions (contact urticaria syndrome). In *Occupational and Industrial Dermatology*, 2nd ed., ed. H. Maibach, Chapter 6, pp. 32–44. Chicago: Year Book Medical.

Lahti, A. and Maibach, H. I. 1987. Immediate contact reactions: Contact urticaria syndrome. *Semin. Dermatol.* 6:313–320.

Lahti, A., Oikarinen, A., Ylikorkala, O. and Viinikka, L. 1983. Prostaglandins in contact urticaria induced by benzoic acid. *Acta. Derm. Venereol. (Stockh.)* 63:425–427.

Lahti, A., McDonald, D. M., Tammi, R. and Maibach, H. I. 1986. Pharmacological studies on nonimmunologic contact urticaria in guinea pig. *Arch. Dermatol. Res.* 279:44–49.

Lahti, A., Väänänen, A., Kokkonen, E.-L. and Hannuksela, M. 1987. Acetylsalicylic acid inhibits non-immunologic contact urticaria. *Contact Dermatitis* 16:133–135.

Larkö, O., Lindstedt, G., Lundberg, P. A. and Mobacken, H. 1983. Biochemical and clinical studies in a case of contact urticaria to potato. *Contact Dermatitis* 9:108–114.

Larmi, E. 1989. Systemic effect of ultraviolet irradiation on non-immunologic immediate contact reactions to benzoic acid and methyl nicotinate. *Acta Derm. Venereol. (Stockh.)* 69:296–301.

Larmi, E., Lahti, A. and Hannuksela, M. 1988. Ultraviolet light inhibits nonimmunologic immediate contact reactions to benzoic acid. *Arch. Dermatol. Res.* 280:420–423.

Larmi, E., Lahti, A. and Hannuksela, M. 1989. Effects of capsaicin and topical anesthesia on nonimmunologic immediate contact reactions to benzoic acid and methyl nicotinate. In *Current Topics in Contact Dermatitis,* eds. P. J. Frosch, A. Dooms-Goossens, J.-M. Lachapelle, R. J. G. Rycroft and R. J. Scheper, pp. 441–447. Berlin: Springer-Verlag.

La Rosa, M., Crea, G. F., Di Francesco, S., Di Paola, M. and Castiglione, N. 1986. Fennel allergy: Case report. Abstr. *3rd Int. Symp. Immunological and Clinical Problems of Food Allergy,* Taormina, Giardini Naxos, Italy, October 1–4.

Larsen, W. G. 1985. Perfume dermatitis. *J. Am. Acad. Dermatol.* 12:1–9.

Leung, D. Y., Schneeberger, E. E., Siraganian, R. P., Geha, R. S. and Bhan, A. K. 1987. The presence of IgE on macrophages and dendritic cells infiltrating into the skin lesion of atopic dermatitis. *Clin. Immunol. Immunopathol.* 42:328–337.

Lewis-Jones, M. S. 1985. Papular urticaria caused by *Dermestes maculatus* Degeer. *Clin. Exp. Dermatol.* 10:181.

Lindskov, R. 1982. Contact urticaria to formaldehyde. *Contact Dermatitis* 8:333.

Lombardi, P., Giorgini, S. and Achille, A. 1983. Contact urticaria from aminophenazone. *Contact Dermatitis* 9:428–429.

Lovell, C. R., Cronin, E. and Rhodes, E. L. 1986. Photocontact urticaria from chlorpromazine. *Contact Dermatitis* 14:290–291.

Lovell, C. R. and Rycroft, R. J. G. 1984. Contact urticaria from winged bean (*Psophocarpus tetragonolobus*). *Contact Dermatitis* 10:310–318.

Löwenfeld, W. 1928. Überempfindlichkeit gegen Iodthion mit gleichzeitiger urtikarieller reaction. *Derm. Wochenschr.* 78:502.

Maibach, H. I. 1976. Immediate hypersensitivity in hand dermatitis: Role of food contact dermatitis. *Arch. Dermatol.* 112:1289–1291.

Maibach, H. I. 1986. Regional variation in elicitation of contact urticaria syndrome (immediate hypersensitivity syndrome): Shrimp. *Contact Dermatitis* 15:100.

Melewicz, F. and Spiegelberg, H. 1980. Fc-receptors for IgE on a subpopulation of human peripheral blood monocytes. *J. Immunol.* 125:1026–1031.

Melino, M., Toni, F. and Riguzzi, G. 1987. Immunologic contact urticaria to fish. *Contact Dermatitis* 17:182.

Mitchell, E. B., Crow, J., Williams, G. and Platts-Mills, T. A. E. 1986. Increase in skin mast cells following chronic house dust mite exposure. *Br. J. Dermatol.* 114:65–73.

Mittelbach, F. 1983. Urticaria and Quincke's edema caused by *Chironomidae (Chironomus thummi thummi)* as fishfood. *Z. Hautkr.* 58:1548–1555.

Monk, B. E. 1988. Contact urticaria to locusts. *Br. J. Dermatol.* 118:707–708.

Morales, C., Basomba, A., Carreira, J. and Sastre, A. 1989. Anaphylaxis produced by rubber glove contact. Case reports and immunological identification of the antigens involved. *Clin. Exp. Allergy* 19:425–430.

Munoz, D., Leanizbarrutia, I., Lobera, T. and de Corres, F. 1985. Anaphylaxis from contact with carrot. *Contact Dermatitis* 13:345–346.

Nagano, T., Kanao, K. and Sugai, T. 1984. Allergic contact urticaria caused by raw prawns and shrimps: Three cases. *J. Allergy Clin. Immunol.* 74:489–493.

Najem, N. and Hull, D. 1989. Langerhans cells in delayed skin reactions to inhalant allergens in atopic dermatitis—An electron microscopic study. *Clin. Exp. Dermatol.* 14:218–222.

Nethercott, J. R., Lawrence, M. J., Roy, A.-M. and Gibson, B. L. 1984. Airborne contact urticaria due to sodium benzoate in a pharmaceutical manufacturing plant. *J. Occup. Med.* 26:734–736.

Niinimäki, A. 1987. Scratch-chamber tests in food handler dermatitis. *Contact Dermatitis* 16:11–20.

Nilsson, E. 1985. Contact sensitivity and urticaria in "wet" work. *Contact Dermatitis* 13:321–328.

Nishioka, K., Doi, T. and Katayama, I. 1984. Histamine release in contact urticaria. *Contact Dermatitis* 11:191.

Paul, E. 1987. Skin reactions to food and food constituents—Allergic and pseudoallergic reactions. *Z. Hautkr. Suppl.* 62:79–87.

Payero, M. L. P., Correcher, B. L. and Garcia-Perez, A. 1985. Contact urticaria and dermatitis from phosphorous sesquisulphide. *Contact Dermatitis* 13:126–127.

Picardo, M., Rovina, R., Cristaudo, A., Cannistraci, C. and Santucci, B. 1988. Contact urticaria from *Tilia* (lime). *Contact Dermatitis* 19:72–73.

Pigatto, P. D., Riva, F., Altomare, G. F. and Parotelli, R. 1983. Short-term anaphylactic antibodies in contact urticaria and generalized anaphylaxis to apple. *Contact Dermatitis* 9:511.

Pinol, J. and Carapeto, F. J. 1984. Contact urticaria to etofenamate. *Contact Dermatitis* 11:132–133.

Reitamo, S., Visa, K., Kähönen, K., Käyhkö, K., Stubb, S. and Salo, O. P. 1986. Eczematous reactions in atopic patients caused by epicutaneous testing with inhalant allergens. *Br. J. Dermatol.* 114:303–309.

Reunala, T., Björksten, F., Förström, L. and Kanerva, L. 1983. IgE-mediated occupational allergy to a spider mite. *Clin. Allergy* 13:383–388.

Rilliet, A., Hunziker, N. and Brun, R. 1980. Alcohol contact urticaria syndrome (immediate type hypersensitivity). *Dermatologica (Basel)* 161:361.

Rivers, J. K. and Rycroft, R. J. G. 1987. Occupational allergic contact urticaria from colophony. *Contact Dermatitis* 17:181.

Rudzki, E. and Rebandel, P. 1985. Occupational contact urticaria from penicillin. *Contact Dermatitis* 13:192.

Rudzki, E., Rebandel, P. and Grzywa, Z. 1985. Incidence of contact urticaria. *Contact Dermatitis* 13:279.

Salo, O. P., Mäkinen-Kiljunen, S. and Juntunen, K. 1986. Milk causes a rapid urticarial reaction on the skin of children with atopic dermatitis and milk allergy. *Acta Derm. Venereol. (Stockh.)* 66:438–442.

Santucci, B., Cristaudo, A. and Picardo, M. 1985. Contact urticaria from papain in a soft lens solution. *Contact Dermatitis* 12:233.

Seifert, H. U., Wahl, R., Vocks. E., Borelli, S. and Maasch, H. J. 1987. Immunoglobulin E-vermittelte Kontakturtikaria bzw. Asthma bronchiale durch Latexenthaltende Haushaltsgummihandschuhe. *Dermatosen* 35:137–139.

Schewach-Millet, M. and Shpiro, D. 1985. Urticaria and angioedema due to topically applied chloramphenicol ointment. *Arch. Dermatol.* 121:587.

Shelley, W. B., Shelley, E. D. and Ho, A. K. S. 1983. Cholinergic urticaria: Acetylcholine-receptor-dependent immediate-type hypersensitivity reaction to copper. *Lancet* i:843–846.

Soschin, D. and Leyden, J. J. 1986. Sorbic acid-induced erythema and edema. *J. Am. Acad. Dermatol.* 14:234–241.

Spaner, D., Dolovich, J., Tarlo, S., Sussman, G. and Buttoo, K. 1989. Hypersensitivity to natural latex. *J. Allergy Clin. Immunol.* 83:1135–1137.

Steinman, H. K., Lovell, C. R. and Cronin, E. 1984. Immediate-type hypersensitivity to *Crataegus monogyna* (hawthorn). *Contact Dermatitis* 11:321.

Sterry, W. and Schmoll, M. 1985. Contact urticaria and dermatitis from self-adhesive pads. *Contact Dermatitis* 13:284–285.

Tachibana, S., Horio, T. and Hayakawa, M. 1977. Contact urticaria and dermatitis due to fluocinonide cream. *Acta Dermatol. (Kyoto)* 72:141.

Tanaka, T., Moriwaki, S. and Horio, T. 1987. Occupational dermatitis with simultaneous immediate and delayed allergy to *Chrysanthemum*. *Contact Dermatitis* 16:152–154.

Tee, R. D., Gordon, D. J., Hawkins, E. R., Nunn, A. J., Lacey, J., Venables, K. M., Cooter, R. J., McCaffery, A. R. and Newman Taylor, A. J. 1988. Occupational allergy to locusts: An investigation of the sources of the allergen. *J. Allergy Clin. Immunol.* 81:517–525.

Temesvari, E. 1984. Contact urticaria from paraphenylenediamine. *Contact Dermatitis* 11:125.

Tigalonowa, M., Braathen, L. R. and Lea, T. 1988. IgE on Langerhans cells in the skin of patients with atopic dermatitis and birch allergy. *Allergy* 43:464–468.

Tosti, A., Bettoli, V., Iannini, G. and Forlani, L. 1986. Contact urticaria from polypropylene. *Contact Dermatitis* 15:51.

Tosti, A., Melino, M. and Veronesi, S. 1987. Contact urticaria to tobacco. *Contact Dermatitis* 16:225–226.

Trunell, T. N., Waisman, M. and Trunell, T. L. 1985. Contact dermatitis caused by *Brucella*. *Cutis* 35:379–381.

Tuer, W. F., James, W. D. and Summers, R. J. 1986. Contact urticaria to O-phenylphenate. *Ann. Allergy* 56:19–21.

Tuft, L. and Blumstein, G. I. 1942. Studies in food allergy II. Sensitization to fresh fruits: Clinical and experimental observations. *J. Allergy* 13:574–581.

Turjanmaa, K. 1987. Incidence of immediate allergy to latex gloves in hospital personnel. *Contact Dermatitis* 17:270–275.

Turjanmaa, K. and Reunala, T. 1988. Contact urticaria from rubber gloves. *Dermatol. Clin.* 6:47–51.

Turjanmaa, K. and Reunala, T. 1989. Condoms as a source of latex allergen and cause of contact urticaria. *Contact Dermatitis* 20:360–364.

Turjanmaa, K., Reunala, T., Tuimala, R. and Kärkkäinen, T. 1988a. Allergy to latex gloves: Unusual complication during delivery. *Br. J. Dermatol.* 297:1029.

Turjanmaa, K., Reunala, T. and Räsänen, L. 1988b. Comparison of diagnostic methods in latex surgical glove contact urticaria. *Contact Dermatitis* 19:241–247.

Turjanmaa, K., Laurila, K., Mäkinen-Kiljunen, S. and Reunala, T. 1988c. Rubber contact urticaria. Allergenic properties of 19 brands of latex gloves. *Contact Dermatitis* 19:362–367.

Turjanmaa, K., Räsänen, L., Lehto, M., Mäkinen-Kiljunen, S. and Reunala, T. 1989. Basophil histamine release and lymphocyte proliferation tests in latex contact urticaria. *Allergy* 44:181–186.

Valdivieso, R., Moneo, I., Pola, J., Muñoz, T., Zapata, C., Hinojosa, M. and Losada, E. 1989. Occupational asthma and contact urticaria caused by buckwheat flour. *Ann. Allergy* 63:149–152.

Valsecchi, R. and Cainelli, T. 1987. Contact urticaria from nickel. *Contact Dermatitis* 17:187.

Valsecchi, R. and Cainelli, T. 1989. Contact urticaria from dog saliva. *Contact Dermatitis* 20:62.

Valsecchi, R., Foiadelli, L., Reseghetti, A. and Cainelli, T. 1986. Generalized urticaria from DNCB. *Contact Dermatitis* 14:254–255.

van der Meeren, H. L. M. and van Erp, P. E. J. 1986. Life-threatening contact urticaria from glove powder. *Contact Dermatitis* 14:190–191.

van Hecke, E. and Santosa, S. 1985. Contact urticaria to DNCB. *Contact Dermatitis* 12:282.

Varigos, G. A. and Nurse, D. S. 1986. Contact urticaria from methyl ethyl ketone. *Contact Dermatitis* 15:259–260.

Veien, N. K., Hattel, T., Justesen, O. and Norholm, A. 1987. Dietary restrictions in the treatment of adult patients with eczema. *Contact Dermatitis* 17:223–228.

von Krogh, G. and Maibach, H. I. 1982. The contact urticaria syndrome—1982. *Semin. Dermatol.* 1:59–66.

Wahl, R. and Kleinhans, D. 1989. IgE-mediated allergic reactions to fruit gums and investigation of cross-reactivity between gelatine and modified gelatine-containing products. *Clin. Exp. Allergy* 19:77–80.

Wallengren, J. and Möller, H. 1986. Effect of capsaicin on some experimental inflammations in human skin. *Acta Derm. Venereol. (Stockh.)* 66:375–380.

Weissenbach, T., Wutrich, B. and Weihe, W. H. 1988. Allergies to laboratory animals. An epidemiological, allergological study in persons exposed to laboratory animals. *Schweiz. Med. Wochenschr.* 118:930–938.

White, I. R. and Cronin, E. 1984. Irritant contact urticaria to diethyl fumarate. *Contact Dermatitis* 10:315.

Wilkin, J. K. and Fortner, G. 1985. Ethnic contact urticaria to alcohol. *Contact Dermatitis* 12:118–120.

Wrangsjö, K., Mellström, G. and Axelsson, G. 1986. Discomfort from rubber gloves indicating contact urticaria. *Contact Dermatitis* 15:79–84.

Wrangsjö, K., Wahlberg, J. E. and Axelsson, I. G. 1988. IgE-mediated allergy to natural rubber in 30 patients with contact urticaria. *Contact Dermatitis* 19:264–271.

Wuthrich, B. and Dietschi, R. 1985. The celery-carrot-mugwort-condiment syndrome: Skin test and RAST results. *Schweiz. Med. Wochenschr.* 115:258–264.

Yodoi, J. and Iskizaka, K. 1979. Lymphocytes bearing Fc-receptors for IgE. 1. Presence of human and rat lymphocytes with Fc-receptors. *J. Immunol.* 122:2577–2583.

Yoshikawa, M. 1985. Skin lesions of papular urticaria induced experimentally by *Chyletus malaccensis* and *Chelacaropsis* sp. (*Acari, Cheyletidae*). *J. Med. Entomol.* 22:115–117.

18

accurate spectral measurements of laboratory sources of optical radiation

■ Robert H. James ■ S. L. Matchette ■

INTRODUCTION

Experiments with biological systems offer an endless host of pitfalls and surprises. In photobiology the interpretation of results is complicated by at least two other potential variables, the radiation source and its measurement system. Meaningful and reproducible research in photobiology demands a knowledge of appropriate sources of optical radiation and the means of accurately measuring the output. This chapter will present a basic introduction to source selection and measurement, emphasizing the ultraviolet (UV) spectral region.

DEFINITIONS AND UNITS OF MEASUREMENT

Electromagnetic radiation is the energy that propagates through space and is sometimes referred to as radiant energy. It can be described as wave motion, which has three basic properties: frequency, wavelength, and velocity. These parameters are related to each other by the expression $v = f\lambda$, where frequency (f) is the number of vibrations per second, wavelength (λ) is the distance between corresponding points in two successive waves, and velocity (v) is the speed that the energy travels through space. An inverse relationship exists for wavelength and frequency. In a vacuum, the velocity of electromagnetic radiation is 3×10^8 m/s. Therefore, a wavelength of 600 nm corresponds to a frequency of 5×10^{14} Hz.

Optical radiation is a form of radiant energy and constitutes a portion of the electromagnetic spectrum, which is formed by arranging radiant energy according to wavelength (or frequency) (Fig. 1). The eye is sensitive only to a narrow region of the spectrum, commonly called "light." Radio waves have some of the longest wavelengths and are correspondingly the least energetic waves. As wavelengths become progressively shorter and more energetic, the following spectral regions are described: television, microwave, infrared (IR), visible light, ultraviolet (UV), x-ray, and gamma radiation.

Optical radiation falls in the middle of the spectrum and is commonly described as including IR radiation, visible light, and UV radiation. Infrared radiation has wavelengths longer than visible light, and ultraviolet radiation has wavelengths shorter than visible light. Infrared and UV radiation are sometimes incorrectly referred to as "light." More correctly, light refers only to that part of the electromagnetic spectrum that can be seen by the human eye. The Com-

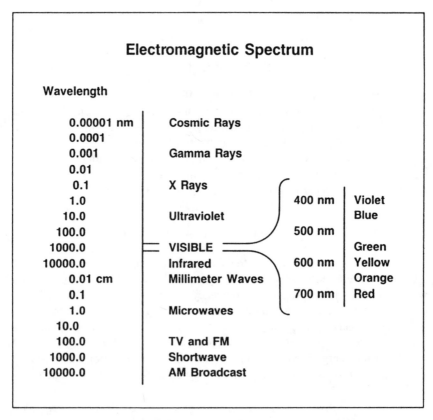

FIGURE 1 Electromagnetic spectrum.

mission Internationale de l'Eclairage (CIE, 1970) has further divided the optical radiation region into various parts (Fig. 2). For the UV region these are UVC (100–280 nm), UVB (280–315 nm), and UVA (315–400 nm). For the IR region the accepted divisions are IRA (760–1400 nm), IRB (1400–3000 nm), and IRC (3 μm to 1 mm). Visible light includes those wavelengths from 400 to 760 nm.

The System International (SI) units (SI Units, 1988) are used for all measurements in photobiology. Table 1 gives selected and commonly used SI units. Radiometric concepts may be used to describe (1) the radiation source, (2) the field surrounding a source, or (3) an irradiated surface. The basic unit of radiant energy emitted by a source is the joule (J). One joule delivered over 1 s constitutes 1 watt (W) of radiant power. Radiant exposure, also known as fluence, is the radiant energy per unit area incident upon a surface and is expressed as joules per square meter (J/m^2). Irradiance, sometimes referred to as fluence rate or optical flux density, is the radiant power per unit area incident upon a surface and is expressed in watts per square meter (W/m^2). Instruments that measure optical radiation are known as radiometers.

The emission spectra of radiation sources are often illustrated in the literature in terms of "relative intensity" versus wavelength. These portrayals can give relative amounts of energy within the various wavelength regions and can demonstrate spectral differences between sources. However, they may be of minimal use for reporting the magnitude of biological exposures. A quantitative and universally accepted way of describing an emission spectrum is the spectral power distribution or spectral irradiance. This is measured in W/m^2 per nanometer of wavelength interval (W/m$^2 \cdot$nm) at a given distance from the source. The most accurate and reproducible exposure data are obtained using information contained in the spectral power distribution of the radiation source. Instruments that measure the spectral power distribution in detail are called spectroradiometers.

The spectral bandpass is defined as the spectral width of a radiation field between those wavelengths where the power is one half maximum value. The spectral output of a source or the spectral sensitivity of a detector can be described in terms of its spectral bandpass.

PHOTOMETRY

We include this discussion on photometry because many suppliers of commercial light sources use photometric quantities to describe the optical radiation output of their products. Many simple, inexpensive light-measuring devices are available that are built and calibrated for photometric applications. It is important to distinguish the difference between photometry and radiometry. Photometry is restricted to the visible region of the spectrum, while radiometry describes the measurement of absolute radiant power or energy throughout the electromagnetic spectrum. The spectral region extending from a wavelength of 400 nm in the deep blue to 760 nm in the red is known as the visible region of

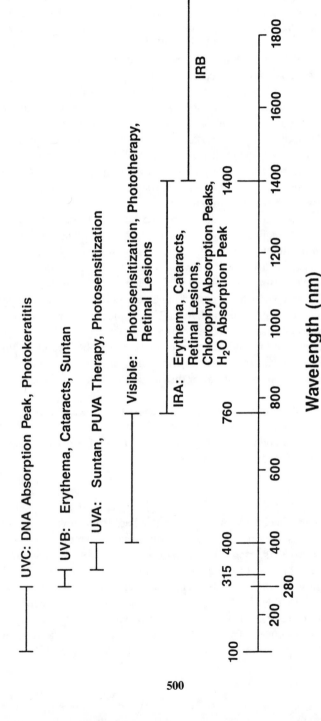

FIGURE 2 Optical radiation spectrum with selected biological end points.

TABLE 1 Relevant S.I. Units

Physical quantity	Unit name	Unit symbol
Energy (work energy)	Joule	J
Power (radiant flux)	Watt	W (J/s)
Radiant exposure (fluence)	Joule per square meter	J/m^2
Irradiance	Watt per square meter	W/m^2
Spectral irradiance	Watt per square meter per nanometer	W/m^2·nm

the spectrum because the energy elicits a visual response in the eye. A specialized science, photometry, has evolved around the measurement of visible light using instruments often referred to as photometers.

We need to define a unit of measurement by which we can quantify the subjective concept of brightness. In order to do this, the relative sensitivity of the eye of an average person has been established by the CIE across the spectrum from 380 to 780 nm. It is known as the relative sensitivity curve for the daylight standard observer, or photopic curve for daylight vision. Each wavelength is assigned a value for sensitivity, or luminous efficacy, and is represented by the symbol V_λ. The value of V_λ is 1 at a wavelength of 555 nm, where the eye is most sensitive in daylight conditions. The value for V_λ decreases for wavelengths shorter than 555 nm and for wavelengths longer than 555 nm, becoming zero at 380 and 780 nm. Detectors have been developed to quantitatively measure the photometric output of a source. They have spectral sensitivity curves designed to closely match the photopic sensitivity curve.

The measure of visual power coming from a source is called the lumen. A lumen is defined by the CIE in terms of the radiometric power coming from a source. One watt of monochromatic radiation at 555 nm provides 683 lumens of light. In order to convert the relative sensitivity curve to photometric values the photopic curve is multiplied by the luminous efficacy at 555 nm, which is 683 lumens/W. Figure 3 contains a graphic representation of this luminous efficacy curve. Fewer lumens of visible light will be produced for each watt of radiometric power at wavelengths either longer or shorter than 555 nm.

When light levels are low, the relative spectral sensitivity of the eye changes. This sensitivity curve is referred to as the scotopic curve for dark-adapted vision. The shape of the curve is similar to the photopic curve, but its peak sensitivity occurs at 512 nm. At 512 nm, 1 W of monochromatic radiation provides 1700 lumens of light (Fig. 3). This provides consistent definitions of the lumen, since at 555 nm, 1 W of radiation provides 683 lumens for both the photopic curve and scotopic curve.

In order to provide a value for the total amount of light being emitted from a source, the contributions from all of the emitted wavelengths are added together. For radiometric measurements, this is simply done by directly adding the output contributions from all emission wavelengths. For photometric mea-

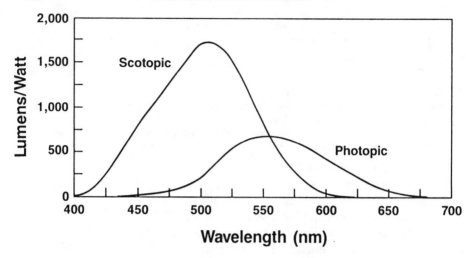

FIGURE 3 Photometric weighting functions.

surements, the spectral power distribution at each wavelength is multiplied by the luminous efficacy at that wavelength, and the results from 380 to 780 nm are added together.

Each radiometric quantity has a corresponding photometric counterpart. All photometric terms have the word "luminous" expressed in one form or another. Table 2 shows important radiometric units and their photometric "equivalents." An often used hybrid unit that has no corresponding unit in the CIE system is the foot-candle, defined to be an illumination of 1 lumen per square foot.

Photometry, then, deals with the measurement of light as perceived by the eye. As such, the sensitivity of photometers is limited to the spectral region from 380 to 780 nm and follows the daylight sensitivity curve established by the CIE as closely as possible. In order to measure UV or IR radiation as well as the radiometric output in the visible region, a radiometer is used. This instrument is designed to measure the absolute quantity of energy being emitted from the source without regard to spectral weighting functions.

SOURCE SELECTION

The two most important criteria in selecting a laboratory exposure source are (1) spectral output appropriate to the biological target to be studied and (2) source intensity. Power requirements, simplicity of operation, maintenance, cost, and lifetime are other considerations. Some lamps provide an almost continuous spectrum of radiation over a broad wavelength range, such as incandescent or xenon arc lamps, while others emit radiation within a narrow spectral region centered around one wavelength, such as germicidal UV lamps or lasers.

Consider the spectrum of a 15-W germicidal UV fluorescent lamp (Fig.

TABLE 2 Comparison of Radiometric and Photometric Units

Radiometric quantity	Unit	Photometric quantity	Unit
Radiant flux	Watt (W)	Luminous flux	Lumen (L)
Radiant intensity	W/sr	Luminous intensity	Candela (L/sr)
Irradiance	W/m²	Illuminance	L/m²

4). Almost all of its energy is emitted in one mercury line at a wavelength of 253.7 nm. The 15 W refers to the electrical input power, not the optical radiation power output, which is about 4 W. Power not emitted as optical radiation is usually dissipated as heat.

The germicidal lamp has become a widely used source of UVC radiation. UV-emitting fluorescent lamps coated with UVC and UVB absorbing phosphors can provide sources of UVA that are acceptable for most experiments involving biological systems. Figure 5 shows, however, that all UVA lamps are not equivalent. While both lamp 1 and lamp 2 emit optical radiation in the UVA spectral region, lamp 1 emits almost half of its energy below 350 nm whereas lamp 2 barely emits in that region. Other sources are available that, by nature of their natural spectra or specialized phosphor coatings, emit in a limited range of wavelengths. One such source is the low-pressure sodium lamp, which emits largely at 589 nm.

Generally, researchers studying the biological effects of UV radiation have relied on mercury-vapor-based lamps. The spectral output of ionized mercury lamps will vary with the lamp pressure, supplied power, and lamp envelope. The germicidal lamp, for example, is a low-pressure mercury vapor lamp. Figure 6 shows the spectral power distribution of a typical high-pressure mercury vapor lamp used to illuminate roadways. These lamps are manufactured with UV-absorbing glass envelopes, which remove all UVC and most UVB wavelengths. High-pressure mercury vapor lamps are also available with quartz envelopes, which allow for high UV transmission. These lamps are powerful sources of UVC as well as other visible wavelengths. In the laboratory, they generally require separate power sources and ventilation to remove the heat and ozone that are also produced.

The high-pressure mercury vapor lamp is a common source of broad-band optical radiation. Broad-band sources are used when specialized sources which emit specific wavelengths are not required or cannot be obtained. Figure 7 shows the spectrum of a xenon arc. Many solar simulators use a xenon arc as the source of radiation. The spectrum is nearly uniform over a wide wavelength range, including the UV, but it also contains wavelengths shorter than those normally present from the sun at the earth's surface. Little, if any, solar radiation at wavelengths shorter than 290 nm reach the surface of the earth due to atmospheric absorption. Xenon arc lamps also have significant IR output.

Other sources of broad-band radiation are metal halide lamps, which pro-

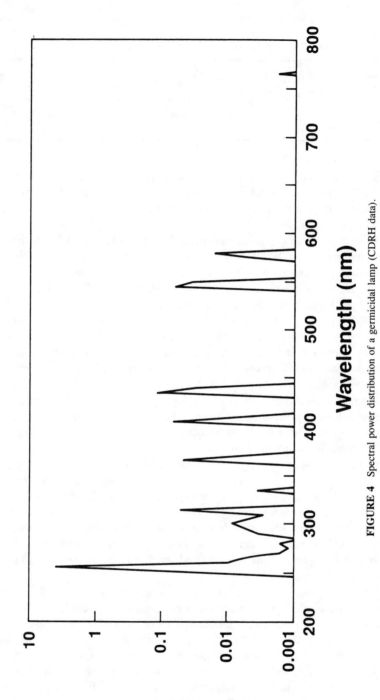

FIGURE 4 Spectral power distribution of a germicidal lamp (CDRH data).

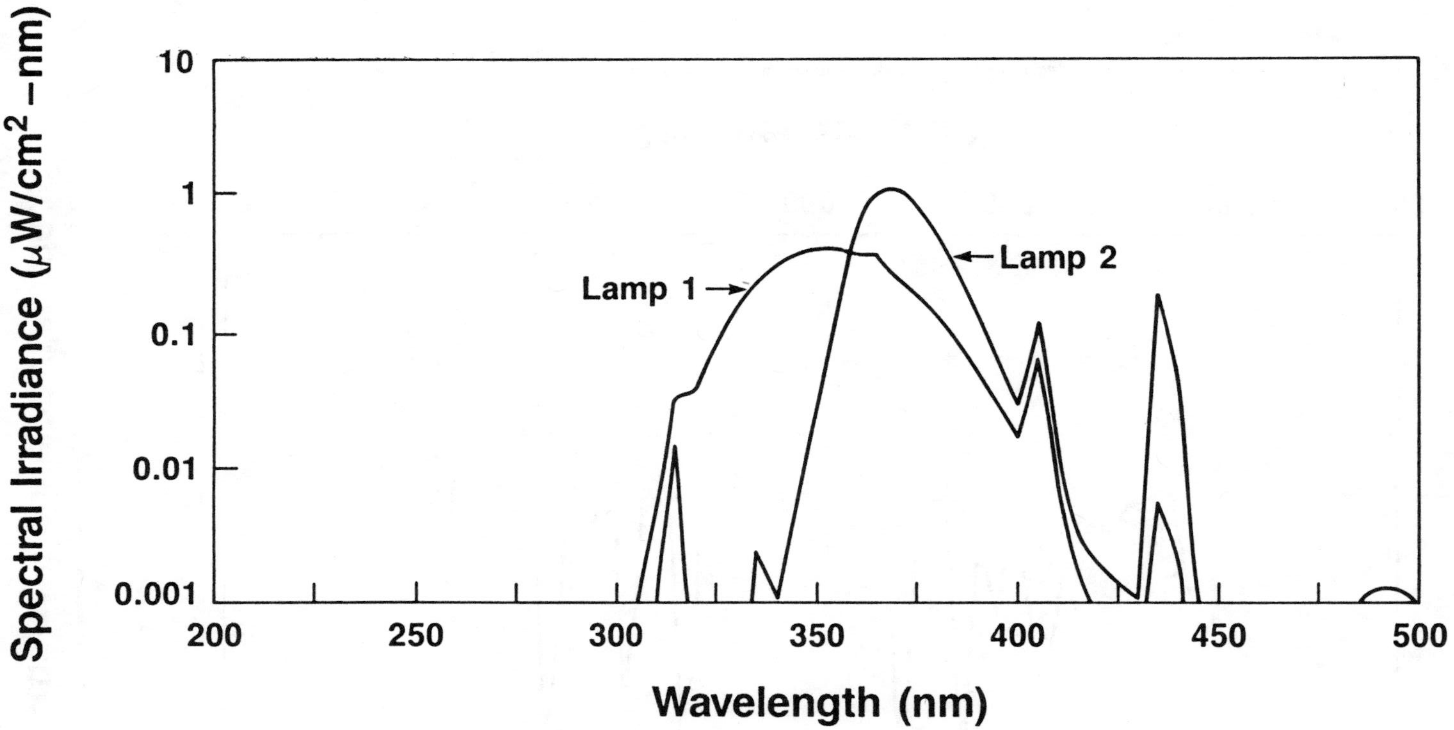

FIGURE 5 Spectral power distribution of UV fluorescent lamps (CDRH data).

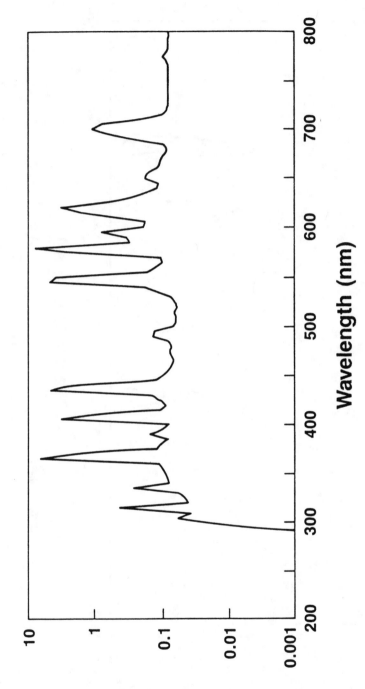

FIGURE 6 Spectral power distribution of a mercury vapor lamp (CDRH data).

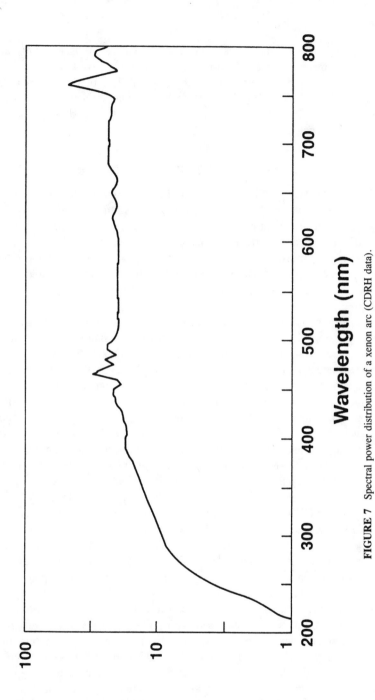

FIGURE 7 Spectral power distribution of a xenon arc (CDRH data).

duce intense UV and visible radiation along with some IR. Tungsten lamps and fluorescent lamps emit primarily in the visible region but have lower intensities than high-pressure mercury or xenon lamps. Regardless of the experimental protocol, some of the energy emitted from broad-band sources is usually not needed or useful. It is therefore desirable to eliminate unnecessary spectral energy before it reaches the sample.

BLOCKING UNWANTED WAVELENGTHS

Filter materials, commonly made of glass or plastic, are available to block unwanted wavelengths while transmitting desired radiation. Less frequently, liquid- or gas-filled cells may be used. It is sometimes difficult, however, to find filters that provide both a narrow wavelength band of transmittance and a high percent transmittance within that band. In addition, all filters reflect some radiation from their surfaces. Most transmit wavelengths other than those within the peak bandpass, and all attenuate the radiation passing through to some degree.

Manufacturers' labels and descriptions of filtering properties may be incomplete. Figure 8 depicts the transmittance curve of a commercially available filter, which, at first glance, transmits radiation from 220 to 500 nm, with wavelengths longer than 500 nm being blocked. However, the filter begins to transmit again at 640 nm and is still transmitting radiation at 1000 nm. Many filters have similar characteristics—transmitting radiation in the UV or visible region, blocking radiation in the red, and then transmitting in the IR. If a xenon arc lamp were being used for exposures, and this filter was chosen for its ability to block red and longer wavelengths, much undesirable IR radiation would be transmitted as well. The entire range of spectral transmittance needs to be evaluated before using a specific filter in an experiment.

Changes in filter transmittance can be induced by high levels (or long exposure times) of UV radiation from a source. Figure 9 shows transmittance curves of Pyrex glass when new and then after a period of UV exposure. Note that the transmittance has decreased and also that the spectral distribution of the transmitted radiation has changed. This illustrates the need to make periodic spectral measurements of filters used in the laboratory to monitor potentially significant changes in transmittance.

Absorbed heat can cause filter materials to crack. This occurs more often when IR-blocking filters are being used with high-intensity sources. Environmental contaminants, such as ozone produced by the source and high humidity, can also induce filter transmittance changes. High-quality filters should generally not be handled by bare hands, to avoid degradation induced by body oils.

Very narrow bands of radiation are transmitted by interference filters. These frequently consist of two metal films evaporated onto glass or quartz plates which are separated by a transparent dielectric material. The thickness of this intermediate layer is comparable to the wavelength to be passed. Figure 10

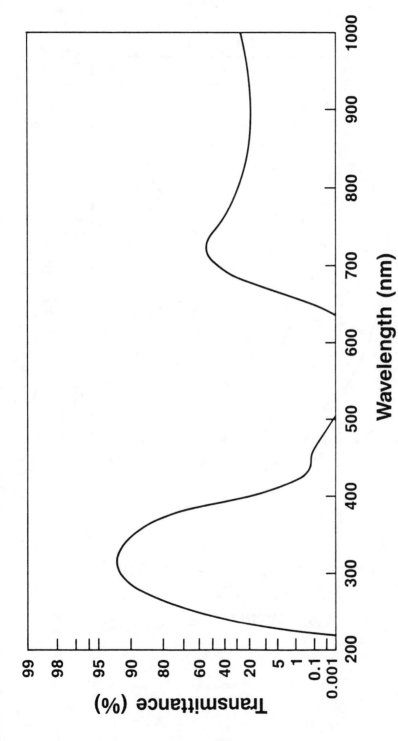

FIGURE 8   Spectral transmittance of Schott UG5 filter.

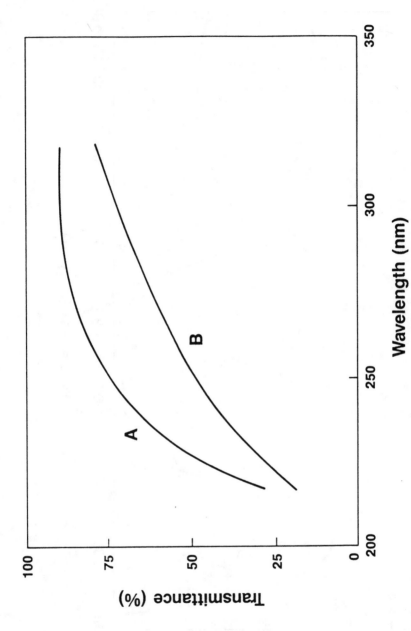

FIGURE 9 Spectral transmittance of Pyrex: A, new; B, following UV exposure.

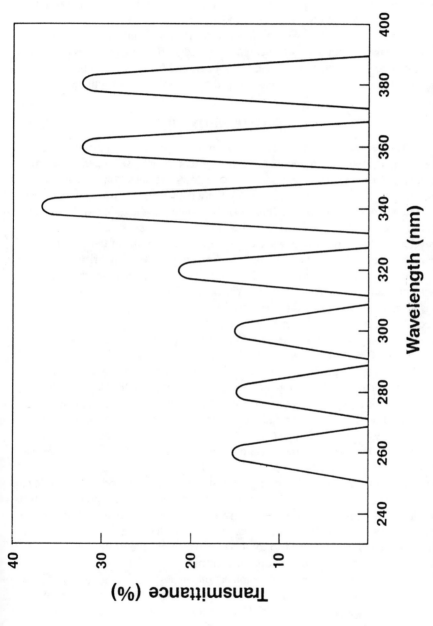

FIGURE 10 Spectral transmittance of UV bandpass filters (Corion Corp., 1983 Catalog, p. 82. Reprinted by permission).

shows transmittance curves of a set of UV bandpass interference filters. Band-pass filters reflect virtually all incident radiation except for the narrow region around the transmittance peak and can provide relatively high transmittance (up to 50%) for very narrow bandwidths (5-20 nm).

A frequently overlooked problem, especially with interference filters, is that the peak transmittance wavelength is dependent on the incident angle of the incoming beam. If the filter surface is not perpendicular to the radiation beam path the transmittance will increase, and the wavelength peak will shift.

THE MONOCHROMATOR

Another method of "filtering" a light source to produce the desired wavelengths is to use a monochromator system, which separates broadband radiation into its spectral components and allows the selection of a particular wavelength. For example, a beam of white light entering a prism will be spread out into its component colors (Fig. 11). The blue wavelengths are bent more than the red because the index of refraction of the prism is higher for shorter wavelengths. Any particular wavelength can be selected from the spectrum by placing narrow slits (on the order of 1 mm) on either side of the prism. One slit, positioned between the source and the prism, serves to narrow the beam of incident white light. The other slit, when placed on the opposite side of the prism, can be used to select a narrow band of the emerging wavelengths. A mechanism can be added to mechanically rotate the prism, which will allow the selection of any desired wavelength. For the UV spectral region, a quartz prism must be used, because glass does not efficiently transmit UV.

A diffraction grating is often used instead of a prism for obtaining mono-chromatic radiation. A grating consists of a substrate, usually glass, ruled with a series of parallel grooves that cover the grating surface, making it resemble a staircase (Fig. 12). Incoming radiation is reflected from each step's reflecting surface. Rays from adjoining steps arrive at a given point in space with different phases. Depending on the angle of incidence, constructive interference occurs only for a narrow band centered around selected wavelengths.

The performance of a grating depends on the quality and spacing of the grooves. The blaze wavelength defines that wavelength where a grating is most efficient. The efficiency falls off at wavelengths both longer and shorter than the blaze wavelength. Blazing is accomplished by changing the groove angle, shape, or depth. When tuned to the blaze wavelength, the grating groove surfaces have just the right orientation to emit radiation by simple specular (mirror) reflection. A more rigorous explanation of how a grating works can be found in many optics texts and reference manuals (Jenkins and White, 1957; Sliney and Wolbarsht, 1980; Oriel Corporation, 1985). Some gratings are engraved by a holographic process. These gratings reduce stray light to 1-10% of that observed for conventionally ruled gratings. To select a particular wavelength region, slits are placed at the input beam to the grating and at the exit

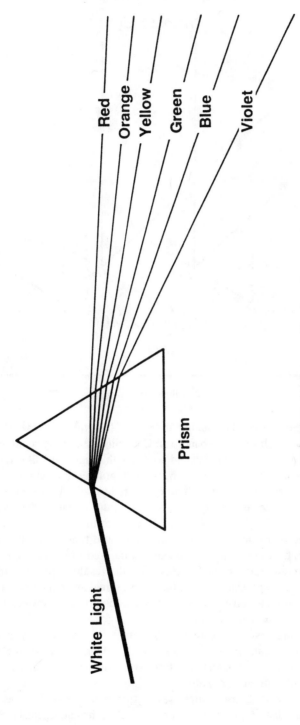

FIGURE 11 Light passage through a prism.

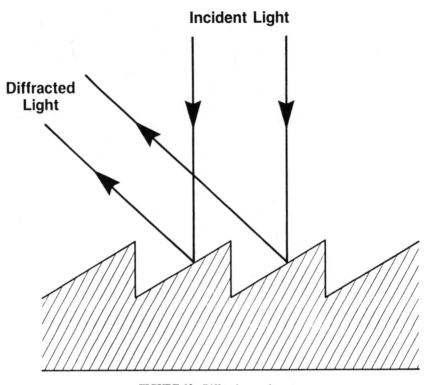

FIGURE 12   Diffraction grating.

reflection from the grating. The quality and size of the grating and width of the slits govern the monochromator's bandpass. Changing the grating rotation angle tunes the monochromator to the desired wavelength. Figure 13 illustrates the components of, and optical path through, a single grating monochromator.

The use of a monochromator significantly reduces the total energy to the sample from the source, especially if a spectrally pure output is desired. This can lead to unacceptably long experimental exposure times. The use of wider slits will produce more intensity and shorter exposure times but will broaden the spectral output. A high-intensity source can be used to increase the output intensity and shorten exposure times. However, the resulting increase in stray light may degrade the spectral purity of the output signal and complicate experimental results. Thus, the investigator must often compromise between desired exposure times and optimal spectral quality.

Delivering the desired radiation to the sample location can be challenging. A series of lenses and mirrors is most often used where on-axis irradiation is difficult or impossible to achieve. Alternatively, an optical fiber coupled to the output slits of a monochromator or other source can be used to direct radiation where needed. Lenses, mirrors, and fibers have optical properties of their own that can distort the desired output wavelengths and intensity. Special lens materials (e.g., quartz, calcium fluoride) are necessary for transmission of UV radiation. Readily available optical fibers may not efficiently transmit, and may be degraded by, UVC.

Finally, most sources require a warm-up period. Spectral quality and output radiation of some sources can vary significantly during the first few minutes of operation. An acceptable warm-up time is usually 20 min to ½ h.

LASERS

Lasers produce very intense monochromatic radiation and are often used in photobiology experiments. Lasers emit energy at specific wavelengths and power levels depending on the type of laser, and operate in either a continuous-wave (CW) or pulsed mode. Average power levels up to several watts and pulses as short as 10 ns are common. Table 3 lists some properties of available

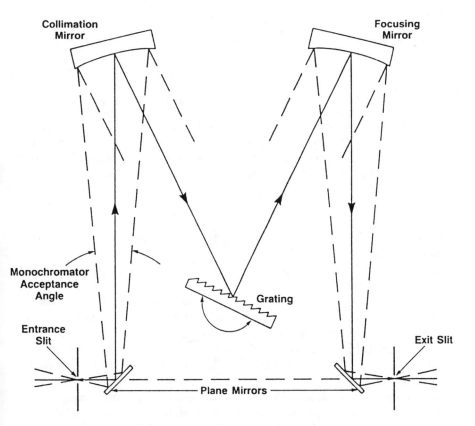

FIGURE 13 Optical path in a typical monochromator.

TABLE 3 Common Lasers

Laser	Wavelength (nm)
Excimer	
ArF	193
KrCl	222
KrF	248
XeF	350
Helium–cadmium	325, 441.6
Nitrogen	337.1
Argon	488, 514.5, other UV/visible
Krypton	568.2, 647.1, other UV/visible
Gold vapor	628
Helium–neon	632.8, IR
Ruby	694.3
Gallium arsenide	850, 905
Neodymium	1060, 530, others
Carbon dioxide	10,600
Tunable dye	UV/Visible/IR

lasers. A more detailed discussion on the use of lasers as light sources can be found in Sliney and Wolbarsht (1980).

SOURCE MEASUREMENTS

The many potential variables associated wtih sources, filters, and other optical components previously described indicate the need for accurate measurements of source parameters such as intensity, beam uniformity, and spectral purity as "seen" by the sample to be irradiated. We should point out here that the term "calibration" is often used in situations where the term "measurement" is more correct. Calibration more correctly refers to the intercomparison of data obtained with a common laboratory measuring instrument against some known standard device. The calibrated instrument is then used to measure the output of the source. The following paragraphs will discuss several generic types of detectors that are used for measuring the output parameters of laboratory light sources.

A calorimeter is a heat-sensing detector that measures total energy output of a source by absorbing the radiation in a receiver, which may be a piece of metal coated with a black surface, usually flat black paint. The absorbed radiation causes a temperature rise, which is converted into an electrical signal by a thermocouple, thermopile, or thermistor. The electrical signal can be used to calculate the energy in joules. This type of detector is equally sensitive to radiation from a wide range of wavelengths, which can cause problems because infrared radiation emitted from persons and objects in the room can also be detected. Other disadvantages include a slow response time and the frequent inability to measure levels of radiation less than 10 mJ. Because of these disadvantages, calorimeters are rarely used in photobiology experiments.

Photodetectors are more commonly used to measure optical power. Examples of these are silicon photodiodes, vacuum photodiodes, and photomultipliers. The spectral sensitivity of these devices depends upon the photosensitive material being used. All of these detectors operate by directly converting photons of optical radiation energy to electrical current. They are typically very sensitive to levels of radiation as low as 1 nW, and will respond rapidly to changes in the level of radiation (less than 1 ns for some detectors). All of these devices have a strong spectral dependence—that is, their sensitivity varies with wavelength. Figure 14 shows the spectral sensitivity curves for three types of photodiodes. Some photodiodes are relatively insensitive in the wavelength region from 200 to 380 nm. A small amount of another substance can be added to the detector material (doping) to make a photodiode more sensitive in the UV region. Some silicon detectors are supplied for use with an appropriate filter to yield a flat spectral response over an extended range. Additionally, there are filter–detector combinations available that utilize spectrally weighted UV filters to match certain biological weighting curves, such as the standard daylight observer curve or the threshold limit values for UV radiation published by the American Conference of Governmental Industrial Hygienists (ACGIH, 1989). Regardless of which photodetector one selects, the instrument must be calibrated at each wavelength where it will be used, unless it has a uniform response over the wavelength range of interest.

Pyroelectric detectors measure the rate of thermal change in a crystalline material. Pyroelectric materials are crystals that have permanent dipoles whose degree of polarization varies with temperature. Any change in polarization results in the generation of a surface charge on the crystal, which is then measured electronically. Response times of 1 ns and sensitivities about 10 μJ are typical. Since pyroelectric detectors can "see" only pulsed signals, a CW beam must be chopped to give a pulsed input to the crystal.

None of the aforementioned detectors can be used to obtain detailed spectral information from the source. A complete characterization of the experimental source needs to include spectral distribution, as well as power and energy. The preferred instrument for measuring the spectral output of a source is the spectroradiometer.

SPECTRORADIOMETRY

As explained before, when used as a radiation source, the monochromator transmits a limited region of the spectrum emitted by a broad-band source of radiation. A spectroradiometer can be described as a monochrometer with a detector attached to measure the output radiation from a source. A typical spectroradiometer consists of four major components: input optics, double-grating monochromator, detector, and electronic controls to operate the system

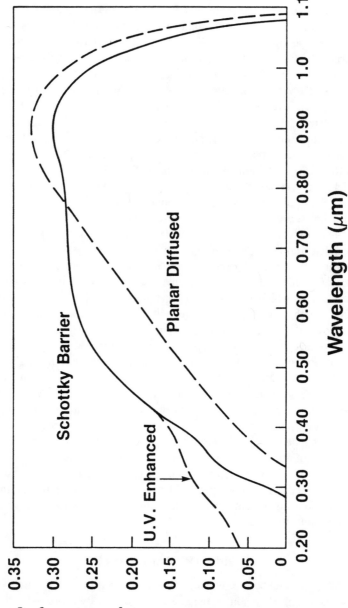

FIGURE 14 Spectral responsivity for silicon pin photodiodes (James, 1976).

and record the data. A high-quality laboratory system will have the capability of measuring radiation from 200 to 800 nm, with a minimum bandpass of 1 nm. The instrument will scan through a spectrum and record the spectral intensity as a function of wavelength.

An input optic collects radiation from the source to be measured and usually consists of an integrating sphere (Fig. 15). This hollow, metal sphere is coated on the inside surface with a reflective material, often barium sulfate, but other materials such as Teflon are also used. These materials reflect fairly uniformly over a broad spectral range from UV to near IR. Examples of other types of input devices are coated reflecting plates or direct field of view optics.

From the integrating sphere, collected radiation usually passes through a

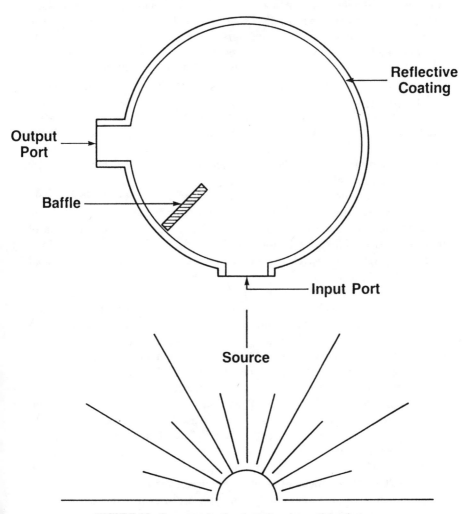

FIGURE 15 Transverse section through an integrating sphere.

quartz lens, which allows UV wavelengths to be transmitted and focuses the radiation onto the input slit of the monochromator. The monochromator, described earlier (Fig. 16), separates broad-based radiation into its spectral components by incorporating a diffraction grating (or prism), which is mechanically rotated to scan through the desired spectral region. Unwanted radiation can pose a serious problem. The exit beam from a spectroradiometer is frequently assumed to be monochromatic. However, even with the best gratings and monochromator designs other wavelengths are usually present as well. One can significantly reduce short-wavelength second-order radiation by positioning a filter wheel before the input slit. These order-sorting filters are automatically inserted at predetermined wavelengths during the scanning operation to block shorter wavelength radiation as the monochromator scans through the spectrum. Stray radiation may also be reduced by using a second monochromator system in tandem with the first. Using a double-grating monochromator system is especially desirable when measuring low levels of UV in the presence of high levels of visible light. Typically, spectroradiometer systems will be supplied as double-grating systems. Figure 17 shows typical scattering curves for a single- and a double-grating system.

Radiation from the double monochromator passes through an output slit and is usually detected by a photomultiplier tube sensitive to wavelengths in the region of 200–800 nm. If the detector is cooled below ambient temperature, thermal electronic noise will be significantly reduced. Cooled photomultiplier housings are available from several vendors.

The output current of the detector is proportional to the radiation incident on the detectors. This current can be input to the signal amplifiers and digitized for processing and recording by computer. The computer will usually control the functions of the spectroradiometer, including reading the voltage of the detector, operating the wavelength drive, and reading and processing the signal output.

All spectroradiometers should be calibrated before they are used. The preferred method of calibration uses a standard of spectral irradiance, or standard lamp, calibrated by the National Institute for Standards and Technology (NIST) (Walker et al., 1987), formerly known as the National Bureau of Standards (NBS). A typical standard lamp consists of a tungsten filament with halogen gas fill and a quartz envelope. It is commonly operated from a regulated direct current power supply. To increase the lifetime of the lamp by eliminating high current shocks when the lamp is turned on, the power supply should have a current ramp feature that gradually increases the current from zero to the operating value. The spectral output of the NIST standard lamps is well characterized over the wavelength region from 250 to 1600 nm, and is accurate to about 5% in the UV and 2% in the visible and IR. For the wavelength region spanning 200–350 nm, deuterium lamps are used as standards.

The spectroradiometer is calibrated by measuring the output of a standard lamp and comparing that output to the known NIST values. The standard lamp

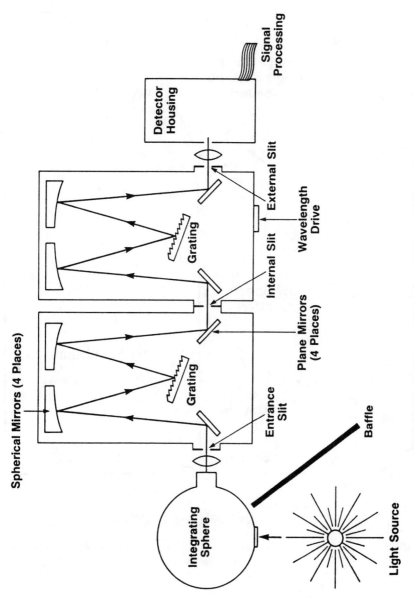

FIGURE 16 Optical path in a double-grating spectroradiometer.

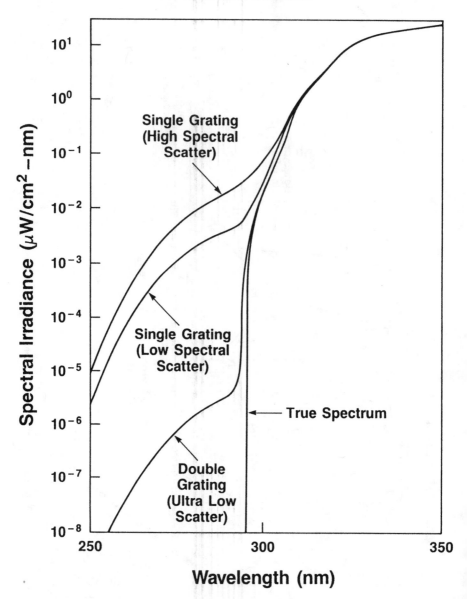

FIGURE 17   Light scatter in a spectroradiometer (Sliney and Wolbarsht, 1980, p. 448. Reprinted by permission).

is normally positioned at a distance of 50 cm from the input aperture of the integrating sphere. After scanning through the desired spectral range, the computer generates a calibration curve by dividing the known lamp output by the detector output signal for each wavelength. The resulting calibration factor is not linear with wavelength, and in the UV changes rather dramatically with a small change in wavelength.

After calibration, the spectroradiometer can be used to measure the output of a laboratory source. The system scans through the desired wavelength region and the computer records the detector current. An absolute output spectrum of the source is generated by multiplying the previously computed calibration curve by the detector current at each individual wavelength. The results can then be interpreted in several ways, including summing the values over a given wavelength range, and weighting the values with various biological action spectra.

FURTHER CAUTIONS

The detector input aperture should be placed as close to the experimental location as possible. Radiation exposure varies with distance from the source. If the source–sample distance is 50 cm, and the detector is placed at 40 cm, the measured irradiance will usually be more than what the sample receives. If it is not possible to place the detector exactly where the experimental sample is located, a distance correction factor can be applied to the measurements. The inverse-square analysis is sometimes used to correct for the effects of distance. However, since most sources are not point sources, this analysis must be applied very carefully. For example, values obtained at a distance of 50 cm do not normally yield the expected factor of 4 greater than the values obtained at 100 cm. Different lamps, reflectors, and lamp housing geometries all have a bearing on how exposure varies with distance. An empirical determination of the exposure variation as a function of distance can be made with a simple broad-band detector. The results can be used to correct any spectral measurements that may be made at a distance different from the sample exposure distance. Each specific exposure configuration will have a different distance correction function.

Considerable intensity variations may be present in the exposure plane. An interesting example of measurements taken of an actual source exposure plane is shown in Fig. 18 (Hitchins et al., 1986). If the sample is placed at one edge of the field, it will receive a different exposure level than if placed at the opposite edge of the field. The intensity distribution over the exposure plane is dependent on the lamp, lamp housing, and other elements in the optical system. The same broad-band detector, mentioned above, equipped with a small aperture at the detector surface, can be used to examine the intensity variations over the exposure plane. A more comprehensive discussion of sources of error in optical radiation measurements can be found in Landry et al. (1987).

The actual exposure to a biological sample will be affected by any sur-

R. H. James and S. L. Matchette

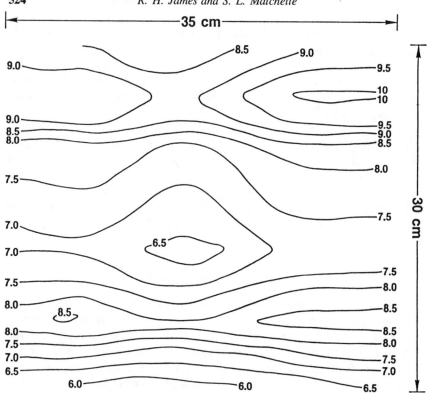

**UVASUN-2000 Exposure Area
Irradiance Contour Map (mW/cm²)**

FIGURE 18 Intensity variation over the exposure plane. Numbers indicate relative intensity (Hitchins et al., 1986. Reprinted by permission).

rounding media. Constituents in media, buffers, culture dish covers, etc., can absorb radiation in the desired spectral region. It is also a mistake to assume that incident energy is the same as absorbed energy. The spectral energy passing through the sample should be measured as well as the incident spectrum. The actual energy absorbed is the difference between the incident energy and the transmitted energy. One should remember, however, that certain experimental conditions may result in a significant quantity of reflected radiation, which is often difficult to measure.

DISCUSSION

The process of making accurate measurements can be expensive and time consuming. If a spectroradiometer is not directly available, there are alternative ways to keep track of exposure parameters. The spectrum of the radiation source must still be measured from time to time, and there are a number of laboratories that can be contracted to do this. A relatively inexpensive, broad-band detector can be used in the local laboratory on a daily basis for routine monitoring of exposure parameters as long as the source spectrum is stable.

All measurements should be performed with all optical elements and types of lamps that will be used during the experiments. After the spectral emission curve has been obtained it can be integrated to obtain the total spectral power. The broad-band detector can then be placed at the same location where the spectral measurements were made. The total spectral power as measured by the spectroradiometer is then divided by the detector reading to obtain the calibration factor to use for daily monitoring of the radiation source.

The calibration factor obtained in this way is valid only for a specific source–detector combination in a given spectral region. For example, if a filter were to be changed on the source, the spectral output distribution could change, and the instrument calibration factor might no longer be valid. In addition, the calibration factor calculated for one spectral region may not be valid for use in another spectral region.

In summary, since the optical components of any experimental exposure situation can change with time and the environment, meaningful and reproducible experimental results depend on frequent, accurate spectral irradiance measurements. The preferred instrument for obtaining such accuracy is a spectroradiometer. A simple broad-band detector may be used for day-to-day monitoring of the sources to track output stability. This detector is calibrated by referencing it to spectroradiometric measurements. The detector itself should be sent back to the manufacturer or to an independent calibration laboratory, for a recalibration on a regular basis to be sure it is operating satisfactorily.

The following checklist may be helpful in designing and executing an experiment. This may avoid some of the problems normally associated with this process. This list is not meant to be all-inclusive, but can serve as a useful starting point.

1. Select a source that emits radiation at the appropriate wavelengths for the experiment. Also be sure that appropriate filter materials or devices are available to block radiation outside of the spectral region of interest. This can be confirmed by spectral measurement of the output. Do not rely on lamp specifications.

2. If using lasers, be sure the emissions are appropriate—that is, CW, pulsed, Q-switched, etc. High peak powers from pulsed lasers should not be measured with an instrument designed for CW only. This will lead to incorrect results.

3. Check filters to be sure they have not deteriorated with long-term UV exposure or other use. Are they continuing to filter out the undesired radiation? It is best to measure the spectrum of the lamp with any filters in place to be sure of this.

4. Check the exposure chamber and ambient environment, including cover glasses, ambient room lights, and shiny or white surfaces for reflections that may alter exposure levels.

5. Be sure the measurement instrument is sensitive to, and calibrated at, the wavelengths and power levels being used. Measurement equipment sensitivity can change dramatically with the wavelength and intensity. If measuring pulsed radiation, be sure the detector and electronics are capable of accurately responding to the temporal variations of the exposure source. Also be sure the calibration is kept up-to-date, ideally at least once a year.

6. Be sure the detector aperture is placed as close to the experimental exposure point as possible in order to measure accurately the actual exposure levels. Also, measure the source output and begin the actual exposures only after the source has warmed up.

7. Determine the uniformity of the radiation over the exposure plane. Changes in exposure level with position can dramatically affect results.

8. Be sure to monitor the exposure parameters on a regular basis—once a day or once a week. Be sure the spectral irradiance at the exposure plane is checked regularly using a spectroradiometer to check for source or filter changes.

REFERENCES

American Conference of Governmental Industrial Hygienists. 1989. Threshold Limit Values for Chemical Substances and Physical Agents in the Work Environment with Intended Changes for 1989–90. Cincinnati: ACGIH.

Commission Internationale de l'Eclairage (International Commission on Illumination). 1970. International Lighting Vocabulary, Publication CIE No. 17.

Hitchins, V. M., Withrow, T. J., Olvey, K. M., Harleston, B. A., Ellingson, O. L. and Bostrom, R. G. 1986. The cytotoxic and mutagenic effects of UVA radiation on L51784 mouse lymphoma cells. *Photochem. Photobiol.* 44:53–57.

James, R. H., ed. 1976. National Conference on Measurements of Laser Emissions for Regulatory Purposes. FDA publication 76-8037.

Jenkins, F. A. and White, H. E. 1957. *Fundamentals of Optics.* New York: McGraw-Hill.

Landry, R. J., Barnes, R. and Mohan, K. 1987. Sources and measurements of optical radiation for medical applications. In *Photomedicine,* vol. 3, eds. E. Ben-Hur, and I. Rosenthal, Chapter 6. Boca Raton, Fla.: CRC Press.

Oriel Corporation. 1985. *Light Sources, Monochromators, Detection Systems,* vol. II, pp. 105–106. Stratford, Conn.:Oriel Corp.

SI Units, Conversion Factors and Abbreviations (Revised). 1988. *Photochem. Photobiol.* 47:1.

Sliney, D. and Wolbarsht, M. 1980. *Safety with Lasers and Other Optical Sources.* New York: Plenum Press.

Walker, J. H., Saunders, R. D., Jackson, J. K. and McSparron, D. A. 1987. Spectral Irradiance Calibrations at NBS. National Bureau of Standards (U.S.) special publication 250-20.

19

light–induced dermal toxicity: effects on the cellular and molecular level

■ Andrija Kornhauser ■ Wayne G. Wamer ■ Lark A. Lambert ■

INTRODUCTION

Die Sonne ist auch da wenn die Wolken schwarz und undurchdringlich scheinen.—Ernst Jucker[1]

Toxicology has evolved as a multidisciplinary field of study and is still in rapid evolutionary development. As such, toxicology overlaps many other basic biomedical disciplines, including biochemistry, pharmacology, and physiology. A recent event in this development has been the intersection of toxicology with photobiology, opening the field of phototoxicology.

Sunlight is the most potent environmental agent influencing life on the earth. Historically, exposure to the sun has been believed to be healthful and beneficial. It has only recently become apparent that many of the effects of solar radiation are detrimental. In a broad sense, therefore, the evolution of life can be regarded as a continuous adaptation to light by simultaneously utilizing solar energy and protecting against its detrimental effects.

Modern civilization presents a challenge for basic phototoxicologic research. This challenge arises from alterations in the life-style of a large portion of the population, including holiday trips, clothing styles, and particularly the fashion of suntanning among Caucasians. It is also possible that environmental factors may change the spectral characteristics of light reaching the earth's

[1] *"The sun is still present even when the clouds seem dark and impenetrable."* From *Ein gutes Wort zur rechten Zeit*, Verlag Paul Haupt, Bern, 1957.

surface. Many of these factors lead to an essentially increased exposure to light for a large segment of the population (Fitzpatrick et al., 1974; Urbach, 1989). Furthermore, in the past decade, phototoxic reactions to drugs, cosmetics, and many industrial and environmental chemicals have become an important health problem.

Definitions of phototoxicity are numerous and frequently inconsistent. In the broadest sense, any toxicity induced by photons can be termed photosensitivity. Photosensitivity may involve either photoallergies or nonimmunologic photoinduced skin reactions. Phototoxicity is used to describe all nonimmunologic light-induced toxic skin reactions. Sunburn is the most frequently occurring phototoxic reaction, requiring only the interaction of ultraviolet (UV) light with skin. In most cases of phototoxicity, however, we deal with an endogenous or exogenous chemical (chromophore) that absorbs light and transfers the energy to, or reacts in the excited state with, cellular components. Such toxic reactions would most properly be termed chemical phototoxicity.

Chronic phototoxic exposure can lead to neoplastic changes. It has been established that the consequence of lifelong enhanced exposure to light is a significant increase in skin tumors (Urbach et al., 1974), including basal and squamous cell carcinomas and, to a certain extent, malignant melanomas. This is confirmed by the pronounced increase in frequency of skin cancers in that part of the population, particularly those Celts and Teutons that in the course of history settled in regions with higher solar irradiation (Africa, Australia, and North America).

Phototoxicity studies, particularly those related to human disorders, have so far been based predominately on gross anatomic or histological procedures. Although our knowledge of the molecular events that occur during these processes is rapidly growing, much basic research remains to be done. In this chapter we discuss some molecular and cellular events that take place on exposure to light.

LIGHT CHARACTERISTICS

Aside from artificial light sources, solar radiation is the primary source of light that elicits biological effects. A portion of the solar spectrum containing the biologically most active region (290–700 nm) is shown in Fig. 1.

The UV part of the spectrum includes wavelengths from 200 to 400 nm. Portions of the UV spectrum have distinctive features from both the physical and medical points of view. The accepted designations for the biologically important parts of the UV spectrum are UVA, 320–400 nm; UVB, 290–320 nm; and UVC, 220–290 nm (Fig. 2).

Wavelengths less than 290 nm (UVC) do not occur at the earth's surface, since they are absorbed, predominantly by ozone, in the stratosphere. The most thoroughly studied photobiological reactions that occur in skin are induced by UVB. Although UVB wavelengths represent only approximately 1.5% of the

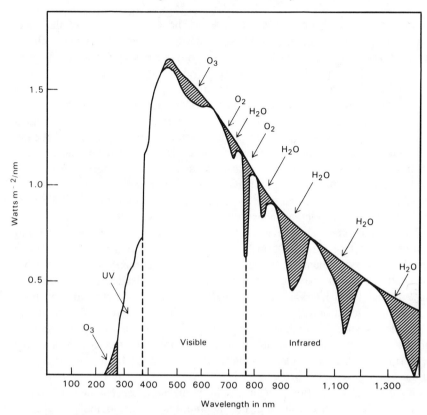

FIGURE 1 Spectrum of solar energy received at the earth's surface. The absorption bands of atmospheric O_2, O_3, and H_2O are shown. Modified from Hynek (1951).

solar energy received at the earth's surface (World Health Organization, 1979), they elicit most of the known biological effects. Light distributed over these wavelengths inhibits cell mitosis, makes vitamin D, and induces sunburn and skin cancer. The UVA region elicits most of the known chemical phototoxic and photoallergic reactions. It has been proposed that the longer wavelengths of the UVA spectrum (UVA I: 340–400 nm) are less detrimental than the shorter UVA wavelengths (UVA II: 320–340 nm) (National Institutes of Health Consensus

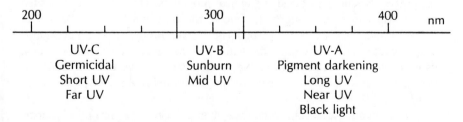

FIGURE 2 Biologically important regions of the UV spectrum.

Development Conference Statement, 1989). The visible portion of the spectrum, representing about 50% of the sun's energy received at sea level, includes wavelengths from 400 to 700 nm. Visible light is necessary for such biological events as photosynthesis, circadian cycles, and vision. Furthermore, visible light in conjunction with certain chromophores (e.g., dyes, drugs, and endogenous compounds) and molecular oxygen induces photodynamic effects.

Understanding the toxic effects of light impinging on the skin requires knowledge of the skin's optical properties. Skin may be viewed as an optically nonhomogeneous medium, composed of three layers that have characteristic refractive indices, chromophore distributions, and light-scattering properties. Light of wavelengths between 250 and 3000 nm entering the outermost layer of the skin, the stratum corneum, is in part reflected approximately 4–7% due to the difference in refractive index between air and stratum corneum (Fresnel reflection) (Anderson and Parrish, 1981). Absorption by urocanic acid (a deamination product of histidine), melanin, and proteins containing the aromatic amino acids tryptophan and tyrosine in the stratum corneum produces further attenuation of light, particularly at shorter UV wavelengths. Approximately 40% of the UVB is transmitted through the stratum corneum to the viable epidermis (Everett et al., 1966). The light entering the epidermis is attenuated by scattering and, predominately, absorption. Epidermal chromophores consist of proteins, urocanic acid, nucleic acids, and melanin. Passage through the epidermis results in appreciable attenuation of UVA and particularly UVB radiation. The transmission properties of the dermis are largely due to scattering, with significant absorption of visible light by melanin, carotenoids, and blood-borne pigments such as bilirubin, hemoglobin, and oxyhemoglobin. Light traversing these layers of the skin is extensively attenuated, most drastically for wavelengths less than 400 nm. Longer wavelengths are more penetrating. It has been noted that there is an "optical window," that is, greater transmission for light at wavelengths of 600–1300 nm, which may have important biological consequences (Anderson and Parrish, 1981). These features are presented in Fig. 3.

Normal variations in the skin's melanin content may result in changes in the attenuation of light, particularly in those wavelengths between 300 and 400 nm, by up to 1.5 times more in Negroes than in Caucasians (Pathak, 1967). Alterations in the amount or distribution of other natural chromophores account for further variations in the skin's optical properties. Urocanic acid deposited on the skin's surface during perspiration (Anderson and Parrish, 1981), and UV-absorbing lipids excreted in sebum (Beadle and Burton, 1981), may significantly reduce UV transmission through the skin. Epidermal thickness, which varies over regions of the body and increases after exposure to UVB radiation, may significantly modify UV transmission (Soffen and Blum, 1961; Parrish and Jaenicke, 1981).

Certain disease states also produce alterations in the skin's optical properties. Alteration of the skin's surface, such as by psoriatic plaques, decreases

Wavelength in Nanometers

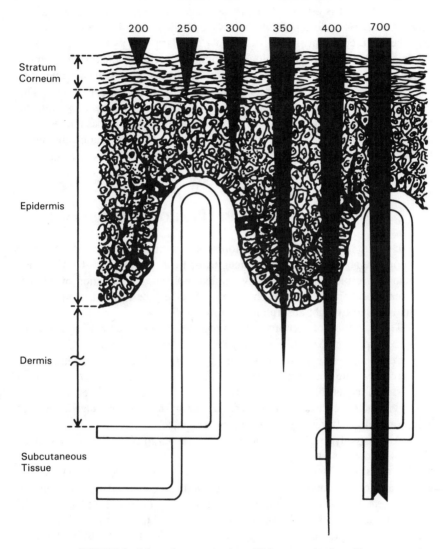

FIGURE 3 Schematic representation of light penetration into skin.

transmitted light. This effect may be lessened by application of oils whose refractive index is similar to that of skin (Anderson and Parrish, 1981). Disorders such as hyperbilirubinemia, porphyrias, and blue skin nevi result in increased absorption of visible light due to accumulation or altered distribution of chromophoric endogenous compounds.

The penetration of light into and through dermal tissues has important consequences. Skin, as the primary organ responsible for thermal regulation, is

A. Kornhauser et al.

overperfused with blood relative to its metabolic requirements (Anderson and Parrish, 1981). It is estimated that the average cutaneous blood flow is 20–30 times that necessary to support the skin's metabolic needs. The papillary boundaries between epidermis and dermis allow capillary vessels to lie close to the skin's surface, permitting the blood and important components of the immune system to be exposed to light. The equivalent of the entire blood volume of an adult may pass through the skin, and potentially be irradiated, in 20 min. This corresponds to the time required to receive 1–2 MEDs.[2] The accessibility of incident radiation to blood has been exploited in such regimens as phototherapy of hyperbilirubinemia in neonates, where light is used as a therapeutic agent. However, in general there is a potential for light-induced toxicity due to irradiation of blood-borne drugs and metabolites.

FUNDAMENTAL CONCEPTS IN PHOTOCHEMISTRY

Damage to cells through a photoreaction is initiated at the site where the chromophore absorbs specific wavelengths of light. Absorption of UV or visible photons results in electronically excited molecules; dissipation of this energy may result in an adverse phototoxic effect on the cell. The sequence of events initiated by light absorption is shown in Fig. 4.

The transition of a ground-state molecule to an excited singlet electronic state accompanies absorption of a visible or UV photon. Molecules in their singlet excited states exist for only about 10^{-8}–10^{-9} s before either returning to the ground state or converting (intersystem crossing) to a long-lived (10^{-4}–10^1 s) metastable triplet state. Both excited singlet and triplet states relax to the ground state through (1) transfer of energy to another molecule and (2) emission of light (fluorescence or phosphorescence) or release of heat.

Alternatively, the excited molecule may undergo photochemistry such as cis-trans isomerization, fragmentation, ionization, rearrangement, and intermolecular reactions. The probability that an excited molecule will choose any given path to the ground state depends on both its molecular structure and its environment and may be determined experimentally (Turro, 1965).

All these factors, such as light absorption, the nature of the excited states, the extent of intersystem crossing, and photochemical reactions, will finally determine the phototoxic potential of an endogenous or exogenous compound. However, we are not yet able to predict the phototoxic potential of a compound from its molecular structure alone. Reliable predictive tests are still required to evaluate suspected compounds. Several lists of compounds that are phototoxic in humans have appeared (e.g., Parrish et al., 1979). Classes of compounds known to be phototoxic in humans are:

[2]The minimal erythema dose (MED) is defined as the minimal dose of UV irradiation that produces definite, but minimally perceptible, redness 24 h after exposure.

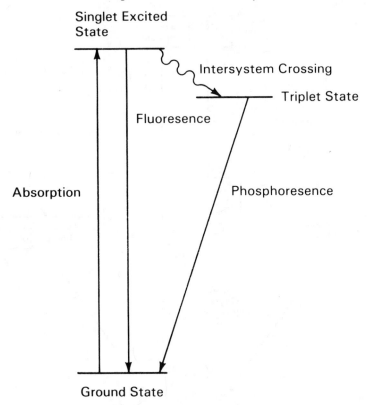

FIGURE 4   Electronic energy diagram of physical events accompanying the absorption of a photon.

Psoralens
Sulfonamides
Sulfonylureas
Phenothiazine
Tetracyclines
Coal tar
Anthracene
Acridine
Phenanthrene

The mechanisms through which absorption of light causes a chemical alteration in the chromophore, eventually resulting in a phototoxic response, are shown in Fig. 5.

Compounds such as psoralens may react directly in their excited states with a biological target. Because of the short lifetimes of most excited states, direct reactions require close association, or complex formation, between the

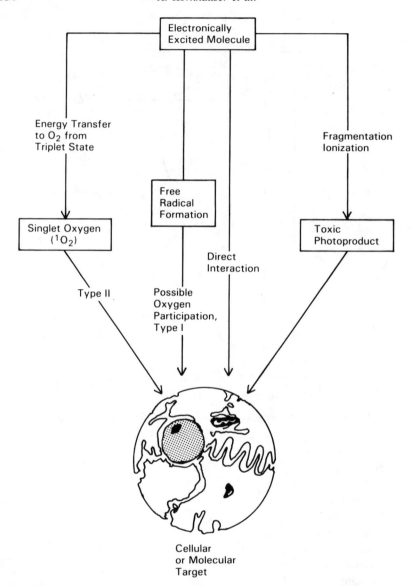

FIGURE 5 Diagram of basic phototoxicity mechanisms. The electronically excited molecule, located within or near a cell, may elicit a phototoxic response through several mechanisms.

chromophore and the target before light absorption. Alternatively, a stable toxic photoproduct may be formed after absorption of light. Chlorpromazine and protriptyline are examples of this mechanism (Kochevar, 1981). The phototoxicity of these compounds is in large part the result of the toxicity of their photoproducts.

The other mechanisms shown in Fig. 5 are frequently categorized as photodynamic mechanisms. Photodynamic reactions usually involve compounds that absorb UVA or visible light. In type I photodynamic reactions the chromophore, in an excited triplet state, is reduced either by an electron or by hydrogen transfer from a compound in the environment. This reduction results in the generation of highly reactive free radicals, whose subsequent attack on biological substrates may result in toxicity. In type II photodynamic reactions the chromophore transfers its energy to O_2, generating singlet oxygen ($^1O_2$), an active oxidizing agent. Although $^1O_2$ has not been directly detected in photodynamic reactions so far investigated *in vivo,* a large body of evidence supports its involvement.

CELLULAR TARGETS AND MECHANISMS OF PHOTOTOXICITY

A vigorous effort is under way to discover the biological targets in phototoxicity. Cellular injury by photons may be studied on either the histological or the molecular level. The characteristic histological change induced by photons is the appearance of the so-called sunburn cell (SBC) (Daniels et al., 1961), a dyskeratotic cell with bright eosinophilic cytoplasm and a pyknotic nucleus. SBCs appear 24–48 h after UVB irradiation (Woodcock and Magnus, 1976) and may persist 1 week or longer (Parrish et al., 1979). The mechanisms of SBC formation are still obscure, although its morphological and biochemical characteristics have been investigated (Danno and Horio, 1980; Olson et al., 1974). The primary chromophore for sunburn-cell production is not known; however, Young and Magnus (1981) found evidence that DNA may be an important chromophore. They detected SBCs in mouse epidermis after administration of 8-methoxypsoralen (8-MOP) followed by UVA irradiation (psoralen + UVA is abbreviated PUVA). They speculated that since the primary molecular lesion in PUVA treatment is in DNA, the fact that PUVA can promote SBC formation supports the view that DNA may be a significant chromophore in SBC induction.

The mechanisms by which photosensitized cells are damaged are in most cases poorly understood. On the subcellular level, the primary targets in a phototoxic reaction include nucleic acids, proteins, and plasma and organelle membranes. Subcellular effects may differ depending on the photosensitizer's structure and intracellular localization. Sensitizers such as rose bengal, porphyrin, and anthracene accumulate selectively in cell plasma membranes (Ito, 1978). Acridine orange and psoralens accumulate in the cell nucleus (Van de Vorst and Lion, 1976; Pathak et al., 1974; Bredberg et al., 1977). Recently, it was reported that psoralens also accumulate in cell membranes. These membrane-bound psoralens may initiate important biological effects (Laskin et al., 1985). Some photosensitizers may become concentrated in lysosomes and on irradiation may induce lysosomal rupture (Allison et al., 1966). Table 1

TABLE 1   Mechanisms and Targets of Selected Groups of Phototoxic Compounds

Compound	Structure	Mechanism of Phototoxicity	Cellular Target	Ref.
Psoralens		Direct Addition	DNA	Pathak et al., 1974.
		Photodynamic	DNA, Proteins, Ribosomes, Membranes	de Mot et al., 1981. Poppe and Grossweiner, 1975. Singh and Vadasz, 1978. Pathak, 1982.
Phenothiazines e.g. Chlorpromazine		Stable (Toxic) Photoproduct	DNA	Kochevar, 1981.
		Photodynamic	DNA, Membranes	Kochevar, 1981. Copeland et al., 1976.
Porphyrins		Photodynamic	Membranes, DNA, Proteins	Spikes, 1975. Verweij et al., 1981. Jori and Spikes, 1981.
Dyes e.g. Acridine Orange		Photodynamic	Proteins, Membranes, DNA	Hass and Webb, 1981. Ito, 1978. Wacker et al., 1964. Wagner et al., 1980.
Kynurenic Acid		Photodynamic	Membranes	Wennersten and Brunk, 1977, 1978. Pileni and Santus, 1978.
Anthracene		Photodynamic	Membranes DNA ·	Allison et al., 1966. Blackburn and Taussig, 1975.

shows results from some studies of the mechanisms of action for several important classes of phototoxic compounds. It includes two endogenous photosensitizers, porphyrins and kynurenic acid. As reflected in Table 1, most compounds
that evoke chemical phototoxicity are thought to act through a photodynamic
mechanism. Further, it appears that a compound may elicit a phototoxic re-

sponse through several modes. Studies are needed to correlate specific molecular alterations (such as DNA cross-linking and photooxidation of enzymes and of DNA) with cell toxicity and mutagenesis. To date, the mechanism of psoralen phototoxicity is relatively well understood. Much more remains to be learned about the mode of action for other groups of photosensitizers.

SPECIFIC MOLECULAR ALTERATIONS IN CELLS

On the molecular level, DNA is the most critical target in a cell exposed to UV light. As previously discussed, other cellular constituents may also be affected, generally with less severe consequences for the cell.

Thymine Photoproducts

Cyclobutane-type pyrimidine dimers in DNA are the best-studied lesions induced in cells by UV. They are formed predominately at wavelengths less than 300 nm (Rothman and Setlow, 1979; Rosenstein and Setlow, 1980; Kantor et al., 1980), although they have also been found in human skin exposed *in situ* to UV wavelengths of 340–400 nm (Freeman et al., 1987a). These dimers result from the formation of covalent bonds between adjacent pyrimidines of the same DNA strand and interfere with normal DNA function. Beukers and Berends (1960) first demonstrated the formation of these dimers *in vitro,* and Wacker et al. (1960) found them in DNA from UV-irradiated bacteria. These findings marked the beginning of a new era in molecular biology. Pyrimidine dimers were later shown to occur in a number of higher systems, including mammalian (Pathak et al., 1972) and human skin (Freeman et al., 1987b) after UV irradiation.

Studies initiated by Cleaver and Trosko (1970) demonstrated the involvement of thymine dimers (TT) (Fig. 6a) in the disorder xeroderma pigmentosum

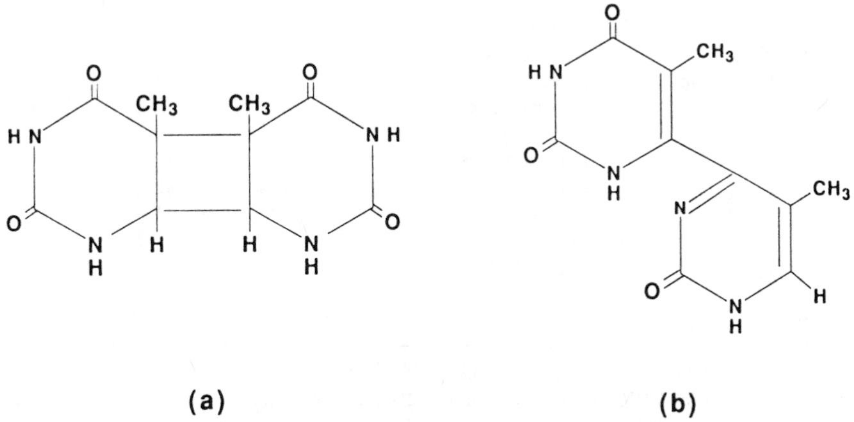

(a)   (b)

FIGURE 6   Structure of (a) the thymine dimer (cis, syn) and (b) the (6-4) photoproduct.

(XP). This finding represents one of the rare cases in which a specific molecular lesion can be correlated with a malignant process. In another approach, Hart et al. (1977) used cell extracts from UV-irradiated Amazon mollies (small fish) and reported evidence that pyrimidine dimers in DNA gave rise to tumors.

Until recently, sensitive assays for pyrimidine dimers required use of radioisotopes. However, additional techniques have now been developed for measuring pyrimidine dimers. These methods include radioimmunoassays (Mitchell and Clarkson, 1981) and endonuclease digestion followed by determination of DNA chain length (D'Ambrosio et al., 1981; Freeman et al., 1986), which have made quantitation of pyrimidine dimers in human biopsies feasible.

Several possible reaction mechanisms for the sensitized photodimerization of pyrimidines have been suggested, including population of the triplet state of a suitable sensitizer (Lamola, 1968). Our previous work showed that a Schenck type of mechanism (Schenck, 1960) involving a complex-forming reaction is highly favored in photosensitized thymine dimer formation (Kornhauser and Pathak, 1972; Kornhauser et al., 1974). Also, we found that only a few of the potential sensitizers caused measurable thymine dimerization. A small amount (1–2%) of thymine dimer was detected after UV irradiation, even in the absence of a sensitizer. Acetone, ethyl acetoacetate, and dihydroxyacetone were more potent sensitizers than acetophenone and benzophenone (Table 2).

TABLE 2   Formation of Thymine Dimers (TT) after Irradiation of [2-^{14}C]Thymine in the Presence of Different Sensitizers

Number	Sensitizer	TT formed (%)
1	None	1–2
2	Acetone	30–40
3	Dihydroxyacetone	25–30
4	Acetophenone	5–10
5	Benzophenone	5–8
6	4-Methoxyacetophenone	2–4
7	Ethyl acetoacetate	35–45
8	Phenyl cyanide	1–3
9	Carbazole	3–6
10	Fluorene	2–3
11	Naphthalene	1–3
12	Xanthene-9-one	1–3
13	Urocanic acid	1–3

Note. Solutions of [2-^{14}C]thymine (2×10^{-3} M) and sensitizer (10^{-4}–10^{-1} M) were irradiated with a total UV (≤ 300 nm) dose of 1.2 J/cm^2. Irradiations were carried out in water (sensitizers 1, 2, 3, and 13), water and ethanol (3 : 1) (sensitizers 4 and 6–12), and water and dioxane (3 : 1) (sensitizers 5 and 12).

The following conclusions can be derived from our results:

1. The sensitized energy transfer taking place during thymine dimerization most likely does not occur through a simple physical mechanism. The ability of the sensitizer in its excited state to form a complex with the pyrimidine molecule appears to be a prerequisite for this type of photosensitization.
2. Ethyl acetoacetate and dihydroxyacetone, molecules that are commonly present in any viable cell and were not previously known to be photosensitizers, proved as effective as acetone or acetophenone. On the other hand, urocanic acid, a major UV-absorbing compound in mammalian skin, did not show sensitizing ability in inducing thymine dimerization. The UV energy absorbed by urocanic acid is believed to induce its cis-trans isomerization (Baden and Pathak, 1967).
3. Topical preparations containing acetone, dihydroxyacetone, or other acetone derivatives should be used cautiously, since they might damage the epidermal DNA when skin is exposed to UV radiation. Interestingly, one of these compounds, dihydroxyacetone, has been used in cosmetics, notably as the active component in "sunless" tanning lotions (Maibach and Kligman, 1960).

The studies discussed above have practical application for correlating the structure of a potential phototoxic agent with its ability to induce pyrimidine dimerization or other molecular lesions in cells.

Recently, some other interesting photoproducts of DNA have been isolated and characterized. When a solution of DNA or a frozen thymine solution is irradiated, a new absorption peak at 320 nm appears. This is due to the photochemical formation of new products, the (6-4) adducts. In the case of thymine, 6,4'-(5'-methylpyrimidin-2'-one)-thymine is formed (Fig. 6b) (Franklin et al., 1982). These compounds cannot be split by reirradiation at short wavelengths as can cyclobutane-type pyrimidine dimers. An additional diagnostic property of these compounds is their instability in hot alkali (Franklin et al., 1982). The (6-4) photoproducts are also generally produced less efficiently than are pyrimidine dimers (Franklin et al., 1982). More recently, there has been an increased interest in the (6-4) adduct type lesions as they have been shown to play a major role in UV-induced mutagenesis at specific sites in DNA (Franklin and Haseltine, 1986). They used the application of DNA sequencing procedures in *Escherichia coli* to demonstrate that the (6-4) adduct was the mutagenic lesion at certain "hot spots" in the *lacI* gene, a mutation that was previously ascribed to cyclobutane pyrimidine dimers. The relative importance of (6-4) adducts in the lethal and mutagenic effects of UV light, as well as current methods for detection and quantitation, have been discussed in a recent review (Mitchell and Nairn, 1989).

DNA-Protein Cross-Links

The previous discussion focused on the reaction between bases, specifically thymine, within a strand of DNA to form an adduct. However, DNA in the cell has a complex and varied environment, making possible additional light-induced reactions.

Heteroadducts of DNA are those adducts formed by the covalent attachment of different types of compounds to DNA. These adducts may involve cellular constituents such as proteins, or exogenous compounds such as drugs, food additives, and cosmetics. Heteroadducts may have profound effects on cells. Artificially produced covalent linkages like DNA-protein cross-links, of the type not observed in normal viable cells, may result in a phototoxic response or be expressed as mutagenic or carcinogenic events.

The chemical nature of the DNA-protein cross-links is not yet known. An *in vitro* photochemical reaction between thymine and cysteine has been observed (Schott and Shetlar, 1974) and may be one of the mechanisms for covalent linking of DNA to protein *in vivo* (Smith, 1974). Similarly, it has been reported that irradiation of thymine-labeled DNA and lysine in aqueous solvent produces a photoproduct that behaves like a thymine-lysine adduct (Shetlar et al., 1975). Furthermore, 11 of the common amino acids combine photochemically with uracil in different model systems (Smith, 1974). These pyrimidine-amino acid adducts are regarded as models for the coupling sites between proteins and DNA. In addition to reactions directly induced by UV, model systems provide evidence that acetone and acetophenone are effective photosensitizers for the covalent addition of amino acids to pyrimidine bases (Fisher et al., 1974). It is reasonable to assume that suitable chromophores present in drugs, cosmetics, etc., will also be able to photosensitize the cross-linking of proteins and nucleic acids *in vitro* and *in vivo*.

The cross-linking of DNA and protein in bacteria was the first *in vivo* photochemical heteroadduct reaction reported (Smith, 1962). Several studies of UV-induced DNA and protein cross-links in mammalian cells *in vitro* have been based mainly on reduced DNA extractability after UV irradiation (Todd and Han, 1976). Evidence that this lesion plays a significant role in killing UV-irradiated cells has been obtained under several experimental conditions.

Mammalian (eukaryotic) cells, in general, represent a suitable model for the cross-linking reaction. Within the nuclei of eukaryotic cells, DNA is in intimate contact with proteins responsible for structurally organizing DNA and controlling macromolecular synthesis. Such a DNA-protein complex is commonly referred to as chromatin. The proximity of nuclear proteins to DNA should facilitate the formation of UV-induced DNA-protein covalent bonds. Todd and Han (1976) studied the general features of UV-induced (254 nm) DNA-protein cross-links in asynchronous and synchronous HeLa cells. Cross-linking was demonstrated by the detection of unextractable DNA in irradiated cells. Fornace and Kohn (1976), using a sensitive alkaline elution assay, measured UV-induced DNA-protein cross-links in both normal and xeroderma pigmentosum human fibroblasts. They noted that normal cells exhibit a repair phase lacking in XP cells. Similarly, Peak and Peak (1989) have reported DNA-protein cross-linking in cells exposed to UVA, UVB, or UVC radiation. These workers reported the relative importance of several DNA lesions (thymine dimers, single strand breaks, and DNA-protein cross-links) for each spectral region. DNA-protein cross-links were found to be the lesion most efficiently produced by UVA irradiation of cells.

No *in vivo* data on DNA-protein cross-linking in mammalian skin, other than our preliminary work, have been reported. To study the possible role of the DNA-protein cross-links in epidermis, we focused on the isolation of chromatin from irradiated and nonirradiated guinea pig skin (Kornhauser et al., 1976a; Kornhauser, 1976). The epilated backs of guinea pigs were irradiated with a moderate physiological dose (80 mJ/cm^2; 290–350 nm) that corresponds to approximately four times the minimal erythema dose in an average fair-skinned Caucasian. Epidermis was obtained from both the irradiated and the control (nonirradiated) sites on the same animal and was homogenized. Chromatin was isolated from the homogenates by using Sepharose B-4 and DEAE cellulose chromatography and density gradient centrifugation. Its biological activity was determined by chemical and biochemical methods (Kornhauser et al., 1976a). We were able to obtain 4–5 mg extractable DNA free of protein from 1 g wet epidermal tissue. Immediately after UV irradiation, the yield of extractable DNA was reduced by 20–30%, presumably as a result of DNA-protein cross-linking and possibly of DNA strand breakage. The latter molecular lesion is consistent with previous findings (Zierenberg et al., 1971). In this experiment we found (1) a significant breakdown of the high-molecular-weight DNA fraction and the presence of low-molecular-weight DNA fragments on top of the sucrose gradient after UV irradiation, and (2) an increment in the high-molecular-weight DNA isolated 60 min after irradiation (the regeneration or repair phase).

The results discussed above can be summarized as follows:

1. UV irradiation, at physiological doses (4 MED) of 290–350 nm, decreased the actual amount of dissociable chromosomal DNA by 20–30% as a result of DNA strand breakage and cross-linking of DNA to protein.
2. A comparison of corresponding elution profiles from Sepharose columns of dissociable DNA isolated from UV-irradiated and nonirradiated epidermal specimens indicated cross-linking of protein to DNA.
3. UV irradiation caused significant breakdown of the high-molecular-weight DNA that was isolated after irradiation.
4. In the regeneration phase, an active repair of strand breaks and possibly DNA-protein heteroadducts was operating in the viable cells of the epidermis.

So far, no other evidence for the cellular repair of DNA-protein heteroadducts has been found *in vivo*. It is conceivable that cells exposed to light have evolved a repair system for eliminating this type of heteroadduct. It is likely that this system is different from photoreactivation, which is specific for pyrimidine dimers (Setlow and Setlow, 1963).

All these findings suggest that UV radiation, even in moderate doses, can induce measurable alterations of the chromosomal material chromatin in mammalian skin. At present, it is not known what biochemical changes accompany light-induced lesions in chromatin. It is possible that damage by photons may alter such important chromatin functions as regulation of gene expression. Thus further studies of lesions in chromatin are indispensable for a complete understanding of light-induced effects on cells.

Psoralen Phototoxicity

In addition to DNA-protein cross-linking, cross-links between DNA strands are possible. Because of the distance between bases in the DNA double helix, light-induced cross-linking is not observed without a bridging molecule such as a drug or component of a cosmetic, etc. Psoralens, a class of furocoumarins, are important cross-linking agents. Psoralens are a group of naturally occurring and synthetic substances that, when added to biological systems and irradiated with UVA, produce various biological effects. These effects are not observed with either psoralens or light alone.

The photobiological reactions of psoralens with DNA have received widespread attention in recent years. On the molecular level, the following facts are known:

1. Psoralens intercalate into DNA, that is, slip in between adjacent base-pairs by forming molecular complexes involving weak chemical interactions ("dark reaction").

2. UV irradiation of the DNA-psoralen complex, *in vivo* or *in vitro*, results in covalent bond formation between a pyrimidine base and the furocoumarin molecule (C_4 cycloaddition). Because of their structure, psoralens in this reaction can react either at their 3,4 double bond or at their corresponding $4',5'$ site, yielding monoadducts (in the former case the product is not fluorescent, and in the latter case it is).

3. The absorption of an additional photon may result in a further chemical reaction, yielding a "cross-linked DNA." Thus psoralens can behave as photoactive bifunctional agents, one psoralen molecule reacting with two pyrimidines in opposite strands of DNA. The structures of psoralen mono- and di-adducts with thymine are shown in Fig. 7. Figure 8 schematically shows DNA cross-linked by a psoralen molecule. The result is a cross-linked DNA in which the individual strands cannot be separated by standard denaturation conditions. Both types of lesions, the monofunctional adduct and the cross-linked product, can be repaired *in vivo* (Pathak and Kramer, 1969; Baden et al., 1972) and *in vitro* (Friedburg, 1988).

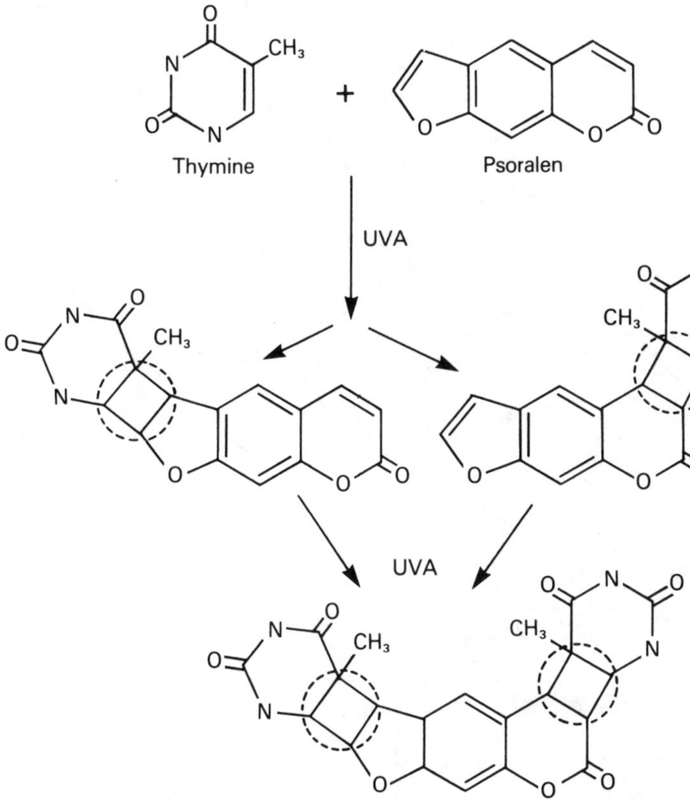

FIGURE 7 Photoaddition products of psoralen with thymine after UV irradiation *in vitro*.

Dall'Acqua (1977) showed that the photoaddition of furocoumarins to DNA is not a random process. Specific sites exist in DNA for the photochemical interaction with psoralens. The sites that can be considered specific receptors for the photobiological activity of psoralens are represented by alternating sequences of adenine and thymine in each complementary strand of the polynucleotide. Psoralen has a greater photoreactivity toward thymine than it has toward cytosine. The receptor sites have a high capacity for intercalation and subsequent photoreaction with psoralens (Dall'Acqua, 1977). It has recently been shown that flanking sequences, in addition to the adenine and thymine content of DNA, determine cross-linking (Boyer et al., 1988).

The covalent addition of psoralens to DNA, particularly the cross-linking reaction, is usually believed to be responsible for the major effects of psoralen photosensitization. These include mutation and lethality in prokaryotic and eukaryotic systems, inhibition of DNA synthesis, sister chromatid exchange, and carcinogenesis. However, the relationship between psoralen photoaddition to DNA and the appearance of erythema remains to be elucidated. From early

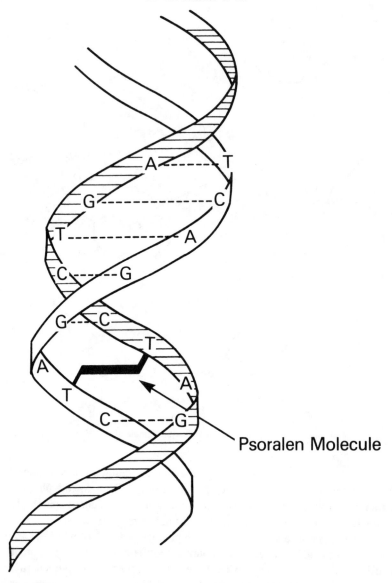

FIGURE 8   Schematic representation of DNA cross-linked by a psoralen molecule.

studies it appeared that erythema, the basic phototoxic effect induced by psoralens, correlated well with the *in vitro* capacity of psoralen derivatives to bind covalently to DNA (Vedaldi et al., 1983). Neither the specific photoproduct(s) required for initiating psoralen-induced erythema nor the subsequent molecular events (e.g., mediators involved) have been definitely established.

    Initially, the ability to sensitize cutaneous tissue appeared to be a unique characteristic of the psoralen ring system; for instance, pyranocoumarins, which have a similar linear tricyclic ring system, are found to lack photosensitizing activity (Pathak, 1967). Furthermore, cutaneous phototoxicity is usually expressed only with linear derivatives; the angular furocoumarin, angelicin, does not photosensitive mammalian skin (Dall'Acqua et al., 1981). Small changes in the structure of psoralen may produce dramatic changes in photosensitizing ability. Unsubstituted psoralen causes the most severe phototoxicity. This photobiological activity is reduced by adding methyl (on carbon 3) or halogen substituents (Pathak, 1967). The structures of some furocoumarins and pyranocoumarin are shown in Fig. 9.

The correlation of the structure of psoralen photoproducts to their photobiological effects has been the topic of several recent investigations. A large number of synthetic and natural furocoumarins have been subjected to systematic studies. From this work it has been concluded that the erythemogenic effect correlates with the capacity of a furocoumarin to form cross-links rather than monoadducts to DNA (Vedaldi et al., 1983). This fact was confirmed by several investigators by preparing a relatively large number of monofunctional furocoumarin derivatives and testing their photobiologic properties (Rodighiero et al., 1984).

In general, the monofunctional compounds do not induce erythema in human and guinea pig skin. Although this fact has been experimentally verified in many cases, exceptions to this rule seem to exist. A few 4-methyl angelicin derivatives are able to strongly photoreact with DNA without forming cross-links. When tested on guinea pig skin they were able, under certain experimental conditions, to induce a mild erythema (Baccichetti et al., 1981, 1984). We must point out, however, that those experiments involved topical application of the compound in a relatively high concentration and with a high UVA dose. Also, great care must be taken in these experiments to ensure that the sample is free from bifunctional psoralen impurities, as they can easily yield false positives. In summary, a simple concept such as cross-links = erythema, monoadduct = no erythema, has yet to be established.

Recently, various derivatives of psoralen, some with photosensitizing activity, have been synthesized. These derivatives include benzopsoralens and their tetrahydroderivatives, pyrrolocoumarins, azapsoralens, and khellin and related methylfurochromones (Dall'Acqua, 1989). Preliminary studies of the photobiological properties of some of these derivatives have been reported; the remaining compounds are being investigated (F. Dall'Acqua, personal communication). The driving force behind these investigations is to find new agents with the potential for improving current photochemotherapeutic treatment regimens.

Alternative mechanisms for the induction of erythema by psoralens and UV light that do not involve photoaddition to DNA have been suggested. One alternative mechanism is derived from the observation that there is a relationship between erythema production and the ability of a compound to form $^1O_2$

(Pathak, 1982). This correlation suggests that $^1O_2$ may be a mediator in psoralen-induced erythema. The involvement of $^1O_2$ in psoralen phototoxicity, however, has yet to be conclusively proven. Indeed, it has been pointed out that both the production of $^1O_2$ and the monoadduct and, particularly, the diadduct formation proceed by way of a common intermediate, the psoralen triplet state (de Mol and Beijersbergen van Henegouwen, 1981). Thus, psoralens that undergo efficient intersystem crossing should readily photosensitize the formation of $^1O_2$ as well as photoreact with DNA, unless low DNA binding or steric constraints predominate. It is therefore understandable that reports of correlation between both $^1O_2$ formation and erythema production (Pathak and Joshi, 1984) as well as DNA photobinding and erythema production (Vedaldi et al., 1983) have appeared. However, the causal relationship between these two photoproducts ($^1O_2$ or DNA adducts) and erythema production is still under active investigation. Another alternative mechanism, not involving direct addition to DNA, has recently been proposed (Laskin et al., 1986). It was demonstrated *in vitro* that 8-MOP binds to a specific cell surface receptor, thus inhibiting epidermal growth-factor binding. This work demonstrated for the first time that 8-MOP in combination with UVA irradiation can modify cell surface receptors in a variety of human and mouse cell lines. This alteration may play an important role in the mechanism of psoralen phototoxicity.

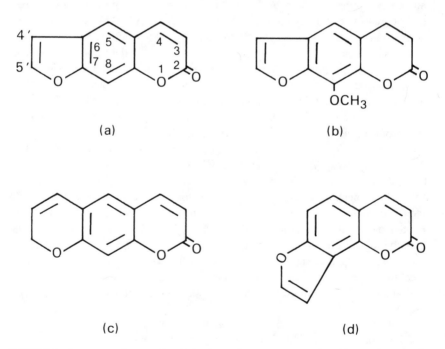

(a)   (b)

(c)   (d)

FIGURE 9   Structures of some furocoumarins and a pyranocoumarin: (a) psoralen; (b) 8-methoxypsoralen (8-MOP); (c) pyranocoumarin; (d) angelicin.

Two studies have been completed in our laboratory that have focused on psoralen + UVA (PUVA) induced phototoxicity. Both involved the micronutrient β-carotene, a naturally occurring pigment and vitamin A precursor found in many green and yellow-orange fruits and vegetables. Beta-carotene is a well-established quencher of $^{1}O_{2}$ and photooxidation (Krinsky and Deneke, 1982).

In the first experiment, we studied the potential of β-carotene to influence PUVA-induced erythema in rats (Giles et al., 1985). The rats were fed a β-carotene-fortified diet for approximately 14 weeks before treatment. Levels of β-carotene accumulated in the skin were measured by high-performance liquid chromatography (HPLC). The rats were then orally dosed with 8-MOP (20 mg/ kg body weight, in corn oil) and were irradiated 2 h later with a single dose of UVA (5 J/cm^{2}). We found that the animals on the β-carotene-fortified diet were significantly protected against PUVA-induced erythema. Furthermore, those rats having the highest β-carotene skin levels showed no perceptible erythema, indicating a correlation between β-carotene skin levels and a protective effect. No such protective effect was observed against UVB-induced erythema.

In the second experiment we investigated the potential of β-carotene for decreasing PUVA-induced melanogenesis (Kornhauser et al., 1989). One of the side effects of PUVA therapy is tanning of the skin caused by an increase in the number of epidermal melanocytes (Blog and Szabo, 1979). Melanin is formed by an oxidative process. Previous *in vitro* studies indicated a role of activated-oxygen species in melanin synthesis (Kornhauser et al., 1976b). Therefore, we reasoned that β-carotene might be able to influence melanogenesis *in vivo*. The animal of choice was the C57 BL/6 mouse, since the tail skin had been found to be a good model for melanogenesis in human skin (Szabo et al., 1982). Mice were fed standard rodent diets supplemented with either 1% β-carotene beadlets or 1% placebo beadlets for 10 week before treatment and throughout the treatment period. Mice were divided into UVA-treated and PUVA-treated groups. PUVA-treated mice received 20 mg/kg body weight doses of 8-MOP in corn oil, followed 2 h later with 3 J/cm^{2} of UVA irradiation. UVA-treated mice received 3 J/cm^{2} of UVA only. Mice received two, four, or five treatments within a 3-week period. Selected mice from each group were euthanized after these treatments and the tail-skin epidermis was removed for dihydroxyphenylalanine (DOPA) histochemical processing (Staricco and Pinkus, 1957). Melanogenesis was evaluated by counting the number of DOPA-positive melanocytes. As expected, the PUVA treatment resulted in an increase in the number of DOPA-positive melanocytes counted in each tail-skin epidermal section. An increase was also observed in the UVA-treated mice. However, mice fed β-carotene in both the UVA and PUVA-treated groups had significantly fewer ($p < .05$, Students's t-test) DOPA-positive melanocytes than the corresponding placebo-fed animals at all three time points. The results are presented in Fig. 10.

The most direct interpretation of the results described in both of these experiments would be that PUVA treatment involves photooxidation via $^{1}O_{2}$ or free radicals. It is well known that β-carotene is an effective quencher of these

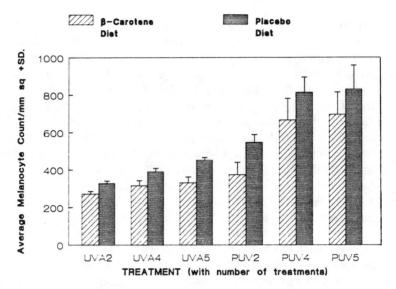

FIGURE 10   Average melanocyte counts as a measure of the effects of diet and treatment on DOPA-processed tail-skin epidermis of C57BL/6 mice. Averages are shown with the corresponding standard deviation. Mice were fed either β-carotene- or placebo-fortified diets. Treatment groups: UVA-treated (UVA), and PUVA-treated (PUV). Mice received two, four, or five treatments. The numbers of DOPA-positive melanocytes were counted using a light microscope.

reactive intermediates (Krinsky and Deneke, 1982; Burton and Ingold, 1984). However, there is an alternative explanation for the observed protective effect, which involves the quenching of the psoralen triplet state by β-carotene (Giles et al., 1985). Further studies are in progress to ascertain the mechanism for the β-carotene protective effect and the role of $^1O_2$ in PUVA-induced phototoxicity. In summary, the role of $^1O_2$ and related species in the induction of PUVA-induced erythema and other photobiological effects needs to be more extensively investigated before definitive conclusions can be drawn.

Skin photosensitization is one of the most widely studied properties of furocoumarins. Several types of photodermatoses occur when skin comes into contact with plant or vegetable products and is later exposed to sunlight. Much less is known about potential adverse cutaneous effects resulting from chronic ingestion of foods that contain furocoumarins, such as figs, limes, parsnips, and cloves.

Although furocoumarins are potent phototoxic compounds, they are also used as therapeutic agents. Because of their ability to induce melanogenesis, psoralen derivatives have been applied clinically to treat vitiligo (leukoderma) and increase the tolerance of human skin to solar radiation. A new clinical discipline, photochemotherapy (PCT), is increasingly being introduced to treat psoriasis and other skin disorders (Parrish et al., 1974; Wolff et al., 1976; Gilchrest et al., 1976).

PCT involves the controlled interaction of light and orally administered drugs in order to produce beneficial effects. Psoralen PCT has entered medical terminology as PUVA. The PUVA regimen is effective, clean, and acceptable to patients. However, some problems persist; these include possible induction of cataracts (Cloud et al., 1960), hematologic effects (Friedmann and Rogers, 1980), alteration of the immune response (Strauss et al., 1980), skin aging (Bergfeld, 1977), and a possible increase of cutaneous cancers (Stern et al., 1979; Stern, 1989; Honigsmann et al., 1980).

The use of psoralens in PCT has raised some additional questions concerning their phototoxicity. The structurally similar psoralens 8-MOP, 5-methoxypsoralen (5-MOP), and 4,5',8-trimethylpsoralen (TMP) have similar topical phototoxicity. However, when they are orally administered, the phototoxicity of TMP and 5-MOP is greatly diminished compared to that of 8-MOP (Mandula et al., 1976; Honigsmann et al., 1979). This has been exploited by two European teams, who introduced 5-MOP as an alternative to 8-MOP in the PCT of psoriasis (Honigsmann et al., 1979; Grupper and Berretti, 1981). Although the clearing of psoriatic lesions was comparable with 5-MOP and 8-MOP, acute side effects (including phototoxicity) were significantly reduced in the 5-MOP regimen. As more has been learned about the biotransformations of psoralens (Mandula et al., 1976), it appears that metabolism may play a central role in determining the relative oral phototoxicity of substituted psoralens. However, it has not been established that reduced delivery of the phototoxic psoralen to the epidermis, due to metabolism or lack of absorption, is the basis for the observed differences in oral phototoxicity.

We have reported serum and epidermal levels of 5-MOP and 8-MOP (Kornhauser et al., 1982). Determinations of psoralen levels in the epidermis, the primary target organ for phototoxicity, had not previously been reported for either humans or an animal model. For this study we chose a guinea pig model system that we and others (Harber, 1969) have found to be reliable for predicting phototoxicity in humans. Our results indicated that, after equivalent oral dosing, metabolism and/or absorption constrains 5-MOP to lower epidermal levels than 8-MOP. Therefore, by orally administering 5-MOP it should be possible to maintain epidermal drug concentrations at lower levels than in an 8-MOP regimen.

Because psoralens, as used in PCT, react covalently with DNA, there is a potential risk of mutagenicity and oncogenicity. Indeed, in an *in vitro* study, 8-MOP and 5-MOP exhibited essentially the same activity in inducing chromosome damage in human cells (Natarajan et al., 1981). Furthermore, it was reported that topical 5-MOP combined with UVA induced carcinogenesis in mice comparable to that observed with 8-MOP (Zajdela and Bisagni, 1981). These two studies suggest that 5-MOP and 8-MOP have a similar oncogenic potential when topically administered.

Extrapolating our findings with orally dosed guinea pigs to clinical applications, we suggest that a 5-MOP therapeutic regimen may minimize damage to epidermal DNA, reducing the risk of carcinogenesis that is suspected in 8-MOP PCT. For this reason, and because of the reduced acute side effects in a 5-MOP regimen, we feel that 5-MOP should be tested further, along with other psoralen derivatives, as alternatives to 8-MOP in PCT.

An additional application of psoralen phototoxicity, extracorporeal photophoresis, is increasingly being used for management of disorders such as cutaneous T-cell lymphoma (Edelson, 1988). Photophoresis involves oral administration of 8-MOP, then withdrawal of 1 unit of blood 2 h later. The blood is separated into its components by centrifugation. Plasma and leukocytes are combined with saline. This suspension is then passed as a thin film between twin banks of high-intensity UVA lamps. After irradiation, the erythrocytes are recombined with the remainder of the blood and retransfused into the patient. Preliminary reports have indicated that photophoresis is an effective treatment in many instances (Edelson et al., 1987). Furthermore, the mechanism of this therapy appears to be complex, involving not merely cytotoxicity but also immunologic effects.

Photosensitized Oxidations

Many phototoxic compounds, such as porphyrins and dyes, affect biological substrates through photosensitized oxidations. These substances absorb light (both in long-wavelength UV and visible regions) and sensitize photooxidization from their triplet excited states. Following excitation, there are two distinct mechanisms (type I and type II) that results in photooxidation (Fig. 11).

Although opinion is divided, type II is probably the more common mechanism producing $^1O_2$, a highly reactive oxidizing agent. A unique feature of $^1O_2$ involvement in photodynamic action is the fact that the generation and reaction sites may be different, the diffusion range of $^1O_2$ in cytoplasm being on the order of 0.1 μm (Moan et al., 1979). In contrast, in the type I (radical) mechanism the sensitizer and substrate must be closer at the time of photon absorption. The major processes involving $^1O_2$ are photooxidative loss of histidine, methionine, tryptophan, tyrosine, and cysteine in proteins; photooxidation of guanine base in DNA; and formation of hydroperoxides with unsaturated lipids.

It has been recognized for decades that membrane damage plays a role in the photoinactivation of cells, especially in the presence of photodynamic sensitizers (Raab, 1900; Blum, 1941). The mechanism of cell membrane damage and disruption has been extensively studied for several photodynamic sensitizers. Photohemolysis of red blood cells sensitized by protoporphyrin (metal-free porphyrin) has been studied extensively, because in several porphyria diseases of abnormal porphyrin metabolism, the red cells contain unusually high levels of photosensitizing porphyrins. Oxygen is required for protoporphyrin-photosensitized red cell lysis. On the molecular level, it is known that $^1O_2$, formed by energy transfer from triplet-state protoporphyrin in red blood cell membranes, oxidizes unsaturated lipids (Lamola et al., 1973; Goldstein and Harber, 1972). Incorporation of cholesterol hydroperoxides, such as those

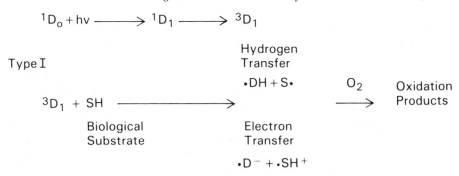

FIGURE 11 Mechanisms of photosensitized oxidation. The ground-state sensitizer ($^1D_0$) is excited to the lowest excited singlet state ($^1D_1$) and undergoes intersystem crossing to the lowest excited triplet state ($^3D_1$).

formed in cholesterol photooxidation by protoporphyrin, leads to increased osmotic fragility and hemolysis of red blood cells (Lamola et al., 1973). Protoporphyrin has also been shown to photosensitize protein cross-linking in membranes (Verweij et al., 1981). It has been suggested that additional, more subtle, membrane functions, such as active transport of small molecules, are altered by membrane protein cross-linking (Kessel, 1977; Lamola and Doleiden, 1980).

Photooxidation of cell membrane components and proteins is not the only mode of photodynamic damage. Various photodynamic sensitizers were found to be mutagenic in bacteria (Gutter et al., 1977), yeast (Kobayasi and Ito, 1976), and mammalian cells (Gruener and Lockwood, 1979). Thus direct photodynamic damage to DNA is suspected, although alternative mechanisms for photodynamic mutagenesis have been proposed (Mukai and Goldstein, 1976).

There is evidence from *in vitro* studies that the bases in DNA, particularly guanosine, are oxidized by photodynamic dyes (Wacker et al., 1964). Photooxidation products of guanosine have been isolated and characterized (Cadet and Teoule, 1978). Further, photooxidation of guanosine has been found in bacteria (Wacker et al., 1964). The detailed mechanism of photooxidation of bases in DNA is not fully understood. When cells are in an environment containing a photodynamically active chromophore, such as a porphyrin or toluidine blue, damage to DNA from $^1O_2$ might be expected to result from an extracellular as well as an intracellular sensitizer. However, it has been found that toluidine blue, which is not taken up by cells, does not damage DNA (Ito and Kobayashi, 1977). Porphyrins, on the other hand, accumulate in cells, and the efficiency of inducing DNA lesions follows the cellular uptake curve (Moan and Christensen, 1981). It is generally felt that accessibility of the sensitizing dye to DNA is a major factor in determining photomutagenic potential.

Both type I and type II mechanisms have been proposed for the photooxidation of DNA. The major pathway will be determined by the structure of the photosensitizing compound, the extent and type of binding to DNA, the oxygen concentration, and the polarity of the cellular environment (Kochevar, 1981; Ito, 1978).

Selective photosensitized oxidative damage to cells has been effectively employed in photodynamic therapy (PDT) of solid tumors including eye, bladder, skin, and endobronchial tumors (Dougherty, 1987). PDT involves the use of hematoporphyrin (HP) derivatives as the photosensitizer. The HP derivatives, when injected, localize in tumors. Tissue is then irradiated with intense visible light, usually obtained by using a dye laser conjoined with fiber optics. The therapy described, which involves light activation of therapeutic agents, has the clear advantage of selectivity, that is, only the irradiated tissue is affected.

Mutations and Changes in Cellular Phenotype

The described classes of light-induced damage [thymine dimers, (6-4) adducts, DNA-protein cross-links, psoralen-DNA adducts, and oxidation of bases] represent potential premutational sites in DNA. High-fidelity repair of these DNA lesions would eliminate adverse cellular effects. As discussed, repair mechanisms have been found for many light-induced changes in DNA. Alternatively, unrepaired (or incorrectly repaired) DNA damage may lead to a range of cellular outcomes, including no effect (if the genetic alteration is unexpressed), cell death, or transformation to a neoplastic phenotype. The complex sequence of molecular events that determine these cellular outcomes is now becoming understood through the techniques of molecular biology.

Errors in DNA repair or replication of a damaged DNA template result in the fixation of a DNA mutation. Several types of light-induced DNA mutations have been reported. Point mutations, involving single nucleotide base pair replacements, have been characterized in bacterial systems (Hutchinson and Wood, 1988; Cebula and Koch, 1990), well-defined plasmid sequences (Drobetsky et al., 1989), and mammalian genes (Bohr and Okumoto, 1988). Frameshift mutations, resulting from the addition or deletion of one or more base pairs, have also been studied (Cebula et al., 1989). Techniques used to define mutational spectra (i.e., types of mutation and specific location) include hybridization with highly specific probes (Cebula and Koch, 1990), direct DNA sequencing (Cebula et al., 1989; Hutchinson and Wood, 1988), and analysis of altered restriction endonuclease sites (Drobetsky et al., 1989). The derived mutation spectra should prove extremely useful for both understanding the mechanism of UV-induced genetic alterations and tracing the etiology of genetic damage.

In the past decade, our understanding of the genetic basis of cancer has dramatically increased. This is in large part due to the discovery of specific genes, proto-oncogenes, whose normal function is vital for appropriate regulation of cellular growth and differentiation. Alteration of proto-oncogene structures or the regulation of their expression may lead to cancer (Bishop, 1983).

It is now well established that DNA damage, such as point mutations, can activate proto-oncogenes. The role of oncogenes in UV-induced carcinogenesis is currently under active investigation. Several animal studies indicate that activation of the *Ha-ras* oncogene is associated with photocarcinogenesis. Strickland et al. (1985) have reported activation of *ras* oncogenes by single treatment of Sencar mice with UVB or PUVA. More recently, Husain et al. (1990) have reported that UVB induces amplification and overexpression of *Ha-ras* proto-oncogenes in mouse skin papillomas and carcinomas. In these animal studies, UV irradiation can definitely be associated with both the formation of morphological changes (i.e., papillomas and carcinomas) and activation of an oncogene(s). Investigators have reported that *ras* oncogene activation in human skin cancers occurred on sun-exposed sites (Ananthaswamy et al., 1988; Gerrit van der Schroeff et al., 1990). However, in studies of human skin carcinogenesis the etiology is less clear. Further studies of the role of oncogene activation in photocarcinogenesis may provide important insights into the mechanism of UV-induced skin cancer and possible approaches for prevention and treatment.

CELLULAR MEDIATORS INDUCED BY LIGHT

We have reviewed various sensitized and unsensitized light-induced reactions, such as pyrimidine dimer formation, DNA-protein cross-linking, and various photooxidations. It is still not known how these molecular events are involved in the complex physiological processes that give rise to erythema in sunburn or phototoxic reactions. Generally, a UV-induced effect in tissue may be a direct photon effect or may be mediated by diffusible substances induced by photons. Such substances include prostaglandins (PGs), histamines, kinins, lysosomal enzymes, and activated oxygen species (e.g., $^1O_2$, superoxide, radical).

PGs have dominated research in this area and have been implicated in many physiological processes. The almost ubiquitous occurrence of the PG synthetase enzyme system and the presence of its substrate fatty acids in membrane phospholipids of mammalian cells suggest that PGs can be formed in most types of cells, where they can act as intracellular messengers (Silver and Smith, 1975).

The role of PGs in cutaneous pathology and inflammation is well estab-

A. Kornhauser et al.

lished (Goldyne, 1975). PGs were found in whole rat skin homogenates; when the epidermis was separated from the dermis, most of the PG activity was located in the epidermis. The realization that PGs are important in cellular control mechanisms has motivated a great deal of research on their possible role in the etiology of cancer (Snyder and Eaglstein, 1974).

A tentative pathway of PG formation and its interrelation with the adenylate cyclase system in cutaneous tissue after UV irradiation is shown in Fig. 12. Tissue (specifically membrane) damage induced by light makes membrane phospholipids "accessible" to the enzyme, phospholipase. This is the first step in inducing the arachidonic acid cascade, which results in PG production.

Prostaglandins E_2 (PGE$_2$) and F_2 (PGF$_2$) are produced in skin irradiated with UVB. PGE$_2$ is believed to play a part in the pathogenesis of UVB-induced tissue injury. This is supported by the observation that inhibitors of PG synthetase such as indomethacin and aspirin can suppress UVB-induced erythema (Snyder and Eaglstein, 1974). On the other hand, erythema due to psoralen phototoxicity (PUVA) cannot be suppressed with indomethacin (Morison et al., 1977), and no increase in PG activity is found in exudate from PUVA-inflamed skin (Greaves, 1978). For these reasons, mediators other than PG are likely to be involved in the pathogenesis of PUVA-induced inflammation.

PGs are rapidly metabolized near the site of their synthesis, which increases the difficulty of studying their role in inflammation. A metabolite of PGE$_2$, 13,14-dihydro-15-keto-PGE$_2$ (PGE$_2$-M), is much more stable and accumulates in plasma, where it can be measured (Tashjian et al., 1977). The introduction of a specific assay for the measurement of PGE$_2$-M provides an opportunity to examine, in a relatively noninvasive manner, the systemic levels of PGE$_2$ after a single acute UV injury.

The systemic effect of UVB and PUVA on PGE$_2$ plasma levels has been investigated in a preliminary study of eight fair-skinned Caucasians. The subjects were divided into two groups. Four were exposed to whole-body UVB irradiation and four to whole-body PUVA irradiation. The aim was to produce the equivalent of a moderate sunburn over most of the body surface. For the PUVA subjects, a less aggressive approach was adopted. It was necessary to monitor the radiant exposure very carefully, since the dose-response curve for PUVA is steep and phototoxic burns are more painful and persistent than sunburns. Plasma samples were obtained from each subject at appropriate time intervals. Plasma PGE$_2$-M concentrations, including a preirradiation baseline for each subject, were determined by radioimmunoassay (H. A. D. White et al., personal communication).

It was found that plasma concentrations of PGE$_2$-M were increased significantly in the four subjects treated with UVB but not in any of the PUVA-treated subjects. This is consistent with data on the effects of indomethacin on PUVA-induced erythema (Morison et al., 1977). Animal studies with an increased dose of UVA could confirm these findings and give valuable information about the proposed different mechanisms of UVB and PUVA phototoxicity.

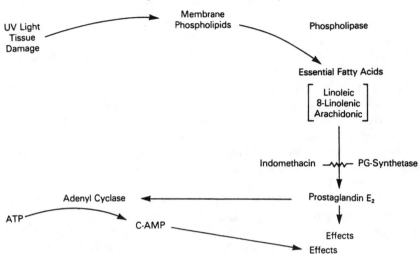

FIGURE 12 Tentative pathway of prostaglandin formation and its interrelation with the adenylate cyclase system in cutaneous tissue following UV irradiation.

PHOTOIMMUNOLOGY

In a broad sense, immunology is the study of how and why the body reacts against anything that is foreign and how an organism can recognize the difference between self and nonself. That UV light can significantly influence the immune system is a relatively recent discovery. As a matter of fact, photoimmunology as a scientific discipline is about 10 years old. The decade has been a time of exceptional activity and development. Of all the sections described in this chapter, photoimmunology has probably made the fastest progress. As a result of this activity, a new understanding of the connection between light, skin, and the immune system has been established. A complete discussion of these findings is beyond the scope of this section; the interested reader is advised to consult recent publications (Streilein, 1983; Kripke, 1986; Edelson and Fink, 1985; Morison, 1989).

The discipline of photoimmunology began with two important observations: (1) UVB induces suppression of contact hypersensitivity (CHS) in mice evoked by dinitrochlorobenzene or similar compounds, and (2) UV-induced alterations in immune functions are involved in the pathogenesis of photocarcinogenesis in mice (Kripke, 1980). UVB-induced tumors in mice are highly antigenic; they are immunologically rejected when transplanted into normal syngeneic recipients, but grow progressively in immunosuppressed animals. Subtumorigenic doses of UVB produce specific systemic alterations, which permit progressive growth of these highly antigenic tumors after transplantation.

The mechanism(s) of these phenomena are far from understood. The available evidence suggests that both CHS responses and tumor rejection processes involve suppressor T lymphocytes that inhibit normal immunologic reactions. UVB-mediated alteration of antigen processing cells (macrophages) has also been suggested (Kripke, 1980).

Evidence for the involvement of the immune system in the etiology of photocarcinogenesis in humans is now established. It is possible that chronic exposure to UV causes nonspecific immunosuppression and thus leads to the development of light-induced skin tumors. Long-term clinical treatment with PUVA also induces immunosuppression (Morison et al., 1979), and this may be one of the mechanisms of PUVA-mediated carcinogenesis.

The immune system involves complex molecular and cellular interactions, which are now being gradually revealed. A major breakthrough, as a result of studies in the fields of photobiology and immunology, has yielded new understanding of the skin as an active element of the immune system. The majority of the cells in the epidermis, Langerhans and Granstein cells, both dendritic populations of the epidermis, and even keratinocytes, have been shown to be active immunologically (Edelson and Fink, 1985). Furthermore, it was shown that certain types of T cells can undergo maturation in the epidermis. To emphasize the connection of these epidermal components to the total immune system, a new term, skin-associated lymphoid tissue (SALT), has been coined (Streilein, 1983). The old concept of immune surveillance, which has undergone ups and downs in its history, can be reformulated today: it is presently believed that immune surveillance does exist but is limited to the lymphoreticular and cutaneous system (Streilein, 1983).

These diverse observations dramatically demonstrate the relevance of photobiology to dermatology and studies of carcinogenesis. An important new insight from these findings is the demonstration that both direct (i.e., DNA damage) and indirect (modification of the immune system) effects influence the development of primary skin cancers. Aside from virus-associated cancers, this remains the only experimental carcinogenesis system in which the immune system has been shown to play a role in the carcinogenic process (Kripke, 1986).

Recently some interesting observations have been made about the mechanism(s) of the photoimmunologic response and the potential mediators involved. One of the experimental models that has attracted widespread attention is the UVB suppression of the CHS response in rodents. In addition this phenomenon has also been studied in various *in vitro* systems (CHS is commonly referred to as contact allergy in humans). Mediators, produced by keratinocytes exposed to UV, may be involved. A soluble mediator isolated from the culture medium of murine keratinocytes exposed to UV mimicked the effect of UV, as evidenced by suppression of the CHS response (Applegate et al., 1989). In addition, a factor present in the plasma of UV-irradiated mice also suppressed the induction of the CHS response (Applegate et al., 1989). The characterization of these factors is being pursued further.

Another important approach to this problem was to identify the chromophore responsible for various photoimmunologic responses. Correlation of the action spectrum for UV-induced suppression of CHS with the absorption spectrum of components in the skin suggests that urocanic acid (UCA), a molecule present in stratum corneum, may play this role (DeFabo et al., 1981). DeFabo and Noonan (1983) presented additional evidence that the UVB-induced immunosuppression in mice is initiated by the photoisomerization of UCA (De-Fabo and Noonan, 1983). They predicted that the cis isomer is the natural immunosuppressant, and as such may play an important role as the "mediator" between the environment (UVB) and the immune system (DeFabo and Noonan, 1983). Since that time, additional support for an immunoregulatory role for *cis*-UCA has been provided in a number of experimental systems. Administration of *cis*-UCA *in vivo* has been found to decrease the function of splenic antigen presenting cells (Noonan et al., 1988). Furthermore, topical application of UCA during UV-induced carcinogenesis resulted in an increase in both the tumor number and the degree of malignancy (Reeve et al., 1989).

The results from the studies on UCA came from experiments performed in *in vitro* systems or in rodents. Although at this time there is no direct evidence that *cis*-UCA is immunosuppressive in humans, the fact that UCA is present in human skin and also isomerizes in response to UVB suggests that it may play the same immunoregulating role in humans. The importance of these findings is increased by the fact that the UV wavelengths (UVB) most affected by depletion of the stratospheric ozone layer are those known to be the most immunosuppressive in animals.

These studies also indicate that light-induced modification of the immune system will be important in the future, with broad applications for managing disorders such as graft rejection, allergies, and autoimmune diseases.

PHOTOTOXICITY TESTING

Because of the proliferation of topically applied compounds in use today, as both drugs and cosmetics, the need has arisen for a rapid and meaningful test for phototoxicity. To date, a uniform test method has not been established. Tests with human subjects are of unique value since they directly predict the clinical behavior of a compound. Several test protocols with human subjects have been reported (Kligman and Breit, 1968; Harber et al., 1974). However, since total reliance on human testing is not practical, we briefly mention some alternative test methods.

Over the past 15 years, the use of microbiological phototoxicity tests has increased. The Daniels test, employing the pathogenic yeast *Candida albicans*, is perhaps the best known example (Daniels, 1965). The test is assayed by inhibition of cell growth in an agar medium. Although simple to perform, this test does not reliably predict the clinical phototoxicity of compounds such as sulfanilamide and demeclocycline (demethylchlortetracycline) (Daniels, 1965). A nonpathogenic yeast, *Candida utilis,* has been suggested as an alternative test organism (Kagen and Gabriel, 1980). Bacterial systems have also been studied (Ashwood-Smith et al., 1980; Harter et al., 1976). A quantitative *in vitro* method of phototoxic evaluation was devised by Tennenbaum et al. (1984). This test procedure used the yeast *Saccharomyces cerevisiae*. An inhibition curve from 8-MOP phototoxicity was constructed as a standard against which test material could be measured.

Phototoxicity tests with animal model systems are potentially more predictive than those with simple organisms. Several test systems are in use, mostly employing hairless mice (Forbes et al., 1976) and guinea pigs (Harber, 1969). Maurer (1987) has briefly reviewed phototoxicity testing in humans, animals, and *in vitro* systems.

Table 3 shows the results of several comparative phototoxicity tests. We have also included results from the guinea pig model for phototoxicity used in our laboratory (Giles et al., 1979). For a number of psoralens, the guinea pig model appears to accurately predict human phototoxicity. The chemical 5,7-dimethoxycoumarin (entry 8 in Table 3), which was reported to be lethal in a bacterial system (Harter et al., 1976), was found to be inactive in humans and guinea pigs (Giles et al., 1979). Carbethoxypsoralen (entry 3), a compound of potential therapeutic importance, was found to be weakly phototoxic in humans (Dubertret et al., 1978) and inactive in guinea pigs (Pathak et al., 1967). The sterically hindered psoralen derivatives (entries 3 and 4) and pyranocoumarins (entry 5) are new, and their phototoxicity has not been completely tested.

5-Methylangelicin (entry 9) is an example of the angelicins being developed for potential use in photochemotherapy (Dall'Acqua et al., 1981). These compounds show strong photobiological activity, yet they do not provoke skin phototoxicity.

EPILOGUE

Since its beginning around the turn of the century, the science of photobiology has had various stages of development. At a very early stage, through the classical experiments by Raab (1900) and others, it was shown that many dyes and pigments can sensitize various cells and organisms to visible light. The introduction of phototherapy by Niels R. Finsen dates from the same period. These developments extended the boundaries of photobiology to physicists, biologists, and clinicians.

The past three decades marked the beginning of molecular photobiology. An early milestone was the isolation of thymine dimers from living systems exposed to UV. Also, the molecular basis of a genetic disease, xeroderma pigmentosum, was established. The rapid expansion of molecular photobiology significantly contributed to the development of molecular biology and related disciplines and led to the advent of a new clinical discipline, photochemotherapy.

One of the objectives of photobiology will be to shed more light on the relation between phototoxicity and photocarcinogenesis, which is poorly established. It is still believed that chronic phototoxicity can lead to carcinogenesis.

TABLE 3 Comparison of Phototoxicity of Selected Compounds in Different Organisms (Topical Phototoxicity Reported for Guinea Pigs and Humans)

Compound	Human	Guinea Pig	Bacteria
 8 methoxypsoralen	+	+	+
 5 methoxypsoralen	+	+	+
 3 carbethoxypsoralen	+	N.D.	N.D. Petite Mutations in Yeast
 3 (α,α-dimethylallyl) psoralen	N.D.	—	N.D.
 pyranocoumarins	N.D.	—	+ *(E. Coli)*
 anthracene	+	+	+
 6 methylcoumarin	(Photo- allergic) —	—	N.D.
 5,7 dimethoxycoumarin	—	—	+ *(B. Subtilis)*

In at least a few cases, however, such as chronic phototoxicity evoked by anthracene or porphyrins, no carcinogenic developments were observed. A possible explanation for this phenomenon is that the primary targets of anthracene and other photodynamic sensitizers are molecules not directly involved in the transmission of genetic information.

One of the major conceptual advances in photobiology in the past few years is the perception that photon toxicity is not limited to skin; it can, and often does, induce significant systemic alterations. Therefore, the significance of photobiology exceeds that of dermatology. Basic photobiology should become common knowledge in all branches of basic and clinical medicine.

In all civilizations humans have worshiped the sun. They have recognized that the sun is the most important of the factors that sustain life on the earth, and that many of our daily rhythms are dependent on the cycles of sunlight. We know today that sunlight is also one of the most potent carcinogens present in the environment. To survive the insult of photons, humans have evolved a group of defense mechanisms. These include keratinization (thickening of the stratum corneum), production of melanin (the most important protective pigment in the skin), and synthesis of urocanic acid (an absorber of UV). The dietary carotenoid pigments also provide some protection by absorbing in the visible region and quenching singlet oxygen and various active radical species.

The protective mechanisms evolved against the detrimental effects of the sun are, in a growing number of cases, inadequate because of our modern lifestyles. We must therefore increase our understanding of light-induced toxic reactions and judiciously use this knowledge to protect the public health.

REFERENCES

Allison, A. C., Magnus, I. A. and Young, M. R. 1966. Role of lysosomes and of cell membranes in photosensitization. *Nature (Lond.)* 209:874–878.

Ananthaswamy, H. N., Price, J. E., Goldberg, L. H. and Bales, E. S. 1988. Detection and identification of activated oncogenes in human skin cancers occurring on sun-exposed body sites. *Cancer Res.* 48:3341–3346.

Anderson, R. R. and Parrish, J. A. 1981. The optics of skin. *J. Invest. Dermatol.* 77:13–19.

Applegate, L. A., Ley, R. D., Alcalay, J. and Kripke, M. L. 1989. Identification of the molecular target for the suppression of contact hypersensitivity by ultraviolet radiation. *J. Exp. Med.* 170:1117–1131.

Ashwood-Smith, M. J., Poulton, G. A., Barker, M. and Midenberger, M. 1980. 5-Methoxypsoralen, an ingredient in several suntan preparations, has lethal mutagenic and clastogenic properties. *Nature (Lond.)* 285:407–409.

Baccichetti, F., Bordin, F., Carlassare, F., Rodighiero, P., Guiotto, A., Peron, M., Capozzi, A. and Dall'Acqua, F. 1981. 4'-Methylangelicin derivatives: A new group of highly photosensitizing monofunctional furocoumarins. *Il Farmaco. Ed. Sci.* 36:585–597.

Baccichetti, F., Carlassare, F., Bordin, F., Guiotto, A., Rodighiero, P., Tamaro, M. and Dall'Acqua, F. 1984. 4,4',6-Trimethylangelicin, a new very photoreactive and non skin-phototoxic monofunctional furocoumarin. *Photochem. Photobiol.* 39:525–529.

Baden, H. P. and Pathak, N. A. 1967. The metabolism and function of urocanic acid in skin. *J. Invest. Dermatol.* 48:11–17.

Baden, H. P., Parrington, J. M., Delhanty, J. D. A. and Pathak, M. A. 1972. DNA synthesis in normal and xeroderma pigmentosum fibroblasts following treatment with 8-methoxypsoralen and long wave ultraviolet light. *Biochim. Biophys. Acta* 262:247–255.

Beadle, P. C. and Burton, J. L. 1981. Absorption of ultraviolet radiation by skin surface lipid. *Br. J. Dermatol.* 104:549–551.

Bergfeld, W. F. 1977. Histopathologic changes in skin after photochemotherapy. *Cutis* 20:504–507.

Beukers, R. and Berends, W. 1960. Isolation and identification of the irradiation product of thymine. *Biochim. Biophys. Acta* 41:550–551.

Bishop, J. M. 1983. Cellular oncogenes and retroviruses. *Annu. Rev. Biochem.* 52:301–354.

Blackburn, G. M. and Taussig, P. E. 1975. The photocarcinogenicity of anthracene: Photochemical binding to deoxyribonucleic acid in tissue culture. *Biochem. J.* 149:289–291.

Blog, F. B. and Szabo, G. 1979. The effects of psoralen and UVA (PUVA) on epidermal melanocytes of the tail in C57BL mice. *J. Invest. Dermatol.* 73:533–537.

Blum, H. F. 1941. *Photodynamic Action and Diseases Caused by Light.* New York: Reinhold.

Bohr, V. A. and Okumoto, D. S. 1988. Analysis of pyrimidine dimers in defined genes. In *DNA Repair,* vol. 3, eds. E. C. Friedburg and P. C. Hanawalt, pp. 347–366. New York: Marcel Dekker.

Boyer, V., Moustacchi, E. and Sage, E. 1988. Sequence specificity in photoreactions of various psoralen derivatives with DNA: Role in biological activity. *Biochemistry* 27:3011–3018.

Bredberg, A., Lambert, B., Swanbeck, G. and Thyresson-Hok, M. 1977. The binding of 8-methoxypsoralen to nuclear DNA of UVA irradiated human fibroblasts *in vitro. Acta Dermatol. Venereol.* 57:389–391.

Burton, G. W. and Ingold, K. U. 1984. β-Carotene: An unusual type of lipid antioxidant. *Science* 224:569–573.

Cadet, J. and Teoule, R. 1978. Comparative study of oxidation of nucleic acid components by hydroxyl radicals, singlet oxygen and superoxide anion radicals. *Photochem. Photobiol.* 28:661–667.

Cebula, T. A. and Koch, W. H. 1990. Analysis of spontaneous and psoralen-induced *Salmonella typhimurium hisG46* revertants by oligodeoxyribonucleotide colony hybridization: Use of psoralens to cross-link probes to target sequences. *Mutat. Res.* 229:79–87.

Cebula, T. A., Koch, W. H. and Lampel, K. A. 1989. Polymerase chain reaction (PCR) amplification of spontaneous and PUVA-induced mutations. *Photchem. Photobiol.* 49(Suppl.):111s.

Cleaver, J. E. and Trosko, J. E. 1970. Absence of excision of ultraviolet-induced cyclobutane dimers in xeroderma pigmentosum. *Photochem. Photobiol.* 11:547–550.

Cloud, T. M., Hakim, R. and Griffin, A. C. 1960. Photosensitization of the eye with methoxsalen. I. Chronic effects. *Arch. Ophthalmol.* 64:346–351.

Copeland, E. S., Alving, C. R. and Grenan, M. M. 1976. Light-induced leakage of spin label marker from liposomes in the presence of phototoxic phenothiazines. *Photochem. Photobiol.* 24:41–48.

Dall'Acqua, F. 1977. New chemical aspects of the photoreaction between psoralen and

562   *A. Kornhauser et al.*

DNA. In *Research in Photobiology,* ed. A. Castellani, pp. 245–255. New York: Plenum Press.

Dall'Acqua, F. 1989. New psoralens and analogs. In *PSORALENS Past, Present and Future of Photochemoprotection and Other Biological Activities,* eds. T. B. Fitzpatrick, P. Forlot, M. A. Pathak and F. Urbach, pp. 237–250. Paris: John Libbey Eurotex.

Dall'Acqua, F., Vedaldi, D., Caffieri, S., Guiotto, A., Rodighiero, P., Baccichetti, F., Carlassare, F. and Bordin, F. 1981. New monofunctional reagents for DNA as possible agents for the photochemotherapy of psoriasis: Derivatives of 4,5'-dimethylangelicin. *J. Med. Chem.* 24:178–184.

D'Ambrosio, S. M., Whetstone, J. W., Slazinski, L. and Lowney, E. 1981. Photorepair of pyrimidine dimers in human skin *in vivo. Photochem. Photobiol.* 34:461–464.

Daniels, F. 1965. A simple microbiological method for demonstrating phototoxic compounds. *J. Invest. Dermatol.* 44:259–263.

Daniels, F., Jr., Brophy, D. and Lobitz, W. C., Jr. 1961. Histochemical responses of human skin following ultraviolet irradiation. *J. Invest. Dermatol.* 37:351–357.

Danno, K. and Horio, T. 1980. Histochemical staining of cells for sulphhydryl and disulphide groups: A time course study. *Br. J. Dermatol.* 102:535–539.

DeFabo, E. C. and Noonan, F. P. 1983. Mechanism of immune suppression by ultraviolet irradiation *in vivo. J. Exp. Med.* 157:84–98.

DeFabo, E. C., Noonan, F. P. and Kripke, M. L. 1981. An *in vivo* action spectrum for ultraviolet radiation-induced suppression of contact sensitivity in BALB/c mice. *9th Annu. Meet. Am. Soc. Photobiol. Program Abstr.* 185.

de Mol, N. J. and Beijersbergen van Henegouwen, G. M. J. 1981. Relation between some photobiological properties of furocoumarins and their extent of singlet oxygen production. *Photochem. Photobiol.* 33:815–819.

Dougherty, T. J. 1987. Photosensitizers: Therapy and detection of malignant tumors. *Photochem. Photobiol.* 45:879–890.

Drobetsky, E. A., Grosovsky, A. J., Skandalis, A., and Glickman, B. W. 1989. Perspectives on UV light mutagenesis: Investigation of the CHO aprt gene carried on a retroviral shuttle vector. *Somat. Cell Mol. Genet.* 16:401–408.

Dubertret, L., Averbeck, D., Zajdela, F., Bisagni, E., Moustacchi, E., Touraine, R. and Latarjet, R. 1978. Photochemotherapy (PUVA) of psoriasis using 3-carbethoxypsoralen, a noncarcinogenic compound in mice. *Br. J. Dermatol.* 101:379–389.

Edelson, L. E. and Fink, J. M. 1985. The immunologic function of skin. *Sci. Am.* June, 46–53.

Edelson, R. L. and 19 other participating investigators. 1987. Treatment of cutaneous T-cell lymphoma by extracorporeal phototherapy. *N. Engl. J. Med.* 316:297–303.

Edelson, R. L. 1988. Light-activated drugs. *Sci. Am.* August, 68–75.

Everett, M. A., Yeargers, E., Sayre, R. M. and Olson, R. L. 1966. Penetration of epidermis by ultraviolet rays. *Photochem. Photobiol.* 5:533–542.

Fisher, G. J., Varghese, A. J. and John, H. E. 1974. Ultraviolet induced reactions of thymine and uracil in the presence of cysteine. *Photochem. Photobiol.* 20:109–120.

Fitzpatrick, T. B., Pathak, M. A., Harber, L. C., Seiji, M. and Kukita, A. 1974. An introduction to the problem of normal and abnormal responses of man's skin to solar radiation. In *Sunlight and Man,* eds. M. A. Pathak, L. C. Harber, M. Seiji, and A. Kukita, pp. 3–14. Tokyo: University of Tokyo Press.

Forbes, P. D., Davies, R. E. and Urbach, F. 1976. Phototoxicity and photocarcinogenesis: Comparative effects of anthracene and 8-methoxypsoralen in the skin of mice. *Food Cosmet. Toxicol.* 14:303–306.

Fornace, A. J. and Kohn, K. W. 1976. DNA-protein cross-linking by ultraviolet radiation in normal human and xeroderma pigmentosum fibroblasts. *Biochim. Biophys. Acta* 435:95–103.

Franklin, W. A., Ming Lo, K. and Haseltine, W. A. 1982. Alkaline lability of fluorescent photoproducts produced in ultraviolet light-irradiated DNA. *J. Biol. Chem.* 257:13535–13543.

Franklin, W. A. and Haseltine, W. A. 1986. The role of the (6-4) photoproduct in ultraviolet light-induced transition mutations in *E. coli. Mutat. Res.* 165:1–7.

Freeman, S. E., Blackett, A. D., Monteleone, D. C., Setlow, R. B., Sutherland, B. M. and Sutherland, J. C. 1986. Quantitation of radiation-, chemical-, or enzyme-induced single strand breaks in nonradioactive DNA by alkaline gel electrophoresis: Application to pyrimidine dimers. *Anal. Biochem.* 158:119–129.

Freeman, S. E., Gange, R. W., Sutherland, J. C., Matzinger, E. A. and Sutherland, B. M. 1987a. Production of pyrimidine dimers in DNA of human skin exposed *in situ* to UVA radiation. *J. Invest. Dermatol.* 88:430–433.

Freeman, S. E., Gange, R. W., Sutherland, J. C. and Sutherland, B. M. 1987b. Pyrimidine dimer formation in human skin. *Photochem. Photobiol.* 46:207–212.

Friedburg, E. C. 1988. Deoxyribonucleic acid repair in the yeast *Saccharomyces cerevisiae. Microbiol. Brief Rev.* 52:70–102.

Friedman, P. S. and Rogers, S. 1980. Photochemotherapy of psoriasis: DNA damage in lymphocytes. *J. Invest. Dermatol.* 74:440–443.

Gerrit van der Schroeff, J., Evers, L. M., Boot, J. M. and Bos, J. L. 1990. Ras oncogene mutations in basal cell carcinomas and squamous cell carcinomas of human skin. *J. Invest. Dermatol.* 94:423–425.

Gilchrest, B., Parrish, J. A., Tannenbaum, L., Haynes, H. and Fitzpatrick, T. B. 1976. Oral methoxsalen photochemotherapy of mycosis fungoides. *Cancer (Philadelphia)* 38:683–689.

Giles, A., Jr., Tobin, P. and Kornhauser, A. 1979. 8-MOP and 5,7-dimethoxycoumarin (DMC) phototoxicity, oral vs. topical. *7th Annu. Meet. Am. Soc. Photobiol. Program Abstr.* 146.

Giles, A., Jr., Warner, W. and Kornhauser, A. 1985. The *in vivo* protective effect of β-carotene against psoralen phototoxicity. *Photochem. Photobiol.* 41:661–666.

Goldstein, B. D. and Harber, L. C. 1972. Erythropoietic protoporphyria: Lipid oxidation and red cell membrane damage associated with photochemolysis. *J. Clin. Invest.* 51:892–902.

Goldyne, M. E. 1975. Prostaglandins and cutaneous inflammation. *J. Invest. Dermatol.* 64:377–385.

Greaves, M. W. 1978. Does ultraviolet-evoked prostaglandin formation protect skin from actinic cancer? *Lancet* i:189.

Gruener, N. and Lockwood, M. P. 1979. Photodynamic mutagenicity in mammalian cells. *Biochem. Biophys. Res. Commun.* 90:460–465.

Grupper, C. and Berretti, B. 1981. 5-MOP in PUVA and RE-PUVA—A monocentric study: 250 Patients with a follow-up of three years. Presented at the 3rd International Symposium on Psoriasis, Stanford, Calif.

Gutter, B., Speck, W. T. and Rosenkranz, H. S. 1977. A study of the photoinduced mutagenicity of methylene blue. *Mutat. Res.* 44:177–182.

Harber, L. C. 1969. Use of guinea-pigs in photobiologic studies. In *The Biologic Effects of Ultraviolet Radiation,* ed. F. Urbach, pp. 291–295. New York: Pergamon Press.

Harber, L. C., Baer, R. L. and Bickers, D. R. 1974. Technique of evaluation of phototoxicity and photoallergy in biologic systems, including man, with particular emphasis on immunologic aspects. In *Sunlight and Man*, eds. M. A. Pathak, L. C. Harber, M. Seiji, and A. Kukita, pp. 515–528. Tokyo: University of Tokyo Press.

Hart, R. W., Setlow, R. B. and Woodhead, A. D. 1977. Evidence that pyrimidine dimers in DNA can give rise to tumors. *Proc. Natl. Acad. Sci. USA* 74:5574–5578.

Harter, M. L., Felkner, I. C. and Song, P. S. 1976. Near-UV effects of 5,7-dimethoxycoumarin in *Bacillus subtilis. Photochem. Photobiol.* 24:491–493.

Hass, B. S. and Webb, R. B. 1981. Photodynamic effects of dyes on bacteria. *Mutat. Res.* 81:277–285.

Honigsmann, H., Jaschke, E., Gschnait, W. B., Fritsch, P. and Wolff, K. 1979. 5-Methoxypsoralen (Bergapten) in photochemotherapy of psoriasis. *Br. J. Dermatol.* 101:369–378.

Honigsmann, H., Wolff, K., Gschnait, F., Brenner, W. and Jaschke, E. 1980. Keratoses and nonmelanoma skin tumors in long-term photochemotherapy (PUVA). *J. Am. Acad. Dermatol.* 3:406–414.

Husain, Z., Yang, Q. and Biswas, D. K. 1990. cHa-ras proto-oncogene: Amplification and overexpression in UV-B-induced mouse skin papillomas and carcinomas. *Arch. Dermatol.* 126:324–330.

Hutchinson, F. and Wood, R. D. 1988. Determination of sequence changes induced by mutagenesis of the cI gene of lambda phage. In *DNA Repair*, vol. 3, eds. E. C. Friedburg and P. C. Hanawalt, pp. 219–233. New York: Marcel Dekker.

Hynek. 1951. *Astrophysics,* p. 272. New York: McGraw-Hill.

Ito, T. 1978. Cellular and subcellular mechanisms of photodynamic action: The $^1O_2$ hypothesis as a driving force in recent research. *Photochem. Photobiol.* 28:493–508.

Ito, T. and Kobayashi, K. 1977. A survey of *in vivo* photodynamic activity of xanthenes, thiazines, and acridine in yeast cells. *Photochem. Photobiol.* 26:581–587.

Jori, G. and Spikes, J. D. 1982. Photosensitized oxidations in complex biological structures. In *Oxygen and Oxy-Radicals in Chemistry and Biology,* eds. M. A. J. Rodgers and E. L. Powers, pp. 441–457. New York: Academic Press.

Kagan, J. and Gabriel, R. 1980. *Candida utilis* as a convenient and safe substitute for the pathogenic yeast *C. albicans* in Daniel's phototoxicity test. *Experientia* 36:587–588.

Kantor, G. J., Sutherland, J. C. and Setlow, R. B. 1980. Action spectra for killing nondividing normal human and xeroderma pigmentosum cells. *Photochem. Photobiol.* 31:459–464.

Kessel, D. 1977. Effects of photoactivated porphyrins at the cell surface of leukemia L1210 cells. *Biochemistry* 16:3443–3449.

Kligman, A. M. and Breit, R. 1968. The identification of phototoxic drugs by human assay. *J. Invest. Dermatol.* 51:90–99.

Kobayashi, K. and Ito, T. 1976. Further *in vivo* studies on the participation of singlet oxygen in the photodynamic inactivation and induction of genetic changes in *Saccharomyces cerevisiae. Photochem. Photobiol.* 23:21–28.

Kochevar, I. 1981. Phototoxicity mechanisms: Chlorpromazine photosensitized damage to DNA and cell membranes. *J. Invest. Dermatol.* 77:59–64.

Kornhauser, A. 1976. UV-induced DNA-protein cross-links *in vivo* and *in vitro. Photochem. Photobiol.* 23:457–460.

Kornhauser, A. and Pathak, M. A. 1972. Studies on the mechanism of the photosensitized dimerization of pyrimidines. *Z. Naturforsch. Teil B* 27:550–553.

Kornhauser, A., Burnett, J. B. and Szabo, G. 1974. Isotope effects in the photosensitized dimerization of pyrimidines. *Croat. Chem. Acta* 46:193–197.

Kornhauser, A., Pathak, M. A., Zimmerman, E. and Szabo, G. 1976a. The *in vivo* effect of ultraviolet irradiation (290–350 nm) on epidermal chromatin. *Croat. Chem. Acta* 48:385–390.

Kornhauser, A., Garcia, R. I., Szabo, G., Stanford, D. and Krinsky, N. I. 1976b. Possible role of singlet oxygen in melanin biosynthesis. *Fourth Annu. Meet. Am. Soc. Photobiology*, Denver, Colo.

Kornhauser, A., Warner, W. G. and Giles, A. L., Jr. 1982. Psoralen phototoxicity: Correlation with serum and epidermal 8-methoxypsoralen and 5-methoxypsoralen in the guinea pig. *Science* 217:733–735.

Kornhauser, A., Warner, W. G., Lambert, L. A. and Koch, W. H. 1989. Are activated oxygen species involved in PUVA-induced biological effects in vivo? In *PSORA-LENS Past, Present and Future of Photochemoprotection and Other Biological Activities*, eds. T. B. Fitzpatrick, P. Forlot, M. A. Pathak, and F. Urbach, pp. 251–260. Paris: John Libbey Eurotex.

Krinsky, N. I. and Deneke, S. M. 1982. Interaction of oxygen and oxy-radicals with carotenoids. *J. Natl. Cancer Inst.* 69:205–210.

Kripke, M. L. 1980. Immunologic effects of UV radiation and their role in photocarcinogenesis. *Photochem. Photobiol. Rev.* 5:257–292.

Kripke, M. L. 1986. Photoimmunology: The first decade. *Curr. Prob. Dermatol.* 15:164–175.

Lamola, A. A. 1968. Excited state precursors of thymine photodimers. *Photochem. Photobiol.* 7:619–632.

Lamola, A. A. and Doleiden, F. H. 1980. Cross linking of membrane proteins and protoporphyrin-sensitized photohemolysis. *Photochem. Photobiol.* 31:597–601.

Lamola, A. A., Yamane, T. and Trozzalo, A. M. 1973. Cholesterol hydroperoxide formation in red cell membranes and photochemolysis in erythropoietic protoporphyria. *Science* 179:1131–1133.

Laskin, J. D., Lee, E., Yurkow, E. J., Laskin, D. L. and Gallo, M. A. 1985. A possible mechanism of psoralen phototoxicity not involving direct interaction with DNA. *Proc. Natl. Acad. Sci. USA* 82:6158–6162.

Laskin, J. D., Lee, E., Laskin, D. L. and Gallo, M. A. 1986. Psoralens potentiate ultraviolet light-induced inhibition of epidermal growth factor binding. *Proc. Natl. Acad. Sci. USA* 83:8211–8215.

Maibach, H. I. and Kligman, A. M. 1960. Dihydroxyacetone: A suntan-stimulating agent. *Arch. Dermatol.* 82:505–507.

Mandula, B. B., Pathak, M. A. and Dudek, G. 1976. Photochemotherapy: Identification of a metabolite of 4,5′,8-trimethylpsoralen. *Science* 193:1131–1134.

Maurer, T. H. 1987. Phototoxicity testing—In vivo and in vitro. *Food. Chem. Toxicol.* 25:407–414.

Mitchell, D. L. and Clarkson, J. M. 1981. The development of a radioimmunoassay for the detection of photoproducts in mammalian cell DNA. *Biochim. Biophys. Acta* 655:40–54.

Mitchell, D. L. and Nairn, R. S. 1989. The biology of the (6-4) photoproduct. *Photochem. Photobiol.* 49:805–820.

Moan, J. and Christensen, T. 1981. Photodynamic effects on human cells exposed to light in the presence of hematoporphyrin. Localization of the active dye. *Cancer Lett.* 11:209–214.

Moan, J., Pettersen, E. O. and Christensen, T. 1979. The mechanism of photodynamic inactivation of human cells in vitro in the presence of hematoporphyrin. *Br. J. Cancer* 39:398–407.

Morison, W. L., Paul, B. S. and Parrish, J. A. 1977. The effects of indomethacin on long-wave ultraviolet-induced delayed erythema. *J. Invest. Dermatol.* 68:120–133.

Morison, W. L., Parrish, J. A., Block, K. J. and Krugler, J. I. 1979. Transient impairment of peripheral blood lymphocyte function during PUVA therapy. *Br. J. Dermatol.* 101:391–397.

Morison, W. L. 1989. Effects of ultraviolet radiation on the immune system in humans. *Photochem. Photobiol.* 50:515–524.

Mukai, F. and Goldstein, B. 1976. Mutagenicity of malonaldehyde, a decomposition product of peroxidized polyunsaturated fatty acids. *Science* 191:868–869.

Natarajan, A. T., Verdegaal-Immerzeel, E. A. M., Elly, A. M., Ashwood-Smith, M. J. and Poulton, G. A. 1981. Chromosomal damage induced by furocoumarins and UVA in hamster and human cells including cells from patients with ataxia telangiectasia and xeroderma pigmentosum. *Mutat. Res.* 84:113–124.

National Institutes of Health Consensus Development Conference Statement. 1989. *Sunlight, Ultraviolet Radiation, and the Skin,* vol. 7, number 8, May 8–10.

Noonan, F. P., DeFabo, E. C. and Morrison, H. 1988. *Cis*-urocanic acid, a product formed by ultraviolet-B irradiation of the skin, initiates an antigen presentation defect in splenic dendritic cells *in vivo. J. Invest. Dermatol.* 90:92–99.

Olson, R. L., Gaylor, J. and Everett, M. A. 1974. Ultraviolet-induced individual cell keratinization. *J. Cutan. Pathol.* 1:120–125.

Parrish, J. A. and Jaenicke, K. F. 1981. Action spectrum for phototherapy of psoriasis. *J. Invest. Dermatol.* 76:359–362.

Parrish, J. A., Fitzpatrick, T. B., Tannenbaum, L. and Pathak, M. A. 1974. Photochemotherapy of psoriasis with oral methoxsalen and long-wave ultraviolet light. *N. Engl. J. Med.* 291:1207–1222.

Parrish, J. A., White, H. A. D. and Pathak, M. A. 1979. Photomedicine. In *Dermatology in General Medicine,* eds. T. B. Fitzpatrick, A. Z. Eisen, K. Wolff, I. M. Freedberg, and K. F. Austen, pp. 942–994. New York: McGraw-Hill.

Pathak, M. A. 1967. Photobiology of melanogenesis: Biophysical aspects. In *Advances in Biology of Skin,* vol. 8, *The Pigmentary System,* eds. W. Montagna and F. Hu, pp. 400–419. New York: Pergamon Press.

Pathak, M. A. 1982. Molecular aspects of drug photosensitivity with special emphasis on psoralen photosensitization reaction. *J. Natl. Cancer Inst.* 69:163–170.

Pathak, M. A. and Kramer, D. M. 1969. Photosensitization of skin *in vivo* by furocoumarins (psoralens). *Biochim. Biophys. Acta* 195:197–206.

Pathak, M. A. and Joshi, P. C. 1984. Production of active oxygen species ($^1O_2$ and O_2) by psoralens and ultraviolet radiation (320–400 nm). *Biochim. Biophys. Acta* 798:115–126.

Pathak, M. A., Kramer, D. M. and Fitzpatrick, T. B. 1974. Photobiology and photochemistry of furocoumarins (psoralens). In *Sunlight and Man,* eds. M. A. Pathak, L. C. Harber, M. Seiji, and A. Kukita, pp. 335–368. Tokyo: University of Tokyo Press.

Pathak, M. A., Kramer, D. M. and Gungerich, U. 1972. Formation of thymine dimers in mammalian skin by ultraviolet radiation *in vivo. Photochem. Photobiol.* 15:177–185.

Pathak, M. A., Worden, L. R. and Kaufman, K. D. 1967. Effect of structural alterations on the potency of furocoumarins (psoralens) and related compounds. *J. Invest. Dermatol.* 48:103–118.

Peak, M. J. and Peak, J. G. 1989. Solar-ultraviolet-induced damage to DNA. *Photodermatology* 6:1–15.

Pileni, M. and Santus, R. 1978. On the photosensitizing properties of *N*-formyl kynurenine and related compounds. *Photochem. Photobiol.* 28:525–529.

Poppe, W. and Grossweiner, L. I. 1975. Photodynamic sensitization by 8-

methoxypsoralen via the singlet oxygen mechanism. *Photochem. Photobiol.* 22:217–219.

Raab, O. 1900. Uber die Wirkung Fluorescierender Stoffe auf Infusoriera. *Z. Biol.* 39:525–535.

Reeve, V. E., Greenoak, G. E., Canfield, P. J., Boehm-Wilcox, C. and Gallagher, C. H. 1989. Topical urocanic acid enhances UV-induced tumor yield and malignancy in the hairless mouse. *Photochem. Photobiol.* 49:459–464.

Rodighiero, G., Dall'Acqua, F. and Pathak, M. A. 1984. Photobiological properties of monofunctional furocoumarin derivatives. In *Topics in Photomedicine*, ed. K. C. Smith, pp. 319–397. New York: Plenum Press.

Rosenstein, B. S. and Setlow, R. B. 1980. Photoreactivation of ICR 2A frog cells after exposure to monochromatic ultraviolet radiation in the 252–313 nm range. *Photochem. Photobiol.* 32:361–366.

Rothman, R. H. and Setlow, R. B. 1979. An action spectrum for cell killing and pyrimidine dimer formation in hamster V-79 cells. *Photochem. Photobiol.* 29:57–61.

Schenck, G. O. 1960. Selektivitat und typische Reaktions-mechanismen in der Strahlenchemie. *Z. Electrochem.* 64:997–1011.

Schott, H. N. and Shetlar, M. D. 1974. Photoaddition of amino acids to thymine. *Biochem. Biophys. Res. Commun.* 59:1112–1116.

Setlow, J. K. and Setlow, R. B. 1963. Nature of the photoreactivable ultra-violet lesion in deoxyribonucleic acid. *Nature (Lond.)* 197:560–562.

Shetlar, M. D., Schott, H. N., Martinson, H. G. and Lin, E. T. 1975. Formation of thymine-lysine adducts in irradiated DNA-lysine systems. *Biochem. Biophys. Res. Commun.* 66:88–93.

Silver, M. J. and Smith, J. B. 1975. Prostaglandins as intracellular messengers. *Life Sci.* 16:1635–1648.

Singh, H. and Vadasz, J. A. 1978. Singlet oxygen: A major reactive species in the furocoumarin photosensitized inactivation of *E. coli* ribosomes. *Photochem. Photobiol.* 28:539–546.

Smith, K. C. 1962. Dose-dependent decrease in extractability of DNA from bacteria following irradiation with ultraviolet light or with visible light plus dye. *Biochem. Biophys. Res. Commun.* 8:157–163.

Smith, K. C. 1974. Molecular changes in nucleic acids produced by ultraviolet and visible radiation. In *Sunlight and Man*, eds. M. A. Pathak, L. C. Harber, M. Seiji, and A. Kukita, pp. 57–66. Tokyo: University of Tokyo Press.

Snyder, D. S. and Eaglstein, W. H. 1974. Intradermal antiprostaglandin agents and sunburn. *J. Invest. Dermatol.* 62:47–50.

Soffen, G. A. and Blum, H. F. 1961. Quantitative measurements of cell change following a single dose of ultraviolet light. *J. Cell. Comp. Physiol.* 58:81–96.

Spikes, J. D. 1975. Porphyrins and related compounds as photodynamic sensitizers. *Ann. N.Y. Acad. Sci.* 44:496–508.

Staricco, R. J. and Pinkus, H. 1957. Quantitative and qualitative data on the pigment cells of adult human epidermis. *J. Invest. Dermatol.* 28:33–45.

Stern, R. S., Thibodeu, L. A., Kleinerman, R. A., Parrish, J. A., Fitzpatrick, T. B., and 22 participating investigators. 1979. Risk of cutaneous carcinoma in patients treated with oral methoxsalen photochemotherapy for psoriasis. *N. Engl. J. Med.* 300:809–813.

Stern, R. S. 1989. PUVA: Its status in the United States, 1988. In *PSORALENS Past, Present and Future of Photochemoprotection and Other Biological Activities*, eds. T. B. Fitzpatrick, P. Forlot, M. A. Pathak, and F. Urbach, pp. 367–376. Paris: John Libbey Eurotex.

Strauss, G. H., Greaves, M., Price, M., Bridges, B. A., Hall-Smith, P. and Vella-

Briffa, D. 1980. Inhibition of delayed hypersensitivity reaction in skin (DNCB test) by 8-methoxypsoralen photochemotherapy. *Lancet* ii:556–559.

Streilein, J. W. 1983. Skin-associated lymphoid tissues (SALT): Origins and functions. *J. Invest. Dermatol.* 80:12–16s.

Strickland, P. T., Kelley, S. M. and Sukumar, S. 1985. Cellular transforming genes in mouse skin carcinomas induced by UVA or PUVA. *Photochem. Photobiol.* 41(suppl).:110S.

Szabo, G., Blog, F. B. and Kornhauser, A. 1982. Toxic effect of ultraviolet light on melanocytes: Use of animal models in pigment research. *J. Natl. Cancer Inst.* 69:245–250.

Tashjian, A. H., Jr., Voelkel, E. F. and Levine, L. 1977. Plasma concentrations of 13,14-dihydro-15-keto-prostaglandin E_2 in rabbits bearing the VX_2 carcinoma: Effects of hydrocortisone and indomethacin. *Prostaglandins* 14:309–317.

Tenenbaum, S., DiNardo, J., Morris, W. E., Wolf, B. A. and Schnetzinger, R. W. 1984. A quantitative *in vitro* assay for the evaluation of phototoxic potential of topically applied materials. *Cell Biol. Toxicol.* 1:1–9.

Todd, P. and Han, A. 1976. UV-induced DNA to protein cross-linking in mammalian cells. In *Aging, Carcinogenesis, and Radiation Biology,* ed. K. C. Smith, pp. 83–104. New York: Plenum Press.

Turro, N. J. 1965. *Molecular Photochemistry.* Reading, Mass.: Benjamin.

Urbach, F. 1989. Potential effects of altered solar ultraviolet radiation on human skin cancer. *Photochem. Photobiol.* 50:507–513.

Urbach, F., Epstein, J. H. and Forbes, P. D. 1974. Ultraviolet carcinogenesis: Experimental, global and genetic aspects. In *Sunlight and Man,* eds. M. A. Pathak, L. C. Harber, M. Seiji, and A. Kukita, pp. 259–283. Tokyo: University of Tokyo Press.

Van de Vorst, A. and Lion, Y. 1976. Indirect EPR evidence for the production of singlet oxygen in the photosensitization of nucleic acid constituents by proflavine. *Z. Naturforsch.* 31C:203–204.

Vedaldi, D., Dall'Acqua, F., Gennaro, A. and Rodighiero, G. 1983. Photosensitized effects of furocoumarins: The possible role of singlet oxygen. *Z. Naturforsch.* 38C:866–869.

Verweij, H., Dubbelman, T., and Van Steveninck, J. 1981. Photodynamic protein cross-linking. *Biochim. Biophys. Acta* 647:87–94.

Wacker, A., Dellweg, H. and Weinblum, D. 1960. Strahlenchemische Veranderung der bakterien-Deoxyribonucleinsaure *in vivo. Naturwissenschaften* 47:477.

Wacker, A., Dellweg, H., Trager, L., Kornhauser, A., Lodenmann, E., Turk, G., Selzer, R., Chandra, P. and Ishimoto, M. 1964. Organic photochemistry of nucleic acids. *Photochem. Photobiol.* 3:369–395.

Wagner, S., Taylor, W. D., Keith, A. and Snipes, W. 1980. Effects of acridine plus near ultraviolet light on *Escherichia coli* membranes and DNA *in vivo. Photochem. Photobiol.* 32:771–780.

Wennersten, G. and Brunk, U. 1977. Cellular aspects of phototoxic reactions induced by kynurenic acid I. *Acta Dermatol. Venereol.* 57:201–209.

Wennersten, G. and Brunk, U. 1978. Cellular aspects of phototoxic reactions induced by kynurenic acid II. *Acta Dermatol. Venereol.* 58:297–305.

Wolff, K., Fitzpatrick, T. B., Parrish, J. A., Gschnait, F., Gilchrest, B., Honigsmann, H., Pathak, M. A. and Tannenbaum, L. 1976. Photochemotherapy for psoriasis with orally administered methoxsalen. *Arch. Dermatol.* 112:943–950.

Woodcock, A. and Magnus, J. A. 1976. The sunburn cell in mouse skin: Preliminary quantitative studies on its production. *Br. J. Dermatol.* 95:459–468.

World Health Organization. 1979. *Ultraviolet Radiation, Environmental Health Criteria 14,* p. 18. Geneva: WHO.

Young, A. R. and Magnus, I. A. 1981. An action spectrum for 8-MOP induced sunburn cells in mammalian epidermis. *Br. J. Dermatol.* 104:541–547.

Zajdela, F. and Bisagni, E. 1981. 5-Methoxypsoralen, the melanogenic additive in suntan preparations, is tumorigenic in mice exposed to 365 nm UV radiation. *Carcinogenesis* 2:121–127.

Zierenberg, B. E., Kramer, D. M., Geisert, M. G., and Kirste, R. G. 1971. Effects of sensitized and unsensitized longwave UV-irradiation on the solution properties of DNA. *Photochem. Photobiol.* 14:515–520.

20

estimating the photoallergenicity of compounds in a mouse model

■ Henry C. Maguire, Jr. ■

HISTORY

The first basic experimental work in photoallergy was done more than 50 years ago, when Epstein, in a straightforward and very perceptive study, demonstrated that sulfanilamide was both a phototoxin and a photoallergen (Epstein, 1939; Maguire and Kaidbey, 1986). He and others had observed patients receiving sulfanilamide who developed a dermatitis in sun-exposed areas. Six naive subjects (one of whom was himself) were chosen and skin sites were injected intradermally with sulfanilamide (0.1 ml of a 1% saline solution). Then theses areas were irradiated with ultraviolet light from a mercury arc lamp (UVA + UVB). In all six subjects, the procedure induced a mild erythema leading to hyperpigmentation at the injected sites, that is, a sulfanilamide-mediated phototoxic reaction. Repetition of the protocol (intradermal sulfanilamide, then UV irradiation) at a different site, some days later, caused a marked dermatitis in two of the six individuals. These two subjects had been photosensitized to sulfanilamide, and with further phototesting they continued to show an altered reactivity to sulfanilamide followed by UVR (but not to sulfanilamide alone); their photoallergy persisted. In later work, Epstein induced photoallergic contact dermatitis to chlorpromazine in human subjects, utilizing the topical application of chlorpromazine for photosensitization and photochallenge (Epstein, 1968). Those results paralleled his findings with sulfanilamide: chlorpromazine was both a phototoxin and a photoallergen. Biopsies of positive chlorpromazine photoallergic reaction sites showed a histopathological picture consistent with that of delayed type hypersensitivity, that is, reactions similar to those of classical experimental allergic contact dermatitis in man.

Over the ensuing years, a considerable number of compounds have been tested in humans for their possible photoallergenicity, and many of the larger dermatology units have phototesting sections for evaluating patients for possible photoallergy to materials with which they come into contact (Harber and Bickers, 1989). Experimental work in humans sometimes followed the lead of clinical impressions, as was the case with chlorpromazine and tetrachlorosalysilanilide (TCSA) (Epstein, 1986; Willis and Kligman, 1968a, 1968b). Kaidbey and Kligman designed a prospective testing scheme in man for evaluating possible photocontact allergens (Kaidbey and Kligman, 1980). Their method requires repeated photosensitizing exposures, that is, application of the test chemical to the skin, followed by ultraviolet light, for photosensitization; photochallenge is done 10–14 d after the last photosensitization at an untreated skin site. This routine, which is a variant of the "maximization" test in man for classical contact allergens, has proven very useful for identifying the photoallergenicity of suspect materials (Kligman, 1966).

Schwartz and Speck were the first to demonstrate photoallergy in an experimental animal, the guinea pig. Their initial investigation was with sulfanilamide and derivatives, and later experiments were with chlorpromazine (Schwarz and Speck, 1957; Schwarz, 1969). Vinson and Borselli studied TCSA, bithionol, and several derivatives in the guinea pig and proposed a testing scheme for identifying photocontact allergens of humans in that laboratory animal (Vinson and Borselli, 1966). Variants of their method are in current use (Harber and Bickers, 1989; Maurer et al., 1980; Maurer, 1984; Jordan, 1982; Ichikawa et al., 1981; Harber et al., 1982). The common theme is to photosensitize by the repeated successive application of prospective allergen, followed by UVR, to a clipped area (sometimes with the injection of complete Freund's adjuvant into the photosensitization site). Photochallenge is done at a different skin site some weeks later and reactions are evaluated by eye, as for classic allergic contact dermatitis in the guinea pig. The technique successfully identifies most known photocontact allergens, although in our experience and that of others, the substance bisphenol-A, by clinical report a photosensitizer of humans, does not photosensitize guinea pigs (Allen and Kaidbey, 1979; Maguire, 1988).

MECHANISMS OF PHOTOALLERGENICITY

The classical explanation of photoallergenicity, originally proposed by Burckhardt, and later developed by Kligman and Willis, is that ultraviolet light causes a photochemical reaction that converts the photoallergen to a stable contact allergen (Burckhardt, 1941; Willis and Kligman, 1968a, 1968b). The UV irradiation could take place in the petri dish, and indeed, there are experiments to that effect. An alternative mechanism has been proposed by Harber and Bickers, namely, that the photoallergen is activated by UV energy to an unstable state and chemically reacts with nearby protein, the entire complex being recognized as nonself by the host's immune system (Harber and Bickers, 1989). These two mechanisms are not exclusive, and one or the other may dominate with a particular photoallergen. For prospective phototesting, it would be very unwise to rely on UV irradiation of the chemical alone to produce stable photoproducts that would then be evaluated for classic contact allergenicity. However, an *in vivo–in vitro* scheme for photohaptenization has been designed by Maguire; this method appears to overcome relevant objections and may prove of use for phototesting in special situations (Maguire, 1990).

Harber and colleagues were the first to formally show that photoallergic contact dermatitis could be adoptively transferred with viable peritoneal exudate cells from guinea pigs actively photosensitized (to TCSA), to naive guinea pigs (Harber et al., 1966). Their investigations, modeled after the experiments of Landsteiner and Chase, provided a firm link between photoallergy and classical contact allergy to simple chemicals and were of considerable theoretical importance (Landsteiner and Chase, 1942).

PHOTOALLERGY IN MICE

The development of the field of experimental photoallergy followed that of delayed-type hypersensitivity to classical contact allergens; experiments were first done in humans, then in guinea pigs, and finally in the mouse (Maguire and Kaidbey, 1986). The seminal observation of Asherson and Ptak that the mouse ear could serve as a conveniently measurable challenge site for contact allergens initiated a flood of investigations of allergic contact dermatitis using the mouse (Asherson and Ptak, 1969). Working independently, Maguire and Kaidbey and Takigawa and Myachi adapted that methodology to photoallergy: photosensitizing on the trunk and photochallenging on the ear. They showed that positive photochallenge reactions evolved with a similar time course and similar histology to those of delayed-type hypersensitivity reactions to classical contact allergens in the mouse. In addition, the photoallergic reactions were specific to the individual photoallergens, and the photoallergy could be adoptively transferred with lymphoid cells from photosensitized to naive mice of the same or appropriately related strain—that is, the hypersensitivity was genetically restricted.

In a typical protocol from our laboratory, groups of six mice are atraumatically clipped on the back with an Oster electric clipper and then anesthetized with intraperitoneal Nembutal. A solution of 20 μl of 1% chlorpromazine (CPZ) is pipetted onto the area and then this sensitization site is irradiated with UVR (UVB + UVA), taking care not to expose the mouse's ears to the UV irradiation (UVB at 0.1 J/cm^2, then UVA at 5 J/cm^2). The procedure is repeated to the same skin site the next day. Five days later, the mice are photochallenged with a solution of 1% chlorpromazine as follows: Baseline measurements are taken of the thickness of both ears utilizing an engineer's micrometer bearing a pressure-sensitive rachet. Chlorpromazine is pipetted on the distal portion of the ear (10μl to the external aspect and 5 μl to the inner aspect), and both ears are irradiated with UVA from a fluorescent source (5 J/cm^2). Following the UVA, 15 μl of chlorpromazine solution is applied to the right ear. Ear thickness is evaluated 1 and 2 d later. This experiment is outlined in Figure 1 (second day readings not shown).

In this prototypical experiment, swelling of the right ear in the experimental group (I) identifies any contact allergenicity of the material that might be superimposed on a reaction of photoallergenicity (left ear). Phototoxic and toxic reactions are seen as left and right ear swelling in the control group II (photochallenge, no photosensitization). We have successfully worked with many of the known common photoallergens in this mouse model (Maguire, 1990; Maguire and Kaidbey, 1982, 1983).

IMMUNOLOGICAL ADJUVANTS

Sometimes immunological adjuvants are employed to heighten the acquisition of the photosensitivity. Cyclophosphamide is frequently used, since pretreatment of the mouse (and of animals of other species) with cyclophosphamide (to diminish T suppressor cells) heightens the acquisition of the induced sensitivity (Maguire and Ettore, 1965; Maguire et al., 1979; Granstein et al., 1983). Cyclophosphamide pretreatment was advocated by Miyachi and Takigawa in a protocol that they recommended for screening compounds for their photoallergenicity in the mouse (Miyachi and Takigawa, 1983). Our laboratory introduced injection of heat-killed (*Corynebacterium parvum* (*Propionibacterium acnes*) into the sensitization site as a means of increasing the acquisition of delayed-type hypersensitivity in mice (and other experimental animals) (Maguire, 1981; Maguire and Cipriano, 1983). In practice, we find that combining these two immunological adjuvants gives the best result.

Laboratory Mice

We have photosensitized mice of a variety of inbred strains (including BALB/c, C3H, DBA/2, C57B1/6, and AKR, and hybrids) as well as randomly

	GROUP	Days 0, 1	Day 6	Day 7	
				Left Ear	Right Ear
(6)	I	CPZ 1% then UVR	CPZ 1%-UVA to Left Ear;	4.3*	0.3
(6)	II	--------------	UVA-CPZ 1% to Right Ear	0.7	0.0

* mm x 10^2; Left ear > right ear, p < 0.02.

FIGURE 1 Outline and results of a typical protocol.

bred mice to different photoallergens, usually using *C. parvum* and/or cyclophosphamide as immunological adjuvants, but sometimes, with less regularly induced photosensitivity, with no adjuvant. Recently, genetic restrictions at the H-2 locus were described for the induction of photosensitivity to TCSA in mice; in those experiments genetic restriction could generally be overcome by treatment with cyclophosphamide prior to photosensitization (Tokura et al., 1990). Considerations of potential genetic restriction of the immune response to unknown compounds suggest that a random-bred mouse, such as the ICR (Hauschke) mouse, be used for prospective phototesting. In addition, the random-bred mouse is cheaper, easier to breed in-house, generally healthier, and has a thicker, more readily measured ear for photochallenge.

We prefer female mice since they are more tractable, and fighting, which can result in ear damage, is less likely with them than with male mice. Pregnant mice are to be avoided, since they give erratic responses. The housing and care of the mice should conform to the best standards: temperature-controlled and light-cycled animal rooms, round-the-clock access to a mouse pellet diet and to water (preferably from a source outside the cage to avoid damp bedding), avoidance of overcrowding, frequent changes of bedding, etc.

The mouse colony should be free of common pathogens, particularly of mouse hepatitis virus, since many microorganisms, especially viruses, downregulate the immune response. This requires sensible reverse isolation, such as purchase of mice from a single source that is certified pathogen free and prohibition of visits by individuals who have recently been at other rodent facilities, etc. If possible, the test mice should be bred in-house. Surveillance for common viral pathogens is usually done by antibody testing of sera from representative mice; there are commercial laboratories that specialize in such antibody testing.

ADVANTAGES OF THE MOUSE FOR PHOTOALLERGENICITY PROSPECTIVE TESTING

As with the prospective testing of substances for common contact allergenicity, the prospective testing of possible photoallergens should first be done in experimental animals rather than in humans (Klecak, 1982). Guinea pigs or mice are possible models. Currently the guinea pig has the benefit of its history, as a model for prospective phototesting for the past 15 or more years by a number of laboratories; experience with the mouse is limited. However, development of the mouse as a standard model for photoallergy testing is worthwhile. The mouse is far cheaper to purchase, and much easier and less expensive to house. Maintaining a large inventory of guinea pigs is difficult, not so with mice. The results of prospective phototesting in guinea pigs takes many weeks, as opposed to about 10 d with the mouse. The gestation time of the guinea pig is 65 d, while that of the mouse is only 20 d, with the litter size and overall fertility of the mouse far exceeding that of the guinea pig. Thus, supplying animals in large numbers by in-house breeding is routine for mice, but next to impossible for guinea pigs.

RECOMMENDED PROTOCOL

Based on an experience that includes the photosensitizing of many thousands of mice, we recommend the following "standards" protocol. Healthy pathogen-free random-bred ICR female mice are pretreated with cyclophosphamide (100 mg/kg intraperitoneally) 2 d before photosensitization. A skin site on the rear dorsal back is gently clipped, with no abrading of skin. The mouse is anesthetized with Nembutal intraperitoneally. The test material is applied and the site is irradiated with UVB at 0.1 J/cm^2 and UVA at 5 J/cm^2 from banks of fluorescent tubes, care being taken to light shield the ears. (UVB is substantially toxic to mouse skin, and radiation with UVB can compromise the ears as a challenge site). This routine is repeated the next day and, additionally, the photosensitization site is injected intradermally with 30 μg of a suspension of C. parvum (P. acnes) in 50 μl saline (Burroughs-Wellcome). Five days later the putatively photosensitized mice, as well as a matched cohort of mice not exposed to the photosensitizing program, are ear-challenged by the application of the test material (15 μl) to the left ear prior to UVA (5 J/cm^2) and to the right ear after the UVA. Baseline, 24-h, and 48-h measurements of the ear thickness are made and compared. The method is outlined in Table 1.

PHOTOALLERGY TO SYSTEMIC DRUGS

Photoallergic reactions have been noted to systemically administered drugs as well as to topically applied medications. Indeed, the sulfanilamide experiments of Stephen Epstein, cited in the beginning of this article, derived from the observation made by a number of clinicians that patients receiving parenteral sulfanilamide could develop a dermatitis on sun-exposed areas (Tedder, 1939). Photosensitivity eruptions have been related to a number of systemic drugs including sulfa drugs, chlorpromazine, quinidine, and thiazide diuretics. We described a mouse model for photoallergy (and phototoxicity) to systemic drugs using the classic photoallergens sulfanilamide and chlorproma-

TABLE 1   Outline of Protocol in Mice for the Predictive Testing of Compounds for Their Photoallergenicity (and Phototoxicity)

Day	Procedure
−2	Cyclophosphamide 100 mg/kg ip
0, 1	Test compound, then UVR to sensitization site
1	C. parvum intradermally to sensitization site
5	Measure ear thickness, photochallenge
6, 7	Measure ear thickness

zine (Maguire and Kaidbey, 1983; Giudici and Maguire, 1989; Wirestrand and Ljunggren, 1988a). Mice were dosed intraperitoneally a few hours before UV irradiating the sensitization site (clipped trunk) or challenge site (ear). Interestingly, mice photosensitized (or photochallenged) in this way reacted to topical photochallenge (or photosensitization) with the homologous compound (Maguire and Kaidbey, 1983). This suggests that screening compounds for systemic photoallergenicity might be done by testing their capacity to induce photoallergenicity by topical application (or intradermal injection for materials that would not otherwise penetrate the skin barrier). Wirestrand and Ljunggren (1988a, 1988b), in their elegant experiments using a mouse model, demonstrated photoallergy in quinidine (Wirestrand and Ljunggren, 1988b).

A number of compounds that are putative photoallergens of man have been evaluated in the mouse assay and shown activity. These compounds are as follows: sulfanilamide, chlorpromazine, tetrachlorosalysilanilide (TCSA), bisphenol A, quinidine, hydrochlorothiazide, musk ambrette, 6-methylcoumarin, and sodium omadine. Salicylanilide, salicylic acid, and 3,4-dichloroaniline, which do not have any apparent photoallergenicity in man, have been reported negative by mouse testing (Miyachi and Takigawa, 1983).

SUMMARY

We have briefly reviewed the history of photoallergy testing. A prospective test for photoallergens in a mouse model is described and some of its advantages are indicated. We predict that this mouse model will have substantial success in identifying photoallergens of humans.

REFERENCES

Allen, H. and Kaidbey, K. 1979. Persistent photosensitivity following occupational exposure to epoxy resin. *Arch. Dermatol.* 115:1307–1310.

Asherson, G. L. and Ptak, W. L. 1969. Contact and delayed hypersensitivity in the mouse. I. Active sensitization and passive transfer. *Immunology* 15:405.

Burckhardt, W. 1941. Untersuchugen über die photoaktivität einiger sulfanilamide. *Dermatologica* 83:63.

Epstein, A. 1939. Photoallergy and primary photosensitivity to sulfanilamide. *J. Invest. Dermatol.* 2:43.

Epstein, S. 1968. Chlorpromazine photosensitivity, phototoxic and photoallergic reactions. *Arch. Dermatol.* 98:354.

Giudici, P. A. and Maguire, H. C., Jr. 1985. Experimental photoallergy to systemic drugs. *J. Invest. Dermatol.* 85:207–211.

Giudici, P. A. and Maguire, H. C., Jr. 1989. Systemic photoallergy. In *Models in Dermatology,* vol. 4, eds. H. I. Maibach and N. J. Lowe, pp. 253–255.

Granstein, R. D., Morison, W. L. and Kripke, M. L. 1983. The role of suppressor cells in the induction of murine photoallergic contact dermatitis and its suppression by prior UVB irradiation. *J. Immunol.* 130:2099–2103.

Harber, L. C. and Bickers, D. R. 1989. *Photosensitivity Diseases, Principles of Diagnosis and Treatment.* Philadelphia: W. B. Saunders.

Harber, L. C., Harris, H. and Baer, R. L. 1966. Photoallergic contact dermatitis due to halogenated salicylanilides and related compounds. *Arch. Dermatol.* 94:225.

Harber, L. C., Armstrong, R. B. and Ichikawa, H. 1982. Current status of predictive animal models for drug photoallergy and their correlation with drug photoallergy in humans. *JNCI* 69:237.

Ichikawa, I., Armstrong, R. B. and Harber, I. C. 1981. Photoallergic contact dermatitis in guinea pigs: Improved induction techniques using Freund's complete adjuvant. *J. Invest. Dermatol.* 76:498.

Jordan, W. P., Jr. 1982. The guinea pig as a model for predicting photoallergic contact dermatitis. *Contact Dermatitis* 8:109.

Kaidbey, K. H. and Kligman, A. M. 1980. Photomaximization for identifying photoallergic contact sensitizers. *Contact Dermatitis* 6:161.

Klecak, G. 1982. Identification of contact allergens: predictive tests in animals. In *Dermatotoxicology,* eds. F. N. Marzulli and H. I. Maibach. New York: Hemisphere.

Kligman, A. M. 1966. The identification of contact allergens by human assay. III. The maximization test. *J. Invest. Dermatol.* 47:393.

Landsteiner, K. and Chase, M. W. 1942. Experiments on transfer of cutaneous sensitivity to simple compounds. *Proc. Soc. Exp. Biol. Med.* 49:688.

Maguire, H. C., Jr. 1981. Immunopotentiation of allergic contact dermatitis in the guinea pig with *C. parvum (P. acnes). Acta Dermatol. Venereol. (Sweden)* 61:565.

Maguire, H. C., Jr. 1988. Experimental photoallergic contact dermatitis to bisphenol A. *Acta Dermatol. Venereol.* 68:408–412.

Maguire, H. C., Jr. 1990. A general method for photohaptenization. *Contact Dermatitis* 22:57–58.

Maguire, H. C., Jr. and Cipriano, D. 1983. Immunopotentiation of cell-mediated hypersensitivity by *C. parvum (P. acnes). Int. Arch. Allergy Appl. Immunol.* 70:34.

Maguire, H. C., Jr. and Ettore, V. 1965. Enhancement of dinitrochlorobenzene (DNCB) contact sensitization by cyclophosphamide in the guinea pig. *J. Invest. Dermatol.* 48:39.

Maguire, H. C., Jr. and Kaidbey, K. 1982. Photoallergic contact dermatitis: Induction of hypersensitivity and of immunological tolerance. *J. Invest. Dermatol.* 78:356.

Maguire, H. C., Jr. and Kaidbey, K. 1983. Studies in experimental photoallergy. In *The Effect of Ultraviolet Radiation on the Immune System,* ed. J. A. Paris, pp. 181–192. Skillman, N.J.: Johnson & Johnson.

Maguire, H. C., Jr. and Kaidbey, K. 1986. Experimental photoallergy. In *Experimental and Clinical Photoimmunology,* vol. III, pp. 167–187. Boca Raton, Fla.: CRC Press.

Maguire, H. C., Jr., Faris, L. and Weidanz, W. 1979. Cyclophosphamide intensifies the acquisition of allergic contact dermatitis in mice rendered B-cell deficient by heterologous anti-IgM antisera. *Immunology* 37:367.

Maurer, T. 1984. Experimental contact photoallergenicity: Guinea pig models. *Photodermatology* 1:221–231.

Maurer, T., Weirich, E. G. and Hess, R. 1980. Predictive animal testing for photocontact allergenicity. *Br. J. Dermatol.* 103:593.

Miyachi, Y. and Takigawa, M. 1982. Mechanisms of contact photosensitivity to tetrachlorosalicylanilide in mice. *J. Invest. Dermatol.* 78:343.

Miyachi, Y. and Takigawa, M. 1983. Mechanisms of contact photosensitivity in mice. III. Predictive testing of chemicals with photoallergenic potential in mice. *Arch. Dermatol.* 119:737.

Schwarz, K. J. 1969. Experimentelle Untersuchungen zur photoallergie gegen sulfanilamid und chlorpromazin. *Dermatologica* 139 (suppl.) 139:7–88.

Schwarz, V. K. and Speck, M. 1957. Experimentelle untersuchungen zur frage der photoallergie der sulfonilamide. *Dermatologica* 114:232–243.

Tedder, J. W. 1939. Toxic manifestations in the skin following sulfanilamide therapy. *Arch. Dermatol. Syphilol.* 39:217–227.

Tokura, Y., Takahiro, S., Takigawa, M. and Yamada, M. 1990. Genetic control of contact photosensitivity to tetrachlorosalicylanilide. I. Preferential activation of suppressor T cells in low responder H-2^k mice. *J. Invest. Dermatol.* 94:471–476.

Vinson, L. J. and Borselli, V. F. 1966. A guinea pig assay of the photosensitizing potential of topical germicides. *J. Soc. Cosmet. Chem.* 17:123.

Willis, I. and Kligman, A. M. 1968a. The mechanism of photoallergic contact dermatitis. *J. Invest. Dermatol.* 51:378.

Willis, I. and Kligman, A. M. 1968b. The mechanism of the persistent light reactor. *J. Invest. Dermatol.* 51:385.

Wirestrand, L.-E. and Ljunggren, B. 1988a. Photoallergy to systemic quinidine in the mouse. *Acta Dermatol. Venereol.* 68:41–47.

Wirestrand, L.-E. and Ljunggren, B. 1988b. Photoallergy to systemic quinidine in the mouse: dose-response studies. *Photodermatology* 5:201–205.

21

phototoxicity of topical and systemic agents

■ Francis N. Marzulli ■ Howard I. Maibach ■

INTRODUCTION

Phototoxicity is a form of chemically induced nonimmunologic skin irritation requiring light (photoirritation). The skin response is likened to an exaggerated sunburn. The involved photoactive chemical may be applied to the skin or reach this target tissue via the blood, following ingestion or parenteral administration. When systemically administered, the chemical may require metabolic conversion to become photoactive, but this is not usually the case. Aftereffects may include erythema, edema, vesiculation, hyperpigmentation, and desquamation. Inflammatory response products that may be released during these processes include histamine and arachidonic acid derivatives such as prostaglandins, leukotrienes, and kinins.

Recent addition of new photoactive therapeutic chemicals to the physicians' armamentarium together with the development of better methods for measuring and delivering solar-simulated radiation have had a stimulating effect on research involving light-related biologic phenomena. This research activity has been accompanied by the development of new test methods and therapies.

Attention of the photobiologist is largely directed at the ultraviolet (UV) area of the electromagnetic spectrum, which is subdivided for convenience into UVA (from 320 to 400 nm), UVB (from 280 to 320 nm), and UVC (below 280 nm). The visible spectrum is important in certain medical conditions such as erythropoietic protoporphyria, porphyria, and light-mediated treatment of solid tumors (Dougherty et al., 1975, 1978; Mathews–Roth, 1981).

Tests for phototoxic potential of topically applied chemicals are usually

581

conducted using UV radiation sources within the UVA range. Some phototoxic substances, however, are activated by wavelengths in the visible spectrum (bikini dermatitis; Hjorth and Moller, 1976), some by UVB (Jeanmougen et al., 1983), and some like doxycycline are augmented by UVB (Bjellerup, 1986).

Accurate measurements of radiation intensity and frequency are important prerequisites for work in phototoxicity. For further details relating to physical measurements of light the reader is directed to Chapter 18. A report by Landry and Anderson (1982) also contains useful information in this regard.

Among animals that have proved useful in predicting phototoxic effects are the mouse (hairless or haired), rabbit, swine, guinea pig, squirrel monkey, and hamster, in that approximate order of effectiveness (Marzulli and Maibach, 1970).

Phototoxic events are initiated when a photoactive drug (a chemical that is capable of absorbing UV radiation) enters the skin (via skin penetration or through blood circulation) and becomes excited by appropriate UV radiation that also penetrates skin. In some cases the photoexcited drug transfers its energy to oxygen, exciting it to the singlet oxygen state, which is cytotoxic. In other cases oxygen may not be involved. Chlorpromazine is thought to be activated by a photodynamic process involving molecular oxygen, whereas psoralens do not require molecular oxygen to produce phototoxic effects. Further discussion of photodynamic action is found in Spikes and Livingston (1969); Kearns (1971), Wennersten (1977), and Kochevar (1981).

The clinical identification of phototoxicity largely resides in morphology, together with clinical suspicion that is based upon knowledge about phototoxic chemicals. Phototoxicity generally begins with erythema (sometimes even large bullae), increased skin temperature, and pruritis. This is followed some time later by hyperpigmentation, which is the chief complaint of patients, as this condition may last for months or years.

The morphology of phototoxic eruptions from skin exposure is not always readily identified by the clinician; the lack of diagnosis in thousands of cases of dimethyl-*para*-aminobenzoic acid (sunscreen) dermatitis, until Emmett et al. (1977) brought this to our attention, provides testimony to this issue. A prepared mind is essential; removing the phototoxics is efficient, as clinical identification is often difficult.

With oral agents, photorelated dermatoses present an even greater challenge. Not only is the entity often not suspected or morphologic grounds, but the criteria for defining which are phototoxic versus photoallergic rests on relatively imprecise grounds.

PHOTOTOXIC AGENTS

Naturally occurring plant-derived furocoumarins, including psoralen, 5-methoxypsoralen (bergapten), 8-methoxypsoralen (xanthotoxin), angelicin, and others, constitute the most important class of phototoxic chemicals. Psoralens occur in a wide variety of plants such as parsley, celery, and citrus fruits (Pathak, 1974; Juntilla, 1976).

The Rutaceae (common rue, gas plant, Persian limes, bergamot) and Umbelliferae (fennel, dill, wild carrot, cow parsnip) are prominent among plant families responsible for phytophotodermatitis (Pathak, 1974). Bergapten (5-methoxypsoralen), psoralen, and xanthotoxin (8-methoxypsoralen) are among the more commonly encountered phototoxic agents. Bergapten is the active component of bergamot oil, a well-known perfume ingredient, whose phototoxic skin effects have been accorded the name berlock dermatitis. Perfume phototoxicity was studied in considerable detail by Marzulli and Maibach (1970). On the basis of these studies, it was suggested that perfumes should contain no more than 0.3% bergamot, which is equivalent of about 0.001% bergapten, to avoid phototoxicity. This study also established that bergapten was the only one of five components isolated from oil of bergamot that were responsible for phototoxic effects of the parent material. Limettin (5,7-dimethoxycoumarin), although more intensely fluorescent than bergapten, did not prove phototoxic. Since publication of this report, the FDA has received few consumer complaints of berlock dermatitis. Bergamot PT continues in some countries where bergapten-free bergamot is not used (Zaynoun et al., 1981). Bergapten has also been implicated as the cause of phototoxicity from skin contact with *Heracleum laciniatum,* a weed that grows in abundance in Norway (Kavli et al., 1983). The giant hogweed (*Heracleum mantegazzianum*) of Denmark is similarly implicated (Knudson, 1983).

Xanthotoxin, or 8-MOP, as it is often called, is the active ingredient of a drug marketed for treatment of vitiligo and psoriasis. It produces photodynamic skin effects both by topical application and by oral ingestion following skin exposure to ultraviolet irradiation. It was used orally in crude form in Egypt since ancient times (El Mofty, 1948); impetus for the use of psoralens in this country in the treatment of vitiligo was provided in large part by the work of Lerner et al. (1953). Chronic use in conjunction with exposure to light may enhance prospects for squamous-cell skin cancer, especially in young patients and those whose skin is genetically predisposed (Stern et al., 1979). This potential provides concern and restraint in the now widespread application of psoralen phototherapy (PUVA) for the management of psoriasis (Parrish et al., 1974).

Phototoxicity reactions to psoralen-containing sweet oranges (Volden et al., 1983) and to *Ruta graviolens* (common rue) have been reported recently (Heskel et al., 1983).

Coal-tar derivatives, another important group of phototoxic agents, produce occupational contact photodermatitis in industrial workers and road workers. Anthraquinone-based disperse blue 35 dye caused such effects in dye process workers. Radiation in the visible spectrum activates the dye (Gardiner et al., 1974). Pyrene, anthracene, and fluoranthene are strongly phototoxic in guinea pigs (Kochevar et al., 1982).

Oral therapeutic use of amiodarone produced phototoxic effects, a cardiac antiarrhythmic agent (Chalmers et al., 1982). Incidence, time course, and recovery from phototoxic effects of amiodarone in humans were studied by Rappersberger et al. (1989).

Quinoline antimalarials appears to be phototoxic, and some of these have been studied *in vitro* and *in vivo* (Moore and Himmens, 1982; Epling and Sibley, 1987; Ljunggren and Wirestrand, 1988). Systemic effects in a 12-yr-old boy, who was treated with a combination of chloroquine and sulfadoxine-pyrimethamine, an oral antimalarial prophylaxis, were probably related to the sulfa component.

Tetracyclines—particularly demethylchlortetracycline, but also doxycycline, chlortetracycline, and tetracycline—are phototoxic when orally ingested by humans (Verbov, 1973; Frost et al., 1972; Maibach et al., 1967). Doxycycline was reported more potent than demethylchlortetracycline or limecycline, in one study involving human volunteers (Bjellerup and Ljunggren, 1987).

Cadmium sulfide, used in tattoos for its yellow color, is phototoxic (Bjornberg, 1963).

Thiazide diuretics (hydrochlorothiazide and bendrofluazide) showed phototoxic potential (decrease in minimal erythema dose) in experiments involving cardiovascular patients (hypertension, heart failure, edema) for whom diuretics were prescribed by medical practitioners (Diffey and Langtry, 1989). The incidence of thiazide-induced photosensitivity in clinical practice, however, is rare.

NONSTEROIDAL ANTI-INFLAMMATORY DRUGS (NSAID)

NSAID have been the subject of extensive recent investigations for phototoxic potential, following reports that benoxaprofen, a suspended British antirheumatic NSAID, has this capability when administered orally or by intradermal injection (Webster et al., 1982; Allen, 1983; Stern, 1983; Anderson et al., 1987). Positive findings have been reported using sheep erythrocytes or human leucocytes in vitro (Anderson et al., 1987; Przbilla, 1987).

NSAID that are structurally related to propionic acid have been shown to possess phototoxic potential, whereas certain other type NSAID such as tenoxicam and piroxicam were not experimentally phototoxic *in vitro* or *in vivo* (Anderson, 1987; Kaidbey et al., 1989; Western et al., 1987). The propionic acid-derived NSAID produce unique immediate wheal and flare in contrast with the much-delayed exaggerated sunburn response that typifies psoralen phototoxicity.

Although piroxicam is not phototoxic under experimental test conditions involving human volunteers (Kaidbey, 1989), it has been implicated as a possible photosensitizer (photoallergic or phototoxic) clinically. One explanation for the unexpected photoactivity of piroxicam in skin is that a metabolite of piroxicam is indeed phototoxic when isolated and tested on human mononuclear cells *in vitro* (Western et al., 1987). These positive findings and likely explanation are related to production of singlet oxygen as indicated by emission at 1270 nm when the suspect metabolite is irradiated with UV *in vitro* (Kochevar, 1989; Western et al., 1987).

Other propionic acid-derived NSAID associated with an immediate phototoxic response are nabumetone, carprofen, naproxen, ketoprofen and tiaprofenic acid (Kaidbey et al., 1989; Merot et al., 1983; Aloman, 1985; Diffey et al., 1983).

HUMAN TESTING

Because of the universal response, testing of humans with topically applied photoactive chemicals can be done with minimal or no hazard on small test areas in a few subjects. For many years there was confusion on the basic pathophysiology of bergamot dermatitis. Burdick (1966) and Marzulli and Maibach (1970) showed that this dermatitis can be produced in almost all subjects. With sufficient light exposure (from a high-output Wood's light) and percutaneous penetration, dermatitis will occur. Obtaining appropriate light sources presents no problem. Penetration is enhanced in several ways: choosing a highly permeable anatomic site such as the scrotum (Feldman and Maibach, 1967), or better still, decreasing the barriers to penetration by removing the stratum corneum by stripping with cellophane tape.

CHEMICAL–SKIN CONTACT TIME BEFORE LIGHT EXPOSURE

With many chemicals there is considerable lag time before significant amounts of percutaneous penetration occurs (Feldman and Maibach, 1970). Bioassays on skin must take this delay factor into consideration, for example, reading the vasoconstrictor corticoid assay at 18–24 h after application. One might expect that light exposure could or should be delayed for many hours after application to the skin. This does not appear to be the case, at least with bermagot. Animals exposed within minutes after application will react; degree and frequency of reaction are increased with light exposure 1–2 h later. By 4 h, animals are less reactive; at 24 h, light exposure will often produce no response. This time factor must be taken into account for predictive assays; it is of considerable interest in terms of the relationship of pharmacokinetics and site of action in skin. The time relationship found optimal for bergamot does not appear to hold for all other phototoxic chemicals. Chemical–skin contact time before light exposure must be altered accordingly.

VEHICLES

Vehicles alter percutaneous penetration. A considerable literature defines chemical and vehicle properties that increase or decrease chemical release and penetration. Much of this work is done with *in vitro* or other model test systems. The experience with vehicles in animal or human *in vitro* test systems is limited. Marzulli and Maibach (1970) showed that reactions to bergamot were greater in the rabbit with 70% than with 95% alcohol. K. John and T. Gressel (personal communications, 1971) noted that in the guinea pig 8-methoxypsoralen produced greater reactions in 70% alcohol than in absolute alcohol; in the rabbit the reverse response occurred. Mineral oil gave a similar response to 70% alcohol, but there was a greatly decreased reactivity in castor and olive oil. Kaidbey and Kligman (1974), in studying the phototoxic properties of coal tar, methoxsalen, and chlorpromazine, found the result strongly influenced by vehicle choice. No single base produced optimal effects for the three chemicals; emulsion-type creams were generally poor vehicles.

It is likely that the effect of vehicle on phototoxicity (and penetration) is more complex than generally stated; until all the variables are understood, it is prudent to employ the vehicle intended for human use in the predictive assay. A more realistic evaluation of potential hazard is obtained by also employing an experimental vehicle (such as alcohol) that is likely to release the test compound.

ANIMAL TESTING

By definition, phototoxicity is a form of light-activated irritation that would occur in almost everyone, following exposure to sufficient chemical and light. In practice this rarely occurs. Even bergamot at the highest commercially used concentrations only occasionally produced dermatitis.

The development of an animal model followed that of a similar model in humans (Marzulli and Maibach, 1970). The basic requisites are adequate non-erythrogenic light and percutaneous penetration of the phototoxic agent. Most conveniently, the known phototoxic agents will produce dermatitis at wavelengths that do not ordinarily yield erythema. For this reason, with light sources such as the Wood's light, the light-irradiated negative control site should be free of dermatitis. This convenience makes for an all-or-none effect on reading.

Under appropriate test conditions, several species have been utilized successfully with oil of bergamot (Marzulli and Maibach, 1970). With bergamot the hairless mouse and rabbit appeared somewhat more sensitive than the guinea pig. The pig (swine) was less reactive, but "stripping" enhanced the responsiveness; the squirrel monkey appeared quite resistant; and the hamster showed histologic changes that were not apparent on gross inspection of the skin. It is possible that alternate anatomic test sites and different treatment schedules might alter these relative rankings. In practical terms this allows for a more than reasonable choice of test animals for laboratories to choose from. Until additional use experience is obtained, new chemicals that will be used widely in humans might also be examined on human skin.

Forbes et al. (1977) tested 160 fragrance raw materials for phototoxicity using the skin of hairless mutant mouse, humans, and swine. Mouse skin was most sensitive; however, humans and swine were more alike in quantitative and qualitative aspects of skin responses. The test methodology was similar to that used by Marzulli and Maibach (1970); however, additional light source and light measurement equipment was used. These results, reported in considerable detail, substantiate the usefulness of the basic test procedure recommended in this report for evaluating phototoxicity in animals. Furthermore, their results support information on the animal models described here.

Stott et al. (1970) used changes in guinea pig ear thickness to establish that chlorpromazine, perchlorperazine, and demethylchlortetracycline are phototoxic by topical application.

Mouse ear swelling, as measured with a caliper, was employed to quantitate phototoxic responses by Sambuco and Forbes (1984), Cole et al. (1984), and Gerberick and Ryan (1989). Maurer (1987) reported a preference for back skin rather than ear skin as a measure of phototoxic response when using calipers.

Ljunggren and Moller (1976, 1977a) produced dermatitis on the tail of the mouse by exposing it to UVA for 5 h after intraperitoneal injection with chlorpromazine. Increase in tissue fluid weight was considered a useful quantitative measure of phototoxicity. Griseofulvin, nalidixic acid imperatorin, kynaurenic acid, and amiodarone were phototoxic, in addition to psoralens and tetracyclines, by this technique (Ljunggren and Moller, 1977b).

Saunders et al. (1972) suggested measuring the photoresistance of the mouse ear to evaluate phototoxic potential of candidate agents. By this technique, chlorpromazine (ip) produced significant effects when tested on albino or black mice.

Gloxhuber (1970) used hairless mice to study phototoxicity. He found chlorpromazine and tetracycline phototoxic when administered ip but not when topically applied. On the other hand, tetrachlorsalicylanilide, acridine, and anthracene were phototoxic by topical application but not by ip administration. Differences in metabolic pathways may account for these different findings.

Bay et al. (1970) reported a reproducible technique for studying phototoxicity using white swine.

PHOTOTOXICITY IN ANIMALS FROM ORALLY ADMINISTERED CHEMICALS

As phototoxicity from orally administered chemicals may involve species-specific differences in absorption and metabolism, a useful animal model for one chemical may not apply to another.

Several animal test systems are in use, hairless mice and albino guinea pigs being animals of choice (Forbes et al., 1970; Kornhauser et al., 1982). As with topical PT, erythema is the toxicological end point. Although simple and convenient, this evaluation is subjective and not always comparable in different laboratories (A. Kornhauser, personal communication, 1984).

Kornhauser et al. (1983) prefer the epilated guinea pig. Results are reliable for extrapolating to certain human (clinical) situations. With 8-MOP, serum concentrations marking the onset of PT were within the range of those accompanying the appearance of PT in humans receiving therapeutic doses of 8-MOP (Kornhauser et al., 1982).

The hairless mouse is less effective in detecting weaker PT substances. This is mainly due to difficulties in quantitating erythema and edema. The hairless mouse is well established, however, as a model of choice for photocarcinogenesis studies (Urbach et al., 1974).

Female albino rats have been used with some success in PT tests. The male, whose dorsal skin is thick, patchy, and not uniform, does not lend itself to this type of evaluation (A. Kornhauser, personal communication, 1984). This is the only model for PT where gender of the animals is a limiting condition.

NONANIMAL TEST METHODS

There is need for nonanimal models for phototoxicity; however, it is important that they be validated prior to extrapolation of results to humans. In some cases, nonanimal tests that have limited direct application to humans may be extremely useful in explaining mechanism of action or other aspects of phototoxicity.

A simple method for screening phototoxic agents, such as *Candida albicans* (Daniels, 1965), gave discrepant results when used by Mitchell (1971). Tetramethyl thiuram monosulfide appeared to be phototoxic by the *C. albicans* test, but these results could not be confirmed when tested by topical application in mice and humans.

Gibbs (1987) has modified the *C. albicans* phototoxicity test to study action spectra of pyrrolocoumarin derivatives.

Weinberg and Springer (1981) used UVA irradiation during diffusion of chemicals from a paper disc placed on agar seeded with baker's yeast to measure phototoxic potential of fragrance materials. Resulting light-specific zones of inhibited yeast growth provided test results within 72 h.

Tennenbaum et al. (1984) similarly used yeast (*Saccharomyces cerevesiae*) to examine phototoxic potential of fragrance materials.

Salmonella typhimurium has been used to study phototoxicity of chlorodiazepoxide (Librium) and its metabolites (De Vries et al., 1983).

Mammalian cells in culture (human red blood cells, mouse peritoneal macrophages, and Chinese hamster lung cells) were used by Lock and Friend (1983) to study phototoxic effects of representative drugs, dyes, and antiseptics. Their work was intended to investigate the nature and site of phototoxic action within isolated cells—specifically to identify and differentiate substances that damage nucleus, plasma membrane, and cytoplasmic organelles.

SPECIAL EFFECTS

Phototoxic reactions sometimes mask or contribute to human photoallergic reaction. Schauder (1985) has proposed a method to distinguish phototoxic from photoallergic reactions with topical chlorpromazine, based on specific test concentrations and UVA doses.

When the skin temperature of human subjects was experimentally raised during exposure to UVA, the erythema component of phototoxicity from topical 8-MOP plus UVA was reduced (Youn et al., 1987). Thus skin temperature may have clinical significance during PUVA treatments for psoriasis, which is reported to increase the skin temperature about 5 °C (Ciafone et al., 1980).

TREATMENT

Acute lesions of human phototoxic dermatitis resolve in days to weeks, whereas recovery from hyperpigmentation is delayed for months or years. Depigmentation therapy is accomplished with 2% hydroquinone. Sunscreens are useful to protect against further hyperpigmentation.

COMMENT

Research was first driven by concerns about topically applied phototoxic substances (bergamot photodermatitis) and attempts to harness the useful aspects of psoralen phototoxicity for therapy of vitiligo and psoriasis. More recently, phototoxic potential of certain nonsteroidal anti-inflammatory drugs for oral use has provided impetus for work in this area.

Insights have been gained from bergamot, whose clinical effects long awaited simple resolution by experimental work with animal and human models.

Phototoxicity (photoirritation) is easy to detect and prevent because of the simplicity of predictive animal and human test methods. With increasing use of predictive assays, phototoxicity in humans is expected to become a minor concern to dermatologists. On the other hand, future work with nonanimal models may provide further insight regarding mechanisms of action of phototoxic chemicals.

REFERENCES

Allen, B. 1983. Benoxaprofen and the skin. *Br. J. Dermatol.* 109:361–364.

Aloman, A. 1985. Ketoprofen photodermatitis. *Contact Dermatitis* 12:112–113.

Anderson, R., Eftychis, H., Weiner, A. and Findlay, G. 1987. An in vivo and in vitro investigation of the phototoxic potential of tenoxicam, a new non-steroidal anti-inflammatory agent. *Dermatologica* 175:229–234.

Bay, W., Gleiser, C. A., Dukes, T. W. and Brown, R. S. 1970. Experimental production and evaluation of drug-induced phototoxicity in swine. *Toxicol. Appl. Pharmacol.* 17:538–547.

Bjellerup, M. 1986. Medium-wave ultraviolet radiation (UVB) is important in doxycline phototoxicity. *Acta Dermatovenereol.* 66:510–514.

Bjellerup, M. and Ljunggren, B. 1985. Photohemolytic potency of tetracyclines. *J. Invest. Dermatol.* 83:179–183.

Bjornberg, A. 1963. Reactions to light in yellow tattoos from cadmium sulfide. *Arch. Dermatol.* 88:267.

Burdick, K. 1966. Phototoxicity of Shalimar perfume. *Arch. Dermatol.* 93:424–425.

Chalmers, R. J. G., Muston, H. L., Srinivas, V. and Bennett, D. H. 1982. High incidence of amiodarone-induced photosensitivity in Northwest England. *Br. Med. J.* 285:341.

Ciafone, R., Rhodes, A., Audley, M., Freedberg, I. and Abelmann, W. 1980. The cardiovascular stress of photochemotherapy (PUVA). *J. Am. Acad. Dermatol.* 3:499–505.

Cole, C., Sambuco, C., Forbes, P. and Davies, R. 1984. Response to ultraviolet radiation: ear swelling in hairless mice. *Photodermatology* 1:114–118.

Daniels, F. 1965. A simple microbiological method for demonstrating phototoxic compounds. *J. Invest. Dermatol.* 44:259–263.

De Vries, H., Van Henegowen, G. and Wouters, P. 1983. Correlations between phototoxicity of some 7-chloro-1, 4-benzodiazepines and their (photo)chemical properties. *Pharmaceutisch Week. Sci. Ed.* 5:302–307.

Diffey, B. L., Daymond, T. J. and Fairgreaves, H. 1983. Phototoxic reactions to piroxicam, naproxen and tiaprofenic acid. *Br. J. Rheumatol.* 22:239–242.

Diffey, B. L. and Langtry, J. 1989. Phototoxic potential of thiazide diuretics in normal subjects. *Arch. Dermatol.* 125:1355–1358.

Dougherty, T., Grindey, G., Fiel, R., Weishaupt, K. and Boyle, D. 1975. Photoradiation therapy. II. Cure of animal tumors with hematoporphyrin and light. *J. Natl. Cancer Inst.* 55:115–129.

Dougherty, T., Kaufman, J., Goldfar, A., Weishaupt, K., Boyle, D. and Mittelman, A. 1978. Photoradiation therapy for treatment of malignant tumors. *Cancer Res.* 38:2628–2635.

El Mofty, A. M. 1948. A preliminary clinical report on the treatment of leukoderma with *Ammi majus*, Linn. *J. R. Egypt. Med. Assoc.* 31:651.

Emmett, E. A., Taphorn, B. R. and Kominsky, J. R. 1977. Phototoxicity occurring during the manufacture of ultraviolet-cured ink. *Arch. Dermatol.* 113:770–775.

Epling, G. and Sibley, M. 1987. Photosensitized Lysis of red blood cells by phototoxic antimalarial compounds. *Photochem. Photobiol.* 46:39–43.

Feldman, R. and Maibach, H. 1967. Regional variation in percutaneous penetration of hydrocortisone in man. *J. Invest. Dermatol.* 48:181–183.

Feldman, R. and Maibach, H. 1970. Absorption of some organic compounds through the skin of man. *J. Invest. Dermatol.* 54:399–404.

Forbes, P. D., Davies, R. E. and Urbach, F. 1970. Phototoxicity and photocarcinogenesis: Comparative effects of anthracene and 8-methoxypsoralen in the skin of mice. *Food Cosmet. Toxicol.* 14:243.

Forbes, P. D., Urbach, F. and Davies, R. E. 1977. Phototoxicity testing of fragrance materials. *Food Cosmet. Toxicol.* 15:55–60.

Frost, P., Weinstein, C. D. and Gomex, E. C. 1972. Phototoxic potential of minacycline and doxycycline. *Arch. Dermatol.* 105:681.

Gardiner, J. S., Dickson, A., MacLeod, T. M. and Frain-Bell, W. 1974. The investigation of photocontact dermatitis in a dye manufacturing process. *Br. J. Dermatol.* 86:264–271.

Gerberick, G. and Ryan, C. 1989. A predictive mouse ear-swelling model for investigating topical phototoxicity. *Food Chem. Toxicol.* 27:813–819.

Gibbs, N. 1987. An adaptation of the Candida albicans phototoxicity test to demonstrate photosensitizer action spectra. *Photodermatology* 4:312–316.

Gloxhuber, C. 1970. Phototoxicity testing of cosmetics. *J. Soc. Cosmet. Chem.* 21:825.

Heskel, N. S., Amon, R. B., Storrs, F. and White, C. R. 1983. Phytophotodermatitis due to *Ruta graveolens. Contact Dermatitis* 9:278–280.

Hjorth, N. and Moller, H. 1976. Phototoxic textile dermatitis (bikini dermatitis). *Arch. Dermatol.* 112:1445–1447.

Jeanmougin, M., Pedreio, J., Bouchet, J. and Civatte, J. 1983. Phototoxicity of 5% benezoyl peroxide in man. Evaluation with a new methodology. *Fra-Dermatologica* 167:19–23.

Juntilla, O. 1976. Allelopathic inhibitors in seeds of Heraculeum laciniatum. *Physiol. Plant* 36:374–378.

Kaidbey, K. and Kligman, A. 1974. Topical photosensitizers: Influence of vehicles on penetration. *Arch. Dermatol.* 110:868–870.

Kaidbey, K. and Mitchell, F. 1989. Photosensitizing potential of certain non-steroidal anti-inflammatory agents. *Arch. Dermatol.* 125:783–786.

Kavli, G., Midelfart, G. V. K., Haugsbo, S. and Prytz, J. O. 1983. Phototoxicity of Heracleum laciniatum. *Contact Dermatitis* 9:27–32.

Kearns, D. R. 1971. Physical and chemical properties of singlet molecular oxygen. *Chem. Rev.* 71:395–427.

Knudsen, E. A. 1983. Seasonal variations in the content of phototoxic compounds in giant hogweed. *Contact Dermatitis* 9:281–284.

Kochevar, I. 1981. Phototoxicity mechanisms: Chlorpromazine photosensitized damage to DNA and cell membranes. *J. Invest. Dermatol.* 76:59–64.

Kochevar, I. 1989. Phototoxicity of non-steroidal and anti-inflammatory drugs. *Arch. Dermatol.* 125:824–826.

Kochevar, I., Armstrong, R. B., Einbinder, J., Walther, R. R. and Harber, L. 1982. Coal tar phototoxicity: Active compounds and action spectra. *Photochem. Photobiol.* 36:65–69.

Kornhauser, A., Wamer, W. and Giles, A. 1982. Psoralen phototoxicity: Correlation with serum and epidermal 9-methoxypsoralen and 5-methoxypsoralen in the guinea pig. *Science* 217:733–735.

Kornhauser, A., Wamer, W. and Giles, A., Jr. 1983. Light-induced dermal toxicity: Effects on the cellular and molecular level. In *Dermatotoxicology,* eds. F. Marzulli and H. Maibach, pp. 323–355. Washington, D.C.: Hemisphere.

Landry, R. and Anderson, F. A. 1982. Optical radiation measurements: Instrumentation and sources of error. *J. Natl. Cancer Inst.* 69:115–161.

Lerner, A. B., Denton, C. H. and Fitzpatrick, T. B. 1953. Clinical and experimental studies with 8-methoxypsoralen in vitiligo. *J. Invest. Dermatol.* 20:299–314.

Ljunggren, B. and Moller, H. 1976. Phototoxic reaction to chlorpromazine as studied with the quantitative mouse tail technique. *Acta Dermatovenereol.* 56:373–376.

Ljunggren, B. and Moller, H. 1977a. Phenothiazine phototoxicity: An experimental study on chlorpromazine and its metabolites. *J. Invest. Dermatol.* 68:313–317.

Ljunggren, B. and Moller, H. 1977b. Drug phototoxicity in mice. *Acta Dermatovenereol.* 58:125–130.

Ljunggren, B. and Wirestrand, L. 1988. Phototoxic properties of quinine and quinidine: Two quinoline methanol isomers. *Photodermatology* 5:133–138.

Lock, S. and Friend, J. 1983. Interaction of ultraviolet light, chemicals and cultured mammalian cells: Photobiological reactions of halogenated antiseptics, drugs, and dyes. *Int. J. Cosmet. Sci.* 5:39–49.

Maibach, H. and Marzulli, F. 1975. Phototoxicity (photoirritation) from topical agents. In *Animal Models in Dermatology*, ed. H. Maibach, pp. 84–89. Edinburgh: Churchill Livingstone.

Maibach, H., Sams, W. and Epstein, J. 1967. Screening for drug toxicity by wavelengths greater than 3100 Å. *Arch. Dermatol.* 95:12–15.

Marzulli, F. and Maibach, H. 1970. Perfume phototoxicity. *J. Soc. Cosmet. Chem.* 21:686–715.

Mathews-Roth, M. 1981. Photosensitization by porphyrins and prevention of photosensitization bt carotenoids. In *Photochemical Toxicity. Proc. Seventh Symp. Food and Drug Administration Science*, pp. 279–285. U. S. Department of Health and Human Services, Public Health Service, FDA, Rockville, Md.

Maurer, T. 1987. Phototoxicity testing—*In vivo* and *in vitro*. *Food Chem. Toxicol.* 25:407–414.

Merot, Y., Harms, M., Sauvat, J. H. 1983. Photosensibilisation au carprofene (Imadyl): Un nouvel anti-inflammatoire non-steroidien. *Dermatologica* 166:301–307.

Mitchell, J. C. 1971. Psoralen-type phototoxicity of tetramethylthiurammono-sulfide for *Candida albicans; Not for man or mouse. J. Invest. Dermatol.* 56:340.

Moore, D. E. and Himmens, V. J. 1982. Photosensitization by antimalarial drugs. *Photochem. Photobiol.* 36:71–77.

Parrish, J. A., Fitzpatrick, T. B., Tannenbaum, L. and Pathak, M. A. 1974. Photochemotherapy of psoriasis with oral methoxsalen and longwave ultraviolet light. *N. Engl. J. Med.* 291:1207–1211.

Pathak, M. A. 1974. Phytophotodermatitis. In *Sunlight and Man: Normal and Abnormal Photobiologic Responses*, eds. M. A. Pathak, L. Harber, M. Seiji and A. Kukita, pp. 495–513. Tokyo: University of Tokyo Press.

Przybilla, B., Schwab-Przybilla, V., Ruzicka, T. and Ring, J. 1987. Phototoxicity of non-steroidal anti-inflammatory drugs demonstrated in vitro by a photobasophil-histamine-release test. *Photodermatology* 4:73–78.

Rappersberger, K., Honigsmann, H., Ortel, B., Tanew, A., Konrad, K. and Wolff, K. 1989. Photosensitivity and hyperpigmentation in amiodarone-treated patients: Incidence, time course and recovery. *J. Invest. Dermatol.* 93:201–209.

Sambuco, C. and Forbes, P. 1984. Quantitative assessment of phototoxicity in the skin of hairless mice. *Food Chem. Toxicol.* 22:233–236.

Saunders, D. R., Miya, T. and Mennear, J. H. 1972. Chlotopromazine-ultraviolet interaction on mouse ear. *Toxicol. Appl. Pharmacol.* 21:260–264.

Schauder, S. 1985. How to avoid phototoxic reactions in photopatch testing with chlorpromazine. *Photodermatology* 2:95–100.

Spikes, J. D. and Livingston, R. 1969. The molecular biology of photodynamic action: Sensitized photooxidation in biological systems. In *Advances in Radiation Biology*, vol. 3, eds. L. G. Augenstein, R. Mason and M. Zelle, pp. 29–121. New York: Academic Press.

Stern, R. S. 1983. Phototoxic reactions to piroxicam and other nonsteroidal antiinflammatory agents. *N. Engl. J. Med.* 309:186–187.

Stern, R. S., Thibodeau, L. A., Klinerman, R. A., Parrish, J. A. and Fitzpatrick, T. B. 1979. Risk of cutaneous carcinoma in patients treated with oral methoxsalen photochemotherapy for psoriasis. *N. Engl. J. Med.* 300:809–813.

Stott, C. W., Stasse, J., Bonomo, R. and Campbell, A. H. 1970. Evaluation of the phototoxic potential of topically applied agents using longwave ultraviolet light. *J. Invest. Dermatol.* 55:335–338.

Tennenbaum, S., DiNardo, J., Morris, W., Wolf, B. and Schuetzinger, W. 1984. A quantitative in vitro assay for the evaluation of phototoxic potential of topically applied materials. *Cell Biol. Toxicol.* 1:1–9.

Urbach, F., Epstein, J. and Forbes, P. D. 1974. Ultraviolet carcinogenesis: Experimental, global and genetic aspects. In *Sunlight and Man,* eds. M. A. Pathak, L. C. Harber, M. Seiji and A. Kukita, pp. 259–283. Tokyo: University of Tokyo Press.

Verbov, J. 1973. Iatrogenic skin disease. *Br. J. Clin. Pract.* 27:310–314.

Volden, G., Krokan, H., Kavli, G. and Midelfart, K. 1983. Phototoxic and contact toxic reactions of the exocarp of sweet oranges: A common cause of cheilitis? *Contact Dermatitis* 9:201–204.

Webster, G., Kaidbey, K. and Kligman, A. 1983. Phototoxicity from benoxaprofen: In vivo and in vitro studies. *Photochem. Photobiol.* 36:59–64.

Weinberg, E. and Springer, S. 1981. The evaluation in vitro of fragrance materials for phototoxic activity. *J. Soc. Cosmet. Chem.* 32:303–315.

Wennersten, G. 1977. Photodynamic aspects of some metal complexes. *Acta Dermatovenereol. (Stockh.)* 57:519–524.

Western, A., Van Camp, J., Bensasson, R., Land, E. and Kochevar, I. 1987. Involvement of singlet oxygen in the phototoxicity mechanism for a metabolite of piroxicam. *Photochem. Photobiol.* 46:469–475.

Youn, S., Maytum, D. and Gange, R. 1987. Effect of temperature on the cutaneous phototoxic reaction to 8-methoxypsoralen in human skin. *Photodermatology* 4:277–280.

Zaynoun, S., Aftimos, B., Tenekjian, K. and Kurban, A. 1981. Berloque dermatitis—A continuing cosmetic problem. *Contact Dermatitis* 7:111–116.

ADDITIONAL PERTINENT REFERENCES

Austad, J. and Kavli, G. 1983. Phototoxic dermatitis cause celery infected by Sclerotinia sclerotiorum. *Contact Dermatitis.* 9:448–451.

Balato, N., Giordano, C., Montesano, M. and Lembo, G. 1984. 8-Methoxypsoralen-induced photo-onycolysis. *Photodermatology* 1:202–203.

Beani, J. C., Gautron, R., Amblarh, P., Bastrenta, F., Harrouch, L., Jardon, P. and Reymond, J. L. 1985. Screening for drug photosensitization activity by the variations in oxygen consumption of *Bacillus subtilis*. *Photodermatology* 2:101–106.

Bjellerup, M. and Ljunggren, B. 1984. Studies on photohemolysis with special references to demethylchlortetracycline. *Acta Derm. Venereol. (Stockh.)* 64:378–383.

Diette, K. M., Gange, R. W., Stern, R. S., Arndt, K. A. and Parrish, J. A. 1983. Coal tar phototoxicity: Kinetics and exposure parameters. *J. Invest. Dermatol.* 81:347–350.

Garge, R., Levins, P., Murray, J., Anderson, R. and Parrish, J. 1984. Prolonged skin photosensitization induced by methoxsalen and subphototoxic UVA irradiation. *J. Invest. Dermatol.* 82:219–222.

Golpashin, F., Weiss, B. and Durr, H. 1984. Photochemische Modell-Studien an lichtdermatoseninduzierenden Pharmaka: Sulfonamide and Sulfonylharnstoffe. *Arch. Pharm. (Weinheim)* 317:906–913.

Jeanmougin, M., Pedreiro, J., Bouchet, J. and Civatt, K. 1983. Phototoxicity of 5% benzoyl peroxide in man. Evakuation with a new methodology (Fren). *Dermatologica* 167(1):19–23.

Kamiole, R., Gigli, I. and Lim, H. W. 1984. Participation of mast cells and complement in the immediate phase of hematoporphyrin-induced phototoxicity. *J. Invest. Dermatol.* 82:485.

Kavli, G. and Volden, G. 1984. The Candida test for phototoxicity. *Photodermatology* 1:204–207.

Keane, J., Pearson, R. and Malkinson, F. 1984. Nalidixic acid-induced photosensitivity in mice: A model for pseudoporphyria. *J. Invest. Dermatol.* 82:210–213.

Knudsen, E. A. 1985. The *Candida* phototoxicity test. The sensitivity of different strains and species of *Candida,* standardization attempts and analysis of the dose-response curves for 5- and 8-methosypsoralen. *Photodermatology* 2:80–85.

Kochevar, I., Hoover, K. and Gawienowski, M. 1984. Benoxaprofen photosensitization of cell membrane disruption. *J. Invest. Dermatol.* 82:214–218.

Ljunggren, B. 1985. Propionic acid-derived non-steroidal antiinflammatory drugs are phototoxic in vitro. *Photodermatology* 1:3–9.

Lock, S. O. and Friend, J. V. 1983. Interaction of ultraviolet light, chemicals and cultured mammalian cells: Photobiological reactions of halogenated antiseptics, drugs and dyes. *Int. J. Cosmet. Sci.* 5:39–49.

Marzulli, F. N. and Maibach, H. I. 1983. Phototoxicity (photoirritation) of topical and systemic agents. In *Dermatotoxicology,* eds. F. Marzulli and H. Maibach, 2d ed., pp. 375–389. Washington, D.C.: Hemisphere.

Rauterberg, A., Jung, E., Burger, R. and Rauterburg, E. 1990. Phototoxic erythema following PUVA treatment: Independence of complement. *J. Invest. Dermatol.* 94:144–149.

Sambuco, C. and Forbes, P. 1984. Quantitative assessment of phototoxicity in the skin of hairless mice. *Food Chem. Toxicol.* 22(3):233–236..

Tennenbaum, S., DiNardo, J., Morris, W., Wolfe, B. A. Schnetzinger, R. W. 1984. A quantitative in vitro assay for the evaluation of phototoxic potential of topically applied material. *Cell Biol. Toxicol.* 1:1–9.

22

the evaluation of photoallergic contact sensitizers in humans

■ Kays Kaidbey ■

INTRODUCTION

Test procedures designed to identify potentially photosensitizing chemicals evolved in the wake of the photosensitivity outbreak caused by the antimicrobial halogenated salicylanilides in the early 1960s (Wilkinson, 1961; Calnan et al., 1961). Photocontact allergy, although relatively uncommon, proved to be particularly troublesome. A minority of affected patients developed a persistent photodermatitis for many years despite avoidance of further contact with the offending chemical (Wilkinson, 1962; Jillson and Baughman, 1963). While removal of the photosensitizing phenolic compounds from the marketplace reduced the incidence of photosensitivity (Smith and Epstein, 1977), it quickly became apparent that other, chemically unrelated substances were also capable of inducing this adverse reaction. There was a clear need for a laboratory test to detect potentially photosensitizing agents.

Most of our knowledge concerning photocontact allergy was, until recently, based on the halogenated salicylanilide class of chemicals. Information was gathered primarily from studies of patients (photopatch testing) and from attempts to induce photosensitization experimentally in guinea pigs (Herman and Sams, 1972). Much remains to be learned about the basic mechanism(s) underlying photocontact sensitivity. It is generally accepted that the process is of the delayed cell-mediated type (Harber et al., 1966; Sams, 1975), although the evidence for this has been criticized (Amos, 1973). The role of ultraviolet (UV) radiation is less clear. Absorption of UV energy by the sensitizer in the skin is required for both induction and elicitation. The most plausible explanation for the role of UV radiation is that absorption of photons of specific energy by the sensitizer leads to the formation of an excited molecule, which, under appropriate conditions, can interact with other molecules normally found in the skin to form an antigen or hapten. Other explanations have been postulated (Amos, 1973). Irradiation of the photosensitizer in vitro followed by repeated topical application of the irradiated solution is ineffective in inducing photocontact sensitization. Hence the formation of stable photoproducts that can act as potential contact sensitizers is an unlikely mechanism (Schmidt and Kingston, 1984).

Test procedures for identifying photocontact allergens have received less attention than methods designed to detect ordinary contact sensitizers. Efforts to induce photocontact sensitivity have involved animals primarily, usually guinea pigs, and have thus far not been standardized. Of the animals tested so far, the mouse ear swelling model appears to be the most sensitive (Maguire and Kaidbey, 1982; Miyachi and Takigawa, 1983; Gerberick and Ryan, 1990). Experience with human testing is even more limited. In theory, the variables that influence ordinary contact-sensitization such as the vehicle, concentration, and frequency of application (Marzulli and Maibach, 1974) can similarly affect the induction of photosensitization. Furthermore, there is the added important factor of UV radiation. The wavelength dependence (action spectrum), energy requirements (dose) for both induction and elicitation, and absorption characteristics of the chemical must be determined. For screening of novel agents with unknown action spectra, however, it is necessary to use a UV source with a broad emission spectrum. The sources commonly used in the past were fluorescent tubes such as the FS-20 sunlamp bulbs, with emission primarily in the UV-B region, or blacklight fluorescent bulbs, which emit primarily in the UV-A range, or a combination of both. More recently, xenon arc solar simulators have been used that offer the advantage of providing spectra similar to sunlight.

PHOTOMAXIMIZATION TEST

This test is conducted in humans and is essentially a repeated insult technique that entails an exaggerated exposure to both chemical and UV (Kaidbey and Kligman, 1980) and follows a design similar to that of the maximization test (Kligman, 1966). The UV source is a 150-W xenon arc solar simulator. The emission spectrum is continuous extending from about 290 to 410 nm with a peak at about 350 nm, and closely resembles the UV-B spectrum of midday sunlight at 41 °N and 70 ° sun elevation (Berger, 1969).

A 5% concentration of the test agent in an appropriate base (such as Hydrophilic Ointment USP) is delivered to the skin by plastic tuberculin syringes at a concentration of 10 $\mu l/cm^2$. The material is spread uniformly with thin glass rods and the sites covered with nonwoven cotton cloth (Webril, Curity) and sealed to the skin with clear occlusive tape (Blenderm, 3M Co.). Twenty-four hours later, the patches are removed and the sites exposed to three minimal erythema doses (MEDs) from the solar simulator. The MED is individually determined beforehand by exposing the skin sites to 25% increments of radiation. The dose required to produce minimal but uniform erythema with a clear border 24 h after exposure is the MED. After a rest period of 48 h, a similar occlusive application is made to the same site for another 24 h, followed again by exposure to three MEDs. This sequence is repeated for a total of six exposures over a period of 3 wk. The subjects are then challenged after a rest period of 14 d by a single exposure to a fresh skin site. An occlusive application is made with the test agent (1.0% concentration) for 24 h, followed by exposure to 4.0 J/cm² UV-A. The UV-A is obtained from the same source by filtering the radiation through a 2-mm Schott WG345 filter (50% transmission at about 345 nm). The sites are examined 48 and 72 h after irradiation. Unirradiated control sites are sealed and then covered with three or four layers of opaque adhesive tape. Development of erythema and edema or a vesicular dermatitis in the irradiated but not the unirradiated sites signifies the induction of photocontact sensitivity. Each substance is usually examined in 25 volunteers.

EVALUATION OF SOME PHOTOCONTACT SENSITIZERS

Halogenated Phenolic Compounds

Several members of this class of compounds, notably those that gave rise to outbreaks of photosensitivity in the past, were identified as photosensitizers by the photomaximization test (Table 1). 3,5-Dibromosalicylanilide (3,5-DBS) and tetrachlorosalicylanilide (TCSA) produced the highest sensitization rates (40 and 32%, respectively). One sample of tribromosalicylanilide (TBS) that contained up to 47% dibrominated derivatives as impurities (sample A) produced photosensitization, while a purer sample (B) containing only 1.2% dibrominated derivative (3,5-DBS) produced no instances of sensitization. TBS

TABLE 1 Induction of Photoallergic Contact Dermatitis by the Photomaximization Test ($n = 25$): Halogenated Phenolic Compounds

Compound	No. of photosensitized subjects
3,3',4',5-Tetrachlorosalicylanilide	8
3,4,5-Tribromosalicylanilide (sample A)	2
3,4,5-Tribromosalicylanilide (sample B)	0
4,5-Dibromosalicylanilide	3
3,5-Dibromosalicylanilide	10
5-Monobromosalicylanilide	0
4-Chloro-2-hydroxybenzoic acid *n*-butylamide (Jadit)	3
Bithionol	3
Trichlorocarbanilide	0
Hexachlorophene	0

may have little or negligible photosensitization potential compared to the dibrominated derivatives. The latter substances have also produced higher sensitization rates than TBS in animals (Morikawa et al., 1974). Jadit and bithionol, which are also known photosensitizers, produced photosensitization, although the rates were lower than with TCSA. Trichlorocarbanilide and hexachlorophene (Hex) were inactive. Rare reports of photocontact allergy to Hex and TCC based on positive photopatch tests could have represented cross-photoreactions to some other primary photosensitizers such as TCSA or bithionol. In one such study, for example, all patients who were positive in photopatch tests to Hex also had strong reactions to other halogenated phenolics (Epstein et al., 1968).

Coumarins

The coumarins, which constitute a large class of synthetic and naturally occurring substances, are potentially strong photosensitizing agents. Certain synthetic derivatives were used as optical bleachers (Calnan, 1973), while others were incorporated in toiletries as fragrances (Opdyke, 1974). The photosensitizing properties of coumarins became apparent after outbreaks of photosensitivity among users of sunscreens containing 6-methylcoumarin as a fragrance (Kaidbey and Kligman, 1978). This potential was readily demonstrated in the photomaximization test (Table 2). Other derivatives such as 5,7-dimethoxycoumarin, which is naturally found in bergamot oil, were less photosensitizing, while coumarin itself had no detectable activity. Individuals photosensitized to any one of these substances can develop cross-reactions to other derivatives, even when the latter are not primary inducers (Kaidbey and Kligman, 1981). This underscores the importance of identifying and eliminating the photosensitizing or offending derivatives. Examination of the chemical structures shows that substitution of a methyl group at position 6 or an alkoxy

TABLE 2   Photosensitization Potential of Courmarin Derivatives
and Other Fragrances ($n = 25$)

Compound	No. of photosensitized subjects
6-Methylcoumarin	15
4-Methyl-7-ethoxycoumarin	13
7-Methoxycoumarin	11
7-Methylcoumarin	6
5,7-Dimethoxycoumarin	5
Coumarin	0
Hexahydrocoumarin	0
Octahydrocoumarin	0
Isoeugenol	0
Phthalide	0
Musk ambrette	0

group at position 7 of the benzopyrone ring confers strong photoallergenic activity (Kaidbey and Kligman, 1981; Opdyke, 1981). The coumarins in general are strong UV absorbers.

Of special interest was the observation that certain healthy individuals with no history of photodermatitis or other adverse reactions to sunlight had a positive photopatch test to coumarins (Kaidbey and Kligman, 1978b). The significance of this finding is not clear, although it is possible that repeated exposure to coumarins in toiletries or elsewhere in the environment could have led to photosensitization. These may be the individuals who are at risk of developing a photodermatitis on their "first" exposure to a coumarin-containing preparation.

Maurer et al. (1980) were unable to induce photosensitization to 6-methylcoumarin in guinea pigs despite concomitant stimulation with Freund's adjuvant. This could have been due to the low concentration (0.1%) used for induction, since Ichikawa et al. (1981) achieved induction with larger concentrations.

Musk Ambrette

This synthetic fragrance, which is used in aftershave lotions, perfumes, and soaps, was recently identified as a photosensitizer (Raugi et al., 1979). Most commonly affected were middle-aged or elderly men using aftershave lotions containing musk. Sporadic cases, some with persistent photosensitivity, have since been reported (Giovinazzo et al., 1980). We have seen three similarly affected males, one of whom had a persistent photodermatitis; all these patients had positive photopatch tests to pure musk ambrette. Some photosensitized patients present with a dermatitis which does not have the clinical features of a "typical" photodermatitis and hence the diagnosis may not be suspected (Ramsay, 1984). Musk ambrette is the most significant photocontact sensitizer in patients with chronic actinic dermatitis (Barber and Cronin, 1982). Efforts to induce photosensitization to this substance in humans have been unsuccessful, even in a trial in which a 10% concentration was employed and the induction phase extended to 6 instead of 3 weeks. Musk ambrette is probably a very weak photosensitizer that cannot be detected by the photomaximization test. Furthermore, shaving may be a factor contributing to induction (Kochevar et al., 1979). Other musk derivatives have not yet been examined for their photosensitizing potential, and it is possible that positive photopatch tests in patients may represent cross-reactions to other nitro-musks that are more potent inducers.

Recently, photosensitization to musk ambrette has been induced in guinea pigs by use of special procedures such as stripping (Kochevar et al., 1979) and intradermal injection of Freund's complete adjuvant before induction (Ichikawa et al., 1981). Without such modifications, induction was unsuccessful even at a concentration of 10%, which supports the contention that this substance has a very low potential for photosensitization compared to the agents previously discussed.

Other Photosensitizers

Several other topically applied agents have occasionally been incriminated as photosensitizers on the basis of positive photopatch tests in patients (Table 3). These include certain essential oils (e.g., sandalwood oil), sunscreens such as p-aminobenzoic acid and benzophenone-3, and drugs such as benzocaine and diphenhydramine. PABA and other commonly used sunscreens such as benzophenone-3 did not induce photosensitization in the photomaximization test, and the other agents have not been examined in humans. It is unlikely that weak photocontact allergens will be identified as such in routine laboratory screens. There have been reports of photocontact allergy to such agents as PABA and less frequently to benzocaine. Sunscreens are now a well recognized cause of photocontact allergy (Thune, 1984) with benzophenone-3 the most frequent sensitizer in this country.

Another substance that was found to induce photocontact allergy by the photomaximization test is sodium omadine. The zinc, magnesium, and sodium compounds of omadine are potentially useful since they have broad-spectrum antibacterial and antifungal properties. Sodium omadine, unlike the zinc derivative, has a significant photoallergenic potential (Table 4). The sodium salt has absorption peaks at about 280 and 330nm, and little or no significant absorption beyond 360nm.

Some photocontact sensitizers are also capable of inducing ordinary contact allergy. The halogenated salicylanilides and certain sunscreens (e.g., PABA) are examples. Contact sensitization developed in 6 of 25 subjects exposed to TCSA in the photomaximization test, while in another 6 a combined contact and photocontact sensitivity was suspected on the basis of a marked accentuation of the patch test reactions by UV-A (Kaidbey and Kligman, 1980). Similar observations were made with DBS and bithionol, although they were far less active. It should be pointed out, however, that the photomaximization test is not designed to assess contact sensitization. Repeated exposures to the chemical and UV during induction may lead to the formation of photoproducts, which can themselves be sensitizing. UV may also alter local reactivity and cellular responses by its well-known effects on lymphoid cells. Nonetheless, the halogenated salicylanilides appear to be strong sensitizers in humans (Marzulli and Maibach, 1973). There is, however, no apparent relation between photocontact potential and ordinary contact sensitization. Thus the substituted coumarins, which are potent photosensitizers, are weak or poor contact allergens in the maximization test in humans (Opdyke, 1976, 1981). No instances of contact sensitization have been reported with musk ambrette, either clinically or in the maximization test.

PHOTOPATCH TESTING

The interpretation of photopatch test results is usually straightforward. Difficulties arise when there is marked enhancement of a positive or weakly

TABLE 3   Topically Applied Substances Reported to Produce
Photoallergic Contact Dermatitis in Humans

Halogenated phenolic compounds
Fentichlor
Dichlorophene
Bromochlorosalicylanilide (Multifungin)
Chloro-2-phenylphenol
   Sunscreens
      p-Aminobenzoic acid (PABA)
      Benzophenone-3
      Glyceryl PABA
      Digalloyl trioleate
      2-Hydroxy-4-methoxybenzophenone (Mexenone)
   Phenothiazines
      Promethazine hydrochloride
      Diphenhydramine
   Others
      Sandalwood oil
      Benzocaine
      8-Methoxypsoralen (rare)
      Quindoxin
      Optical brighteners

positive reaction to a chemical in the unirradiated site by UV. This has been observed in patients and in experimentally photosensitized humans. In these cases, photopatch testing should be carefully repeated by quantitative methods. Measured amounts of the chemical in a suitable vehicle should be delivered to the skin and the unirradiated site quickly and rigorously sealed with several layers of opaque material to prevent stray radiation. Small amounts of UV-A can reach the skin surface through ordinary tape and trigger a reaction in the

TABLE 4   Induction of Photoallergic Contact Dermatitis
Miscellaneous Compounds ($n = 25$)

Compound	No. of photosensitized subjects
Chlorpromazine[a]	6
Benzoyl peroxide	0
5-Fluorouracil	0
p-Aminobenzoic acid	0
Sulfanilamide	0
Chlorothiazide	0
Sodium omadine[b]	6
Zinc omadine	0

[a]Chlorpromazine was tested in 12 volunteers.
[b]Sodium omadine was tested at 2.5% because of irritancy at higher concentrations.

unirradiated patch test sites in highly sensitive individuals. This was observed years ago by Epstein (1963), who termed the reaction a "masked" photopatch test and noted that it can lead to an erroneous diagnosis of contact sensitivity. That exceedingly small doses of UV-A are sufficient to provoke a response in photosensitized individuals has been amply demonstrated, especially when relatively large concentrations of the sensitizers (1.0 or 0.1%) are employed (Epstein et al., 1968; Osmundsen, 1968; Willis and Kligman, 1969). If a definite and clear enhancement is still observed after the above procedures, other explanations must be invoked. These include nonspecific enhancement of contact allergy by UV, as through effects on the vasculature, release of inflammatory mediators, modification of local cellular immunologic responses, formation of cross-reacting photoproducts, and so on. Such possibilities have not been adequately investigated. Another explanation is the existence of dual sensitivity: i.e., contact and photocontact allergy. Photopatch testing with serial dilutions of the sensitizer should then be performed. A positive photopatch test at a drug concentration that fails to elicit a response in the unirradiated test site is suggestive of dual sensitization.

ACTION SPECTRUM

Few detailed studies have been made of the action spectrum for elicitation of photocontact allergic dermatitis in sensitized humans. Freeman and Knox (1968) and Cripps and Enta (1970), using narrow wavebands, showed that responses to the halogenated salicylanilides in pretreated skin could be elicited over a relatively wide portion of the UV-A spectrum. Furthermore, a reduction of the threshold erythema dose was found with UV-B wavelengths. Essentially similar findings were obtained with two subjects who were photosensitive to 6-methylcoumarin (Kaidbey and Kligman, 1981), although no responses could be provoked with wavelengths longer than 360 nm. In rare cases, there is narrower spectral reactivity-for example, to UV-B wavelengths in a case of photocontact allergy to diphenhydramine (Emmett, 1974).

Studies involving the wavelength dependence for induction of photocontact allergy are also very few, and only studies in animals have been reported. Cripps and Enta (1970) found that UV-B was necessary for induction with TCSA, while Horio (1976) was able to induce photosensitivity to TCSA and TBS with UV-A only after pretreating the skin with 20% sodium lauryl sulfate (SLS). In the mouse ear model, induction to TCSA was most effective with UV-A wavelengths (Brown et al., 1987). UV-A + UV-B and solar simulated radiation are more effective than UV-A alone in inducing photocontact allergy to 6-methylcoumarin (Gerberick and Ryan, 1990). When solar simulated radiation was used during induction, 15 to 25 subjects were sensitized. When UV-B was filtered out from the irradiation system and an equivalent dose of UV-A was used, only 4 of 25 were sensitized (Table 5). For the coumarins, at least, it appears that shorter wavelengths are more efficient for induction. Spectral ef-

TABLE 5 Influence of UV Waveband on Induction
on Photocontact Allergy to 6-Methylcoumarin

Wave band	Incidence of photosensitization (%)
Simulated solar radiation	60
UV-A	16

fectiveness for induction will most probably be found to depend on the absorption characteristics of the chemical in the skin.

CONCLUSIONS

The photomaximization test is a useful laboratory procedure for identifying substances that are potentially capable of producing photoallergic contact sensitivity in humans. The test combines exaggerated exposure to the drug and simulated solar radiation. Agents suspected of being photosensitizers on clinical grounds or from photopatch testing can be evaluated for this potential in the laboratory. This is necessary to determine whether the chemical can act as an inducer or merely as a cross-reactant. Although substances can be ranked for their photosensitizing under a defined set of laboratory conditions, the possible incidence of photoallergic reactions with normal usage cannot be predicted. Furthermore, this test has the same limitations as other predictive laboratory methods, such as those designed to evaluate ordinary contact sensitization potential. Very weak or marginally active chemicals may not be detected. Systemically administered photosensitizers cannot be evaluated in this test.

Experience with human testing has been limited. Factors that influence induction, such as concentration, vehicle, and UV dose, need to be further investigated.

REFERENCES

Amos, H. E. 1973. Photoallergy. A critical survey. *Trans. St. John's Hosp. Dermatol. Soc.* 59:147–151.

Barber, K. A. and Cronin, E. 1982. Patch and photopatch testing in chronic actinic dermatitis. *Contact Dermatitis.* 10:69–73.

Berger, D. S. 1969. Specification and design of solar ultraviolet simulators. *J. Invest. Dermatol.* 53:192–199.

Brown, W. R., Shivji, G. M., Furukawa, D. R. and Ramsay, C. A. 1987. Studies of the action spectrum for induction of photosensitivity to tetrachlorosalicylanilide in mice. *Photodermatology* 4:196–200.

Calnan, C. D., Harman, R. R. M. and Wells, G. C. 1961. Photodermatitis from soaps. *Br. Med. J.* 2:1266.

Calnan, C. D. 1973. Hazards of optical bleachers. *Trans. St. John's Hosp. Dermatol. Soc.* 59:275–282.

Cripps, D. J. and Enta, T. 1970. Absorption and action spectra studies on bithionol and halogenated salicylanilide photosensitivity. *Br. J. Dermatol.* 82:730-742.

Emmett, E. A. 1974. Diphenhydramine photoallergy. *Arch. Dermatol.* 110:249-252.

Epstein, S. 1963. "Masked" photopatch test. *J. Invest. Dermatol.* 41:369-370.

Epstein, J. H., Wuepper, K. D. and Maibach, H. I. 1968. Photocontact dermatitis to halogenated salicylanilides and related compounds. *Arch. Dermatol.* 97:236-244.

Freeman, R. G. and Knox, J. M. 1968. The action spectrum of photocontact dermatitis. *Arch. Dermatol.* 97:130-136.

Gerberick, G. F. and Ryan, C. A. 1990. Use of UVB and UVA to induce and elicit contact photoallergy in the mouse. *Photodermatol. Photoimmunol. Photomed.* 7:13-19.

Giovinazzo, V. J., Harber, L. C., Armstrong, R. B. and Kochevar, I. E. 1980. Photoallergic contact dermatitis to musk ambrette. *J. Am. Acad. Dermatol.* 3:384-393.

Harber, L. C., Harris, H. and Baer, R. L. 1966. Photoallergic contact dermatitis. *Arch. Dermatol.* 94:255-262.

Herman, P. S. and Sams, W. M., Jr. 1972. *Soap Photodermatitis: Photosensitivity to Halogenated Salicylanilides.* Springfield, Ill.: Thomas.

Horio, T. 1976. The induction of photocontact sensitivity in guinea pigs without UV-B radiation. *J. Invest. Dermatol.* 67:591-593.

Ichikawa, H., Armstrong, R. B. and Harber, L. C. 1981. Photoallergic contact dermatitis in guinea pigs: Improved induction technique using Freund's complete adjuvant. *J. Invest. Dermatol.* 76:498-501.

Jillson, O. F. and Baughman, R. D. 1963. Contact photodermatitis from bithionol. *Arch. Dermatol.* 88:409-416.

Kaidbey, K. H. and Kligman, A. M. 1978a. Contact photoallergy to 6-methyl-coumarin in proprietary sunscreens. *Arch. Dermatol.* 114:1709-1710.

Kaidbey, K. H. and Kligman, A. M. 1978b. Photocontact allergy to 6-methyl-coumarin. *Contact Dermatitis* 4:277-282.

Kaidbey, K. H. and Kligman, A. M. 1980. Photomaximization test for identifying photoallergic contact sensitizers. *Contact Dermatitis* 6:161-169.

Kaidbey, K. H. and Kligman, A. M. 1981. Photosensitization by coumarin derivatives: Structure-activity relationships. *Arch. Dermatol.* 117:258-263.

Kligman, A. M. 1966. The identification of contact allergens by human assay. III. The maximization test. A procedure for screening and rating contact sensitizers. *J. Invest. Dermatol.* 47:393-409.

Kochever, I. E., Zaler, G. L., Einbinder, J., and Harber, L. C. 1979. Assay of contact photosensitivity to musk ambrette in guinea pigs. *J. Invest. Dermatol.* 73:144-146.

Maguire, H. C. and Kaidbey, K. H. 1982. Experimental photoallergic contact dermatitis: A mouse model. *J. Invest. Dermatol.* 79:147-152.

Marzulli, F. and Maibach, H. 1973. Antimicrobials. Experimental contact sensitization in man. *J. Soc. Cosmet. Chem.* 24:399-421.

Marzulli, F. and Maibach, H. 1974. Use of graded concentrations in studying skin sensitization in man. *Food Cosmet. Toxicol.* 12:219-277.

Maurer, T. H., Weirich, E. G. and Hess, R. 1980. Evaluation of the photocontact allergenic potential of 6-methylcoumarin in the guinea pig. *Contact Dermatitis* 6:275-278.

Miyachi, Y. and Takigawa, M. 1983. Mechanisms of contact photosensitivity in mice. III. Predictive testing of chemicals with photoallergenic potential in mice. *Arch. Dermatol.* 119:736-739.

Morikawa, F., Nakayama, Y., Fukuda, M., Hamano, M., Yokoyama, Y., Nagura, T., Ishihara, M. and Toda, K. 1974. Techniques for evaluation of phototoxicity and photoallergy in laboratory animals. In *Sunlight and Man*, eds. T. B. Fitzpatrick, M. A. Pathak, L. C. Harber, M. Seiji and A. Kukita, pp. 529–557. Tokyo: Univ. of Tokyo Press.

Opdyke, D. L. 1974. Monographs on fragrance raw materials: Coumarin. *Food Cosmet. Toxicol.* 12:385–405.

Opdyke, D. L. 1976. Monographs on fragrance raw materials: 6-Methyl-coumarin. *Food Cosmet. Toxicol.* 14:605.

Opdyke, D. L. 1981. The structure activity relationships of some substituted coumarins with respect to skin reactions. *Dragoco Rep. (Engl. Ed.)* 2:43–48.

Osmundsen, P. E. 1968. Contact photodermatitis due to tribromosalicylanilide. *Br. J. Dermatol.* 80:228–234.

Ramsay, C. A. 1984. Transient and persistent photosensitivity due to musk ambrette. Clinical and photobiological studies. *Br. J. Dermatol.* 111:423–429.

Raugi, G. J., Storrs, F. J. and Larsen, W. G. 1979. Photoallergic contact dermatitis to men's perfume. *Contact Dermatitis* 5:251–260.

Sams, W. M., Jr. 1975. The immunology of photocontact dermatitis. *Int. J. Dermatol.* 14:251–253.

Schmidt, R. J. and Kingston, T. 1984. Testing with musk ambrette and congeners in a case of photosensitivity dermatitis and actinic reticuloid syndrome (PD/AR) *Photodermatology* 1:195–198.

Smith, S. Z. and Epstein, J. H. 1977. Photocontact dermatitis to halogenated salicylanilides and related compounds. *Arch. Dermatol.* 113:1372–1374.

Thune, P. 1984. Contact and photocontact allergy to sunscreens. *Photodermatology* 1:5–9.

Wilkinson, D. S. 1961. Photodermatitis due to tetrachlorosalicylanilide. *Br. J. Dermatol.* 73:213–219.

Wilkinson, D. S. 1962. Patch test reactions to certain halogenated salicylanilides. *Br. J. Dermatol.* 74:302–306.

Willis, I. and Kligman, A. M. 1969. Photocontact allergic reactions. Elicitation by low doses of long ultraviolet rays. *Arch. Dermatol.* 100:535–539.

23

photocontact allergy
in humans

■ John H. Epstein ■

INTRODUCTION

Adverse photocutaneous reactions to exogenous chemicals have become increasingly prevalent in the last few decades due to enhanced opportunities for sun exposure and the rapidly increasing numbers of photosensitizing chemicals available. The present discussion is concerned primarily with photoallergic reactions induced by topically applied materials in humans. However, a few definitions would appear to be in order before entering into this specific aspect of photoreactivity.

DEFINITIONS

Action Spectrum and Absorption Spectrum

The wavelengths that are responsible for a photobiological response are termed the *action spectrum* for that particular response. Since nonionizing radiation must be absorbed to act, as described by the Grotthuss-Draper law, a chromophore must be present that will absorb this energy to initiate the photoreaction. The wavelengths that any individual molecule or material will absorb is termed its *absorption spectrum*. Thus the action spectrum for a photoreaction induced by a particular molecule or chemical would be expected to parallel its

This study was supported in part by USPHS grant CA 15605-01.

absorption spectrum. Although this is generally true, it is not essential. It is only necessary that the action spectrum be included in at least some part of the absorption spectrum. An example of this discrepancy occurs with a number of psoralen compounds that have peak absorption characteristics of wavelengths shorter than 300 nm but produce their phototoxic effects by absorbing rays in the longer UV range (Pathak et al., 1974).

Sun's Spectrum and Photobiological Reactions

The sun's rays that reach the earth's surface range from 290 nm (or 286 nm) in the UV spectrum through the visible (400-700 nm), into the infrared, and beyond (>700 nm). Almost all of the photobiological reactions that occur in the skin on absorption of sunlight are produced by rays between 290 and 320 nm (UV-B), which make up about 0.1-0.2% of the total sun's energy that reaches the earth. These are the rays that inhibit DNA, RNA, and protein synthesis, interrupt mitoses, make vitamin D, cause skin cancer, and produce the delayed erythema response that we call "sunburn" (J. H. Epstein et al., 1970; Daniels, 1974). The longer UV rays between 320 and 400 nm (UV-A) produce a few minor photobiological reactions such as immediate pigment darkening and immediate transient erythema responses (Bacheim, 1956). However, these wavelengths are of great importance because they markedly augment the photoinjury induced by the UV-B spectrum (Willis et al., 1972; Parrish et al., 1974), and they are responsible for the vast majority of exogenously photosensitized reactions (both phototoxic and photoallergic) that occur in human skin. UV rays shorter than 290 nm (<280 nm = UV-C) emitted by artificial light sources do produce a delayed erythema, alter DNA, RNA, and proteins, cause cancer under experimental conditions, and may enter into photosensitivity problems on occasion.

Photosensitivity

Photosensitivity (J. H. Epstein, 1972) is the broad term that is used to describe abnormal or adverse reactions to the sun or artificial light sources. These responses may be phototoxic or photoallergic in nature.

Phototoxicity. The vast majority of adverse cutaneous reactions induced by the sun and/or artificial light sources are phototoxic in nature and are independent of immune or allergic mechanisms. They can occur in everybody if enough light energy and, in the case of photosensitized responses, enough of the photosensitizer is present in the skin. The clinical picture usually consists of a delayed erythema followed by hyperpigmentation and desquamation. Thus they tend to resemble the usual "sunburn" reaction, which is in itself the most common of all the known phototoxic responses. The mechanisms of these reactions are quite complex and vary greatly with the etiology. In certain instances the presence of oxygen is essential, as in the so-called photodynamic reactions (Blum, 1941). In others, photoproducts with nucleic acids are formed or membrane damage is produced. These responses will be dealt with in a subsequent chapter.

Photoallergy. Unlike phototoxicity, photoallergy is uncommon. It represents an acquired altered reactivity to irradiation that is dependent on an antigen-antibody or a cell-mediated hypersensitivity response. Clinically it is characterized by unusual lesions ranging from immediate urticarial (Fig. 1) to delayed papular and eczematous reactions (Fig. 2). Involvement extending beyond the exposed site frequently occurs. A biopsy of the urticarial response usually reveals very little specific change, whereas the delayed reactions show dense perivascular round cell infiltrates in the dermis (Fig. 3). In general, less energy is required to produce photoallergic than phototoxic reactions.

In addition to the clinical and histological features the following criteria are used to help define the presence of a photoallergic reaction: (1) flares of previously exposed sites following irradiation of a distant site, (2) passive and reverse passive transfer of the reactions with serum for antigen-antibody responses, (3) passive transfer with white blood cells for cell-mediated immunity, and (4) the demonstration of an incubation period and spontaneous flare response when the process is produced under controlled conditions.

Photoallergic reactions may be produced by irradiation alone without the presence of known photosensitizers or may be due to exogenous chemicals. "Solar urticaria" responses are immediate, transient wheal and flare reactions to irradiation alone, which clinically suggest the presence of an antigen-

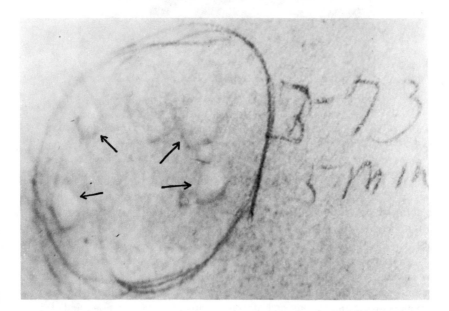

FIGURE 1 Clinical picture of solar urticaria with multiple wheals (J. H. Epstein et al., 1963; reprinted with permission of the American Medical Association).

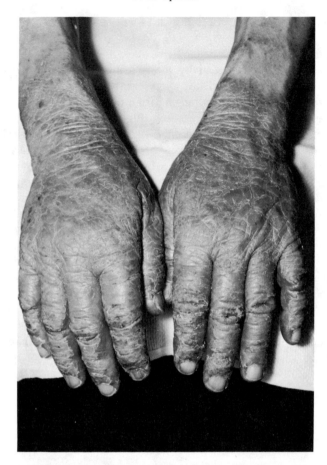

FIGURE 2 Clinical picture of an eczematoid photocontact dermatitis induced by a halogenated salicylanilide (3,5-dibromosalicylanilide) (J. H. Epstein, 1972; reprinted with permission of the American Medical Association).

antibody reaction. In certain of these responses, induced primarily by UV-B rays, passive transfer and reverse passive transfer studies have confirmed this relationship (Harber et al., 1963; Sams, 1970). In addition, the clinical and histologic patterns of the polymorphous light eruptions (PMLEs) strongly suggest possible CMI responses to UV-B alone (J. H. Epstein, 1966).

Photoallergic reactions induced by exogenous photosensitizers, when they occur, usually are characterized by delayed reactions, which appear to depend on cell-mediated immune (CMI) mechanisms. However, Horio (1975) reported a patient with immediate and delayed photoallergic reactions induced by chlorpromazine and UV-A. Thus immediate antibody-mediated reactions may occur. They are very uncommon.

PHOTOALLERGIC CONTACT DERMATITIS

Clinical Picture

Photoallergic contact reactions are clinically identical to any other type of allergic contact dermatitis. Thus the spectrum of the possible responses may range from a simple erythema to a severe vesiculobullous eruption. The most common picture is eczematous in nature (Figs. 2 and 3). When the process is chronic, lichenification results from repeated mechanical trauma (rubbing and scratching). The sun-exposed areas of the skin are involved primarily as would be expected. However, the eruption may extend to unexposed parts of the body and even become generalized due to conditioned irritability and autoeczematization reactions. Even when this occurs the dermatitis is most notable in the exposed sites.

Adults are much more commonly affected than children. Obviously the reactions will occur in populations that are exposed to sunlight and the photo-contactants. Thus reactions to the optical brighteners would more likely be seen in persons who use them, those to chlorpromazine would more likely occur in people who work in mental institutions, and so on. Perhaps the most extensive statistical data have been compiled on the eruptions induced by the halogenated salicylanilides and related antibacterial compounds because of the large number

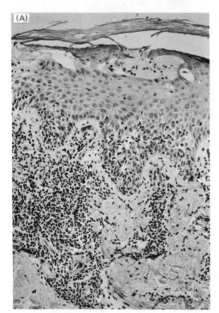 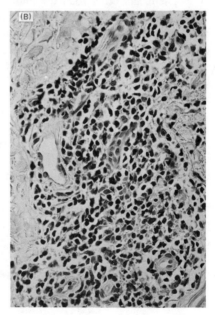

FIGURE 3 (A) Histological appearance of an allergic photocontact reaction showing epidermal edema and vesicle formation and a dense perivascular round cell infiltrate. (B) Higher magnification of the dense perivascular infiltrate. (J. H. Epstein, 1972; reprinted with the permission of the American Medical Association).

of people photosensitized by these agents between 1960 and 1970 (Herman and Sams, 1972). The reactions occurred predominantly in men past the age of 40 yr. The reason for this age and sex distribution is unknown. Skin color and race apparently have little influence on the problem, which occurs readily in blacks and Orientals as well as Caucasians.

In general, removal of the offending photosensitizer and related compounds will eliminate the problem once the eruption has subsided. A small percentage of patients who have developed this process will eventuate as persistent light reactors (Jillson and Baughman, 1963). These are people who continue to develop the dermatitis on sun-exposed areas without apparent further contact with the offending agent or related structures. These patients tend to be exquisitely sensitive to the sun and usually have very low UV-B minimal erythema doses. The incidence of this most disturbing problem is unknown, but it probably represents only a small percentage of those who become contact photosensitive. However, up to 25% of patients with photocontact reactions to the halogenated salicylanilides severe enough to necessitate consultation at medical centers have been persistent light reactors. In our studies with the antibacterial halogenated salicylanilides we found two types of persistent light reactors: a mild variety that loses its reactivity within 1 1/2 years and a severe type that appears to persist indefinitely (J. H. Epstein et al., 1968).

Chemicals other than the antibacterial halogenated salicylanilides have induced persistent light reactions, including the related antifungal compounds buclosamide (Jadit) (Burry, 1970; Burry and Hunter, 1970), chlorpromazine (Wiskemann and Wulf, 1959; Burdick, 1969), and promethazine (Sidi et al., 1955). Persistent light reactions induced in guinea pigs with sulfonamides have been noted (Schwarz and Speck, 1957), and I have observed a phototoxic persistent light reaction induced by systemic dimethylchlortetracycline that has persisted 3 yr. The mechanism or mechanisms of this persistent light reactivity are not clear. Cross-reactions to unknown photocontactants have been considered. Willis and Kligman (1968a) presented evidence suggesting that the reactions could result from the retention of small amounts of the photosensitizer in the dermis. These authors also reported that the lowered MED in persistent light reactors was a photoallergic reaction, which resembled a sunburn. Other possibilities include the persistence of a sensitized mononuclear infiltrate in the dermis, which will react on minimal antigenic exposure; hypersensitivity to the protein component of the complete antigen, which then becomes an independent photoallergen; or the development of clones of cells that are persistently sensitive to a number of photoallergens (Herman and Sams, 1972). Also, a possible relationship to the chronic eczematous type of polymorphous light eruption (PMLE) has been reported (J. H. Epstein et al., 1968).

Histology

The microscopic anatomy of photocontact reactions is characteristic but not diagnostic. In general, there is some intercellular edema in the epidermis with or without vesicle formation, depending on the clinical pattern. However, the characteristic finding is present in the dermis and consists of a dense perivascular round cell infiltrate, which is identical to that found in any allergic contact dermatitis response (Fig. 3).

Differential Diagnosis

The differential diagnosis includes essentially any eruption that may involve the sun-exposed skin. However, for practical purposes, allergic contact dermatitis, the eczematous type of PMLE, and phototoxic reactions are by far the most important.

Airborne allergens will contact exposed skin primarily. Unlike photocontact reactions, the airborne contact eruption will be accentuated in fold areas such as the upper eyelids, antecubital fossae, flexural areas of the wrists, and the like because of concentration of the airborne material in these areas. Differentiation from allergic contact reactions to sunscreens, "suntanning" lotions and creams, and medications used to relieve the discomfort of a sunburn is more difficult since they are confined to the sun-exposed areas and are indistinguishable clinically and histologically. The same is true for the eczematous type of PMLE.

Phototoxic reactions induced by topical or systemic exogenous photosensitizers will have the same distribution as the photoallergic reactions. The clinical picture and lack of the dermal round cell infiltrate histologically will usually serve to make this differentiation. However, the most useful diagnostic tools available are the patch, photopatch, and phototesting procedures.

Diagnosis

The diagnosis of photocontact dermatitis is suspected by the clinical picture, including the character and distribution of the eruption and the histology. Confirmation and identification of the offending chemical depend on photopatch testing. This is accomplished by the application in duplicate of nonirritating concentrations of the potential photosensitizers in appropriate vehicles (i.e., a 1% concentration of the halogenated salicylanilides in petrolatum). The use of an extra layer of black paper over the patches will help prevent a "masked" positive reaction to the photopatch test (S. Epstein, 1963). This is unnecessary with the use of aluminum patches. Twenty-four hours later one set of patches is irradiated with the UV-A rays. Any light source that emits sufficient amounts of these rays can be utilized, including the sun, hot quartz lamps, fluorescent tubes, xenon arcs, carbon arcs, and monochromatic sources (Harber et al., 1974). Window glass filtration is necessary if there is a significant amount of UV-B emitted by the lamp, as in the case of the hot quartz source. Twenty-four hours after the irradiation, the closed and exposed sites are compared. The reading techniques are identical to those used in evaluation of ordinary patch tests. A positive reaction to the photopatch tests reproduces the clinical lesions morphologically and histologically (Fig. 4). Certain difficulties with patch testing may occur. If the patient is contact allergic to a chemical it may be difficult

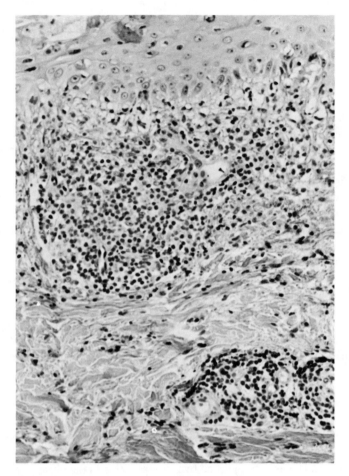

FIGURE 4   Histological appearance of a positive phototest demonstrating
the dense perivascular round cell infiltrate.

to determine if he or she is photocontact allergic as well. However, in general,
the photopatch test site will be much more reactive than the patch test area in a
patient with dual sensitivity.

Another significant problem concerns identifying the potential photoallergen. The history may be helpful in this determination. Unfortunately the
patients often do not know what they contacted (except for suntan oils or
the like). This is especially true of preservatives and ingredients in soaps.

Since the halogenated salicylanilides and photoreactive-related compounds have been essentially removed from the market, we no longer photopatch test to the extreme list of such agents noted in the second edition of this
test. At present we routinely photopatch test with the following compounds, and
add whatever can be determined from the patient's history: 5% PABA, 8.6%

amyl dimethyl PABA, and glyceryl PABA, in 70% alcohol; and 5% musk ambrette, 10.5% octyl dimethyl PABA, 8.3% oxybenzone, 5% dioxybenzone, 0.025% TCSA, and 1% TBS, in petrolatum.

We also routinely patch test with the screening materials suggested by the North American Contact Dermatitis Group (NACDG, 1974) to evaluate other potential contactants and phototest to examine for PMLE (J. H. Epstein, 1966).

Photocontactants

Photoallergic reactions to a number of topically contacted chemicals have been reported. These include sulfonamides (S. Epstein, 1962, Storck, 1965, Schwarz and Speck, 1957), phenothiazines (Sidi et al., 1955; S. Epstein and Rowe, 1957; S. Epstein, 1960a, 1968; Polano, 1964; Storck, 1965; Burdick, 1969) sulfonylcarbamides (Burckhardt and Schwarz-Speck, 1957), men's colognes and after-shave lotions (Starke, 1967), blankophores (optical brighteners) (Burckhardt, 1957), Persian lime rind (S. Epstein, 1956), ragweed (S. Epstein, 1960b; Burley et al., 1983; Burley et al., 1973; Thune and Solberg, 1983), sunscreens (Satulsky, 1950; Sams, 1956; Fitzpatrick et al., 1963; Goldman and Epstein, 1969; Schauder and Ippen, 1986; Thune, 1984), diphenhydramine (Emmett, 1974), and psoralens (Sidi and Bourgeois-Cavardin, 1953; Fulton and Willis, 1968).

However, the halogenated salicylanilides and related antibacterial and antifungal compounds represented the most important group of allergic contact photosensitizers. In the 1960s these chemicals were responsible for almost an epidemic of photoallergic reactions. perhaps tetrachlorosalicylanilide (TCSA) was the most potent photosensitizer of this type. Between 1960 and 1961 it was responsible for an estimated 10,000 cases in England (Wilkinson, 1961) before it was removed from general use. Subsequently, a number of related phenolic compounds were incorporated into soaps and other vehicles to combat infection, reduce body odor, act as preservatives, and destroy fungi. Photocontact reactions were induced by many of these agents, including bithionol, the brominated salicylanilides, hexachlorophene, dichlorophene, the carbanilides, Fentichlor [bis(2-hydroxy-5-chlorophenyl)sulfide], Multifungin (bromochlorosalicylanilide), Jadit (a mixture of buclosamide and salicylic acid) (Herman and Sams, 1972; J. H. Epstein, 1972), and chloro-2-phenylphenol (Adams, 1972).

There has been a rapid decline in the induction of photocontact dermatitis by the halogenated salicylanilides and related compounds since 1968 (Smith and Epstein, 1977). This is most likely due to the removal of the more potent of these photosensitizers from general use. However, within the past 5 yr two new contactants appear to produce primarily, if not exclusively, photoallergic responses. These are the two widely used fragrance compounds 6-methylcoumarin (Kaidbey and Kligman, 1978; Jackson et al., 1980) and musk ambrette (Raugi et al., 1979; Giovinazzo et al., 1980). In addition, musk ambrette has been reported to be responsible for the induction of a persistent-light reactor state similar to that noted with the halogenated salicylanilides (Giovinazzo et al., 1980). The action spectrum for the photoallergic reactions to these fragrances appears to fall in the UV-A range (Giovinazzo et al., 1981; Kaidbey and Kligman, 1978; Jackson et al., 1980).

Predictive Photopatch Testing

Although animal models are readily available for phototoxicity studies, their use in evaluating photoallergic reactions has presented a more complicated problem. Predictive testing in human skin is even less definitive. In the 1960s identifications of TCSA and related phenolic compounds was accomplished by photopatch testing clinically involved patients. Subsequently, Willis and Kligman (1968b) induced contact photoallergy to certain of these agents in normal human subjects using a modification of the maximization test, which was developed for evaluating the potential of chemicals to produce contact dermatitis (Kligman, 1966).

Kaidbey and Kligman (1980) and Kaidbey (1983) modified the photomaximization procedure. With their test they were able to photoallergic contact sensitize normal human volunteers relatively readily to certain methylated coumarin derivatives, e.g., TCSA, 3,5-DBS, chlorpromazine, and sodium omadine. A lesser number of positive induction responses were noted with TBS contaminated with 47% DBS, 4,5-DBS, Jadit, and bithionol.

Negative results, however, were noted with para-aminobenzoic acid (PABA) and musk ambrette, which have produced photoallergic contact reactions clinically. The authors considered them weak photosensitizers. Thus, to date, there is no proven effective predictive testing model for photoallergic contact dermatitis.

Mechanism

The clinical appearance, histology, and photopatch test responses strongly suggest that the photoreactions described in this discussion are dependent on a cell-mediated immunity (CMI) process. A number of experimental studies utilizing animal and human models have supported this concept. The present discussion will be limited to human investigations.

Immediate or antibody-mediated hypersensitivity. Herman and Sams (1972), using micro-ouchterlony immune diffusion techniques, could not demonstrate antibodies to 3,5-dibromosalicylanilide (3,5-DBS) protein complexes in the serum of patients photocontact sensitive to this chemical. No binding of fluorescein-tagged goat antihuman IgG, IgA, IgM, complement, or fibrin was noted in positive photopatch test sites with the direct immunofluorescence methods. In addition, immunoglobulins in serum from patients photosensitive to TCSA and 3,5-DBS did not bind to cutaneous tissues bathed in these chemicals. Thus no evidence of antibody-mediated hypersensitivity was discovered in patients with photocontact reactions to the halogenated salicylanilides.

Cell-mediated immunity. Photoallergic reactions in human skin characteristic of CMI responses have been induced to a number of agents, including sulfonamides (S. Epstein, 1939), phenothiazines (Burdick, 1969), and the halogenated salicylanilides (Willis and Kligman, 1968b). Perhaps the most extensive studies have been accomplished with the last of these chemical agents; that is, the halogenated salicylanilides. Willis and Kligman utilized UV-B as well as UV-A exposures plus the chemicals to induce the photosensitivity, but only UV-A and the halogenated salicylanilides were used to elicit the contact allergy.

As noted, animal and human studies have confirmed the CMI mechanism for the photocontact allergy reactions, which appears to be identical to the mechanism of contact allergy itself. However, the nature of the antigen has not been settled. The studies of Schwarz and Speck (1957), Burckhardt and Schwarz-Speck (1957), and Jung and Schwarz (1965) with sulfonilamide and related compounds; Willis and Kligman (1968b, 1969), S. Epstein and Enta (1965), and Jung and Schültz (1968) with the halogenated salicylanilides; and Fulton and Willis (1968) with methoxypsoralen suggested that the haptens were stable photoproducts of these chemicals. Also, *in vitro* binding studies have supported this concept.

An alternative concept was proposed by Jenkins et al. (1964). They concluded that the photoproducts might well be short-lived free radicals, which would attach to the protein carrier within microseconds to form the complete antigen. Support for this theory has developed from clinical observations (Osmundsen, 1969; J. H. Epstein, 1972; Herman and Sams, 1972).

In addition, Jung's studies of postirradiation free radical formation and subsequent binding to albumin and beta-globulin of chlorpromazine (Jung, 1970) and triplet state induction by radiation of triacetyldiphenolisatin (TDI) with deactivation by binding to albumin, γ-globulin, and skin protein (Jung, 1967) present further evidence in favor of the latter concept. The studies of Jung et al. (1968a, 1968b) with Jadit were even more supportive of this second theory immunologically. They were able to demonstrate protein binding *in vitro* after irradiation. This *in vitro* protein complex then acted as a full antigen on plain patch testing of Jadit-photosensitive patients.

As one can see, there is a significant amount of discrepancy in the theories concerning the origin of the antigen in photocontact reactions. Most probably both theories are correct under different circumstances; that is, it is likely that at least some of the subjects experimentally photosensitized by Willis and Kligman (1968b) were actually contact sensitized by stable photoproducts of the chemicals. In contrast, the available evidence suggests that the haptens in the clinically acquired disease are unstable photoproducts, perhaps free radicals, which must be in close proximity to the protein carrier at the time of irradiation.

SUMMARY

Photoallergic contact allergic reactions have become increasingly prevalent over the past several years because of increased opportunities for sun exposure and increasing numbers of photosensitizing chemicals available. The clinical process presents as delayed papular to eczematous eruptions, and histologically it is characterized by a dense perivascular round cell infiltrate in the dermis. The diagnosis is confirmed with photopatch testing techniques, and the action spectrum is usually found in the UV-A range. The clinical picture, histology, and test responses suggest that these reactions are dependent on cell-mediated immunity mechanisms. *In vivo* and *in vitro* experimental studies have confirmed this concept. However, there is a great deal of discrepancy concerning the nature of the antigen at present. It seems likely that both stable and unstable photoproducts may play a role under different circumstances.

REFERENCES

Adams, R. M. 1972. Photoallergic contact dermatitis to chloro-2-phenyl-phenol. *Arch. Dermatol.* 106:711–714.

Allen, H. and Kaidbey, K. H. 1979. Persistent photosensitivity following occupational exposure to epoxy resin. *Archives of Dermatology* 115:1307–1310.

Amblard, P., Beani, J. C. and Reymond, J. L. 1982. Persistent light reaction due to phenothiazinges in atopic disease. *Annals of Dermatology and Venerology* 109:225–228.

Bacheim, A. 1956. Ultraviolet action spectrum. *Am. J. Phys. Med.* 35:177–190.

Blum, H. F. 1941. *Photodynamic Action and Diseases Caused by Light.* New York: Rhinehold.

Burckhardt, W. 1957. Photoallergy eczema due to blankophores (optic brightening agents). *Hautarzt* 8:486–488.

Burckhardt, W. and Schwarz-Speck, M. 1957. Photoallergische Ekzeme durch Nadisan. *Schwiez. Med. Wochenschr.* 87:954–956.

Burdick, K. H. 1969. Prolonged sensitivity to intradermal chlorpromazine. *Cutis* 5:1113–1114.

Burley, C. L., Beltzer-Garelly, E., Kaufman, P., Binet, O. and Robin, J. 1986. Allergy and photoallergy to frollania. *Photodermatology* 3:49–50.

Burry, J. N. 1970. Persistent light reactions from buclosamide. *Arch. Dermatol.* 101:95–97.

Burry, J. N. and Hunter, G. A. 1970. Photocontact dermatitis from Jadit. *Br. J. Dermatol.* 82:244–249.

Burry, J. M., Kuchel, R., Reid, J. G. and Kirk, J. 1973. Australian bush dermatitis: compositae dermatitis in South Australia. *Med. J.* 1:110–116.

Daniels, F., Jr. 1974. Physiological and pathological extracutaneous effects of light on man and mammals not mediated by pineal or other neuroendocrine mechanisms. In *Sunlight and Man,* eds. T. B. Fitzpatrick et al., pp. 247–258. Tokyo: Univ. of Tokyo Press.

Davies, M. G., Hawk, J. L. and Rycfort, R. J. 1982. Acute photosensitivity from the sunscreen 2-ethoxyethyl-P-methoxycinnamate, *Contact Dermatitis* 8:190–200.

Emmett, E. A. 1974. Diphenhydramine photoallergy. *Arch. Dermatol.* 110:249–251.

Epstein, J. H. 1966. Polymorphous light eruption. *Ann. Allergy* 24:397–405.

Epstein, E. 1969. Perfume dermatitis in men. *J. Amer. Med. Assoc.* 209:911–913.

Epstein, J. H. 1972. Photoallergy: A review. *Arch. Dermatol.* 106:741–748.

Epstein, J. H., Vandenberg, J. J. and Wright, W. L. 1963. Solar urticaria. *Arch. Dermatol.* 133–145.

Epstein, J. H., Wuepper, K. D. and Maibach, H. I. 1968. Photocontact dermatitis to halogenated compounds and related compounds. *Arch. Dermatol.* 97:236–244.

Epstein, J. H., Fukuyama, K. and Fye, K. 1970. Effects of ultraviolet radiation on the mitotic cycle, DNA, RNA and protein synthesis in mammalian epidermis in vivo. *Photochem. Photobiol.* 12:57–65.

Epstein, S. 1939. Photoallergy and primary phototoxicity to sulfanilamide. *J. Invest. Dermatol.* 243–251.

Epstein, S. 1956. Discussion of Sams, W. M. (1956).

Epstein, S. 1960a. Allergic photocontact dermatitis from promethazine (Phenergan). *Arch. Dermatol.* 81:175–180.

Epstein, S. 1960b. Role of dermal sensitivity in ragweed contact dermatitis. *Arch. Dermatol.* 82:48–55.

Epstein, S. 1962. Photoallergy versus phototoxicity. In *Dermatoses Due to Environmental and Physical Factors,* ed. R. B. Rees, pp. 119–135. Springfield, Ill.: Thomas.

Epstein, S. 1963. "Masked" photopatch tests. *J. Invest. Dermatol.* 41:369–370.

Epstein, S. 1968. Chlorpromazine photosensitivity: Phototoxic and photoallergic reactions. *Arch. Dermatol.* 98:354–363.

Epstein, S. and Enta, T. 1965. Photoallergic contact dermatitis. *J. Am. Med. Assoc.* 194:1016–1017.

Epstein, S. and Rowe, R. J. 1957. Photoallergy and photocross-sensitivity to Phenergan. *J. Invest. Dermatol.* 29:319–326.

Epstein, S., Enta, T. and Mehregan, A. H. 1968. Photoallergic contact dermatitis from antiseptic soaps. *Dermatologica* 136:457–476.

Ertle, T. 1982. Work-related contact and photocontact allergy in a farmer caused by chlorpromazine. *Dermatosen in Beruf und Umwelt* 30:120–122.

Fitzpatrick, T. B., Pathak, M. A., Magnus, I. A., et al. 1963. Abnormal reactions of man to light. *Annu. Rev. Med.* 14:195–214.

Frain-Bell, W. 1986. Photosensitivity and Compositae dermatitis. *Clin. in Dermatol.* 4:122–126.

Fulton, J. E., Jr. and Willis, I. 1968. Photoallergy to methoxsalen. *Arch. Dermatol.* 98:455–450.

Giovinazzo, V. J, Harber, L. C., Bickers, D. R., Armstrong, R. B. and Silvers, D. N. 1980. Photoallergic contact dermatitis to musk ambrette. *J. Amer. Acad. Dermatol.* 3:384–393.

Giovinazzo, V. J., Ichikawa, H., Kochevar, I. E., Armstrong, R. B. and Harber, L. C. 1981. Photoallergic contact dermatitis to musk ambrette: Action spectrum in guinea pigs and man. *Photochem. Photobiol.* 33:773–777.

Goldman, G. C. and Epstein, E., Jr. 1969. Contact photosensitivity dermatitis from sunprotective agent. *Arch. Dermatol.* 100:447–449.

Harber, L. C., Holloway, R. M., Wheatley, V. R. and Baer, R. L. 1963. Immunologic and biophysical studies in solar urticaria. *J. Invest. Dermatol.* 41:439–443.

Harber, L. C., Harris, H. and Baer, R. L. 1966. Structural features of photoallergy to salicylanilides and related compounds. *J. Invest. Dermatol.* 46:303–305.

Harber, L. C., Bickers, D. R., Epstein, J. H., Pathak, M. A. and Urbach, F. 1974. Report on ultraviolet light sources. *Arch. Dermatol.* 109:833–839.

Herman, P. S. and Sams, W. M., Jr. 1972. *Soap Photodermatitis.* Springfield, Ill.: Thomas.

Horio, T. 1975. Chlorpromazine photoallergy. *Arch. Dermatol.* 111:1469–1471.

Hozle, E. and Plewig, G. P. 1982. Photoallergic contact dermatitis by benzophenone containing sunscreening preparations. *Hautarzt* 33:391–393.

Jackson, R. T., Nesbitt, L. T. and DeLeo, V. A. 1980. 6-Methyl coumarin photocontact dermatitis. *J. Amer. Acad. Dermatol.* 2:124–127.

Jenkins, F. P., Welti, D. and Baines, D. 1964. Photochemical reactions of tetrachlorosalicylanilide. *Nature (Lond.)* 201:827–828.

Jillson, V. F. and Baughman, R. D. 1963. Contact photodermatitis from bithionol. *Arch. Dermatol.* 88:409–418.

Jung, E. G. 1967. Photoallergie durch Triacetyldiphenolisatin (TDI) II. Photochemische Untersuchungen zur Pathogenese. *Arch. Klin. Exp. Dermatol.* 231:39–49.

Jung, E. G. 1970. In Vitro-Untersuchungen zur Chlorpromazine (CPZ) Photoallergie. *Arch. Klin. Exp. Dermatol.* 237:501–506.

Jung, E. G. and Schültz, R. 1968. Kontakt- und Photoallergien durch Desinfizienzien. *Dermatologica* 137:216–226.

Jung, E. G. and Schwarz, K. 1965. Photoallergy to "Jadit" with photo cross-reactions to derivatives of sulfanilamide. *Int. Arch. Allergy Appl. Immunol.* 27:313–317.

Jung, E. G., Dümmler, U. and Immich, H. 1968a. Photoallergic durch 4-Chlor-2-hydroxy-benzoesäure-butylamid. I. Lichtbiologische Untersuchungen zur Antigenbildung. *Arch. Klin. Exp. Dermatol.* 232:403–412.

Jung, E. G., Hornke, J. and Hajdu, P. 1968b. Photoallergie durch 4-Chlor-2-hydroxy-benzoesäure-n-butylamid. II. Photochemische Untersuchungen. *Arch. Klin. Exp. Dermatol.* 233:287–295.

Kaidbey, K. H. 1983. The evaluation of photoallergic contact sensitizers in humans. In *Dermatotoxicology,* 2d ed., eds. F. N. Marzulli and H. I. Maibach, pp. 405–414. Washington, D.C.: Hemisphere.

Kaidbey, K. H. and Kligman, A. M. 1978. Contact photoallergy to 6-methyl coumarin in proprietary sunscreens. *Arch. Dermatol.* 114:1709–1710.

Kaidbey, K. H. and Kligman, A. M. 1980. Photo-maximization test for identifying photoallergic contact sensitizers. *Contact Dermatitis* 6:161–169.

Kligman, A. M. 1966. Identification of contact allergens by human assay. III. The maximization test. A procedure for screening and rating contact sensitizers. *J. Invest. Dermatol.* 47:393–409.

Lonker, A., Mitchell, J. C. and Calnan, C. D. 1974. Contact Dermatitis from Parthenium hysterophorus, Trans. St. Johns' Hosp. *Dermatol. Soc.* 60:43–53.

NACDG (North American Contact Dermatitis Group) of the National Program for Dermatology. 1974. *The Role of Patch Testing in Allergic Contact Dermatitis.* New Brunswick, N.J.: Johnson & Johnson.

Osmundsen, P. E. 1969. Contact photoallergy to tribromsalicylanilide. *Br. J. Dermatol.* 81:429–434.

Parrish, J. A., Ying, C. Y., Pathak, M. A. and Fitzpatrick, E. 1974. Erythemogenic properties of long-wave ultraviolet light. In *Sunlight and Man,* eds. M. A. Pathak, L. C. Harber, M. Seiji and A. Kukita, pp. 131–141. Tokyo: Univ. of Tokyo Press.

Pathak, M. A. 1986. Phytophotodermatitis. *Clin. in Dermatol.* 4:102–121.

Pathak, M. A., Kramer, D. M. and Fitzpatrick, T. B. 1974. Photobiology and photochemistry of furocoumarins (psoralens). In *Sunlight and Man,* eds. M. A. Pathak, L. C. Harber, M. Seiji and A. Kukita, pp. 335–368. Tokyo: Univ. of Tokyo Press.

Polano, J. K. 1964. Photosensitivity due to drugs. *Excerpta Med. Int. Congr. Ser.* 85:102–107.

Raugi, G. J., Storrs, F. J. and Larsen, W. G. 1979. Photoallergic contact dermatitis to men's perfume. *Contact Dermatitis* 5:251–260.

Sams, W. M. 1956. Contact photodermatitis. *Arch. Dermatol.* 73:142–148.

Sams, W. M., Jr. 1970. Solar urticaria: Studies of the active serum factor. *J. Allergy Clin. Immunol.* 45:295–301.

Satulsky, E. M. 1950. Photosensitization induced by monoglycerol paraminobenzoate. *Arch. Dermatol.* 62:711–713.

Schauder, S. and Ippen, H. 1986. Photoallergic and allergic contact dermatitis from dibenzoylmethanes. *Photodermatology* 3:140–147.

Schwarz, K. and Speck, M. 1957. Experimentelle Untersuchungen zur Frage der Photoallergie der Sulfonamide. *Dermatologica* 114:232–243.

Sidi, E. and Bourgeois-Cavardin, J. 1953. Mise au point due traitment du vitiligo par l'Ammi Majus. *Presse Med.* 61:436–440.

Sidi, E., Hincky, M. and Gervais, A. 1955. Allergic sensitization and photosensitization to Phenergan cream. *J. Invest. Dermatol.* 24:345–352.

Smith, S. Z. and Epstein, J. H. 1977. Photocontact dermatitis to halogenated salicylanilides and related compounds. *Arch. Dermatol.* 113:1372–1374.

Starke, J. C. 1967. Photoallergy to sandlewood oil. *Arch. Dermatol.* 96:62–63.

Storck, H. 1965. Photoallergy and photosensitivity: Due to systemically administered drugs. *Arch. Dermatol.* 91:469–482.

Torinukl, W., Kumai, N. and Miura, T. 1982. Chronic photosensitive dermatitis due to phenethiazines. *Tohoku J. Exp. Med.* 138:223–226.

Thune, P. 1984. Contact and photocontact allergy to sunscreens. *Photodermatology* 1:5–9.

Thune, P. and Eeg-Larsen, T. 1984. Contact and photocontact allergy in persistent light reactivity. *Contact Dermatitis* 11:98–107.

Thune, P. O. and Solbery, Y. 1983. Photosensitivity and allergy to aromatic lichen acids, compositae oleoresins and other plant substances. *Contact Dermatitis* 6:81–87.

Wilkinson, D. S. 1961. Photodermatitis due to tetrachlorosalicylanilide. *Br. J. Dermatol.* 73:213–219.

Willis, I. and Kligman, A. M. 1968a. The mechanism of the persistent light reactor. *J. Invest. Dermatol.* 51:385–394.

Willis, I. and Kligman, A. M. 1968b. The mechanism of photoallergic contact dermatitis. *J. Invest. Dermatol.* 51:378–384.

Willis, I. and Kligman, A. M. 1969. Photocontact allergic reactions: Elicitation by low doses of long ultraviolet rays. *Arch. Dermatol.* 110:535–539.

Willis, I., Kligman, A. M. and Epstein, J. H. 1972. Effects of long ultraviolet rays on human skin: Photoprotective or photoaugmentative? *J. Invest. Dermatol.* 59:416–420.

Wiskemann, A. and Wulf, K. 1959. Untersuchungen über den auslösenden Spektralbereich und die direkte Lichtpigmentierung bei chronischen und akuten Lichtausschlägen. *Arch. Klin. Exp. Dermatol.* 209:443–453.

24

uvb-induced immunosuppression is mediated through effects on immunocompetent epidermal cells

■ Ponciano D. Cruz, Jr. ■ Paul R. Bergstresser ■

INTRODUCTION

The immune system constitutes our primary defense mechanism for protection against infectious and neoplastic disease. It is a complex and interactive system that is designed to maintain homeostasis, in the process ridding the body of foreign substances (antigens). In this process, immune responses are tightly controlled by a network of regulatory lymphocytes that either activate (helper cells) or inactivate (suppressor cells) our response to antigens.

Like many other tissues, the skin can be considered an integral part of the immune system because it contains both resident cells of immunologic consequence and circulating white blood cells. However, in contrast with other tissues (with the possible exception of the lung and gut), skin is unique in that is serves as an interface with the external environment, a peripheral location that allows several exogenous agents to impinge directly upon its functions.

Electromagnetic radiation from the sun is a ubiquitous agent that is encountered often in the environment. It has beneficial effects (e.g., synthesis of previtamin D) as well as adverse consequences (e.g., cutaneous carcinogenesis and aging). Radiation from within the ultraviolet (UV) B (280–320 nm) spectrum, in particular, is a focus of concern since it is principally responsible for the induction and the promotion of skin cancer (Blum, 1976). In addition, UVB radiation can alter directly the biology of immunocompetent epidermal cells, leading to the suppression of immune responses (Romerdahl et al., 1989).

UVB RADIATION AND SKIN CANCER

On the basis of clinical and epidemiological evidence in humans and experimental studies in laboratory animals, there can be little doubt that UVB radiation is a carcinogen.

In humans, the prevalence of basal-cell cancer correlates inversely with the degree of melanogenic pigmentation and the geographic latitude away from the equator (Doll et al, 1970). There is an increased skin cancer prevalence in Celts who have migrated from the British Isles to Australia (Urbach 1972). More than 90% of skin cancers in whites occur on sun-exposed areas of the body, and such lesions occur more frequently in individuals who receive sun exposure (Urbach, 1972). Finally, skin cancer is markedly increased in patients with albinism, in whom there is a genetic deficiency in melanin pigmentation (Mosher et al., 1987), and in patients with xeroderma pigmentosum, in whom there is an inability to repair UVB-induced DNA damage (Kraemer et al., 1987).

In animal studies, chronic exposure to UVB has been shown to be both a tumor initiator and tumor promoter for epidermal cells (Penn, 1984). In this respect, it has been demonstrated that UV radiation will also convert photochemically naturally occurring sterols to carcinogenic substances and will induce the polyamine biosynthetic enzyme ornithine decarboxylase (Penn, 1985).

In association with its direct carcinogenic effects, UVB radiation also impairs immunosurveillance for skin cancer. In humans, the best evidence is circumstantial but strong: the high frequency of squamous-cell cancer in patients who receive immunosuppressive drugs during the course of organ transplantation (Penn, 1975). In laboratory mice, this concept was verified further in several studies conducted by Fisher and Kripke and by Daynes and their colleagues in the 1970s (Fisher and Kripke, 1977; Daynes et al., 1979). Summarily, they showed that mice exposed chronically to relatively high doses of UVB would develop skin cancers. When these tumors were transplanted into genetically identical (syngeneic) recipients, they were rejected vigorously, indicating these UVB-induced cancers are highly antigenic. By contrast, when tumor recipients were immunosuppressed, whether by exposure to sublethal doses of x-radiation, or subcarcinogenic doses of UVB radiation, or, most importantly, by transfer of spleen and lymph node cells from UVB-irradiated mice, these cancers would grow progressively (Daynes and Spellman, 1977; Fisher and Kripke, 1977, 1982).

Thus, UVB radiation not only induces skin cancers, but it also promotes their development and causes the emergence of tumor-specific suppressor cells that prevent their immunologic destruction (Fisher and Kripke, 1982). A striking parallel to this phenomenon is a second form of UVB-induced immune suppression—mice exposed to UVB radiation fail to mount immune responses to chemicals applied to their skin (Kripke, 1986). This inhibition of contact hypersensitivity is also associated with the emergence of antigen-specific T suppressor cells (Jessup et al., 1978).

UVB RADIATION AND IMMUNOSUPPRESSION

Because UVB radiation penetrates no farther than the superficial layers of skin, it stands to reason that its immunologic effects should be mediated initially through elements of the epidermal compartment, in which the major portion of this radiation is absorbed. Indeed, available evidence points to at least three mechanisms, all involving epidermal cells, by which UVB irradiation may lead to immunosuppression: (1) production by keratinocytes of soluble mediators of immunosuppression (Table 1), (2) abrogation of the normal antigen presentation function of Langerhans cells (LC), thus permitting the generation of immuno-suppression by alternative antigen presenting cells (Table 2), and (3) conversion of LC from immunogenic to tolerogenic antigen-presenting cells. The first mechanism is supported by studies that have employed UVB in fluences that range from low to relatively high doses ($>10^3$ J/m^2). By contrast, the second and third mechanisms have been illuminated by studies that have used low doses of UVB ($<10^3$ J/m^2) exclusively. These latter studies have been referred to as the low-dose model of UVB-induced immunosuppression (Cruz et al, 1988). The significance of this low-dose UVB model arises from the fact that the fluences used are comparable to those commonly encountered by humans (1–4 minimum erythema dose). Thus, unlike its high-dose counterpart, the low-dose model more closely simulates physiologic exposure to UVB radiation.

Production by Keratinocytes of Soluble Mediators of Immunosuppression

Keratinocytes comprise the vast majority of epidermal cells *in situ* and are capable of secreting an array of biologically active inflammatory and immuno-modulatory substances. Among these substances, several have been suggested as mediators of immunosuppression (Table 1), including prostaglandin E$_2$ (Jun et al., 1988), interleukin-1 (IL-1) (Robertson et al., 1987), a recently isolated protein (termed contra IL-1) that is capable of inhibiting both IL-1 effects and

TABLE 1 Keratinocyte-Derived Products That Have Been Implicated as Mediators of UVB-Induced Immunosuppression

---

Prostaglandin E2 (PGE2)
Interleukin-1 (IL-1)
Contra-IL-1
cis-Urocanic acid
Tumor necrosis factor α (TNFα)
Pre-vitamin D3

TABLE 2   Cells in Epidermis That Have Been Implicated as Sources of the Suppressor Signal during the Induction of Contact Hypersensitivity

Mice
Low-dose UVB-irradiated Langerhans cell
γ/σ T cell receptor-expressing Thy-1$^+$ dendritic epidermal cell
IJ$^+$/Ia$^+$ epidermal cell
Humans
CD1$^-$/DR$^+$/OKM5$^+$ cell that migrates into epidermis following UVB irradiation

contact hypersensitivity (Schwartz et al., 1988), the cis isomer of urocanic acid (Noonan et al., 1988), tumor necrosis factor α (TNFα) (Yoshikawa and Streilein, 1989), and pre-vitamin D_3. The mechanistic linkage between UVB-induced production by keratinocytes of these substances and the evocation of immunosuppression has not yet been established.

Abrogation of the Normal Presentation Function of Langerhans Cells

LC act as antigen presenting cells for T-cell-mediated responses. This has been demonstrated repeatedly *in vitro* for allogeneic responses as well as syngeneic responses to soluble antigens (Stingl, 1981), and *in vivo* for delayed-type hypersensitivity reactions such as contact hypersensitivity and skin graft rejection (Toews et al., 1980; Streilein et al., 1982; Streilein et al., 1984).

Studies that have employed low-dose UVB protocols *in vivo* have demonstrated an abrogation of the antigen presenting capacity of LC. Low-dose UVB irradiation (equivalent to <4 MED in humans) causes a substantial diminution in the density of ATPase$^+$ or Ia$^+$ LC in irradiated mouse skin (Toews et al., 1980; Aberer et al., 1981). Such treatment also results in an inhibition of the capacity of locally irradiated skin to mediate induction of contact hypersensitivity to reactive haptens such as dinitrofluorobenzene (DNFB), trinitrochlorobenzene (TNCB), fluorescein isothiocyanate (FITC), and oxazolone (Toews et al., 1980; Cruz and Bergstresser, 1988; Okamoto and Kripke, 1987). (Fig. 1). Furthermore, suppressor T cells that act on the afferent limb of the contact hypersensitivity response have been shown to be responsible for this inhibition (Elmets et al., 1983). Equally important, *in vitro* UVB exposure also abrogates the capacity of LC-containing epidermal cell populations to stimulate primed T-cell proliferation to soluble antigens, such as PPD and dinitrophenylated ovalbumin (Stingl, 1981).

One consequence of UVB-induced abrogation of normal LC function may be the unmasking of inherent suppressive effects induced by alternative antigen presenting cells in epidermis. Among the cells that have been proposed to play this role are two residents of mouse epidermis, the γ/Δ receptor-expressing dendritic T cell (Thy-1$^+$EC) (Sullivan et al., 1986; Cruz, 1989) and an Ia$^+$/I-J$^+$ cell (Granstein et al., 1987), and a CD1$^-$/DR$^+$/OKM$^+$ cell that migrates into human epidermis following UVB exposure (Table 2) (Baadsgaard et al., 1988).

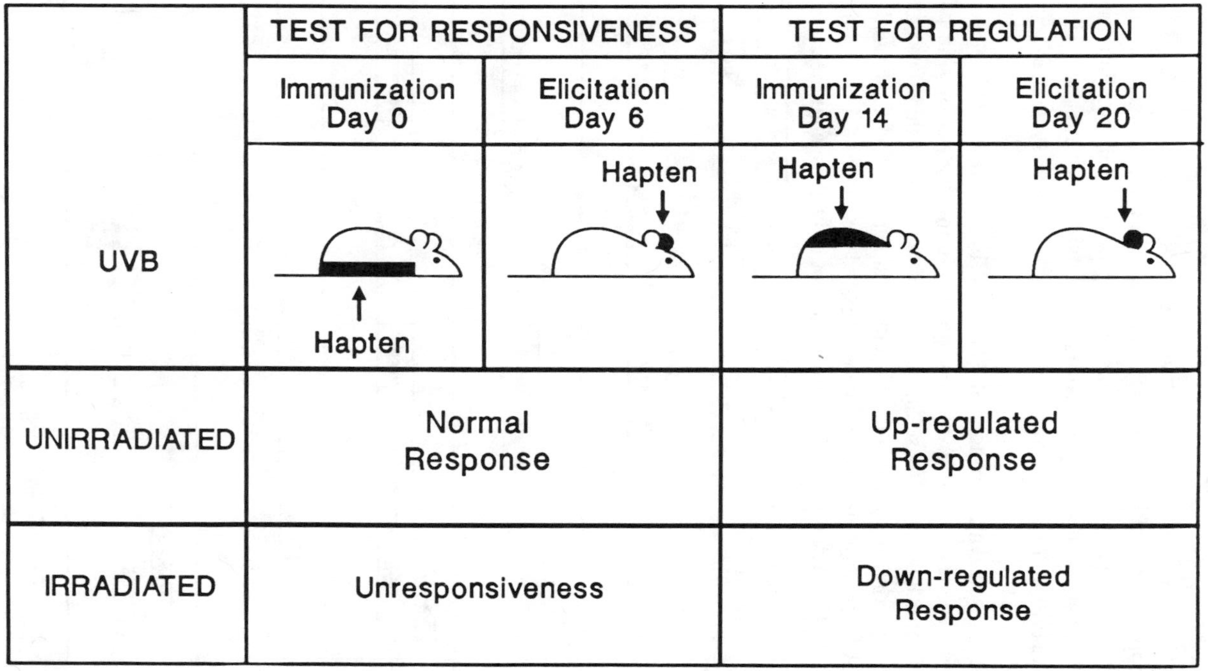

FIGURE 1 Contact hypersensitivity assays following hapten-painting with and without low-dose UVB pretreatment.

Conversion of Langerhans Cells from Immunogenic to Tolerogenic Antigen-Presenting Cells

To identify the relevant epidermal cell target of low-dose UVB-induced immunosuppression, we have compared the capacities of unirradiated and low-dose UVB-irradiated, sorter-purified mouse epidermal cell populations to induce and regulate contact hypersensitivity following derivatization with trinitrophenol (TNP) and then intravenous immunization into syngeneic recipients (Cruz et al., 1989).

Mice infused with unirradiated TNP-LC (Fig. 2, panel 1) displayed normal contact hypersensitivity responses; upon reimmunization by skin painting with TNCB at a later date, these animals exhibited exaggerated (up-regulated) responses. By contrast, mice injected with irradiated TNP-LC showed initial unresponsiveness and subsequent down-regulated responses. Thus, a single exposure to 200 J/m^2 UVB (1 MED in humans) not only abrogated the capacity of

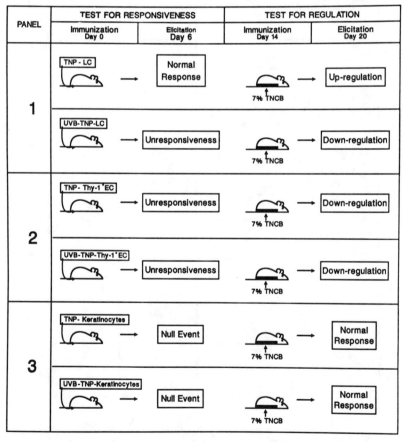

FIGURE 2 Contact hypersensitivity assays following intravenous immunization of hapten-derivatized purified epidermal cell populations with and without low-dose UVB pretreatment.

LC to induce contact hypersensitivity, but also incited LC to initiate a tolerogenic response (Cruz et al., 1989). These findings are significant in at least two ways: (1) they constitute the first direct evidence that UVB can reverse the immunologic attributes of LC, and (2) they support the hypothesis that low-dose UVB can perturb events that occur during antigen presentation.

On the other hand, UVB irradiation had not significant effect on either the inherent down-regulatory property mediated by Thy-1$^+$EC (Fig. 2, panel 2) or the immunologically null event produced by keratinocyte cells (Fig. 2, panel 3) (Cruz et al., 1989). Taken together, these data indicate that LC are a relevant epidermal cell target of low-dose UVB-induced suppression of contact hypersensitivity.

UVB RADIATION AND ANTIGEN PRESENTATION BY LANGERHANS CELLS

Several loci in the antigen presentation pathway of LC are potential sites of perturbation by low-dose UVB (Table 3). These loci include steps involved in antigen processing (e.g., internalization and acidification of antigen, and the association of processed antigen with the MHC class II molecule) and in T-cell activation (e.g., association of MHC/antigen with the T-cell receptor, interaction of adhesion molecules on LC with their ligands on T cells, production and secretion of costimulatory signals, and selective activation of T-cell subsets). In addition, low-dose UVB may disrupt the migration of LC.

SUMMARY AND CONCLUSIONS

The suppressive effects of UVB radiation on the immune system may be viewed in at least two ways. Immunosuppression produced by chronic and/or high doses of UVB irradiation are detrimental to the host since it initiates the

TABLE 3 Possible Loci of Perturbation of Langerhans Cell Function by Low-Dose UVB Leading to Immunosuppression

Antigen processing
  Internalization (endocytosis)
  Acidification (unfolding and degradation)
  Association of processed antigen with MHC molecule
T-Cell activation
  Association of MHC/antigen with the T-cell receptor
  Interaction of adhesion molecules (on LC) with their ligands
    (on T cells)
  Production and secretion of costimulatory signals
  Selective activation of T-cell subsets
Migration
  From blood into skin
  From skin into peripheral lymph nodes

growth and promotes the development of skin cancers. On the other hand, immunosuppression induced by transient and/or low doses of UVB irradiation may be an efficient means of protection against the development of cutaneous autoimmune disease. In either case, it is clear that immunosuppression evoked by UVB is mediated initially through influences on immunocompetent cells in skin. On the basis of recent scientific evidence, three mechanisms have been proposed: (1) production by keratinocytes of cytokines that can suppress immune responses, (2) unopposed suppressive action of non-LC, accessory cells, and (3) conversion of LC from immunogenic to tolerogenic antigen-presenting cells. The molecular and biochemical basis of these models of immunosuppression await future clarification.

REFERENCES

Aberer, W., Schuler, G., Stingl, G., Honigsmann, H. and Wolff, K. 1981. Ultraviolet light depletes surface markers of Langerhans cells. *J. Invest. Dermatol.* 76:202–210.

Baadsgaard, O., Fox, D. A. and Cooper, K. D. 1988. Human epidermal cells from ultraviolet light-exposed skin preferentially activate autoreactive CD4$^+$2H4$^+$ suppressor-inducer lymphocytes and CD8$^+$ suppressor-inducer lymphocytes. *J. Immunol.* 140:1738–1744.

Blum, H. F. 1976. Ultraviolet radiation and skin cancer: In mice and men. *Photochem. Photobiol.* 24:249–254.

Cruz, P. D., Jr. and Bergstresser, P. R. 1988. The low-dose model of UVB-induced immunosuppression. *Photodermatology.* 5:151–161.

Cruz, P. D., Jr., Nixon-Fulton, J., Tigelaar, R. E. and Bergstresser, P. R. 1988. Local effects of UV radiation on immunization with contact sensitizers: I. Down-regulation of contact hypersensitivity by application of TNCB to UV-irradiated skin. *Photodermatology.* 5:126–132.

Cruz, P. D., Jr., Nixon-Fulton, J., Tigelaar, R. E. and Bergstresser, P. R. 1989. Disparate effects of in vitro low-dose UVB irradiation on intravenous immunization with purified epidermal cell subpopulations for the induction of contact hypersensitivity. *J. Invest. Dermatol.* 92:160–165.

Daynes, R. A. and Spellman, C. W. 1977. Evidence for the generation of suppressor cells by ultraviolet radiation. *Cell. Immunol.* 31:182–187.

Daynes, R. A., Schmitt, M. K., Roberts, L. K. and Spellman, C. W. 1979. Phenotypic and physical characteristics of the lymphoid cells involved in the immunity to syngeneic UV-induced tumors. *J. Immunol.* 122:2458–2464.

Doll, R., Payne, P. and Waterhouse, J. 1970. *Cancer Incidence in Five Continents.* New York: Springer-Verlag.

Elmets, C. A., Bergstresser, P. R., Tigelaar, R. E., Wood, P. J. and Streilein, J. W. 1983. Analysis of the mechanism of unresponsiveness produced by haptens painted on skin exposed to ultraviolet radiation. *J. Exp. Med.* 158:781–794.

Fisher, M. S. and Kripke, M. L. 1977. Systemic alteration induced in mice by ultraviolet radiation and its relationship to ultraviolet carcinogenesis. *Proc. Natl. Acad. Sci. USA* 74:1688–1692.

Fisher, M. S. and Kripke, M. L. 1982. Suppressor T lymphocytes control the development of primary skin cancer in ultraviolet-irradiated mice. *Science* 216:1133–1134.

Granstein, R. D., Askari, M., Whitaker, D. and Murphy, G. F. 1987. Epidermal cells in activation of suppressor lymphocytes: further characterization. *J. Immunol.* 138:4055–4062.

Harber, L. C. and Bickers, D. R. 1989. Non-melanoma skin cancer and melanoma. In *Photosensitivity Diseases,* Toronto: B.C. Decker.

Jessup, J. M., Hanna, N., Palaszynski, E. and Kripke, M. L. 1978. Mechanisms of depressed reactivity to dinitrochlorobenzene and ultraviolet-induced tumors during ultraviolet carcinogenesis in BALB/c mice. *Cell. Immunol.* 38:105–115.

Jun, B. D., Roberts, L. K., Cho, B. H., Robertson, B. and Daynes, R. A. 1988. Parallel recovery of epidermal antigen-presenting cell activity and contact hypersensitivity responses in mice exposed to ultraviolet irradiation: The role of a prostaglandin-dependent mechanism. *J. Invest. Dermatol.* 90:311–316.

Kraemer, K. H., Lee, M. M. and Scotto, J. 1987. Xeroderma pigmentosum. Cutaneous, ocular, and neurologic abnormalities in 830 published cases. *Arch. Dermatol.* 123:241–250.

Kripke, M. L. 1986. Immunology and photocarcinogenesis. *J. Am. Acad. Dermatol.* 14:149–155.

Mosher, D. B., Fitzpatrick, T. B., Ortonne, J.-P. and Hovi, Y. 1987. Disorders of pigmentation. In *Dermatology in General Medicine,* eds. T. B. Fitzpatrick, A. Z. Eisen, K. Wolff, I. M. Freedberg and K. F. Austen, pp. 794. New York: McGraw-Hill.

Noonan, F. P., DeFabo, E. C. and Morrison, H. 1988. *Cis*-urocanic acid, a product formed by ultraviolet B irradiation of the skin, initiates an antigen presentation defect in splenic dendritic cells in vivo. *J. Invest. Dermatol.* 90:92–99.

Okamoto, H. and Kripke, M. L. 1987. Effector and suppressor circuits of the immune response are activated in vivo by different mechanisms. *Proc. Natl. Acad. Sci. USA* 84:3841–3845.

Penn, I. 1975. The incidence of malignancies in transplant recipients. *Transplant Proc.* 7:323–326.

Penn, I. 1984. Depressed immunity and skin cancer. *Immunol. Today* 5:291–293.

Penn, I. 1985. Ultraviolet light and skin cancer. *Immunol. Today* 6:206–208.

Robertson, B., Gahring, L., Newton, R. and Daynes, R. 1987. In vivo administration of interleukin-1 to normal mice depresses their capacity to elicit contact hypersensitivity responses: prostaglandins are involved in this modification of immune function. *J. Invest. Dermatol.* 88:380–387.

Romerdahl, C. A., Okamoto, H. and Kripke, M. L. 1989. Immune surveillance against cutaneous malignancies in experimental animals. In *Immune Mechanisms in Cutaneous Disease,* ed. D. A. Norris, pp. 749–767. New York: Marcel Dekker, Inc.

Schwartz, T., Urbanski, F., Kirnbauer, R., Kock, A., Gschnait, F. and Luger, T. A. 1988. Detection of a specific inhibitor of interleukin-1 in sera of UVB-treated mice. *J. Invest. Dermatol.* 91:536–540.

Stingl, G., Gazze-Stingl, L. A., Aberer, W. and Wolff, K. 1981. Antigen presentation by murine epidermal Langerhans cells and its alteration by ultraviolet B light. *J. Immunol.* 127:1707–1713.

Streilein, J. W., Lonsberry, L. W. and Bergstresser, P. R. 1982. Depletion of epidermal Langerhans cells and Ia immunogenicity from tape-stripped mouse skin. *J. Exp. Med.* 155:863–871.

Streilein, J. W., Wood, P. J., Lonsberry, L. W. and Bergstresser, P. R. 1984. Induction of H-2 restricted contact hypersensitivity by hapten-derivatized skin grafts: Evidence that the immunologic signal includes H-2 determinants derived from skin. *Transplantation.* 37:195–201.

Sullivan, S., Bergstresser, P. R., Tigelaar, R. E. and Streilein, J. W. 1986. Induction and regulation of contact hypersensitivity by resident, bone marrow-derived, dendritic epidermal cells: Langerhans cells and Thy-1[+] epidermal cells. *J. Immunol.* 137:2460–2467.

Toews, G. B., Bergstresser, P. R., Tigelaar, R. E. and Streilein, J. W. 1980. Epidermal Langerhans cell density determines whether contact hypersensitivity or unresponsiveness follows skin painting with DNFB. *J. Immunol.* 124:445–453.

Urbach, F. 1972. *Environment and Cancer.* Baltimore, Md.: Williams & Wilkins.

Yoshikawa, T. and Streilein, J. W. 1989. Concerning a possible link between the effect of UVB on contact hypersensitivity and the gene that dictates LPS responsiveness. *J. Invest. Dermatol.* 92:547.

25

photocarcinogenesis

■ Frederick Urbach ■

INTRODUCTION

The high-energy, short-wavelength portion of the solar electromagnetic spectrum (wavelengths shorter than 320 nm) is potentially very detrimental to living cells and tissues. A low concentration of ozone formed in the stratosphere absorbs most of the photons of ultraviolet (UV) radiation and thus prevents most of them from reaching the earth. However, even in the presence of this ozone layer, which varies in thickness at different latitudes and different seasons, a biologically significant amount of UV radiation reaches the surface of the earth.

The major effects on humans of ultraviolet radiation in the UVB range (320–280 nm) are on the skin and eyes. Acute effects consist of "sunburn," and inflammatory response of the tissues that may be no more than mild redness or slight stinging of the eyes, or may develop into the equivalent of second-degree (blistering) burns. The acute effects of single overdoses of UVB are transient, heal without scarring, and in the skin lead to adaptive changes of skin thickening and pigmentation, which afford some degree of protection. The only established positive (beneficial) effect of UVB in humans is the production of vitamin D precursors in the skin, which are absorbed into the bloodstream and prevent rickets, a serious vitamin deficiency disease. Most work has been done on the harmful effects of UVB, but relatively little attention has been given to possible beneficial effects.

Repeated UVB exposure, prolonged over years, can result in chronic degenerative changes in skin, characterized by skin "aging" and the development of premalignant and malignant skin lesions.

EXPERIMENTAL SKIN CARCINOGENESIS

Effects of Long-Term Exposure of Skin to Ultraviolet Radiation

Ultraviolet irradiation induces an inflammatory response and ulceration in the epidermis and the dermis, the latter being infiltrated with leukocytes in the region of the lesions, and to a much lesser extent between them. These lesions ulcerate and the epidermis may disappear for a time in the center. However, peripherally there is particularly active hyperplasia. The basal membranes (between the epidermis and the dermis) may disappear for a time in the regions of these "open" lesions. Between the lesions, the infiltration of leukocytes is relatively slight.

Injury to the epidermis and dermis, brought about by long-term exposure to UV, leads to dermal alteration. fibrosis and elastosis, and to epidermal atrophy. Experimental production of cutaneous elastotic changes in animals by artificial UV irradiation has been reported. Using histochemical methods, Sams et al. (1964) demonstrated focal dermal elastosis in mice after prolonged exposure to artificial UV radiation. UV-induced changes in connective tissue were seen in rat skin by Nakamura and Johnson (1968). The most extensive studies are those of L. and A. Kligman (1985; L. Kligman, 1988).

TUMOR TYPES

The first visible step in UV-induced epidermal tumor formation in animal skin consists of cell proliferation, that is, an increase in the number of squamous cells and cell layers, which gradually become papillomatous in character (Stenback, 1978). This is accompanied by an increase in cellular atypia, nuclear enlargement, hyperchromatism, indentation, and prominence of nucleoli. This basically proliferative response is frequently replaced by a dysplastic pleomorphism, occasionally with pseudoepitheliomatous hyperplasia-like features, which ultimately invade the dermis. The tumors first seen are acanthomatous papillomas, with a predominantly epithelial component.

Among malignant tumors that ultimately develop are squamous-cell carcinomas of different types, including solid keratin-containing moderately differentiated tumors, individually keratinizing tumors with distinct intercellular bridges, and less differentiated, nonkeratinizing spindle-cell tumors in which ultrastructural analysis reveals squamous-cell patterns.

Another type of neoplastic progression is seen in mice, particularly after intensive treatment with large doses of UVR over a short time. It consists of ulceration, scarring, and the subsequent formation of dermal tumors. These tumors begin as aggregates of regularly built, elongated cells with small monomorphic nuclei. Epithelial proliferation is occasionally observed as a secondary phenomenon. The tumors rarely extend grossly through the surface. In the early stages, they appear to be papillomas, although they consist entirely of fibroblastic cells (Stenback, 1975a). Sarcoma induction is partly species-specific, as such tumors are not seen in UV-irradiated Syrian golden hamsters (Stenback, 1975b) or in hairless mice (Epstein and Epstein, 1963) or guinea pigs, all of which are susceptible to chemical sarcoma induction (Stenback, 1969, 1975b).

Adnexal tumor formation is not as common in UV-treated animals (Stenback, 1975b) as in, for example, carcinogen-treated rats (Zackheim, 1963; Stenback, 1969). Hyperplasia and cystic disorganization of hair follicle walls are common, but rarely progress to grossly visible neoplasia. Even more common are hamartomatous tumors, hair follicle-derived trichofolliculomas, and sebaceous-gland tumors.

ACTION SPECTRUM FOR PHOTOCARCINOGENESIS

Determination of the effective wavelengths or "action spectrum" is one of the primary objectives in the study of photobiological responses. However, data are not available for the action spectrum of UV-induced cancer formation. The paucity of this information for one of the most extensively studied photobiological reactions is due to a number of factors, including the large number of potential wavelengths, the difficulties in immobilizing experimental animals, and the need for an especially good monochromator with practically no stray light contamination. Although the complete curve of the carcinogenic spectrum is not known, certain aspects have been determined by less sophisticated methods. Roffo (1933) reported that window glass filtration eliminated the carcinogenic effects of sunlight on white rats. Thus the offending rays of the sun would be found approximately between 290 and 320 nm. Investigators using mercury arc and fluorescent sunlamps with filters confirmed that, under their experimental conditions, 320 nm represented the longer wavelength limit for cancer formation (Griffin et al., 1955; Blum, 1969). Furthermore, carcinogenic responses have been produced by radiation as short as 230 nm (Roffo, 1933), and skin cancer has been induced by UVC and UVB. Thus the action spectrum appears to include wavelengths between 230 and 320 nm, but wavelengths between 290 and 320 nm have significantly greater carcinogenic effects than those shorter than 260 nm (Rusch et al., 1941, Blum, 1943, Blum and Lippincott, 1943; Kelner and Taft, 1956).

Freeman (1978) performed experiments to provide more specific comparative data by testing the hypothesis that the action spectrum for carcinogenesis paralleled that for erythema. Squamous-cell carcinomas developed at approximately the same rate and frequency, when UV exposure was proportional to that for erythema, with decreasing potency from 300 to 320 nm. No tumors occurred in mice exposed to 290 nm.

Extensive studies on the action spectra for two biologic effects, acute skin erythema in humans and skin carcinogenesis in animal models, have been performed. Based on these studies it has been shown that there is a precipitous, practically semilogarithmic drop in biologic effectiveness of wavelengths from 290 to 330 nm (Cole et al., 1986; Sterenborg and van der Leun, 1987).

A modern skin erythema action spectrum has been proposed by McKinlay and Diffey (1987) and accepted by both Comitè Internationale de l'Eclairage (CIE) and International Electrical Commission (IEC). It has been found to predict accurately the erythemal effectiveness of several polychromatic light sources differing greatly in spectral composition (Urbach, 1987).

Review of extensive photocarcinogenesis experiments in animals performed with light sources of differing UVB content by Cole et al. (1986) suggests that, as long as a light source contains 2% or more UVB, radiation of wavelengths longer than 330 nm provides no measurable incremental contribution to photocarcinogenesis. That action spectrum closely simulates the older erythema action spectra. However, detailed experimental work in animals by Sterenborg and van der Leun (1987) showed that the action spectrum for mouse skin cancer carcinogenesis is very similar to the new (McKinlay–Diffey) human erythema action spectrum; that is, wavelengths longer than 330 nm are measurably effective for skin cancer production.

While it cannot be assumed that the action spectra for human skin erythema and mouse skin photocarcinogenesis are necessarily identical, it appears reasonable that they would be similar. Setlow (1974) proposed that the common denominator was the action spectrum for affecting DNA. Making some allowance for the skin transmission of UV radiation, he showed that the shapes of action spectra for DNA, erythema, and possibly skin cancer production were similar and could be made to coincide.

PHYSICAL FACTORS INFLUENCING PHOTOCARCINOGENESIS

Although the tumor-promoting properties of such physical factors as freezing, scalding, and wounding have been described for chemical carcinogenesis systems, little information is available about the effects of these factors on UV-induced cancer formation. Bain and Rush (1943) reported that increasing the temperature to 35–38 °C accelerated the tumor growth rate. The stimulating effects of heat on UV carcinogenesis were confirmed by Freeman and Knox (1964). Heat also enhanced the acute injury response to UV.

Temperature does not affect the photochemical reactions that follow UV irradiation, but it does affect many of the biochemical reactions that follow the initial photochemical change (Blum, 1943, 1969). Although it is known that heat adversely affects photosensitivity (Lipson and Baldes, 1960) and other phenomena of light injury (Bovie and Klein, 1919; Hill and Eidenow, 1923) and the heat alters the effect of X-rays (Carlson and Jackson, 1959), the influence of heat on burns produced by sunlight or UV has rarely been considered (Freeman and Knox, 1964).

High winds and high humidity significantly increase tumor incidence (Zilov, 1971; Owens et al., 1977).

INTERACTION OF UVR AND CHEMICALS IN CARCINOGENESIS

Photomodification of Chemical Carcinogenesis

The interrelationships between light and chemicals in skin carcinogenesis were first noted by Findlay (1928). This early study of chemically induced skin cancer using coal tar drew attention to the earlier observation of Lewin (1913) that coal tars display photodynamic toxicity of various polynuclear aromatic hydrocarbons—principal agents, responsible for the photodynamic effects of coal tar—toward the test organism *Paramecium caudatum* (e.g., Epstein et al., 1964), using UVR. Although the photodynamic assay cannot identify a particular polynuclear compound as being carcinogenic or noncarcinogenic, compounds with high photodynamic activity have four times greater odds of being carcinogenic than compounds with low activity (Epstein et al., 1964).

Combined UVR and visible radiation together with polynuclear aromatic hydrocarbon carcinogen treatment of mouse skin have produced somewhat conflicting results. Clark (1964) showed that irradiation with UVA, immediately following painting with 3-methylcholanthrene, decreased the latent period of the appearance of papillomas, but without affecting the incidence of carcinomas. This effect was to some extent dose related; however, prolonged or intense UVR inhibited tumorigenesis. Stenback (1975c) found that pretreatment of mouse skin with UVB caused a marked increase of the incidence of skin tumors induced by 7,12-dimethylbenz[a]anthracene (DMBA), whereas irradiation *following* application of the carcinogen significantly decreased the tumor incidence.

The potency of DMBA is reduced by UVA in accord with the demonstrable photochemical activity of the compound (Davies et al., 1972). Either preirradiating DMBA *in vitro,* or treating animals with DMBA and immediately irradiating them with blue light, resulted in much lower incidence of tumors than was observed in animals treated with unexposed DMBA and maintained under red light. On the other hand, if animals pretreated with DMBA were exposed to intense UVR, a phototoxic reaction was induced, accompanied by a somewhat increased tumor yield.

The decreased biological activity was shown to be due to the photochemical transformation and degradation of DMBA. Irradiation at 360 nm produced a transannular peroxide, whereas shorter wavelengths brought about degradation to multiple products. Each of the five major products, as well as the mixture of all photoproducts, was shown to have negligible carcinogenic activity.

Depending on the UV wavelengths used, polynuclear aromatic hydrocarbon carcinogens may be photograded to less carcinogenic compounds or can induce phototoxicity, which may enhance carcinogenicity. Irradiation may also cause such a severe local phototoxic reaction that most epithelial cells are destroyed at the irradiation site. Thus, depending on the nature of the carcinogen and the wavelength of light used, either enhancement or inhibition of carcinogenesis may occur.

Photochemical Carcinogenesis

Photoinduced carcinogenesis has been observed following topical application of agents that are phototoxic, but not by themselves carcinogenic. The introduction of 8-methoxypsoralen (8-MOP) as a therapeutic agent for psoriasis and some other human skin disease was followed by reports that it enhances photocarcinogenesis in mice. It was shown that skin cancer can be induced by the interacting effects of 8-MOP and irradiation with UVA; neither of these agents alone was a primary carcinogen under the conditions of the test.

Forbes et al. (1976) investigated the relative enhancing effect of two widely recognized photoactive compounds, 8-MOP and anthracene, on photocarcinogenesis (neither compound per se is a chemical carcinogen). Compared with the vehicle alone, topical treatment with 8-MOP but not with anthracene markedly enhanced photocarcinogenesis under conditions in which neither compound was acutely phototoxic. This suggests that the phototoxicity of a compound is a property distinct from the capacity to enhance photocarcinogenesis.

Chemical Promotion of Photocarcinogenesis

Epstein and Roth (1968) showed that croton oil promotes the induction of tumors initiated by exposing skin to UVR. Similarly, Epstein reported the promotion of photocarcinogenesis by *trans*-retinoic acid (RA). Just as promotion in chemical carcinogenesis—implying that, following initiation with a subthreshold dose of carcinogen, treatment with the promoter agent is continued to bring about tumor emergence—photocarcinogenesis promotion studies involve delivery of a subthreshold or minimally carcinogenic dose of radiation in a limited time (typically 3–10 wk); the animals are then exposed to a second agent (retinoic acid, phorbol ester, benzoyl peroxide, or a different radiation source) to promote the tumor-initiating stimulus. For example, simulated sunlight irradiation, followed by topical application of RA in methanol, resulted in marked enhancement of skin photocarcinogenesis in two strains of mice, and in a strain of nonhaired rats (Forbes et al., 1979). We have also examined the effect of RA and tetradecanoyl phorbol acetate (TPA) on hairless mice pretreated with either UVR or DMBA. Groups receiving each initiating regimen were treated for 20 wk with the vehicle alone or with RA or with TPA. Both TPA and RA accelerated the appearance of tumors initiated by DMBA as well as those initiated by UVR. Virtually all tumors were pedunculated papillomas typically induced in chemical carcinogenesis, but were unlike the squamous-cell carcinomas produced by chronic UV irradiation alone. Thus RA was found to be an effective promoter of skin tumors initiated by either UVR or DMBA.

PHOTOIMMUNOLOGY

Following the recognition that skin disturbances caused by light may be due to an allergic (immunologic) mechanism, Merklen (1904) established solar urticaria as a clinical entity. Blum et al. (1937) showed that the symptoms of urticaria solare could be elicited by different wavelength ranges in different patients. The field was reviewed by Epstein (1939) and Rajka (1942), who demonstrated subsequently the existence of a specific antibody or solar urticaria by showing that it is transferable with serum. In addition to this immediate type of solar urticaria, Epstein (1939) induced a delayed, eczematous type of photoallergic reaction by the intradermal administration of sulfanilamide, and Burckhardt (1941) confirmed the presence of delayed photoeczematous dermatitis and introduced the photopatch test. The observation by Fisher and Kripke (1977) that relatively minor UVB irradiation suppresses the immune response of animals to highly antigenic UVR-induced skin tumors has opened a new field of investigation, termed *photoimmunology.*

Collective evidence accumulating in recent years has shown the skin to be an immune organ with features unique to this protective barrier, and markedly affected in this function by exposure to UVR (reviewed in Parrish, 1983). Probably the most interesting finding of photoimmunology has been that systemic alterations occur in the host following local skin exposure to UVR. Circulating cells and cells of the internal lymphoid organs are altered, as well as unexposed skin. Local exposure of skin to UVR induces specific tolerance for UV-induced tumors, which tolerance is transferable with suppressor T cells. The sensitization (induction) step of contact sensitization is more easily affected than the elicitation (challenge) phase. The effects are highly antigen-specific and apparently due to suppressor T cells. Similar observations have been made with UVR affecting the reaction to injected antigens (Parrish 1983). Recently while studying the action spectrum of the suppression of contact hypersensitivity, Noonan and DeFabo (1985) noted that this action spectrum resembles the absorption spectrum of urocanic acid; indeed, removal of the stratum corneum, which contains urocanic acid, interferes with the development of immunosuppression.

In contrast to immunosuppression by UVB, exposure to large doses of UVA produces enhancement of the contact hypersensitivity response. The reason for this striking difference in the effects of UVA and UVB is not clear.

HUMAN SKIN CARCINOGENESIS

Nonmelanoma Skin Cancer (NMSC)

Examination of the sun's role in the production of human skin cancer does not lend itself to direct experimentation. However, extensive astute observations have strongly suggested the etiologic significance of light energy in the induction of these tumors. Skin cancers in Caucasians in general, are most prevalent in the geographic areas of greatest insolation and among people who receive the most exposure, that is, men who work outdoors. They are rare in Negroes and other deeply pigmented individuals, who have the greatest protection against UV light injury. Further, the lightest complexioned individuals, such as those of Scottish and Irish descent, appear to be most susceptible to skin cancer formation when they live in geographic areas of high UV exposure. When skin cancers do occur in the darkly pigmented races, they are not distributed primarily in the sun-exposed areas as they are in light-skinned people. The tumors in these pigmented individuals are more commonly stimulated by other forms of trauma, such as chronic leg ulcers, irritation due to lack of wearing shoes, use of kangri (an earthenware pot filled with burning charcoal and strapped to the abdomen for warmth), wearing of a dhoti (loincloth), and so on. In contrast, the distribution of skin cancer in the Bantu albino and in patients with xeroderma pigmentosum follows sun exposure patterns.

Blum (1959), Urbach et al. (1972), and Emmett (1974) reviewed the evidence supporting the role of sunlight in human skin cancer development. Briefly, the main arguments are:

1. Superficial skin cancers occur most frequently on the head, neck, and hands, parts of the body habitually exposed to sunlight.
2. Pigmented races, who sunburn much less readily than people with light skin, have very much less skin cancer, and when skin cancer does occur it affects areas not exposed to sunlight most frequently.
3. Among Caucasians there appears to be a much greater incidence of skin cancer in those who spend more time outdoors than those who work predominantly indoors.
4. Skin cancer is more common in light-skinned people living in areas where insolation is greater.
5. Genetic diseases resulting in greater sensitivity of skin to the effect of solar UV radiation are associated with marked increases in and premature skin cancer development (albinism, xeroderma pigmentosum).
6. Superficial skin cancers, particularly squamous-cell carcinomas of the skin, occur predominantly on the areas that receive the maximum amounts of solar UV radiation and where histological changes of chronic UV damage are most severe.
7. Skin cancer can be produced readily on the skin of mice and rats with repeated doses of UV radiation, and the upper wavelength limit of the most effective cancer-producing radiation is about 320 nm—that is, the same spectral range that produces erythema solare in human skin.

Though these arguments do not constitute absolute proof, there is excellent epidemiologic evidence supporting the role of sunlight in three types of skin cancers: basal-cell carcinomas, squamous-cell carcinomas, and malignant melanomas.

Together the first two types of skin cancer add up to the most frequently detected cancer in humans, and they show an increased incidence over the last decade. They are also the most easily and most successfully treated human cancers. The quantitative extent to which agents other than UV exposure cause NMSC in the white population has not been established; it is, however, believed to be small. Some NMSC are caused by exposure to arsenic, pitch, and x-rays, often as occupational/industrial exposure, sometimes following treatment of skin disorders. This latter group of tumors is found among patients of all degrees of skin pigmentation who happen to be exposed to these agents.

Nonmelanoma skin cancer is at present a serious problem because of disfigurement and the significant economic burden associated with its treatment, particularly in the United States, Europe, and Australia, and to emigrants from these regions to other parts of the world.

Malignant Melanoma

Malignant melanoma (MM) is a relatively uncommon tumor, primarily occurring in humans. The sex ratio varies from 1:1 to 1:1.2 (males:females). In contrast to nonmelanoma skin cancer (NMSC), the anatomic distribution of MM does not follow the most UV-exposed sites. About 10% of MM are on the head and neck. This type of lesion most often represents lentigo maligna melanoma (LMM) and has basically the same characteristics as squamous-cell carcinoma: location on the most exposed sites of the head and neck, low incidence before age 50, rapid and progressive rise in frequency with advancing age, almost uniform presence of solar elastosis in the adjacent skin, and low aggressiveness (Magnus, 1977).

While NMSC is extremely uncommon in pigmented races, MM occurs about one-fifth as frequently in such people as in light-skinned patients and is mostly found (75–85%) on the foot and lower leg (Oettle, 1963).

Another 6–11% of MM appear to be of genetic origin, as evidenced by familial and multiple lesions and peculiar precursors found early in life (B-K mole, dysplastic nevus) (Clark et al., 1978).

The remaining approximately 75–80% of MM in whites have interesting attributes. The incidence rises sharply from adolescence to early adult life (particularly on the legs of women), levels off through middle age, and rises again in old age (because of the appearance of LMM). The incidence in males and females shows a preponderance of young females (less than 40 yr old), and the sites of greatest incidence differ, being the trunk in males and the lower leg in females (Magnus, 1977). Of interest is the observation that, although the various populations studied live in such disparate areas as Finland (north of 60°N) (Teppo et al., 1978) and Queensland, Australia (25–15°S) (Beardmore, 1972) and thus are exposed to very different amounts of solar UVR, the relative proportions of MM affecting various body sites remained quite stable until recently. In at least two areas (Norway and Hawaii) the differences in incidence of MM between males and females on the most affected sites (back in men and legs in women) seem to have been decreasing in the past decade (Hinds and Kolonel, 1980).

Latitude gradients for incidence (and mortality) of MM exist in some countries but not in others. Thus there are real latitude gradients for MM in Norway, Sweden, Great Britain, and the United States (Lee, 1977); less striking or even reversed gradients in Western Australia and central Europe (Crombie, 1979); and partial latitude gradient in Eastern Australia, where in Queensland the incidence of MM is less in the tropics than in the subtropical areas (Holman et al., 1980).

In contrast to NMSC, the populations most affected are not the outdoor workers, but the white-collar, more educated, more affluent people (Lee and Strickland, 1980). The concentration of MM in large cities cancels out a latitude gradient in such places as Finland and Western Australia, where this has been investigated (Holman et al., 1980).

The worldwide rapid increase in the incidence of MM (and much slower increase in mortality rates, as if MM were becoming less aggressive) has been attributed to changes in life-style, as greater exposure to solar UV occurs during leisure activities and vacations (Magnus, 1977). The more affluent are considered more likely to participate in such activities, and it is reasoned that men removing their shirts outdoors and women wearing shorter skirts account for the peculiar anatomic distribution of MM (Fears et al., 1976).

The lack of evidence for chronic solar damage of skin in which MM appears, young age of the majority of patients, variation in latitude gradients, anatomic distribution not matching the most exposed skin areas, and the preponderance of city dwellers suggest strongly that there is a significant difference in pathogenesis between NMSC and MM, at least as far as the significance of solar UVR is concerned.

Except for LMM, MM are certainly not related to chronic, repeated solar UV damage resulting from accumulated dose. Whether acute, intermittent exposure to solar UV, intensity of irradiation, or some interaction of UV with chemicals or precursor lesions is the basis of MM etiology remains to be determined. The absence of a good animal model for MM, at least for the relation of UV to MM, makes such studies difficult.

SUMMARY

Human skin cancers, particularly basal-cell and squamous-cell carcinomas, are closely associated with chronic, repeated exposure of the skin to solar UV radiation. Individuals who sunburn easily and have considerable exposure to solar UV have a much higher incidence of nonmelanoma skin cancer than those who sunburn rarely, tan easily, and have little exposure to the sun. Pigmented peoples rarely develop such skin cancers in light-exposed areas unless pigment is missing (albinos).

In addition to natural UV exposure, the interaction of UV and certain photosensitizing chemicals (psoralens, coal tar, etc.) can augment photocarcinogenesis.

Skin tumors similar to squamous-cell carcinoma in humans can be regularly induced in rodents by using UV similar to that present in sunlight.

Malignant melanoma, which is considerably rarer than nonmelanoma skin cancer, is more serious because of its capacity to metastasize and cause death. There has been a consistent, worldwide increase in the incidence of MM of about 3–7% per year, leading to a doubling of incidence rates in 10–15 yr.

There are striking differences in anatomic distribution between MM and NMSC by sex and site. MM is a disease of younger adults; NMSC occurs primarily in the older population. A relation to chronic insolation, which is so striking in NMSC, is less certain in MM.

REFERENCES

Bain, J. and Rush, H. P. 1943. Carcinogenesis with UV radiation of wavelengths 2800–3400 Å. *Cancer Res.* 3:425–430.

Beardmore, G. L. 1972. The epidemiology of malignant melanoma in Australia. In *Melanoma and Skin Cancer*, pp. 39–64. Sydney: New South Wales Government Printer.

Black, H. S. and Douglas, D. R. 1973. Formation of a carcinogen of natural origin in the etiology of UV carcinogenesis. *Cancer Res.* 33:2094–2096.

Blum, H. F. 1943. Wavelength dependence of tumor induction by ultraviolet radiation. *J. Natl. Cancer Inst.* 3:533–537.

Blum, H. F. 1959. *Carcinogenesis by Ultraviolet Light.* Princeton, N.J.: Princeton University Press.

Blum, H. F. 1969. Quantitative aspects of cancer induction by UV light. In *The Biological Effects of Ultraviolet Radiation*, ed. F. Urbach, pp. 543–549. Oxford: Pergamon.

Blum, H. F. and Lippincott, S. W. 1943. Carcinogenic effectiveness of UV radiation of wavelength 2537 Å. *J. Natl. Cancer Inst.* 3:211–216.

Blum, H. F., Allington, H. and West, R. D. 1937. Studies of an urticarial response to blue and violet light in man. *J. Invest. Dermatol.* 16:261–277.

Bovie, W. T. and Klein, A. 1919. Sensitization to heat due to exposure to light of short wavelengths. *J. Gen. Physiol.* 1:331–336.

Burckhardt, W. 1941. Untersuchungen uberohe photoaktivitat einiger Sulfonilamiolen. *Dermatologica* 83:63–68.

Carlson, L. D. and Jackson, B. H. 1959. Combined effects of ionizing radiation and high temperature on longevity of Sprague-Dawley rats. *Radiat. Res.* 11:509–519.

Clark, J. H. 1964. The effect of longwave ultraviolet radiation on the development of tumors induced by 20-methylcholanthrene. *Cancer Res.* 24:207.

Clark, W. H., Jr., Reiner, R. R., Greene, M., Ainsworth, A. M. and Mostrongelo,

M. J. 1978. Origin of familial malignant melanoma from heritable melanocytic lesions. *Arch. Dermatol.* 114:732–738.

Cole, C. A., Forbes, P. D. and Davies, R. E. 1986. An action spectrum for photocarcinogenesis. *Photochem. Photobiol.* 43, 275–284.

Crombie, I. K. 1979. Variation of melanoma with latitude in North America and Europe. *Br. J. Cancer* 40:774–781.

Davies, R. E., Dodge, H. A. and DeShields, L. H. 1972. Alteration of the carcinogenicity of DMBA by light. *Proc. Am. Assoc. Cancer Res.* 13:14 (abstract).

Emmett, E. A. 1974. Ultraviolet radiation as a cause of skin tumors. *Crit. Rev. Toxicol.* 2:211.

Epstein, J. H. and Epstein, W. L. 1963. A study of tumor types produced by UV light in hairless and hairy mice. *J. Invest. Dermatol.* 41:463–473.

Epstein, J. H. and Roth, H. L. 1968. Experimental ultraviolet carcinogenesis: A study of croton oil promoting effects. *J. Invest. Dermatol.* 50:387.

Epstein, S. 1939. Photoallergy against sulfanimides. *J. Invest. Dermatol.* 2:43–51.

Epstein, S., Small, M., Falk, H. L. and Monk, L. 1964. On the association between photodynamic and carcinogenic activities in polycyclic compounds. *Cancer Res.* 24:855–862.

Fears, T. R., Scotto, J. and Schneiderman, M. A. 1976. Skin cancer, melanoma and sunlight. *Am. J. Public Health* 66:461–464.

Findley, G. M. 1928. Ultraviolet light and skin cancer. *Lancet* 215:1070–1073.

Fisher, M. S. and Kripke, M. L. 1977. Systemic alteration induced in mice by ultraviolet light irradiation and its relationship to ultraviolet carcinogenesis. *Proc. Natl. Acad. Sci. USA* 74:1688.

Forbes, P. D., Davies, R. E. and Urbach, F. 1976. Phototoxicity and photocarcinogenesis: Comparative effects of anthracene and 8-methoxypsoralen in the skin of mice. *Food Cosmet. Toxicol.* 14:303–306.

Forbes, P. D., Davies, R. E. and Urbach, F. 1979. Aging, environmental influences and photocarcinogenesis. *J. Invest. Dermatol.* 73:131.

Freeman, R. G. 1978. Data on the action spectrum for ultraviolet carcinogenesis. *Natl. Cancer Inst. Monogr.* 50:27–30.

Freeman, R. G. and Knox, J. M. 1964. Ultraviolet-induced corneal tumors in different species and strains of animals. *J. Invest. Dermatol.* 43:431–436.

Griffin, A. C., Dolman, V. S., et al. 1955. The effect of visible light on the carcinogenicity of ultraviolet light. *Cancer Res.* 15:523.

Hill, L. and Eidenow, A. 1923. Biological action of light. I. Influence of temperature. *Proc. R. Soc. Lond. Ser. B.* 95:163–180.

Hinds, M. W. and Kolonel, L. N. 1980. Malignant melanoma of the skin in Hawaii, 1960–1977. *Cancer* 45:811–817.

Holman, C. D. J., Mulroney, C. D. and Armstrong, P. K. 1980. Epidemiology of pre-invasive and invasive malignant melanoma in Australia. *Int. J. Cancer* 25:317–323.

Kelner, A. and Taft, E. B. 1956. The influence of photoreactivating light on the type and frequency of tumors induced by UV radiation. *Cancer Res.* 16:860–866.

Kligman, L. H. 1988. The hairless mouse as a model for photocarcinogenesis. *J. Cut. Aging Cosmet. Dermatol.* 1:61–69.

Kligman, L. H. and Kligman, A. 1985. A cutaneous photoaging by ultraviolet radiation. In *Models in Dermatology,* eds. H. I. Maibach and N. J. Lowe, vol. 1, pp. 59–68. Basel: S. Karger.

Lee, J. A. H. 1977. Current evidence about the causes of malignant melanoma. *Prog. Clin. Cancer* 7:151.

Lee, J. A. H. and Strickland, D. 1980. Malignant melanoma: Social status and outdoor work. *Br. J. Cancer* 41:757–763.

Lewin, L. 1913. Uber photodynamische wirkungen von inhaltstoffen des steinkohsenteer Pech's am Menschen. *Muench. Med. Wochenschr.* 60: 1529–1530.

Lipson, R. L. and Baldes, E. J. 1960. Photosensitivity and heat. *Arch. Dermatol.* 82:517–520.

Magnus, K. 1977. Incidence of malignant melanoma of the skin in the five Nordic countries. *Int. J. Cancer* 20:477–485.

McKinley, A. F. and Diffey, B. L. 1987. A reference action spectrum for ultraviolet-induced erythema in skin. In *Human Exposure to Ultraviolet Radiation: Risks and Regulations,* eds. W. F. Passchier and B. F. M. Bosnajkovic, pp. 83–87. Amsterdam: Elsevier.

Merklen, P. 1904. *Pratique Dermatogique.* Paris: Masson.

Nakamura, K. and Johnson, W. C. 1968. Ultraviolet light induced connective tissue changes in rat skin. *J. Invest. Dermatol.* 51:253–258.

Noonan, F. and DeFabo, E. 1983. Mechanisms of immune suppression by UVR. In *The Effect of Ultraviolet Radiation on the Immune System,* ed. J. A. Parrish, pp. 291–298. Skilman, N.J.: Johnson & Johnson.

Oettle, C. H. 1963. Skin cancer in Africa. *Natl. Cancer Inst. Monogr.* 10:197–214.

Owens, D. W., Knox, J. H., Hudson, H. T., Rudolph, A. H. and Troll, D. 1977. The influence of wind on chronic ultraviolet light-induced carcinogenesis. *Br. J. Dermatol.* 97:285.

Parrish. J. E., ed. 1983. *The Effect of Ultraviolet Radiation on the Immune System.* Skilman, N.J.: Johnson and Johnson Baby Products Co.

Rajke, E. 1942. Passive transfer in light urticaria: Pathomechanism of physical allergy. *J. Allergy* 13:327–345.

Roffo, A. H. 1933. Cancer y sol. *Boll. Inst. Med. Exp. Estud. Trata Cancer* 10:417–439.

Rusch, H. P., Kline, B. Z. and Bauman, C. A. 1941. Carcinogenesis by UV rays with reference to wavelength and energy. *Arch. Pathol.* 371:135–146.

Sams, W. M., Jr., Smith, J. G. and Burk, P. G. 1964. The experimental production of elastosis with ultraviolet light. *J. Invest. Dermatol.* 43:467.

Setlow, R. B. 1974. The wavelengths in sunlight effective in producing skin cancer: A theoretical analysis. *Proc. Natl. Acad. Sci. USA* 71:3363–3366.

Stenback, F. 1969. Promotion in the morphogenesis of chemically inducible skin tumors. *Acta Pathol. Microbiol. Scand. Suppl.* 208:1–116.

Stenback, F. 1975a. Cellular injury and cell proliferation in skin carcinogenesis by UV light. *Oncology* 31:61–65.

Stenback, F. 1975b. Species-specific neoplastic progression by ultravioletlight on the skin of rats, guinea pigs, hamsters and mice. *Oncology* 31:209–225.

Stenback, F. 1975c. Studies on the modifying effect of ultraviolet radiation on chemical skin carcinogenesis. *J. Invest. Dermatol.* 64:253.

Stenback, F. 1978. Life history and histopathology of ultraviolet light induced skin tumors. *Natl. Cancer Inst. Monogr.* 50:37–70.

Sterenborg, H. C. M. and van der Leun, L. C. 1987. Action spectra for tumorigenesis by ultraviolet radiation. In *Human Exposure to Ultraviolet Radiation: Risks and Regulations,* eds. W. F. Passchier and B. F. M. Bosnajkovic, pp. 173–190. Amsterdam: Elsevier.

Teppo, L., Pakkanen, M. and Hakulinen, T. 1978. Sunlight as a risk factor of malignant melanoma of the skin. *Cancer* 41:2018–2027.

Urbach, F. 1987. Man and Ultraviolet Radiation. In *Human Exposure to Ultraviolet*

Radiation: Risks and Regulations, eds. W. R. Passchier and B. P. M. Busnojo-kovic, pp. 3–17. Amsterdam: Elsevier.

Urbach, F., Rose, D. B. and Bonnem, M. 1972. Genetic and environmental interactions in skin carcinogenesis. In *Environment and Cancer,* pp. 355–371. Baltimore, Md.: Williams & Wilkins.

Zackheim, H. S. 1963. Origin of the human basal cell epithelioma. *J. Invest. Dermatol.* 40:283–297.

Zilov, J. N. D. 1971. In *Ultraviolet Radiation,* pp. 237–241. Moscow: Medicina.

26

chloracne (halogen acne)

■ **K. D. Crow**[†] ■ **S. Madli Puhvel** ■

DEFINITION

Chloracne is defined as an acneform cutaneous eruption resulting from exposure to polyhalogenated aromatic hydrocarbons of specific molecular configuration (Poland and Glover, 1977). The chemicals that induce chloracne are referred to as chloracnegens. In human subjects chloracne appears to be the most sensitive indicator of exposure to such chemicals (Moore, 1978), and should therefore always be considered a symptom of possible systemic poisoning (Goldmann, 1973), even though in most cases the systemic levels of chloracnegen are insufficient to cause clinical symptoms. Conversely, it must also be stressed that although presence of chloracne is an excellent indicator of exposure to polyhalogenated aromatic hydrocarbons, evidence has shown that its absence does not preclude the possibility of other toxic manifestations (Scarisbrick and Martin, 1981; Martin, 1984).

CHLORACNEGENS

The substances listed in Table 1 have been proved unequivocally to have caused chloracne in humans. As can be seen, most are polychlorinated compounds. Biphenyls have induced human chloracne also when polybrominated. This occurred in Michigan in 1973 when, as a result of a shipping error, cattle feed was accidentally contaminated with hexabromobiphenyl manufactured as a

[†]Deceased.

TABLE 1 Chloracnegens

Chloronaphthalenes (CNs)
Polychlorinated biphenyls (PCBs)
Polybrominated biphenyls (PBBs)
Polychlorinated dibenzodioxins (PCDDs)
Polychlorinated dibenzofurans (PCDFs)
Tetrachloroazobenzene (TCAB)
Tetrachloroazoxybenzene (TCAOB)

flame retardant (Firemaster) (Landrigan et al., 1979). Widespread human exposure through contact with contaminated feed and from consumption of polybrominated biphenyls (PBBs) in dairy foods resulted in chloracne in 3% of the exposed farm populations (Kay, 1977). It is generally believed that bromination renders compounds as acnegenic as chlorination (Ecobichon et al., 1977) and for that reason halogen acne may be a more specific term than chloracne, but the terms chloracne and chloracnegens are too well established to be abandoned at this point.

During the early part of this century chlorinated naphthalenes (CNs) were the primary causes of chloracne. CNs have many useful physical properties, such as being excellent dielectric agents, chemically very stable, inherently fire retardant, resistant to oxidation, antifungal, and antimagnetic (Brinkman and Reymer, 1976). CNs were used extensively in the electrical, rubber, paint, wood, and asphalt industries as separators for batteries, flame-resistant seals for condensers and coils, insulating material for cables, and impregnants of wood, paper, and textiles in order to make these waterproof and flame and fungus resistant. Polychlorinated biphenyls (PCBs) were introduced into industry in 1929. Their primary use was as dielectric fluids in capacitors and transformers. Without proper precautions, industrial manufacture and use of both CNs and PCBs was potentially hazardous to the workers involved. Inhalation of toxic fumes generated during heating of these compounds was particularly damaging. During the 1930s and 1940s several incidents of fatal intoxication of industrial workers occurred in PCB and CN production plants (Drinker et al., 1937; Jones, 1941; Flinn and Jarvik, 1936). During the Second World War, CNs and PCBs were used in the ship building industry to neutralize ships against magnetic contact mines. In the United States CNs were manufactured under the trade name Halowaxes, PCBs under the trade name Aroclors. By the late 1970s stringent safety regulations for their manufacture and use made synthesis of these compounds unprofitable in the United States and their function in industry was gradually replaced by less toxic compounds. Even though Aroclors are no longer manufactured in the United States for industrial use, considerable amounts of PCBs are still around, primarily in the form of dielectric fluids in electrical capacitors and transformers.

The chloracnegens of primary concern presently are not synthesized intentionally for commercial purposes, but are formed inadvertently as accidental byproducts during the synthesis of di-, tri-, and pentachlorophenol and dichloroaniline-based herbicides and pesticides. Thus polychlorinated dibenzodioxins (PCDDs) and polychlorinated dibenzofurans (PCDFs) are formed during the synthesis of chlorinated phenols, and the chlorinated azo and azoxybenzenes during the synthesis of chloroanilines (Taylor, 1974; Taylor et al., 1977).

In pure form, the active congeners of PCDDs, PCDFs, TCAB, and TCAOB are up to 100,000-fold more potent chloracnegens in the rabbit ear bioassay than were CNs and PCBs. In all likelihood much of the chloracnegenicity formerly attributed to the latter class of compounds may have resulted from contamination with the more potent PCDFs and PCDDs.

Current understanding of the chemistry of chloracnegens is derived from studies carried out in the 1970s and later. Technical advances in analytical chemistry provided the tools for separating and purifying individual congeners of the different classes of chloracnegens. Only when these were available in pure form, could biologic activity be related to chemical structure. Poland et al., using 15 different purified congeners of PCDDs, were the first to demonstrate that a similarity in specific molecular structure of the five most toxic congeners correlated with their ability to induce the enzyme aryl hydrocarbon hydroxylase (AHH) in chick embryo livers (Poland and Glover, 1973). Further analysis of the structure-activity relationships revealed that the most active congeners from all classes of chloracnegens are approximate stereoisomers with halogen atoms occupying at least three, and for maximal potency four, of the lateral ring positions. At least one ring position is nonsubstituted (Kende et al., 1974; Poland et al., 1976). The degree of planarity of the molecule can be correlated with biological activity. Substitution of halogen atoms to positions that lead to molecular nonplanarity has been found to reduce biological activity.

The stereospecificity required for biological activity suggested the involvement of specific receptors at the cellular level. Poland et al. (1976), using radiolabled TCDD, were the first to demonstrate the presence of a binding protein in the cytosol of livers of responsive strains of mice and a relative absence of this protein in nonresponsive animals. The degree of affinity of various chloracnegens for this binding protein, termed the *Ah* receptor (for aromatic hydrocarbon), correlated with their biological potency (Poland and Knutson, 1982). It is now thought that *Ah* receptors act in much the same manner as steroid hormone receptors in translocating chloracnegenic ligands to the cell nucleus where they bind to DNA and alter the translation of a battery of genes, possibly via promoter and inhibitor domains. Ultimately these molecular changes are thought to be responsible for the range of biological effects seen (Greenlee and Neal, 1985).

In humans the skin is the most sensitive target organ to express chloracnegen-induced toxicity, regardless of whether exposure has occurred via skin contact, inhalation, or ingestion. In most animals the skin is not similarly sensitive, and cutaneous changes, when reported, have generally been late manifestations of severe intoxication. It should be noted that despite variations in potency between different classes of chloracnegens, within each species all chloracnegenic chemicals induce very similar patterns of toxic effects. The target organs for expressing toxicity vary from species to species, but are identical within a species for all classes of chloracnegens. The explanation for the differences in species response to these chemicals remains unelucidated.

During the past 15 yr, one particular chloracnegen, 2,3,7,8-tetrachlorodibenzo-p-dioxin, or TCDD, has been the subject of an immense amount of research. TCDD is recognized as the most potent prototype of the entire group of chloracnegenic chemicals, all of which appear to trigger similar, species-specific biological pathways. Interest in the mechanism of action of TCDD is only peripherally related to its chloracnegenic effect in humans. Rather, it is recognized that understanding the mechanisms of action of this prototype, which has been referred to as a "molecular probe" (Poland and Kende, 1976), could help to elucidate many unanswered questions about the basic regulatory mechanisms of cell growth and differentiation. TCDD is the topic for a separate chapter (Chapter 27) in this volume.

Sources and Routes of Chloracnegen Exposure

Manufacture (primary). The formation of halogenated dioxins, dibenzofurans, and azo- and azoxybenzenes during chemical manufacture of chlorinated phenols and chlorinated biphenyls has already been mentioned. Although these are closed processes, they have certain well-known points at which exposure can occur. Thus spillage during the repair and servicing of pipework, valves, and reactors, the laboratory checks of reaction masses, and the removal of highly toxic reaction residues may all entail contact, often at points in the reaction where there are high contaminant levels. There have also been instances where laboratory workers have been poisoned while synthesizing highly toxic chloracnegens (Oliver, 1975).

Manufacture (secondary). Some materials, such as chlorophenols (containing PCDDs and PCDFs) and 3,4-dichloroaniline (3,4-DCA) (containing TCAB and traces of TCAOB), are used as chemical intermediates. Thus 2,4,5-trichlorophenoxyacetic acid (2,4,5-T) can be reacted to form numerous herbicidal esters; 3,4-DCA may be further reacted to form the herbicides diuron, linuron, and propanil and others. Depending on the reaction, the final products may contain small amounts of the chloracnegenic contaminant. Linuron and 3,4-DCA may have high TCAB levels.

Use of final product. Chloracne in users of final products is extremely rare. Moderate but prolonged heating, as when PCBs are used as heat exchange fluids, may increase the PCDF content, posing a toxic risk if they are subsequently handled or ingested (Meigs et al., 1954).

Pyrolysis. Fire, either accidental or deliberate (such as in municipal incinerators), may form PCDDs from chlorophenols and PCDFs from PCBs. The first accidental fire involving PCB-containing transformers occurred in the 18-

story Binghamton State Office Building in Binghamton, N.Y., in 1981. A surge of excess electricity led to an electrical panel malfunction, and resulted in intense electrical arcing for about 30 min. Dense smoke containing PCDFs and PCDDs billowed through the air shafts and contaminated all areas of the building (Schechter, 1986). By 1986 more than 30 different incidents involving capacitor explosions, capacitor fires, or transformer accidents, all resulting in the release of PCBs, PCDDs and PCDFs, had been recorded (Rappe et al., 1986).

CUTANEOUS MANIFESTATIONS OF CHLORACNE

The distribution of chloracne lesions is of considerable diagnostic importance. The areas of the human skin that are most sensitive to chloracnegens are below and to the outer side of the eye (the so-called malar crescent) and behind the ear. These may frequently be affected when the rest of the skin is normal. Furthermore, these are the areas most likely to show residual lesions years after more extensive chloracne has disappeared. Next in sensitivity are the cheeks, forehead, and neck, but the nose is almost invariably spared. The genitalia—both penis and scrotum, but particularly the latter—are sensitive regions. With increasing exposure, the lesions spread to the shoulders, chest and back, and eventually to the buttocks and abdomen. The hands, forearms, feet, legs, and thighs are usually only involved in the worst cases. Axillary lesions have only been seen in patients for whom ingestion or inhalation was the major route of chloracnegen absorption, as in Japan in 1968 (Yusho poisoning), or at Seveso, Italy, in 1976, where axillary lesions were seen only in the few children who were actually enveloped in the toxic cloud.

HISTOPATHOLOGY AND MORPHOLOGY OF PRIMARY CUTANEOUS LESIONS

Histopathology of chloracne has been studied experimentally by Hambrick (1957), Shelley and Kligman (1957), and by Plewig (1970), using topical application of CNs (Halowaxes) to human volunteers. These studies demonstrated that initial microscopic changes in the skin could be detected within 5 d after cutaneous exposure, although overt follicular accentuation took a minimum of 2 wk to develop. In cases of accidental exposure to chloracnegens, the time frame for developing visible lesions typical of chloracne has varied from 3–4 wk to even longer periods. The initial change observed in experimental studies was hyperplasia of the epithelium lining the ducts of sebaceous follicles. Subsequently the hyperplastic follicular epithelium underwent abnormal keratinization, and eventually the follicular lumen became distended by lamellae of tightly adhering layers of abnormally keratinized epithelial cells. Simultaneously the number of lipid-forming cells in the acini of the sebaceous glands decreased as these cells underwent squamous metaplasia. Gradually all the affected sebaceous follicles were transformed into comedones, tiny keratinous sacs attached to the epidermis, with only vestiges of lipid-forming glandular elements attached to their base.

Squamous metaplasia may also occur in meibomian glands, the modified sebaceous glands lining the eyelids. This was reported particularly in patients exposed to PCBs via ingestion (Kuratsune et al., 1972). This process, so similar to that of the sebaceous follicles in skin, is clearly an extension of chloracne. The rapid and total transformation of all types of sebaceous glands into comedones appears to be pathognomonic to poisoning with chloracnegens and is therefore of diagnostic value.

As described above, the basic lesion of chloracne is the comedo, and in the mildest cases these may be the only lesions present (Fig. 1). If so, they are likely to involve only the most sensitive areas of skin, that is, the malar crescents and behind the ears. As few as a dozen lesions on each side may be diagnostic. One must be careful in older patients to distinguish the so-called senile comedones that are often seen in the malar areas. In younger patients comedonal acne vulgaris may exactly mimic chloracne. The distinction may be clinically impossible, but consideration of other factors should decide the issue. Thus, apart from the distribution of lesions, a history of exposure to a possibly chloracnegenic chemical is of utmost importance in making the diagnosis of chloracne.

In all but the mildest cases, pale yellow cysts, from the size of a pinhead to a lentil, mingling with the comedones, make up the characteristic picture of typical chloracne (Fig. 2) (Crow, 1970). As the severity of the disease increases, the lesions become more numerous, and in the worst cases, comedones, some no larger than pinpoints, may involve every follicle, giving the appearance of grayish sheets. These lesions are to be distinguished from the equally profuse, but pale, follicular hperkeratoses, to be described in following sections.

In the most severe cases of chloracnegen exposure, inflammatory lesions develop with large cysts and cold abscesses (Fig. 3). As ever wider areas become involved the picture may resemble that of severe cystic acne or acne conglobata, but with less inflammation than in the latter diseases. Such gross lesions are most often seen on the back of the neck, on the trunk and buttocks (Fig. 4).

Additional Cutaneous Changes

Pigmentation. Development of cutaneous pigmentation in association with chloracne has been seen primarily following ingestion of chloracnegen. This was true of the Japanese victims of the Yusho incident of 1968, a mass poisoning in which over 1000 individuals ingested a rice-based cooking oil that had been accidentally contaminated with large amounts of transformer fluid containing PCBs (Kuratsune et al., 1972). Later it was established that the PCBs in turn were heavily contaminated with PCDFs (Nagayama et al., 1976). About 70% of the victims exhibited pigmentation affecting the nails, lips, and the gingival, buccal, and conjunctival mucosae. In a similar mass poisoning in Taiwan in 1979 (Wong and Hwang, 1981) the same distribution of pigmentation was reported.

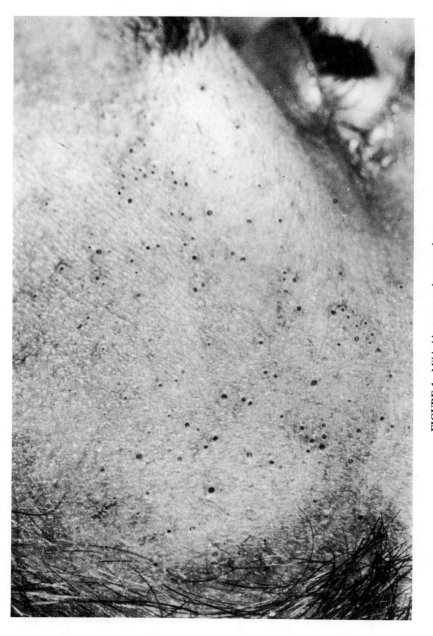

FIGURE 1 Mild chloracne: malar comedones.

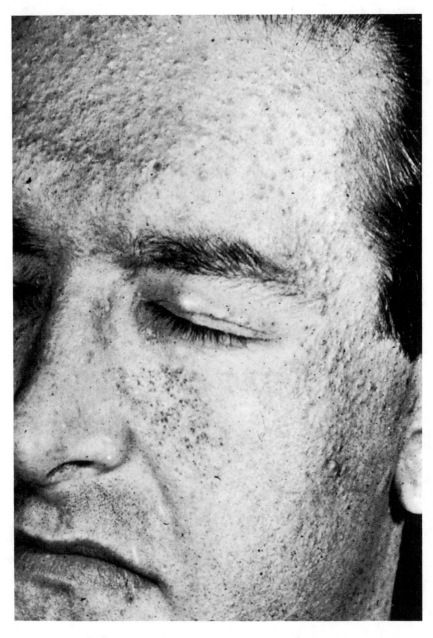

FIGURE 2 Classic chloracne: Comedones and small cysts.

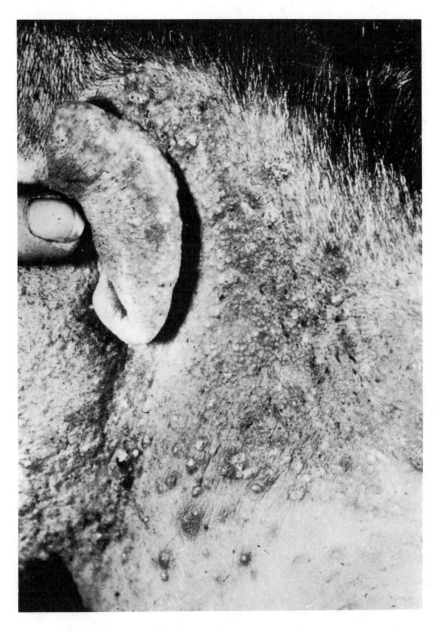

FIGURE 3 Severe chloracne: comedones, cysts, and inflammatory lesions.

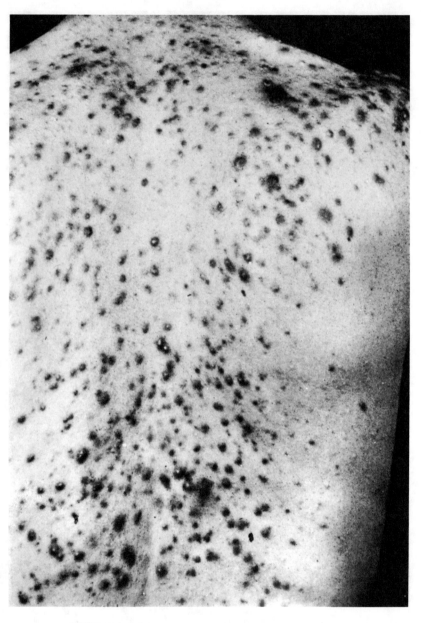

FIGURE 4 Very severe chloracne resembling acne conglobata.

Fischbein et al. (1979) have also reported the development of pigmentation affecting nails and conjunctivae in cases of industrial PCB poisoning, but only involving 2–3% of the cases. It is not known whether the route of exposure (i.e., ingestion vs. skin contact), racial differences, specificity of the chloracnegen, or the dose was instrumental in the development of the pigmentary changes.

Skin of the stillborn infants and of neonates born to Yusho and Taiwanese mothers poisoned with PCBs and PCDFs was hyperpigmented and covered with grayish scales. Histologically the epidermas appeared atrophic with hyperkeratosis and dilation of follicles with keratin. In surviving infants the skin became normal within several months after birth (Higuchi, 1976; Wong and Hwang, 1981).

Hypertrichosis. Hypertrichosis in association with chloracne is a rare finding, mainly confined to the temples. It may be secondary to hepatic porphyria, but it has also been described in patients whose uroporphyrin levels have been normal (Jirasek et al., 1974).

Phrynoderma. Follicular hyperkeratosis, to be distinguished from comedones, may be widespread and even generalized in rare cases of severe chloracne (Crow, 1978). Despite its rarity, no fewer than 70% of the Japanese Yusho and 20% of the Taiwanese victims developed a fine follicular hyperkeratosis of the upper trunk, neck, and most unusual of all, the flexural areas (Goto and Higuchi, 1969; Cheng and Liu, 1981). Again, it is unknown whether the route of exposure (i.e., ingestion) was related to the development of this response.

Erythema. The erythematous changes that have occasionally been associated with the onset of chloracne (Jirasek et al., 1974; May, 1973) have been a source of confusion. Because such erythema has been confined to exposed areas of skin, it has been wrongly ascribed to photosensitivity. Telegina and Biklulatuva (1970), describing an outbreak of severe chloracne and systemic poisoning during the manufacture of 2,4,5,-trichlorophenoxy acetic acid esters, established that the affected individuals had a reduced, rather than an increased, sensitivity to ultraviolet light. A few cases of erythema preceding the severe chloracne resulting from massive internal exposure to chloronaphthalenes are genuine. All other recorded cases have occurred during chlorophenol manufacture. Erythema has never been recorded to have resulted from PCB exposure, even in the massive Yusho and Taiwan poisonings, nor from TCAB or TCAOB exposure. It is therefore much more likely that the erythema reported to have developed as a result of chloracnegen exposure during chlorophenol manufacture is the result of sodium chlorophenate burns of exposed areas of skin, rather than the result of chloracnegen exposure.

DURATION OF CHLORACNE

The duration of chloracne has been correlated with the severity of the disease, which in turn is usually a reflection of the degree of intoxication. Generally the greater the exposure, the more severe and long lasting the chloracne. Suskind (1985), in a follow-up of 436 employees in a 2,4,5-T manufacturing plant who had been exposed to TCDD during an accidental runaway reaction in 1949, found that 86% of the exposed persons originally developed chloracne, and on examination 20–30 yr after the initial exposure, 52.7% still had some minimal residual lesions.

Of the 193 cases of chloracne that resulted from the Seveso explosion in June 1976, there were 8 cases of very severe disease, and in these 8 subjects new lesions continued to develop for 18 mo after the initial exposure. Regression of lesions by the end of 1978 was followed by the appearance of atrophic scars in the affected areas (Caputo et al., 1988).

The chloracne lesions induced in the Yusho incident in 1968 were followed on a yearly basis at least until 1984 (Urabe and Asahi, 1984). In most cases the skin symptoms improved with time; however, in the severely intoxicated group, lesions characteristic of chloracne remained even 14 yr after the original exposure. In many cases regression of chloracne was followed by development of atrophic pit-like scars. Comparison of cutaneous symptoms of Yusho patients with serum PCB levels indicated that with time the correlation between these two parameters disappeared. Initially highly intoxicated subjects had high serum levels of PCBs as well as the most severe grades of chloracne. With time the acne lesions regressed, even though the serum PCB levels remained elevated (Urabe and Asahi, 1984).

TREATMENT OF CHLORACNE

There are no known effective methods for treating chloracne. Unlike acne vulgaris, in which inflammation is a major component of the disease process, inflammatory lesions are rare in chloracne. Because chloracne does not involve cutaneous bacteria, the antimicrobial agents that have been found to be beneficial in the treatment of acne vulgaris are of no use in treating chloracne.

Topical retinoic acid, which is effective in preventing the development of comedones in acne vulgaris, may be useful in treating mild residual comedonal chloracne (Plewig and Braun-Falco, 1971). However, typically the keratinizing (i.e., comedogenic) effect of chloracnegenic chemicals far outweighs the normalizing effect of retinoic acid on follicular hyperkeratinization, and for that reason this agent is of little use in cases of severe exposure.

Accutane (13-*cis*-retinoic acid, isotretinoin) is an extremely effective therapeutic for treating severe cystic acne. This drug, taken orally at a dose of 1–2 mg/kg body weight for 4–5 mo, often results in permanent remission from cystic acne (Peck et al., 1979). One of the mechanisms of action of 13-*cis*-retinoic acid is normalization of abnormal follicular epithelial keratinization (Zelickson et al., 1985). Accutane has been reported to be temporarily helpful in treating chloracne, but in severe cases lesions have returned when treatment has been discontinued (J. S. Taylor, personal communication). It seems that as long as the lipophilic chloracnegenic chemicals are present in sufficiently high levels in the skin, little can be done to reverse their hyperkeratinizing, comedogenic effect. One suggestion for speeding the mobilization of the chemicals from the skin is to put exposed subjects on low-calorie diets to mobilize fat depots.

SYMPTOMS IN NONCUTANEOUS SYSTEMS

Numerous clinical side effects, indicative of systemic poisoning, have been reported in patients with chloracne. Studies to date have failed to establish a consistent pattern of systemic effects; however, it is advisable that patients in whom chloracne has been diagnosed undergo careful clinical and laboratory examinations to make sure that systemic poisoning has not occurred. The following abnormalities have been reported in patients known to have been exposed to chloracnegens.

Hepatic Effects

Liver damage was formerly considered one of the classic signs of systemic poisoning by chloracnegens (Jirasek et al., 1973, 1974; Goldmann, 1973). This was particularly true in the early cases of industrial exposure to CNs and PCBs, where cases of fatal jaundice were reported (Drinker et al., 1937) but not always in association with chloracne. In some of the earlier reports, workers had been exposed to carbon tetrachloride and trichlorobenzene solvents, in addition to the CNs and PCBs. More recent investigations (Homberger et al., 1979), particularly following episodes of acute exposure, such as following the trichlorophenol plant explosion in Seveso, Italy, in 1976, have described a transient rise in values of hepatic enzymes that reflect hepatocellular damage (e.g., gamma-glutamyl transferase and alanine aminotransferase). However, alkaline phosphatase and serum bilirubin levels have not been found to be increased, and no jaundice or other overt or extensive signs of liver insufficiency have been found. It could therefore be that the degree of liver involvement is dependent on the specificity of the toxicant involved, rather than a consistent consequence of all forms of chloracnegen exposure.

Porphyria

Development of porphyria cutanea tarda has been described at least twice in humans following TCDD exposure. (Bleiberg et al., 1964; Jirasek et al., 1974), but to date it has not been found to be a common sequela of chloracne. Urinary porphyrin levels have been monitored in several different groups of subjects involved in incidents of severe chloracnegen exposure, and have been found to be normal (Strik, 1979).

On the other hand, experimental administration of halogenated aromatic hydrocarbons to laboratory animals has been shown to increase uroporphyrin levels, probably as a result of inhibition of uroporphyrinogen decarboxylase (UDP) activity (Jones and Sweeney, 1977). Inhibition of UDP activity in humans has also been associated with the development of porphyria cutanea tarda (Benedetto et al., 1978).

Lipid Abnormalities

There have been numerous reports of long-term elevations in serum triglyceride, cholesterol, and low-density lipoprotein levels following chloracnegen exposure, particularly in association with TCDD-induced chloracne (Baxter, 1984; Walker and Martin, 1979; Martin, 1984).

Peripheral Neuropathy and Other Neurological Effects

Painful peripheral neuropathy, particularly in the lower extremities, may be a long-lasting sequela of chloracnegen poisonings. Following the ingestion of PCBs by Yusho patients this diagnosis was confirmed by biopsies that demonstrated demyelination of peripheral sensory nerves. In addition to neuritis, patchy areas of numbness were also reported to have developed. Nerve conduction velocities were demonstrably lowered in the affected limbs (Murai and Kuroiwa, 1971). Motor nerves were rarely affected, and then only after sensory involvement. Peripheral neuropathy was also found in follow-up studies of populations exposed to TCDD in the Seveso incident (Filippini et al., 1981), and in populations exposed during the runaway reaction at the 2,4,5-T manufacturing plant in Nitro, W. Va. in 1949 (Suskind, 1978).

In addition to the peripheral nervous system changes described above, numerous reports of central nervous system effects have been described in patients acutely poisoned with chloracnegens. Headache, fatigue, irritability, insomnia, impotence, and loss of libido have been reported so often that they are unquestionably genuine symptoms. It must be stressed however, that these have always been found to be acute effects, reported at the height of the poisoning, and only in cases of severe intoxication (Suskind, 1978; Jirasek et al., 1974; Goldmann, 1973).

Immunologic Effects

The effects of the different classes of chloracnegens on the human immune system have not been fully analyzed to date. Animal studies with halogenated aromatic hydrocarbons (particularly with TCDD) suggest that these chemicals may be effective immunosuppressors (Faith and Luster, 1979), although the actual response induced varies not only with the species of animal used, but in several instances is also age dependent. Involution of the thymus gland is one of the most sensitive indicators in many animal species of exposure to TCDD. However, effects of all chloracnegens are very species specific and therefore experimental findings with animals cannot be extrapolated to clinical expectations in humans. To date the few reports that have monitored immunologic parameters in humans known to have been exposed to chloracnegens do not suggest any alarming effects (e.g., Jennings et al., 1988, Mocarelli et al., 1986), although a decrease in T-lymphocyte counts has been reported (Bekesi et al., 1978).

Teratogenicity and Fetotoxicity

In view of animal studies indicating that chloracnegens have teratogenic and fetotoxic effects, these potential sequelae in particular have been investigated in cases of known accidental human exposure. Exposure to TCDD during the Seveso incident did not result in an increase in the rate of spontaneous abortions, or of birth defects (Skene et al., 1989). There were 13 babies delivered of mothers who had ingested PCB- and PCDF-contaminated rice oil during the Yusho incident. Most babies showed some of the same cutaneous symptoms as adults (already described earlier). Some were small at birth and grew more slowly initially but later resumed normal growth rates (Yoshimura and Ikeda, 1978). There were no birth defects. Of two stillbirths, one was autopsied; it showed minor signs of chloracnegen exposure, but death was due to asphyxia from a twisted umbilical cord (Kikuchi et al., 1969).

Cancer

One of the major unanswered concerns about chloracnegenic chemicals is whether they are potentially carcinogenic for humans. This concern of course is greatest for populations who have been victims of accidental exposure to large quantities during industrial or environmental accidents that have resulted in episodes of acute poisoning, but it is also of relevance to the population as a whole. Due to the chemical stability of chloracnegens and their resistance to biodegradation, our entire ecosystem is contaminated with detectable amounts of many of these materials. The effect of such long-term, low-dose, chronic exposure is therefore also relevant.

To date, follow-up studies of subjects who have been acutely exposed have been somewhat equivocal. Seventy men who suffered chloracne and severe poisoning with TCDD during 2,4,5-T manufacture were followed up for 25 yr and showed an increase in stomach cancer in one age group only (Goldmann, 1973). Seventy-nine cases of chloracne from TCDD following the explosion of a 2,4,5-T reactor in 1968 had, 10 yr later, no excessive evidence of malignant neoplasms (May, 1982). Yusho victims have shown an increased mortality from malignant neoplasms. A review of 79 male and 41 female deaths found a significant overall cancer death only for males (33 observed vs. 15.5 expected) accounted for largely by liver and lung cancer (Kuratsune et al., in press). In another follow-up of 121 men who had severe chloracne and poisoning from TCDD, again after the explosion of a 2,4,5-T reactor, 9 cancer deaths were recorded, compared to an expected figure of 9.04, 29 yr later (Zack and Suskind, 1980).

ANIMAL MODELS FOR CHLORACNE

Unlike humans in whom skin is the most sensitive organ to express the effect of exposure to the chloracnegenic group of chemicals, skin of most furred animals generally does not exhibit a similar sensitivity. In most species, cutaneous changes are seen as late manifestation of severe systemic toxicity. Known exceptions to this are skin of the inner surface of the rabbit ear (Adams et al., 1941), facial skin of monkeys (McConnell et al., 1978), and skin of hairless mice (Inagami et al., 1976; Knutson and Poland, 1982; Puhvel et al., 1982).

Prior to the development of sensitive analytical technology for detection and identification of chloracnegenic compounds, suspicious substances were identified on the basis of their effect in the rabbit ear bio-assay. Topical application of a chloracnegenic compound, dissolved in acetone or in propylene glycol, induced significant follicular hyperkeratosis in rabbit ears within 2 wk (Adams et al. 1941). More recently the hairless mouse has been used as the animal model for experimental chloracne. Topical application of chloracnegens induces epidermal hyperplasia and hyperkeratinization in skin of hairless mice, but has little effect on skin of haired counterparts. The dose and time-course for the production of chloracne in hairless mouse skin depends on the potency of the chloracnegen used. Less than 1 μg of topically applied TCDD will induce the typical cutaneous changes within 2 wk after application.

REFERENCES

Adams, E. M., Irish, D. D., Spencer, H. C. and Rowe, V. K. 1941. The response of rabbit skin to compounds reported to have caused acneform dermatitis. *Ind. Med. Ind. Hyg. Sect.* 2:1–4.

Baxter, R. A. 1984. Biochemical study of pentachlorophenol workers. *Ann. Occup. Hyg.* 28:429–438.

Bekesi, J. G., Holland, J. F., Anderson, H. A., Fischbein, A. S., Wolff, M. S. and Selikoff, I. J. 1978. Lymphocyte function of Michigan dairy farmers exposed to polybrominated biphenyls. *Science* 199:1207–1209.

Benedetto, A. V., Kushner, J. P. and Taylor, J. S. 1978. Porphyria cutanea tarda in three generations of a single family. *N. Eng. J. Med.* 298:358–362.

Bleiberg, J., Wallen, M., Brodkin, R. and Applebaum, I. L. 1964. Industrially acquired porphyria. *Arch. Dermatol.* 89:793–797.

Brinkman, U. A. T. and Reymer, H. G. M. 1976. Polychlorinated naphthalenes. *J. Chromatography,* 127:203–243.

Caputo, R., Monti, M., Ermacora, E., Carminati, G., Gelmetti, C., Gianotti, R., Gianni, E. and Puccinelli, V. 1988. Cutaneous manifestations of tetrachlorodibenzo-p-dioxin in children and adolescents. *J. Am. Acad. Dermatol.* 19:812–819.

Cheng, P. C. and Liu, K. Y. 1981. PCB poisoning. Special issue. *Clin. Med. (Taipei)* 7:41–45 (Chinese).

Crow, K. D. 1970. Chloracne: A critical review including a comparison of two series of cases of acne from chloronaphthalene and pitch fumes. *Trans. St. John's Hosp. Dermatol. Soc.* 56:79–99.

Crow, K. D. 1978. Chloracne: The chemical disease. *New Sci.* April 13:78–80.

Drinker, C. K., Warren, M. F. and Bennett, G. A. 1937. The problem of possible systemic effects from certain chlorinated hydrocarbons. *J. Ind. Hyg. Toxicol.* 19:283–311.

Ecobichon, D. J., Hansell, M. M. and Safe, S. 1977. Halogen substituents at the 4 and 4' positions of biphenyl: influence on hepatic function in the rat. *Toxicol. Appl. Pharmacol.* 42:359–366.

Faith, R. E. and Luster, M. I. 1979. Investigations on the effect of 2,3,7,8-tetrachlorodibenzo-*p*-dioxin (TCDD) on parameters of various immune functions. *Ann. NY Acad. Sci.* 320:564–571.

Filippini, G., Bordo, B., Masetto, N., Musicco, M. and Boeri, R. 1981. Relationship between clinical and electrophysiological findings and indicators of heavy exposure to 2,3,7,8-tetrachlorodibenzo-*p*-dioxin. *Scand. J. Work Environ. Health* 7:257–262.

Fischbein, A., Wolff, M. D., Lilis, R., Thornton, J. and Selikoff, I. J. 1979. Clinical findings among PCB-exposed capacitor manufacturing workers. *Ann. NY Acad. Sci.* 320:703–715.

Flinn, F. B. and Jarvik, D. E. 1936. Action of certain chlorinated naphthalenes on the liver. *Proc. Soc. Exp. Biol. Med.* 35:118–120.

Goldmann, P. J. 1973. Severe acute chloracne, a mass intoxication by 2,3,6,7-tetrachlorodibenzodioxin. *Hautarzt* 24:149–152.

Goto, M. and Higuchi, K. 1969. The symptomatology of Yusho (chlorobiphenyl poisoning) in dermatology. *Fukuoka Acta Med.* 60:409–431.

Greenlee, W. F. and Neal, R. A. 1985. The *Ah* receptor: A biochemical and biologic perspective. In *The Receptors,* vol. II, ed. M. Conn, pp. 89–129. Orlando, Fla.: Academic Press.

Hambrick, G. S. 1957. The effect of substituted naphthalenes on the pilosebaceous apparatus of rabbit and man. *J. Invest. Dermatol.* 28:89–103.

Higuchi, K. 1976. *PCB Poisoning and Pollution.* London: Academic Press.

Homberger, E., Reggiani, G., Sambeth, J. and Wipf, H. K. 1979. The Seveso accident: Its nature, extent and consequences. *Ann. Occup. Hyg.* 22:327–367.

Inagami, K., Koga, T., Kikuchi, M., Hashimoto, M., Takahashi, H. and Wada, K. 1969. Experimental study of hairless mice following administration of rice oil used by "Yusho" patient. *Fukuoka Acta Med.* 60:548–553.

Jennings, A. M., Wild, G., Ward, J. D. and Ward, A. M. 1988. Immunological abnormalities 17 years after accidental exposure to 2,3,7,8-tetrachlorodibenzo-*p*-dioxin. *Br. J. Ind. Med.* 45:701–704.

Jirasek, L., Kalensky, J. and Kubec, K. 1973. Acne chlorina, porphyria cutanea tarda during the manufacture of herbicides. Part I. *Cesk. Dermatol.* 48:306–315.

Jirasek, L., Kalinsky, J., Kubec, K. and Pazderova, J., et al. 1974. Acne chlorina, porphyria cutanea tarda and other manifestations of general intoxication during the manufacture of herbicides. Part II. *Cesk. Dermatol.* 49:145–157.

Jones, T. A. 1941. The etiology of acne with special reference to acne of occupational exposure. *J. Ind. Hyg. Toxicol.* 23:290–312.

Jones, K. G. and Sweeney, G. D. 1977. Association between induction of aryl hydrocarbon hydroxylase and depression of uroporphyrinogen decarboxylase activity. *Res. Commun. Chem. Pathol. Pharmacol.* 17:631–637.

Kay, K. 1977. Polybrominated biphenyls (PBBs) environmental contamination in Michigan, 1973–1976. *Environ. Res.* 13:74–93.

Kende, A. S., Wade, J., Ridge, D. and Poland, A. 1974. Synthesis and fourier transform carbon-13 nuclear magnetic resonance spectroscopy of new toxic polyhalodibenzo-*p*-dioxins. *J. Org. Chem.* 39:931–937.

Kikuchi, M., Hashimoto, M., Hozumi, M., Koga, A., et al. 1969. An autopsy case of stillborn of chlorobiphenyls poisoning. *Fukuoka Acta Med.* 60:489–495.

Knutson, J. C. and Poland, A. 1982. Response of murine epidermis to 2,3,7,8-tetrachlorodibenzo-*p*-dioxin: Interaction of the Ah and hr loci. *Cell* 30:225–234.

Kuratsune, M., Yoshimura, T., Matsuzaka, J. and Yamaguchi, A. 1972. Epidemiologic study of Yusho, a poisoning caused by ingestion of a rice oil contaminated with a commercial brand of polychlorinated biphenyls. *Environ. Health Perspect.* 1:119–128.

Kuratsune, M., Nakamure, Y., Ikeda, M. and Hirohata, T. Analysis of deaths seen among patients with Yusho: A preliminary report. *Chemosphere*, in press.

Landrigan, P. J., Wilcox, K. R., Silva, J., Jr., Humphrey, H. E. B., et al. 1979. Cohort study of Michigan residents exposed to polybrominated biphenyls: Epidemiologic and immunologic findings. *Ann. NY Acad. Sci.* 320:284–294.

Martin, J. V. 1984. Lipid abnormalities in workers exposed to dioxin. *Br. J. Ind. Med.* 40:87–89.

May, G. 1973. Chloracne from the accidental production of tetrachlorodibenzodioxin. *Br. J. Ind. Med.* 30:276–283.

May, G. 1982. Tetrachlorodibenzodioxin: A survey of subjects ten years after exposure. *Br. J. Ind. Med.* 39:128–135.

McConnell, E. E., Moore, J. A. and Dalgard, D. W. 1978. Toxicity of 2,3,7,8-tetrachlorodibenzo-*p*-dioxin in rhesus monkeys (*macaca mulatta*) following a single oral dose. *Toxicol. Appl. Pharmacol.* 43:175–187.

Meigs, J. W., Albom, J. J. and Kartin, B. L. 1954. Chloracne from an unusual exposure to Arochlor. *J. Am. Med. Assoc.* 154:1417–1418.

Mocarelli, P., Marocchi, A., Brambilla, P., Gerthoux, P., Young D. S. and Mantel, N. 1986. Clinical laboratory manifestations of exposure to dioxin in children: A six-year study of the effects of an environmental disaster near Seveso, Italy. *J. Am. Med. Assoc.* 256:2687–2695.

Moore, J. A . 1978. Toxicity of 2,3,7,8-tetrachlorodibenzo-*p*-dioxin. In Chlorinated phenoxy acids and their dioxins, ed. by C. Ramel. *Ecol. Bull (Stockh.)* 27:134–144.

Murai, Y. and Kuroiwa, Y. 1971. Peripheral neuropathy in chlorobiphenyl poisoning. *Neurology* 21:1173–1176.

Nagayama, J., Kuratsune, M. and Masuda, Y. 1976. Determination of chlorinated dibenzofurans in Kanechlors and "Yusho oil". *Bull. Environ. Contam. Toxicol.* 15:9–13.

Oliver, R. M. 1975. Toxic effects of 2,3,7,8-tetrachlorodibenzo-1,4 dioxin in laboratory workers. *Br. J. Ind. Med.* 32:49–53.

Peck, G. L., Olsen, T. G., Yoder, F. W., Strauss, J. S., Downing, D. T., Pandya, M., Butkus, D. and Arnaud-Battandier, J. 1979. Prolonged remission of cystic and conglobate acne with 13-cis retinoic acid. *N. Engl. J. Med.* 300:329–333.

Plewig, G. 1970. Kinetics of the formation of comedos in chloracne (Halowax acne). *Arch. Klin. Exp. Dermatol.* 238:228–241.

Plewig, G. and Braun-Falco, O. 1971. Behandlung von Comedonen bei Morbus Favre-Racouchot und Acne venenata mit Vitamin A-Säure. *Hautarzt* 22:341–345.

Poland, A. and Glover, E. 1973. Chlorinated dibenzo-*p*-dioxins. Potent inducers of δ-aminolevulinic acid synthetase and aryl hydrocarbon hydroxylase II. A study of structure-activity relationships. *Mol. Pharmacol.* 9:736–747.

Poland, A. and Glover, E. 1977. Chlorinated biphenyl induction of aryl hydrocarbon hydroxylase activity: A study of the structure activity relationships. *Mol. Pharmacol.* 13:924–938.

Poland, A. and Kende, A. S. 1976. 2,3,7,8-Tetrachlorodibenzo-*p*-dioxin; environmental contaminant and molecular probe. *Fed. Proc.* 35:2404–2418.

Poland, A. and Knutson, J. C. 1982. 2,3,7,8-Tetrachlorodibenzo-*p*-dioxin and related halogenated aromatic hydrocarbons: Examination of the mechanisms of toxicity. *Annu. Rev. Pharmacol. Toxicol.* 22:517–554.

Poland, A., Glover, E. and Kende, A. S. 1976. Stereospecific high affinity binding of 2,3,7,8-tetrachlorodibenzo-*p*-dioxin by hepatic cytosol. *J. Biol. Chem.* 251:4936–4946.

Puhvel, S. M., Sakamoto, M., Ertl, D. C. and Reisner, R. M. 1982. Hairless mice as models for chloracne: Study of cutaneous changes induced by topical application of established chloracnegens. *Toxicol. Appl. Pharmacol.* 64:492–503.

Rappe, C., Kjeller, L.-O., Marklund, S. and Nygren, M. 1986. Electrical PCB accidents, an update. *Chemosphere* 15:1291–1295.

Scarisbrick, D. A. and Martin, J. V. 1981. Biochemical changes associated with cloracne in workers exposed to tetrachloroazobenzene and tetrachloroazoxybenzene. *J. Soc. Occup. Med.* 31:158–163.

Schechter, A. 1986. the Binghamton state office building PCB, dioxin and dibenzofuran electrical transformer incident: 1981–1986. *Chemosphere* 15:1273–1280.

Shelley, W. B. and Kligman, A. M. 1957. The experimental production of acne by penta and hexachloronaphthalenes. *Arch. Dermatol.* 75:689–695.

Skene, S. A., Dewhurst, I. C. and Greenberg, M. 1989. Polychlorinated dibenzo-*p*-dioxins and polychlorinated dibenzofurans: The risks to human health. A review. *Hum. Toxicol.* 8:173–203.

Strik, J. J. T. W. A. 1979. Porphyrins in urine as an indication of exposure to chlorinated hydrocarbons. *Ann. NY Acad. Sci.* 320:308–310.

Suskind, R. R. 1978. Chloracne and associated health problems in the manufacture of 2,4,5,-T. Report of the Joint Conferences, National Institute of Environmental Health Sciences and International Agency for Research on Cancer, Lyon, France, Jan. 11.

Suskind, R. R. 1985. Chloracne, "the hallmark of dioxin intoxication". *Scand. J. Work Environ. Health* 11:165–171.

Taylor, J. S. 1974. Chloracne—A continuing problem. *Cutis* 13:585–591.

Taylor, J. S., Wuthrich, R. C., Lloyd, K. M. and Poland, A. 1977. Chloracne from manufacture of a new herbicide. *Arch. Dermatol.* 113:616–619.

Telegina, K. A. and Biklulatuva, M. 1970. Affection of the follicular apparatus of the skin in workers occupied in production of butyl ester of 2,4,5-trichlorophenoxy acetic acid. *Vestn. Dermatol. Venerol.* 44:35–39.

Urabe, H. and Asahi, M. 1984. Past and current dermatological status of Yusho patients. *Am. J. Ind. Med.* 5:5–12.

Walker, A. E. and Martin, J. V. 1979. Lipid profiles in dioxin exposed workers. *Lancet* i:446–447.

Wong, G. C. and Hwang, M. Y. 1981. PCB poisoning. Special issue. *Clin. Med* (Taipei) 7:83–88 (Chinese).

Yoshimura, T. and Ikeda, M. 1978. Growth of school children with polychlorinated biphenyl poisoning or Yusho. *Environ. Res.* 17:416–425.

Zack, J. A. and Suskind, R. R. 1980. The mortality experience of workers exposed to tetrachlorodibenzodioxin in a trichlorophenol process accident. *J. Occup. Med.* 22:11–14.

Zelickson, A. S., Strauss, J. S. and Mottaz, I. 1985. Ultrastructural changes in open comedones following treatment of cystic acne with isotretinoin. *Am. J. Dermatopathol.* 7:241–244.

27

dioxin: a case study in chloracne

■ Ellen K. Silbergeld ■

INTRODUCTION

Among the recognized chloracnegenic compounds found in occupational and environmental settings, the chlorinated dibenzodioxins have been the best studied. These chemicals appear to be solely of anthropogenic origin arising from combustion of phenolic or benzoic precursors in the presence of chlorine or as byproducts of synthetic chemical production (U.S. EPA, 1980; Czuzcwa et al., 1984). They are hence of relatively recent toxicological concern. Nevertheless, exposures of humans to the chlorinated dioxins in general and in specific environmental and occupational circumstances have provoked extraordinary controversy. The nature of their health risks to humans is still a matter of scientific investigation and public policy debate. The general issues of dioxin toxicity and human health risk assessment will not be discussed in this chapter, which focuses on one of the less disputed aspects of dioxin toxicity, its property as a chloracnegen.

"Dioxin" is a general term for the halogen-substituted molecule shown in Fig. 1; toxicologically, only the halogenated forms appear to be active, and, like the polychlorinated biphenyls, the greatest biological potency is associated with halogenation at three or more positions that place the molecule in a more or less planar position within the dimensions of 8 by 14 Å (Safe, 1987). The greatest body of clinical and experimental studies has concerned one dioxin isomer, the 2,3,7,8-tetrachlorodibenzo-*para*-dioxin molecule, but studies have also been done on polyhalogenated dibenzofurans, polyhalogenated biphenyls, axoxybenzenes, azobenzenes, and structurally similar molecules. In this paper,

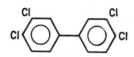

2,3,7,8 TETRACHLORODIBENZO-p-DIOXIN (TCDD)

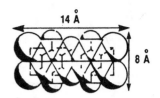

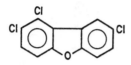

3,4,3',4' TETRACHLOROBIPHENYL

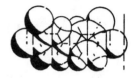

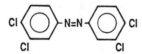

2,3,7,8, TETRACHLORODIBENZOFURAN

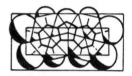

TRICHLORONAPHTHALENE

β - NAPHTHOFLAVONE

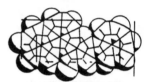

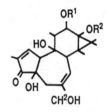

3,4,3',4' TETRACHLOROAZOBENZENE (TCAB)

$R^1 = CO - (CH_2)_{12} - CH_3$
$R^2 = COCH_3$

12,- O - TETRADECANOYLPHORBOL - 13 ACETATE (TPA)

FIGURE 1 Structures and space-filling models of 2,3,7,8-TCDD and compounds. The first three molecules are the most toxic isomers of the polychlorinated dibenzo-*p*-dioxins, polychlorinated biphenyls, and polychlorinated dibenzofurans, respectively. Also shown are three other compounds that have been shown to bind to the *Ah* receptor and/or induce P-450 enzymes. As indicated, a molecular size of 14 by 8 Å appears to confer optimal binding and biological potency; in addition, arrangement of the chlorine atoms at the positions indicated confers a quasi-planar structure that appears to produce increased biological activity as well as resistance to degradation and metabolism. See Silbergeld and Gasiewicz (1989) and Safe (1987) for further discussion of molecular structure-activity relationships.

668

"dioxin" will be used to refer to any dioxin isomer, "PCDD" to any chlorinated dioxin with three or more chlorines, and "TCDD" will be used only to refer to 2,3,7,8-tetrachlorodibenzo-*p*-dioxin. Similarly, "PCDF" will be used to refer to any chlorinated dibenzofuran with three or more chlorines.

Despite the relatively low rates and unintended nature of dioxin production in the world since the late nineteenth century (Hay, 1982), at present it is likely that all organisms carry levels of the persistent dioxins, primarily in lipid compartments, in excess of one part per quadrillion (U.S. EPA, 1985; Patterson et al., 1989). This has an impact upon the design and evaluation of epidemiological studies, since there are no true controls available for comparison to an exposed group. Under these conditions, accurate exposure ascertainment becomes critical, since comparisons can only be relative, not absolute. If outcomes are used as surrogates for exposure there can be complicating effects upon data interpretation.

The sources of dioxins for human exposure include both general and specific inputs, from both proximate and ultimate sources. The largest general proximate source of dioxin exposure for humans is the food supply (Travis et al., 1989). Human breast milk is also a ubiquitous dietary source of dioxins for nursing infants. Contamination of food and breast milk reflects the stability of many dioxins in the biosphere and their propensity to be bioaccumulated in specific food chains leading to top-level consumers such as humans.

The main ultimate sources of dioxins are industrial processes and combustion. The synthesis reactions for certain organic chemicals are known to yield dioxins (U.S. EPA, 1980); use of products contaminated with dioxins and waste disposal from these production processes are the two major past and ongoing sources of dioxin inputs (U.S. EPA, 1987). Some of these products have been controlled or discontinued, and waste management practices in the United States have been greatly improved since 1980, but prior to that time millions of pounds of these products were made and used in inherently dispersive ways (e.g., for pest control and weed eradication) for several decades around the world. Some chlorophenoxyacetic acid herbicides contained between 10 and 100 ppm TCDD (U.S. EPA, 1980). Recently, analyses have shown that dioxins, including TCDD, are produced by many combustion processes, including incineration of household wastes and the use of gasoline with lead scavenger additives (Olie et al., 1977). These combustion sources are likely to be significant contributors to the ubiquitous "background" level of human exposure, but in terms of intensity they are dwarfed in specific situations by sources in the organic chemical industry. This is important since most of the clinical and epidemiological studies of TCDD, including dermatotoxicity, have examined cohorts and individuals exposed to TCDD through the manufacture, use, or waste disposal of chlorinated phenols and chlorinated phenoxyacetic acids. Inferences as to likely effects at lower levels of exposure are necessarily less than certain.

This chapter will review the clinical and experimental studies on dioxin-induced dermatotoxicity with an emphasis on mechanisms, dose response, and the relationships between chloracne and other systemic and cellular responses to dioxin. It is the main thesis of this chapter that the effects of dioxin represent a common set of mechanistic cellular responses that vary in their specific expression according to organ system, due to the higher-order functioning of each specific organ system. In addition, there may be genetic determinants that govern the expression of toxicity in organisms. While the focus of this chapter is on human dermatotoxicity, the role of genetic determinants of response is relevant to evaluating the validity of both animal models and mechanistic hypotheses largely based upon experimental research.

Dermatotoxicity of the Dioxins

Clinical: An epidemic of chloracne.   The phenomenon of chemically acquired dermatotoxicity was described in workers soon after the development of the synthetic organic chemical industry in Germany in the 1890s (Herxheimer, 1899; for reviews of this early literature see Greenburg et al., 1939; Thelwell Jones, 1941; Crow, 1982; Hay, 1982). The *inferential* identification of the generation of potent chloracnegenic factors in specific production processes was made by observant physicians long before the *analytic* identification of 2,3,7,8-TCDD as the agent responsible in 1957 by Kimmig and Schulz and its unambiguous isomer-specific quantification by Bauer et al. in 1961 (Kimmig and Schulz, 1957; Bauer et al., 1961). These two papers are sometimes cited as the first identification of TCDD as the toxic agent, but it would be incorrect to assume that before their publication there were no data supporting the reasonable conclusion that an unidentified byproduct of chlorophenol and chlorobiphenyl production processes was the agent responsible for occupational disease and fatality, including dermatotoxicity (Drinker, 1939; Greenberg et al., 1939).

Thelwell Jones, for one, reported extensively upon dermatologic and other manifestations in workers employed in polychlorinated biphenyl manufacture (Thelwell Jones, 1941). He observed that at two factories in England about 6% of production workers had persistent acne, among other signs. In total, about 14% had manifestations of skin toxicity; moreover, among younger workers (whom Thelwell Jones considered most susceptible), the incidence was between 29 and 32% at both factories. He correctly proposed that these toxic effects were not due to the main product but to a contaminant whose yield of unintended production was related to the heat of the synthesis reaction. [This contaminant was probably a mixture of PCDFs, which are now known to be present in most PCBs (Silbergeld, 1983).] He also concluded on the basis of his clinical observations and toxicological data that the responses to the contaminant were systemic rather than topical, a conclusion reached by other early observers (see also review by Dunagin, 1984). He deduced that the toxic agent was exceedingly potent and resistant to degradation. Even more remarkably, he proposed that its mechanism of action was likely to be similar to that of a steroid hormone. Almost 50 yr later, it is hard to find many major errors in his observations or conclusions.

Recognition of dioxin dermatotoxicity was also advanced by investigations of the sequelae in workers exposed to an industrial accident at the Monsanto trichlorophenol works in Nitro, W. Va. In 1949, a runaway process reaction resulted in an explosion with a relatively large release of TCDD likely (Hay, 1982; Suskind and Hertzberg, 1984). Over 100 workers were heavily exposed, particularly during the immediate response and cleanup. They were evaluated periodically by Suskind and Ashe in consultation with Monsanto. Of 36 workers evaluated in 1953, 35 had signs of cutaneous lesions; most had other signs as well (Table 1). Other reports were made by the West Virginia Department of Public Health. Although these reports have not been completely published, they have been widely circulated by the Environmental Protection Agency (EPA) (U.S. EPA, 1985), and some studies based upon them have been published (see below). Dermatotoxic signs were very widespread in the Monsanto workforce after 1949; in 1953, the medical officer for Monsanto headquarters in St. Louis wrote to the plant manager in Nitro, "Is there anyone [at Nitro] who does *not* have chloracne?" Dermatotoxicity was also described in a child exposed indirectly to residues from the explosion when his father removed a truck from the premises; this was quite reminiscent of Thelwell Jones's account of a case of chloracne in a child exposed to contamination on his father's work clothes (Thelwell Jones, 1941).

Two long-term follow-up studies on dermatotoxicity and other health effects in members of the Monsanto cohort have been published (Suskind and Herzberg, 1984; Moses et al., 1984). In these reports, persistent chloracne was found in some workers as long as 30 yr after the explosion. The presence of other health effects in this cohort remains controversial.

Other major episodes of relatively intense human exposure to TCDD and other dioxins occurred at industrial facilities in the United States, Germany, England, Czechoslovakia, the Netherlands, and Italy (for historical narratives on these episodes see Hay, 1982; U.S. EPA, 1985). In every instance, dermatologic manifestations were reported as prevalent. Unfortunately, published reports on all these cohorts are not available so that it is not clear how dermatotoxicity is correlated with exposure, work history, or other symptoms of toxicity. The Diamond Shamrock workforce was studied by Bleiberg in the 1960s and many manifestations of systemic toxicity, including chloracne, were reported (Bleiberg et al., 1964).

Two environmental exposures associated with relatively large releases of TCDD occurred during the 1970s, one at Seveso, Italy, and the other at several sites of waste disposal in Missouri (Caramaschi et al., 1981; Webb et al., 1986). In these two situations, exposures were probably less intense than those in the industrial situations discussed above. They have been less clearly defined, although recent analyses of human samples may reduce some of the uncertainties (Patterson et al., 1989). In this study, persons with no production experience had in all cases lower adipose tissue levels of TCDD than those found in production workers. In Missouri, relatively few cases of frank chlor-

TABLE 1   Exposures and Symptoms in 36 Workers Exposed to TCDD at Nitro

Type of Exposure	Number of workers
Accident in building 41	10
Regular operations, building 34	12
Regular operations, building 51	4
Hauling 2,4,5-T	2
Maintenance of equipment, buildings 51 and 34	3
Combined exposures	
Buildings 34 and 51	2
Buildings 40 (adjacent to 41), 46	
(for drying 2,4,5-T), and 34	1
Buildings 79, 16, 34—grinding and drying	1
Buildings 46 and 79, drying 2,4,5-T	1
Total subjects	36
Clinical Symptoms	
Cutaneous lesions	35*
Fatigue	21
Aches and pains	27
Dyspnea	9
Nervousness and irritability	17
Loss or decrease of libido	13
Vertigo	4

Note. From Ashe and Suskind (1953), quoted by U.S. EPA (1985).
[a]One subject complained of pains, fatigue, and irritability, but never developed acne.

acne were diagnosed (Ayres et al., 1988). In Seveso, in contrast, a large number of persons, particularly children, exhibited chloracne, among other acute toxic reactions to exposure via direct dermal contact, inhalation and ingestion (Tindall, 1985). A decade later, almost all cases of chloracne had subsided (Assennato et al., 1989). Exposure assessment of the Seveso cohort is currently underway (Stehr-Green, personal communication).

Another large cohort with potential TCDD exposure is the Vietnam veteran group (including the Ranch Handers, Air Force personnel directly involved in the offensive use of herbicides and ground troops in the areas of herbicide use). In this group a very low frequency of chloracne has been reported (Tindall, 1985).

There are also two cohorts in Taiwan and Japan, exposed to PCDFs and PCBs by ingesting contaminated cooking oil (Kuratsune et al., 1972; Hsu et al., 1984). Chloracne has not been reported in these people, but a range of other dermatotoxic manifestations was found, including hyperpigmentation, conjunctivitis, scaly skin (in infants), and follicular hyperkeratosis (Rogan, 1982; Tindall, 1985).

Thus the clinical studies confirm that human exposure to TCDD can cause chloracne and other types of dermatotoxicity. The importance of route of exposure and of dose-response for these signs of dermatotoxicity is still unclear. Tindall (1985) suggests that dermal contact appears to increase the risks and severity of chloracne, citing occupational studies, but it is very likely that there was concomitant inhalation exposure in all these incidents. In the Yusho and Yucheng incidents in Japan and Taiwan, where exposure was predominantly by ingestion, there was a relatively low incidence of chloracne; however, other severe dermatologic changes have been described in these populations.

Even less is known about dose. Chloracne has come to be considered almost pathognomic for dioxin exposure, with the converse assumption that the absence of chloracne is evidence of lack of exposure (or exposure above background) (Dunagin, 1984; Webb et al., 1986). To accept this requires an understanding of the dose-response relationship for chloracne, and a quantitative understanding of the dose-response relationships for other toxic effects of dioxin, including its long-term manifestations of toxicity. This issue can only be fully resolved with complete understanding of dioxin toxicology. In the absence of that, at present, an examination of some clinical studies supports the conservative conclusion that while chloracne *when it occurs* is a reliable clinical marker for dioxin exposure, its absence is *not* proof that no toxicologically significant exposure has taken place. Moreover, it appears clear that the dermatotoxic effects of dioxins are not limited to chloracne, but include other systemic effects manifested in dermal tissue. The potency of chloracnegenic chemicals is similar to their potency as systemic toxins (Knutson and Poland, 1982, 1984; Crow, 1982). Chloracne may be "the most sensitive clinical indicator of exposure," as concluded by Dunagin (1984); however, this may reveal more about the sensitivity of clinical examinations (in the absence of biochemistry) than about TCDD toxicity. This lack of complementarity is shown in the data from one of the followup studies of the Monsanto workforce at Nitro.

A substantial number of workers whose employment histories substantiated exposure to TCDD did not have any record of chloracne (Moses et al., 1984).

The dose response for chloracne is uncertain. Information on exposures in almost all situations involving TCDD is rather imprecise, and the factor of exposure duration may be as important as total dose. The condition with the closest approximation of intake dose, the Yusho and Yucheng exposures, was not associated with chloracne, as noted above, although other skin changes have been described. As noted by Webb et al. (1986) in considering the Missouri situation, it is likely that exposures to TCDD in solids and soils at levels above 1 ppm can produce chloracne. However, as the authors note, this estimate (which is not a dose estimate but an exposure measurement) is highly inferential since "it is almost impossible to determine whether chloracne is a universal sign or if a reproducible threshold exists." Moreover, the presence of TCDD in soils does not define actual dose, given the great variability in human interactions with surface dusts and soils (LaGoy, 1987). It is possible that the ongoing NIOSH study of TCDD-exposed workers, which combines some measurements of body burdens of TCDD with assessment of health status, may refine our understanding of dose response.

Experimental studies. Soon after the clinical observations of dermato-toxicity in the chlorophenol industry, attempts were made to develop animal models of chloracne. As will be discussed below, these studies have been most useful in increasing our understanding of the mechanisms of TCDD dermato-toxicity and its relationship to other manifestations of cellular response to this agent. The early experimental studies were primarily undertaken as bioassays to monitor on a relative basis the presence of potential chloracnegens in industrial materials. For this purpose, the rabbit was widely used by industry toxicologists and others (Adams et al., 1941; Jones and Krizele, 1962). Some human experi-mentation was also done, by self-administration and by tests on prisoners and volunteers (Hambrick, 1957). Aside from their qualitative value, these early studies were not useful for refining information on dose response or improving mechanistic hypotheses. Prior to the identification of the toxic constituent of the process-related condition, it is not surprising that relatively little knowledge of this type was gained. These early studies were also limited by the failure to produce recognizable "chloracne" in rats or mice, so that no investigation of dermatotoxicity was undertaken in these accessible species, and the connection between dermatotoxicity and other toxic effects of TCDD was not drawn until substantially later (see below).

The *in vivo* experimental studies also failed to provide much information on overall dose response. In rabbits, these applications to the inner ear surface produced chloracne when the amount of TCDD applied exceeded 0.1 μg (Webb et al., 1986). It should be noted that the early experimental literature also indicated that chloracnegenic mixtures also produced severe, persistent sys-temic toxicity, including death (for a discussion of this forgotten literature, see Greenburg et al., 1939). Most of the early studies utilized direct skin applica-tion of incompletely characterized mixtures containing undetermined amounts of TCDD. Little attempt was made to determine uptake or target organ dose. Recently, Brewster et al., (1989) have shown that roughly 6% of the dose applied to skin is found in subsurface (washed) skin 72 h after application.

Recent research by Puhvel, among others, has focused on specific cellular events involved in dermatotoxicity. This will be discussed below in terms of understanding mechanisms of action of TCDD as a dermatotoxin.

Mechanisms of Dioxin Dermatotoxicity

Dioxins and other chloracnegens are distinguished by a broad range of organ-specific toxic manifestations, often occurring at relatively low dose and persisting well beyond the time of active exposure. The dermatotoxicity of these agents is unlikely to be a unique phenomenon, distinct from other toxic events in terms of dose or mechanism. As discussed by Silbergeld and Ga-siewicz (1989), the spectrum of dioxin toxicity possesses certain common elements, regardless of the species, developmental stage, or organ system involved.

1. Cell death is not a prominent feature of cellular response to TCDD *in vivo* or *in vitro*; overt morphological changes do not generally occur early after TCDD exposure.
2. Nearly all of the cells affected by TCDD are epithelial. This is another reason why the response of skin is unlikely to be unique. In epithelial cells, the primary response to TCDD at the cellular level appears to be hyperplasia and/or altered differentiation. Fundamentally similar phenomena can be discerned in TCDD-induced dermatotoxicity, teratogenicity, immunotoxicity, and possibly carcinogenicity.
3. Many of the toxic effects of TCDD appear to be sensitive to genotype as well as species, although within a species genotype confers only relative and not absolute resistance to toxicity.
4. Although TCDD does not appear to be mutagenic or to bind directly to DNA, many of its cellular actions involve alterations in gene expression consequent to its translocation to the cell nucleus through a receptor-mediated process. The number of genes that may respond to TCDD is unknown (Whitlock, 1987), but recent studies suggest that more than one gene is likely to be involved and that these genes may function independently in response to a dioxin-responsive promotor element (Sutter et al., 1990).
5. The toxic effects of PCDDs are highly dependent upon structure, although this structure-activity relationship is relative rather than absolute in that sufficiently prolonged exposure even to the fully substituted molecule octachlorodibenzodioxin can induce toxic effects. Based upon these observations, it has been proposed that the toxicity of dioxin and related compounds involves highly specific interactions between the toxic molecule and an endogenous intracellular protein that serves to translocate dioxin to specific dioxin-responsive elements within the genome (Silbergeld and Gasiewicz, 1989; Whitlock, 1987; Safe, 1986). This endogenous protein has been called the dioxin or *Ah* receptor. Whether or not all toxic manifestations of dioxin involve this specific receptor-mediated process is not known with certainty; some of the metabolic and immunologic effects of TCDD have not been as clearly linked to the so called dioxin receptor (Dencker, 1984).

Mechanistic research on dioxin dermatotoxicity was greatly advanced in the early 1980s by the demonstration that mice could be used for investigation, thus linking the large body of research on the molecular and genetic aspects of TCDD toxicology with the skin as a target organ. Although mice do not develop a condition that exactly mimics human chloracne, the response of murine skin in terms of altered differentiation and proliferation has been accepted as an appropriate analogous experimental model for TCDD dermatotoxicity (Knutson and Poland, 1980, 1982; Puhvel et al., 1982). Multiple doses as low as 0.6 μg of TCDD (repeated doses of 0.01 μg/dose) and single doses as low as 1.0 μg applied cutaneously to hairless mice produce hyperplasia, altered protein synthesis, and hyperkeratinization, signs that are similar to the cellular changes observed in human chloracne (Puhvel and Sakamoto, 1988; Molloy et al., 1987). Gierthy and Crane (1985) have adapted this model for *in vitro* bioassay studies of complex mixtures and poorly characterized environmental samples. Using a transformed cell line derived from a mouse teratoma (XB cells), they have been able to induce a characteristic response in the morphology of cell culture indicative of toxicity. As shown in Table 2, at concentrations of TCDD as low as 10^{-11} M, this response can be observed. Moreover, structurally similar compounds (see Fig. 1) also induce this response. In a slightly different system using human keratinocytes from squamous-cell carcinoma, Rice and Cline (1984) reported that TCDD inhibited cell growth at about the same concentration and Knutson and Poland (1984) reported that TCDD at 5×10^{-11} M induced keratinization in XB cells. These studies establish that dermatologic changes appear to be very sensitive responses to low cellular doses of TCDD. Using this model, Poland has shown that cellular response to TCDD involves the presence of the dioxin receptor and coordinate expression of at least one other gene, expressed in the hairless HRS/J hr/hr mouse (Poland and Knutson, 1982; Knutson and Poland, 1982; Poland et al., 1984). The gene-level and posttranslational events involved in this response are not fully understood. They appear to be separate from, although strongly parallel to, the action of TCDD to induce certain P-450 enzymes, as shown in Table 3 (Poland et al., 1984). Puhvel has observed that TCDD-induced morphologic changes in skin cells in culture are accompanied by increased protein synthesis and induction of epidermal transglutaminase activity, an enzymatic signal of terminal differentiation (Knutson and Poland, 1984; Puhvel et al., 1984). How these and other posttranslational events are triggered by TCDD remains to be determined. Four current hypotheses are discussed below; as will be noted, they are highly provisional in nature and based in large part upon comparisons drawn with endogenous regulators of epithelial cell growth and differentiation.

1. TCDD dermatotoxicity involves steroid hormone mechanisms. The similarity of chloracne to steroid-dependent acne was first suggested by Thelwell Jones in 1941. More recently, at the molecular level, Evans (1987) has reviewed the similarity between many of the cellular events involved in TCDD response and those associated with glucocorticoids (see also Okret et al., 1985). The dioxin receptor may be appropriately considered as a member of the superfamily of steroid hormone receptors and genes. At the molecular level, TCDD interacts with glucocorticoid receptors and glucocorticoid-mediated events in liver and muscle (Max and Silbergeld, 1987; Sunahara et al., 1990).

TABLE 2 Association of Dermatotoxicity and Enzyme Induction in Mouse Strains Carrying the Hairless Mutation: Phenotypes of the *Ah* and *Es* 10 Loci

Mouse strain	*Hr* locus	Esterase 10 locus	*Ah* locus	Hepatic AHH activity (pmol/mg/min)		Histologic changes in skin		Keratinized Cyst formation
				Control	Induced (BNF)[a]	Keratinization	Hyperplasia	
HRS/J	hr/hr	b/b	Ah^b	2.4	44	+++	++	+++
	hr/+	b/a		2.7	42	0	0	0
C57BL/6J	hr/hr	a/a	Ah^b	8.1	118	±	+	+
	hr/+	a/a				0	0	0
C3H/HeN	hr/hr	b/b	Ah^b	1.9	20	++	+	++
	hr/+	b/b		4.2	33	0	0	0
DBA/2J	hr/hr	b/b	Ah^b	4.7	5.9	±	+	++
	hr/+	b/b				0	0	0
HRA/Skh	hr/hr	b/b	Ah^b	5.2	27	+	++	++
Skh/hr-1	hr/hr	b/b	Ah^b	3.4	18	+	+	++
HR/DeHfcr	hr/hr	a/a	Ah^b	7.4	42	++	++	+++
	hr/+	a/b						
WLHR/Le	hr/hr	c/c	Ah^b	11.5	41	+	+++	+++
	hr/+	c/c						

Note. Data from Poland et al. (1984).
[a]Beta-naphthoflavone.

TABLE 3   Concentrations Required for *In Vitro* Effect on XB Cells

Compound	Minimum concentration (ppb)
2,3,7,8-Tetrachlorodibenzo-*p*-dioxin	0.0032
1,2,4,7,8-Pentachlorodibenzo-*p*-dioxin	0.359
2,3,7,8-Tetrachlorodibenzofuran	0.032
2,3,4,6,7,8-Hexachlorodibenzofuran	0.378
Octachlorodibenzofuran	4.48
3,4,3',4'-Tetrachlorobiphenyl	100
2,4,5,2',4',5'-Hexachlorobiphenyl	1000
Aroclor 1254	10,000
Dibenzo[a,h]anthracene	10
Benz[a]anthracene	100
3-Methylcholanthrene	>100
Benzo[a]pyrene	>100
β-Napthoflavone	1000

Note. Data from Gierthy and Crane (1985).

While these interactions have not been directly studied in skin, there is indirect evidence for an hypothesis of steroid mechanisms in TCDD dermatotoxicity. In human keratinocytes, TCDD effects *in vitro* were modulated by the presence or absence of steroids. Addition of corticosteroids (hydrocortisone or dexamethasone) antagonized TCDD-induced inhibition of cell growth, while TCDD itself antagonized hydrocortisone-induced markers of differentiation in these cells (Rice and Cline, 1984).

2. TCDD dermatotoxicity involves vitamin A mechanisms. The importance of retinoic acid in cell differentiation is well known (Kublis, 1983). Retinoic acid has been used to treat chloracne (Tindall, 1985; Taylor, 1979). TCDD and vitamin A show strong similarities in their effects on skin (Puhvel et al., 1984) and other target organs (Thunberg, 1984; Hakansson and Ahlborg, 1985). Retinoic acid is more generally a powerful regulator of cell differentiation and organ development. *In vivo*, TCDD affects organ storage of vitamin A, as shown in Table 4. However, *in vitro*, neither the presence or absence of vitamin A or retinyl acetate affected TCDD-induced growth inhibition of keratinocytes (Rice and Cline, 1984).

3. TCDD dermatotoxicity involves epidermal growth factor mechanisms. Epidermal growth factor (EGF) is a regulator of cell status in many organ systems, including skin. EGF, like TCDD, is very potent in inducing keratinization in cells in culture (Knutson and Poland, 1984). *In vivo* treatment of rodents with TCDD reduces the amount of EGF binding to liver plasma membranes (Madhukar et al., 1984). *In vitro*, TCDD also downregulates EGF receptors in epidermal cells with an EC50 of 1–2 n*M* (Hudson et al., 1986). The decrease in ligand binding

TABLE 4 Effect of TCDD (10 mg/kg) on Vitamin A Storage in Rat Tissue

Tissue	1 h	24 h	72 h	192 h
Liver, mg				
Control	1.54 ± 0.31[a]	1.57 ± 0.12	1.65 ± 0.16	1.91 ± 0.22
TCCD	0.78 ± 0.10	0.96 ± 0.11	1.00 ± 0.10	0.89 ± 0.26
Kidney, μg				
Control	11.70 ± 5.27	11.82 ± 6.09	10.14 ± 5.44	4.03 ± 2.07
TCDD	28.35 ± 15.02*	82.72 ± 9.68*	49.53 ± 21.46*	108.67 ± 43.33*
Intestine, μg				
Control	7.20 ± 2.04	5.13 ± 1.52	5.57 ± 2.05	5.25 ± 1.22
TCDD	2.73 ± 1.15*	3.43 ± 1.15	2.08 ± 0.38*	4.27 ± 2.09
Testes, μg				
Control	1.03 ± 0.57	0.81 ± 0.19	1.04 ± 0.19	0.45 ± 0.09
TCDD	0.76 ± 0.29	0.65 ± 0.28	0.47 ± 0.08*	0.41 ± 0.20
Epididymis, μg				
Control	—	1.04 ± 0.12	1.08 ± 0.30	1.15 ± 0.16
TCDD	0.63 ± 0.04	0.58 ± 0.13*	0.71 ± 0.14*	0.82 ± 0.15*
Thymus, μg				
Control	0.54 ± 0.16	0.38 ± 0.14	0.25 ± 0.07	0.22 ± 0.13
TCDD	0.92 ± 0.44	0.29 ± 0.05	0.15 ± 0.09*	0.16 ± 0.11
Spleen, μg				
Control	0.16 ± 0.07	0.09 ± 0.07	0.08 ± 0.04	0.09 ± 0.03
TCDD	0.09 ± 0.02*	0.17 ± 0.06*	0.09 ± 0.03	0.08 ± 0.03
Serum, μg/ml				
Control	0.20 ± 0.04	0.42 ± 0.18	0.44 ± 0.12	0.31 ± 0.08
TCDD	0.37 ± 0.04*	0.35 ± 0.13	0.32 ± 0.06	0.45 ± 0.09*

Note. Data from Hakansson and Alburg (1985).

[a]Values are means ± SD for 5 control and 5 TCDD-pretreated rats. Asterisk indicates significant differences from the controls, $p < .05$.

679

was accompanied by an inhibition of EGF-stimulated DNA synthesis. It may be noted that the EGF hypothesis may be part of the vitamin A hypothesis. Abbott et al. (1988) have shown that retinoic acid changes the expression of EGF during development, as does TCDD (Abbott and Birnbaum, 1989).

4. TCDD dermatotoxicity involves porphyrin-related mechanisms. TCDD and several related chlorinated hydrocarbons can produce a clinical condition of acquired porphyria, or chemically induced chronic hepatic porphyria, using the nomenclature suggested by Doss (1987). Biochemically, this condition is distinguished by an accumulation of uroporphyrin and 7-carboxyporphyrin compounds (Bonkovsky et al., 1987). The chemically induced porphyrias are caused by the great induction of hepatic P-450 enzymes by TCDD and other chemicals, with a resulting derangement in porphyrin biosynthesis as shown in Fig. 2. Uroporphyrin decarboxylase is inhibited, although not in all cases, so that the role of enzyme inhibition is not clear in clinical conditions (Bonkovsky et al., 1987; Cantoni et al., 1987; Elder et al., 1987). TCDD is also reported to cause the overt expression of hereditary porphyria in persons carrying a latent gene defect (Doss, 1987). Porphyrins are well-known photosynthesizers, and cutaneous symptoms are characteristic of several porphyrinopathic conditions (Bickers, 1987). While chloracne is not one of the manifestations of porphyria, other expressions of dermatotoxicity in dioxin-exposed persons may involve porphyrinopathic mechanisms. Among these are increased skin fragility, elactinosis, hyperpigmentation, and hypertrichosis (Tindall, 1985).

TCDD is known to induce P-450 enzymes in epithelial cells, including skin (Hudson et al., 1983; Harper et al., 1988; Uziel et al., 1985). The role of these porphyrinopathic effects in dermatotoxicity has not been explicitly addressed. It is highly likely that some of the dermatotoxic manifestations of dioxin exposure are manifestations of porphyrinopathy at the cellular level, which may interact with other toxic effects specific to dioxin and other chloracnegens.

CONCLUSIONS

TCDD is one of the best studied chloracnegens in exposed human populations and in defined experimental systems. Nevertheless, considerable uncertainties remain in both clinical and mechanistic understanding. The dose response for inducing chloracne and other dermatotoxic effects in humans is not known, and as a consequence, the status of chloracne as a "sentinel" or sensitive clinical marker for exposure cannot be evaluated. It is probably inappropriate to use chloracne as the sine qua non for dioxin exposure, in terms of

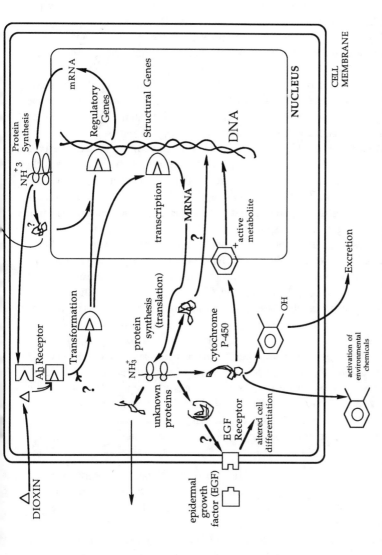

FIGURE 2 Schematic representation of the molecular mechanisms in cellular response to TCDD and similar molecules. Based upon current understanding, TCDD enters cells primarily through its lipophilic properties; once inside the cell it associates with high affinity with an endogenous protein, termed the *Ah* receptor. The TCDD:receptor complex is then translocated to the nucleus, where it binds to specific genes (dioxin-responsive elements) that appear to regulate transcription of several downstream genes, including the gene for certain P-450 enzymes. The binding of TCDD to its receptor is linearly related to the amount of mRNA for these enzymes. Similar gene-regulated events probably result in other cellular changes, such as alterations in receptor number and affinity for EGF, estrogen, and glucocorticoids. The role of these events in dermatotoxicity is not clear; however, there is good evidence (discussed in the text) for genetic control of skin response [see Silbergeld and Gasiewicz (1989) and Whitlock (1988) for further discussion of general mechanisms of TCDD toxicity].

ruling out exposure in its absence, although its presence may indeed be a relatively specific indicator of such exposure. Because it is a more immediate and visible response than carcinogenicity or hepatotoxicity, chloracne has been considered the distinguishing feature of human response to dioxin and related compounds. Chloracne may depend upon route of exposure and duration, as well as amount. In heavily exposed occupational cohorts, chloracne is frequently but not invariably found. The possibility of genetic differences in human susceptibility has not been explored, although these are clearly important in determining murine response.

The mechanisms of TCDD-induced chloracne (and other dermatotoxic responses) are not known. Most evidence suggests that it is associated with the dioxin receptor, although this is not conclusive (see Dencker, 1984). In defined mouse strains, the coordinate expression of a battery of genes is likely to be involved (Molloy et al., 1987; Whitlock, 1987). In cell culture systems derived from murine or human cells, dermatologic responses are produced by relatively low exposures, in the order of pico- and femtomolar concentrations. These are the same concentrations (K_d) for the binding of TCDD to its intracellular receptor, which reinforces the hypothesis that dermatotoxicity is not a more sensitive sign than other target organ responses.

In cell systems, using both transformed and nontumorigenic cell lines, some of the cellular events related to TCDD dermatotoxicity have been further explicated. Hyperplasia and altered differentiation appear to be fundamental responses of exposed cells (Osborne and Greenlee, 1985). Alterations in the expression of specific keratins are observed in mouse epidermis. The mechanisms for these responses are not fully understood; observations of similarities to steroid-, vitamin A-, and EGF-induced effects have been cited in support of hypotheses associating glucocorticoids, retinoic acid, and EGF with TCDD toxicity in skin and other organ systems. Some of the dermatotoxic manifestations associated with exposure to dioxins and related compounds may involve their capacity to cause an acquired form of chronic porphyria, but porphyrinopathic conditions do not involve the characteristic signs of chloracne.

It is possible to propose several conclusions, nevertheless, at this stage:

1. TCDD-induced dermatotoxicity, broadly defined, is likely to be an early response to relatively low levels of TCDD. The specific clinical manifestation of chloracne may be a less sensitive indicator of exposure and early response.
2. TCDD-induced dermatotoxicity is likely to represent an organ-specific expression of toxic responses that involve many of the same mechanisms involved in other organ system responses to TCDD, including a cytosolic steroid hormone-like receptor and receptor-regulated alterations in gene expression.
3. Like these other organ system responses, particularly those involving

epithelial cells, TCDD-induced dermatotoxicity may demonstrate genetic and age-dependent modulation of response.

4. The reversibility of TCDD-induced dermatotoxicity is not known, nor is it easy to separate irreversibility in biological terms from the persistence of TCDD in skin and other organs long after external exposure has been reduced.

5. Further research on TCDD-induced dermatotoxicity may be useful in understanding mechanisms of TCDD toxicity, including carcinogenicity and developmental toxicity. Because of the commonality of responses to TCDD involving the growth and differentiation of epithelial cells, it is likely that common mechanisms may be involved. On an epidemiological basis, however, research is needed on the association of dermatotoxicity with other longer-term responses such as cancer.

6. The reactions of skin, in defined systems, like those of other organs, confirm the great potency of TCDD as an environmental and occupational hazard. Human exposure to TCDD and similar molecules should be minimized to the maximum extent possible.

REFERENCES

Abbott, B. D. and Birnbaum, L. S. 1989. Cellular alterations and enhanced induction of cleft palate after coadministration of retinoic acid and TCDD. *Toxicol. Appl. Pharmacol.* 99:287-301.

Abbott, B. D., Adamson, E. D., and Pratt, R. M. 1988. Retinoic acid alters EGF receptor expression during palatogenesis. *Development* 102:853-967.

Adams, E. M., Irish, D. D. and Spencer, H. C. 1941. The respone of rabbit skin to compounds reported to have caused acneform dermatitis. *Ind. Med. Surg.* 2:1-4.

Assennato, G., Cervino, D., Emmett, E. A., Longo, G. and Merlo, F. 1989. Follow-up of subjects who developed chloracne following TCDD exposure at Seveso. *Am. J. Ind. Med.* 16:119-125.

Bauer, H., Schulz, K. H. and Spiegelsberg, U. 1961. Occupational intoxication in manufacturing chlorophenol compounds. *Arch. Gewerbepath.* 18:538-555.

Bickers, D. R. 1987. The dermatologic manifestations of human porphyria. *Ann. NY Acad. Sci.* 514:261-267.

Bleiberg, J., Wallen, M., Brodkin, R. and Applebaum, I. 1964. Industrially acquired porphyria. *Arch. Dermatol.* 89:793-797.

Bonkovsky, H. L., Sinclair, P. R., Bement, W. J., Lambrecht, R. W. and Sinclair, J. F. 1987. Role of cytochrome P-450 in porphyria caused by halogenated aromatic compounds. In Silbergeld and Fowler, pp. 96-112.

Brewster, D. W., Banks, Y. B., Clark, A. M. and Birnbaum, L. S. 1989. Comparative dermal absorption of 2,3,7,8-tetrachlorodibenzo-*p*-dioxin and three polychlorinated dibenzofurans. *Toxicol. Appl. Pharmacol.* 97:156-166.

Cantoni, L., Rizzardini, M., Graziani, A., Carugo, C. and Garattini, S. 1987. Effects of chlorinated organics on intermediates in the heme pathway and on uroporphyrinogen decarboxylase. *Ann. NY Acad. Sci.* 514:128-140.

Caramaschi, R., DelCorno, G., Favaretti, C., Giambelluca, E., S. E., Montesarchio, E. and Fara, G. M. 1981. Chloracne following environmental contamination by TCDD in Seveso, Italy. *Int. J. Epidemiol.* 10:135-143.

Crow, K. D. 1982. Chloracne. *Semin. Dermatol.* 1:305–314.

Czuczwa, J. M., McVetty, B. D., and Hites, R. A. 1984. Polychlorinated dibenzo-*p*-dioxins and dibenzofurans in sediments from Siskiwit Lake, Isle Royale. *Science* 226:568–572.

Dencker, L. 1985. The role of receptors in 2,3,7,8-tetrachlorodibenzo-*p*-dioxin (TCDD) toxicity. *Arch. Toxicol. Suppl.* 8:43–60.

Doss, M. 1987. Porphyrinurias and occupational disease. *Ann. NY Acad. Sci.* 514:204–218.

Drinker, C. K. 1939. Further observations on the possible systemic toxicity of certain of the chlorinated hydrocarbons with suggestions for permissible concentrations in the air of workrooms. *J. Ind. Hyg. Toxicol.* 21:155.

Dunagin, W. G. 1984. Cutaneous signs of systemic toxicity due to dioxins and related chemicals. *J. Am. Acad. Dermatol.* 10:688–700.

Elder, G. H., Roberts, A. G. and Urquhart, A. J. 1987. Alterations of uroporphyrinogen decarboxylase by chlorinated organics. *Ann. NY Acad. Sci.* 514:141–147.

Evans, R. M. 1988. The steroid and thyroid hormone receptor superfamily. *Science* 240:889–895.

Gierthy, J. F. and Crane, D. 1985. *In vitro* bioassay for dioxinlike activity based on alterations in epithelial cell proliferation and morphology. *Fundam. Appl. Toxicol.* 5:754–759.

Greenburg, L., Mayers, M. R. and Smith, A. R. 1939. Systemic effects resulting from exposure to certain chlorinated hydrocarbons. *J. Ind. Hyg. Toxicol.* 21:29–38.

Hakansson, H. and Ahlborg, U. G. 1985. The effect of TCDD on the uptake, distribution and excretion of a single oral dose of [11,12-^{3}H]retinyl acetate and on the vitamin A status in the rat. *J. Nutr.* 115:759–771.

Hambrick, G. S. 1957. The effect of substituted naphthalenes on the pilosebaceous apparatus of rabbit and man. *Acta Dermatol. Venereol.* 55:211–214.

Harper, P. A., Golas, C. L. and Okey, A. B. 1988. Characterization of the *Ah* receptor and aryl hydrocarbon hydroxylase induction by 2,3,7,8-tetrachlorodibenzo-*p*-dioxin and benz(*a*)anthracene in the human A431 squamous cell carcinoma line. *Cancer Res.* 48:2388–2395.

Hay, A. 1982. *The Chemical Scythe.* New York: Plenum Press.

Herxheimer, K. 1899. Ueber Chlorakne. *Munch. Med. Wochenschr.* 46:278.

Hsu, S. T., Ma, C. L., Hsu, Sk. H., Wu, S. S., Hsu, N. M. and Yeh, C. C. 1984. Discovery and epidemiology of PCB poisoning in Taiwan. *Am. J. Ind. Med.* 5:71–80.

Hudson, L. G., Shaikh, R., Toxcano, W. A., and Greenlee, W. R. 1983. Induction of 7-ethoxycoumarin o-deethylase activity in cultured human epithelial cells by 2,3,7,8-tetrachlorodibenzo-*p*-dioxin (TCDD): Evidence for TCDD receptor. *Biochem. Biophys. Res. Commun.* 115:611–617.

Hudson, L. G., Toscano, W. A., and Greenlee, W. F. 1986. 2,3,7,8-tetrachlorodibenzo-*p*-dioxin (TCDD) modulates epidermal growth factor (EGF) binding to basal cells from a human keratinocyte cell line. *Toxicol. Appl. Pharmacol.* 82:481–492.

Jones, E. L. and Krizek, H. 1962. A technique for testing acnegenic potency in rabbits, applied to the potent acnegen, 2,3,7,8-tetrachlorodibenzo-*p*-dioxin. *J. Invest. Dermatol.* 39:511–517.

Kimmig, J. and Schulz, K. H. 1957. Berufliche Akne (sog. Chlorakne) durch chlorierte aromatische zyklische Aether. *Dermatologica* 115:540–546.

Knutson, J. C. and Poland, A. 1980. Keratinization of mouse teratoma cell line XB produced by 2,3,7,8-tetrachlorodibenzo-*p*-dioxin: An in vitro model of toxicity. *Cell* 22:36.

Knutson, J. C. and Poland, A. 1982. Response of murine epidermis to 2,3,7,8-tetrachloridibenzo-*p*-dioxin: Interaction of the *Ah* and *hr* loci. *Cell* 30:225–234.

Knutson, J. C. and Poland, A. 1984. 2,3,7,8-Tetrachlorodibenzo-*p*-dioxin: Examination of biochemical effects involved in the proliferation and differentiation of XB cells. *J. Cell. Physiol.* 121:143–151.

Kublis, J. 1983. Modulation of differentiation by retinoids. *J. Invest. Dermatol.* 81:55–58.

Kuratsune, M., Yoshimura, J., Mutsuzaka, J., et al. 1972. Epidemiologic study on Yusho. *Environ. Health Perspect.* 1:119–128.

LaGoy, P. K. 1987. Estimated soil ingestion rates for use in risk assessment. *Risk Anal.* 7:355–359.

Madhukar, B. V., Brewster, D. W. and Matsumura, F. 1984. Effects of *in vivo*-administered 2,3,7,8-tetrachlorodibenzo-*p*-dioxin on receptor binding of epidermal growth factor in the hepatic plasma membrane of rat, guinea pig, mouse and hamster. *Proc. Natl. Acad. Sci. USA* 81:7407–7411.

Max, S. R. and Silbergeld, E. K. 1987. Skeletal muscle glucocorticoid receptor and glutamine synthetase activity in the wasting syndrome in rats treated with 2,3,7,8-tetrachlorodibenzo-*p*-dioxin. *Toxicol. Appl. Pharmacol.* 87:523–527.

Molloy, C. J., Gallor, M. A. and Laskin, J. D. 1987. Alterations in the expression of specific epidermal keratin markers in the hairless mouse by the topical application of the tumor phorbol promoters 2,3,7,8-tetrachlorodibenzo-*p*-dioxin and the phorbol ester 12-*O*-tetradecanoylphorbol-13-acetate. *Carcinogen.* 8:1193–1199.

Moses, M., Lilis, R., Crow, K. D., et al. 1984. Health status of workers with past exposure to 2,3,7,8-tetrachlorodibenzo-*p*-dioxin in the manufacture of 2,4,5-trichlorophenoxyacetic acid: Comparison of findings with and without chloracne. *Amer. J. Ind. Med.* 5:161–182.

Okret, S., Carlstedt-Duke, J., Wistrom, A. C., Radojcic, M. and Gustafsson, J. A. 1985. Glucocorticoid receptor structure and function. In *Interaction of Steroid Hormone Receptors with DNA,* ed. M. Sluyser, pp. 155–189. Chichester (UK):Ellis Horwood.

Olie, K., Verneulen, P. and Hutzinger, O. 1977. Chlorodibenzodioxins and chlorodibenzofurans are components of fly ash and flue gas of some municipal incinerators in the Netherlands. *Chemosphere* 6:455–459.

Osborne, R. and Greenlee, W. F. 1985. TCDD enhances termnal differentiation of cultured human epidermal cells. *Toxicol. Appl. Pharmacol.* 77:434–443.

Patterson, D. G., Fingerhut, M. A., Roberts, D. W., et al. 1989. Levels of polychlorinated dibenzo-*p*-dioxins and dibenzofurans in workers exposed to 2,3,7,8-tetrachlorodibenzo-*p*-dioxin. *Am. J. Ind. Med.* 16:135–146.

Poland, A. and Knutson, J. C. 1982. 2,3,7,8-Tetrachlorodibenzo-*p*-dioxin and related halogenated aromatic hydrocarbons: Examination of the mechanism of toxicity. *Ann. Rev. Pharmacol. Toxicol.* 22:517–554.

Poland, A., Knutson, J. C. and Glover, E. 1984. Histologic changes produced by 2,3,7,8-tetrachlorodibenzo-*p*-dioxin in the skin of mice carrying mutations that affect the integument. *J. Invest. Dermatol.* 83:454–459.

Puhvel, S. M. and Sakamoto, M. 1988. Effect of 2,3,7,8-tetrachlorodibenzo-*p*-dioxin on murine skin. *J. Invest. Dermatol.* 90:354–358.

Puhvel, S. M., Sakamoto, M., Ertle, D. and Reisner, R. M. 1982. Hairless mice as models for chloracne: A study of cutaneous changes induced by topical application of established chloracnegens. *Toxicol. Appl. Pharmacol.* 64:492–503.

Puhvel, S. M., Ertl, D. C. and Lynberg, C. A. 1984. Increased epidermal transglutaminase activity following 2,3,7,8-tetrachlorodibenzo-*p*-dioxin: *In vivo* and *in vitro* studies with mouse skin. *Toxicol. Appl. Pharmacol.* 73:42–47.

Rice, R. H. and Cline, P. R. 1984. Opposing effects of 2,3,7,8-tetrachlorodibenzo-*p*-dioxin and hydrocortisone on growth and differentiation of cultured malignant human keratinocytes. *Carcinogen* 5:367–371.

Rogan, W. J. 1982. PCBs and cola-colored babies: Japan, 1968, and Taiwan, 1979. *Teratology* 26:259–261.

Safe, S. H. 1986. Comparative toxicology and mechanism of action of polychlorinated dibenzo-*p*-dioxins and dibenzofurans. *Ann. Rev. Pharmacol. Toxicol.* 26:371–399.

Schwartz, L. 1936. Dermatitis from synthetic resins and waxes. *Am. J. Public Health.* 26:586–592.

Silbergeld, E. K. 1984. Health effects of PCBs: Review of occupational exposure. In *PCB Seminar Proceedings,* eds. M. Barros, H. Konneman and R. Visser, pp. 136–151. The Hague: OECD.

Silbergeld, E. K. and Gasiewicz, T. A. 1989. Dioxins and the *Ah* receptor. *Am. J. Ind. Med.* 16:455–474.

Sunahara, G. I., Lucier, G. W., McCoy, Z., Bresnick, E. H., Sanchez, E. R. and Nelson, K. R. 1990. 2,3,7,8-TCDD medicated decrease in dexamethasone binding to hepatic cytosolic glucocorticoid receptor is not accompanied by a decrease in immunodetectable glucocorticoid receptor protein concentrations: The role of adrenal steroids. *J. Biol. Chem.,* in press.

Suskind, R. R. and Hertzberg, V. S. 1984. Human health effects of 2,4,5-T and its toxic contaminants. *J. Am. Med. Assoc.* 251:2372–2380.

Sutter, T. R., Dold, R. M., Guzman, K. and Greenlee, W. R. 1990. Isolation of TCDD-responsive genes by differential hybridization. *Toxicology* 10:30.

Taylor, J. S. 1979. Environmental chloracne: update and review. *Ann. NY Acad. Sci.* 320:295–307.

Thelwell Jones, A. 1941. The etiology of acne with special reference to acne of occupational origin. *J. Ind. Hyg. Toxicol.* 23:290–312.

Thunberg, T. 1984. Effects of TCDD on vitamin A and its relation to TCDD toxicity. In *Biological Mechanisms of Dioxin Action,* eds. A. Poland and R. D. Kimbrough, pp. 333–344. Cold Spring Harbor, N.Y.: Banbury Report 18.

Tindall, J. P. 1985. Chloracne and chloracnegens. *J. Am. Acad. Dermatol.* 13:539–558.

Travis, C., Hattemer-Frey, H. and Silbergeld, E. K. 1989. Dioxin, dioxin, everywhere. *Environ. Sci. Technol.* 16:1061–1063.

Uziel, M., Griffin, G. D. and Walsh, P. J. 1985. Aryl hydrocarbon hydroxylase tissue-specific activities: Evidence for baseline levels in mammalian tissues. *J. Toxicol. Environ. Health* 16:727–742.

U.S. Environmental Protection Agency. 1980. *Dioxins.* Cincinnati: U.S. EPA ORD.

U.S. Environmental Protection Agency. 1985. *Health Assessment Document for Polychlorinated Dibenzo-p-Dioxins.* Washington, D.C.: U.S. EPA OHEA.

Webb, K. B., Ayres, S. M., Mikes, J. and Evans, R. G. 1986. The diagnosis of dioxin-associated illness. *Am. J. Prev. Med.* 2:103–108.

Whitlock, J. P. 1987. The regulation of gene expression by 2,3,7,8-tetrachlorodibenzo-*p*-dioxin. *Pharmacol. Rev.* 39:147–161.

28

retinoids: a specific example in dermatotoxicology

■ William J. Powers, Jr. ■ Gerard J. Gendimenico ■
Basil E. McKenzie ■ James A. Mezick ■ E. George Thorne ■

INTRODUCTION

Retinoids are a class of natural/synthetic compounds that have profound effects on cell differentiation of many cell types. Because they have diverse pharmacological effects, retinoids are being used and investigated as therapeutic agents in a variety of dermatologic conditions including acne, psoriasis, other disorders of keratinization, photoaging, and skin cancer (Orfanos et al., 1987; Goldfarb et al., 1989). The purpose of this chapter is to discuss how retinoids can be tested and developed as safe dermatotherapeutic agents. Although retinoids exhibit toxicity under certain conditions, preclinical and clinical methods are available to determine these toxicities so that retinoids can be used safely and effectively. In this chapter we discuss retinoids, specifically, when used as topical therapeutic agents.

Cellular and Molecular Mechanisms of Retinoid Actions

Retinoids (Fig. 1) are molecules that modulate cell growth, differentiation, and proliferation of skin cells of different embryological origin including keratinocytes, fibroblasts, melanocytes, sebocytes, endothelial cells, and skin-associated immune cells (Sporn and Roberts, 1984a). In cases where abnormal cells are present, retinoids can reverse the abnormal phenotype of cells and cause them to function in a normal fashion, which explains why retinoids are effective in different skin disorders.

Tretinoin   Retinoic Acid
                                                  Vitamin A Acid

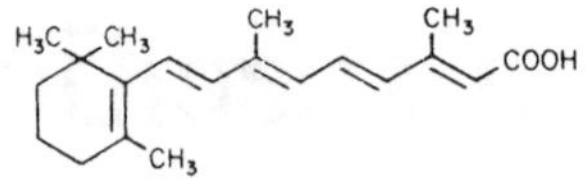

Isotretinoin   13-*cis*-Retinoic Acid

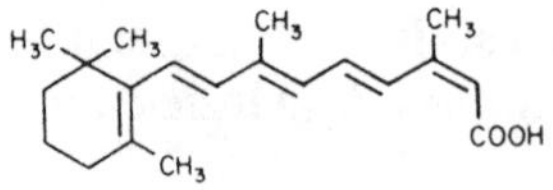

FIGURE 1   Retinoids.

Until 1988, the molecular mechanisms of retinoid actions in cells were uncertain. The discovery of specific nuclear receptors for all-*trans*-retinoic acid (tretinoin), which are homologous to steroid and thyroid hormone nuclear receptors, demonstrated that retinoids act by a specific mechanism to alter gene expression by a process known as DNA transcription activation (Evans, 1988). When a retinoid enters the cell and binds to its nuclear receptor, a portion of the receptor binds to a region of the DNA known as the retinoid-responsive element (RRE). The binding of the retinoid-receptor complex to the RRE triggers a change in the transcription rate of retinoid-responsive genes (Evans, 1988). A number of gene products influenced by tretinoin have been identified and include cytoskeletal proteins, enzymes and receptors (Chytil, 1986). These changes in gene expression thus influence the differentiation state of cells and tissues.

Three subtypes of the retinoic acid receptors are known, designated as retinoic acid receptor (RAR)-alpha, RAR-beta, and RAR-gamma (Green and Chambon, 1988; Krust et al., 1989). They differ slightly in amino acid content in various functional regions of the receptor, and there are also some differences in the tissue distribution of each receptor subtype. Skin contains a high amount of RAR-gamma and some RAR-alpha and RAR-beta (Krust et al., 1989; Zelent, et al., 1989). In fact, RAR-gamma is almost exclusively located in skin whereas other tissues lack it, except for spleen and lung, which contain smaller amounts than skin (Zelent et al., 1989). The functional significance of the three RAR subtypes is uncertain; however, they probably account for the diverse pharmacological and toxicological effects of retinoids, possibly by interacting with different target genes.

Cutaneous Pharmacology of Retinoids

Retinoids, when applied topically, have many prominent pharmacologic effects on skin. The most notable of these are reversal and prevention of abnormal follicular keratinization, induction of epidermal hyperplasia, and repair of connective tissue in photodamaged skin. These effects can be evaluated quantitatively in animal models, in which the abnormal cutaneous processes preexist or can be induced.

Abnormal Follicular Keratinization. The effects of retinoids on abnormal follicular keratinization can be studied in the skin of hairless rhino mice (hr^{rh}hr^{rh} strain), which contains numerous pilosebaceous structures ("horn-filled utriculi") with excess amounts of keratin. Retinoids reverse the abnormal follicular keratinization by causing exfoliation of the keratinized material and marked reductions in the size of the utriculi (Kligman and Kligman, 1979; Mezick et al., 1984). This effect can be quantitated in whole mount sections of epidermis. Using this method, all-*trans*-retinoic acid (tretinoin), 13-*cis*-retinoic acid (isotretinoin), etretinate and motretinide all cause dose-related reductions of utricular size when applied topically to rhino mice (Mezick et al., 1984).

The epidermis of the rhino mouse also undergoes changes in the pattern of cytoskeletal protein expression when treated with retinoids (Eichner et al., 1986, 1987; Mezick et al., 1989). Tretinoin and other retinoids induce expression of epidermal 50-kD and 58-kD keratin proteins and a 190-kD glycoprotein. In contrast, the amount of the histidine-rich protein filaggrin decreases dramatically with retinoid treatment. The amounts of three stratum corneum keratins (57 kD, 63 kD, and 65kD) are reduced after retinoid treatment. Normally, these three keratins are derived by proteolysis of keratins from the epidermis (living layers). A 52-kD keratin, which is near-completely degraded in normal stratum corneum, is elevated in retinoid-treated skin. Thus, retinoids alter these stratum corneum keratins possibly by interfering with their proteolytic degradation.

The external ear canal of the rabbit can be used to induce abnormal follicular keratinization by applying coal tar, acetylated lanolin alcohol (Polylan), or other comedogenic substances for 2 wk. In the coal tar model, tretinoin applied after comedones are induced causes a dose-related comedolytic effect (Mezick et al., 1983). Also, tretinoin and isotretinoin prevent the formation of comedones induced by Polylan (Mezick et al., 1987).

The reversal of abnormal follicular keratinization by retinoids is a major factor in the therapeutic effect of topical tretinoin in acne, where it acts by normalizing the function of the thickened, poorly desquamating sebaceous follicle stratum corneum cells. During tretinoin treatment, the stratum corneum cells are more easily extruded from the follicle, thereby causing existing comedones to resolve and preventing the formation of new comedones (Kligman, 1987a).

Epidermal Hyperplasia. A prominent effect of retinoids on skin is their capacity to induce epidermal hyperplasia. This effect has been observed in normal mouse, guinea pig, and human skin. In the hairless mouse (Skh-1 strain), a number of structurally different retinoids, applied once to dorsal trunk skin, cause dose-related increases in the number of epidermal cell layers, with a peak effect at 4–5 d after retinoid is applied (Connor et al., 1986). Epidermal hyperplasia is also induced in the rhino mouse after retinoids are applied topically to dorsal trunk skin, once daily, 5 times per week for 2 wk (Ashton et al., 1984). In the guinea pig ear, tretinoin induces epidermal hyperplasia when applied once daily for 8–10 d (Christophers and Braun-Falco, 1970).

Epidermal hyperplasia has also been observed in human skin treated topically with tretinoin. In acne patients given 0.1% tretinoin, epidermal hyperplasia is observed after only 10 d of treatment and maintained for up to 50 d of treatment (Plewig and Braun-Falco, 1975). Patients with solar damaged (photoaged) skin who have been treated with 0.1 and 0.05% tretinoin creams for 16 and 12 wk, respectively, also have significant epidermal hyperplasia (Weiss et al., 1988; Lever et al., 1990).

The induction of epidermal hyperplasia appears to be due to stimulation of keratinocyte proliferation, as demonstrated by increased epidermal DNA synthesis in hairless mouse skin treated topically with retinoids (Connor and Lowe, 1983).

Photodamaged Skin. Topical retinoids are effective in repairing photodamaged skin. Photodamage can be induced in hairless mouse skin by subchronic exposure to UVB radiation. When tretinoin or isotretinoin is applied topically to these mice for 10 wk, a new zone of connective tissue is formed (Kligman et al., 1984; Bryce et al., 1988). Biochemically, new collagen and new elastin are synthesized in photodamaged hairless mouse skin, as demonstrated for tretinoin (Kligman et al., 1989, 1990). These results demonstrate that the dermis is also an important site of retinoid action in the skin.

Topical tretinoin has been shown to reduce fine wrinkles and to produce increased blood flow and lightening of hyperpigmented lesions (Kligman et al., 1986; Weiss et al., 1988; Lever et al., 1990). The marked epidermal hyperplasia, stratum corneum compaction, and accumulation of epidermal glycosaminoglycans induced by tretinoin in these subjects may contribute in part to the improved appearance and texture of their skin (Weiss et al., 1988).

Local Skin Reactions from Retinoids. A local erythema and scaling is a common finding with the use of some topical retinoids. It differs from primary skin irritation because it does not develop until after four consecutive daily treatments have been given. The time course of the reaction is similar in rabbit and human skin (Shroot, 1986). This retinoid reaction is not a prerequisite for its therapeutic effects. As an example, in acne, irritation subsides after treatment with topical tretinoin after the first few weeks, but the antiacne efficacy of the retinoid continues (Kligman, 1987a).

The appearance of redness, peeling, and itching after application of retinoids has been studied by a number of investigators. There still is no clear cause for this cutaneous retinoid effect. Previous hypotheses have included prostaglandin release (Ziboh, 1975), or lysosomal and cell membrane labilization (Lucy et al., 1961) releasing inflammatory mediators. Recent work from a University of Michigan research team suggests that retinoid irritation is a cell-poor immune reaction, distinct from the reaction seen with common irritants (Fisher et al., 1990).

Preclinical Toxicology

The increased use of topical retinoids in acne, psoriasis, actinic keratosis, and photodamage has promoted interest in retinoid toxicity (Kamm et al., 1984). Tretinoin (all-*trans*-retinoic acid) is currently the only widely marketed topical retinoid; however, hundreds of new retinoid compounds have been synthesized, by modification of the vitamin A molecule, and screened for therapeutic activity. Because of the potential for systemic absorption of topical retinoids, acute and long-term animal studies are conducted to evaluate the potential for both localized and systemic toxicity.

ACUTE

In general, most retinoids are not potent acute toxins. The acute oral LD50 of tretinoin, isotretinoin, and etretinate (rats and mice) each exceeds 2000 mg/kg (Kamm et al., 1984; Kamm, 1982; Ehmann and Cheripko, 1984; Klaassen, 1986) classifies most retinoids as slightly toxic by acute administration. Localized irritation and sensitization potential of development retinoids are evaluated in standard *in vivo* assays. Tretinoin, for example, produces dermal changes that include erythema, alopecia, hyperkeratosis, and epidermal hyperplasia, which are actually exaggerated pharmacologic effects. Tretinoin is not a sensitizer in guinea pigs, but some of the synthetic retinoids show a weak sensitization potential.

SUBCHRONIC

Subchronic administration of tretinoin, isotretinoin, or etretinate to mice, rats, or dogs produces "classical signs of retinoid toxicity." The effects of retinoid overdosage are generally referred to as "hypervitaminosis A-syndrome" (Teelman, 1989). The effects in rodents involve several organ systems in addition to reduced food consumption, decreased body weight gain or weight loss, lethargy, and decreased motor activity. The main target-organ systems in laboratory animals are the skin, skeleton, hematopoietic system, liver, testes, and the nervous system.

Common or classical signs of retinoid toxicity in rats and mice include cartilage and bone resorption, bone fracture, subcutaneous and internal hemorrhage, elevations in cerebral spinal fluid pressure, fatty infiltration in hepatic parenchyma, and epithelial drying and scaling. Similar to the toxicity observed in humans, reductions in body weight, hair thinning, dermatitis, mucocutaneous lesions, elevated alkaline phosphatase, albumin, hemoglobin, erythrocyte count, triglyceride levels, and transaminase activity in animals were common.

Hepatic pathology and testicular atrophy with interruption of spermato-genesis also occurred. Bone fractures, corneal opacity, epiphora, cardiovascular lesions, and erythrophagocytosis in lymph nodes were observed after ingestion of relatively high levels for prolonged periods. For example, oral administra-tion of 150–250 mg/kg of tretinoin induced alopecia, weight loss, and mucocu-taneous disorders. Oral or ip treatment with tretinoin or isotretinoin for 21 d was associated with epidermal and dermal inflammation and hyperkeratosis in male and female mice. Testicular necrosis and suppression of spermatogenesis occurred in males (Howard and Wilhite, 1986).

Retinoid-induced hematologic changes included a dose-dependent periph-eral anemia, erythrocytopenia, and decreased hemoglobin and packed cell vol-umes. Orally administered retinoids decreased serum albumin and increased plasma alkaline phosphatase. Testicular toxicity included coagulation necrosis and arrested development of spermatogonia, spermatocytes, and spermatids. Sertoli cells were the last testicular cell population to be affected. In ad-dition, thymic and cardiac lesions were also reported (Howard and Wilhite, 1986).

Systemic Toxicity

Skeletal System.   Some of the most striking effects in retinoid tolerance testing *in vivo* are bone alterations in rodents with rats being more sensitive than mice (Teelman, 1989). Acute, subchronic, and chronic toxicities of retinoids on bone and other connective tissues in laboratory animals are related to dose and duration of treatment. Intubation of tretinoin and other naturally occurring reti-noids induced disturbances in calcium metabolism as evidenced by bone thin-ning, osteoporosis, and calcification of soft tissues (Howard and Wilhite, 1986; Kamm, 1982). Oral administration of up to 10 mg/kg/d tretinoin to rats for 17 wk produced osteocytic osteolysis, subperiosteal and osteoclastic resorption, and dissolution of bone matrix (Howard and Wilhite, 1986). Doses of 0.4–10 mg/kg po to rats for 90 d or dietary administration of 300–1500 IU of tretinoin for 84 d increased the concentration of serum alkaline phosphatase. Administra-tion of tretinoin or isotretinoin for 21 d induced dose-dependent fractures of the long bones, dermal and epidermal abnormalities, cartilage degeneration, and elevations in plasma alkaline phosphatase. However, changes in alkaline phos-phatase were not always associated with bone fractures because alkaline phos-phatase is also associated with both resorption and deposition of bone in addi-tion to its distribution in other tissues such as liver and prostate gland. Changes in connective tissues are often observed in concert with hepatic toxicity, such as dose-related decreases in plasma albumin.

Circulating triglyceride and cholesterol concentrations were increased af-ter chronic retinoid treatment as well. Administration of tretinoin or isotretinoin to rats induced hypertriglyceridemia in addition to changes in the composition of liver fatty acids (Howard and Wilhite, 1986). Whereas skeletal alteration in laboratory rodents is a major finding, bone changes in nonrodent species, such as the dog, are much less prominent, and fractures have not been reported to date. Indicators of bone involvement in the hypervitaminosis-A syndrome in dogs are clinical signs of reduced motor activity, lameness, and/or increased pain sensitivity during manipulations.

Liver and Lipid Disorders. The naturally occurring retinoids are transported from the gut in chylomicrons via the portal system and concentrate in hepatocytes (Howard and Wilhite, 1986).

Synthetic retinoids tend to concentrate in the liver, where a number of pathological and biochemical alterations can occur. Administration of tretinoin or isotretinoin to rats induced hypertriglyceridemia in addition to changes in the composition in liver fatty acids (Howard and Wilhite, 1986; Teelman, 1989).

MUTAGENICITY

The mutagenic potential of tretinoin was evaluated in the Ames assay at a maximum plate concentration of 2.0 mg/plate of tester strains TA1535, TA1537, TA1538, TA98, and TA100 with and without metabolic activation (Howard and Wilhite, 1986; Kamm, 1982; Teelman, 1989; David et al., 1988). Tretinoin was nonmutagenic in this assay and several others. The retinoid class in general is nonmutagenic; however, synthetic retinoids as new chemical entities should be evaluated for this potential.

CARCINOGENICITY/PHOTOCARCINOGENICITY

Tsubura and Yamamoto (1979) applied 0.1% tretinoin in a cream or lotion to female SLC:ICR mice either 1 or 3 times per week for 2 yr and found no indication of a carcinogenic response. Epstein (1986) observed that tretinoin has antineoplastic activity in chemically induced tumors in experimental animals, but not in transplantable tumors. It has also been found to inhibit and enhance experimental photocarcinogenesis.

In human skin, tretinoin has proved to be of therapeutic value in the treatment of premalignant actinic keratosis on the face. There is no evidence that tretinoin is carcinogenic in either experimental animals or humans. Furthermore, there is no indication that it promotes UVB-induced carcinogenesis or any other type of tumor formation in humans.

Forbes et al. (1979) reported that topical application of tretinoin solutions enhanced the response of hairless mice to a dose of simulated sunlight. Skin tumors appeared earlier and in greater number in animals treated daily with 1 or 10 μg of tretinoin in methanol immediately after a 2-h exposure to a xenon arc lamp filtered through 2 mm of Schott WG 320 glass, compared to mice treated with light and methanol only. The higher amount of tretinoin, in combination with light, produced moderate epidermal hyperplasia and some scaling and transient erythema, but no gross dermal ulceration or inflammation. The lower amount of tretinoin, though about equally effective in enhancement of photocarcinogenesis, produced minimal epidermal hyperplasia compared to the ultraviolet radiation plus methanol.

Kligman (1987b) published a critical review on the subject of retinoic acid and photocarcinogenesis. She points out that there is considerable evidence that retinoic acid can exert an anticarcinogenic effect. Eight photocarcinogenicity studies conducted in five different laboratories are reviewed. No study completely duplicated any other. The studies differed in the light source, UV dose per exposure, retinoic acid concentrations, vehicles, and animal and treatment schedules, consequently producing divergent results that are difficult to interpret. Furthermore, the validity of the hairless mouse model is questioned in view of the lack of DNA repair capability, lack of melanin, and thinness of the stratum corneum and epidermis allowing for greater penetration of test material and UV light (Ley et al., 1977; Kligman et al., 1981; Lowe et al., 1982; Davies and Forbes, 1988; Steinel et al., 1988).

From a comprehensive review of the results of twelve photocarcinogenicity studies of topical tretinoin, four studies suggest that tretinoin inhibits photocarcinogenicity, six suggest an enhancement, and two suggest no effect of tretinoin on photocarcinogenicity (Forbes et al., 1979; Kligman and Kligman, 1981a, 1981b; Hartmann et al., 1981; Conner et al., 1983; Epstein and Grekin, 1981; M. Davies et al., 1988; R. E. Davies et al., 1980; Epstein, 1986, 1977; Kligman, 1987b; Forbes, 1981). Enhancement of photocarcinogenesis by tretinoin was never demonstrated in a study conducted exclusively in pigmented animals. There is no evidence in animals or humans that topical tretinoin is itself carcinogenic. Furthermore, there is no indication that topical tretinoin, after more than 25 yr of use on human skin, promotes UVB-induced carcinogenesis in humans. If topical tretinoin were a human carcinogen or an enhancer or promoter of photocarcinogenicity, it should have been observed after almost 30 yr of use on human skin. While the extreme vulnerability of the hairless mouse to UV radiation makes it a valuable model for photobiologic studies, this makes extrapolation of photocarcinogenicity data to humans of questionable significance. Therefore, a cautious extrapolation to humans of results from the photocarcinogenicity studies with tretinoin using albino hairless mice is warranted.

REPRODUCTIVE TOXICITY

Vitamin A and the majority of retinoids tested so far are embryotoxic and teratogenic in laboratory animals when high doses are administered at susceptible stages during pregnancy (Kamm, 1982; Teelman, 1989). The malformations induced in the animals' offspring affect various organ systems such as the central nervous system, cranio-facial alterations, including cleft palate, and defects of the eye and ear, the axial skeleton, and the extremities.

Various *in vitro* and *in vivo* test systems have been used to evaluate a large variety of retinoids more or less closely related to the parent vitamin A molecule. A number of retinoids are teratogenic without preceding bioactivation, particularly those with free carboxylic acids in the polar end group; others appear to require metabolic conversion to the free acid before they become teratogenic. Furthermore, an important factor in the teratogenic potential of retinoids has been attributed to the length of the side chain; a polyene chain of greater than five carbon atoms appeared to be necessary for retinoid teratogenic activity.

The doses required to induce teratogenic effects vary from species to species. Rabbits are often more susceptible than mice or rats. Major factors contributing to differences in species sensitivity may be intestinal absorption and transfer of the retinoid via the placenta into the developing embryo. The lower teratogenicity of isotretinoin as compared to tretinoin in mice could be attributed to minimal placental transfer of isotretinoin, in contrast to extensive transfer of tretinoin, and the corresponding metabolites (Kraft et al., 1989).

Although it has long been believed that the biological activity and teratogenicity of retinoids are closely related, new evidence suggests that this may not necessarily be true. Retinoids belonging to the class of *N*-ethyl-retinamides appeared to bear almost no teratogenic risk, although good chemopreventive activity could be demonstrated in chemically induced cancer in laboratory rodents. There are other classes of retinoids that appear to hold similar promise.

In animal studies designed to evaluate fertility and general reproductive performance, as well as in peri- and postnatal studies, the main adverse effects recorded are increased numbers of stillbirths and decreased neonatal survival. The doses needed to induce these changes are on the average close to or in the range of those producing maternal toxicity. The pathophysiology behind the reduced rate of survival remains to be elucidated.

The question has been repeatedly raised whether retinoid exposure of males can induce teratogenicity in the offspring of untreated females. All retinoids tested so far have only been teratogenic when the dam was exposed to sufficiently high doses of active retinoids during the susceptible stages of pregnancy. Neither earlier treatment of dams nor treatment of males at any dose level has shown a relationship to teratogenicity. Thus a direct teratogenic or embryotoxic effect in the traditional sense caused by sperm of males exposed to retinoids has not been demonstrated.

Theoretically, there are two ways in which the indirect adverse effects via the male's sperm could operate. The first is vaginal resorption of retinoids from sperm during the susceptible stages of pregnancy. Since teratogenicity of retinoids is clearly dose dependent, a number of major barriers must be passed before this mode of action could become effective. These are absorption from the male gastrointestinal tract, secretion into sperm, vaginal resorption in the female, and transplacental transfer to the developing embryo. All these barriers contain major diluting steps—particularly with regard to the small sperm volume (the highest human etretinate sperm content measured was 2–5 ng/ml as compared to plasma levels of 300–500 ng/ml)—which reduced the retinoid content of the various fluids involved to a substantial degree. Thus, this type of indirect teratogenicity can be regarded as extremely improbable.

A second possible mechanism is mutation of the male germ cells by retinoids. Since the underlying mechanisms of teratogenicity and mutagenicity are basically different, they are not to be confused with each other. As earlier mentioned, in general, retinoids are not mutagenic.

A number of reports indicate that oral tretinoin produces a broad spectrum of congenital defects in rodents including craniofacial, cardiovascular, and central nervous system and skeletal tissue of the limbs and other regions (Kochhar et al., 1988; Kochhar et al., 1984; Yasuda et al., 1986). The level of teratogenic activity of tretinoin has been repeatedly confirmed in several species, including nonhuman primates. There have been no reports, however, of tretinoin's teratogenicity in humans, since it is used only topically, with minimal systemic absorption. In mouse teratogenicity studies, tretinoin seems to be a more potent teratogen than isotretinoin. Isotretinoin is known to be a potent human teratogen when ingested; however, data following human oral ingestion of tretinoin are unavailable. This species difference may be related to a difference in placental transfer and pharmacokinetic disposition of retinoids (Kochhar et al., 1988; Kraft et al., 1989; Kochhar and Penner, 1987). In the mouse tretinoin is readily transferred into the embryo with a relatively long half-life. On the contrary, the isotretinoin isomer is less readily transferred into the mouse embryo and has a much shorter half-life. The serum half-life of isotretinoin in mice is about 20 min., versus 20 h in humans. Species differences in response may make a direct extrapolation from mouse to humans difficult.

The teratogenic potential of tretinoin was evaluated in pigtail monkeys (Fantel et al., 1977; Newell-Morris et al., 1980). Daily oral administration of 10 mg/kg/d tretinoin to pregnant *Macaca nemestrina* on d 20–44 gestation resulted in a high frequency of craniofacial and musculoskeletal malformations. Craniofacial defects including cleft palate and anomalies of the pinna were common as were ectrodactyly, kyphosis, and muscular-joint contractures. Shorter treatment periods with similar or higher dosages (up to 40 mg/kg/d) were not teratogenic and were less fetotoxic. Although only relatively long treatment courses were teratogenic, the defects that resulted were morphologically similar to those induced with tretinoin or other retinoids in other animal orders. Similar findings were reported in animals receiving 7.5 mg/kg/d on gestational d 20–44 (Yip et al., 1980).

Oral administration of tretinoin to Wistar rats at doses of either 1.0 or 2.5 mg/kg/d throughout organogenesis (gestational d 6–15) produced no maternal toxicity (Zbinden, 1975). The higher dose produced only a modest increase in intrauterine death. There was a treatment-related but not dose-related increase in the anatomical variations of increased thoracic rib or sternebrae. Tretinoin treatment at either dose did not interfere with implantation or fetal weight, and did not produce a teratogenic response. A review of the literature confirms an oral dose of 1.0 mg/kd/d as the nonteratogenic dose of tretinoin in animals that can be used in calculating margins of safety in humans (Kochhar, 1967; Kamm, 1982; Teratology Society, 1987; Kamm et al., 1984). Similarly, a topical dose of up to 0.5 mg/kg/d has been shown to be a nonteratogenic dose in rats.

A recent report on a topical teratogenicity study suggested that 20 mg/kg administered on gestational d 12 produced skeletal anomalies and plasma tretinoin levels of up to 300 ng/ml (Chahoud et al., 1989). A topical dose of 20 mg/kg is approximately 4000 times the estimated clinical dose and the plasma levels reached in this study were roughly 150 times endogenous plasma levels. Seegmiller et al. (1989) reported that up to 250 mg/kg/d tretinoin in dimethyl sulfoxide (DMSO) applied topically to Sprague-Dawley rats on gestational d 11–14 was both maternal and fetotoxic, but not teratogenic. The data to date suggest that a dose of tretinoin sufficient to significantly elevate plasma levels above endogenous levels is required to produce terata.

The results of a clinical percutaneous absorption study indicate that topical application of a tretinoin cream (single or multiple) produces peak plasma levels of approximately 20 pg Eq/ml, which compares to an endogenous level of approximately 2000 pg Eq/ml, which compares to more than 200,000 pg Eq/ml in the Chahoud topical teratogenicity study. These data support the argument that the dose and resultant tretinoin blood levels in the Chahoud study are unrealistically high in terms of clinical relevance.

Clinical Toxicology

The most commonly used assay for human irritation is the repeat insult patch test (RIPT) (Kligman, 1982). It is a phase I safety study required for approval of a topical drug. Other studies in this category are contact sensitization, phototoxicity, and photosensitization. None of the numerous retinoids we have tested in these studies have shown sensitization, phototoxicity, or photosensitization potential. However, the RIPT has consistently provided positive responses usually in a dose-response manner. We have used occluded and semi-occluded patches for 14 or 21 d. The patches are changed daily 5 d/wk. Total scores are determined using standard scoring techniques. The occluded sites generally yield a 10-fold increase in irritation scoring, which helps magnify any difference between treatment groups.

In our experience with tretinoin, the difference between 0.025 and 0.05% creams is significant. This difference is also seen in acne studies where 0.05% is approximately half as irritating as 0.025% (Thorne, 1988).

CONCLUSION

The retinoids are an exciting class of compounds. They present a diverse repertoire of effects on the biology of cells and tissues, that is, regulating differentiation (Sporn and Roberts, 1984b), stimulating wound healing (Hung et al., 1989), and antitumor effects (Lippman et al., 1987). Associated with these effects come toxicity questions regarding teratogenicity, chronic toxicity, photo-carcinogenicity, and irritation. Techniques to evaluate retinoid pharmacology and those to test their toxicity must be developed in parallel. Additionally, the tests should be adaptable for testing in the context of clinical usage. By blending pharmacology and toxicology these important compounds will fulfill their high expectations in the treatment of diseases of the skin and other organs.

REFERENCES

Ashton, R. E., Connor, M. J. and Lowe, N. J. 1984. Histologic changes in the skin of the rhino mouse (hr^{rh}hr^{rh}) induced by retinoids. *J. Invest. Dermatol.* 82:632–635.

Bryce, G. F., Bogdan, N. J. and Brown, C. C. 1988. Retinoic acids promote the repair of the dermal damage and the effacement of wrinkles in the UVB-irradiated hairless mouse. *J. Invest. Dermatol.* 91:175–180.

Chahoud, I., Lofberg, B., Mittmann, B. and Nau, H. 1989. Teratogenicity and pharmacokinetics of vitamin A acid (tretinoin, all-*trans*-tretinoin) after dermal application in the rat. *Naunyn-Schmeideberg's Arch. Pharmacol.* 339(suppl.):119.

Christophers, E. and Braun-Falco, O. 1970. Mechanisms of parakeratosis. *Br. J. Dermatol.* 82:268–275.

Chytil, F. 1986. Retinoic acid: Biochemistry and metabolism. J. Am. Acad. Dermatol. 15:741–747.

Connor, M. J., Lowe, N. J., Breeding, J. H. and Chalet, M. 1983. Inhibition of ultraviolet-B skin carcinogenesis by all-*trans*-retinoic acid regimens that inhibit ornithine decarboxylase induction. *Cancer Res.* 43:171–174.

Connor, M. J. and Lowe, N. J. 1983. Induction of ornithine decarboxylase and DNA synthesis in hairless mouse epidermis by retinoids. *Cancer Res.* 43:5174–5177.

Connor, M. J., Ashton, R. E. and Lowe, N. J. 1986. A comparative study of the induction of epidermal hyperplasia by natural and synthetic retinoids. *J. Pharmacol. Exp. Ther.* 237:31–35.

David, M., Hodad, E. and Lowe, N. J. 1988. Adverse effects of retinoids. *Med. Toxicol.* 3:273–288.

Davies, R. E., Kripke, M. L. and Glassman, H. W. 1980. Retinoic acid and photocarcinogenesis workshop. *J. Am. Acad. Dermatol.* 2:439–442.

Davies, R. E. and Forbes, P. D. 1988. Retinoids and photocarcinogenesis: A review. *J. Toxicol. Cut. Ocular Toxicol.* 7:241–253.

Ehmann, C. W. and Cheripko, J. A. 1984. Retinoids: An update. In *Cutaneous Toxicity,* eds. V. A. Drill and P. Lazar, pp. 239–251. New York: Raven Press.

Eichner, R., Mezick, J. A. and Capetola, R. J. 1986. Effects of topical all-*trans*-retinoic acid on cytoskeletal proteins in rhino mouse epidermis. *J. Invest. Dermatol.* 86:473.

Eichner, R., Mezick, J. A., Kissner, D. M., Shea, L. M. and Capetola, R. J. 1987. Biochemical effects of topical all-*trans*-retinoic acid on protein expression in rhino mouse epidermis. *J. Invest. Dermatol.* 88:486.

Epstein, J. H. 1977. Chemicals and photocarcinogenesis. *Australas. J. Dermatol.* 18:57–61.

Epstein, J. H. 1986. All-*trans*-retinoic acid and cutaneous cancers. *J. Am. Acad. Dermatol.* 15(4):772–778.

Epstein, J. H. and Grekin, D. A. 1981. Inhibition of ultraviolet induced carcinogenesis by all-*trans*-retinoic acid. *J. Invest. Dermatol.* 76:178–180.

Evans, R. M. 1988. The steroid and thyroid hormone receptor superfamily. *Science* 240:889–894.

Fantel, A. G., Shepard, T. H. and Newell-Morris, L. L. 1977. Teratogenic effects of retinoic acid in pigtail monkeys (*Macaca nemestrina*) I. General Features. *Teratology* 15:65–72.

Fisher, G. J., Esmann, J., Griffiths, C. M., et al. 1990. Cellular, immunological and biochemical characterization of topical retinoic acid treated skin. *Clin. Res.* 38:677A.

Forbes, P. D. 1981. Photocarcinogenesis: An overview. *J. Invest. Dermatol.* 77:139–143.

Forbes, P. D., Urbach, F. and Davies, R. E. 1979. Enhancement of experimental photocarcinogenesis by topical retinoic acid. *Cancer Lett.* 7:85–90.

Goldfarb, M. T., Ellis, C. N., Weiss, J. D. and Voorhees, J. J. 1989. Topical tretinoin therapy: Its use in photoaged skin. *J. Am. Acad. Dermatol.* 21:645–650.

Green, S. and Chambon, P. 1988. Nuclear receptors enhance our understanding of transcription regulation. *Trends Genet.* 4:309–314.

Hartmann, H. R. and Teelmann, K. 1981. The influence of topical and oral retinoid treatment on photocarcinogenicity in hairless albino mice. In *Retinoids: Advances in Basic Research and Therapy,* ed. C. E. Orfanos, pp. 447–451. Berlin: Springer-Verlag.

Howard, W. B. and Wilhite, C. C. 1986. Toxicity of retinoids in humans and animals. *J. Toxicol. Toxin Rev.* 5(1):55–94.

Hung, V. C., Yu-Yun Lee, J., Lee, J. Y., Zitelli, J. A. and Hebda, P. A. 1989. Topical tretinoin and epithelial wound healing. *Arch. Dermatol.* 125:65–69.

Kamm, J. J. 1982. Toxicology, carcinogenicity and teratogenicity of some orally administered retinoids. *J. Am. Acad. Dermatol.* 6:652–663.

Kamm, J. J., Ashenfelter, K. O. and Ehmann, C. W. 1984. Preclinical and clinical toxicology of selected retinoids. In *The Retinoids,* vol 2, ed. M. B. Sporn, A. B. Roberts and D. S. Goodman, pp. 287–326. London: Academic Press.

Klaassen, C. D. 1986. Principles of toxicology. In *Casarett and Doull's Toxicology: The Basic Science of Poisons,* 3rd ed., eds. C. D. Klaassen, M. O. Amdur and J. Doull, pp. 11–32. New York: Macmillan.

Kligman, A. M. 1982. Assessment of mild irritants. In *Principles of Cosmetics for the Dermatologists,* eds. P. Frost and S. N. Horwitz, pp. 265–276. St. Louis, Mo.: C. V. Mosby.

Kligman, A. M. 1987a. Topical tretinoin: Indications, safety, and effectiveness. *Cutis* 39:486–488.

Kligman, L. 1987b. Retinoic acid and photocarcinogenesis—A controversy. *Photodermatology* 4:88–101.

Kligman, L. H. and Kligman, A. M. 1979. The effect on rhino mouse skin of agents which influence keratinization and exfoliation. *J. Invest. Dermatol.* 73:354–358.

Kligman, L. H. and Kligman, A. M. 1981a. In *Lack of Enhancement of Experimental Photocarcinogenesis by Retinoic Acid,* eds. C. E. Orfanos, O. Braun-Falco, E. M. Farber, M. K. Polano and R. Schuppli, pp. 411–415. Berlin: Springer-Verlag.

Kligman, L. H. and Kligman, A. M. 1981b. Lack of enhancement of experimental photocarcinogenesis by topical retinoic acid. *Arch. Dermatol. Res.* 270:453–462.

Kligman, L. H., Duo, C. H. and Kligman, A. M. 1984. Topical retinoic acid enhances the repair of ultraviolet damaged dermal connective tissue. *Connective Tissue Res.* 12:139–150.

Kligman, A. M., Grove, G. L., Hirose, R. and Leyden, J. J. 1986. Topical tretinoin for photoaged skin. *J. Am. Acad. Dermatol.* 15:836–859.

Kligman, L., Cruickshank, F., Mezick, J. and Schwartz, E. 1989. Retinoic acid increases collagen synthesis in ultraviolet-irradiated hairless mice. *J. Invest. Dermatol.* 92:460.

Kligman, L., Cruickshank, F., Mezick, J. and Schwartz, E. 1990. Quantitative assessment of elastin and fibronectin in tretinoin treated photoaged hairless mouse skin. *J. Invest. Dermatol.* 94:543.

Kochhar, D. M. 1967. Teratogenic activity of tretinoin. *Acta Pathol. Microbiol. Scand.* 70:398–404.

Kochhar, D. M., Penner, J. D. and Tellone, C. I. 1984. Comparative teratogenic activities of two retinoids: Effects on palate and limb development. *Teratogen. Carcinogen. Mutagen.* 4:377–387.

Kochhar, D. M. and Penner, J. D. 1987. Developmental effects of isotretinoin and 4-oxo-isotretinoin: The role of metabolism in teratogenicity. *Teratology* 36:67–75.

Kochhar, D. M., Kraft, J. and Nau, H. 1988. Teratogenicity and disposition of various retinoids *in vivo* and *in vitro*. In *Pharmacokinetics in Teratogenesis: Vol. II Experimental aspects in Vivo and in Vitro,* eds. H. Nau and W. J. Scott. Boca Raton, Fla.: CRC Press.

Kraft, J. C., Lofberg, B., Chahoud, I., Bochert, G. and Nau, H. 1989. Teratogenicity and placental transfer of all-*trans*-, 13-*cis*-, 4-oxo-all-*trans*-, and 4-oxo-13-*cis*-retinoic acid after administration of a low oral dose during organogenesis in mice. *Toxicol. Pharmacol.* 100:162–176.

Krust, A., Kastner, P., Petkovich, M., Zelent, A. and Chambon, P. 1989. A third human retinoic acid receptor, hRAR-gamma. *Proc. Natl. Acad. Sci. USA* 86:5310–5314.

Lever, L., Kumar, P. and Marks, R. 1900. Topical retinoic acid for treatment of solar damage. *Br. J. Dermatol.* 122:91–98.

Ley, R. E., Sedita, B. A., Grube, D. D. and Fry, R. J. 1977. Induction and persistence of pyrimidine dimers in the epidermal DNA of two strains of hairless mice. *Cancer Res.* 37:3243–3248.

Lippmann, S. M., Kessler, J. F. and Meysken, F. L. 1987. Retinoids as preventive and therapeutic anticancer agents (Part III). *Cancer Treat. Rep.* 71:493–515.

Lowe, N. J. and Breeding, J. 1982. Retinoic acid modulation of ultraviolet light-induced epidermal ornithine decarboxylase activity. *J. Invest. Dermatol.* 78(2):121–124.

Lucy, J. A., Dingle, J. J. and Fell, H. B. 1961. Studies of the mode of action of excess Vitamin A. *Biochem. J.* 79:500.

Mezick, J. A., Bhatia, M. C., Shea, L. M. and Capetola, R. J. 1983. Evaluation of topical antiacne agents in animal models of keratinization. *Clin. Res.* 31:588A.

Mezick, J. A., Bhatia, M. C. and Capetola, R. J. 1984. Topical and systemic effects of retinoids on horn-filled utriculus size in the rhino mouse. A model to quantify "antikeratinizing" effects of retinoids. *J. Invest. Dermatol.* 83:110–113.

Mezick, J. A., Thorne, E. G., Bhatia, M. C., Shea, L. M. and Capetola, R. J. 1987. The rabbit ear microcomedo prevention assay: A new method to evaluate anti-acne agents. In *Models in Dermatology,* vol. 3, eds. H. I. Maiback and N. J. Lowe, pp. 68–73. Basel: Karger.

Mezick, J. A., Exner, R. E., Loughney, D. A., Capetola, R. J. and Eichner, R. 1989. Topical effects of various retinoids on utriculus reduction and cytoskeletal protein expression in rhino mouse epidermis. *J. Invest. Dermatol.* 92:481.

Newell-Morris, L., Sirianni, J. E., Shepard, T. H., Fantel, A. G. and Moffett, B. C. 1980. Effects of retinoic acid in pigtail monkeys (*Macaca nemestrina*) II. Craniofacial features. *Teratology* 22:87–101.

Orfanos, C. E., Ehlert, R. and Gollnick, H. 1987. The retinoids. A review of their clinical pharmacology and therapeutic use. *Drugs* 34:459–503.

Plewig, G. and Braun-Falco, O. 1975. Kinetics of epidermis and adnexa following vitamin A acid in the human. *Acta Dermatovenereol.* 55(Suppl 74):87–98.

Seegmiller, R. E., Carter, M. W., Ford, W. H. and White, R. D. 1989. Induction of prenatal toxicity in the rat by dermal application of retinoic acid. *Teratology* 39(5):480–481.

Shroot, B. 1986. Pharmacology of topical retinoids. *J. Am. Acad. Dermatol.* 15:748–756.

Sporn, M. B. and Roberts, A. B. 1984a. Biological methods for analysis and assay of retinoids—Relationships between structure and activity. In *The Retinoids,* vol. 1, eds. M. B. Sporn, A. B. Roberts and D. S. Goodman, pp. 235–279. Orlando, Fla.: Academic Press.

Sporn, M. B. and Roberts, A. B. 1984b. Role of retinoids in differentiation and carcinogenesis. *J. Natl. Cancer Inst.* 73:1381–1387.

Steinel, H. H. and Baker, R. S. U. 1988. Sensitivity of HRA/Skh hairless mice to initiation/promotion of skin tumors by chemical treatment. *Cancer Lett.* 41:63–68.

Teelman, K. 1989. Retinoid: Toxicology and teratogenicity to date. *Pharmacol. Ther.* 40(1):29–43.

Teratology Society. 1987. Teratology Society position paper: Recommendations for Vitamin A use during pregnancy. *Teratology* 35:269–275.

Thorne, E. G. 1988. Topical tretinoin 0.025% cream: A new treatment for acne vulgaris. Presented at the 49th Annual Meeting of the American Academy of Dermatology, Washington, D.C.

Tsubura, Y. and Yamamoto, H. 1979. Effect of long-term dermal application of retinoic acid on mice with special reference to the solvent and application interval. *J. Nara Med. Assoc.* 30:55–67.

Weiss, J. S., Ellis, C. N., Headington, J. T., Tincoff, T., Hamilton, T. A. and Voorhees, J. J. 1988. Topical tretinoin improves photoaged skin. A double-blind vehicle-controlled study. *J. Am. Med. Assoc.* 259–527–532.

Yasuda, Y., Okamoto, M., Konishi, H., Matsuo, T., Kihara, T. and Tanimura, T. 1986. Developmental anomalies induced by all-trans-retinoic acid in fetal mice: I. Macroscopic findings. *Teratology* 34:37–49.

Yip, J. E., Kokich, V. G. and Shepard, T. H. 1980. The effects of high doses of retinoic acid on prenatal craniofacial development in *Macaca nemestrina. Teratology.* 21:29–38.

Zbinden, G. 1975. Pharmacology of Vitamin A acid (B-all-*trans*-retinoic acid). *Acta Derm. Venereol (Stockh.).* 55(suppl. 74):25–28.

Zelent, A., Krust, A., Petkovich, M., Kastner, P. and Chambon, P. 1989. Cloning of murine alpha and beta retinoic acid receptors and a novel receptor gamma predominantly expressed in skin. *Nature (Lond.)* 339:714–717.

Ziboh, V. A. 1975. Regulation of prostaglandin E_2 biosynthesis in guinea pig skin and retinoic acid. *Acta Dermatovenereol. Suppl.* 74:57.

29

reproductive hazards from chemicals absorbed through the skin

■ Susan M. Barlow ■

INTRODUCTION

In 1983, dermatologists became acutely aware of potential reproductive hazards from drugs that they might prescribe when the U.S. Food and Drug Administration (FDA) announced it had received a number of reports of adverse outcome of pregnancy associated with isotretinoin exposure (Rosa, 1983). Isotretinoin, a 13-cis derivative of retinoic acid, was marketed in the United States in 1982 as an oral preparation for treatment of severe acne. By 1984, in 2 series of 18 and 16 women who took isotretinoin in the first trimester of pregnancy, there were 10 reports of congenital malformations, 19 reports of spontaneous abortions, and only 5 normal outcomes (Rosa, 1984). Further isotretinoin cases have since been identified, and another retinoid, etretinate, used orally for treatment of psoriasis, has also been implicated as a human teratogen (Rosa et al., 1986). Etretinate has a very long half-life, persisting in the body for several years after cessation of treatment. An analog, acetretin, originally reported to have a shorter half-life may also persist. The types of malformation seen in those who have taken isotretinoin or etretinate are similar; they comprise one or more components of a syndrome of central nervous system, cardioaortic, ear, facial, and palatal defects. The number and circumstances of the reports are such that there is now general agreement that the vitamin A congeners, isotretinoin and etretinate, are teratogenic in humans at therapeutic doses.

Tretinoin, the all-trans derivative of retinoic acid, is available as topical preparations for the treatment of acne and has been proposed as a cosmetic to prevent aging of skin. It has not yet been adequately investigated for its teratogenic potential in humans. Tretinoin is absorbed through the skin and is absorbed to a greater extent when skin is damaged by acne. Tretinoin, isotretinoin, and etretinate are all teratogenic in several species of animals, including primates, producing a spectrum of abnormalities similar to those reported in humans exposed to isotretinoin (Biesalski, 1989). In rodents tretinoin is more teratogenic, dose for dose, than the other two congeners, and it is likely that it is the active teratogen, since there is ready interconversion between isotretinoin and tretinoin in the body.

The possibility that topically applied drugs absorbed through the skin might have an adverse effect on reproduction has received little attention until recently. Indeed, of those agents known to affect human reproduction, the majority are either therapeutic drugs given by the oral route, or industrial chemicals or pesticides to which there has been excessive exposure by inhalation or accidental ingestion. However, for some chemicals, particularly those encountered in the occupational or domestic environments, the skin may be a major route of entry into the body. One such example is mercury in soaps and creams used for skin lightening. A case of renal tubular dysfunction, cataract and anemia has been reported in a 3-mo-old boy exposed prenatally and for 1 mo postnatally via breast milk to high levels of inorganic mercury. The kidney, lens, and bone marrow are known target organs for mercury in adults exposed to high levels of inorganic mercury. The mother regularly used mercury-containing cream and soap during pregnancy and lactation, and high levels of mercury were found in the blood and urine of both mother and son (Lauwerys et al., 1987).

RANGE OF REPRODUCTIVE EFFECTS IN HUMANS

In considering the range of possible reproductive effects of chemicals, it is important to remember that it is not only exposure during pregnancy itself that may be hazardous, but that exposure of males or females at any time up to the end of their reproductive years may cause abnormalities in the germ cells, resulting in infertility or an adverse outcome for a subsequent conceptus. Subfertility or infertility may be caused by any one of the following effects: mutation or poor maturation of male or female germ cells, menstrual-cycle disorders, decreases in libido or potency, interferences with fertilization or implantation of the embryo, or unnoticed early spontaneous abortion. Similarly, reproductive outcomes affecting the fetus, such as abortion, perinatal death, structural or functional abnormalities, growth retardation, or cancer, can be caused by one or several of the following mechanisms: chromosome abnormalities contributed by the male or female parent, effects on the mother such as hormonal disturbances, enhanced toxicity of a chemical in pregnancy that may indirectly affect the fetus, nonchromosomal effects on the father's sperm, or direct effects of a chemical on the fetus. Finally, there is the possibility of postnatal developmental disorders in the offspring, including effects on growth, physical or mental development, or the induction of cancer, by exposure to chemicals in the breast milk or contaminants brought home on the parent's work clothes.

EXTRAPOLATION OF ANIMAL DATA TO HUMANS

The predictive value of animal tests for reproductive toxicity in humans has been discussed extensively elsewhere (Council on Environmental Quality, 1981; Barlow and Sullivan, 1982). In summary, many of the agents known to affect human reproduction can be shown to have qualitatively similar effects in animals, at quantitatively similar doses to those that affect humans (see Table 1). In some instances, humans appear to be rather more sensitive than animals to particular agents, as is the case with alcohol and spontaneous abortions, the pesticide dibromochloropropane and male sterility, the drug thalidomide and reduction deformities of the limbs, and the industrial pollutant methylmercury and congenital functional abnormalities of the central nervous system.

While most drugs, food additives, and pesticides have generally been tested orally in animals for effects on reproduction, testing of chemicals encountered in the workplace has been very limited and testing via the percutaneous route rare. Even with pesticides, where dermal exposure of sprayers in particular may be substantial, reproductive toxicity testing is generally carried out using only oral administration by gavage or in the diet.

TABLE 1 Comparison of Doses of Chemicals Causing Similar Reproductive Effects in Animals and Humans

Chemical	Effects	Ratio of lowest effective dose animal/human
Drugs		
Aminopterin	Absorption, malformation	2
Thalidomide	Limb reduction	5–2.5
Diphenylhydantoin	Cleft palate	25
Industrial chemicals/pollutants		
Polychlorinated biphenyls/dibenzofurans	Menstrual disturbances, abortion, stillbirth, low birth weight, skin hyperpigmentation	1.8
Methylmercury	Functional central nervous system abnormalities	50
Carbon disulfide	Testicular damage, sperm abnormalities	5.5–2.7
Pesticides/fungicides		
Dibromochloropropane	Testicular damage, sterility	18
Hexachlorobenzene	Stillbirth, postnatal death	4–2

Note. Adapted from Council on Environmental Quality (1981).

In general, this is not a major drawback since data on reproductive effects, no matter how derived, coupled with a knowledge of percutaneous bioavailability, may be used to make some assessment of the potential for reproductive effects from materials penetrating the skin. However, this approach may occasionally be misleading. When, for example, the reproductive toxicity of the compound is due to transient high peak blood levels that would not be attained by administration in the diet, then rapid absorption through the skin could be hazardous. Similarly, when reproductive effects are caused by a parent compound that is rapidly metabolized by the liver and loses its activity before it reaches the reproductive organs after oral administration, then percutaneous exposure might show no such first-pass effect, provided the compound is not metabolized in the skin (see Chapter 9 by Kao).

POTENTIAL REPRODUCTIVE TOXIC AGENTS THAT MAY BE ABSORBED THROUGH THE SKIN

A wide range of solvents encountered in the occupational environment can readily penetrate the skin. For the majority there is little or no information on their potential for reproductive toxicity. However, there is evidence, for example, that carbon tetrachloride, epichlorohydrin, glycol ethers, tetrachloroethylene, toluene, and xylene may have adverse reproductive effects in animals, including testicular damage, estrous-cycle changes, intrauterine growth retardation, intrauterine death, congenital malformation, and alterations in postnatal development. However, there is no clear evidence of adverse reproductive effects in humans from exposure to any of these solvents (see Barlow and Sullivan, 1982, for review of comparative data).

A few examples of chemicals, including some solvents, that have been associated with reproductive casualty in animals and/or humans after dermal exposure are discussed next. In many cases involving human exposure, the epidemiological or anecdotal evidence is insufficient to conclude that there is a causal relationship between the chemical exposure and the adverse reproductive effects observed.

Formamides

Toxicity tests have been carried out in animals on a series of formamides, including formamide (F), monomethylformamide (MMF), and dimethylformamide (DMF). Formamide and DMF are solvents, the latter being in widespread use. MMF does not have any industrial applications. Both F and MMF, when given by a variety of routes including percutaneously, are highly embryolethal and teratogenic, causing similar malformations in rats and mice including exencephaly, encephalocele, spina bifida, cleft palate, and rib abnormalities. Teratogenicity occurs at doses below those lethal to the mother and, in the case of MMF, in the absence of any overt signs of toxicity in the mother.

Only very small quantities of F and MMF given cutaneously were required to produce intrauterine deaths and malformations. In the mouse, 0.1 ml of F (about one-fourth of the LD50 dose) dropped onto the skin on 1 or 2 d of embryogenesis was sufficient to cause death of half the embryos and malformation of all the survivors (Oettel and Frohberg, 1964; Gleich, 1974). In the rat, cutaneous application of F, at doses of 600 mg/kg body weight (about one-twenty-eighth of the average lethal dose), on 1 or 2 d during embryogenesis, was weakly embryotoxic, causing intrauterine deaths but not malformations (Stula and Krauss, 1977).

MMF is more embryolethal and teratogenic than F; as little as 0.01 ml or 20 mg applied cutaneously on 1 or 2 d of embryogenesis in the mouse caused 50–60% embryomortality with 37–89% of survivors malformed (Oettel and Frohberg, 1964; Roll and Bär, 1967; Gleich, 1974). In the rat, cutaneous application of 600 mg/kg body weight of MMF (about one-eighteenth of the average lethal dose), or "3 drops" on 1 or more days of pregnancy again resulted in very high embryomortality with the majority of survivors malformed (Tuchmann-Duplessis and Mercier-Parot, 1965; Stula and Krauss, 1977). In the rabbit, application of 200 mg/kg body weight (about one-seventh of the average lethal dose) on d 8–16 of pregnancy caused 100% embryomortality.

Thus F and particularly MMF are highly teratogenic when absorbed percutaneously. DMF does not appear to be teratogenic in mice, rats, or rabbits when given cutaneously at doses up to or close to doses lethal to the mothers (Oettel and Frohberg, 1964; Stula and Krauss, 1977). There are no case reports or epidemiological studies on the effects of formamides on reproductive function in humans.

Glycol Ethers

The glycol ethers are a widely used group of solvents with many industrial and consumer applications, including paints, varnishes, polishes, cleaning products, and inks. In animal studies, four of the glycol ethers have been shown to be teratogenic and six have been shown to cause testicular atrophy or infertility in males (Hardin, 1983). These effects have been shown in a variety of species (mice, rats, and rabbits) and by a variety of routes of exposure (oral, inhalational, cutaneous, and subcutaneous). When given by inhalation, reproductive toxicity occurs at exposure levels lower than those necessary to produce the other known toxic effects of glycol ethers.

The teratogenicity of one of the glycol ethers, ethylene glycol monoethyl ether (EGEE), applied to the skin of rats has been investigated (Hardin et al., 1982). Volumes of 0.25 for 0.5 ml of undiluted EGEE were applied 4 times daily to the skin of rats on d 7–16 of pregnancy. In those treated with 0.5 ml there were signs of slight maternal toxicity (ataxia) and all the embryos died. In the 0.25 ml group, intrauterine deaths were significantly increased with an increased incidence of cardiovascular malformations and skeletal anomalies in survivors.

Thus, as with formamides, embryotoxicity was readily produced with application via the cutaneous route, although larger volumes were required. It is not known whether repeated applications are necessary to produce these effects. There are no human studies on the reproductive effects of exposure to glycol ethers alone. Syrovadko and Malysheva (1977) reported an increased incidence of menstrual disorders and low-birth-weight babies in women working in the production of enamel-coated wires using a variety of solvents, including EGEE, where skin contact did occur. Pastides et al. (1988) have reported an increased incidence of spontaneous abortion among women working in semiconductor manufacture when there is exposure to glycol ethers, but also to other solvents, gases, acids, and metals.

Hexachlorophene

The antiseptic hexachlorophene (HCP) can be absorbed through the skin resulting in measurable blood concentrations. In 1978, a U.S. FDA Drug Bulletin carried an interim warning to health-care personnel to avoid HCP scrubs, especially if they were pregnant. This warning was based partly on data from France, where infants accidentally exposed to high concentrations of up to 6% HCP in talcum powder suffered damage to the central nervous system and in some cases died (Powell et al., 1973; Shuman et al., 1975).

Subsequently, two epidemiological studies on pregnancy outcome in relation to HCP use have appeared, with conflicting results. Halling (1979) reported on a retrospective study carried out in six hospitals for chronic diseases in Sweden. Clusters of severe congenital malformations occurred more frequently in offspring born to mothers who used HCP soaps 10–60 times/d in hand washing or as hand creams in the first trimester of pregnancy. Overall, 25 of 460 infants had severe malformations in the HCP group compared with 0 out of 233 in controls. However, the malformation rate in the control group was very low (0 versus 7 expected), and this study has been criticized for bias in the selection of exposed and control groups.

Baltazar et al. (1979) carried out a national study in two parts in Sweden. In the first part, they studied a cohort of 1500 women exposed to HCP soaps and disinfectants, working in 31 hospitals for chronic diseases from 1965 to 1975. No general increase in malformations was observed compared with controls matched from existing data registers. In the second part of the study, they looked at a cohort of Swedish women doctors, nurses, and allied professionals who had 29,000 deliveries in the years 1973–1975. HCP use varied in different subgroups of the cohort. Perinatal mortality was increased in certain subgroups but was not related to HCP use. The overall malformation rate was not increased, though the clusters reported by Halling (1979) were detected.

Thus, if there is any risk from dermal exposure to HCP, then it is likely to be very low and not involve major malformations. The possibility that prenatal exposure might cause subtle neurological defects cannot yet be excluded.

Solvents Used in Specific Industries

The major route of exposure to solvents in occupational environments is generally via inhalation. However, in particular industries there may be considerable dermal exposure to solvents. It should be noted that many of the reports on reproductive effects of mixed solvent exposure come from eastern Europe and are difficult to evaluate due to inadequate methodology and reporting. In particular, the matching of controls with exposed subjects for variables other than chemical exposure, which is critical for reliable reproductive epidemiology, is sometimes questionable in these studies.

Syrovadko and co-workers (Syrovadko, 1977; Syrovadko and Malysheva, 1977; Syrovadko et al., 1973) have reported an increased incidence of menstrual disorders and low-birth-weight babies in women working with a variety of solvents and solvent-containing resins and varnishes in the production of electrical insulating materials. Exposure occurred through inhalation and by direct skin contact of the hands and forearms when varnish was applied by hand.

Mukhametova and Vozovaja (1972) have studied menstrual function and pregnancy outcome in glueing operatives in a mechanical rubber products factory. The gluers were exposed to petroleum and chlorinated hydrocarbons, particularly dichloroethane and dichloromethane. Exposure was by inhalation and by skin contact. Concentrations of the various solvents in the air were said to be usually within the maximum permissible levels. The incidences of gynecological and menstrual disorders, spontaneous abortions, premature births, pregnancy and birth complications, and perinatal mortality were all higher in gluers than in controls. Menstrual disorders and premature births in the solvent-exposed group were related to the duration of employment.

Michon (1965) found an increased incidence of prolonged and/or heavy menstrual bleeding in women working in a Polish factory producing leather and rubber shoes and exposed to benzene, toluene, and xylene. Inhalational exposure levels were said to be within permissible workplace limits. Dermal exposure to the solvents was not discussed but was likely to have been considerable, bearing in mind conditions generally prevalent in boot and shoe manufacturing industries at that time. Historically, chronic benzene poisoning has been associated with menorrhagia (Hunt, 1979).

Spontaneous abortion rates were examined in a study from Finland, based on workers identified from the membership register of the Union of Rubber and Leather Workers and from the personnel records of a large rubber factory (Lindbohm et al., 1983). Among union and factory workers generally, there were no increases in spontaneous abortions during employment compared with rates before or after employment in rubber work. However, spontaneous abortions were increased among the 1000 women working in the first 2 mo of pregnancy in the footwear-manufacturing department of the factory, but not among the 450 women in the tire-manufacturing plant. Both groups were exposed to rubber chemicals, but it was suggested that the difference between the two departments might be due to the additional exposure to solvents in the footwear department.

A study on women working in the tire-manufacturing department of a large Swedish rubber plant, where there was opportunity for absorption of chemicals through the skin, confirmed that a cluster of abnormal pregnancies (threatened abortion, spontaneous abortion, or malformation) had occurred in the plant (Axelson et al., 1983).

Further indications that leather workers may be at reproductive risk has come from studies in the United Kingdom and Canada. One study showed an increased risk of perinatal death, due to congenital malformation or macerated stillbirth (Clarke and Mason, 1985), and the other showed an increased incidence of stillbirths (McDonald and McDonald, 1986) among women leather workers. Exposure to glues, silicone, or the leather itself could be involved.

These studies suggest that dermal exposure to certain solvents may be involved in the production of adverse effects on reproductive function, but they require confirmation by other well-controlled studies. While dermal exposure may have been considerable in these industries, the likely contribution of percutaneous absorption, as opposed to inhalation, to the total body burden of solvents was unknown.

CONCLUSIONS

In the present state of knowledge, it is impossible to estimate the extent to which dermal exposure to chemicals may be a hazard to reproduction. Few animal studies have been carried out utilizing agents known to be toxic to male or female reproductive systems with administration by the cutaneous route. However, assessment of the reproductive function of workers is becoming increasingly acknowledged as an important facet of occupational health, and some epidemiological studies have already focused attention on skin absorption as a route of exposure to chemicals that may affect reproduction.

REFERENCES

Axelson, O., Edling, C. and Andersson, L. 1983. Pregnancy outcome among women in a Swedish rubber plant. *Scand. J. Work. Environ. Health* 9:79.

Baltazar, B., Ericson, A. and Kallen, B. 1979. Delivery outcome in women employed in medical occupations in Sweden. *J. Occup. Med.* 21:543.

Barlow, S. M. and Sullivan, F. M. 1982. *Reproductive Hazards of Industrial Chemicals.* London: Academic Press.

Biesalski, H. K. 1989. Comparative assessment of the toxicology of vitamin A and retinoids in man. *Toxicology* 57:117.

Clarke, M. and Mason, E. S. 1985. Leatherwork: A possible hazard to reproduction. *Br. Med. J.* 290:1235.

Council on Environmental Quality. *Chemical Hazards to Reproduction.* Washington, D.C.: U.S. Government Printing Office.

Gleich, J. 1974. The influence of simple acid amides on fetal development of mice. *Naunyn-Schmiedeberg's Arch. Pharmakol.* 282:R25.

Halling, H. 1979. Suspected link between exposure to hexachlorophene and malformed infants. *Ann. NY Acad. Sci.* 320:426.

Hardin, B. D. 1983. Reproductive toxicity of the glycol ethers. *Toxicology* 27:91.

Hardin, B. D., Niemeier, R. W. and Smith, R. J. 1982. Teratogenicity of 2-ethoxyethanol by dermal application. *Drug Chem. Toxicol.* 5:277.

Hunt, V. R. 1979. *Work and the Health of Women.* Boca Raton, Fla.: CRC Press.

Lauwerys, R., Bonnier, Ch., Evrard, P., Gennart, J. P. and Bernard, A. 1987. Prenatal and early postnatal intoxication by inorganic mercury resulting from the maternal use of mercury containing soap. *Hum. Toxicol.* 6:253.

Lindbohm, M.-L., Hemminki, K., Kyyronen, P., Kilpikari, K. and Vainio, H. 1983. Spontaneous abortions among rubber workers and congenital malformations in their offspring. *Scand. J. Work Environ. Health* 9:85.

McDonald, A. D. and McDonald, J. C. 1986. Outcome of pregnancy in leatherworkers. *Br. Med. J.* 292:979.

Michon, S. 1965. Disturbance of menstruation in women working in an atmosphere polluted with aromatic hydrocarbons. *Pol. Tyg. Lek.* 20:1648.

Mukhametova, I. M. and Vozovaja, M. A. 1972. Reproductive power and the incidence of gynecological effects in female workers exposed to the combined effect of benzine and chlorinated hydrocarbons. *Gig. Tr. Prof. Zabol.* 16:6.

Oettel, H. and Frohberg, H. 1964. Teratogene Wirkung einfacher Saureamide in Tieversuch. *Arch. Exp. Pathol. Pharmakol.* 247:363.

Pastides, H., Calabrese, E. J., Hosmer, D. W. and Harris, D. R. 1988. Spontaneous abortion and general illness symptoms among semiconductor manufacturers. *J. Occup. Med.* 30:543.

Powell, H., Swarner, O., Gluck, L. and Lampert, P. 1973. Hexachlorophene myelinopathy in premature infants. *J. Pediatr.* 82:976.

Roll, R. and Bär, F. 1967. Teratogenic effect of monomethylformamide in pregnant mice. *Arzneim. Forsch.* 17:610.

Rosa, F. W. 1983. Teratogenicity of isotretinoin. *Lancet* ii:513.

Rosa, F. W. 1984. Isotretinoin—A newly recognized human teratogen. *Morbidity Mortality Weekly Rep.* 13:171.

Rosa, F. W., Wilk, A. L. and Kelsey, F. O. 1986. Teratogen update: Vitamin A congeners. *Teratology* 33:355.

Shuman, R. M., Leech, R. W. and Alvord, E. C., Jr. 1975. Neurotoxicity of hexachlorophene in humans. II. A clinicopathologic study of 46 premature infants. *Arch. Neurol.* 32:320.

Stula, E. F. and Krauss, W. C. 1977. Embryotoxicity in rats and rabbits from cutaneous application of amide-type solvents and substituted ureas. *Toxicol. Appl. Pharmacol.* 41:35.

Syrovadko, O. N. 1977. Working conditions and health status of women handling organosilicon varnishes containing toluene. *Gig. Tr. Prof. Zabol.* 12:15.

Syrovadko, O. N. and Malysheva, Z. V. 1977. Work conditions and their influence on some specific functions of women engaged in the manufacture of enamel-insulated wires. *Gig. Tr. Prof. Zabol.* 4:25.

Syrovadko, O. N., Skornin, V. F., Pronkova, E. N., Sorkina, N. S., Izyumova, A. S., Gribova, I. A. and Popova, A. F. 1973. Effect of working conditions on the health status and some specific functions of women handling white spirit. *Gig. Tr. Prof. Zabol.* 17:5.

Tuchmann-Duplessis, H. and Mercier-Parot, L. 1965. Production of anomalies in the rat after cutaneous applications of an industrial solvent: Monomethylformamide. *C. R. Acad. Sci. [D] (Paris)* 261:241.

30

risk assessment
in dermatotoxicology

- Claire A. Franklin ▪ Diana A. Somers ▪
  ▪ Daniel Krewski ▪

As the number and volume of chemicals used increase, there are demands that the associated health risks be identified. In the past, the emphasis was more on identifying the presence or absence of hazard or danger, and governments were called upon to ban a product or eliminate its danger. Currently, with the advent of increasingly more sensitive analytical tools, capable of detecting extremely low levels of chemicals, the task is much more complex. The result is that the risk assessment process has become formalized and the testing requirements more stringent.

Humans can be exposed to chemicals in the food they eat, the water they drink, the air they breathe, and through the products they contact daily. Chemicals may enter the body following absorption through the gastrointestinal tract, the lungs, and the skin. Under some circumstances, these sites of absorption may also be adversely affected by the agent of interest.

The importance of the skin as a target tissue and as a route of entry has led to increased emphasis on the development of tests to aid in the diagnosis of the dermatoses resulting from exposure and to the prediction of the dermal systemic hazard of chemicals prior to marketing. Risk assessment procedures for dermal exposure to chemical hazards are the focus of this chapter.

The use of a structured approach for assessing the health risks associated with exposure to environmental and workplace chemicals is relatively new. The first publications on risk assessment/risk management as a formal discipline did not appear until the mid to late 1970s (Lowrance, 1976; Kates, 1978). The lack of a standard set of risk-related definitions and of a corresponding risk assessment/risk management model led to confusion in oral and written scientific communications.

In an attempt to alleviate the problem, several models have been proposed (Krewski and Birkwood, 1987). A generalized scheme outlining the steps that should be taken when doing a risk assessment is presented in Figure 1. The first step involves the identification of the adverse effect on health through toxicity testing in animals, controlled human studies, epidemiological studies, case reports, and, in some instances, structure-activity relationships to known toxic compounds. The second step, risk estimation, involves quantitative estimation of the risks associated with the hazards identified through testing. This requires a knowledge of the shape of the dose response curve, of the level at which no adverse toxic effects are observed (NOAEL), and the level of human exposure. Simple models to relate the effects seen in animals to those likely to occur in humans can be used, or complex mathematical models can be employed to extrapolate data obtained using high doses to low doses in animals, and from animals to humans. Once the risks have been estimated, the third stage is to develop options to deal with the risk at hand. These options could include reducing exposure through controls or removal of the product from the market. Option analysis often involves a risk/benefit analysis and a determination of the feasibility of various options. These steps constitute the formal risk assessment process. Risk management involves decisions about which option to implement, monitoring and evaluating the situation after implementation, and critically reviewing outcomes to ensure that the management process is successful.

The purpose of this chapter is to acquaint the reader with the steps in risk assessment, and to illustrate how they are utilized in the field of dermatotoxicology. This chapter is written from a Canadian regulatory perspective using pesticides as the primary example. However, the basic principles of toxicology and risk assessment applied to this group of chemicals should be applicable for most xenobiotics to which the public is exposed via the dermal route.

RISK ASSESSMENT WHEN SKIN IS THE TARGET TISSUE

A variety of mechanical, physical, and biological agents can cause occupational and nonoccupational skin diseases. The resulting dermatoses can be placed into two broad categories: inflammatory conditions and tumors. Inflammatory conditions can be caused by (1) infections (viral, bacterial, mycobacterial, fungal, scabies, helminths, and arthropods); (2) chemicals that can cause irritant dermatitis, allergic contact dermatitis, or contact urticaria syndrome; (3) sunlight (the most common cause of bullous diseases); (4) diseases, connective tissue diseases, and granulomatous and fibrotic processes are additional inflammatory responses. The second major category of dermatoses is skin cancer,

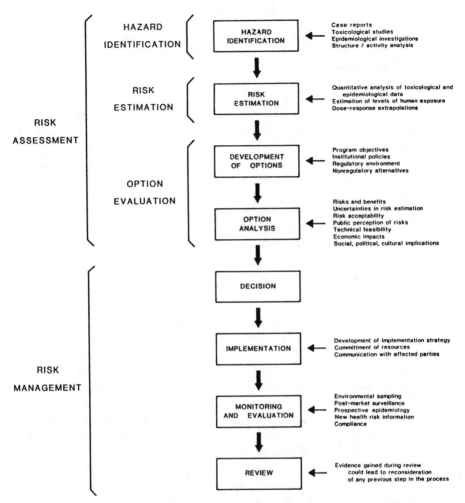

FIGURE 1 Summary of the steps in risk assessment/risk management. (Canada Health Protection Branch, 1990a).

which can occur as either benign or malignant lesions, and specific chemicals and radiation are known causes.

Since chemicals are responsible for many occupational dermatoses, a wide range of tests has been developed that can be used to determine the potential for a chemical to cause a specific effect. These tests may be required to assess the hazard of a chemical before it is used, or they can be used to diagnose dermatoses observed in people using the chemicals. Predictive tests can be used to assess the potential of the chemical to cause irritation, sensitization, phototoxicity, contact urticaria syndrome, and skin cancer.

Dermal Irritation

Description.   Irritant dermatitis is a nonimmunological, local inflammatory response at the site of application following single, repeated, or continuous
contact with a chemical. It is characterized by erythema (reddening of the skin)
and edema (accumulation of fluid). Corrosion is the result of irreversible damage at the application site. Organic and inorganic acids, alkalies, metal salts,
solvents, resins, and soaps can act on the keratin, dissolve surface lipids, denat-
ure protein, or induce enzymes in the skin. The immune system is not involved
in these responses.

A distinguishing characteristic of an irritant response is the decline in the
intensity of the response with time (usually 24–72 h). The time course of this
decline may vary with the chemical substance, the exposure concentration, and
variability of individual thresholds for irritation responses. Irritant dermatitis is
classified into three types according to exposure parameters and irritant potential of the chemical. Type 1 is the acute response observed after a single skin
exposure to a strong chemical substance. Skin etching/chemical burns are typical of this response. Type 2 is the response observed following repeated low-
grade irritation. This response can be induced by environmental factors such as
repeated exposure to cold dry atmospheres. When chemically induced, there is
usually no visible reaction after a single exposure. The condition in its mildest
form presents itself as a chapping reaction involving only the horny layers of
the skin. In its severest form, hemorrhagic fissures (cracks in the dermis) occur.
The condition is generally reversed when exposure to the irritant ceases. A
reaction of this type is the most common form of occupational dermatitis observed. Type 3 is also a reaction to repeated low-grade irritation. However, for
unknown reasons the reaction progresses to a chronic spongiotic dermatitis,
similar in appearance to eczema. The condition is not easily reversed and
presents a significant occupational problem when it occurs.

Predictive tests for dermal irritation.   A wide variety of predictive tests
has been developed based on testing a small surface area on animals or the
immersion of the animal in the test solution. The wide divergence of results has
led to the development of a wealth of experimental procedures that attempt to
reduce the variability of the data (U.S. EPA, 1982a; Ritter and Franklin, 1990).

Animal testing.   The Organization for Economic Co-operation and Development (OECD) test guideline for acute dermal irritation testing is widely
used for a variety of chemicals including industrial chemicals and pesticides. It
is based on the Draize test (1955), and employs applying a patch to the shaved
skin of a rabbit. Many other test guidelines use a similar procedure. The guinea
pig immersion test is also used for certain types of chemicals (Jackson and
Goldner, 1990). Repeat exposure protocols are utilized in many cases, and the
duration and frequency of dosing vary. In general, the animal tests reliably
predict nonirritant and severe-irritant chemicals, but they often fail to discriminate between mild and moderate irritants (Phillips et al., 1972; U.S. EPA,

1982a). The rabbit generally overpredicts the reaction observed in humans (Nixon et al., 1975). This may be advantageous in some situations but is a flaw in the test. The guinea pig test seems to correlate better with human tests for certain types of chemicals, and it serves as a useful adjunct for screening chemicals (EPA, 1982a). Other animal tests such as the mouse ear swelling test and the rabbit ear assay are useful alternatives for studying irritant effects in animals (Jackson and Goldner, 1990).

Human testing. The same general principles applied to animal predictive tests are used in human testing. Patch tests or arm immersion tests varying in exposure duration of 2 h to 21 d for single applications and from 2 to 21 repeated exposures have been used. The application sites may be occluded or not, and the skin abraded or intact. If the intent is to maximize the irritant response, the skin is abraded and the site occluded. At least 29 different procedures have been used on humans and the results have been extremely variable (U.S. EPA, 1982a). Human tests are generally used to diagnose dermatoses seen in people exposed to chemicals, but these tests may be used for premarket predictive purposes to determine potential for reactions to cosmetics and dermally applied medicaments.

Structure-activity relationships. The use of structure/activity relationships to predict irritation potential of chemicals has been examined. However, there is no consistency among reported findings. Some studies demonstrate poor predictive capabilities, while other studies show good correlation in the intensity of irritation of chemicals and activity (Björnberg, 1987).

In Vitro tests. In an attempt to minimize the use of animals in irritation testing, *in vitro* approaches have been examined. Test systems using human keratinocyte cultures are actively being explored for predictive potential. Fibroblast cultures have been developed to study the irritant properties of synthetic detergents (De Leo et al., 1982). Artificial skin products based on cocultured fibroblasts and keratinocytes in a collagen matrix are also being tested for predictive irritation capacity (*Biotechnology News,* April 27, 1990, p. 8).

Risk assessment for dermal irritation. Most of the tests utilized in both animals and humans rely on visual scoring of the irritant response (Table 1). In a collaborative study involving over 20 laboratories, there were many discrepancies in the resulting data, and it was concluded that the Draize test should not be used to classify materials to avoid inconsistent data (Weil and Scala, 1971). Attempts have been made to incorporate other end points into irritation testing, including histological examination of the skin (Ingram and Grasso, 1975), histopathologic examination (Brown, 1971), dermal respiration, and other parameters (Lansdown, 1972), or simply the presence or absence of erythema (Kligman and Wooding, 1967). Despite many modifications to testing protocols there is still no standardized, objective procedure for assessing skin irritancy.

Although the rabbit may not accurately predict the magnitude and mechanism of response identically to humans, it does serve as a useful tool to screen chemicals prior to use in humans. The rabbit is more sensitive to irritants than

TABLE 1 Summary of Predictive Tests Used to Assess Toxic Effects on the Skin

Dermatosis	Test species	Predictive test	Risk assessment
Irritant dermatitis	Rabbits	Draize Test in Rabbit (OECD, FIFRA, TSCA, IRLG)	Numerical score for erythema and edema on abraded and intact skin Primary irritation of 0 (negligible) to 8 (severe)
	Rabbits	5-d dermal test	Same as Draize test
	Guinea pig	Immersion	Numerical score for skin changes Guinea pig immersion grading scale 10 (normal) 0 (death)
	Humans	2-h to 21-d continuous exposure irritation test	Numerical code 1 (mild) to 4 (severe)
		Arm immersion test Repeat exposure	Ranked on number of days to reach initial reaction for index of irritation potential
Allergic contact dermatitis	Guinea pig	Draize patch test	Intensity of erythema is scored Not very predictive for weak or moderately weak compounds
		Freund's complete adjuvant	Varying doses used Scored at + or −
		Open epicutaneous	Several concentrations (dose/response) Scored as + or −
		Closed patch test	Varying concentrations Occluded site Scored 1 (slight) to 3 (marked erythema)
		Maximization test	Varying concentrations Scored 1 (weak) to 8 (extreme redness and swelling) Good for weak allergens but gives false positives
		Split adjuvant	Good screening Scored 0 (normal) to 5+ (bright pink marked thickening)
		Foot pad test	Scored for 1 (slight) to 4 (red) erythema, and 1 (slight) to 3 (marked thickening)
Allergic contact dermatitis	Humans	Predictive tests (maximization test)	Identify allergens singly
		Diagnostic (standard screening kit)	Identify substances that are posing clinical problems
		Use tests	Assess safety of ingredients in product

718

humans; therefore, a negative response would certainly indicate that there would likely be no response in humans. While it is true that some chemicals cause a positive response in rabbits but are negative in humans, there are few examples of the converse (Calabrese, 1983).

Given these observations, there is no attempt to determine if the irritation effect is dose dependent and to establish the margin of safety between effect and exposure. Rather, the approach is to ensure that the hazard potential is identified so that steps can be taken to reduce exposure to a minimum. As a result, the emphasis is on gathering information on the potency of the irritant, the intended use (occupational, cosmetic, medicinal, pesticidal), population likely to be exposed (workers, adults, children), and the exposure frequency, duration, and condition.

This type of assessment can result in the development of measures to reduce exposure such as changes in formulation from liquid to granular, reduction of concentration of the product, use of closed systems in the case of pesticides or industrial chemicals, and use of protective clothing, barrier creams, and stringent labeling. When the chemical is a severe skin irritant, restricted use or elimination of use of the product may be considered.

Dermal Sensitization

Description. Sensitization or allergic contact dermatitis is a delayed, immunologically mediated response to a chemical. Initial contact with the chemical does not appear to have any effect on the skin. After a short delay (about 5 d), reexposure to the chemical causes an acute inflammatory reaction. The sensitization reaction is a T-lymphocyte-mediated immune response to chemical haptens that conjugate with protein components of skin to form a complete antigen. Clinically, the dermatitis may be similar to an irritant response. Symptoms include erythema and infiltration. Papules, vesicles, and coalescing vesicles may develop. In contrast to an irritation response, which is often irregular and patchy, an allergic contact dermatitis reaction on the skin is generally homogeneous in nature. Under test conditions the reaction often extrudes beyond the test patch whereas irritant responses generally manifest at site of contact. In contrast to an irritant response, which may diminish fairly quickly with time, an allergic contact dermatitis usually takes longer to develop and to resolve after exposure. In animals (guinea pig), the condition is distinguishable histologically from an irritant response by increased numbers of tissue basophils in the allergic cell infiltrate and by the presence of the Ia markers on keratinocytes in the late phases of the reaction (Fisher and Maibach, 1987).

Chemicals that elicit allergic contact dermatitis often have the following characteristics: generally simple substances, molecular weight (MW) rarely exceeds 500, water soluble, permeable to skin, form conjugates with skin protein, and usually form strong covalent bonds. The most common contact allergic sensitizers are botanical in origin (poison ivy, poison oak). However, industrial chemicals such as nickel sulfate, phenols, and potassium dichromate are well-known sensitizers. Tests used to predict or diagnose sensitization are outlined in Table 1.

Predictive tests for dermal sensitization. *Animal testing.* Numerous animal species (mouse, rat, rabbit, hamster, dog, chicken, guinea pig) have been studied for their capacity to predict the human dermal sensitization potential of chemicals for humans (Maguire, 1973). The mouse and dog can usually be sensitized with strong allergens, but they respond erratically to moderate and weak sensitizers. The rabbit and chicken have been observed to be generally resistant to even the strong sensitizers. Consistently, the young, adult guinea pig responds more often in a manner similar to humans. Most chemicals known to be strong sensitizers in human subjects have been readily detected as positive in the guinea pig assay. However, there are instances, especially with weak sensitizers, when the guinea pig assay was not predictive of results in humans, suggesting humans are more sensitive to contact sensitizers (Buehler, 1965). The value of the guinea pig as a good animal model for screening the potential of moderate/strong sensitizers has resulted in a proliferation of guinea pig assays to more than a dozen different assays. The protocols are generally grouped according to the following methods of administration of the test chemical:

1. Topical application used in closed patch test and the open epicutaneous test.
2. Intradermal injection used in the Draize and Freund complete adjuvant tests.
3. Combination of topical application and intradermal injection used in the guinea pig maximization test, optimization, split-adjuvant, and the footpad tests.

Human testing. Several human tests have been developed to examine chemicals for their potential for causing allergic contact dermatitis. For the most part, the human tests are used clinically to define the causative agents for a reported dermatitis (Marzulli and Maibach, 1987). As with animal testing, the human tests are specifically designed to maximize exposure and likelihood of reaction. Occlusive conditions are generally employed, and in some cases sodium lauryl sulfate is used to damage the skin and facilitate penetration of the test substances.

The two most frequently used human tests are (1) the modified Draize test (Marzulli and Maibach, 1974) and (2) the modified maximization test (Kligman and Epstein, 1975). In brief, these tests involve human exposure to test substances at concentrations as large as possible without inducing irritation. Induction exposure is conducted under occlusive conditions for 24- to 48-h periods, several days per week for a period of 2–3 consecutive weeks. The protocols then incorporate a 2- 3-wk rest phase. Challenge patches (with the highest nonirritating dose of test material possible) are applied for 24–48 h, and the dose site is graded for reaction generally at 72–96 h after exposure. At this time, any mild irritant reaction will have faded and slow allergens will have had time to elicit a reaction.

For human diagnostic purposes, a variety of screening trays containing numerous combinations of well-known allergens in petrolatum at nonirritant concentrations have been developed to test humans for contact sensitization reactions. Trays of preservatives, perfumes, metals, epoxy resins, plastics, solvents, and rubber are available for testing.

A human predictive screening test has been used for testing fragrance materials. Briefly, 25 individuals are exposed to the fragrance material at 10 times the normal use concentration. A positive reaction in any one individual necessitates further investigation of the material for contact sensitization potential.

All of the human bioassays require care and experience to administer properly (Marzulli and Maibach, 1987). False negatives due to a variety of causes (inadequate patch contact, insufficient test material, decreased summer sensitization rate) are frequent. False positives due to confusion between an irritation response or hyperirritable skin and a true contact sensitization response have also been described (Marzulli and Maibach, 1987; Epstein, 1966).

Structure-activity relationships. Despite the common characteristics noted for many chemicals that may induce allergic contact dermatitis, structure-activity relationships do not reliably predict if a chemical will combine with skin proteins. For some groups of related chemicals (e.g., chrysanthemum family), the responsible chemical group that binds with skin protein has been determined and activity can be predicted. For other groups of chemicals (heavy metals), it is not known why some (nickel, chromium) will induce an allergic contact dermatitis response while others (gold) do not (Hjorth, 1987).

In vitro methods. Because contact allergic dermatitis is a cell-mediated response to a chemical–skin protein conjugate and requires interaction of a number of different cell types, direct *in vitro* methodologies have been difficult to develop. However, indirect assays to evaluate activity of lymphocytes, macrophages, polymorphonuclear leukocytes have been established (Luster et al., 1982). As well, experimental studies in humans have demonstrated that eosinophilia (5–20% of circulating leukocytes) is a common observation during dermal sensitization to multiple antigens (Kligman, 1966a, 1966b).

Risk assessment for dermal sensitization. In many countries regulatory requirements include premarket testing of chemicals (drugs, pesticides) for contact dermal sensitization potential. Predictive tests in animals and humans facilitate only comparative (not absolute) grading of test chemicals into weak or strong sensitizers. The grading is based on the number of test subjects that become sensitized and not the severity of the skin reaction. The ranking into weak and strong sensitizers should be applied with caution since there are chemicals (lanolin) that fail to sensitize significantly in bioassays but have an extensive history of contact sensitization in clinical practice. Other chemicals such as gold and cobalt show sensitization potential in bioassays but rarely result in clinical problems. Despite the inherent subjectivity in grading responses in sensitization tests and the apparently small number of test subjects (25–200), all of the common allergens have been identified in a well-designed and executed multiple insult patch test (Marzulli and Maibach, 1987).

Risk assessment for potential contact dermal sensitizers is qualitative rather than quantitative in recognition of the fact that under appropriate conditions all chemicals have the potential to become sensitizers. Many factors are therefore considered during the risk assessment process for chemicals identified as contact dermal sensitizers. These include potency of sensitizer, concentration of sensitizer in use product, availability of alternative products, use (occupational, cosmetic, drug, pesticide, environmental), exposure (frequency of use, duration of contact when used, transient/continuous use, exposure site, normal/abnormal skin, voluntary/involuntary exposure), and population exposed (adult, children, aged, sensitive subgroups).

Dependent on the weighting of the above variables, even strong sensitizers have been made available to consumers. For instance, some hair dyes are strong sensitizers. Risk assessment indicated normal use to be limited to adult hair and normal scalp skin that is known to be a poor site for eliciting sensitization reactions. Exposure would likely be voluntary, transient, and of short contact duration. Under such circumstances risk management may include label warnings of sensitization potential or label suggestions to perform some form of pre-use patch test. In contrast, the risk management approach for a mild to moderate sensitizer such as a residual pesticide intended for use in nursing homes or schools may be completely different. In this use scenario, the exposed population is primarily children and the elderly whose skin absorption properties may be enhanced (Schalla and Schaffer, 1982; Shah et al., 1987, 1988). Furthermore, exposure is involuntary and is expected to be continuous. Under such circumstances, simply labeling the product as a potential skin sensitizer may not be sufficient. Risk management options include restriction of use to exclude such settings (schools, nursing homes), change in use from broadcast to crack and crevice treatment only, or change in concentration of the sensitizing chemical in the formulation. For topical drugs, the risk assessment may take yet another approach, which includes a strong consideration for benefit and the availability of alternative drugs. Reducing the concentration of the drug in a formulation has been a successful means of reducing the hazard of some sensitizers such as neomycin.

Phototoxic Dermal Irritation

Description. Phototoxic dermal irritation is a nonimmune dermatitis induced by a chemical or its metabolites after it has undergone light-induced molecular changes. Most photosensitive chemicals are activated by ultraviolet (UV) radiation in the range of 315–400 nm (UVA). The mechanism of irritation is thought to occur through UV excitation of the exogenous chemicals/

metabolites in the skin and subsequent dissipation of energy as heat, vibrations, fluorescence, free radical formation, or photochemical alteration (generally oxidative) resulting in oxidation of membranes and other cellular components. The resultant dermatitis can be acute or chronic in nature. The clinical response is generally mild, although severe reactions have been reported. As well, chronic repeated phototoxic reactions can result in persistent hyperpigmentation of the skin. The extent of the irritation response is dependent on the concentration of photosensitive chemical in the skin and the number of photons of UV exposure. Exposure may occur directly following topical contact or indirectly after chemical delivery to the skin following oral or parenteral intake. The reaction can occur with first exposure to a phototoxic chemical; an incubation period is not required (Emmett, 1987).

Predictive tests for phototoxic dermal irritation. *Animal testing.* Numerous animals have been tested for their ability to predict phototoxicity in humans. In order of decreasing sensitivity they include hairless mouse, rabbit, swine, guinea pig, squirrel monkey, hamster. Most animal tests are based on the same experimental design: percutaneous localization of the phototoxic agent and exposure to nonerythemogenic light. Most known phototoxic agents will induce dermatitis at wavelengths that generally do not produce erythema. For topical agents there may be a lag time (particularly for slowly penetrating compounds) before sufficient concentration of chemical is attained in the skin. Accordingly, the choice of vehicle has a strong influence, and it has been suggested that predictive tests include testing the vehicle intended in the formulation for human use. The tests have been summarized (U.S. EPA, 1982a).

Human testing. Human testing for phototoxic dermal irritation is a simple process. Few subjects are needed and a small area on the body can be tested with and without exposure to UV radiation. For chemicals that penetrate poorly, absorption can be enhanced by choosing highly permeable skin sites or by stratum corneum stripping with cellophane tape. The methods currently used are summarized (U.S. EPA, 1982a).

In vitro tests. There are a few *in vitro* tests that have been developed to predict phototoxicity (Jackson and Goldner, 1990). These include the *Candida* test, RBC photohemolysis test, histidine photomediation test, mouse peritoneal macrophage test, and human peripheral lymphocyte test adapted as a phototoxic screen test. All of these tests are based on observable cellular changes following chemical and UV exposure.

Risk assessment for phototoxic dermal irritation. Premarket predictive testing for phototoxic irritation potential is not routinely required for chemicals such as pesticides unless the chemical is structurally related to a known phototoxic irritant. As a result, except for fragrance materials, few chemicals have been examined extensively for phototoxic potential. For chemicals identified as phototoxic irritants the risk assessment process is generally conducted as described above for irritants.

Contact Photoallergy

Description. Analogous to contact allergic dermatitis, contact photoallergic dermatitis is a T-lymphocyte-mediated, delayed hypersensitivity response to a chemical after activation by UV light (Harber et al., 1987). Postulated mechanisms of action include alteration of the haptenic group by UV light (generally UVA; 315–400 nm) or UV-induced changes in the avidity with which the hapten combines with the carrier protein to form a complete antigen. Symptoms often include an eczematous reaction of acute onset 1–2 d after sun exposure. Generally, the dermatitis is mild and the reaction is usually confined to light-exposed skin such as the face, v of neck, and extensor surface of the arms. Contact photoallergic reaction may result in long-term adverse responses to sun exposure (Emmett, 1987; Harber et al., 1987).

Predictive tests for contact photoallergy. Animal testing. Similar to recommendations for contact sensitization testing, the animal of choice for predicting contact photoallergic reactions in humans is the guinea pig (Harber et al., 1987). Briefly, the chemical is applied to the shaved, depilated back of guinea pigs. Following a short wait (~30 min), the treated area is irradiated with an adequate dose of nonerythemogenic ultraviolet radiation (generally between 315 and 400 nm; UVA). The procedure is repeated daily for varying periods of time. Following a rest period of about 2 w, the challenge dose is applied at 2 previously untreated sites. One site is exposed to UVA light while the other site is kept occluded from light. Adequate controls (areas receiving light only, areas receiving chemical only) are necessary to differentiate between responses due to light alone, light-activated chemical, or unrelated toxic effect of the chemical.

Human testing. A maximization test for detecting photoallergy potential has been developed for human studies. The testing procedure is similar to that described for animals. The test chemical in a petrolatum vehicle is applied to the back of volunteers. Prior to the first application only, the skin site is tape stripped to glistening. Following application of the chemical the site is irradiated and occluded for 24–48 h. A minimum of five induction exposures is recommended. Challenge exposure occurs about 2 wk after the last induction treatment. As per the animal studies, two skin sites should be treated with the chemical but only one site receives irradiation. Treated sites are usually evaluated 48–72 h after irradiation.

Risk assessment for contact photoallergens. Predictive tests for photoallergic potential are not normally required by regulatory agencies unless the chemical is structurally similar to known photoallergens. For suspect chemicals the risk determination approach is identical to that for potential contact sensitizers. However, because exposure to UV is a requirement for the photosensitization reaction, the risk management may include avoidance of sunlight following chemical exposure. It is recognized that this option may be difficult to achieve.

Contact Urticaria

Description. Contact urticaria is a specific dermal reaction resulting from exposure to a chemical. Itching, tingling, or burning sensations, erythema/edema, and urticaria (itching wheals) are common symptoms that usually appear within minutes to an hour after contact and disappear by 24 h. The reaction is thought to result from chemically induced release of inflammatory mediators such as histamines, leukocytes, and prostaglandins. It is often difficult to differentiate between contact urticaria and an irritation reaction. Contact urticaria can be either immunologically or nonimmunologically based. The nonimmunological form is most common and symptoms generally present as a localized reaction with no systemic involvement. The reaction can vary depending on the chemical substance, concentration, and skin site. Immunologically based contact urticaria is an immediate reaction observed in previously sensitized individuals. The contact urticant penetrates through the skin to interact with antibodies on mast cells, resulting in release of vasoactive compounds including histamine. Immunologically based urticarial reactions often extend beyond the contact site. In addition to the skin symptoms, clinical manifestations may occur, including rhinitis, conjunctivitis, asthma, or anaphylactic shock. Specific antibodies to the chemical antigen may be detectable in the serum of patients with symptoms.

Predictive tests for contact urticaria. *Animal testing.* Animal tests for predicting urticarial potential are not well developed, although the guinea pig ear thickness test has been proposed as a reproducible, quick model for quantification of edema (Lahti and Maibach, 1984).

Human testing. Human predictive testing for urticarial potential is not normally conducted unless symptoms appear and diagnostic investigation is warranted.

In Vitro *methods.* Predictive *in vitro* tests are usually not conducted to detect urticarial potential of chemicals. *In vitro* tests are available to detect release of vasoactive compounds from cells. Tests include the rat peritoneal mast cell test, rabbit polymorphonuclear leukocyte test, and human neutrophil test (Jackson and Goldner, 1990). Serum immunoglobulin E (IgE) measurements have also been used for diagnostic purposes.

Risk assessment for contact urticaria. Unless structure-activity relationships warrant investigation, predictive studies for urticarial potential are usually not done. Accordingly, risk estimation is not routinely conducted. Risk estimation for chemicals demonstrating nonimmunological urticarial potential is approached in a manner similar to that for dermal irritants, keeping in mind that the responses are often mild and dissipate quickly. The magnitude of immunologically based responses can be severe and may be life threatening. Because such responses are usually characteristic to the exposed individual, the risk estimation is tailored to the individual circumstances. Risk management approaches include avoidance of contact dermal exposure.

Skin Carcinogenesis

Description. The skin is the primary barrier to xenobiotics and represents the first target for action of chemicals with carcinogenic potential. The skin and associated glands also contain a variety of enzymes capable of metabolizing precarcinogens to active compounds. These observations were exemplified by the link between scrotal cancer and dermal exposure to soot.

A considerable amount of information on skin carcinogenesis has been derived from studies conducted on compounds containing polycyclic aromatic hydrocarbons (PAH), benzo[*a*]pyrene in particular (Shubik, 1975). The concept of cocarcinogenesis and promoting action arose from studies conducted initially by Berenblum (1941). Prolonged and repeated exposure to UVB radiation is associated with development of skin cancer. Alone, UVA radiation is generally not associated with carcinogenic effects. However, UVA radiation is responsible for most phototoxic and photoallergic reactions, which can cause repeated skin injury. Animal studies have shown that phototoxic injuries plus UVA exposure can result in skin cancer if the insult is repeated for an extensive period of time. Some animal studies have also demonstrated that the effects of chemicals that cause skin cancer and effects of UVB radiation are additive. Furthermore, synergistic effects of radiation and chemical promoters have also been demonstrated in animal studies.

Predictive tests for skin cancer. Animal testing. For most chemicals there is little or no emphasis on conducting predictive quantitative dermal studies to determine the potential for skin carcinogenicity because these studies are expensive and technically difficult to do (Schubik, 1975). Predictive dermal animal carcinogenic studies may be required for topically applied drugs, depending on the proposed duration of administration of the product to humans, when structure-activity relationships to known skin carcinogens are noted or when epidemiological data suggests cause/effect relationships. Traditionally, the *rabbit* has been the animal of choice for predictive studies of prolonged dermal administration, although mouse, rat, dog, hamster, monkey, and pig may be used.

Human testing. For obvious ethical and technical reasons, predictive studies for skin carcinogens are not conducted in humans. Epidemiological studies may be conducted to correlate rates of skin cancer development and exposure to specific chemicals. From such studies, predictive risks or odds ratios may be obtained for an exposed population.

Risk assessment for skin cancer. For chemicals identified as potential skin carcinogens (creosote), and where adequate animal studies are available, a quantitative skin cancer risk assessment may be conducted using an acceptable mathematical model, as will be discussed in the following section on systemic effects.

Summary of Risk Assessment Approaches for Dermatoses

Data from animal tests to predict the potential of a chemical to cause irritant dermatoses are used generally in a semiquantitative manner. The scoring of effects is subjective and some end points are difficult to interpret. Nevertheless, these tests are valuable to screen out chemicals that are strong irritants or sensitizers. For pesticides, there are usually only data from a single irritation study and a single sensitization study. The identification of positive responses in animal tests leads to labeling of the product to warn workers of potential problems. Extremely strong positive results might result in restricted uses. For cosmetics and drugs that are not strongly positive in animal tests, predictive testing in humans is usually the next step. Positive results in clinical trials are usually taken seriously because of the limits on predictive capacity of human trials involving relatively few volunteers. Positive sensitization data may result in premarket restriction or elimination of the product. When dermal predictive tests are performed as diagnostic tools to identify the etiology of a dermatosis in a worker, positive results may lead to control measures on exposure to specific workers or groups of workers to minimize disease.

Improvements in our capability to quantitatively predict health effects should be sought especially for products that have significant exposure to humans.

RISK ASSESSMENT WHEN SKIN IS THE ROUTE OF ENTRY INTO THE BODY (SYSTEMIC TOXICITY)

Because humans are exposed to such a wide variety of chemicals with potential for causing adverse health effects, many countries have established legislation under which manufacturers are required to assess the toxicity of their products. Most of the information is obtained through toxicity studies in animals, using the tests outlined in Table 2. Detailed protocols for these tests are available (U.S. EPA, 1982b; National Research Council, 1977a; OECD, 1981). Many regulatory agencies require that studies submitted to them in support of registration be conducted according to these specific protocols, or they may have their own test guidelines. Not all products have to be supported by an extensive data package, but, in general, the requirements are more stringent for products to which the general public is exposed through food and water than those that are used under controlled conditions (industrial chemicals).

The purpose of the battery of required toxicology tests is to identify the toxic potential of the test chemical following single and repeated exposure to both sexes of animals, to determine whether the route of exposure (oral, dermal, inhalation) modifies the response, and to determine the dose response. For many years, it was presumed that the skin was an impenetrable barrier protecting the body from systemic exposure. This, of course, is not true, and a wide

TABLE 2 Types of Predictive Toxicity Tests Used to Assess Health Hazards

Acute		Subchronic		Chronic	
Test	Species[a]	Test	Species	Test	Species
LD50/Acute oral	Rats, dogs	Oral, 90 d	Rats	Oral,[d] 2 yr toxicity	Rats
		Oral, 6 mo	Dogs	Oral,[d] 2 yr oncogenicity	Rats, mice
Dermal	Rabbits	Dermal, 14–90 d	Rats	[b]	
Inhalation	Rats	Inhalation 90 d	Rats	[b]	
		Developmental/teratology, period of organogenesis	Rats, rabbits		
Dermal irritation; eye irritation[c]	Rabbits			Two generation reproduction	Rats
Skin sensitization	Guinea pigs				
Delayed neurotoxicity	Domestic hens	Delayed neurotoxicity	Domestic hens		
		Mutagenicity			

[a]Predominantly used, others are allowed.
[b]Occasionally inhalation, dermal, and dermal skin painting tests are done.
[c]May be required if dermal irritation is negative or mildly positive.
[d]May be combined into one study.

728

range of chemicals are known to enter, via the skin, the systemic circulation for distribution to target tissues following dermal exposure. Despite this, most toxicity tests are conducted using the oral route of exposure, although there may frequently be a requirement for dermal acute studies to ascertain whether there is significant absorption and systemic toxicity.

Predictive Dermal Systemic Tests

Acute dermal toxicity tests. Acute dermal toxicity studies are a premarket, regulatory requirement for many chemicals for which human exposure by the dermal route is likely. Acute dermal studies are conducted to determine whether a substance can be absorbed in quantities sufficient to elicit a systemic effect. Historically, these tests were based on the determination of acute lethality (LD50 test), but due to concerns over animal welfare, many regulatory agencies no longer require this test. Some regulatory groups incorporate limit tests that obviate the need for further investigation if animals receiving a topical dose of at least 2000 mg/kg body weight demonstrate no adverse effects.

Although recommended methods suggest use of rabbit, rat, or guinea pig, most acute dermal studies are performed on the rabbit. Young adult animals of both sexes are used. Females should be nulliparous and nonpregnant. Normally, the test chemical is administered on intact skin, although some regulatory groups stipulate use of abraded skin. A minimum exposure time of 4 h is considered a realistic simulation to expected exposure in humans.

Risk assessment for acute tests. Data from acute oral or dermal studies are used in the risk assessment process to rank chemicals into toxicity categories (Table 3). In Canada, for certain types of chemicals such as pesticides, the toxicity category dictates commercial channels for the product and, in effect, may restrict access. Chemicals that cause no adverse systemic effects following acute dermal administration of high concentrations likely penetrate so poorly that they present little appreciable risk for systemic effects. For chemicals that are readily absorbed dermally causing systemic effects, restrictions minimizing dermal exposure could be put in place. These might include label warnings, use

TABLE 3 Toxicity Hazard Categories and Product Classification Based on Acute Oral and Dermal Testing

	LD50 (mg/kg body weight)		
Toxicity rating[a]	Oral[a]	Dermal[b]	Product classification[b]
Extremely toxic	<50	100	Restricted
Very toxic	50–500	101–1000	Commercial
Moderate toxicity	500 +	1000 +	Domestic

[a]Oral LD50 classification according to Klaassen et al. (1986).
[b]Dermal rating, product classification codes according to regulations in *Guidelines for Registering Pesticides and Other Control Products* under the Pest Control Products Act in Canada.

restrictions, volume and/or concentration restrictions, protective clothing requirements, and/or formulation changes.

Repeat dose exposure tests. Many regulatory agencies require repeated
dosing dermal studies for products that are likely to repeatedly come in contact
with human skin. Repeated dose studies include short-term dermal exposure
studies (repeated dermal exposure up to 90 d), dermal developmental studies
(repeated dermal exposure of pregnant animals), or chronic dermal studies (dermal dosing over most of an animal's lifetime). Short-term dermal toxicity studies are usually required for products intended for prolonged, repeated application to large areas of the human body. Typical products include sun screens and
topical drugs. Short-term limit tests with a single high dose administration have
been used to rule out further dermal testing of chemicals with very low percutaneous absorption.

For developmental toxicity testing, almost universally the chemical is first
tested in at least two species via oral exposure (gavage) to maximize systemic
dose and better define developmental toxicity potential. Chemicals identified as
developmental toxicants by the oral route and that are likely to result in dermal
exposure may require dermal developmental toxicity studies. Recently, however, some chemical companies have attempted to supply only dermal developmental toxicity studies for products for which the sole route of human exposure
is dermal. Advantages to this approach include the fact that dermal studies are
often the sole studies in which the material formulated with other chemicals
such as carriers and solvents is examined. Dermal testing also avoids the problem inherent in extrapolating from oral exposure in animals to dermal exposure
in humans.

However, the lack of sensitivity of dermal testing, coupled with problems
of species extrapolation, dictates that at least one of the studies be conducted by
the oral route to fully determine the potential for developmental toxicity.

Chronic dermal studies are not routinely conducted due to technical difficulties and excessive costs of labor when performing such studies. However,
systemic effects can be examined by oral dosing, which usually provides a more
accurate means of attaining a quantifiable systemic dose. Drugs that are intended for chronic human use, however, may need data from chronic dermal
animal studies to facilitate risk estimates.

Animal testing. There are clearly defined protocols available for short-
term dermal testing in animals. Most regulatory agencies recommend use of
rats, rabbits, or guinea pigs. Briefly, three dose groups (including the highest
maximum tolerated dose) and a control group should be tested. Exposure times
of at least 5 h/d, 5–7 d/wk, for up to 90 d, are recommended. Specific physical,
biochemical, and histopathological data are gathered from the studies to characterize systemic toxicity from dermal exposure. The dose level at which no
adverse effects are observed (NOAEL) is subsequently used in the risk estimation process.

For developmental toxicity studies, well-defined animal protocols are available for oral tests, which are usually conducted in rats or mice and rabbits as the two required species. Dermal testing should incorporate the most sensitive species identified in oral testing. As per the generally accepted protocol in oral testing, three dosages and a control group are recommended for testing, with the highest dose producing some evidence of systemic maternal toxicity. Test material should be administered at minimum 6 h/d, and some agencies insist on 24-h dosing throughout the period of organogenesis for the chosen species. Prior to conducting dermal developmental toxicity studies, extensive pharmacokinetic data are necessary to ensure a steady state exists during the period of organogenesis. Accordingly, for dermal developmental toxicity studies, the dosing period may need to be started prior to the period of organogenesis, depending on the dermal penetration rate of the chemical.

During all dermal testing, appropriate restraint should be used to prevent exposure via other routes and allow meaningful interpretation of results. The method of restraint should be minimally stressful especially for developmental toxicity studies because effects caused by stress may confound effects caused by the test chemical.

Also, there are several factors unique to dermal testing that must be taken into consideration when extrapolating from animal data to humans. It has been shown that there are differences in percutaneous penetration of chemicals with permeability increasing in the following order: humans, miniature pig, rat, and rabbit (Bartek et al., 1972). The rhesus monkey appears to be a good model for estimating absorption in humans (Sidon et al., 1988; Franklin, 1985; Wester and Maibach, 1975). These species differences complicate the extrapolation of animal data to humans, since systemic effects are related to the amount of chemical absorbed percutaneously.

Human exposure assessment. In addition to establishing the dose response that includes toxicological effects and no-adverse-effect level (NOAEL) in test animals, the amount of chemical that humans are exposed to must be known before a risk assessment can be done. For drugs and cosmetics where a known amount of chemical is applied, the task is relatively straightforward. In the case of worker exposure to chemicals, the task is more complicated. Measurement of exposure to industrial chemicals in the workplace has generally been accomplished by monitoring the concentration of the chemical in the air or by placing samplers at various locations in the workplace. Extrapolation of dose from this type of environmental monitoring may be inaccurate, depending on how representative the sampling is. Furthermore, environmental monitoring does not take dermal exposure into consideration and therefore does not allow full body burden estimates. Pesticide applicators pose a different problem since they are generally working outdoors, precluding workplace monitoring.

It has been shown that the dermal route of exposure is important in agricultural workers (Durham et al., 1972). An estimate of exposure can be made by having the worker wear absorbent patches attached over and under his clothing or taped onto his body. Patches are usually located on the regions of the body outlined in Table 4. After exposure, the patches are removed and extracted. The concentration of the chemical on the patch is then extrapolated to the exposed body surface area represented by the patch (Table 4) and corrected for efficiency of the field sampling matrix (field recovery) to arrive at a dermally deposited dose, usually expressed in micrograms or milligrams. Some researchers analyze the entire item of work clothing, thus eliminating the need to extrapolate from the patch to the body surface area (U.S. EPA, 1987; Chester and Hart, 1986). Hands are difficult to monitor, and sometimes the worker wears thin cotton gloves, which are removed after the exposure and extracted. The total concentration in the eluate is then equated to the hand exposure. Alternatively, rinsing the workers' hands in a suitable solvent after the exposure and analysis of the rinsate may provide good quantitative hand measurement. Since the hands generally account for most of the dermal deposition exposure, it is important to get as accurate an estimate as possible.

A newer technique involving the use of fluorescent tracers added to the pesticide has helped increase awareness of how much dermal exposure occurs in pesticide application (Franklin et al., 1981). Further developments to quantify exposure using this technique is promising (Fenske, 1989).

Estimates of exposure from such studies represent the amount of material that impinges on the skin (contact exposure), not the amount of material absorbed into systemic circulation. The NOAEL from animal studies is generally derived after oral dosing, and it is assumed (sometimes erroneously) that the administered dose and the systemic dose are equivalent. In order to properly conduct the risk assessment, the estimate of dose from toxicity studies and from the exposure study should be equivalent. This can be achieved if the predictive

TABLE 4 Surface Areas for Regions of the Adult Body and Locations of Dermal Exposure Pads That Represent These Regions

Region of the body	Surface area (cm^2) of region	Location of pads representing region
Head	1300[a]	Shoulder, back, chest
Face	650	Chest
Back of neck	110	Back
Front of neck	150[b]	Chest
Chest/stomach	3550	Chest
Back	3550	Back
Upper arms	2910	Shoulder, forearm, upper arm
Hands	820	—
Thighs	3820	Thigh
Lower leg	2380	Shin
Feet	1310	—

Note. From U.S. EPA (1987).
[a]Includes face.
[b]Includes V of chest.

animal testing is done using the dermal route of exposure in an appropriate animal model. Alternatively, the contact dermal exposure estimate can be corrected by a percutaneous absorption factor to give an estimate of systemic dose.

Rather than using environmental monitoring to measure the amount of chemical in air or on patches and then estimating absorbed dose, biological monitoring can be used (Ashford et al., 1984). It involves analysis of the chemical and its metabolites or biotransformation products in body tissues such as urine, blood, fat, hair, nails, sweat, saliva, and expired air. The major advantage of biological monitoring is that it provides an integrated estimate of dermal, inhalation, and oral exposure. The disadvantage at this time is that the relationship between concentration in body fluids and health effects is known for only a few chemicals.

There are other problems associated with the discordance between the estimate of exposure to humans and the dose (exposure) to animals. In workers, exposure is often characterized by intermittent, short, peak exposure. This makes comparison with animal data where dosing is continuous and the level constant, tenuous. As a result, numerous assumptions have to be made when doing quantitative risk assessments. The case study that is presented later in the chapter illustrates these issues.

Percutaneous absorption. Percutaneous absorption studies have been used to determine the bioavailability of topically applied medication and have also been used to establish testing priorities for cosmetics. Their use to estimate a systemic dose following dermal contact and exposure is relatively new, and this approach has been applied primarily in pesticide registration when assessment of risk to workers, applicators, and users is conducted.

Whatever the ultimate use of the absorption data, it is imperative that an accurate estimate of absorption be derived. The two general approaches available utilize *in vivo* studies in a variety of species including humans, and *in vitro* studies using skin from several species. *In vivo* estimates are affected by:

1. Site of application. Studies on volunteers have shown that there are differences in the amount of pesticide absorbed from various sites on the body (Maibach et al., 1971; Wester et al., 1980). Since the forehead of pesticide applicators is heavily contaminated during spraying and since it is one of the more penetrable sites, it is important that the absorption through the forehead be used to factor the contact dose.

2. Species variation. It has been shown that there is considerable variation in the amount of chemical absorbed by different species (Bartek et al., 1971; Moody and Franklin, 1987; Moody et al., 1987; Sidon et al., 1988). It is important that the estimate of absorption used in the risk assessment be done in a species that is predictive of humans. Some feel that the rat is acceptable since it overpredicts the absorption in humans and leads to an overestimate of systemic dose, which adds an additional measure of safety. The problem with this approach is that

the comparative database is relatively small and that this wide margin may not always exist.

3. Dosing characteristics. The number of applications, the size of the application site, washing of the site, dosing vehicle, and occlusion all affect the amount of chemical that penetrates the skin (Franklin et al., 1989). It is important that these factors be taken into consideration when deriving the dermal penetration to be used for risk assessment.

4. Other factors. Age, sex, race, skin decontamination procedures, and skin damage are all known to affect percutaneous penetration and should be considered.

In vitro systems have been developed to measure the penetration of chemicals through the skin and offer the advantage that they are faster and cheaper to use than *in vivo* systems. One additional factor is that human skin can be used, thereby eliminating the need to compare absorption from one species to another. However, there are several limitations to their use by regulatory agencies for risk assessment. There seems to be reasonable concordance between *in vivo* and *in vitro* data when the chemical is hydrophilic. This is not always the case for lipophilic compounds (Bronaugh and Stewart, 1984; Bronaugh et al., 1985).

Regulatory agencies are using appropriately derived *in vivo* data to adjust deposited dose and are using *in vitro* data to set priorities for further testing. However, there needs to be considerable research done to validate *in vitro* data before they can be more widely used.

Risk assessment for subchronic and chronic studies. Toxicological risk assessment proceeds along different lines depending on whether or not a threshold exists for the induction of the toxic response of interest. In the absence of a threshold dose, any level of exposure will result in some level of risk, so that zero risk can only be assured by eliminating all possible exposure. When a threshold dose exists, exposures below the threshold will result in no increased risks.

It is possible that threshold levels may vary among exposed individuals, in which case the population threshold will be the minimum of the individual thresholds. The challenge of regulatory toxicology is to estimate this threshold for the health effect or effects of interest, and to establish exposure guidelines to ensure that the threshold is not exceeded.

According to prevailing toxicological views, a threshold dose may well exist for nonstochastic toxic phenomena that occur in a predictable fashion following exposure to a control dose of the toxicant of interest. The existence of thresholds is supported by the apparent capacity of many toxicants to exert their effects only at doses at which the homeostatic physiological processes responsible for normal biological function are overwhelmed. Mammalian organisms are often able to repair or sustain a certain degree of damage such as cytotoxicity or enzyme inhibition without experiencing apparent adverse effects.

The existence of a threshold is less well established for stochastic processes such as carcinogenesis that occur as a consequence of a series of random genetic events such as DNA damage. In this case, there are certain numeric probabilities that any level of exposure may lead to neoplastic conversion of cancer progenitor cells within the target tissue.

Uncertainty factors and thresholds. The establishment of guidelines for acceptable levels of human exposure in the presence of a threshold dose is traditionally done by applying a suitable safety or uncertainty factor to the dosage observed to induce no adverse effects (NOAEL) in toxicological tests.

Historically, this concept was first introduced by Lehman and Fitzhugh (1954), who proposed that an "acceptable daily intake" or ADI could be estimated for contaminants in food. This concept was endorsed by the Joint FAO/WHO Expert Committee on Food Additives (JECFA) in 1961 and subsequently adopted by the Joint FAO/WHO Meeting of Experts on Pesticide Residues (JMPR) in 1962 (Lu, 1988). The acceptable daily intake assumes 100% of gut absorption and was estimated from the equation ADI = NOAEL/SF, where the NOAEL is the most sensitive no-observed-adverse-effect level in toxicological studies, and the safety factor (SF) is selected to allow for differences in sensitivity to the test agent in humans as compared to animals, and for variation in sensitivity within the human population. These two sources of variation have often been accommodated through the use of a $10 \times 10 = 100$-fold safety factor (McColl, 1990). An additional 10-fold margin of safety has also been recommended in the presence of only limited toxicological tests (National Research Council, 1977b). Although these concepts were originally applied to risk assessment from exposure to chemicals in food, the same principles apply to exposure via other routes. If the same presumption of 100% absorption through the skin is used, the approaches are parallel. Thus ADI could also be applied to exposures from dermal or inhalation routes and called acceptable daily exposure. Unfortunately, because of the numerous variables in skin absorption, this assumption may unduly overestimate absorbed dose.

Although the use of safety factors is now accepted practice in toxicological risk assessment, the limitations of these approaches should also be emphasized. Since the ADI is only an estimate of the population threshold or true no-effect level (NOAEL), it does not provide absolute assurance of safety (Crump, 1984a, 1984b). The size of the safety factor is not directly related to sample size, so that smaller experiments would tend to lead to larger ADIs than would larger, more sensitive studies (Mantel and Schneiderman, 1975). Although factors of 10-fold are used to accommodate both inter- and intraspecies variation in sensitivity, it cannot be guaranteed that a 100-fold safety factor will afford adequate protection in this regard in all cases. For these reasons, the ADI should not be viewed as possessing a high degree of mathematical precision, but rather as a guide to human exposure levels that are not expected to present serious health risks.

Recently, the term "uncertainty factor" (UF) rather than "safety factor" has been used in recognition that the ADI is a reference dose or RfD (U.S.

EPA, 1988; Barnes and Dourson, 1988). The Environmental Protection Agency has also introduced the concept of a modifying factor (MF) to be applied to the UF in recognition of the specific circumstances surrounding the establishment of the RfD. The estimated ADI for specific chemicals allowed the assumption that food containing the chemical could be safely consumed daily by humans, including sensitive subgroups, for a lifetime without inducing harmful effects. Thus, the RfD is determined by use of the equation RfD = NOAEL/(UF × MF). When the data do not demonstrate a NOAEL, a LOAEL (lowest-observed-adverse-effect level) may be used. This is the lowest dose at which a statistically significant adverse effect is observed.

Carcinogenic risk assessment. The apparent absence of a threshold dose for carcinogenic effects calls for a different approach to risk assessment for carcinogens and mutagens than is used for threshold toxicants. The direct estimation of small risks associated with low levels of exposure is not feasible due to a limitation in the sensitivity of tests for carcinogenic effects at very low doses. However, it is possible to extrapolate results obtained at higher doses to individual estimates of low dose cancer risks. Although our level of knowledge of the precise mechanisms of neoplastic development necessarily confers a degree of uncertainty on estimates of risk obtained in this fashion, such estimates can play an important role in establishing exposure standards for carcinogens. Although the choice of the dose-response model to be used for extrapolation purposes can have a marked impact on estimates of low dose risk (Krewski and Van Ryzin, 1981), such differences are small when attention is restricted to models that are linear in the low dose region.

The assumption of low dose linearity for chemical carcinogens that act through direct interaction with genetic material is supported by both theoretical considerations in carcinogenesis (Krewski and Van Ryzin, 1981) and the linearity of DNA binding observed at very low doses with a number of chemical carcinogens (Lutz et al., 1990). Although perhaps not applicable in cases where carcinogenesis occurs subsequent to toxic tissue injury, the assumption of low dose linearity is widely made in regulatory applications of low dose risk assessment in the absence of clear information to the contrary (Office of Science and Technology Policy, 1985).

The linearized multistage model (LMS) is used by many regulatory agencies to obtain estimates of low dose risk. This is done by obtaining an upper confidence limit q star (q_1^*) on the linear term in the model (Crump, 1984b). The value of q_1^* represents the slope of the dose-response curve (changes in tumor incidence/change in dose) in the low dose region, and corresponds to the risk associated with a unit measure of dose (such as the number of tumors/mg chemical/kg body weight or 1 ppm in the diet). Only an upper confidence limit on this low dose slope is used since point estimates of risk based on this model are highly uncertain. Other models for linear extrapolation may also be used (Krewski et al., 1990), although the results obtained are generally comparable with those based on the LMS.

Other measures of carcinogenic potency have also been proposed (for recent reviews see Barr, 1985; Krewski et al., 1991). One of the most widely used indices is the TD50, which is defined as the dose which will reduce by 50% the proportion of animals not developing the lesion of interest spontaneously under control conditions (Peto et al., 1984). Gold et al. (1984, 1989) have established a carcinogenic potency database (CPDB) containing the TD50 values for nearly 900 animal carcinogens, with all results expressed in units of mg/kg body weight/d and standardized to a typical 2-yr rodent lifetime. The TD50 values for these compounds vary by more than 100-million-fold, demonstrating the wide variation in carcinogenic potency of these compounds.

In contrast to q_1^*, which is intended to provide a measure of carcinogenic potency at two doses, the TD50 provides an indication of carcinogenic potential at high doses. The latter measure underlies the human exposure risk potential (HERP) index proposed by Ames et al. (1987), defined as the percentage of the TD50 accounted for by the anticipated level of human exposure. Wartenburg and Gallo (1991) point out that the relative potency of two carcinogens measured at high doses need not reflect their relative potency at much lower levels of exposure, thereby limiting the utility of the HERP index as a measure of relative risk. While there are examples where this occurs, the TD50 is highly correlated with the values of q_1^*(Krewski et al., 1989), so that the two measures of potency are to some extent providing similar information.

The use of simple measures of carcinogenic potency such as the TD50 or q_1^* may be criticized on the grounds that they do not take into account all of the information that may be available on the mechanisms by which neoplastic transformation occurs among cells in the target tissues. Currently, there exists a considerable body of evidence that suggests that malignant transformation is influenced by cell kinetics as well as genotoxic damage to cells in the target tissue (Moolgavkar, 1986). This has resulted in the development of theoretical models of carcinogenesis that are based on initiation of stem cells by means of genetic damage, clonal expansion of such initiated cells by nongenotoxic means, and finally malignant transformation by a second genetic event. Although biologically appealing, applications of this two-stage clonal expansion model have been limited due to the need for information on both cell kinetics and mutation rates (Cohen and Ellwein, 1990).

In a similar vein, the use of pharmacokinetic data on the uptake, metabolism, distribution, and elimination of chemical substances in the body has been proposed as a means of improving estimates of carcinogenic risk (National Research Council, 1987). Pharmacokinetic studies provide information on the dose delivered to the target tissue, which may be used as a dose "metameter" for risk assessment rather than the external level of exposure to which the host organism is exposed. This is important since the tissue dose will not be proportional to the external level of exposure when one or more pharmacokinetic pathways is saturable. When this occurs, estimates of risk based on external measures of exposure may be biased (Hoel et al., 1983).

In an attempt to determine the dose delivered to the target tissue, complex physiologic pharmacokinetic models have been developed for several carcinogens, including methylene chloride (Anderson et al., 1987) and benzene (Belisles and Totman, 1989). Such models envisage the body as being comprised of a small number of physiologically relevant compartments, such as fat or muscle tissues, or critical organs such as the liver or kidney. In practice, a physiologically based pharmacokinetic model (PBPK) is described by a number of parameters characterizing the anatomy and physiology of the host, the solubility of the test chemical or its metabolites in various organs and tissues, and pharmacokinetic coefficients governing metabolism in specific organs such as the lung and liver. Since each of these parameters will be known only to within a certain degree of error, it has been argued that the cumulative effect of such errors over a moderately large number of PBPK parameters will be to instill more uncertainty in estimates of risk than was present prior to the incorporation of pharmacokinetic data into the risk estimation process (Portier and Kaplan, 1989). While this argument is of some merit, the judicious use of pharmacokinetic information can still be of value in cancer risk assessment.

One area in which pharmacokinetic data can play an important role is in extrapolation of bioassay results from one route of exposure to another. This is of particular importance when inferring potential risks associated with dermal exposure, since experiments on which an assessment of risk must be made frequently are conducted using oral or inhalation exposures. To illustrate, consider the PBPK model shown in Fig. 2, in which the route of entry of the test chemical into the body is absorption through the skin. With the exception of the parameters governing dermal absorption, all of the parameters in the PBPK model may be estimated from studies based on other routes of exposure. Once the rate of absorption is determined, it is possible to use this model to predict the dose of the reactive metabolite reaching the target tissue under conditions of dermal exposure.

Another complication in carcinogenic risk assessment arises from the fact that human exposure to toxicants present in the environment is often not constant over time. This can occur as a result of changes in occupation, dietary and lifestyle practices, and in levels of environmental contamination. If the available toxicological data has been acquired under conditions of constant lifetime exposure, as is standard practice in long-term laboratory studies of carcinogenicity, there exists a need to translate these results to conditions of variable exposure.

One approach to carcinogenic risk assessment with variable exposure levels is to base estimates of risk on a time-weighted average daily dose, calculated by averaging the cumulative dose experienced over the period during which exposure occurs over a lifetime (U.S. EPA, 1986). While this approach is appropriate in the absence of dose rate effects, it should not be applied in cases where the cumulative lifetime dose does not characterize risk. Conditions under which the use of time-weighted average doses will lead to reasonable estimates

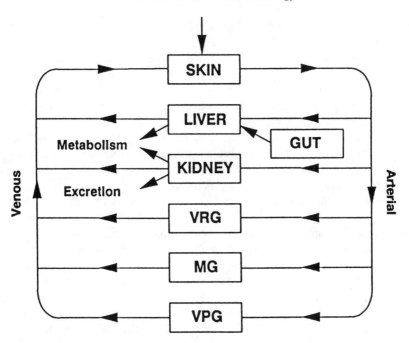

FIGURE 2 Physiologically-based pharmacokinetic model: VRG, vessel-rich group; MG, muscle group; VPG, vessel-poor group. From Withey and Murdoch in *Pesticide Science and Biotechnology,* Blackwell Scientific Publications (1987).

of risk have been identified by Crump and Howe (1984) and Kodell et al. (1987) within the context of the multistage model of carcinogenesis. Briefly, these investigators demonstrated that the error associated with using a time-weighted average dose for risk estimation purposes was less than a factor of k, the number of stages in the model. Unfortunately, a similar bound on the possible error in predicting risks under variable exposure patterns does not hold with the two-stage clonal expansion model (Chen et al., 1988; Murdoch and Krewski, 1988). Thus caution is advised when using time-weighted average doses for risk assessment, particularly in situations where cellular proliferation is thought to represent an important component of carcinogenesis. Ideally, experiments with variable exposure patterns should be conducted to explore the relative effectiveness of dosing at different points in time (Krewski and Murdoch, 1990).

Ultimately, the application of measures of carcinogenic potency derived from toxicological studies requires extrapolation from animals to humans. The use of animal bioassay data to infer carcinogenic hazards to humans is supported by the 74% concordance in test results for rats and mice achieved with 266 chemicals tested by the U.S. National Toxicology Program (Haseman and Huff, 1987) and by the fact that, with the exception of ethanol, all known human carcinogens are also effective in one or more animal species (Interna-

C. A. Franklin et al.

tional Agency for Research on Cancer, 1987). Although there is a fair correlation between measures of carcinogenic potency in rats and mice (Gaylor and Chen, 1986; Chen and Gaylor, 1987), the basis for the quantitative extrapolation of laboratory data on carcinogenicity to humans is less well established (Allen et al., 1988; Kaldor, 1990). Nonetheless, quantitative interspecies conversion of measures of carcinogenic potency has traditionally been done on the basis of either body weight or body surface area (Krewski et al., 1991). These two methods of species conversion can differ by a factor of approximately sixfold when extrapolating from rats to humans, with surface area leading to greater potency than body weight conversion. Travis and White (1988) have recently suggested that species conversion should be done on a scale based on body weight to the $3/4$ power. Because surface area varies roughly in proportion to the $2/3$ power of body weight, this proposal will lead to potency measures intermediate to those based on either body weight or surface area.

   Application of risk assessment techniques.   To illustrate the application of the risk assessment techniques discussed in the previous section, we now consider the case of the pesticide alachlor. This product is a preemergent herbicide used extensively for weed control in corn crops. Alachlor has recently been under regulatory review in Canada (Report of the Alachlor Review Board, 1987).

   Alachlor was registered for use in Canada on the basis of invalid toxicology data. To comply with regulatory requirements, the manufacturer conducted several animal bioassays to replace the invalid data. Results of these new studies demonstrated dose-related increases in the occurrence of tumors in various organs. Furthermore, one of the animal studies demonstrated that tumors could be induced following short-term exposure (5–6 mo) to the herbicide. These toxicological findings necessitated assessment of the potential risk to humans occupationally exposed via the dermal route. Accordingly, the manufacturer conducted a worker exposure study providing quantitative values of dermally deposited dose for workers wearing protective clothes and gloves (protected) and workers wearing protective clothes and no gloves (unprotected). The exposure study demonstrated the dermally deposited dose for unprotected workers was comparable to the orally administered "systemic" dose that induced tumors in experimental animals. Because there was no dermal penetration data available to adjust deposited dose in the worker study to systemic dose, 100% dermal penetration was assumed for risk assessment purposes.

   A complication in evaluating the human risk was the nature of human exposure. Alachlor is typically applied for about 3–15 d each year. In contrast, the laboratory studies involved daily exposure for 5–6 mo in one study and throughout the lifetimes in other studies. This difference between animals and humans in the pattern of temporal exposure presents serious problems in evaluating risk. In an effort to accommodate intermittent exposure patterns, a time-weighted average dose has been suggested (U.S. EPA, 1986). However, this approach was considered to be inappropriate in the presence of dose rate effects, such as those observed when tumors formed following short-term dosing.

In the interest of prudence, government officials took the view that even a single day's exposure to Alachlor could conceivably result in neoplastic conversion of stem cells in the target tissue. Thus the dermal dose experienced on 1 d (uncorrected for dermal penetration) was used to obtain an upper limit on risk. For applications at the rate of 3 d/yr over a 40-yr period, this approach to exposure evaluation leads to risk estimates approximately 18,000 higher than does the use of a time-weighted average daily dose. It was recognized, however, that had dermal penetration data been available, a better estimate for systemic dose could have been used in the risk assessment. Furthermore, the use of a single day's exposure for risk assessment purposes may overstate risk, but it was felt that a less stringent approach could not offer assurances of not understating the risk to workers exposed for short periods of time. Accordingly, on the basis of the toxicological data and worker dermal dose, it was concluded that the continued use of Alachlor could pose an unacceptable risk to workers, and the product was removed from the Canadian market.

In the future, the risk assessment for Alachlor may need to be readdressed in light of new information such as dermal penetration data or biological monitoring data that will provide better quantitative estimates of systemic dose than that available for the original risk assessment.

SUMMARY

The fact that the skin can be affected by the chemicals that come into contact with it has been known for centuries. The utilization of predictive tests to identify the potential of a chemical to do so prior to marketing was established by Draize et al. (1944). Since then, there have been numerous methods developed to elucidate the toxic behavior of chemicals toward skin. New chemicals are usually tested in animals first to eliminate very toxic ones. The next step involves predictive testing in humans, and despite small numbers of volunteers used, the tests seem to reliably predict those chemicals that are irritants and sensitizers to humans. That is not to suggest that there is no room for improvement in the tests. More objective measures of effects would greatly assist in the quantification of toxicity and allow more precise risk assessment. There are also many end points that are not routinely tested, such as phototoxicity. This may have to change since current prediction of increased levels of UV radiation, particularly UVA, due to depletion of stratospheric ozone have resulted in concern over the potential for increased incidence of skin cancer and cataracts.

Recognition of the skin as a significant route of entry of chemicals to workers has been more recent. It was not until the 1970s that regulatory agencies started to assess the risk to applicators and bystanders in any consistent fashion. The problems involved in doing these have been outlined. Further recognition that people are exposed to chemicals in many different media (food, air, water, consumer products) by multiple routes of exposure (oral, dermal, inhalation) has led to a multiple media approach to risk assessment. Simply stated, it is no longer reasonable to apportion acceptable levels in one medium when the chemical occurs in others as well. Dioxin, PCBs, and lead are examples of chemicals that should be assessed this way. This has put growing emphasis on being able to quantify exposure from the dermal route.

The steps in risk assessment/risk management as outlined in this chapter are generally utilized by regulatory agencies. The specific application and use of quantitative risk assessment for carcinogens differs from one agency to another. Some rely almost totally on it, whereas others rely more heavily on total weight of evidence. Whatever the case, the use of a systematic approach ensures that all possible variables are factored into the decision.

REFERENCES

Allen, B., Crump, K. and Shipp, A. 1988. Carcinogenic potency of chemicals in animals and humans. *Risk Anal.* 8:531–544.

Ames, B. N., Magaw, R. and Gold, L. S. 1987. Ranking possible carcinogenic hazards. *Science* 236:271–280.

Anderson, M. E., Clewell, H. J., Gargas, W. L., Smith, F. A. and Reitz, R. H. 1987. Physiologically based pharmacokinetics and the risk assessment process for methylene chloride. *Toxicol. Appl. Pharmacol.* 87:185–205.

Ashford, N. A., Spadafor, C. J. and Caldart, C. C. 1984. Human monitoring: Scientific, legal, and ethical considerations. *Harvard Environ. Law Rev.* 263–363.

Barnes, D. G. and Dourson, M. L. 1988. Reference dose (RfD): Description and use in health risk assessments. *Reg. Toxicol. Pharmacol.* 8:471–486.

Barr, J. T. 1985. The calculation and use of carcinogenic potency: a review. *Reg. Toxicol. Pharmacol.* 5:432–459.

Bartek, M., Labudde, J. and Maibach, H. I. 1971. Skin permeability *in vivo*: Comparison in rat, rabbit, pig, and man. *J. Invest. Dermatol.* 58:114–123.

Belisles, R. P. and Totman, L. C. 1989. Pharmacokinetically based risk assessment of workplace exposure to benzene. *Reg. Toxicol. Pharmacol.* 9:186–195.

Berenblum, I. 1941. The cocarcinogenic action of croton resin. *Cancer Res.* 1:44–48.

Björnberg, A. 1987. Irritant dermatitis. In *Occupational and Industrial Dermatology*, eds. H. I. Maibach, pp. 15–21. Chicago: Yearbook Medical Publishing.

Biotechnology News, April 27, 1990, p. 8.

Bronaugh, R. L. and Stewart, R. F. 1984. Methods for *in vitro* percutaneous absorption studies III: Hydrophobic compounds. *J. Pharm. Sci.* 73(9):1255–1258.

Bronaugh, R. L., Stewart, R. F., Wester, R. C., Bucks, D., Maibach, H. I. and Anderson, J. 1985. Comparison of percutaneous absorption of fragrances by humans and monkeys. *Food Chem. Toxicol.* 23(1):111–114.

Brown, V. K. H. 1971. A comparison of predictive irritation tests with surfactants on human and animal skin. *J. Soc. Cosmet. Chem.* 22:411–442.

Buehler, E. V. 1965. Delayed contact hypersensitivity in the guinea pig. *Arch. Dermatol.* 91:171–177.

Calabrese, E. 1983. *Principles of Animal Extrapolation,* pp. 403–414. New York: Wiley.

Canada Health Protection Branch. 1981. *Bureau of Human Prescription Drugs. Predictive Toxicology Guidelines.* Ottawa: Minister of Supply and Services.

Canada Health Protection Branch. 1990a. *Risk Management in the Health Protection Branch.* Ottawa: Minister of Supply and Services.

Canada Health Protection Branch. 1990b. *Health Risk Determination: The challenge of Health Protection.* Ottawa: Minister of Supply and Services.

Chen, J. J. and Gaylor, D. W. 1987. Comparison of estimated safe doses for rats and mice. *Environ. Health Perspect.* 72:305–309.

Chen, J. J., Kodell, R. L. and Gaylor, D. W. 1988. Using the biological two-stage model to assess risk from short-term exposures. *Risk Anal.* 6:223–230.

Chester, G. and Hart, B. 1986. Biological monitoring of a herbicide applied through backpack and vehicle sprayers. *Toxicol. Lett.* 33:137–148.

Cohen, S. M. and Ellwein, L. B. 1990. Cell growth dynamics and DNA alterations in carcinogenesis. In *Scientific Issues in Quantitative Cancer Risk Assessment*, eds. S. H. Moolgavkar, pp. 116–135. Boston: Birkhaüser.

Crump, K. S. 1984a. A new method for determining allowable daily intakes. *Fundam. Appl. Toxicol.* 4:854–871.

Crump, K. A. 1984b. An improved procedure for low-dose carcinogenic risk assessment from animal data. *J. Environ. Pathol. Toxicol. Oncol.* 6:339–348.

Crump, K. S. and Howe, R. B. 1984. The multistage model with a time-dependent exposure pattern: applications to carcinogenic risk assessment. *Risk Anal.* 4:163–176.

De Leo, V. A., Harber, L. C., Kong, B. M. and De Salva, S. J. 1982. Surfactant-induced alteration of arachidonic acid metabolism of mammalian cells in culture. *Proc. Soc. Exp. Biol. Med.* 184:477–482.

Draize, J. H. 1955. V111. Dermal Toxicity. *Food Drug Cosmet. Law J.* 10:722–732.

Durham, W. F., Wolfe, H. R. and Elliot, J. W. 1972. Absorption and excretion of parathion by spraymen. *Arch. Environ. Health* 24:381–387.

Emmett, E. A. 1987. Photobiologic effects. In *Occupational and Industrial Dermatology*, ed. H. I. Maibach, pp. 94–104. Chicago: Yearbook Medical Publishing.

Epstein, E. 1966. Allergy to dermatologic agents. *J. Am. Med. Assoc.* 198:103.

Fenske, R. A. 1989. Validation of environmental monitoring by biological monitoring. In *Biological Monitoring for Pesticide Exposure*, eds. R. G. M. Wang, C. A. Franklin, and J. C. Reinert, pp. 70–84. Washington, D.C.: ACS Symposium Series 382.

Fisher, T. and Maibach, H. I. 1987. Patch testing in allergic contact dermatitis, an update. In *Occupational and Industrial Dermatology*, eds. H. I. Maibach, pp. 94–104. Chicago: Yearbook Medical Publishing.

Franklin, C. A. 1985. Occupational exposure to pesticides and its role in risk assessment procedures used in Canada. In *Dermal Exposure Related to Pesticides Use*, eds. R. C. Honeycutt, G. Zweig, and N. Ragsdale, pp. 429–444. Washington, D.C.: ACS Symposium Series 273.

Franklin, C. A., Fenske, R. A., Greenhalgh, R., Mathieu, L., Denley, H. V. Leffingwell, J. T. and Spear, R. C. 1981. Correlation of urinary metabolite excretion with estimated dermal contact in the course of occupational exposure to guthion. *J. Toxicol. Environ. Health* 7:715–781.

Franklin, C. A., Somers, D. A. and Chu, I. 1989. Use of percutaneous absorption data in risk assessment. *J. Am. Coll. Toxicol.* 8(5):815–827.

Gaylor, D. W. and Chen, J. J. 1986. Relative potency of chemical carcinogens in rodents. *Risk Anal.* 6:283–290.

Gold, L. S., Sawyer, C. B., Magan, R., Backman, G. M., de Veciana, M., Levinson, R., Hooper, N. K., Havender, W. R., Bernstein, L., Peto, R., Pike, M. C. and Ames, B. N. 1984. A carcinogenic potency database of the standardized results of animal bioassays. *Environ. Health Perspect.* 58:9–322.

Gold, L. S., Slone, T. H. and Bernstein, L. 1989. Summary of the carcinogenic potency and positivity for 492 rodent carcinogens in the carcinogenic potency database. *Environ. Health Perspect.* 79:259–272.

Guidelines for Registering Pesticides and Other Control Products Under the Pest Control Products Act in Canada. 1984. Agriculture Canada, Pesticide Division, Ottawa.

Harber, L. C., Shalita, A. R., Armstrong, R. B. 1987. Immunologically mediated contact photosensitivity in guinea pigs. In *Dermatotoxicology,* 3rd ed., eds. F. N. Marzulli and H. Maibach, pp. 413–429. New York: Marcel Dekker.

Haseman, J. K. and Huff, J. E. 1987. Species correlation in long-term carcinogenicity studies. *Cancer Lett.* 37:125–132.

Hjorth, N. 1987. The allergens. In *Occupational and Industrial Dermatology,* ed. H. I. Maibach, pp. 94–104. Chicago: Yearbook Medical Publishing.

Hoel, D. G., Kaplan, N. L. and Anderson, M. W. 1983. Implication of nonlinear kinetics on risk estimation in carcinogenesis. *Science* 219:1032–1037.

Ingram, A. J. and Grasso, P. 1975. Patch testing in the rabbit using a modified human patch test method. Application of histological and visual assessment. *Br. J. Dermatol.* 92:131–142.

International Agency for Research on Cancer. 1987. Overall evaluation of carcinogenicity: An updating of IARC monographs volumes 1–42. *IARC Monogr. Eval. Carcinogen. Risk Hum.* Supplement 7. Lyon: IARC.

Jackson, E. M. and Goldner, R. eds. 1990. *Irritant Contact Dermatitis.* New York: Marcel Dekker.

Kaldor, J. 1990. Carcinogenic drugs: A model database for human risk quantification. In *Scientific Issues in Quantitative Cancer Risk Assessment,* ed. S. H. Moolgavkar, pp. 286–305. Boston: Birkhaüser.

Kates, R. W. 1978. On the quantitative definition of risk. *Risk Anal.* 1:11–28.

Klassen, C. D., Amdur, M. O. and Doull, J. 1986. *Casarett and Doull's Toxicology,* 3rd ed. Toronto: Collier MacMillan.

Kligman, A. M. 1966a. The identification of contact allergens by human assay. II Factors influencing the induction and measurement of allergic contact dermatitis. *J. Invest. Dermatol.* 47(5):375–392.

Kligman, A. M. 1966b. The identification of contact allergens by human assay. III The maximization test. A procedure for screening and rating contact sensitizers. *J. Invest. Dermatol.* 47(5):393–410.

Kligman, A. M. and Epstein, W. 1975. Updating the maximization test for identifying the contact allergens. *Contact Dermatitis* 1:231–239.

Kligman, A. M. and Wooding, W. M. 1967. A method for the measurement and evaluation of irritants on human skin. *J. Invest. Dermatol.* 49:78–94.

Kodell, R. L., Gaylor, D. W. and Chen, J. J. 1987. Using average life-time dose rate for intermittent exposures to carcinogens. *Risk Anal.* 7:339–345.

Krewski, D. and Birkwood, P. 1987. Risk assessment and risk management. *Risk Abstr.* 4:53–61.

Krewski, D. and Murdoch, D. J. 1990. Cancer modelling with intermittent exposures. In *Scientific Issues in Quantitative Cancer Risk Assessment,* ed. S. H. Moolgavkar, pp. 196–214. Boston: Birkhaüser.

Krewski, D. and Van Ryzin, J. 1981. Dose response models for quantal response toxicity data. In *Statistics and Related Topics,* eds. M. Csorgo, D. Dawson, J. N. K. Rao and E. Saleh. Amsterdam: North Holland.

Krewski, D., Murdoch, D. and Withey, J. R. 1989. Recent developments in carcinogenic risk assessment. *Health Phys.* 57:313–325.

Krewski, D., Gaylor, D. W. and Szyszkowicz, M. 1990. A model-free approach to low dose extrapolation. *Environ. Health Perspect.,* in press.

Krewski, D., Goddard, M. J. and Withey, J. R. 1991. Carcinogenic potency and interspecies extrapolation. In *Proc. Fifth International Conf. Environmental Mutagens,* eds. M. L. Mendelsohn. New York: Alan R. Liss.

Lahti, A. and Maibach, H. I. 1984. An animal model for non-immunologic contact urticaria. *Toxicol. Appl. Pharmacol.* 76:219–224.

Lansdown, A. B. G. 1972. An appraisal of methods for detecting primary skin irritants. *J. Soc. Cosmet. Chem.* 23:739–772.

Lehman, A. J. and Fitzhugh, O. G. 1954. 100-Fold margin of safety. *Assoc. Food Drug Off. U.S.Q. Bull.* 18:33–35.

Lowrance, W. 1976. *Of Acceptable Risk.* Los Altos, Calif.: W. Kaufman.

Lu, F. 1988. Acceptable daily intake: Inception, evolution, and application. *Reg. Toxicol. Pharmacol.* 8:45–60.

Luster, M. I., Dean, J. N. and Boorman, G. A. 1982. Cell-mediated immunity and its application in toxicology. *Environ. Health Perspect.* 43:31–36.

Lutz, W. K., Buss, P., Baertsch, A. and Caviezel, M. 1990. Evaluation of DNA binding *in vivo* for low dose extrapolation in chemical carcinogenesis. In *Genetic Toxicology of Complex Mixtures,* eds. M. D. Waters, S. Nesnow, J. Lewtas, N. M. Moore and F. B. Daniel. New York: Plenum Press.

Maguire, H. C. 1973. The bioassay of contact allergens in the guinea pig. *J. Soc. Cosmet. Chem.* 24:151–162.

Maibach, H. I., Feldmann, R. J., Milby, T. H. and Serat, W. F. 1971. Regional variation in percutaneous penetration in man. *Arch. Environ. Health* 23:208–235.

Mantel, N. and Schneiderman, N. A. 1975. Estimating safe levels, a hazardous undertaking. *Cancer Res.* 35:1379–1386.

Marzulli, F. and Maibach, H. 1974. The use of graded concentrations in studying skin sensitizers: Experimental contact sensitization in man. *Food Cosmet. Toxicol.* 12:219–227.

Marzulli, F. N. and Maibach, H. I. 1987. Human predictive tests for allergic contact dermatitis. In *Occupational and Industrial Dermatology,* eds. (H. I. Maibach, pp. 227–240. Chicago: Yearbook Medical Publishing.

McColl, S. 1990. *Biological Safety Factors in Toxicological Risk Assessment.* Ottawa: Department of National Health and Welfare.

Moody, R. P. and Franklin, C. A. 1987. Percutaneous absorption of the insecticides fenitrothion and aminocarb in rats and monkeys. *J. Toxicol. Environ. Health* 20:209–218.

Moody, R. P., Riedel, D., Ritter, L. and Franklin, C. A. 1987. The effect of DEET (*N,N*-diethyl-*m*-toluamide) on dermal persistence and absorption of the insecticide fenitrothion in rats and monkeys. *J. Toxicol. Environ. Health* 22:471–479.

Moolgavkar, S. H. 1986. Carcinogenesis modelling: From molecular biology to epidemiology. *Annu. Rev. Public Health* 7:151–169.

Murdoch, D. J. and Krewski, D. 1988. Carcinogenic risk assessment with time-dependent exposure patterns. *Risk Anal.* 8:521–530.

National Research Council. 1977a. *Drinking Water and Health.* Washington, D.C.: National Academy Press.

National Research Council. 1977b. *Principles and Procedures for Evaluating the Toxicity of Household Chemicals.* Washington, D.C.: NAS Pub. 1138.

National Research Council. 1987. *Pharmacokinetics in Risk Assessment. Drinking Water and Health,* vol. 8. Washington, D.C.: National Academy Press.

Nixon, G. A., Tyson, C. A. and Wertz, W. C. 1975. Interspecies comparisons of skin irritancy. *Toxicol. Appl. Pharmacol.* 31:481–490.

OECD Guidelines for Testing of Chemicals. 1981. Acute dermal irritation/corrosion.

Organization for Economic Cooperation and Development. OECD Publications and Information Centre, Washington, D.C.

Office of Science and Technology Policy. 1985. Chemical carcinogens: a review of the science and its associated principles. *Fed. Reg.* 50:10372–10442.

Peto, R., Pike, M. C., Bernstein, L., Gold, L. S. and Ames, B. N. 1984. The TD50: A proposed general convention for the numerical description of the carcinogenic potency of chemicals in chronic-exposure animal experiments. *Environ. Health Perspect.* 58:1–8.

Phillips, L. H., Steinberg, M., Maibach, H. I. and Akers, W. A. 1972. A comparison of rabbit and human skin response to certain irritants. *Toxicol. Appl. Pharmacol.* 21:369–382.

Portier, C. J. and Kaplan, N. L. 1989. The variability of safe dose estimates when using complicated models of the carcinogenic process. A case study: methylene chloride. *Fundam. Appl. Toxicol.* 13(3):533–544.

Report of the Alachlor Review Board. 1987. Argiculture Canada, Sir John Carling Building, Ottawa. October.

Ritter, L. and Franklin, C. A. 1990. Dermal toxicity testing: Exposure and absorption. In *Handbook of In Vivo Toxicity Testing,* eds. D. Arnold, H. Grice, and D. Krewski, pp. 247–270. San Diego: Academic Press.

Schalla, W. and Schaefer, H. 1982. Mechanisms of penetration of drugs into the skin. In *Dermal and Transdermal Absorption,* eds. R. Brandeu and B. H. Lippoid. MBH Stuttgart: Wissenschaftliche Verlagsgesellschaft.

Shah, P. V., Fisher, H. L., Sumler, M. R., Monroe, R. J., Chernoff, N. and Hall, L. L. 1987. Comparison of the penetration of 14 pesticides through the skin of young and adult rats. *J. Toxicol. Environ. Health* 21:353–366.

Shah, P. V., Fisher, H. L., Sumler, M. R. and Hall, L. L. 1989. Dermal absorption and pharmacokinetics of pesticides in rats. In *Biological Monitoring for Pesticide Exposure,* eds. R. G. M. Wang, C. A. Franklin, R. C. Honeycutt, and J. C. Reinert, pp. 169–187. Washington, D.C.: ACS Symposium Series 382.

Shubik, P. 1975. Skin carcinogenesis in animal models. In *Dermatology,* ed. H. I. Maibach, pp. 146–155. Edinburgh: Churchill Livingstone.

Sidon, E., Moody, R. P. and Franklin, C. A. 1988. Percutaneous absorption of *cis*- and *trans*-permethrin in rhesus monkeys and man. Anatomic site and intraspecies variation. *J. Toxicol. Environ. Health* 23:207–216.

Travis, C. C. and White, R. K. 1988. Interspecific scaling of toxicity data. *Risk Analy.* 8:119–125.

U.S. Environmental Protection Agency. 1982a. Dermatotoxicity, Selected Issues in Testing for Dermal Toxicity, Including Irritation, Sensitization, Phototoxicity, and Systemic Toxicity. Washington, D.C. EPA 660/11-82-002.

U.S. Environmental Protection Agency. 1982b. Pesticides Assessment Guidelines. Subdivision F Hazard Evaluation: Human and Domestic Animals. Report EPA 540/9-82-025.

U.S. Environmental Protection Agency. 1986. Guidelines for the health assessment of suspect developmental toxicants. *Fed. Reg.* 34028.

U.S. Environmental Protection Agency. 1987. Pesticides Assessment Guidelines. Subdivision U. Applicator Exposure Monitoring Report. Washington, D.C. EPA PB 87-133286.

U.S. Environmental Protection Agency. 1988. Reference dose (RfD): Description and use in health risk assessments. Integrated risk information system (IRIS). Online. Intra-agency reference dose (RfD) work group. Office of Health and Environmental Assessment. Cincinnati: Environmental Criteria and Assessment Office.

Wartenburg, D. and Gallo, M. A. 1991. The fallacy of ranking possible carcinogen hazards using the TD50. *Risk Anal.,* in press.

Weil, C. S. and Scala, R. A. 1971. Study of intra- and interlaboratory variability in results of rabbit eye and skin irritation tests. *Toxicol. Appl. Pharmacol.* 19(2):276–360.

Wester, R. C. and Maibach, H. I. 1975. Percutaneous absorption in the rhesus monkey compared to man. *Toxicol. Appl. Pharmacol.* 32:394–398.

Wester, R. C., Noonan, R. K. and Maibach, H. I. 1980. Variation in percutaneous absorption of testosterone in the rhesus monkey due to anatomic site of application and frequency of application. *Arch. Dermatol. Res.* 267:229–235.

Withey, J. R. and Murdoch, D. 1987. Application of pharmacokinetics in risk assessment for pesticides. In *Pesticide Science and Biotechnology,* eds. R. Greenhalgh and T. R. Roberts, pp. 569–572. Boston: Blackwell Scientific Publications.

31

eye irritation

■ **Robert B. Hackett** ■ **T. O. McDonald** ■

INTRODUCTION

Ocular irritation testing represents an important step in the safety evaluation of many substances. Significant advances in reliability, predictability, and reproducibility have been made and are presented herein.

Historical Perspective on Eye Irritancy Evaluation

In 1944, two groups of investigators described methods for grading reactions of eyes to ocular irritants. Friedenwald et al. (1944) studied the effect of various acidic and basic solutions on eyes of rabbits and recorded their observations using a numerical grading system in which reactions of cornea, conjunctiva, and iris were evaluated. Brief descriptions were provided that correlated the nature of the reaction with the number used for scoring. Lesions of increasing severity received higher scores. Carpenter and Smyth (1946) also described an ocular scoring system for grading and comparing ocular lesions in rabbits. The system was devised independently of Friedenwald et al., but was similar to their system in some respects. Since Carpenter and Smyth tested many indus-

The assistance of the Word Processing Center of Alcon Laboratories is gratefully acknowledged.

The contents of this chapter represent the individuals' viewpoint and not that of any federal agency.

trial materials, their scores were designed for recording corneal necrosis, and conjunctival changes were not scored.

Draize et al. (1944) described an eye irritancy grading system for use in evaluating the potential ocular irritative effect of drugs and other materials intended for use in or around the eye. Numerical scores (somewhat different from those of Friedenwald et al.) were given for reactions of cornea, conjunctiva, and iris. Brief verbal descriptions were provided to guide the observer in converting the changes noted to the numerical score. The authors also specified the number of animals (albino rabbits) to be used and provided techniques for application (frequency and route of administration) of the irritants. This paper had a profound influence on ocular irritation testing and subsequently became the official Food and Drug Administration (FDA) test method (Falahee et al., 1982).

The Draize scoring system (Draize et al., 1944) provided numerical equivalents for brief subjective statements of ocular reactions observed in the cornea, conjunctiva, and iris. For example, corneal reactions were scored according to the density of corneal opacities and the area of the cornea involved on a scale of 0–4. Iridal reactions and conjunctival responses had similar numerical scores. The total ocular irritation score was calculated by a formula that gave very heavy weight (80–110 points) to corneal changes. The evaluation of ocular responses by Draize et al. (1944) was performed without the aid of magnification devices, although Friedenwald et al. (1944) employed a loupe or slit-lamp to grade corneal edema.[1]

Studies of ocular irritation induced by many different substances have subsequently been reported. Hazelton (1952) used the Draize scoring system to evaluate the irritative effect of several surfactants. Hazelton demonstrated that wetting agents that foamed well would probably be irritants. Cationic materials appeared to precipitate protein and were accompanied by generalized irritation and a high incidence of corneal opacity. The non-protein-coagulating surfactants, primarily in the nonionic groups, produced less severe corneal opacities. The data were interpreted as indicating that the order of irritation for detergents was cationic > anionic > nonionic detergents (Carter et al., 1973).

Kay and Calandra (1962) evaluated the Federal Hazardous Substances Act (FHSA) criteria of pass or fail. They used the ocular scoring scheme of Draize et al. (1944) to devise descriptive eye irritation ratings for nonirritating to maximally irritating in a total of eight grades. They noted that many cosmetic

---

[1]It should be noted here that Draize et al. (1944) not only described a scoring system but also gave several regimens for applying materials and recommended the number of rabbits to be used. We use the term "Draize scoring system" here to refer to the scoring system without implying that other parts of the original methods were used.

products would require labeling as eye irritants by the FHSA criteria, but in their system some separation of various levels of severity was possible. They stressed the difficulty of devising a totally adequate numerical system for scoring or classifying eye irritants.

Russell and Hoch (1962) submitted shampoos for ocular irritation testing in rabbits to several laboratories and noted marked variability among the results reported. There was some disagreement for two sets of rabbits treated with identical test samples at the same laboratory. The scores for the cornea, iris, and conjunctiva covered wide ranges when one laboratory was compared to another laboratory. Verbal descriptions of the effects induced by the same formulation were variable among laboratories, with ratings of the same sample ranging from a mild to a moderate ocular irritant. Russell and Hoch suggested that results would be improved if standard methods were available to instill materials into eyes and if a "standard irritant" existed against which to compare other materials.

Gaunt and Harper (1964) concluded that a fairly consistent pattern of ocular responses was obtained regardless of the test method used. They noted that dilution was a critical factor, and substantial dilution with water prior to instillation into the eye could prevent expression of the full irritancy of the formulation. They recommended that eyes should be irrigated with water after ocular instillation of the test irritant.

Battista and McSweeney (1965) developed approaches for quantitation of methods for testing of eye irritation. They noted that substances that were quite severely irritating were damaging to the rabbit eye and were readily recognized. It was more difficult to test materials that were nonirritating or mildly irritating or to compare the eye irritancy of related formulations. The methods available were unreliable and yielded erroneous or ambiguous data. In an attempt to partially control this, they developed a corneal applicator for the dispensing of the test formulation onto the cornea in a uniform manner.

Battista and McSweeney (1965) noted that inclusion of discharge and chemosis in conjunctiva scores was a source of variation. Numerical scores for these lesions were of little value unless it was clearly established that the results were not influenced by factors such as ocular infection. The authors concluded that iris, cornea, and conjunctiva should be considered individually and the maximum response alone, rather than the area involved, should be used in estimating the severity of ocular injury.

Beckley (1965a) reviewed the literature and sent questionnaires to various laboratories and manufacturers of drugs, cosmetics, and household products asking for methods used to perform and interpret tests for eye irritancy. This paper summarized the results obtained from his questionnaire and contained a list of comments and recommendations for improving the FHSA for eye irritancy evaluation. Beckley and more recently Gloxhuber (1985) have recommended the use of a set of reference standards for irritation. Beckley also concluded that at least two animal species, the rabbit and either the dog or the monkey, should be included in eye irritancy testing.

Alexander (1965) reported one incident in 1951 in which a product was marketed that had passed eye irritation tests in rabbits and yet produced minor ocular lesions in some persons.

Bonfield and Scala (1965) evaluated 13 shampoos. Only one shampoo was free of ocular irritative effects 14 d after instillation, and even it produced irritation in irrigated eyes 7 d after instillation. They considered the Draize eye test as a useful tool in screening materials for eye irritancy but suggested that other means or methods should be utilized before new material is thoroughly evaluated in humans.

In an attempt to standardize the assignment of numerical scores to chemically induced ocular changes, the *Illustrated Guide for Grading Eye Irritation by Hazardous Substances* appeared in 1965 (FDA, 1965). It provided color illustrations and short descriptions of the effects noted in rabbit eyes following instillation of an irritant. The color photographs provided an important reference for standardization of ocular irritation test scores. Scores for individual ocular changes were based on Draize's system (Draize, 1959) but were recorded individually and not summed.

Weltman et al. (1965) combined the Draize (1959) procedures and additional techniques such as photographic collection of data and ophthalmoscopic and histologic observations. The objective was to reduce subjective errors and improve evaluation and assessment of eye irritation. They also considered the role of population size, the time of release of the lids after topical ocular instillations, and other factors that might affect the course of the eye irritation. They observed that the individual scoring or subjective errors were a relatively minor influence, but could not rule out the possibility that variations among scores recorded by differently trained individuals from two laboratories may be considerable. The study also demonstrated that one could have considerable differences between total mean scores of various test groups with studies containing 4, 8, or 24 eyes. Statistical analysis demonstrated the greater validity of values based on samples of sufficient population size. Weltman et al. felt that increasing the number of rabbits used in the standard Draize test would be helpful in avoiding the pass–fail errors that can occur by chance when small populations are employed. They concluded that eight eyes was a sufficient number. Their data indicated that early release of the lids had an ultimately beneficial effect, which was attributed to eye wash by lacrimation. They noted that the techniques of different laboratories relative to the release of the lids after topical ocular instillation varied and this could contribute to the variability noted among laboratories.

Variability among laboratories employing subjective ocular scoring schemes has not been resolved. Weltman et al. (1965) stated that the greatest variability was due to the animal itself. Unfortunately there were (and still are) no standard strains of rabbit used for eye tests. In the rabbit, they felt that age, sex, and strain differences could affect the resistance of the laboratory animal to either chemical or physical states of stress. This aspect has yet to be investigated and still warrants attention. In attempting to interpret the usefulness of photographic, ophthalmoscopic, and histologic methods for assessing eye irritation, they noted that the photographic method could permanently record the external appearance and the physical state of the eye within certain limits. The slit-lamp assisted in determining location, extent, and depth of corneal, iridal, and lens damage, and also permitted observation of changes in the anterior and posterior chambers of the eye. The use of the slit-lamp has long been advocated by others (Marzulli, 1968; Baldwin et al., 1973; Marzulli and Ruggles, 1973). Weltman et al. (1965) also noted that histologic procedures could more fully ascertain and permanently record the structural damage done to tissues and cells of the eye.

Ballantyne and Swanston (1972) pointed out that ocular scores published in the literature were uninformative about responses of individual tissues and this was a major limitation of the Draize system (Draize et al., 1944). Identical mean Draize scores could result from two entirely different reactions. Investigators, they felt, must keep ocular scores separate for each ocular tissue, as indicated in the *Illustrated Guide for Grading Eye Irritation by Hazardous Substances* (FDA, 1965). In contrast, Ashford and Lamble (1974) pointed out that their method of assigning numerical values to a number of suitable symptoms and totaling them to give an overall description of the syndrome is valid if it correctly arranges the eyes in order of clinical severity. Shuster and Kaufman (1974), however, noted that addition of the scores assigned to different tissues or responses was statistically improper since some lesions or signs are more important than others. For example, mild but persistent corneal lesions are more ominous than severe but transient conjunctival hyperemia.

Ocular irritation is now evaluated routinely for a wide variety of materials. Some aspects of potential importance have received relatively little attention. For example, Aronson et al. (1966) demonstrated that the prolonged topical ocular instillation of allergenic materials could result in ocular lesions. Studies are currently underway in the author's laboratory to determine whether an allergenic or sensitizing response can be observed by the topical instillation of materials.

Schuck et al. (1966) devised a procedure for evaluating the ocular irritation potential of atmospheric pollutants in human eyes. A dose-response study of the major pollutants was performed to determine the level at which an irritation response was observed.

MECHANISMS OF OCULAR RESPONSE
TO IRRITANTS

An understanding of the origin and significance of ocular lesions is central to their recognition and correct interpretation. A brief summary of the pathogenesis of topical ocular injury is presented below, together with a brief description of the normal histology of each tissue (Prince et al., 1960; Marzulli and Simon, 1971; Hogan et al., 1971; Fine and Yanoff, 1972; Leibowitz, 1984).

Conjunctiva

The conjunctiva is squamous, nonkeratinized epithelium that contains numerous mucus-secreting cells. The bulbar conjunctival epithelium has fewer goblet cells and is less glandular than the palpebral conjunctival epithelium. More polyhedral cells appear in the palpebral conjunctiva and the surface cells are more stratified, like those of corneal epithelium. The outermost cell surfaces are covered by numerous microvilli (Phister, 1975). Melanophores are frequently present in the conjunctiva, particularly the bulbar conjunctiva near the limbus. They are, of course, absent in albino rabbits.

Visible through the conjunctiva on the posterior surface of the lids are the Meibomian glands (specialized sebaceous glands), which are parallel rows of lobulated glands with ducts opening into the rims of the eyelids. Modified sweat glands (of Moll) are also present in the eyelid and open near the cilia (eyelashes) somewhat anterior to the outlets of the Meibomian glands. Many of the ducts of the glands of Moll also empty into the ciliary follicles. In some species there are also rudimentary sebaceous glands (of Zeiss), which open into the ciliary follicles. Rabbits also have accessory lacrimal glands in the conjunctiva around the Meibomian glands.

The nictitating membrane or third eyelid is a prominent and important structure in many common animal species and is especially prominent in rabbits. It is attached in the medial canthus of the eye and moves laterally or diagonally across the eye behind the external lids. The membrana nictitans consist of a T/shaped skeleton of cartilage covered by a layer of squamous epithelium. There are small lymphoid follicles and a prominent secretory gland, which is similar in many ways to accessory lacrimal glands. In rabbits, the gland of the nictitating membrane and Harder's glands are very similar histologically. The nictitating gland may be continuous with Harder's gland, which lies adjacent to the globe at the depth of the medial canthus (Prince et al., 1960). Harder's gland is present in rabbits but not in humans and nonhuman primates. The lacrimal gland is very large in the rabbit. It nearly encloses the globe near the orbital rim. The lacrimal gland is serous, while the glans nictitans and Harder's glands of the rabbit secrete lipid materials. Each of these glandular structures can affect ocular irritation scores, either directly by contributing to exudates and discharge or indirectly by altering the properties or concentrations of materials applied to the eye. Despite the relatively large size of the ocular glands, tearing in the rabbit is much less than in humans (Beuhler and Newmann, 1964).

Vessels of the conjunctiva are prominent. They generally run in two layers, a deep and a more superficial group. The deep vessels are direct branches of the anterior ciliary arteries, while the superficial vessels are derived from the branches of this artery that supply the fornix. The vascular supply is greatest on the bulbar conjunctiva and less on the conjunctiva of the lids. There are two systems of lymphatics. The one within the fibrous layer contains larger vessels, while the one adjacent to the more superficial capillary blood vessels contains smaller lymphatic channels.

The various secretory cells and glands of the lids and orbit contribute significantly to normal corneal function. In addition to the washing and sweeping actions alluded to earlier, secretions of serous, fatty, and mucinous materials contributed to the tear film (precorneal film). This thin layer of liquid covers the cornea under normal circumstances and plays a vital role in the wettability of corneal epithelium. In particular, glycoproteins from the conjunctiva contribute to the stability and effectiveness of the tear film (Holly and Lemp, 1971). Materials that interfere with the stability or sources of the components of the film can seriously affect the corneal epithelium and may eventually result in corneal ulcers (Dohlman, 1971).

There is frequently a rather rapid response following topical administration of irritants. The subject often blinks rapidly, tearing may occur, and a sudden increase in the apparent vascularity of the conjunctiva is observed. It is difficult to evaluate accurately the effect these responses play in diluting and changing the pH, ionic concentration, and so forth of ocular irritants.

If the irritant persists or if it elicits a more prolonged reaction, more dramatic changes occur. They include continued secretion from the various conjunctival and orbital glands and accumulation of these materials on lid margins, at the medial canthus, and even on the haired skin of the lower lid. Continued irritation results in continued dilation of the conjunctival vascular bed. This is recognized clinically as increased redness and vascular injection (congestion). Intravascular stasis and/or injury to endothelial cells of the microcirculation (directly by the irritant or indirectly by release of chemical mediators of inflammation) results in escape of intravascular fluids and their accumulation in the loose subjunctival connective tissues. This results in edema (chemosis) and is recognized by bulging of the conjunctiva, especially of the palpebral conjunctiva, which may eventually prevent normal lid closure (Hogan and Zimmerman, 1962).

Cornea

The cornea consists of five layers; from without inward they are epithelium, Bowman's membrane, stroma, Descemet's membrane, and endothelium. The epithelial layer is made up of several layers of cells and is approximately 10% of the total corneal thickness in humans and most other mammals. The innermost layer of cells is a basal cell layer, which is columnar and closely packed. Middle layer cells are more flattened and become thinner and wider, until finally in the superficial layers the outermost cells are flat and squamoid. Cell membranes are markedly intedigitated and connected by desmosomes. Interdigitation becomes less tortuous and intercellular spaces widen between the desmosomes as the surface is approached (Phister, 1973). Cytoplasmic projections exist on the outer surfaces of the superficial epithelial cells. The density of these projections per unit surface area and their organization vary from area to area on the cornea. Shifts in the organization occur apparently as part of normal metabolic events. On the outermost surface there is an osmophilic layer of material, which constitutes the lipid film on the surface of the corneal epithelium.

Stroma makes up about nine-tenths of the thickness of the cornea in most mammals. It is divided into sheets of collagenous material, which lie parallel to the surface and have numerous cells (corneal keratocytes) scattered throughout them. Blood vessels and lymphatics are absent except at the extreme periphery. The lamellae are formed of fibrous bands of collagen that run uninterruptedly from limbus to limbus, with the possible exception of the most superficial layer of the stroma, which appears to be slightly interdigitated. The most anterior portion of the stromal zone forms Bowman's membrane in humans and nonhuman primates. This is a sheet approximately 12 μm thick that is distinguishable under ordinary light microscopic conditions. In most other mammals this zone is very thin (in rabbits it is about 2μm thick) or suggested only as a condensation of the stromal surface. The transparency of the cornea is afforded by the spatial configuration of the collagen fibrils. These fibrils are arranged in a regular array separated by less than one-half the wavelength of light. Each fibril is surrounded by glycosaminoglycans, which are very hydroscopic. Separation of the fibrils due to water imbibition (edema) from their normal array of less than one-half of the wavelength of light results in light scattering, that is, corneal cloudiness.

In addition to the specialized organization in sheets or lamellae and the relatively smaller diameters of the collagen fibrils, the other unique feature of the corneal stroma that contributes to transparency is its relative degree of hydration in comparison to the sclera. The water content of the stroma is approximately 78% in most species, while, in comparison, the sclera is approximately 68% water (Maurice, 1969).

The endothelium is a single layer of cells, which completely covers the posterior surface of the cornea and forms a hexagonal matrix when viewed from the flat surface or via the slit-lamp. The cells vary slightly in thickness from species to species, being approximately 4–5 μm thick in humans but somewhat thinner in other species. Nuclei are large, flat, and oval or round. There are intracellular spaces, although the passageways between the anterior chamber and basement membrane are very tortuous. On the apical surfaces the cells are attached by zonula occludentes.

Descemet's membrane is an elastic sheet, which is 5–10 μm thick in humans (7 or 8 μm in the rabbit) and bounds the inner surface of the stroma. It is the exaggerated basement membrane of the endothelium. While appearing structureless under light microscopy, in the electron microscope it has some organization, particularly in the anterior zone.

The transitional zone (limbus) is the region in which the cornea adjoins the sclera; it is important in the study of corneal injury because one of the sources of fluid and cells is the blood vessel meshwork lying in the limbus. As one approaches the limbus the number of cells in the epithelial layer of the cornea increases and their morphologic appearance varies to approach that of conjunctival epithelium. Descemet's layer splits and begins to merge with the trabeculae of the angle of the anterior chamber together with the endothelium. The collagen fibrils continue into the scleral stroma. In the limbus the diameter of the fibrils is greater than that in the cornea, and they begin to assume the appearance of twisted bundles of fibers. There is a rich vascular plexus, and capillary loops enter a short distance into the stroma, particularly in the superficial layers. This is quite prominent in albino rabbits (Prince et al., 1960).

Animal corneas differ from those of humans in several ways. Those in the rabbit and other common infrahuman species are thinner than those of humans. Beckley (1965b) compared the corneal thickness and relative area of the corneal surface to the total area of the globe for the mouse, rat, rabbit and human.

Species	Corneal thickness (mm)	Area (%)
Mouse	0.1	50
Rat	0.15	50
Rabbit	0.4	25
Human	0.52–0.54	7

Epithelial layers are usually somewhat thinner, although usually 5 or 6 layers can be seen in rabbits and 7–10 layers occur in humans. Major differences occur in the structure of Bowman's membrane, which is essentially unrecognizable in rabbits but is prominent in human and nonhuman primate eyes. Thicknesses are given as 8–12 μm (human) and 1.75–2.0 μm (rabbit) in histological sections (Carpenter and Smyth, 1946; Prince et al., 1960). The stromal thickness accounts for the bulk of the difference in corneal thickness among most mammals. The stromal lamellae are more loosely arranged in the rabbit than the human eye. Descemet's membrane and the endothelial layer are quite similar among various mammals.

The cornea maintains its normal state of transparency in part by maintaining the peculiar arrangement of lamellae of collagen fibers. Destruction of either of the limiting cell layers will result in swelling of the corneal stroma. The swelling is the result of imbibition of fluid through the damaged epithelial or endothelial cell layers. Fluid can also enter from the capillary plexus at the limbus, particularly in situations where inflammatory changes of the vascular endothelium occurs. Swelling appears to take place first in the anterior, more irregular layers of the stroma. The expansion takes place within lamellae and may be the result of fluid imbibition into the glycosaminoglycan ground substance around the collagen fibers. In the grossly swollen cornea of the rabbit, stroma appears to be divided sharply into anterior and posterior zones. The posterior zones show lamination into alternate sheets of greater or lesser cloudiness, suggesting that the lamellae are separating.

The corneal epithelium is highly resistant to fat-insoluble substances. Since it is probable that many substances penetrate at the epithelium largely by way of intracellular spaces, the outer layers of cells may offer great resistance to the movement, because the flattened cell forms increase the path distance from one face to the other, while at the same time the total area into which ions may penetrate is very much reduced.

Examination of the cornea includes evaluation of endothelial and stromal lesions as well as epithelial lesions. Corneal cloudiness is contributed to by edema of the stroma and infiltration of inflammatory cells into the cornea. Increases in intensity or severity of corneal cloudiness indicate increasingly severe stromal swelling. Epithelial lesions may occur independently of corneal opacity (cloudiness), provided the basal cell layer of the corneal epithelium is not destroyed. Careful examination is necessary to detect these changes, and fluorescein is frequently recommended as an aid in detecting small epithelial defects. Careful examination of the cornea with magnification and various light sources will also often reveal fine opacities associated with mild epithelial injury. Materials that cause denudation of epithelium and exposure of the stroma are of much greater consequence. Corneal epithelium can rapidly migrate across epithelial defects and cover even denuded but otherwise intact Bowman's membrane. Rabbit cornea seems to reepithelialize much more slowly than human cornea (Carpenter and Smyth, 1946). Injuries that affect large areas of the corneal surface and penetrate to Bowman's membrane significantly interfere with this process. Even punctate lesions that penetrate into and damage Bowman's membrane are serious because of the vital role played by the superficial stromal layers in affecting epithelization.

It should be noted that ocular irritants can induce corneal stromal edema by their action on the prominent vessels at the limbus and that this can occur without substantial injury to corneal epithelium. Prolonged damage to the cornea, especially persistent corneal edema, results in endothelial proliferation from limbal vessels and the extension of vascular loops toward the center of the cornea (pannus). Vascularization of the cornea occurs readily in rats and rabbits. Permanent corneal opacities may result from the more severe lesions of the stroma and epithelium.

Iris

There are close anatomic relationships involving both nerves and blood vessels between the cornea and the iris. In addition, the posterior surfaces of the cornea and the anterior aspects of the iris communicate directly via the aqueous humor, which bathes them both. Therefore, ocular irritants applied topically may produce alterations in the iris.

The iris is an extremely vascular structure that is heavily pigmented (except in albinos). The bulk of the iris is made up of loose connective tissue stroma in which the vessels, muscles, and pigmented cells are included. Vascular patterns vary. In humans a major arterial circle is recognized at the root of the iris, from which vessels extend in a radial pattern toward the pupil. They join to form a lesser vascular circle at the collarette. Small vessels then continue to supply the thinner portion of the iris between the collarette and the pupillary margin.

The New Zealand albino rabbit usually employed in ocular irritation studies allows one to observe the iris vessels easily. Beginning from the 3 and 9 o'clock positions there are four vessels, two going to the upper part of the iris, while two others go to the lower part of the iris (Fig. 1; Figs. 1–12, reproduced in full color, are found between pages 766 and 767). These vessels are referred to as primary vessels. Branches coming off the primary vessels that are parallel to each other in a line in the direction of the pupillary border are referred to as secondary vessels. Branching off from the secondary vessels are very small tertiary vessels.

The surface topography of the iris is characterized by a series of radiating furrows, which run from base to pupillary margin. The posterior surface is covered by a layer of cuboidal epithelial cells, which are heavily pigmented except in albinos.

Injury to the iris is detected by observing changes in the vessels of the iris, the thickness of the iridal stroma, and aqueous flare. As in the conjunctiva, the vessels of the iris become hyperemic following chemically induced irritation. This change can be observed directly. Additional fluid may leak from the vessels and be imbibed by the iris stroma, causing swelling (edema) of the stroma. More severe injury may result in exudation of high-molecular-weight proteins and cells, resulting in more severe iridal stromal edema and aqueous flare in the anterior chamber.

The Tyndall phenomenon observed in the anterior chamber is known as aqueous flare. In the normal anterior chamber, there is the absence of an observable light beam as it passes through the aqueous humor. Release of proteinaceous material or cells from iridal vessels in response to chemically induced irritation contributes to changing the refractive index of light in the anterior chamber and gives rise to the Tyndall phenomenon. The presence of aqueous flare is presumptive evidence of breakdown of the blood–aqueous barrier. An interesting phenomenon of direct importance for eye irritation studies is known as "consensual breakdown" of the blood–aqueous barrier (Davson, 1969). It has been observed that a highly irritative substance applied topically to one eye potentiates the breakdown of the barrier by a less irritating substance in the opposite eye. This can be detected by observing an increase in the aqueous level of intravenously administered Evans blue. This phenomena has been attributed to an arterial connection between the two internal ophthalmic arteries (Forster et al., 1979). The importance of this phenomenon in conventional ocular irritation testing has not been determined. However, it seems possible that a highly irritative substance in one eye could give an artificially high reading in the iritis and flare scores of a less irritative substance in the opposite eye.

Although the term iritis is sometimes used to describe all changes in the iris, it should be recognized that iritis correctly refers to inflammation of the iris. Other, less severe, changes such as injection of iridal vessels (hyperemia) and leakage of fluids into the iris stroma (edema) precede frank iritis.

Marzulli and Simon (1971) reviewed many of the factors that influence animal responses to ocular irritants. In addition to the anatomical features reviewed above, methods of application of irritants and the chemical nature of the material are important. The physicochemical properties of the test substance will influence the rate of corneal penetration. Penetration is related to the lipoidal and hydrophilic properties of the material, since substances must first mix with the fatty precorneal film and then penetrate the hydropic corneal tissue. Penetration is achieved best by substances with maximum aqueous and lipid solubility (Havener, 1966; Akers et al., 1977). Osmolarity of the materials bathing the cornea and their ability to combine with corneal fluid and structural components also influence the action of these materials as irritants (Marzulli and Simon, 1971).

ANIMAL TESTS AS PREDICTORS OF HUMAN RESPONSES

One of the major issues in any test conducted to evaluate hazard to humans is how nearly the test animals actually predict the human response.

Probably the single most important factor in preclinical safety testing is selection of the test animal. Ideally, the animal would be neither more nor less sensitive than the human, would predict human response accurately over a wide range of materials, and would be readily available, inexpensive, and yield consistently reproducible data. In ocular irritation testing the albino rabbit has been used most frequently. However, other species, especially dogs and nonhuman primates (rhesus monkey), have also been suggested as suitable animals in some circumstances (Beckley, 1965b; Swanston, 1985).

The albino rabbit has obvious advantages for testing ocular irritants. The animal itself is readily available; it is docile, easily handled, relatively inexpensive, and easy to maintain. The eye is large and the corneal surface and bulbar conjunctival areas are both large and easily observed. The iris is unpigmented, allowing ready observation of the iridal vessels.

There are also deficiencies in the rabbit model. Some anatomic differences between rabbit and human eyes have already been mentioned. In addition, despite the general marked improvement in standardization of laboratory animals over the last few years, there are still significant variations among laboratory rabbits. Age, strain, and sex differences as well as variations in general health status can be expected to influence ocular irritation tests (Weltman et al., 1965).

Limited experience with rhesus monkeys (Beckley et al., 1969) or the cynomolgus monkey (Hackett, 1989) indicated that these animals more nearly reflected human responses than did rabbits. However, there are very real problems in using monkeys. They are very costly and are now very difficult to obtain. Restraint can be difficult, and the ocular responses are less uniform than rabbits. Their pigmented irises make observation of some irritation responses more difficult to evaluate, although as early as 1942 it has been suggested that rabbits with pigmented irises are more appropriate than albinos for studying ocular responses to chemical induced changes (Mann and Pullinger, 1942). Absorption and distribution of a drug can be influenced by binding to melanin pigments and this important factor cannot be ignored in the drug development process.

Another important problem in selecting an animal model that will accurately predict the nature of the human response is lack of adequate information on how humans can be expected to react. Thus, it is not entirely clear what the animal model is expected to predict. McLaughlin (1946) did a retrospective study on industrial accidents which resulted in ocular damage in humans. A total of 602 cases of ocular injury were recorded among 3566 patients referred to the dispensary of a manufacturing plant. Of these, 458 cases demonstrated mild, reversible (by 48 h) ocular lesions, 37 cases required up to 10 d to heal, and 7 involved loss of vision. The majority of the offending agents were alkalis, but many details were not provided. Clinical studies of this type are helpful, but information on the irritating substance, its concentration, and the exposure conditions would enhance their value.

A number of studies have been made in which the ocular irritative effects of various materials in humans and animals can be compared. The bulk of these studies were performed in rabbits. Despite the relative lack of studies in which animal and human responses have been carefully compared under comparable, controlled conditions, there are a number of instances in which reactions in rabbits have generally predicted the observed effects in humans. Leopold (1945) observed that benzalkonium chloride concentrations of 0.03% or greater were irritating in rabbits. A similar reaction has been noted in humans, and several ophthalmic formulations that contain 0.02% benzalkonium chloride have not had any obvious effects. Our own experience is that 0.02% causes no conjunctival irritation in the rabbit, but 0.04% produces obvious ocular irritation (conjunctival congestion, swelling, discharge, and occasional corneal cloudiness).

Slight conjunctival hyperemia was observed after topical ocular instillation in rabbits of propylene glycol (Carpenter and Smyth, 1946). It is noninjurious for human eyes but does produce a transient stinging, blepharospasm, and lacrimation followed by mild conjunctiva hyperemia (Grant, 1986). A 70% concentration has been used as a treatment for corneal edema (Bietti and Giraldi, 1969).

Several liquid hydrocarbons of petroleum, including kerosene, Deo-Base, Stoddard solvent, and petroleum oil, were not harmful to the rabbit and human cornea after direct external contact (Carpenter and Smyth, 1946; Grant, 1986). Similar threshold concentrations (0.5%) for conjunctival irritation were noted for phenethyl alcohol in humans and rabbits (Nakano, 1958; Barkman et al., 1969). Comparable evidence of blepharospasm without ocular damage was noted for rabbit and human eyes after ocular exposure to a commercial preparation of dimercaprol (Grant, 1986).

Human and rabbit eyes reacted similarly to topical ocular administration of oxalic acid (Suker, 1913; McLaughlin, 1946; Grant, 1986). It produced a corneal burn with loss of epithelium but recovery followed in a few days.

No ocular effects were noted in monkeys, humans, and rabbits when 0.1% cytarabine HCl was topically instilled 6 times a day for 6–10 d (Elliott and Schut, 1965). However, 0.5 and 1.0% solutions produced transient speckling, which resembled fine dust particles as seen on retroillumination of rabbit, monkey, and human corneas. McLaughlin (1946) and Grant (1986) reported that humans exhibited only slight corneal epithelial disturbances (clearing within 24–48 h) after a splash of 5% sodium hypochlorite. There was transient corneal haze and conjunctival edema in rabbits, with a return to normal by a day or less (Grant, 1986). Carter and Griffith (1965) reported that monkey eyes healed faster than rabbit eyes after exposure to 5.5% sodium hypochlorite.

The threshold irritation concentration for tetraethoxysilane was 700 ppm for rabbit, guinea pig, and human eyes (Grant, 1986; Smyth and Seaton, 1940). Friemann and Overhoff (1956) and Grant (1986) noted that local application of a 1:5000 (0.02%) solution of colchicine in humans produced very little ocular change, whereas serious reactions were noted with a 1% solution. The 1% solution caused clouding of the stroma with reduced vision, but the cornea cleared in a few weeks. In rabbit eyes, the same solution caused cellular infiltration in the cornea and vascularization which required several weeks before the eyes began to clear.

Full-strength polysorbate 80 (Tween 80) was nonirritating for rabbits. It was well tolerated and nonirritating at 20% concentration in several ophthalmic formulations and at a 9:1 ratio in castor oil for prolonged daily clinical use in humans (Hagiwara and Sugiwia, 1953; Treon, 1965). In our laboratories, we observed comparable minimal to moderate conjunctival congestion in rabbits and humans for 1 and 10% tetracycline ointments.

Podophyllum (Grant, 1986) in humans can produce discomfort, epiphora, and conjunctival hyperemia with slight exposure, but greater exposures may involve loss of the corneal epithelium, severe keratitis, and deposits on the posterior aspects of the cornea associated with wrinkling of Descemet's membrane. Application of podophyllum as a dry powder to the rabbit eye caused an immediate painful reaction, blepharospasm, and a rapid progressive inflammatory reaction (Estable, 1948).

Grant and Kern (1956) evaluated the actions of various alkalis in the corneal stroma, since these are among the most common and the most devastating of chemical injuries to the eye. They noted that the severity of the injury to the corneal stroma by alkalis is governed by the pH rather than the nature of the base. However, they observed certain exceptions to this rule, including long-chain quaternary ammonia compounds, certain dyes, and beryllium. Regardless of the type of alkali used, as long as the pH was greater than 12.0 severe ocular damage was noted. Similarly, Murphy et al. (1982) reported that there is not a very good correlation between acidic pH of solutions and the ocular response in rabbits; however, all alkalis above a pH of 11.5 produce predictable opacities and ocular damage. Grant (1986) generally confirms that alkalis above this pH in humans can cause severe ocular damage that is usually irreversible. A comprehensive study of human ocular injury (McLaughlin, 1946) included reports on six or seven eyes lost in industrial accidents due to exposure to alkalis. Accidental ocular exposure of humans to pure thioglycolic acid produced ocular changes corresponding to that observed for rabbits (Grant, 1986; Butscher, 1953). The eyes progressively deteriorated with the presence of conjunctival edema, hyperemia and discharge, and diffuse corneal opacity requiring several weeks to months to clear.

Turpentine vapors were irritating to human eyes at 720–1100 ppm and to cat eyes at 540–720 ppm (Flury and Zernik, 1931; Clayton and Clayton, 1981). Accidental splash caused comparable conjunctival hyperemia and slight transient injury of the corneal epithelium but no corneal stromal damage for humans and rabbits (Lewin and Guillery, 1913).

Ooka (1967) concluded from rabbit studies and data available for industry workers that Blasticidin-S induced similar ocular reactions for humans and rabbits. Experimental and clinical use of 0.4% chlorobutanol in a 1.4% sodium chloride solution produced comparable keratitis epithelialis for anesthetized (0.5% tetracaine) rabbit and human corneas (Grant, 1986).

Concentrated phenol produced comparable, instantaneous clouding of the cornea with subsequent conjunctival necrosis and scarring for humans and rabbits (D'Asaro Biondo, 1933; Carter, 1906). Polyethylene glycol ethers (2%) in an ointment caused corneal anesthesia, keratitis epithelialis, loss of epithelium, and corneal edema with wrinkling of Descemet's membrane in humans, while it caused conjunctivitis and long-lasting corneal ulceration and vascularization in rabbits (Popp, 1955).

In contrast to the results noted above in which rabbits generally predicted the results in humans, there have been other studies in which results were disparate in the two species. Estable (1948) noted that a solution of 1:200 histamine biphosphate immediately produced a sensory reaction with slight but acute conjunctival vasodilatation that disappeared very soon in the rabbit eye. He noted that the slight conjunctival reaction with a highly concentrated solution in rabbits was in contrast to the potent vasodilatory effect produced in the human eye by 1:40,000 and 1:50,000 solutions (Gartner, 1944). Grant and Loeb (1948) noted that several antihistamine drugs that were noninjurious to the rabbit eye could not be employed in the treatment of human eyes because they produced considerable pain. The concentrations in the rabbit eye that were noninjurious had to be reduced by one-half to cause no pain or slight conjunctival congestion in human eyes. This finding is not surprising, however, since the rabbit appears to possess a higher threshold to pain than the human (Maurice, 1985).

McDonald et al. (1973b) demonstrated that concentrations of ethylene glycol as high at 80% caused only moderate conjunctivitis and mild swelling, discharge, flare, and iritis in the rabbit eye, even when instilled over a 6-h period. Accidental exposure of 100% ethylene glycol in the eye of a man produced marked edema, considerable chemosis, substantial conjunctival congestion, considerable flare, diminished light reflex, and marked keratitis; it was 4 wk before the eye became clear (Skyowski, 1951). No ocular damage in rabbits was noted for topical ocular use of 0.5% selenium sulfide (Rosenthal and Adler, 1962), but an occasional irritation or transient keratitis was noted in human eyes (Bahn, 1954; Cohen, 1954). Ozone at 2–37 ppm caused irritation in human eyes, but similar concentrations were not injurious to rabbits and dogs (Hine et al., 1960; Stokinger et al., 1957).

Conjunctival congestion and swelling with opacification and superficial vascularization of the human cornea after a splash of 2.5% cresol was recorded (Lewin and Guillery, 1913). Only a mild epithelial defect was caused by topical ocular use of 2.5% cresol in rabbits, guinea pigs, and monkey eyes, while a 10–12% solution caused marked conjunctival and corneal changes for rabbits (Lewin and Guillery, 1913).

Marsh and Maurice (1971) reported the influence of nonionic detergents and other surfactants on human corneal permeability. They used 1% concentrations of various nonionic detergents and noted that the most severe symptoms in humans were associated with 1% Brij 58, which caused discomfort, blurred vision, and halos with corneal epithelial bedewing, although these changes disappeared within 24 h. Duponol (1%) caused severe and immediate pain. Grant (1986), on the other hand, has noted that these surfactants are generally nondamaging to the rabbit eye when administered at high concentrations. Marsh and Maurice (1971) also observed that Tween 20 caused no untoward effect in human eyes in concentrations up to 40%, while Brij 35 caused delayed irritation and punctate staining at concentrations above 3%. Hazelton (1952) considered both substances to be nonirritating to the rabbit eye when administered undiluted.

In another study, eye irritation evaluation was conducted on a male hairdressing formulation in rabbits prior to marketing (Van Abbe, 1973). The data indicated that the substance was nonirritating. When the product was marketed there was a high number of eye irritancy reports. The irritancy test in the laboratory for both monkey and rabbit had failed to indicate the likelihood of an adverse effect in humans. However, if the material was placed on the hair and then eluted, the concentrated aqueous eluant caused an immediate slight conjunctivitis and pitting of the corneal epithelium in the human eye but failed to do so in animal eyes.

Harris et al. (1975) demonstrated that some soaps and surfactants induce prolonged and profound corneal anesthesia in rabbits but not in humans. They indicated that studies of corneal anesthesia in rabbits may not be extrapolated to the human eye. Concentrations greater than those that produced corneal anesthesia in the rabbits were not tested in humans. It may be that the dose response for corneal anesthesia in humans is substantially larger than that in rabbits.

Test animals other than rabbits have also been used in eye irritation tests with variable results. Fairhall (1957) showed that piperonyl butoxide (undiluted) was nondamaging but irritating when tested on eyes of rabbits, cats, rats, and dogs. Phosphorus trichloride vapors were irritating to human eyes, while mild conjunctivitis was observed in cats at 2–4 ppm and corneal cloudiness at 23–90 ppm (von Oettingen, 1958; Flury and Zernik, 1931). A splash of liquid phosgene in the eyes of one human patient caused complete opacification of the cornea and subsequent loss of the eyes (D'Osvaldo, 1928), and high concentrations of the gas caused corneal opacification in cats (Laquer and Magnus, 1921).

One of the most comprehensive studies to compare the eye irritation potential of monkeys and rabbits was conducted by Buehler and Newmann (1964). They noted that materials that were moderately irritating to the monkey (primarily superficial changes such as edema and slight surface alterations) produced more severe ocular reactions in rabbits, including various degrees of corneal opacity, pannus formation, and conjunctivitis. They felt that the different degrees of irritation produced in monkey and rabbit eyes may be due in part to anatomical differences. Bowman's membrane is thin in the rabbit eye, and Buehler and Newmann postulated that this might have been the reason for the type of response noted in the monkey eye. However, Hood et al. (1971) compared the responses to rabbit eyes and monkey eyes with Bowman's membrane removed, and demonstrated that Bowman's membrane and the superficial stroma in the monkey eye had no protective or enhancing effect against the irritating effects of iodine.

Buehler and Newmann (1964) mentioned that the nictitating membrane might be responsible for keeping irritating substances in close contact with the eye and might therefore provide a reservoir for an irritating substance. However, they could not demonstrate that surgical removal of the nictitating membrane affected the healing rates of damaged corneas. A study by Mann and Pullinger (1942) implicated the nictitating membrane to the extent that damage to the membrane will result in prolongation of the ocular healing time. Further evidence that the prominent nictitating membrane of this rabbit eye may play a

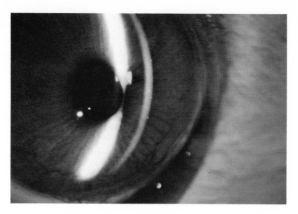

FIGURE 1 Normal albino rabbit eye.

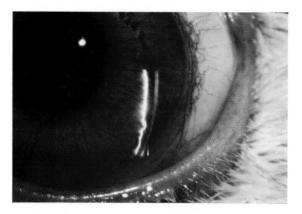

FIGURE 2 +2 Conjunctival congestion: bright red color with perilimbal injection.

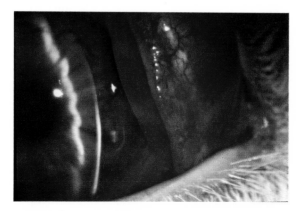

FIGURE 3 +3 Conjunctival congestion: dark, beefy red color, perilimbal injection, and petechia.

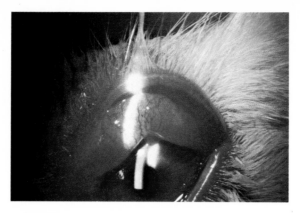

FIGURE 4 +2 Conjunctival swelling: partial eversion of upper eyelid.

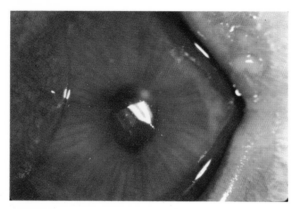

FIGURE 5 +2 Conjunctival discharge: grayish white precipitate on lids.

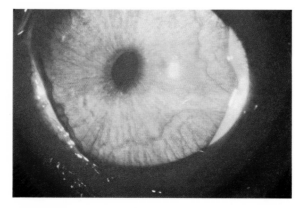

FIGURE 6 +2 Iris involvement: moderate injection of secondary vessels and minimal injection of tertiary vessels.

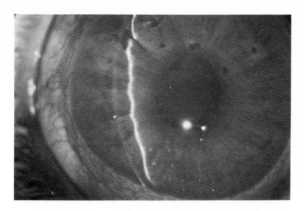

FIGURE 7 +4 Iritis: marked injection of vessels and marked swelling of iris muscle fibers.

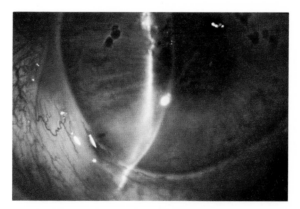

FIGURE 8 Corneal cloudiness (+1 intensity; +1 area): edema of anterior half of stroma; >25% area.

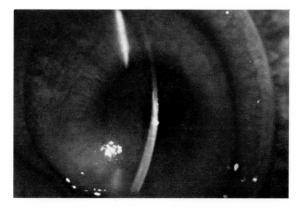

FIGURE 9 Corneal cloudiness (+2 intensity; +2 area): edema of entire stroma, 25–50% area.

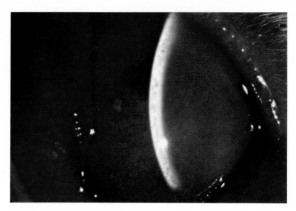

FIGURE 10 Corneal cloudiness (+4 intensity; +4 area): underlying structures obscured, 75–100% area.

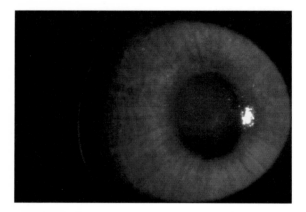

FIGURE 11 Fluorescein staining (+1 intensity; +1 area): diffuse and common in normal rabbit population, >25% area.

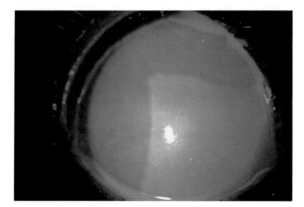

FIGURE 12 Fluorescein staining (+4 intensity; +3 area): obscures underlying structures, 75–100% area.

role in the production of corneal changes observed in rabbits but not in the dog or cynomolgus monkey employing a similar treatment regimen has been presented by Durand-Cavagna et al. (1989) and Hackett (1989), respectively.

Buehler and Newmann (1964) also postulated that the difference in tear flow volume from the rabbit and human eye could account for the differences noted in irritation potential of the various substances. However, no studies have been conducted to date to determine whether this mechanism plays a role. They also observed that the rabbit blinked much less frequently than the human. Our experience has been that the rabbit may blink on the order of 20 times in a 5-min period, which is less frequently than humans. However, it must be pointed out that when an irritant is applied to the rabbit's eye the animal quickly begins to lacrimate and to blink very frequently. To date, there have been no well-controlled studies to focus on whether the blink rate may effect a difference in irritation potential among rabbits, monkeys, and humans.

Pannus formation is very readily apparent in rabbits after a corneal injury (much more so than in humans). Usually it occurs approximately 4–7 d following an ocular insult, and if the corneal injury is substantial it will envelop the entire cornea within a 14-d period. Generally speaking, the pannus does not disappear and remains throughout the lifetime, although it may regress somewhat (Buehler and Newmann, 1964). Pannus response when observed in humans is usually associated with a chronic disease and is not an acute irritative effect. Pannus generally disappears in humans following healing of the cornea.

Rabbit eyes have a rich vascular plexus at the limbus, which responds rapidly and vigorously to ocular injury. This, combined with the looser stromal lamellae of the cornea, may account for the fact that neovascularization and pannus are common responses in the rabbit but occur less readily in human and monkey eyes (Mann and Pullinger, 1942; Buehler and Newmann, 1964).

Other functional and anatomic differences that may contribute to differences in response include pH of the tears (7.1–7.3, human; 8.2, rabbit; 7.4, monkey); looser lids in the rabbit, which may allow irritants to remain in contact with the globe longer; and differences in tear secretion (Buehler and Newmann, 1964; Lee and Robinson, 1986). Rabbits also require more time to repair corneal epithelial lesions than do humans and monkeys (Carpenter and Smyth, 1946; Buehler and Newmann, 1964).

Another factor that influences the response of the rabbit cornea to irritants is the effect of the conjunctival response. Buehler and Newmann (1964) noted that application of irritants to rabbit corneas by means of a cup that confined the material to the cornea resulted in less severe ocular responses, which were more similar to those of humans and monkeys.

Beckley (1965b) conducted comparative eye irritation tests on humans, dogs, rabbits, and monkeys. In a limited number of animal trials (six rabbits, six dogs, and four monkeys) he observed that corneal effects caused by a liquid detergent were most severe in the dogs, while iridal and conjunctival responses were most pronounced in the rabbits. Monkeys were generally less responsive than the other species but exhibited more corneal lesions than humans. Test methods used in the human subjects did not duplicate those used in the animals. In the human subjects the detergent was applied in increasing concentrations and eyes were washed 12 min following exposure. Human subjects experienced burning, mild pain, and conjunctival erythema, and 8 (of 45) exhibited conjunctivitis. The study did not permit direct correlation between the results in animals and humans. In a recent study by Freeberg et al. (1986), groups of 8 human volunteers and 8 albino rabbits under controlled conditions were exposed to the same concentrations and volumes of 4 prototype consumer products using dose volumes of 0.1 or 0.01 ml. The rabbit eyes required a longer time period to clear and the ocular changes observed in the rabbits were more severe than the changes observed in humans receiving the same test material. The results of this study demonstrate that the Draize rabbit test using a volume of 0.1 ml does not predict the effects in humans; however, use of a lower test volume of 0.01 ml was shown to be fully predictive for the consumer products tested.

Battista and McSweeney (1965) reviewed the literature on comparative results for ocular irritants in rabbits, monkeys, and humans. Battista and McSweeney (1965) and Gershbein and McDonald (1977) concluded that the rabbit elicits a more uniform response to ocular irritants as compared to the variable responses observed in humans, and the rabbit should be considered a more sensitive species. In a later study, Beckley et al. (1969) compared the use of the rhesus monkey for predicting human response to eye irritancy. In their study, the instillation of a 5% soap solution in rabbit eyes produced almost no effect on corneal epithelium. However, the same material caused corneal epithelial damage in both monkeys and humans. The lesions were not visible without slit-lamp examination. These studies indicated the potential usefulness of nonhuman primates in predicting human ocular responses to irritating substances. Harris et al. (1975) did not observe a similar relationship of epithelial defects for rabbits and humans for soap solutions.

Swanston (1985) has suggested the mouse, dog, and monkey as alternatives to the rabbit. Experience with these species is limited, and although the monkey presumably would be most representative of humans, the cost of procurement and maintenance presents significant hurdles. Perhaps acute ocular irritation testing in the nonhuman primate should be reserved for special cases to confirm/negate the rabbit test in cases of product liability. Despite the many problems associated with using rabbits as test animals in which to predict human responses, they remain a good test animal. In some instances, the more difficult and expensive tests in monkeys or other species may be justified.

REGULATORY GUIDELINES

Various governmental bodies have published guidelines for eye irritancy procedures. These guidelines are for ophthalmic containers, cosmetics, chemicals, ophthalmic formulations, and other materials that may accidentally or intentionally contact the eye during use.

Ophthalmic Plastic Containers

The *United States Pharmacopeia XXII* sets forth two stages of testing: the first stage is *in vitro* testing, which can be either an agar diffusion test, a direct contact test, or an elution test. Materials that meet the requirements of these tests are then evaluated according to USP-defined procedures in the systemic injection test, intracutaneous test, and eye irritation test. The eye irritation test is a 72-h ocular irritation test in rabbits with saline and cottonseed oil extracts of plastic containers used for packaging ophthalmic formulations. The plastic strips are cleansed and sterilized as per intended use before the extracts are prepared. After topical ocular instillation of the extracts and respective blanks, ocular changes are graded by macroscopic examination. A plastic is rated satisfactory if the ocular changes for the extract-treated eyes are equivalent to or less than those for the blank.

Eye Irritancy

Five federal agencies (Consumer Product Safety Commission, Occupational Safety and Health Administration, Food and Drug Administration, Environmental Protection Agency, and Food Safety and Quality Service of the Department of Agriculture) formed the Interagency Regulatory Liaison Group (IRLG) (*Fed. Reg.*, 1977, 1979). One task was the development of a testing standard including eye irritancy studies. The guidelines for eye irritation (*Fed. Reg.*, 1981) delineated test procedures for liquids, solids, aerosols, and liquids under pressure in order to place in perspective ocular irritancy to laboratory animals. For humane reasons, substances known to be corrosive may be assumed to be eye irritants and should not be tested in the eye. Substances shown to be severe irritants in dermal toxicity tests may be assumed to be eye irritants and need not be tested in the eye.

The guidelines are summarized below:

1. General Considerations
   a. Good laboratory practices. Studies should be conducted according to Good Laboratory Practice regulations (CFR 21, Part 58).
   b. Test substance. As far as is practical, composition of the test substance should be known and should include the names and quantities of all major components, known contaminants and impurities, and the percentages of unknown materials. The lot of the substance should be stored under conditions that maintain its stability, strength, quality, and purity from the date of its production until the tests are complete.
   c. Animals. Healthy animals, without eye defects or irritation and not subjected to any previous experimental procedures, must be used. The test animal shall be characterized as to species, strain, sex, weight, and/or age. Each animal must be assigned an appropriate identification number. Recommendations contained in DHEW publication (NIH) 74–23, entitled "Guide for the Care and Use of Laboratory Animals," should be followed for the care, maintenance, and housing of animals.
   d. Documentation. Color photographic documentation may be used to verify gross and microscopic findings.
2. Specific Considerations
   a. Test preparation. Testing should be performed on young, adult, albino rabbits (male or female) weighing approximately 2.0–3.0 kg. Other species may also be tested for comparative purposes. For a valid eye irritation test, at least six rabbits must survive the test for each test substance. A trial test on three rabbits is suggested. If the substance produces corrosion, severe irritation, or no irritation, no further testing is necessary. However, if equivocal responses occur, testing in at least three additional animals should be performed. If the test substance is intended for use in or around the eye, testing on at least six animals should be performed.
   b. Test procedure. Both eyes of each animal in the test groups must be examined by appropriate means within 24 h before substance administration. For most purposes, anesthetics should not be used; however, if the test substance is likely to cause significant pain, local anesthetics may be used prior to instillation of the test substance for humane reasons. In such cases, anesthetics should be used only once, just prior to instillation of the test substance; the eye used as the control in each rabbit should also be anesthetized. The test substance is placed in one eye of each animal by gently pulling the lower lid away from the globe (conjunctival cul-de-sac)

to form a cup into which the test substance is dropped. The lids are then gently held together for 1 s and the animal is released. The other eye, remaining untreated, serves as a control. Vehicle controls are not included. If a vehicle is suspected of causing irritation, additional studies should be conducted using the vehicle as the test substance. For testing liquids, 0.1 ml is used. For solid, paste, or particulate substances (flake, granule, powder, or other particulate form), the amount used must have a volume of 0.1 ml weighing not more than 100 mg. For aerosol products, the eye should be held open and the substance administered in a single, short burst for about 1 s at a distance of about 4 in directly in front of the eye. The dose should be approximated by weighing the aerosol can before and after each treatment for liquids. After the 24-h examination, the eyes may be washed, if desired. Tap water or isotonic saline solution of sodium chloride (USP or equivalent) should be used for all washings.

c. Observations. The eyes should be examined 24, 48, and 72 h after treatment. At the option of the investigator, the eyes may also be examined at 1 h and at 7, 14, and 21 d. In addition to the required observations of the cornea, iris, and conjunctivae, serious lesions such as pannus, phlyctena, and rupture of the globe should be reported. The grades of ocular reaction (Table 1) must be recorded at each examination. Evaluation of reactions can be facilitated by using a binocular loupe, hand slit-lamp, or other appropriate means. After the recording of observations at 24 h, the eyes of any or all rabbits may be further examined after applying fluorescein stain. An animal has exhibited a positive reaction if the test substance has produced at any observation one or more of the following signs:

   i. Ulceration of the cornea (other than a fine stippling).
   ii. Inflammation of the iris (other than slight deepening of the rugae or light hyperemia of the circumcorneal blood vessels).
   iv. An obvious swelling in the conjunctivae (excluding the cornea and iris) with partial eversion of the eyelids or a diffuse crimson color with individual vessels not easily discernible.

d. Evaluation. The test result is considered positive if four or more animals in either test group exhibit a positive reaction. If only one animal exhibits a positive reaction, the test result is regarded as negative. If two or three animals exhibit a positive reaction, the investigator may designate the substance an irritant. When two or three animals exhibit a positive reaction and the investigator does not designate the substance an irritant, the test shall be repeated

TABLE 1. Grades for Ocular Lesions

Description	Grade
Cornea	
Opacity: degree of density (area most dense taken for reading)	
No ulceration or opacity	0
Scattered or diffuse areas of opacity (other than slight dulling of normal luster), details of iris clearly visible	1[a]
Easily discernible transluent areas, details of iris slightly obscured	2
Nacreous areas, no details of iris visible, size of pupil barely discernible	3
Opaque cornea, iris not discernible through opacity	4
Iris	
Normal	0
Markedly deepened rugae, congestion, swelling, moderate circumcorneal hyperemia, or injection, any of these or any combination thereof, iris still reacting to light (sluggish reaction is positive)	1[a]
No reaction to light, hemorrhage, gross destruction (any or all of these)	2
Conjunctivae	
Redness (refers to palpebral and bulbar conjunctivae excluding cornea and iris)	
Blood vessels normal	0
Same blood vessels definitely hyperemic (injected)	1
Diffuse, crimson color, individual vessels not easily discernible	2[a]
Diffuse beefy red	3
Chemosis: lids and/or nictitating membranes	
No swelling	0
Any swelling above normal (includes nictitating membranes)	1
Obvious swelling with partial eversion of lids	2[a]
Swelling with lids about half closed	3
Swelling with lids more than half closed	4

[a]Readings at these numerical values or greater indicate positive responses.

with a different group of six animals. The second test result is considered positive if three or more of the animals exhibit a positive reaction. Opacity grades 2–4 and/or perforation of the cornea are considered to be corrosive effects or when opacities persist to 21 d. If only one or two animals in the second test exhibit a positive reaction, the test should be repeated with a different group of six animals. When a third test is needed, the substance will be regarded as an irritant if any animal exhibits a positive response.

3. Data Reporting
   a. Identification. Each test report should be signed by the persons responsible for the test, identify the laboratory where the test was performed by name and address, and give inclusive dates of the test.
   b. Body of report. The test report must include all information necessary to provide a complete and accurate description and evaluation of the test procedures and results in the following sections:
   i. Summary and conclusions.
   ii. Materials, including the identification of the test substance (chemical name, molecular structure, and a qualitative and quantitative determination of its chemical composition), manufacturer and lot number of the substance tested, and specific identification of diluents, suspending agents, emulsifiers, or other materials used in administering the test substance. Specific animal data are to be included in the report. This includes species and strain, source of supply of the animals, description of any pretest acclimation, and number, age, and condition of animals of each sex in each test group.
   iii. Methods, such as deviation from guidelines, specifications of test methods, data on dosage administration, and data on observation methods.
   iv. Results, such as tabulation of data and individual, must accompany each report in sufficient detail to permit independent evaluation of results, including summaries and tables that show relation of effects to time of dosing, etc.

Testing of Ophthalmic Therapeutic Formulations

The basic guideline for ocular irritancy evaluation of ophthalmic formulations was a 20-d test recommended by Draize (1959). Goldenthal (1968) set forth more complete general guidelines for toxicity evaluation of ophthalmic formulations (over-the-counter or prescription). The guidelines are not for contact lenses or lens solutions. Goldenthal's guidelines are somewhat dated but remain the only published guidelines for ophthalmic drugs from the FDA, and these guidelines are summarized in Table 2.

An acute ophthalmic safety test is recommended on each manufactured lot of an ophthalmic product. This test is designed to check on gross misformulation during manufacture. A single instillation in two eyes is followed by macroscopic examination at 30 min and 24 h postadministration. Eyes with congestion (greater than 2 +) or any other ocular change (chemosis, discharge, iris involvement, or corneal cloudiness) would warrant a retest. A rejection of the lot would follow if the above ocular changes are noted in the four retest eyes.

CONTACT LENS PRODUCTS

The FDA has provided guidelines for testing new contact lenses (substances other than polymethyl methacrylate) (1988) and solutions (1985) used with new contact lenses. These guidelines were developed as a consequence of interest in soft contact lenses and the unique problems associated with good daily hygiene. The ophthalmic guidelines for testing new contact lenses are reproduced herein.

TABLE 2. Guidelines for Toxicity Evaluation of Ophthalmic Formulations from Goldenthal (1968)

Category	Duration of human administration	Phase[a]	Subacute or chronic toxicity[b]
Ophthalmic	Single application	I	
	Multiple application	I, II, III	One species; 3 wk daily applications, as in clinical use
		NDA	One species; duration commensurate with period of drug administration

[a]Phases I, II, and III are defined in section 130.0 of the New Drug Regulations.

[b]Acute toxicity should be determined in three to four species; subacute or chronic studies should be by the route to be used clinically.

Recommended Toxicology Test Procedures
for Contact Lens Materials

1. Systemic Injection Test (USP):

   The purpose of this study is to assess the potential of leachable chemical constituents from a contact lens material to produce an acute systemic toxicity in mice. Extracts of the lens material are prepared in two types of solvents (polar and nonpolar), injected into mice, and the mice observed for acute systemic toxicity.

   *United States Pharmacopeia XXI/National Formulary XVI (or current update)—Containers for Ophthalmics–Plastics–Biological Test Procedures.

2. Eye Irritation Test (USP):

   The purpose of this study is to evaluate the potential for ocular irritation resulting from the residual chemical leachables in contact lens materials. The effects are assessed *in vivo* using rabbits.

   *United States Pharmacopeia XXI/National Formulary XVI (or current update)—Containers for Ophthalmics–Plastics–Biological Test Procedures.

3. Cytotoxicity Test:

   The purpose of this study is to evaluate the potential for cytotoxicity resulting from residual chemical leachables in contact lens materials. The effects are assessed *in vitro* using cytotoxicity studies, such as tissue culture-agar overlay method (Guess et al., 1965) or a suitable alternative.

4. Sensitization Tests:

   These tests are required, especially for uniquely new monomers, or for new additives used in contact lens polymers, or to assess the sensitization from interaction between new lens materials and preservatives in contact lens solutions. The purposes of these tests are to evaluate the *in vitro* and/or *in vivo* potential for the induction of a sensitivity/allergic response resulting from an uptake and release of preservatives used in lens care solutions or from residual chemical leachables, such as residual unreacted monomers, additives, or other impurities, in contact lens materials.

5. Three Week Ocular Irritation Test in Rabbits:

   The *in vivo* test of the contact lenses in rabbits may be used as a biocompatibility test as well as a toxicity test of the lens material to assess the *in vivo* effects of the ocular environment on the lens material as well as the *in vivo* effects of the lens material on the ocular tissues.

Presented in this section is an example of a test design that can be used as general guidance in developing an appropriate *in vivo* ocular irritation test of a contact lens made of a material other than plastic. It is the responsibility of the sponsor to design an appropriate *in vivo* test using a sufficient number of animals to assess the safety and biocompatibility when using the recommended lens care regimen proposed for use in the clinical investigation.

The Center for Devices and Radiological Health (CDRH) suggests that this *in vivo* ocular irritation test be performed in the rabbit model. Test lenses for the test should be the thickest lenses in the product line or lenses of the greatest mass (with and without the use of the recommended lens care regimen) as they are to be used in a clinical investigation. Appropriate controls, such as eyes receiving no lens or eyes receiving a control lens, should be included in the test design. A minimum of 12 rabbits, determined to be free of corneal defects by initial slit-lamp examination for fluorescein staining, should be distributed into groups similar to the proposed groupings outlined in the example below:

12 Rabbits—6 male/6 female (24 total eyes).

Group 1 (males)—three normal eyes fitted with the test lenses that have been treated with disinfection procedures proposed for patient use.

Group 2 (females)—three normal eyes fitted with the test lenses that have been treated with disinfection procedures proposed for patient use.

Group 3 (males)—three normal eyes fitted with the test lenses that have *not* been treated with disinfection procedures proposed for patient use.

Group 4 (females)—three normal eyes fitted with the test lenses that have *not* been treated with disinfection procedures proposed for patient use.

When appropriate, all lenses used in the test should be retrieved for purposes of assessing the *in vivo* effects of the ocular environment on the lens material when using the recommended lens care regimen. The information submitted in the report should include, but not be limited to, data that compare the physical and optical parameters of the lens, such as physical appearance, lens decolorization, protein deposits, chipped or pitted lenses, center thickness, and lens powers as measured before starting the test and after termination of the test.

Recommended Toxicology Test Procedures
for Contact Lens Solutions

1. Acute oral toxicology assessment. The purpose of this study is to assess the potential of a contact lens solution to produce acute oral

toxicity in rodents. While the Division of Ophthalmic Devices (DOD) believes that acute oral toxicity studies should be performed, the division recognized that alternative testing to the classic LD50 assay may be appropriate under certain circumstances for assessing risks to humans from the proper or improper use (i.e., accidental misuse) of a contact lens solution. DOD will accept for review oral toxicity test data for a contact lens solution as formulated that does not show signs of toxicity, that is, mortality, morbidity and/or pathogenesis, if the solution has been given orally to a group of test animals in a single large dose, generally referred to as the maximum tolerable dose. For rodent testing, the maximum volume of an aqueous solution generally should not exceed 2 ml/100 g body weight. These data will be considered sufficient for predicting with reasonable assurance that a contact lens solution does not present an acute oral concern. This interpretation is based on the division's historical experience with toxicology test data from OTC solutions for contact lens use and is consistent with current trends in safety evaluation testing. However, should signs of toxicity be demonstrated at the maximum tolerable dose, further testing consistent with accepted toxicological practices is recommended in order for DOD to complete its risk/benefit assessment of the contact lens solution.

2. Acute systemic toxicity assessment. The purpose of this study is to assess the potential of the solutions as formulated to produce acute systemic toxicity in mice. The individual solutions are injected into mice, and the mice are observed for acute systemic toxicity.

3. Acute ocular irritation and cytotoxicity assessment. The purpose of this assessment is to evaluate the potential for ocular irritation or cytotoxicity resulting from the solutions as formulated. The effects are assessed *in vitro* using cytotoxicity studies (i.e., tissue culture–agar overlay method or a suitable alternative) and *in vivo* using the 3-wk ocular safety study in rabbits.

4. Sensitization/allergic response assessment. The purpose of this assessment is to evaluate the *in vitro* and/or *in vivo* potential for the induction of a sensitivity/allergic response resulting from an uptake and release of preservatives used in lens care solutions when used in conjunction with a representative lens from each polymer group.

   a. Preservative uptake and release test. All contact lens polymers will either adsorb or absorb preservatives or other chemical components used in lens care solutions. Manufacturers should provide FDA with the amount of preservative uptake per lens, the amount released, and the time course of release. This study is a quantitative analysis that should be conducted with the lens care solutions. At FDA, the toxicologist will evaluate the quantitative findings of the study once the chemist has determined that the methodology used to perform the study is appropriate and the data are accurate for toxicology review. The results of these test data will be used to predict the potential for a preservative related toxicity, as well as the potential for inducing a sensitivity/allergic response associated with the lens group. The suggested test procedures have been established for the quantitative analysis of the uptake of the preservatives thimerosal and chlorhexidine in contact lenses. If preservatives other than thimerosal or chlorhexidine are used in the recommended lens care solutions (sorbic acid, quaternary ammonium compound, etc.), it is the responsibility of the sponsor to select an appropriate chemical method for the quantitative analyses of the uptake and release of the preservative from the lens material for each group.

b. Guinea pig maximization test. The purpose of this test is to grade or rank the active ingredients of the lens solution on a scale of I–V as to their potential for inducing sensitivity response in the guinea pig model. The grades or rankings are based on the number of animals sensitized, and the results are classified on an ascending scale from a weak sensitizing agent (grade I) to an extreme sensitizing agent (grade V). It is FDA's intent to use this test primarily to assess the sensitization potential of *new* preservatives for contact lens solutions.

c. Container/accessory testing requirements. The purpose of these testing requirements is to assess the potential toxicity of any constituent(s) that may be extractable from the solution container and accessories when the solution as formulated will come in contact with the container or accessory for a prolonged period of time. The following *in vitro* and *in vivo* test procedures are recommended by FDA and are consistent with USP XXII Tests for Plastic Ophthalmic Containers.

(1) *In vitro* cytotoxicity testing. Tissue culture–agar overlay (cytotoxicity) test, or an alternate test agreed to by FDA and manufacturer.

(2) Systemic toxicity testing. Systemic toxicity studies using extracts obtained from container/accessory components, utilizing USP XXII Tests for Plastic Ophthalmic Containers. The acute systemic toxicity study in mice is performed using extracts with polar and nonpolar solvents of the lens material obtained

according to procedures outlined in USP XXII Tests for Plastic Ophthalmic Containers.

(3) Primary ocular irritation testing. Primary ocular irritation studies using extractives obtained from container/accessory components, utilizing USP XXII Tests for Plastic Ophthalmic Containers. The following methodologies should be observed: (a) Physiologic saline accessory material extracts should be tested with three healthy albino rabbits for each test extract. Animals determined to be free of eye lesions by slit-lamp examination for fluorescein staining should be used. (b) A volume of 0.2 ml saline accessory material extract will be instilled into the cup formed by gently pulling the lower eye lid away from the eye. The lids will then be held together for 30 s. Similarly, 0.2 ml of blank saline will be instilled into the other eye which will serve as a control. Both eyes should be observed at 24 and 48 h with a hand ophthalmoscope and fluorescein staining. At 72 h, both eyes in each animal should be examined with a slit-lamp and fluorescein stain. In addition, both eyes should be scored for gross signs of eye irritation at the same intervals using the Draize or McDonald—Shadduck method. (McDonald et al., 1987).

APPLIED OCULAR IRRITATION TESTING

In addition to directly applying the test protocols prescribed by various regulatory bodies, it is often necessary to interpret regulatory guidelines and devise additional protocols for a variety of circumstances. Here we present one approach for applied ophthalmic toxicology.

Ocular Examination and Slit-Lamp Scoring Procedure

The most critical feature of eye irritation tests in animals and humans is the ocular examination, since data produced by such examinations form the basis for subsequent evaluation, interpretation, and extrapolation.

In addition to scoring materials as irritants or nonirritants, it is often desirable to compare similar materials in various combinations in order to select a preparation with the least potential for producing human eye irritation. To assist in this endeavor, the Draize (1959) scoring system was modified to include routine slit-lamp examination. By regularly using a magnifying instrument that is also used with humans, we hope to correlate more precisely ocular irritation events in humans and animals. This method also assists in increasing the reproducibility of ocular irritation scores and permits inclusion of some changes in the anterior chamber for monitoring irritation.

McDonald et al. (1987) discussed the techniques and types of illumination that can be utilized with the biomicroscopic slit-lamp when studying the normal and irritated rabbit eye. Adjuncts to conventional slit-lamp microscopy include attachments to ascertain fluorescein staining, measure corneal thickness, determine anterior chamber depth, measure intraocular pressure, and take slit-image or anterior segment photographs.

McDonald et al. (1987) briefly described an ocular scoring system for rabbits based on slit-lamp examination. The following scoring system is an updated version.

Conjunctiva. A normal rabbit eye is shown in Fig. 1. Conjunctival changes can be divided clinically into congestion, swelling (chemosis), and discharge. Generally, the sequence of events for these changes is congestion, discharge, and swelling.

Conjunctival congestion.

0 = Normal. May appear blanched to reddish pink without perilimbal injection (except at 12 and 6 o'clock positions) with vessels of the palpebral and bulbar conjunctiva easily observed (Fig. 2).

+1 = A flushed, reddish color predominantly confined to the palpebral conjunctiva with some perilimbal injection but primarily confined to the lower and upper parts of the eye from the 4 and 7 and 11 and 1 o'clock positions.

+2 = Bright red color of the palpebral conjunctiva with accompanying perilimbal injection covering at least 75% of the circumference of the perilimbal region (Fig. 3).

+3 = Dark, beefy red color with congestion of both the bulbar and the palpebral conjunctiva along with pronounced perilimbal injection and the presence of petechia on the conjunctiva. The petechiae generally predominate along the nictitating membrane and the upper palpebral conjunctiva (Fig. 4).

Conjunctival swelling. There are five divisions from 0 to +4.

0 = Normal or no swelling of the conjunctival tissue.

+1 = Swelling above normal without eversion of the lids (can be easily ascertained by noting that the upper and lower eyelids are positioned as in the normal eye); swelling generally starts in the lower cul-de-sac near the inner canthus, which requires slit-lamp examination.

+2 = Swelling with misalignment of the normal approximation of the lower and upper eyelids; primarily confined to the upper eyelid so that in the initial stages the misapproximation of the eyelids begins by partial eversion of the upper eyelid (Fig. 2). In this stage, swelling is confined generally to the upper eyelid, although it exists in the lower cul-de-sac (observed best with the slit-lamp).

+3 = Swelling definite with partial eversion of the upper and lower eyelids essentially equivalent. This can be easily ascertained by looking at the animal head-on and noticing the positioning of the eyelids; if the eye margins do not meet, eversion has occurred.

+4 = Eversion of the upper eyelid is pronounced with less pronounced eversion of the lower eyelid. It is difficult to retract the lids and observe the perilimbal region.

Conjunctival discharge. Discharge is defined as a whitish-gray precipitate, which should not be confused with the small amount of clear, inspissated, mucoid material that can be formed in the medial canthus of a substantial number of rabbit eyes. This material can be removed with a cotton swab before the animals are used.

0 = Normal. No discharge.

+1 = Discharge above normal and present on the inner portion of the eye but not on the lids or hairs of the eyelids. One can ignore the small amount that is in the inner and outer canthus if it has not been removed prior to starting the study.

+2 = Discharge is abundant, easily observed, and has collected on the lids and around the hairs of the eyelids (Fig. 5).

+3 = Discharge has been flowing over the eyelids so as to wet the hairs substantially on the skin around the eye.

Aqueous flare. The intensity of the Tyndall phenomenon is scored by comparing the normal Tyndall effect observed when the slit-lamp beam passes through the lens with that seen in the anterior chamber. The presence of aqueous flare is presumptive evidence of breakdown of the blood–aqueous barrier.

0 = Absence of visible light beam light in the anterior chamber (no Tyndall effect).

+1 = The Tyndall effect is barely discernible. The intensity of the light beam in the anterior chamber is less than the intensity of the slit beam as it passes through the lens.

+2 = The Tyndall beam in the anterior chamber is easily discernible and is equal in intensity to the slit beam as it passes through the lens.

+3 = The Tyndall beam in the anterior chamber is easily discernible; its intensity is greater than the intensity of the slit beam as it passes through the lens.

Light reflex. The pupillary diameter of the iris is controlled by the radial and sphincter muscles. Contraction of the radial muscle due to adrenergic stimulation results in mydriasis while contraction of the sphincter muscle due to cholinergic stimulation results in miosis. As an ophthalmic drug can exert potential effects on these neural pathways it is important to assess the light reflex of an animal as part of the ophthalmic examination. Using full illumination with the slit-lamp, the following scale is used:

0 = Normal pupillary response.
1 = Sluggish pupillary response.
2 = Maximally impaired (i.e., fixed) pupillary response.

Iris involvement. In the following definitions the primary, secondary, and tertiary vessels are utilized as an aid to determining a subjective ocular score for iris involvement. The assumption is made that the greater the hyperemia of the vessels and the more the secondary and tertiary vessels are involved, the greater the intensity of iris involvement. The scores range from 0 to +4.

   0 = Normal iris without any hyperemia of the iris vessels. Occasionally around the 12 to 1 o'clock position near the pupillary border and the 6 and 7 o'clock position near the pupillary border there is a small area around 1–3 mm in diameter in which both the secondary and tertiary vessels are slightly hyperemic.
   +1 = Minimal injection of secondary vessels but not tertiary. Generally, it is uniform, but may be of greater intensity at the 1 or 6 o'clock position. If it is confined to the 1 or 6 o'clock position, the tertiary vessels must be substantially hyperemic.
   +2 = Minimal injection of tertiary vessels and minimal to moderate injection of the secondary vessels (Fig. 6).
   +3 = Moderate injection of the secondary and tertiary vessels with slight swelling of the iris stroma (this gives the iris surface a slightly rugose appearance, which is usually most prominent near the 3 and 9 o'clock positions.
   +4 = Marked injection of the secondary and tertiary vessels with marked swelling of the iris stroma. The iris appears rugose; may be accompanied by hemorrhage (hyphema) in the anterior chamber (Fig. 7).

Cornea. The scoring scheme measures the severity of corneal cloudiness and the area of the cornea involved. Severity of corneal cloudiness is graded as follows.

0 = Normal cornea. Appears with the slip-lamp adjusted to a narrow slit image as having a bright gray line on the epithelial surface and a bright gray line on the endothelial surface with a marblelike gray appearance of the stroma.

+1 = Some loss of transparency. Only the anterior half of the stroma is involved as observed with an optical section of the slit-lamp. The underlying structures are clearly visible with diffuse illumination, although some cloudiness can be readily apparent with diffuse illumination (Fig. 8).

+2 = Moderate loss of transparency. In addition to involving the anterior stroma, the cloudiness extends all the way to the endothelium. The stroma has lost its marblelike appearance and is homogeneously white. With diffuse illumination, underlying structures are clearly visible (Fig. 9).

+3 = Involvement of the entire thickness of the stroma. With optical section, the endothelial surface is still visible. However, with diffuse illumination the underlying structures are just barely visible (to the extent that the observer is still able to grade flare and iritis, observe for pupillary response, and note lenticular changes).

+4 = Involvement of the entire thickness of the stroma. With the optical section, cannot clearly visualize the endothelium. With diffuse illumination, the underlying structures cannot be seen. Cloudiness removes the capability for judging and grading flare, iritis, lenticular changes, and pupillary response (Fig. 10).

The surface area of the cornea relative to the area of cloudiness is divided into five grades from 0 to +4.

0 = Normal cornea with no area of cloudiness.
+1 = 1–25% Area of stromal cloudiness (Fig. 8).
+2 = 25–50% Area of stromal cloudiness (Fig. 9).
+3 = 51–75% Area of stromal cloudiness.
+4 = 76–100% Area of stromal cloudiness (Fig. 10).

Pannus is vascularization or the penetration of new blood vessels into the corneal stroma. The vessels are derived from the limbal vascular loops. Pannus is divided into three grades.

0 = No pannus.
+1 = Vascularization is present but vessels have not invaded the entire

corneal circumference. Where localized vessel invasion has occurred, they have not penetrated beyond 2 mm.

+2 = Vessels have invaded 2 mm or more around the entire corneal circumference.

The use of fluorescein is a valuable aid in defining epithelial damage (Norn, 1971). For fluorescein staining, the area can be judged on a 0 to +4 scale using the same terminology as for corneal cloudiness. The intensity of fluorescein staining can be divided into a 0 to +4 scale.

0 = Absence of fluorescein staining.

+1 = Slight fluorescein staining confined to a small focus. With diffuse illumination the underlying structures are easily visible (Fig. 11). (The outline of the pupillary margin is as if there were no fluorescein staining.)

+2 = Moderate fluorescein staining confined to a small focus. With diffuse illumination the underlying structures are clearly visible, although there is some loss of detail.

+3 = Marked fluorescein staining. Staining may involve a larger portion of the cornea. With diffuse illumination underlying structures are barely visible but are not completely obliterated.

+4 = Extreme fluorescein staining. With diffuse illumination the underlying structures cannot be observed (Fig. 12).

Interpretation is facilitated by rinsing the eye with an isotonic irrigating solution in order to remove excess and nonabsorbed fluorescein.

Slit-lamps are equipped with cobalt blue filters, which can be placed in front of the light from the slit illuminator in order to excite fluorescence of the fluorescein. Photographs utilizing fluorescein staining require the use of this filter, and fluorescence will be enhanced by a yellow filter placed in front of the objectives of the corneal microscope.

Fluorescein staining is an indication of corneal epithelial damage, which may precede underlying stromal damage. Kikkawa (1972) reported that 10–20% of rabbits examined exhibited focal, punctate fluorescein staining normally. There may be involvement of the whole cornea, or the foci may be limited to one area.

Lens. The crystalline lens is readily observed with the aid of the slit-lamp biomicroscope, and the location of lenticular opacity can readily be discerned by direct and retroillumination. The location of lenticular opacities can be arbitrarily divided into the following lenticular regions beginning with the anterior capsule:

Anterior capsular
Anterior subcapsular
Anterior cortical
Nuclear
Posterior cortical
Posterior subcapsular
Posterior capsular

The lens should be evaluated routinely during ocular evaluations and graded as either N (normal) or A (abnormal). The presence of lenticular opacities should be described and the location noted as defined above.

Reproducing Ocular Scores

Draize and Kelley (1952) noted variation of toxicity scores among different lots of the same surfactant and believed that this was due to investigator variability. Russell and Hoch (1962) reported variability of ocular scores for various shampoos submitted to several contract laboratories. Weil and Scala (1971), in a collaborative study, documented substantial variation in ocular scores within and among 24 laboratories (regulatory, contract, and industrial) and concluded that variability could be related to investigator training, rabbit strain differences, test procedures, and interpretation of ocular changes. Marzulli and Ruggles (1973) reported a similar collaborative study, and they concluded that laboratory variability was reduced to insignificance if the laboratory was asked only to distinguish an irritant from a nonirritant and if all four criteria (cornea, iris, conjunctival congestion, and conjunctival swelling) were used. Weil and Scala (1971) and Marzulli and Ruggles (1973) recommended additional collaborative studies in order to identify and eliminate sources of variability in eye irritancy studies.

We attempted to address this problem by devising a statistically based experimental procedure to measure, monitor, and correct variability among investigators (analyst precision) and within the same investigator (analyst uniformity). We are collecting ocular irritation data for several substances that were evaluated on numerous occasions and have used only one source of rabbits. Later the data base will be expanded to include several rabbit sources. This approach is designed to isolate what many have thought are the two major causes (investigator and animal) of laboratory variability of eye irritancy studies.

The experimental design for the statistically based procedure is presented in Table 3. The previously described semiquantitative, slit-lamp ocular scoring system is used. The design provides a sufficient number of eyes for statistical

TABLE 3. Experimental Design for Reproducibility Test

Animals: 48 New Zealand albino rabbits
Test groups: 24 Eyes, not irritated
           24 Eyes, slight irritation
              24 Eyes, moderate irritation
              24 Eyes, severe irritation
Ocular scoring systems: Modifications of Draize (1955) and
   Baldwin et al. (1972) (0 to 3 or 4+)
Observations: (1) Each eye observed twice, (2) rabbits randomly
   selected, (3) ocular scores assigned under blind conditions, (4)
   scores maintained separately for each ocular parameter
Statistical evaluation:
   (1) Analyst uniformity (between investigators), method of
       correlation
   (2) Analyst precision (within the investigator), ratio of trial 1 to
       trial 2 matches for total possible matches (96); assumed 80%
       reproducibility

evaluation of analyst precision (intervariability) and analyst uniformity (intravariability). Four treatment groups of 24 eyes per group are used. Each group receives a topical ocular treatment, providing groups with a range of changes from nonirritating to severe. Half of the eyes are tested in the morning and the other half in the afternoon. One hour is allowed for observation of each group of 24 rabbits (48 eyes) in order to minimize the effect of time on ocular reactions. Also, careful selection of test materials can minimize this time influence. Other important features of the experimental design are that (1) each eye is observed twice without prior knowledge of treatment, (2) each eye is randomly selected for observation, and (3) scores are maintained and evaluated separately for each ocular parameter. This last feature permits one to determine weak areas of reproducibility for each investigator.

Frequency counts are made for each ocular parameter. An example of a frequency count for conjunctival swelling by three observers is shown in Table 4. The frequency counts compare trial 1 (first observation for an eye) to trial 2 (second observation for the same eye). On seven occasions investigator A gave a score of 3 in the first trial and a score of 2 in the second trial. This tabulation provides a basis for statistical evaluation.

An example of analyst uniformity is shown in Table 5. Here R values (correlation coefficients) are used to evaluate uniformity. The maximum value is 1. Table 4 indicates that analyst uniformity for the three investigators is very good for swelling, light reflex, flare, iritis, and corneal cloudiness (intensity and area). Higher R values for congestion and discharge would be desirable.

TABLE 4. Example of Tabulation of Ocular Scores (Frequency Counts) for Conjunctival Swelling

Trial 2	Trial 1				
	0	1	2	3	4
	Investigator A				
0	48	1	0	0	0
1	2	7	3	0	0
2	0	5	12	7	0
3	0	0	3	8	0
4	0	0	0	0	0
	Investigator B				
0	52	1	0	0	0
1	1	0	0	0	0
2	3	6	33	0	0
3	0	0	0	0	0
4	0	0	0	0	0
	Investigator C				
0	48	0	0	0	0
1	2	14	3	0	0
2	0	9	11	6	0
3	0	1	1	1	0
4	0	0	0	0	0

TABLE 5. Analyst Uniformity for Three Observers

Parameter	R values[a]		
	A vs. B	A vs. C	C vs. B
Congestion	0.63	0.59	0.61
Discharge	0.79	0.60	0.20
Swelling	0.82	0.95	0.81
Light reflex	0.94	0.95	0.99
Flare	0.82	0.94	0.86
Iritis	0.86	0.91	0.94
Corneal cloudiness (intensity)	0.90	0.97	0.92
Corneal cloudiness (area)	0.96	0.95	0.96

[a] R = correlation coefficient.

Analyst precision is shown in Table 6. For conjunctival congestion, percentages ranged from 73 to 88% for the 3 analysts. This is, in our opinion, good reproducibility for a subjective scoring system. For discharge, percentages ranged from 57 to 79% for the 3 analysts, suggesting that the investigators need more training in evaluating this parameter in order to improve their precision. For swelling, light reflex, corneal intensity, iritis, and flare, reproducibility was generally 80% or better. This amount of precision for an investigator is considered good, since it demonstrates that an investigator can reproduce a score 8 out of 10 times.

During the time this system has been used in our laboratory (8 yr), reproducibility between and within investigators improved substantially. Demonstrated reproducibility within and between investigators increases the reliability of tests, even when the data have been collected several months apart or by separate investigators or laboratories. This test provides a means of introducing new investigators to the ocular scoring system, monitoring their progress, and permits corrective instruction.

Adaptation of Guidelines and Experimental Models

As noted before, the FHSA method of the Draize test indicates the amount and mode of administration for solutions, pastes, powders, and aerosols. Materials whose application includes use with water are routinely diluted (one part of the formulation plus one part of water) prior to topical ocular instillation. In this manner, the investigator obtains an ocular irritation potential perspective for the effects of water on the formulation. The dilution is still near the concentrated form, so the data can be rationally extrapolated for the concen-

TABLE 6. Analyst Precision for Three Observers

Parameter	Ratio of trial 1 — trial 2 matches to total possible matches (96)		
	A	B	C
Congestion	73	84	88
Swelling	78	86	77
Discharge	74	57	79
Flare	74	78	83
Iritis	70	79	83
Corneal cloudiness			
Intensity	82	80	87
Area	80	87	85

TABLE 7. Conjunctival Congestion, Swelling, Discharge, and Corneal Cloudiness
for Rabbits 24 Hr after Single Topical Ocular Instillation
of a Gel-Type Shampoo (Undiluted or Diluted 1 : 2)

Treatment		Conjunctiva			Corneal cloudiness	
		Congestion	Swelling	Discharge	Severity	Area
Undiluted shampoo	Mean[b]	6.0	4.0	5.3	4.0	3.7
	Incidence[c]	6/6	6/6	6/6	6/6	6/6
Diluted shampoo[a]	Mean	6.0	3.3	4.3	3.7	3.7
	Incidence	6/6	6/6	6/6	6/6	6/6
Untreated controls	Mean	0.3	0.0	0.0	0.0	0.0
	Incidence	1/6	0/6	0/6	0/6	0/6

[a]One part shampoo diluted with one part water.
[b]Maximum scores: congestion, 6; swelling, 8; discharge, 6; corneal cloudiness (severity and area), 4.
[c]Number of eyes with response/number of eyes in test group.

trate. Data to support this view are shown in Table 7. Too high a dilution (1:10) may prevent the investigator from gaining a true perspective of the ocular damaging potential. Such products as hand lotions and sunscreens are evaluated undiluted since undiluted products are used.

We have combined and modified the FHSA method and the Draize test for evaluation of "dermatologic-type" products following demonstration that the product does not produce dermal irritation. Any test material that elicits dermal irritation is assumed to likewise be an ocular irritant and is not evaluated in the eye. The purpose of the test is to provide information to poison control centers and for material safety data sheets should accidental or intentional ocular exposure occur with these products. The procedure is as follows:

1. Six eyes per test group.
2. Six eyes treated, washed at 20 s.
3. Six eyes treated, washed at 5 min.
4. Six eyes treated, washed at 24 h.
5. Wash with 200 ml tap water for 1 min.
6. Include marketed product control (use the three wash times as above).
7. Examine and grade eyes by slit-lamp scoring system at 1, 24, 48, and 72 h and on d 7 and 14 (test may be terminated at any point if all treated eyes have returned to normal).
8. Use albino rabbits (about 2 kg).

9. Six sham control eyes washed on d 0.
10. Six sham control eyes washed at 24 h.
11. Six untreated controls.

The control groups are important in ascertaining the incidence of normal fluorescein staining of the rabbit cornea, the incidence of normal conjunctival congestion, and the effect of washing of the eye. Both eyes of each rabbit are used.

These wash times were selected because ocular changes for different types of products were different depending on the wash period. For about 80% of the 75 shampoos tested, the ocular reaction was more severe, of a higher incidence, and of longer duration for the 5-min wash group compared to the 20-s and 24-h wash group. Examples of this are shown in Table 8. For some products the earlier washing produced more marked ocular change (Table 9), while other products gave less severe ocular changes when the eyes were washed early.

TESTING OF OPHTHALMIC THERAPEUTIC FORMULATIONS

Guidelines by Goldenthal (1968) and Weissinger (1989) are used in designing the experimental protocol. Screening protocols have been developed and ophthalmic formulations have been evaluated according to the following scheme.

1. One-day acute (short-term) ocular irritation test. Use multiples of the active ingredients when possible and include a similar marketed product, if available, for comparison. This test is used prior to release of an ophthalmic formulation for ingredients that have been placed by Category I by FDA ophthalmic panel(s).
2. Five-day ocular irritation test. When possible, use multiples of the active ingredients and include marketed products. The dosing regimen should be similar to the clinical regimen. This study is an extension of the 1-d test and may be in addition to or in lieu of the 1-d test for ingredients placed in Category I by FDA ophthalmic panel(s).
3. Although the guidelines state a 21-d topical ocular irritation test for establishing safety, subchronic evaluation of drugs for clinical use of up to 3 mo necessitated similar duration of evaluation preclinically. Likewise, drugs intended for chronic therapy should be evaluated in a preclinical test system for a minimum of 1 yr. Use of multiples of the active ingredients, when possible, is essential, as well as inclusion of a marketed product, when available. Dosing is according to the antici-

TABLE 8. Conjunctival Congestion and Swelling in Rabbits after Single Topical Ocular Instillations of Shampoos

Test formulation	Wash time[a]		Congestion					Swelling				
			1 hr	24 hr	48 hr	72 hr	7 days	1 hr	24 hr	48 hr	72 hr	7 days
Nondandruff shampoo	20 sec	Intensity[b]	6.0	3.0	2.3	1.0	0.0	1.3	0.3	0.0	0.0	0.0
		Incidence[c]	6/6	5/6	4/6	1/6	0/4[d]	4/6	1/6	0/6	0/6	0/4[d]
	5 min	Intensity	6.0	5.3	4.7	0.7	0.0	3.3	1.0	0.0	0.0	0.0
		Incidence	6/6	6/6	5/6	2/6	0/6	6/6	3/6	0/6	0/6	0/6
	24 hr	Intensity	5.3	5.7	1.3	0.0	0.0	0.7	0.3	0.0	0.0	0.0
		Incidence	6/6	6/6	4/6	0/6	0/6	2/6	1/6	0/6	0/6	0/6
Mild shampoo	20 sec	Intensity	4.0	1.7	0.0	0.0	0.0	0.0	0.0	0.0	0.0	0.0
		Incidence	6/6	4/6	0/6	0/6	0/6	0/6	0/6	0/6	0/6	0/6
	5 min	Intensity	5.3	1.7	0.7	0.3	0.0	0.0	0.0	0.0	0.0	0.0
		Incidence	6/6	4/6	2/6	1/6	0/6	0/6	0/6	0/6	0/6	0/6
	24 hr	Intensity	4.3	1.7	0.3	0.7	0.0	0.0	0.0	0.0	0.0	0.0
		Incidence	6/6	3/6	1/6	2/6	0/6	0/6	0/6	0/6	0/6	0/6
Dandruff shampoo	20 sec	Intensity	5.3	4.7	2.7	1.0	1.3	2.7	0.0	0.0	0.0	0.0
		Incidence	6/6	6/6	4/6	3/6	4/6	5/6	0/6	0/6	0/6	0/6
	5 min	Intensity	6.0	6.0	4.7	4.0	1.7	4.0	1.7	1.3	0.0	0.0
		Incidence	6/6	6/6	6/6	6/6	5/6	6/6	5/6	4/6	0/6	0/6
	24 hr	Intensity	6.0	4.7	3.7	1.0	2.0	3.3	0.7	1.3	0.0	0.0
		Incidence	6/6	6/6	6/6	3/6	4/6	6/6	2/6	1/6	0/6	0/6

[a]Interval of time after dosing until eye was washed.
[b]Parameter scored by the method of Draize (1955). Maximum scores: congestion, 6; swelling, 8. Total score for the observation period(s). Mean score calculated by multiplying each individual score by 2, adding, and dividing the number of observations.
[c]Number of eyes with response/number of eyes in test.
[d]Rabbit died in test.

791

TABLE 9. Conjunctival Congestion and Swelling after Single Topical Ocular Instillations of Acne Scrub Product

Test formulation	Wash time[a]	Parameter	Congestion					Swelling				
			1 hr	24 hr	48 hr	72 hr	7 days	1 hr	24 hr	48 hr	72 hr	7 days
Acne scrub product	20 sec	Intensity[b]	5.7	6.0	6.0	6.0	1.3	2.0	2.0	1.3	0.7	0.3
		Incidence[c]	6/6	6/6	6/6	6/6	4/6	6/6	6/6	4/6	1/6	1/6
	5 min	Intensity	6.0	6.0	4.0	4.0	1.3	3.3	2.0	0.3	0.0	0.0
		Incidence	6/6	6/6	6/6	6/6	4/6	6/6	6/6	1/6	1/6	0/6
	24 hr	Intensity	5.3	5.3	3.3	2.0	0.0	2.7	1.0	0.0	0.0	0.0
		Incidence	6/6	6/6	6/6	5/6	0/6	6/6	2/6	0/6	0/6	0/6
Sham control[d]	0	Intensity	2.3	0.7	0.0	0.0	0.7	0.0	0.0	0.0	0.0	0.0
		Incidence	6/6	2/6	0/6	0/6	2/6	0/6	0/6	0/6	0/6	0/6
	24 hr	Intensity	2.0	0.0	0.7	0.2	0.0	0.0	0.0	0.0	0.0	0.0
		Incidence	4/6	0/6	2/6	1/6	0/6	0/6	0/6	0/6	0/6	0/6
Untreated control		Intensity	1.0	0.0	0.0	0.0	0.0	0.0	0.0	0.0	0.0	0.0
		Incidence	3/6	0/6	0/6	0/6	0/6	0/6	0/6	0/6	0/6	0/6

[a]Interval of time after dosing until eye was washed.
[b]Parameter scored by the method of Draize (1955). Maximum scores: congestion, 6; swelling, 8. Total score for the observation period(s). Mean score calculated by multiplying each individual score by 2, adding, and dividing the number of observations.
[c]Number of eyes with response/number of eyes in test.
[d]Sham control; eyes were not treated but washed with water as per treated eyes.

pated clinical regimen. This study is used for ingredients that have not been previously used by the topical ocular route. Hematology, clinical chemistry, urinalysis, and histopathology are not included if the ingredients have adequate published safety data or an FDA panel has placed them in a Category I rating by some other route of administration.

4. Subchronic (i.e., 1–3 mo) and chronic (1–2 yr) topical ocular irritation test with systemic toxicologic studies. Multiples of the active ingredient are used, if possible, as well as a comparable marketed product, if available. The regimen should be similar to the clinical dosing regimen. Since the ingredients have not been investigated by any route and have no category rating by any FDA ophthalmic panel, or there are no published toxicology data, systemic toxicity is monitored by including hematology, clinical chemistry, urinalysis, and histopathology of tissues, including the eyes.

In the 1-d test, the test materials are instilled at 0.03–0.05 ml every 30 min for 6 consecutive hours, using at least 6 eyes. This is considered to be essentially continuous exposure for 6 h. For tetracycline ointment, ethylene glycol, and ethylene chlorohydrin, the concentrations that were irritating in similarly designed 1-d acute tests were less than or equal to the concentrations that were irritating in the 21-d test. A typical comparison of ocular changes produced by ethylene glycol is shown in Table 10. Histology confirmed these observations. The 1-d acute model does not reflect human usage, since most, if not all, OTC and prescription ophthalmic formulations are instilled 3, 4, or several times per day. The dosing frequency can be adjusted and the investigator must make a judgment on what is appropriate, keeping in mind the clinical dosing regimen and the concept that one wishes to enhance the chance of observing toxicity and thus predicting human risk.

The 5-d test is an extension of the 1-d test and is used to confirm findings from the 1-d test. In the 5-d test, 6 eyes are used and the animals are dosed at a regimen similar to that to be used clinically. The eyes are evaluated every day for 5 consecutive days by slit-lamp observation. Examinations are usually done 1 h after the last dose of the afternoon.

The subchronic or chronic test dosing regimen should be analogous to that used clinically. For instance, in studying an antifungal or antiviral product, the formulations might be instilled quite frequently (generally at 1- or 2-h intervals) in the first few days since this is the usual clinical regimen in humans. One might also decrease dosing frequency in a way that might be expected to be recommended clinically.

It seems reasonable to omit hematology, clinical chemistry, urinalysis, and histopathology if the substance has a published or known toxicity profile or

TABLE 10. Comparison of Rabbit Ocular Scores Elicited after 6-Hr Acute Topical Ocular Instillation[a] and 21-Day Topical Ocular Instillation[b] of Ethylene Glycol

Ethylene glycol (%)	Parameter	Ocular scores[c]				
		6 hr[a]	Day 3[b]	Day 7[b]	Day 14[b]	Day 21[b]
80	Conjunctival congestion	3.0 (6/6)	1.3 (8/10)	2.0 (10/10)	1.7 (8/9)	2.0 (9/9)
	Conjunctival discharge	3.0 (6/6)	0.3 (3/10)	0.6 (6/10)	0.7 (6/9)	1.0 (9/9)
	Conjunctival swelling	3.0 (6/6)	0.1 (1/10)	0.4 (4/10)	0.2 (2/9)	0.2 (2/9)
	Iritis	2.2 (6/6)	0.0 (0/10)	0.0 (0/10)	0.0 (0/9)	0.0 (0/9)
	Flare	1.0 (4/6)	0.0 (0/10)	0.0 (0/10)	0.0 (0/9)	0.0 (0/9)
	Corneal cloudiness	2.5 (6/6)	0.0 (0/10)	0.0 (0/10)	0.0 (0/9)	0.1 (1/9)
20	Conjunctival congestion	2.8 (6/6)	0.8 (7/10)	1.5 (9/10)	0.9 (6/10)	0.8 (6/10)
	Conjunctival discharge	0.5 (6/6)	0.0 (0/10)	0.0 (0/10)	0.0 (0/10)	0.0 (0/10)
	Conjunctival swelling	0.3 (3/6)	0.0 (0/10)	0.0 (0/10)	0.0 (0/10)	0.0 (0/10)
	Iritis	1.0 (3/6)	0.0 (0/10)	0.0 (0/10)	0.0 (0/10)	0.0 (0/10)
	Flare	0.3 (2/6)	0.0 (0/10)	0.0 (0/10)	0.0 (0/10)	0.0 (0/10)
	Corneal cloudiness	0.2 (1/6)	0.0 (0/10)	0.0 (0/10)	0.0 (0/10)	0.0 (0/10)
5	Conjunctival congestion	0.8 (4/6)	0.4 (3/10)	0.4 (4/10)	0.3 (3/10)	0.5 (5/10)
	Conjunctival discharge	0.0 (0/6)	0.0 (0/10)	0.0 (0/10)	0.0 (0/10)	0.0 (0/10)
	Conjunctival swelling	0.0 (0/6)	0.0 (0/10)	0.0 (0/10)	0.0 (0/10)	0.0 (0/10)
	Iritis	0.0 (0/6)	0.0 (0/10)	0.0 (0/10)	0.0 (0/10)	0.0 (0/10)
	Flare	0.0 (0/6)	0.0 (0/10)	0.0 (0/10)	0.0 (0/10)	0.0 (0/10)
	Corneal cloudiness	0.0 (0/6)	0.0 (0/10)	0.0 (0/10)	0.0 (0/10)	0.0 (0/10)

[a] 0.05 ml/dose at 20 min intervals for 6 hr, grade ocular reactions at 6 hr.

[b] 0.1 ml/dose five times per day for 21 days, grade ocular reaction on days 3, 7, 14, and 21.

[c] Mean ocular score; incidence in parentheses; maximum scores: congestion, 3; discharge, 3; swelling, 4; iritis, 4; corneal cloudiness, 4.

has been given a safe, effective rating by the FDA (McDonald et al., 1970b). However, if the material is a novel drug those parameters cannot be eliminated. Histopathology is of value when it is needed to characterize the nature of reactions cytologically and is important for toxicity evaluation of the vitreous chamber and retina as well as the potential for systemic changes on major organs or tissues.

TESTING OF CONTACT LENSES
AND SOLUTIONS

FDA guidelines for contact lenses and solutions were presented earlier. Corneal physiology under contact lenses has been emphasized by Mishima (1972) and Morrison et al. (1972). The effects of a potential soft contact lens on corneal metabolism were measured by using histochemical methods for LDH and glycogen (de la Iglesia et al., 1974, 1976). Kikkawa (1975) suggested that only corneal thickness be included as a measurement for corneal effects of hydrogel (soft) contact lenses. Corneal thickness measurements (pachymetry) provide a rough measure of corneal metabolism. Corneal metabolism is disrupted if the lids are sutured to keep the lens on the eye (Kikkawa, 1975). Driefus and Wobmann (1975) observed that several bacteriostatic solutions intended for soft contact lenses, as well as water and saline, produced conjunctival edema, hyperemia, and corneal epithelial lesions (by electron microscopy) in rabbits, but the eyes for this study were structured. Other investigators (Bailey and Carney, 1973; Davies, 1972; Uniacke et al., 1972) have used or proposed procedures for assessing the safety of soft contact lenses. Rucker et al. (1972) used corneal epithelial regeneration as an index for assessing the safety of hard contact lens wetting solutions. Some solutions inhibited epithelial regeneration while others did not.

Screening protocols for evaluating soft and hard contact lenses and support solutions have been briefly discussed (McDonald et al., 1973d). The protocol for the soft contact lens test follows.

1. Albino rabbits (3.5–4 kg).
2. Lens dimensions: diameter, 12–15 mm; base curve, 7.5–8.4; center thickness, no greater than 0.5 mm.
3. Treat lens with support solutions as per intended clinical use; as an option, the disinfecting solution may or may not be rinsed prior to insertion on the rabbit eye.
4. A minimum of six eyes per test group.

5. Lenses worn for an intended 8 h/d. Lens retention is checked at appropriate intervals to provide adequate lens wear.
6. Remove lenses and grade ocular changes by slit-lamp scoring system.
7. Ocular changes can be graded at appropriate intervals throughout the duration of the study.
8. Corneal thickness measurements can be made.
9. Controls: eyes with lenses, without solutions; untreated eyes.

Three potential disinfecting solutions caused no ocular damage other than minimal conjunctival congestions when instilled topically without lenses (Table 11). When the solutions were tested with lenses, either rinsed or unrinsed, in the soft contact lens screening protocol a variety of ocular changes were noted. Moderate congestion, minimal swelling, discharge, flare, iritis, and corneal cloudiness were observed for solutions 1 and 2, while solution 3 produced only minimal conjunctival congestion (Table 12). The ocular reactions for solution 3 were similar to those for soft contact lenses sterilized by boiling in saline (without solutions).

TABLE 11. Ocular Changes of Rabbit Eyes during 6-Hr Acute Topical Ocular Instillation of Soft Contact Lens Disinfecting Solutions

Test formulation		Conjunctiva			Flare	Iritis	Corneal cloudiness	
		Congestion	Swelling	Discharge			Intensity	Area
Solution 1	$\bar{X}^a$	1.6	0.0	0.0	0.0	0.0	0.0	0.0
(n = 18; 3 exp.)	Inc.[b]	83%	0%	0%	0%	0%	0%	0%
Solution 2	$\bar{X}$	1.4	0.0	0.0	0.0	0.0	0.0	0.0
(n = 18; 3 exp.)	Inc.	78%	0%	0%	0%	0%	0%	0%
Solution 3	$\bar{X}$	1.4	0.0	0.0	0.0	0.0	0.0	0.0
(n = 12; 2 exp.)	Inc.	75%	0%	0%	0%	0%	0%	0%
Untreated control	$\bar{X}$	0.3	0.0	0.0	0.0	0.0	0.0	0.0
eyes (n = 42; 8 exp.)	Inc.	17%	0%	0%	0%	0%	0%	0%

[a]Each individual score multiplied by 2; added; divided by number of observations for conjunctiva. For remaining each score added and divided by number of observations. Maximum score = 6 for congestion; 8 for swelling; 6 for discharge; and 4 for flare, iritis, and corneal opacity.

[b]Incidence = number of observations with response/number of observations.

TABLE 12. Ocular Changes of Rabbit Eyes Exposed to Soft Contact Lens Processed in Sanitizing Solutions

Formulation	Time (hr)	Congestion	Swelling	Discharge	Flare	Iritis	Corneal cloudiness	
							Intensity	Area
Solution 1	20	3.8[a] (100%)[b]	0.5 (22%)	1.0 (33%)	0.2 (23%)	0.3 (27%)	1.0 (64%)	1.6 (64%)
(n = 27; 9 exp.)	48	1.6 (48%)	0	0.2 (8%)	0	0	0.4 (41%)	0.7 (41%)
(unrinsed)	96	0.3 (11%)		0			0.1 (4%)	0.1 (4%)
	144	0.2 (8%)					0.1 (4%)	0.1 (4%)
Solution 1	20	3.5 (100%)	0.1 (7%)	1.2 (50%)	0	0.1 (14%)	0.7 (57%)	1.6 (57%)
(n = 14; 5 exp.)	48	1.6 (42%)	0	0.1 (7%)	0	0	0.1 (14%)	0.3 (14%)
(rinsed)	96	0		0			0	0
Solution 2	20	4.7 (100%)	1.1 (44%)	3.1 (89%)	0.3 (33%)	0.4 (44%)	1.2 (56%)	1.8 (56%)
(n = 9; 3 exp.)	48	3.1 (78%)	0	0.9 (22%)	0	0	0.8 (56%)	1.2 (56%)
(unrinsed)	96	1.3 (67%)		0			0	0
	144	0.4 (11%)						
Solution 3	20	2.7 (100%)	0	0	0	0	0	0
(n = 5; 2 exp.)	48	0.7 (40%)						
(unrinsed)	96							
Soft lens control	20	1.5 (76%)	0	0	0	0	0	0
(n = 21; 7 exp.)	48	0.4 (19%)						
(in saline)	96	0						

[a]Mean score.
[b]Incidence.

The protocol for the hard contact lenses with solutions is given below.

1. Albino rabbits (3.5–4 kg).
2. Lens dimensions: diameter, 9.0–10.0 mm; base curve 7.1–8.1; center thickness, 0.2 mm.
3. A minimum of six eyes per test group.
4. Lenses are worn for an intended 8 h/d. Lens retention is verified at appropriate intervals (i.e., every 1 or 2 h) to establish adequate lens wear times.
5. Ocular changes graded by slit-lamp scoring system at appropriate intervals, up to 21 d (i.e., d 1, 4, 7, 14 and 21).
6. During lens wearing, topically instill (0.1 ml/dose) test solutions at 2-h intervals and check animals for lens retention.
7. Corneal thickness measurements can be made.
8. Controls: untreated eyes; eyes with lenses, without solutions; eyes treated with solutions but without lenses.

An example of the ocular changes observed in animals wearing lenses continuously for 3 d with instillation of the test solution every 4 h is shown in Table 13 for the same contact lens solutions evaluated in the 1-d acute study (Table 14). In the 1-d acute protocol, contact lens solution 1 produced congestion, swelling, discharge, iritis, and corneal cloudiness. These were enhanced and increased in intensity in the hard contact lens protocol. Contact lens solutions 2 and 3 produced minimal conjunctival congestion in the 1-d acute test. With the hard contact lens protocol, congestion, swelling, discharge, flare, iritis, and corneal cloudiness were associated with contact lens solution 2. These were generally of minimal intensity and at a high incidence. Contact lens solution 3 did not produce any swelling or flare, but there were rare instances of minimal iritis and discharge and a moderate incidence of minimal corneal cloudiness and conjunctival congestion. The ocular reactions for contact lens solution 3 were substantially less than for the contact lens control group. The ocular changes for the contact lens control group were substantial and comparable to those for contact lens wetting solution 1. Contact lens wetting solution 3 appeared to protect the rabbit eye from harmful effects of a hard contact lens.

An example of the value of corneal thickness measurements is shown in Fig. 13. These represent the corneal thickness measurements for both experiments for the hard contact lens procedure. The test formulation with the highest ocular irritative change produced the greatest increase in corneal thickness, while the formulation with the minimal ocular change produced the least change in corneal thickness.

TABLE 13. Ocular Changes of Rabbit Eyes during 6-Hr Acute Topical Ocular Instillation of Hard Contact Lens Wetting Solutions

Test formulation		Conjunctiva			Flare	Iritis	Corneal cloudiness	
		Congestion	Swelling	Discharge			Intensity	Area
CLS 1	$\bar{X}^a$	2.1	0.1	0.6	0.0	0.3	0.7	0.1
(n = 66; 11 exp.)	Inc.[b]	100%	4%	30%	0%	21%	56%	56%
CLS 2	$\bar{X}$	0.9	0.0	0.0	0.0	0.0	0.0	0.0
(n = 18; 3 exp.)	Inc.	61%	0%	0%	0%	0%	0%	0%
CLS 3	$\bar{X}$	1.7	0.0	0.0	0.0	0.0	0.0	0.0
(n = 42; 7 exp.)	Inc.	83%	0%	0%	0%	0%	0%	0%
Untreated control	$\bar{X}$	0.3	0.0	0.0	0.0	0.0	0.0	0.0
eyes (n = 42; 8 exp.)	Inc.	17%	0%	0%	0%	0%	0%	0%

[a]Each score multiplied by 2; added; divided by number of observations for conjunctiva. For remaining each score added and divided by number of observations. Maximum score = 6 for congestion; 8 for swelling; 6 for discharge; and 4 for flare, iritis, and corneal opacity.

[b]Incidence = number of observations with response/number of observations.

At present, there are no published guidelines for evaluating the ocular irritation potential of drug delivery ocular inserts. Perhaps the general guidelines for soft contact lenses can be used, with modification of the protocols to fit the specific use condition of the insert.

CORNEAL WOUND HEALING

While not strictly ocular irritation, the effects of materials on corneal wound healing may be important since many ophthalmic formulations are used in injured eyes. Wounds may be induced, as by surgery or trauma, or may be the result of a disease, such as herpetic, fungal, or bacterial keratitis. Corneal wounds are stromal and/or epithelial in nature. Corneal epithelial wound healing has been discussed and reviewed by several authors (Association for Research in Vision and Ophthalmology, 1975; Bellows, 1943; Hanna, 1966; Sigelman et al., 1954; McDonald et al., 1970a; McDonald, 1973c). The kinetics of epithelial regeneration and an epithelial growth factor have been discussed by Ho et al. (1974).

TABLE 14. Ocular Changes of Rabbit Eyes Exposed to Hard Contact Lens and Topical Ocular Instillations of Contact Lens Wetting Solutions

Test formulation	Time (hr)	Conjunctiva				Iritis	Corneal cloudiness	
		Congestion	Swelling	Discharge	Flare		Intensity	Area
Test 1	24	3.3[a] (6/6)[b]	0.0 (0/6)	1.3 (2/6)	0.5 (3/6)	0.5 (3/6)	1.1 (6/6)	2.8 (6/6)
	72[c]	5.0 (6/6)	1.3 (4/6)	3.0 (6/6)	0.3 (2/6)	0.7 (4/6)	2.3 (6/6)	3.5 (6/6)
CLS 1	120	3.0 (5/6)	0.0 (0/6)	0.0 (0/6)	0.0 (0/6)	0.0 (0/6)	0.5 (3/6)	1.7 (3/6)
Test 2	24	4.5 (6/6)	0.0 (0/0)	2.4 (4/6)	0.0 (0/6)	0.2 (1/6)	1.1 (6/6)	2.3 (6/6)
	72	5.7 (6/6)	1.7 (4/6)	4.4 (6/6)	0.3 (2/6)	0.8 (4/6)	2.3 (6/6)	3.5 (6/6)
	120	3.0 (5/5)[d]	0.0 (0/5)	1.2 (2/5)	0.0 (0/5)	0.0 (0/5)	0.6 (2/5)	1.0 (2/5)
Test 1	24	3.0 (5/6)	0.3 (1/6)	1.3 (3/6)	0.2 (1/6)	0.3 (1/6)	0.7 (3/6)	0.8 (3/6)
	72	4.7 (6/6)	0.0 (0/6)	2.3 (5.6)	0.0 (0/6)	0.2 (1/6)	1.7 (6/6)	2.5 (6/6)
CLS 2	120	0.3 (1/6)	0.0 (0/6)	0.0 (0/6)	0.0 (0/6)	0.0 (0/6)	0.0 (0.6)	0.0 (0.6)
Test 2	24	3.3 (6/6)	0.0 (0/6)	1.3 (3/6)	0.0 (0/0)	0.0 (0/6)	0.5 (3/6)	0.8 (3/6)
	72	4.0 (6/6)	0.3 (1/6)	1.3 (2.6)	0.2 (1/6)	0.2 (1/6)	1.2 (5/6)	2.0 (5/6)
	120	0.4 (1/5)[d]	0.0 (0/5)	0.0 (0/5)	0.0 (0/5)	0.0 (0/5)	0.0 (0/5)	0.0 (0/5)
Test 1	24	2.0 (4/6)	0.0 (0/6)	0.0 (0/6)	0.0 (0/6)	0.0 (0/6)	0.3 (2/6)	0.3 (2/6)
	72	3.7 (6/6)	0.0 (0/6)	0.0 (0/6)	0.0 (0/6)	0.2 (1/6)	0.3 (1/6)	0.3 (1/6)
CLS 3	120	0.7 (2/6)	0.0 (0/6)	0.0 (0/6)	0.0 (0/6)	0.0 (0/6)	0.0 (0.6)	0.0 (0/6)
Test 2	24	2.7 (6/6)	0.0 (0/6)	0.3 (1/6)	0.0 (0/6)	0.0 (0/6)	0.3 (2/6)	0.5 (2/6)
	72	3.3 (6/6)	0.0 (0/6)	2.0 (4/6)	0.0 (0/6)	0.3 (2/6)	1.3 (4/6)	1.5 (4/6)
	120	1.0 (3/6)	0.0 (0/6)	0.0 (0/6)	0.0 (0/6)	0.0 (0/6)	0.0 (0/6)	0.0 (0/6)
Test 1	24	3.3 (6/6)	0.0 (0/6)	0.7 (2/6)	0.2 (1/6)	0.2 (1/6)	0.5 (2/6)	1.0 (2/6)
	72	4.7 (6/6)	0.3 (1/6)	1.7 (5/6)	0.5 (3/6)	0.8 (5/6)	1.7 (6/6)	2.7 (6/6)
Contact lens control	120	2.0 (4.6)	0.0 (0/6)	0.0 (0/6)	0.0 (0/6)	0.0 (0/6)	0.0 (0/6)	0.0 (0/6)
Test 2	24	2.7 (6/6)	0.0 (0/6)	0.0 (0/6)	0.0 (U/6)	0.0 (0/6)	0.7 (2/6)	0.5 (2/6)
	72	5.3 (6/6)	0.3 (1/6)	3.3 (4/6)	0.2 (1/6)	0.8 (4/6)	1.7 (5/6)	2.3 (5/6)
	120	2.0 (3/5)[c]	0.0 (0/5)	0.8 (2.5)	0.0 (0/5)	0.0 (0/5)	0.4 (2/5)	0.8 (2/5)

[a] Mean score.
[b] Incidence.
[c] Topical ocular instillation terminated.

800

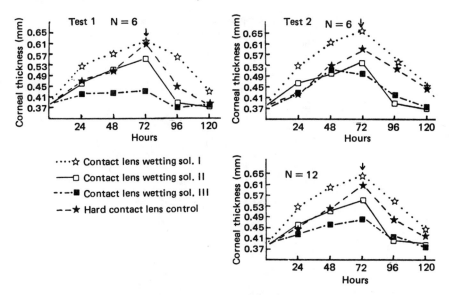

FIGURE 13 Change in corneal thickness of rabbit eyes exposed to hard contact lens and topical ocular instillation of contact lens wetting solutions. Two experiments: test 1 and test 2. Lower right graph represents combination of data for experiments 1 and 2.

SPECULAR MICROSCOPY

The use of the *in vitro* specular microscope has enabled toxicity studies to be conducted on isolated corneas of rabbit, monkey, and human (Maurice, 1968; McCarey et al., 1973; Schimmelpfenning, 1979). Once the cornea has been isolated and the endothelium perfused with a physiological salt solution that is known to maintain the corneal endothelial structure and function for extended periods of time (Dickstein and Maurice, 1972; Edelhauser et al., 1975, 1976, 1978), a chemical or substance to be evaluated can be either added to the corneal endothelial perfusion medium or topically applied to the epithelial surface. During the perfusion, the corneal thickness can be measured with an accuracy of 5 μm, the endothelial cells visualized, and at various times or at the end of a perfusion the cornea can be fixed for scanning and transmission electron microscopy. Corneal toxicity would be measured as a change in corneal thickness and/or ultrastructural damage to the component layers of the cornea that may ultimately lead to corneal opacity.

This technique has been used to evaluate intraocular irrigation solutions (Edelhauser et al., 1975, 1976, 1978), the establishment of pH and osmotic

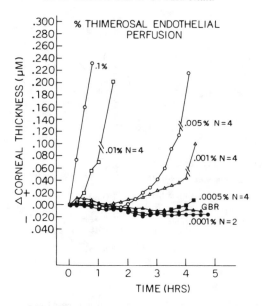

FIGURE 14 Changes in corneal thickness with time during perfusion of the endothelium of rabbit corneas with various concentrations of thimerosal in glutathione bicarbonate Ringer solution (GBR) (*N* = number of corneas).

tolerance of intraocular tissues (Gonnering et al., 1979; Edelhauser et al., 1981), and the effect of preservatives (Van Horn et al., 1977; Edelhauser et al., 1979a) (Figs. 14 and 15), drugs (Hull et al., 1975; Staatz et al., 1980), and potential residues from gas sterilization (i.e., ethylene oxide, ethylene chlorhydrin and ethylene glycol) (Edelhauser et al., 1983) on corneal endothelium.

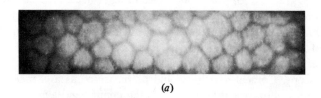

(*a*)

FIGURE 15 (*a*) Specular photomicrograph of rabbit cornea during 4 h of GBR perfusion, ×400.

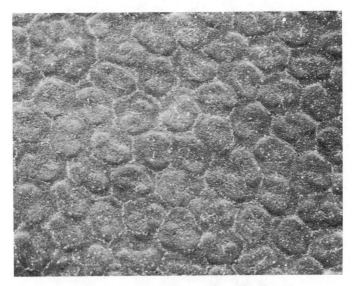

(b)

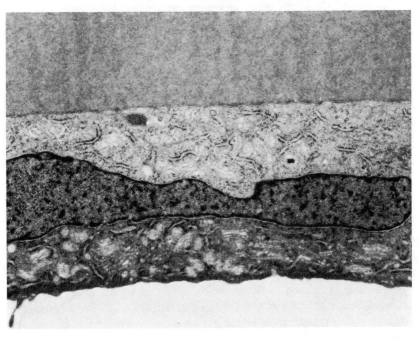

(c)

FIGURE 15 *(Continued)* *(b)* Scanning electron microscopy of same corneal endothelium after 4 h of GBR perfusion; normal mosaic pattern of endothelial cells is present and the posterior surface is smooth, × 800. *(c)* Transmission electron microscopy of same cornea; cell ultrastructure and subcellular organelles are normal, × 10, 300.

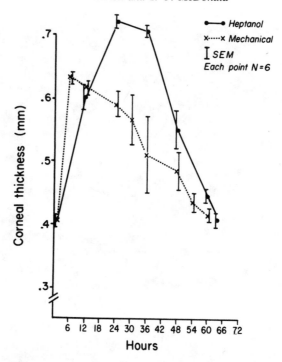

FIGURE 16 Corneal thickness following removal of 6 mm central corneal epithelium as measured with a pachometer. Note the initial swelling upon epithelial removal and the greater increase in corneal thickness in the heptanol group, indicating a degree of stromal damage. Corneal thickness does return to the initial thickness after 66 h.

CORNEAL THICKNESS

The use of a pachymeter (Mishima, 1968; Mishima and Hedbys, 1968) attached to a slit-lamp also allows for an accurate determination of the effect of chemicals topically applied to the eye. This measurement is easy to determine and highly reproducible; for example, a 2.2-kg rabbit exhibits a corneal thickness of 0.400 ± 0.02 mm (mean $\pm$ SD). Figure 16 illustrates the effect of epithelial removal by scraping and heptanol on corneal thickness. This technique has also been used to determine the effect of topical drugs on corneal thickness (Staatz et al., 1980; Edelhauser et al., 1979b). The advantage of corneal thickness measurement is that it is a noninvasive procedure to assess the physiological state of the cornea, and it provides a measure of wound repair following a topical insult. Corneal thickness in conjunction with the Draize scoring method to determine eye irritation would allow a precise measurement of corneal toxicity and repair. Morgan et al. (1987) reported that corneal pachymeter performed 3 d after application of a variety of test materials to the rabbit eye was as predictive of the eye irritation classification determined by observing the ocular response for 21 d. Kennah et al. (1989) utilized changes in corneal thickness as a means of providing an objective quantitation of ocular irritation. The authors state that the use of changes in corneal thickness possesses a greater sensitivity or detection of corneal healing than subjective scoring using the Draize scale.

CORNEAL PHOTOGRAPHY AND REEPITHELIALIZATION

Anterior segment photography with fluorescein staining provides a permanent record for eye irritation and complements the standard scoring method. It also provides uniformity between the various laboratories used to evaluate chemicals for irritation. Figure 17 illustrates corneal reepithelialization following a 6-mm mechanical debridement of the epithelium. The degree of reepithelialization can be assessed by fluorescein staining and measuring the healing rate [area (mm^2/h) or perimeter]. The rate of reepithelialization following epithelial scraping and heptanol removal is shown in Fig. 18. Other investigators used this model to study the normal reepithelialization of the cornea and the effect of growth factors (Ho et al., 1974; Friend and Thoft, 1978; Cintron et al., 1979; Moses et al., 1979; Jumblatt et al., 1980; Ubels et al., 1985). The regeneration rate of rabbit corneal epithelium can be effectively used to evaluate the toxicity of chemicals and substances of the normal wound repair process of the cornea following chemical insult. Simmons et al. (1987) recently evaluated various test agents on the ability of cultured rabbit corneal epithelial cells to migrate and re-cover a wound. This *in vitro* reepithelialization model ranked the test agents in an order similar to that described in the literature for both *in vivo* and *in vitro* tests.

POTENTIALLY USEFUL TECHNIQUES

Electron microscopy has contributed to an understanding of corneal epithelial architecture (Harding et al., 1974; Sheldon, 1956; Hoffman, 1972; Rosen and Brown, 1974). The fingerprinting phenomenon of corneal epithelial surfaces has been detected by scanning electron microscopy (Rosen and Brown, 1974). Harding et al. (1974) observed a variety of corneal epithelial architectures for different animal species. Scanning and transmission electron micros-

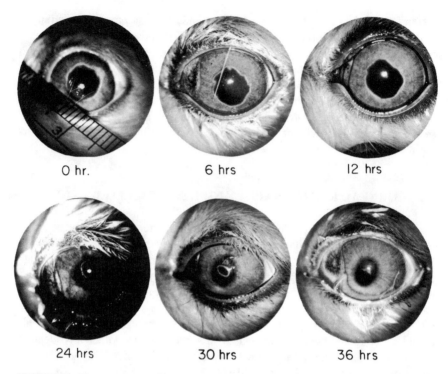

O hr.	6 hrs	12 hrs
24 hrs	30 hrs	36 hrs

FIGURE 17   Fluorescein staining of the central corneal epithelium following 6-mm mechanical debridement. Note the progressive re-epithelialization throughout the 36-h period.

copy may prove useful for evaluating cellular toxicity of topically instilled products.

Maurice described the specular microscope in 1968; as an *in vitro* instrument in which the cornea is isolated and perfused from the endothelial surface. The endothelial surface can be observed easily and corneal thickness measurements can be made accurately. McCarey et al. (1973) have included the specular microscope in a study using transmission and scanning electron microscopy. *In vitro* specular microscopy can also be used to evaluate epithelial surfaces of isolated rabbit corneas (Maurice, 1974). An *in vivo* wide-field specular microscope can be used as part of the routine ophthalmic evaluations to assess changes in the endothelial cell density, percent hexagonality and mean cell size. Yee et al. (1987) recently conducted an extensive comparative study of several vertebrate species with respect to the endothelial morphology.

Gasset et al. (1974) combined the techniques of enzyme histochemistry (NADH$_2$-oxidoreductase), electron microscopy, conventional histology, and *in vitro* specular microscopy to compare the effects of three ophthalmic preservatives on rabbit eyes. They showed that benzalkonium chloride (0.05 and 0.1%) was significantly more cytotoxic to corneal endothelial cells than 2% chlorobutanol or 2% thimerosal.

Ashford and Lamble (1974) noted that increased ocular inflammatory changes were correlated with increased ocular temperatures. Measurement of changes in ocular temperatures with an infrared thermometer may prove valuable in ophthalmic toxicology (Shuster and Kaufman, 1974).

Other quantitative techniques that can be used include corneal thickness measurements to quantitate corneal edema, and determination of corneal edema and amount of vascular leakage in the conjunctiva and aqueous humor by dye diffusion after intravenous injection of Evans blue (Laillier et al., 1975; Conquet et al., 1975).

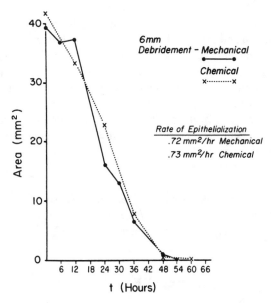

FIGURE 18 Rate of corneal re-epithelialization following mechanical and chemical epithelial debridement.

SUMMARY

A large number of materials are subjected to ocular irritation tests. Significant advances have been made over the past 30 yr, and several useful methods now exist for evaluating the ocular irritancy of materials in animals and predicting their effects in humans. However, several problems still exist that include selection of appropriate test animals, accuracy and reproducibility of observations made in animals, and identifying test animals and protocols that more precisely predict human reactions.

In this chapter we have briefly reviewed the major papers that have influenced the direction of ocular irritation testing. The anatomical similarities and differences among the commonly used test animals have been described, with emphasis on the comparison of albino rabbits and humans. Despite significant anatomical dissimilarities, the rabbit eye appears to be the most useful system for most purposes, although use of other animals (e.g., monkeys) may be justified in special circumstances.

The predictive value for humans of irritation tests in animals (usually rabbits) has been discussed. The rabbit eye is often equally sensitive or more sensitive to a particular irritant than the human eye. However, there are also several examples of cases in which rabbit tests have failed to alert investigators to problems that appeared later in humans. Thus, as in most toxicologic studies, continued evaluation and improved methods are needed in eye irritation testing.

Because various test guidelines must often be adapted and applied to specific situations, some examples of specific protocols, with results obtained during tests of several materials, have been presented. A 1-d acute test, a 5-d test, and two types of subchronic/chronic tests have been discussed. The 1-d test is useful for rapid screening of the ocular irritation potential of numerous materials. The 5-d and subchronic/chronic tests allow longer application to simulate anticipated clinical usage of the materials and evaluation of lesions that evolve more slowly. Modifications of these tests for contact lenses have also been discussed.

A few new techniques, such as specular microscopy, measurement of ocular temperature with an infrared thermometer, and measurement of vascular damage by leakage of dyes, have been mentioned briefly.

REFERENCES

Akers, M. J., Schoenwald, R. B. and McGinty, J. W. 1977. Practical aspects of ophthalmic drug development. *Drug Dev. Ind. Pharm.* 3:185–217.

Alexander, P. 1965. Evaluation of the irritation potential of shampoos and conditioning rinses. *Specialities* 9:33–37.

Aronson, S. B., Martenet, A. C., Yamamoto, E. A. and Bedford, M. J. 1966. Mechanisms of the host response in the eye. II. Variations in ocular diseases produced by several different antigens. *Arch. Ophthalmol.* 76:266–273.

Association for Research in Vision and Ophthalmology. 1975. Smelser symposium on corneal wound healing, Sarasota, Fla., April 28 to May 2.

Ashford, J. J. and Lamble, J. W. 1974. A detailed assessment procedure of anti-inflammatory effects of drugs on experimental immunogenic uveitis in rabbits. *Invest. Ophthalmol.* 13:414–421.

Bahn, G. C. 1954. The treatment of seborrheic blepharitis. *South. Med. J.* 47:749–753.

Bailey, I. L. and Carney, L. G. 1973. Corneal changes from hydrophilic contact lenses. *Am. J. Optom.* 50:299–304.

Baldwin, H. A., McDonald, T. O. and Beasley, C. H. 1973. Slit examination of experimental animal eyes. II. Grading scales and photographic evaluation of induced pathological conditions. *J. Soc. Cosmet. Chem.* 24:181–195.

Ballantyne, B. and Swanston, D. W. 1972. Ocular irritation tests. *Br. J. Pharmacol.* 46:577–578.

Barkman, R., Germanis, M., Karpe, G. and Malmborg, A. S. 1969. Preservatives in drops. *Acta Ophthalmol.* 47:461–475.

Battista, S. P. and McSweeney, E. S., Jr. 1965. Approaches to a quantitative method of testing eye irritation. *J. Soc. Cosmet. Chem.* 16:119–131.

Bayard, S. and Hehir, R. 1976. Evaluation of proposed changes in the modified Draize rabbit eye irritation test. Soc. Toxicol. 15th Meeting, Atlanta, Ga., March, paper 225.

Beckley, J. H. 1965a. Critique of the Draize eye test. *Am. Perfum. Cosmet.* 80:51–54.

Beckley, J. H. 1965b. Comparative eye testing: Man vs animal. *Toxicol. Appl. Pharmacol.* 7:93–101.

Beckley, J. H., Russell, T. J. and Rubin, L. F. 1969. Use of rhesus monkey for predicting human response to eye irritants. *Toxicol. Appl. Pharmacol.* 15:1–9.

Bellows, J. G. 1943. Local toxic effects of sulfanilamide and some of its derivatives. *Arch. Ophthalmol.* 36:65–69.

Bietti, G. B. and Giraldi, J. P. 1969. Topical osmotherapy of corneal edema. *Ann. Ophthalmol.* 1:40–49.

Bonfield, C. T. and Scala, R. A. 1965. The paradox in testing for eye irritation, a report on thirteen shampoos. *Proc. Sci. Sect. Toilet Goods Assoc.* 43:34–43.

Buehler, E. V. and Newmann, E. A. 1964. A comparison of eye irritation in monkeys and rabbits. *Toxicol. Appl. Pharmacol.* 6:701–710.

Butscher, P. 1953. Beitrag zur Therapie von Augenschadigunen durch Thioglykolsaur bei der Herstellung der songenannten Kaltwelle. *Klin. Monatsbl. Augenheilkd.* 122:349–350.

Carpenter, C. P. and Smyth, H. F. 1946. Chemical burns of the rabbit cornea. *Am. J. Ophthalmol.* 29:1363–1372.

Carter, J. C. 1906. Instillation of pure carbolic acid into the eye. *J. Am. Med. Assoc.* 47:37–39.

Carter, L. M., Duncan, G. and Rennie, G. K. 1973. Effects of detergents on the ionic balance and permeability of isolated bovine cornea. *Exp. Eye Res.* 17:490–496.

Carter, R. O. and Griffith, J. G. 1965. Assessment of eye hazard. *Toxicol. Appl. Pharmacol.* 7(Suppl. 2):60–73.

Cintron, C., Hassinger, L., Kablin, C. L., and Friend, J. 1979. A simple method for the removal of rabbit corneal epithelium utilizing *n*-heptanol. *Ophthalmic Res.* 11:90.

Clayton, G. D. and Clayton, F. E., eds. 1981. *Patty's Industrial Hygiene and Toxicology.* New York: Wiley-Interscience.

Code of Federal Regulations. 21, Part 58.

Cohen, L. B. 1954. Use of selsun in blepharitis marginalia. *Am. J. Ophthalmol.* 38:560–562.

Conquet, P., Durand, G., Laillier, J. and Plazonnet, B. 1975. Evaluation of ocular irritation in the rabbit. II. Objective versus subjective assessment. 17th Meeting Eur. Soc. Toxicol., Montpellier, France, June 16–18.

D'Asaro Biondo, M. 1933. Lesioni dell'occhio da catrame di carbon fossile e soui derivati. *Rass. Ital. Ottalmol.* 2:259–335.

Davies, M. 1972. Evaluating the toxicity of soft lens material. *Ophthalmic Optician* 12:939–947.

Davson, H. 1969. The intraocular fluids. In *The Eye,* ed. H. Davson, vol. 1, pp. 217–218. New York: Academic Press.

de la Iglesia, F. A., Mitchell, L. and Schwartz, E. 1974. Soft contact lens studies in rabbit eyes. 13th Meeting Soc. Toxicol., March 10–14.

de la Iglesia, F. A., Mitchell, L., Kayal, M. and Schwartz, E. 1976. Evaluation of hydrophilic contact lens effects on rabbit eyes. *Contacto* 20:18–24.

Dickstein, S. and Maurice, D. M. 1972. The metabolic basis to the fluid pump in the cornea. *J. Physiol.* 221:29.

Dohlman, C. H. 1971. The function of the corneal epithelium in health and disease. *Invest. Ophthalmol.* 10:376–407.

D'Osvaldo, 1928. Contributo clinico all'azione dei gas di guerra (fosgene). *Ann. Ottalmol.* 56:154.

Draize, J. H. 1959. *Appraisal of the Safety of Chemicals in Foods, Drugs and Cosmetics,* pp. 49–51. Austin, Tex.: Association of Food and Drug Officials of the United States.

Draize, J. H. and Kelley, E. A. 1952. Toxicity to eye mucosa of certain cosmetic preparations containing surface-active agents. *Proc. Sci. Sect. Toilet Goods Assoc.* 17:1–4.

Draize, J. H., Woodard, G. and Calvery, H. O. 1944. Methods for the study of irritation and toxicity of substances applied topically to the skin and mucous membranes. *J. Pharmacol. Exp. Ther.* 82:377–390.

Driefus, M. and Wobmann, P. 1975. Influence of soft contact lens solutions on rabbit corneae. *Ophthalmic Res.* 7:140–151.

Durand-Cavagna, G., Delort, D., Duprat, P., Bailly, Y., Plazonnet, B. and Gordon, L. R. 1989. Corneal toxicity studies in rabbits and dogs with hydroxyethyl cellulose and benzalkonium chloride. *Fundam. Appl. Toxicol.* 13:500–508.

Edelhauser, H. F., Van Horn, D. L., Hyndiuk, R. A. and Schultz, R. O. 1975. Intraocular irrigating solutions: Their effect on the corneal endothelium. *Arch. Ophthalmol.* 93:648.

Edelhauser, H. F., Van Horn, D. L., Schultz, R. O. and Hyndiuk, R. A. 1976. Comparative toxicity of intraocular irrigating solutions on the corneal endothelium. *Am. J. Ophthalmol.* 81:473.

Edelhauser, H. F., Gonnering, R. and Van Horn, D. L. 1978. Intraocular irrigating solutions: A comparative study of BSS plus and lactated Ringer's solution. *Arch. Ophthalmol.* 96:516.

Edelhauser, H. F., Van Horn, D. L. and Miller, P. M. 1979a. Modification of sulfhydryl groups in the corneal endothelium with organic mercurials. *Docum. Ophthalmol. Proc. Ser.* 18:271.

Edelhauser, H. F., Hine, J. E., Pederson, H. J., Van Horn, D. L. and Schultz, R. O. 1979b. The effect of phenylephrine on the cornea. *Arch. Ophthalmol.* 97:937.

Edelhauser, H. F., Hanneken, A. M., Pederson, H. J. and Van Horn, D. L. 1981. Osmotic tolerance of rabbit and human corneal endothelium. *Arch. Ophthalmol.* 99:1281.

Edelhauser, H. F., Antoine, M. E., Pederson, H. J., Hiddemen, J. W. and Harris, R. G. 1983. Intraocular safety evaluation of ethylene oxide and sterilant residues. *Journal of Cutaneous and Ocular Toxicology.* 2(1):7–39.

Elliott, G. A. and Schut, A. L. 1965. Studies with cytarabine HCl (CA) in normal eyes of man, monkey and rabbit. *Am. J. Ophthalmol.* 60:1074–1082.

Estable, J. L. 1948. The ocular effect of several irritant drugs applied directly to the conjunctiva. *Am. J. Ophthalmol.* 31:837–844.

Fairhall, L. T. 1957. *Industrial Toxicology,* 2d ed. Baltimore: Williams & Wilkins.

Falahee, F. J., Rose, C. S., Olin, S. S. and Seifried, H. E. 1982. Eye irritation testing: An assessment of methods and guidelines for testing materials for eye irritancy. EPA–560/11–82–001, October 1981, Office of Pesticides and Toxic Substances. Washington, D.C.: U.S. Environmental Protection Agency.

Fine, B. S. and Yanoff, M. 1972. *Ocular Histology. A Text and Atlas.* New York: Harper & Row.

Flury, F. and Zernik, F. 1931. *Schadliche Gase.* Berlin: Springer.

Food and Drug Administration. 1965. *Illustrated Guide for Grading Eye Irritation by Hazardous Substances.* Washington, D.C.: Government Printing Office.

Forster, S., Mead, A. and Sears, M. 1979. An interophthalmic communicating artery as explanation for the consensual irritative response of the rabbit eye. *Invest. Opthamol. Visual Sci.* 18(2):161–165.

Freeberg, F. E., Nixon, G. A., Reer, P. J., Weaver, J. E., Bruce R. D., Griffith, J. F. and Sanders, L. W. 1986. Human and rabbit eye responses to chemical insult. *Fund. Appl. Toxicol.* 7:626–634.

Friedenwald, J. S., Hughes, W. F. and Herrmann, H. 1944. *Arch. Ophthalmol.* 31:379–383.

Friemann, W. and Overhoff, W. 1956. Keratitis als Berufserkrankung in der Ölheringsficherei. *Klin. Monatsbl. Augenheilkd.* 128:425–438.

Friend, J. and Thoft, R. A. 1978. Functional competence of regenerating ocular surface epithelium. *Invest. Ophthalmol.* 17:134.

Gartner, S. 1944. Blood vessels of the conjunctiva. *Arch. Ophthalmol.* 36:464–471.

Gasset, A. R., Ishii, Y., Kaufman, E. and Miller, T. 1974. Cytotoxicity of ophthalmic preservatives. *Am. J. Ophthalmol.* 78:98–105.

Gaunt, I. F. and Harper, K. H. 1964. The potential irritancy to the rabbit eye mucosa of certain commercially available shampoos. *J. Soc. Cosmet. Chem.* 15:230–290.

Gershbein, L. L. and McDonald, J. E. 1977. Evaluation of the corneal irritancy of test shampoos and detergents in various animal species. *Food Cosmet. Toxicol.* 15:131–134.

Goldenthal, E. I. 1968. Current views on safety evaluation of drugs. *FDA Pap.* 2:13–18.

Gonnering, R., Edelhauser, H. F., Van Horn, D. L., and Durant, W. 1979. The pH tolerance of rabbit and human corneal endothelium. *Invest. Ophthalmol. Vis. Sci.* 18:373.

Grant, W. M. 1986. *Toxicology of the Eye,* 3rd ed. Springfield, Ill.: Charles C. Thomas.

Grant, W. M. and Kern, H. L. 1956. Action of alkalies on the corneal stroma. *Arch. Ophthalmol.* 54:931–939.

Grant, W. M. and Loeb, D. R. 1948. Effect of locally applied antihistamine drugs on normal eyes. *Arch. Ophthalmol.* 39:553–554.

Guess, W. L., Rosenbluth, S. A., Schmidt, B. and Autian, J. 1965. Diffusion method for toxicity screening of plastics on cultured cell monolayers. *J. Pharm. Sci.* 54:1545.

Hackett, R. R. 1989. Species selection on the preclinical development of ophthalmic drugs: The rabbit versus the nonhuman primate. Presented at the DruSafe East Meeting, Cherry Hill, N.J., November 30.

Hagiwara, H. and Sugiwia, S. 1953. The use of caster-oil and Tween 80 as an ophthalmic base. *Acta Soc. Ophthalmol. Jpn.* 57:1–5.

Hanna, C. 1966. Proliferation and migration of epithelial cells during corneal wound repair in the rabbit and the rat. *Am. L. Ophthalmol.* 61:55–63.

Harding, C. V., Bagchi, M., Weinsieder, A. and Peters, V. 1974. A comparative study of corneal epithelial cell surfaces utilizing the scanning electron microscope. *Invest. Ophthalmol.* 13:906–912.

Harris, L. S., Kahanowica, Y. and Shimmyo, M. 1975. Corneal anesthesia induced by soaps and surfactants, lack of correlation in rabbits and humans. *Ophthalmologica* 170:320–325.

Havener, W. H. 1966. *Ocular Pharmacology.* Saint Louis, Mo.: Mosley.

Hazelton, L. W. 1952. Relation of surface active properties to irritation of the rabbit eye. *Proc. Sci. Sect. Toilet Goods Assoc.* 17:5–9.

Hine, C. H., Hogan, M. J. and McEwen, W. K. 1960. Eye irritation from air pollution. *J. Air Pollut. Control Assoc.* 10:17–20.

Ho, P. C., Davis, W. H., Elliott, J. H. and Cohen, S. 1974. Kinetics of corneal epithelial regeneration and epidermal growth factor. *Invest. Ophthalmol.* 13:804–809.

Hoffman, F. 1972. The surface of epithelial cells of the cornea under the scanning electron microscope. *Ophthalmol. Res.* 3:207–213.

Hogan, M. J. and Zimmerman, L. E. 1962. *Ophthalmic Pathology: An Atlas and Textbook,* 2d ed. Philadelphia: Saunders.

Hogan, M. J., Alvarado, J. A. and J. E. Weddell. 1971. *Histology of the Human Eye; An Atlas and Textbook.* Philadelphia: Saunders.

Holly, F. J. and Lemp, M. A. 1971. Wettability and wetting of corneal epithelium. *Exp. Eye Res.* 11:239–250.

Hood, C. I., Gasset, A. R., Ellison, E. D. and Kaufman, H. E. 1971. The corneal reaction to selected chemical agents in the rabbit and squirrel monkey. *Am. J. Ophthalmol.* 71:1009–1017.

Hull, D. S., Chemotti, T., Edelhauser, H. F., Van Horn, D. L., and Hyndiuk, R. A. 1975. Effect of epinephrine on the corneal endothelium. *Am. J. Ophthalmol.* 79:245.

Jumblatt, M. M., Fogle, J. A. and Neufeld, A. H. 1980. Cholera toxin stimulates adenosine $3',5'$-monophosphate synthesis and epithelial wound closure in the rabbit cornea. *Invest. Ophthalmol. Vis. Sci.* 19:1321.

Kay, J. H. and Calandra, J. C. 1962. Interpretation of eye irritation tests. *J. Soc. Cosmet. Chem.* 13:281–289.

Kennah, H. E., Hignet, S., Laux, P. E., Dorko, J. D. and Barrow, C. S. 1989. An objective procedure for quantitating eye irritation based on changes of corneal thickness. *Fundam. Appl. Toxicol.* 12:258–268.

Kikkawa, Y. 1972. Normal corneal staining with fluorescein. *Exp. Eye Res.* 14:13–20.

Kikkawa, Y. 1975. A procedure for evaluating corneal side-effects of the hydrogel contact lens. *Contacto* 19:5–11.

Laillier, J., Plazonnet, B. and LeDouarec, J. C. 1975. Evaluation of ocular irritation in the rabbit. I. Development of an objective methodology to study eye irritation. 17th Meeting Eur. Soc. Toxicol. Montpellier, France, June 16–18.

Laquer, E. and Magnus, R. 1921. Über Kampfagasvergiftung. V. Experimentelle und Theoretische Grundlagen zur Therapie der Phosgenerkrankung. *Z. Gesamte Exp. Med.* 13:200–205.

Lee, V. H. L. and Robinson, J. R. 1986. Review: Topical ocular drug delivery. Recent developments and future challenges. *J. Ocul. Pharmacol* 2:67–108.

Leibowitz, H. M. and Laing, R. A. 1984. Specular microscopy. In *Corneal Disorders: Clinical Diagnosis and Managment,* ed H. M. Leibowitz. Philadelphia: W. B. Saunders.

Leopold, I. H. 1945. Local toxic effect of detergents on ocular structures. *Arch. Ophthalmol.* 34:99–102.

Lewin, L. and Guillery, H. 1913. *Die Wirkungen von Arzneimitteln und Giften auf das Auge,* 2d ed. Berlin: Hirschwald.

Mann, I. and Pullinger, B. D. 1942. A study of mustard gas lesions of the eyes of rabbits and men. *Proc. R. Soc. Med.* 35:229–244.

Marsh, R. J. and Maurice, D. M. 1971. The influence of non-ionic detergents and other surfactants on human corneal permeability. *Exp. Eye Res.* 11:43–48.

Marshall, F. 1968. Ocular side effects of drugs. *Food Cosmet. Toxicol.* 6:221–224.

Marzulli, F. N. and Ruggles, D. I. 1973. Rabbit eye irritation test: Collaborative study. *J. Am. Assoc. Anal. Chem.* 56:905–914.

Marzulli, F. N. and Simon, M. E. 1971. Eye irritation from topically applied drugs and cosmetics: Preclinical studies. *Am. J. Optom.* 48:61–79.

Maurice, D. M. 1968. Cellular membrane activity in the corneal endothelium of the intact eye. *Experientia* 24:1094–1095.

Maurice, D. M. 1969. The cornea and sclera. In *The Eye,* ed. H. Davson, vol. 1, pp. 489–600. New York: Academic Press.

Maurice, D. M. 1974. A scanning slit optical microscope. *Invest. Ophthalmol.* 13:1033–1037.

McCarey, B. E., Edelhauser, H. F. and Van Horn, D. 1973. Functional and structural changes in the corneal endothelium during *in vitro* perfusion. *Invest. Ophthalmol.* 12:410–417.

McDonald, T. O. 1973. Experimental ocular studies with polyinosinic acid: polycytidlylic acid. *Eye Ear Nose Throat Mon.* 52:27–34.

McDonald, T. O., Borgmann, A. R., Roberts, M. D. and Fox, L. G. 1970a. Corneal wound healing I. Inhibition of stromal healing by three dexamethasone derivatives. *Invest. Ophthalmol.* 9:703–709.

McDonald, T. O., Roberts, M. D. and Borgmann, A. R. 1970b. Intraocular safety of carbamylcholine chloride (carbachol) in rabbit eyes. *Ann. Ophthalmol.* 2:878–883.

McDonald, T. O., Baldwin, H. A. and Beasley, C. H. 1973a. Slit-lamp examination of experimental animal eyes. I. Techniques of illumination and the normal animal eye. *J. Soc. Cosmet. Chem.* 24:163–180.

McDonald, T. O., Kasten, K., Hervey, R., Gregg, S., Borgmann, A. R. and Murchison, T. 1973b. Acute ocular toxicity of ethylene oxide, ethylene glycol, and ethylene chlorohydrin. *Bull. Parenter. Drug Assoc.* 27:153–164.

McDonald, T. O., Kasten, K., Hervey, R., Gregg, S., Smith, D. and Robb, C. A. 1973c. Comparative toxicity of dexamethasone and its tertiary butyl acetate ester after topical ocular instillation in rabbits. *Am. J. Ophthalmol.* 76:117–125.

McDonald, T. O., Kasten, K., Hervey, R., Gregg, S., Kellogg, M., Borgmann, A. R. and Hecht, G. 1973d. An animal model for toxicity evaluation of contact lens solutions. Assoc. Res. Vision Ophthalmol., Sarasota, Fla., May 1–5, abstract.

McDonald, T. O., Seabaugh, V., Shadduck, J. A. and Edelhauser, H. F. 1987. Eye irritation. In *Dermatotoxicology,* eds. F. N. Marzulli and H. E. Maibach. Cambridge: Hemisphere.

McLaughlin, R. S. 1946. Chemical burns of the human cornea. *Am. J. Ophthalmol.* 29:1355–1362.

Mishima, S. 1968. Corneal thickness. *Survey Ophthalmol.* 13:57.

Mishima, S. 1972. Corneal physiology under contact lenses. In *Soft Contact Lenses,* eds. A. R. Gasset and H. E. Kaufman, pp. 19–36. St. Louis, Mo.: Mosby.

Mishima, S. and Hedbys, B. O. 1968. Measurements of corneal thickness with the Haag-Streit pachometer. *Arch. Ophthalmol.* 80:710.

Morgan, R. L., Sorenson, S. S. and Castles, T. R. 1987. Prediction of ocular irritation by corneal pachymetry. *Food Chem. Toxicol.* 25(8):609–613.

Morrison, D. R., Capella, J. A. and Schaefer, I. 1972. Dynamics of oxygen utilization under a soft contact lens. In *Soft Contact Lenses,* eds. A. R. Gasset and H. Kaufman, pp. 44–58. St. Louis, Mo.: Mosby.

Moses, R. A., Parkinson, G. and Schuchardt, R. 1979. A standard large wound of the corneal epithelium in the rabbit. *Invest. Ophthalmol.* 18:103.

Murphy, J. C., Osterberg, R. E., Seabaugh, V. M. and Bierbower, G. W. 1982. Ocular irritancy responses to various pH of acids and bases with and without irrigation. *Toxicology* 23:281–291.

Nakano, M. 1958. Effect of various antifungal preparations on the conjunctiva and cornea of rabbits. *Yakuzaigaku* 18:94.

Norn, M. S. 1971. Vital staining of cornea and conjunctiva. *Eye Ear Nose Throat Mon.* 50:294–299.

Ooka, R. 1967. Agricultural chemicals, blasticidin and the eyes. *Ophthalmology (Tokyo)* 9:166–175.

Phister, R. R. 1973. The normal surface of corneal epithelium: A scanning electron microscopic study. *Invest. Ophthalmol.* 12:654–668.

Phister, R. R. 1975. The normal surface of conjunctiva epithelium. A scanning electron microscopic study. *Invest. Ophthalmol.* 14:267–279.

Popp, C. 1955. Kornaerosionen durch Polyäthyleneglykole. *Klin. Monatsbl. Augenheilkd.* 126:76–77.

Prince, J. H., Diesem, C. D., Eglitis, I. and Ruskell, G. L. 1960. *Anatomy and Histology of the Eye and Orbit in Domestic Animals.* Springfield, Ill.: Charles C. Thomas.

Rosen, J. and Brown, S. 1974. Scanning microscopy of healing corneal epithelium. Assoc. Res. Vision Ophthalmol., Sarasota, Fla., April 25–29.

Rosenthal, J. W. and Adler, H. 1962. Effect of selenium disulfide on rabbit eyes. *South. Med. J.* 55:318–320.

Rucker, I., Kettrey, R., Bach, F. and Zeleznick, L. 1972. A safety test for contact lens wetting solutions. *Ann. Ophthalmol.* 4:1000–1006.

Russell, K. L. and Hoch, S. G. 1962. Product development and rabbit eye irritation. *Proc. Sci. Sect. Toilet Goods Assoc.* 37:27–32.

Schimmelpfenning, B. H. 1979. Long-term perfusion on human corneas. *Invest. Ophthalmol. Vis. Sci.* 18:107.

Schuck, E. A., Stephens, E. R. and Middleton, J. T. 1966. Eye irritation response at low concentrations of irritants, *Arch. Environ. Health* 13:570–575.

Sheldon, H. 1956. An electron microscope study of the epithelium in the normal mature and immature mouse cornea. *J. Biophys. Biochem. Cytol.* 2:253–260.

Shuster, J. and Kaufman, H. E. 1974. *Invest. Ophthalmol.* 13:892–893 (letter).

Sigelman, S., Dohlman, C. H. and Friedenwald, J. S. 1954. Miotic and wound healing activities in the rat corneal epithelium. *Arch. Ophthalmol.* 52:751–757.

Simmons, S. J., Jumblate, M. M. and Neufeld, A. H. 1987. Corneal epithelial wound closure in tissue culture: An *in vitro* model of ocular irritancy. *Toxicol. Appl. Pharmacol.* 88:13–23.

Skyowski, P. 1951. Ethylene glycol toxicity. *Am. J. Ophthalmol.* 34:1599–1600.

Smyth, H. F. and Seaton, J. 1940. Acute response of guinea pigs and rats to inhalation of vapors of tetraethyl orthosilicate (ethyl silicate). *J. Ind. Hyg.* 22:288–296.

Staatz, W. D., Edelhauser, H. F., Lehner, R. and Van Horn D. L. 1980. Cytotoxicity of pivalylphenylephrine and pivalic acid to the corneal endothelium. *Arch. Ophthalmol.* 98:1279.

Stokinger, H. E., Wagner, W. D. and Dobrogoski, O. J. 1957. Ozone toxicity studies. *Arch. Ind. Health* 16:514–522.

Suker, G. F. 1913. Injury to cornea from oxalic acid. *Ophthalmol. Rec.* 23:40–47.

Swanston, D. W. 1985. Assessment of the validity of animal techniques in eye-irritation testing. *Fd. Chem. Toxic.* 23:169–173.

Treon, J. F. 1965. Physiological properties of selected nonionic surfactants. *Soap Perfum. Cosmet.* 38:47–54.

Ubels, J. L., Edelhauser, H. F., Foley, K. M., Liao, J. C. and Gressel, P. 1985. The efficacy of retinoic acid ointment for treatment of xerophthalmia and corneal epithelial wounds. *Current Eye Res.* 4(10), pp. 1049–1057.

Uniacke, C. A., Hill, R. M., Greenberg, M. and Seward, S. 1972. Physiological tests for new contact lens material. I. Quantitative effects of selected oxygen atmospheres on glycogen storage, LDH concentration and thickness of the corneal epithelium. *Am. J. Optom.* 49:329–335.

Van Abbe, N. Y. 1973. Eye irritation: Studies relating to responses in man and laboratory animals. *J. Soc. Cosmet. Chem.* 24:685–692.

Van Horn, D. L., Edelhauser, H. F., Prodanovich, G., Eiferman, R. and Pederson, H. J. 1977. Effect of the ophthalmic preservative thimerosal on rabbit and human corneal endothelium. *Invest. Ophthalmol. Vis. Sci.* 16:273.

von Oettingen, W. F. 1958. *Poisoning*, 2d ed. Philadelphia: Saunders.

Weil, C. S. and Scala, R. A. 1971. Study of intra- and interlaboratory variability in the results of rabbit eye and skin irritation tests. *Toxicol. Appl. Pharmacol.* 19:276–360.

Weissinger, J. 1989. Nonclinical pharmacologic and toxicologic considerations for evaluating biologic products. *Reg. Toxicol. and Pharmacol.* 10:255–263.

Weltman, A. S., Sparber, S. B. and Jurtshuk, T. 1965. Comparative evaluation and the influence of various factors on eye-irritation scores. *Toxicol. Appl. Pharmacol.* 7:308–319.

Yee, R. W., Edelhauser, H. F. and Stern, M. E. 1987. Specular microscopy of vertebrate corneal endothelium: A comparative study. *Exp. Eye Res.* 44:703–714.

32

alternatives to acute ocular and dermal toxicity tests in animals

■ John M. Frazier ■

INTRODUCTION

During the last decade, significant scientific attention has been directed toward the development of alternative (non-whole-animal) testing methods for the evaluation of acute ocular and dermal irritation. This attention has been motivated by several factors, including economics, technological developments, and animal welfare activism. The desire to have rapid, inexpensive testing methods to evaluate the hazard associated with chemicals, drugs, and household products is always an important consideration in product development. In the area of acute ocular and dermal irritation, existing whole-animal testing is not particularly expensive and the economic argument for developing new testing methods is not as compelling as in other areas of toxicity testing, for example, carcinogenicity testing, where traditional testing methods are extremely expensive and time consuming. Technological developments are certainly another important factor in the development of alternative testing methods. Within the last decade, significant advancements in cell culture and the availability of cells, as well as advances in instrumentation for measuring biological responses, have allowed for the development of new testing methods that provide a diverse range of toxicological data concerning cellular responses to pure chemicals and finished products. In spite of the influence of economics and technological advances in promoting the evolution of new toxicity testing strategies, it is clear that societal pressure to reduce or eliminate toxicity testing in sentient animals has catalyzed the rapid progress seen in recent years. However, the universal desire for humane treatment of animals and for the reduction, or if possible the elimination of, the use of whole animals in toxicity testing must be considered in the context of why toxicity testing is performed in the first place—to protect the health and safety of humans. New methods for safety evaluation can only be implemented when their reliability and scientific relevance have been established, that is, only when they have been appropriately validated.

Historically, acute ocular and dermal irritation testing developed in response to regulatory needs. Specific guidelines for conducting and interpreting *in vivo* tests have been established by regulatory authorities. Current irritation testing procedures can be traced back to early regulatory concerns in the late 1930s and early 1940s, which culminated in the classical report of Draize, et al. (1944). In more recent years, modifications to the Draize eye and skin tests have resulted in several versions of the tests being used for various purposes. Serious considerations of alternatives to the standard *in vivo* irritation tests began to appear in the late 1970s. Early in the 1980s several reviews of the status of alternative testing methods indicated only a handful of possibilities (U.S. EPA, 1981; Cosmetics, Toiletry and Fragrance Association, 1980). A review of alternatives for acute ocular irritation testing in 1986 identified 35 potential alternative tests (Frazier et al., 1987). At the time of publishing this volume, more than 50 tests (including variations of earlier tests) are available for acute ocular irritation testing. None of these tests have been fully validated in the rigorous sense; however, several tests have received considerable attention and based on the weight of evidence may be considered validated for certain restricted purposes (see below for a discussion of purposes of testing). Progress in alternatives for dermal irritation testing has been slower than for ocular testing, and fewer alternative tests have been proposed for acute dermal irritation testing compared to acute ocular irritation testing.

Toxicity testing is used to provide important toxicological information at many stages of product development from early stages of candidate product selection to regulatory approval. As a consequence, the essential characteristics of a particular toxicity test system will vary depending on its intended purpose. In order to classify potential new tests, the intended purposes can be categorized on the basis of two factors: (1) the type of test (screening, adjunct or replacement) and (2) the level of toxicological information provided (toxic potential, potency, or hazard/risk). With respect to the first classification factor, the type of test, the three categories proposed are defined in relation to their use in decision making. *Screening tests* are designed to provide limited information at early stages of product development for internal, corporate decision making. As the term screening implies, more definitive toxicological evaluations will be conducted at later stages of product development. *Adjunct tests* are methods that can provide information that is acceptable to regulatory agencies for product registration. Adjunct tests do not provide sufficient information in and of themselves, but are useful in the regulatory decision process in conjunction with more traditional *in vivo* toxicological data. One strategy currently proposed for toxicological evaluations is a tier testing approach where adjunct tests would be used initially to classify highly dangerous materials, thus eliminating these materials from later stages involving animal testing. Under this strategy, only materials of low potential toxicity would ever be tested *in vivo*. Finally, replacement tests are designed to totally replace an existing *in vivo* testing procedure for regulatory acceptance. Due to the complexity of any toxicological issue, a single alternative test will not be adequate to completely replace an existing *in vivo* toxicity testing procedure, such as the Draize eye or skin test. In all likelihood, a battery of alternative tests will be required to provide sufficient toxicological data to make definitive safety decisions in the absence of *in vivo* test data. With respect to test classification on the basis of type of testing, it is feasible that a particular test would progress from one category to another as experience with the test expands. For example, a particular test initially may be used by a corporation to select candidate materials for product development. The same test, after further validation and if it meets appropriate criteria, could be classified as an adjunct test if it is accepted or used as the first stage of a regulatory tier testing strategy. Finally, if the test proves to be a particularly good predictive test, it might be used as a component of a test battery as a replacement for an *in vivo* test procedure. Note that the characteristics of a good test and the criteria that the test must meet depend on the type of testing being conducted.

A second factor that can be used to classify toxicity tests is the level of toxicological data provided. The three levels that can be used for this classification are toxic potential, potency, and hazard/risk. If the objective is to merely determine whether or not a chemical has the potential to produce a particular effect, independent of a knowledge of its dose-response relationship, then it is possible to utilize testing methods that provide purely qualitative results (basically yes or no answers). Testing for *toxic potential* is the lowest level of toxicological evaluation, that is, hazard identification. The second level of evaluation determines the relative toxicity of a chemical when compared to other toxic agents, that is, a measurement of *potency*. Since various test systems use different measures to evaluate toxic effects, the absolute value of the end-point measurements, such as the ED50, will depend on the particular test employed. Therefore, potency is a relative measure that can be calibrated by benchmark chemicals. Potency testing systems can be used to rank toxic materials, and such rankings can form the basis of a toxicity classification system for regulatory purposes. However, such test systems cannot be used to predict hazard and/or risk to the target organisms (humans, domesticated or feral animals) directly. The highest level of toxicological evaluation is *hazard/risk*. At this level, the toxicological data provided by the test systems are incorporated into a full safety evaluation using various extrapolation procedures to make direct estimates of the toxicological implications of products under conditions of expected use. At this level, understanding of the mechanistic relationship between observations in the test system and the expected/predicted toxicological responses in the target organism is essential in order to provide confidence in predicted outcomes and safe levels of exposure. Again, the scientific criteria for a test to perform at each of these levels of toxicological evaluation vary from one level to the next, with the degree of sophistication increasing from toxic potential to hazard/risk evaluations.

The objective of this chapter is to briefly summarize the existing alternative tests for acute ocular and dermal toxicity using this classification scheme. A few comments will be directed toward the current state of validation of these methods, and the chapter will conclude with a discussion of future directions in alternative toxicity testing.

ACUTE OCULAR IRRITATION TESTING

Use and Classification of Tests

The overall objective of acute ocular irritation testing is to provide toxicological data that can be used in the evaluation of the possible detrimental effects to the eye when a simple, direct exposure to the anterior surface of the eye occurs. The possible scenarios in which this information becomes important range from labeling chemicals for transportation, so that safety measures can be taken in case of an accident, to evaluation of safe levels of dosages for ophthalmic drugs that are intended to be placed in the eye for therapeutic purposes. In the first case, a crude classification scheme is needed to warn emergency workers of the need for safety precautions. In the past, ocular toxicity labeling has been accomplished on the basis of several variations of the Draize eye test. This classification is strictly determined by the *in vivo* animal test data with no additional consideration of modifying factors that may be important in human responses. In the case of ophthalmic drugs, extensive and detailed toxicological evaluations are conducted, which may include primate studies, to determine safe levels of dosage in humans reliably. For this purpose, complete hazard/risk assessments are performed before the drug is ever used in clinical trials. These two examples illustrate the diverse range of testing requirements for acute ocular toxicity. Alternative testing methods for acute ocular irritation can play a role in many testing situations by providing useful toxicological data at various stages of product development and registration. In fact, a single alternative test (or possibly small battery of alternative tests) could potentially replace the use of the Draize eye test for toxicity labeling purposes, thus significantly reducing the use of animals for ocular irritation testing, yet still not be adequate for ophthalmic drug safety evaluation. Each of these testing needs must be considered separately with respect to the possible role of alternative testing methods currently available.

In this chapter, existing tests are classified according to the two factors previously described (type of testing × level of toxicity testing) as well as the potential mechanistic basis of the test. This latter factor is introduced to provide some guidance in interpreting the potential relationship between *in vitro* test results and implications for human ocular toxicity. Classification and interpretation of tests on the basis of mechanisms will continue to improve as knowledge of both the toxicity test systems and ocular pathological processes increases.

The subdivision of currently existing alternative toxicity tests on the basis of proposed mechanisms is derived from the scheme used by Frazier et al. (1987) with some modifications. The five major categories are (A) cell toxicity, (B) tissue physiology, (C) inflammation and irritation, (D) recovery and repair, and (E) other. Category A, cell toxicity, refers to tests which evaluate either cellular lethality or metabolic dysfunction. This category is further subdivided into tests that evaluate (1) cell adhesion/cell proliferation, (2) cell membrane integrity, (3) cell function impairment, and (4) morphology. Category B, tissue physiology, encompasses tests that evaluate alterations in tissue structure or function which are relevant to evaluating acute ocular irritation. The third category, inflammation and immunity, consists of tests that provide information concerning release of mediators of inflammation that act at the immunological level of tissue response. Category D includes tests that determine various characteristics of the tissue repair process and impairment of that process. Finally, the last category, "other," includes tests that are difficult to classify as to their mechanistic basis and/or are only distantly related to ocular tissues in terms of the mechanistic similarity.

Existing Tests

The number of potential alternative tests for acute ocular irritation testing is rapidly increasing and will continue to do so into the foreseeable future. At any given time, the listing of these tests will necessarily be incomplete, in terms of the actual existing methods as well as their classification within the categories that have been defined above. For this reason the reader should view this summary as a slightly unfocused photograph of a single time point in an evolving process. With this caveat in mind, existing tests are listed in Table 1. This table is a modification and update of Table 11 in Frazier et al. (1987).

Due to the large number of tests it is impossible to describe each test individually. The interested reader is referred to the references, which provide adequate descriptions of the test protocols as well as information concerning test performance for specific materials. As is clear from the table, most existing tests are classified as *screening tests* for *potency evaluation*. The first descriptor, screening test, is based on the fact that no non-whole-animal alternative toxicity tests have been accepted by regulatory agencies as adjuncts, much less replacements. However, it should be noted that a subset of existing tests has been demonstrated by widespread experience to have the potential to be upgraded to the class of adjuncts, particularly in the context of a tier testing strategy. The second descriptor (i.e., most tests are classified for *potency evaluation)* is based on the observation that any test that provides an objective concentration-response relationship can be quantified, thus providing a measur-

TABLE 1. *In Vitro* Toxicity Tests for Acute Ocular Irritation Testing

Name	Biological component	Type of testing[a]	Level of testing[b]	References[d]
A. Cell toxicity				
1. Cell adhesion/cell proliferation				
a. Growth inhibition	BKH cells	S	B	(51)
b. Colony formation inhibition	(1) BKH cells	S	B	(51)
	(2) SIRC cells	S	B	(46, 47)
c. Cell detachment	BKH cells	S	B	(51)
d. Total cellular protein	(1) BALB/c T3 cells	S	B	(58, 62)
	(2) BCL-D1 cells	S	B	(2, 32)
e. Agar overlay assay	L929	S	A	(26, 65)
2. Member integrity				
a. Dual dye staining	(1) LS cells	S	B	(45, 52)
	(2) Thymocytes	S	B	(1)
b. ^{51}Cr release	RCE-SIRC/PB15/YAC1	S	B	(15, 54)
c. Hemolysis	Bovine RBC	S	B	(44, 55)
3. Cell function impairment				
a. Plasminogen activator inhibition	Rabbit corneal cell	S	B	(10–12)
b. ATP levels	LS cells	S	B	(30)
c. Uridine uptake inhibition	BALB/c 3T3	S	B	(56, 57, 59)
d. Neutral red uptake	(1) BALB/c 3T3	S	B	(4, 5, 38, 64)
	(2) NHEK	S	B	(14)
e. Metabolic inhibition test (MIT-24)	HeLa cells	S	B	(53)
f. Silicone microphysiometer	NHEK	S	B	(31)
g. Epithelial permeability	NDCK cells	S	B	(23, 63)
4. Morphology				
a. Highest tolerated dose (HTD)	BALB/c 3T3	S	B	(3–6)
B. Tissue physiology				
1. Electrical conductivity assay	Epidermal slice	S	B	(48)
2. Muscle contraction assay	Rabbit irium	S	B	(44, 45)
3. Corneal opacity	Bovine cornea	S	B	(42, 43)
4. Corneal permeability test	Proptosed mouse eye	S	B	(7)
5. Corneal thickness	Enucleated rabbit eye	S	B	(9, 33, 49, 66)

822

C. Inflammatory/immunity
  1. Chorioallantoic membrane assays

a. CAM	Hen's egg	S	(34–38, 41, 50)
b. HET-CAM	Hen's egg	S	(39, 40)
c. CAM-VA	Hen's egg	S	
2. Mediator release assay			
a. Leukocyte chemotactic factors	Bovine corneal	B	(17, 18)
b. Histamine release	Rat peritoneal macrophages	B	(25)
c. Serotonin release	Rat peritoneal mast cells	B	(13)
d. Prostaglandin release	Rat vaginal explant	B	(16)
D. Recovery and repair			
1. Wound repair	Rabbit corneal epithelial cell	B	(27, 28)
E. Other			
1. EYTEX assay	[c]	S	(8, 24, 61)
Computer-based structure-activity relationship	[c]	A	(19–22)
Motility	Tetrahymena	B	(60)
Microtox assay	Bacteria	B	(8)
Liposomes	[c]	B	(29)

[a]S = screening, A = adjunct, R = replacement.

[b]A = toxic potential, B = potency, C = hazard/risk.

[c]No living biological component.

[d]References: 1, Aeschbacher et al. (1986); 2, Balls and Horner, (1985); 3, Borenfreund and Puerner (1984); 4, Borenfreund and Puerner (1985); 5, Borenfreund and Puerner (1987); 6, Borenfreund and Shopsis (1985);7, Brooks and Maurice (1987); 8, Bruner and Parker (1989); 9, Burton et al. (1981); 10, Chan (1985); 11, Chan (1986a); 12, Chan (1986b); 13, Chasin et al. (1979); 14, Clonetics (1989); 15, Douglas and Spillman (1990); 16, Dubin et al. (1985); 17, Elgebaly et al (1987a); 18, Elgebaly et al. (1987b); 19, Enslein (1984); 20, Enslein and Craig (1982); 21, Enslein et al. (1984); 22, Enslein et al. (1983); 23, Gabriels et al. (1989); 24, Gordon and Bergmen, (1986); 25, Jacaruso et al. (1985); 26, Jackson et al. (1988); 27, Jumblatt and Neufeld (1985); 28, Jumblatt and Neufeld (1986); 29, Kato et al. (1988); 30, Kemp et al. (1983); 31, Kercso et al. (1989); 32, Knox et al. (1986); 33, Koeter and Prinsen (1985); 34, Kong et al. (1987); 35, Lawrence et al. (1986); 36, Leighton et al. (1985a); 37, Leighton et al. (1983); 38, Leighton et al. (1985b); 39, Leupke (1985a); 40, Leupke, (1985b); 41, McCormick et al. (1984); 42, Muir (1984); 43, Muir (1985); 44, Muir et al. (1983); 45, Muir et al. (1986); 46, North-Root et al. (1985); 47, North-Root et al. (1982); 48, Oliver and Pemberton (1985); 49, Price and Andrews (1985); 50, Price et al. (1986); 51, Reinhardt et al. (1985); 52, Scaife, (1982); 53, Selling and Ekwall (1985); 54, Shadduck et al. (1985); 55, Shadduck et al. (1987); 56, Shopsis (1984); 57, Shopsis et al. (1985); 58, Shopsis and Eng (1985); 59, Shopsis and Sathe (1984); 60, Silverman (1983); 61, Soto et al. (1989); 62, Stark et al. (1986); 63, Tchao (1988); 64, Thomson et al. (1989); 65, Wallin et al. (1987); 66, York et al. (1982).

able basis for toxicity ranking (e.g., an EC50, LC50). Some tests cannot be objectively quantitated and therefore are classified as toxicity potential measurements. Finally, no test, or battery of tests, is currently available to fully replace *in vivo* testing, nor can they serve as the sole basis for hazard assessment.

Validation

Before any new toxicity testing method can be accepted for use, it must undergo an extensive evaluation of its reproducibility under practical testing conditions and its relevance to the particular toxicological issue under consideration. This process of evaluation is referred to as validation. The scientific basis of the validation process has been ill defined in the past, and the resulting confusion has slowed the acceptance of new tests for toxicological evaluations. Recently, attempts have been made to more rigorously define this process (Frazier, 1990; Balls et al., 1990). However, until scientists involved in these issues reach an agreement on the definition of validation and the essential steps in the process to validate a method, acceptance of new tests, particularly by regulatory agencies, will remain a confused and time-consuming effort.

Several coordinated programs have been conducted by individuals, corporations, trade associations, and governmental organizations to evaluate new tests for acute ocular irritation testing. Individual research groups have evaluated specific tests for their potential application to acute ocular irritation testing. For example, the Rockefeller group has developed and evaluated several tests, such as the neutral red uptake assay, which is being utilized in many laboratories world wide (Borenfreund and Puerner, 1984, 1985, 1987; Borenfreund and Shopsis, 1985). FRAME (The Fund for the Replacement of Animals in Medical Experimentation) has conducted a multiuniversity evaluation of the total cellular protein assay, which has applications not only in ocular irritation testing, but acute toxicological testing in general (Balls and Horner, 1985). At the corporate levels, individual companies have developed new tests as commercial ventures (EYTEX) and have evaluated selections of proposed tests for their potential for acute ocular irritation testing (Bruner and Parker, 1989). Trade associations have supported some of the more ambitious evaluations. Both the Soap and Detergent Association (SDA) and the Cosmetic, Toiletries and Fragrance Association (CTFA) have conducted programs to evaluate multiple tests using a selection of test chemicals relating to commercial products. The SDA program has progressed through several stages, although no definitive conclusions have been reached (Booman et al., 1988, 1989). The CTFA project is somewhat more recent than the SDA project, and publication of its results are expected in the summer of 1990. In Europe, the German federal government is sponsoring a multilaboratory evaluation of several tests. When the results of these various evaluations are made available, it should be possible to obtain a more complete perspective on the role new tests can play in the toxicological evaluation process. The expectation is that several existing tests can be accepted as adjunct tests, which can be used in regulatory accepted tier testing strategies.

ACUTE DERMAL IRRITATION TESTING

Use and Classification of Tests

As in the case with acute ocular irritation testing, acute dermal irritation testing is conducted for many purposes ranging from classification of chemicals for interstate shipping to safety evaluation of topical medicinals. Classically such testing has been conducted using whole animal tests. Alternative (non-whole-animal) approaches for dermal irritation testing have not developed as rapidly as for ocular irritation testing.

In general, the existing test can be classified into two categories on the basis of the biological component of the test system—either cells in culture or skin/synthetic skin culture. Note that the classification of alternative tests for acute dermal irritation testing is not mechanically based, as was true for acute ocular irritation testing, due to the lack of appropriate tests for many mechanistic categories. In general, many cell culture based dermal toxicity test systems have evolved by incorporating relevant cell types (keratinocytes, dermal fibroblasts, etc.) into classical cytotoxicity test protocols, such as neutral red uptake or [^{3}H]uridine uptake. Overall, a wide range of end-point measurements are being investigated to evaluate toxicological responses in these test systems.

Existing Tests

The existing tests currently available are listed in Table 2. A limited number of these methods has been extensively developed; thus the majority of tests listed should be considered as proposed methods. At the current stage of development, most tests can be classified *screening tests* for *potency evaluation,* as is the case for ocular irritation testing. However, some tests show potential as adjuncts, for example, as initial stages in a tier testing strategy. For example, the electrical conductivity assay of Oliver and Pemberton (1985) has been proposed as a screen for highly corrosive chemicals as a first level of evaluation. Thus, chemicals giving a highly positive response in this assay can be labeled as corrosive without additional animal testing. With further validation, it seems feasible that other tests may be developed to serve a similar function.

Validation

Formal validation of alternative toxicity tests for acute dermal irritation evaluation needs further development. One collaborative study of *in vitro* alternatives for acute dermal irritation testing was conducted by the Commission of the European Community. The performances of several *in vitro* tests were compared to the primary irritation index determined *in vivo.* Due to the limited

TABLE 2. Existing *In Vitro* Toxicity Tests for Acute Dermal Irritation Testing

Name	Biological component	Type of testing[a]	Level of testing[b]	References[d]
A. Cell culture assays				
1. Neutral red uptake	(1) BALB/c 3T3 cells	S	B	(1, 3, 4)
	(2) NHEK	S	B	(1, 17)
	(3) 3T3 Swiss mouse fibroblast	S	B	(7)
2. Uridine incorporation	BALB/c 3T3 cells	S	B	(16)
3. Total cellular protein	(1) BALB/c 3T3 cells	S	B	(15)
	(2) NHEK	S	B	(7)
4. Keratinization	XB-2 cells	S	B	(7)
5. MTT assay	3T3 Swiss mouse fibroblast	S	B	(7, 11)
6. Enzyme leakage	3T3 Swiss mouse fibroblast	S	B	(6)
7. Arachidonic acid metabolism	NHEK	S	B	(6, 10)
B. Skin culture assays				
1. Protein synthesis assay	Human skin	S	B	(12)
	Rabbit skin	S	B	(12)
	Guinea pig skin	S	B	(12)
2. Nuclear vacuole formation	Human skin	S	B	(12)
	Rabbit skin	S	B	(12)
	Guinea pig skin	S	B	(12)
3. MTT assay	(1) TESTSKIN (organogenesis)	S	B	(2, 5)
	(2) Human skin model (Marrow-Tech)	S	B	(5)
4. Release of inflammatory mediators	TESTSKIN (organogenesis)	S	B	(13)

5. Neutral red uptake	S	B	(2, 5)
Human skin model (Marrow-Tech)			
Epidermal slice			
6. Electrical conductivity assay	S	B	(14)
C. Other			
1. SKINTEX[c]	S	B	(9)
2. Computer-based structure-activity relationships[c]	S	A	(8)

[a]S = screening, A = adjunct, R = replacement.

[b]A = toxic potential, B = potency, C = hazard/risk.

[c]No living biological component.

[d]References: 1, Babich et al. (1989); 2, Bell et al. (1988); 3, Borenfreund and Puerner (1984); 4, Borenfreund and Puerner (1985); 5, Center for Animals and Public Policy (1989); 6, DeLeo et al. (1987); 7, Duffy et al. (1986); 8, Enslein et al. (1987); 9, Gordon et al. (1989); 10, Lamont et al. (1989); 11, Mol et al. (1986); 12, More et al. (1986); 13, Naughton et al. (1989); 14, Oliver and Pemberton (1985); 15, Shopsis and Eng (1985); 16, Shopsis (1984); 17, Triglia et al. (1989).

number of chemicals tested, it is not possible at this stage to adequately evaluate the methods under consideration. The validation of alternative methods for acute dermal irritation testing requires significant efforts in order to establish the validity of most proposed methods.

CONCLUSIONS

The status of alternative toxicity tests for acute ocular and dermal irritation is rapidly changing. New tests are being introduced and old tests are being more fully evaluated. Many tests are currently utilized by industry to assist in internal decision making, but acceptance of alternative tests as adjuncts in the regulatory process has not occurred. Barriers to regulatory acceptance are mainly related to an imprecise definition of validation as well as the lack of an administrative mechanism at the governmental level to make decisions concerning the acceptability of alternative tests for toxicological evaluations.

Major research and development efforts are needed in several areas:

1. Basic research is needed into the mechanisms of ocular and dermal toxicity of chemicals to identify specific mechanisms by which damage to tissues occurs.
2. New tests should be developed that can evaluate specific mechanisms of ocular and dermal toxicity identified by basic research efforts.
3. A universally accepted definition of the validation process should be agreed on and an administrative framework to conduct validation studies established.
4. Technical personnel to conduct alternative toxicity test procedures are required and training programs to provide these personnel established.
5. Application of new technological developments to the automation of testing methods should be encouraged.

Given adequate research and development efforts, batteries of alternative tests that can serve as replacements for *in vivo* ocular and dermal tests can be defined and specific research needs to validate these batteries can be implemented. Over the next decade, the practicality of the alternative approach to acute ocular and dermal irritation testing will, in all likelihood, be resolved.

REFERENCES

Aeschbacher, M., Reinhardt, C. A. and Zbinden, G. 1986. A rapid cell membrane permeability test using fluorescent dyes and flow cytometry. *Cell Biol. Toxicol.* 2:247–255.

Babich, H., Martin-Alguacil, N. and Borenfreund, E. 1989. Comparisons of the cytotoxicities of dermatoxicants to human keratinocytes and fibroblasts in vitro. In *In Vitro Toxicology: New Directions—Alternative Methods in Toxicology,* vol. 7, ed. A. M. Goldberg, pp. 153–168. New York: Mary Ann Liebert.

Balls, M. and Horner, S. A. 1985. The FRAME interlaboratory programs on in vitro cytotoxicity. *Food Chem. Toxicol.* 23:209–213.

Balls, M., Blaauboer, B., Brusick, O., Frazier, J., Lamb, D., Pemberton, M., Reinhardt, C., Roberfroid, M., Rosenkranz, H., Schmid, B., Spielmann, H., Stammati, A.-L. and Walum, E. 1990. Report and recommendations of the CAAT/ERGATT workshop on the validation of toxicity tests procedures. *ATLA* 18:313–337.

Bell, E., Parenteau, N. L., Haimes, H. B., Gay, R. J., Kemp, P. D., Fofonoff, T. W., Mason, V. S., Kagan, D. T. and Swiderek, M. 1988. Testskin: A hybrid organism covered by a living human skin equivalent designed for toxicity and other testing. In *Progress in In Vitro Toxicology—Alternative Methods in Toxicology,* vol. 6, ed. A. M. Goldberg, pp. 15–25. New York: Mary Ann Liebert.

Booman, K. A., Cascieri, T. M., Demetulias, J., Driedger, A., Griffith, J. F., Grochoski, G. T., Kong, B., McCormick, W. C. III, North-Root, H., Rozen, M. G. and Sedlak, R. I. 1988. In vitro methods for estimating eye irritancy of cleaning products phase I: Preliminary assessment. *J. Toxicol. Cut. Ocular Toxicol.* 7(3):173–185.

Booman, K. A., De Prospo, J., Demetrulias, J., Driedger, A., Griffith, J. F., Grochoski, G., Kong, B., McCormick, W. C. III, North-Root, H., Rozen, M. G. and Sedlak, R. I. 1989. The SDA alternatives program: Comparison of in vitro data with Draize test data. *J. Toxicol. Cut. Ocular Toxicol.* 8(1):35–49.

Borenfreund, E. and Puerner, J. A. 1984. A simple quantitative procedure using monolayer cultures for cytotoxicity assays (HTD/NR-90). *J. Tissue Culture Methods* 9:7–9.

Borenfreund, E. and Puerner, J. A. 1985. Toxicity determined in vitro by morphological alterations and neutral red absorption. *Toxicol. Lett.* 24:119–124.

Borenfreund, E. and Puerner, J. A. 1987. Short-term quantitative in vitro cytotoxicity assay involving an S-9 activating system. *Cancer Lett.* 34:243–248.

Borenfreund, E. and Shopsis, C. 1985. Toxicity monitored with a correlated set of cell-culture assays. *Xenobiotica* 15:704–711.

Brooks, D. and Maurice, D. 1987. A simple fluorometer for use with a permeability screen. In *In Vitro Toxicology—Approaches to Validation. Alternative Methods in Toxicology,* vol. 5, ed. A. M. Goldberg, pp. 173–177. New York: Mary Ann Liebert.

Bruner, L. H. and Parker, R. D. 1989. Evaluation of the EYTEX system as a screen for predicting the ocular irritancy potential of consumer products. *Abstr. 2nd Int. Conf. Practical in Vitro Toxicology* 8.

Burton, A. B. G., York, M. and Lawrence, R. S. 1981. The in vitro assessment of severe eye irritants. *Food Chem. Toxicol.* 19:471–480.

Center for Animals and Public Policy. 1989. Testskin: An analysis. *Alternatives Rep.* 1:1–5.

Chan, K. Y. 1985. An in vitro alternative to the Draize test. In *In Vitro Toxicology. Alternative Methods in Toxicology,* vol. 3, ed. A. M. Goldberg, pp. 407–422. New York: Mary Ann Liebert.

Chan, K. Y. 1986a. Chemical injury to an in vitro ocular system: Differential release of plasminogen activator. *Clin. Eye Res.* 5:357–365.

Chan, K. Y. 1986b. Release of plasminogen activator by cultured corneal epithelial cells during differentiation and wound closure. *Exp. Eye Res.* 42:417–422.

Chasin, M., Scott, C., Shaw, C. and Persico, F. 1979. A new assay for the measurement of mediator release from rat peritoneal mast cells. *Int. Arch. Allergy Appl. Immunol.* 48:1–10.

Clonetics. 1989. Multiple applications of the neutral red bioassay. *Cellular Commun.* 1–3.

Cosmetics, Toiletry and Fragrance Association, 1980. *Proc. CTFA Ocular Safety Testing Workshop: In Vivo and In Vitro Approaches.*

DeLeo, V. A., Harber, L. C., Kong, B. M. and DeSalva, S. J. 1987. Surfactant-induced alteration of arachidonic acid metabolism of mammalian cells in culture. *Proc. Soc. Exp. Biol. Med.* 184:477–482.

Douglas, H. J. and Spillman, S. D. 1990. In vitro ocular irritancy testing. In *Product Safety Evaluation. Alternative Methods in Toxicology,* ed. A. M. Goldberg, pp. 205–230. New York: Mary Ann Liebert.

Draize, J. H., Woodward, G. and Calvery, H. O. 1944. Methods for the study of irritation and toxicity of substances applied topically to the skin and mucus membranes. *J. Pharmacol. Exp. Ther.* 82:377–390.

Dubin, N. H., Wolff, M. C., Thomas, C. L. and DiBlasi, M. C. 1985. Prostaglandin production by rat vaginal tissue, in vitro response to ethanol, a mild mucosal irritant. *Toxicol. Appl. Pharmacol.* 78:458–463.

Duffy, P. A., Flint, O. P., Onton, T. C. and Fursey, M. J. 1986. Initial validation of an in vitro test for predicting skin irritancy. *Food Chem. Toxicol.* 24:517–518.

Elgebaly, S. A., Downes, R. T., Foronhar, F., O'Rourke, J. and Kreutzer, D. L. 1987a. Inflammatory mediators in alkali-burned corneas: Inhibitory effects of citric acid. *Current Eye Res.* 6:1263–1274.

Elgebaly, S. A., Herkert, N., O'Rourke, J. and Kreutzer, D. L. 1987b. Characterization of neutrophil and monocyte specific chemotactic factors derived from the cornea in response to hydrogen peroxide injury. *Am. J. Pathol.* 126:22–32.

Enslein, K. 1984. Estimation of toxicology enpoints by structure-activity relationships. *Pharmacol. Rev.* 36:131–134.

Enslein, K. and Craig, P. N. 1982. Carcinogenesis: A predictive structure-activity model. *J. Toxicol. Environ. Health* 10:521–530.

Enslein, K., Tomb, M. E. and Lander, W. G. 1983. Mutagenicity (Ames): A structure-activity model. *J. Teratogen. Carcinogen. Mutagen.* 3:503–514.

Enslein, K., Tomb, M. E. and Lander, T. R. 1984. Structure-activity models of biological oxygen demand. In *QSAR in Environmental Toxicology,* ed. K. L. E. Kaiser. Dordrecht: D. Reidel.

Enslein, K., Borgstedt, H. H., Blake, B. W. and Hart, J. B. 1987. Prediction of rabbit skin irritation severity by structure-activity relationships. *In Vitro Toxicol.* 1:129–147.

Frazier, J. M. 1990. Scientific criteria for validation of in vitro toxicity tests. *Environment Monograph* 36:62. Paris: Organization for Economic Co-Operation and Development.

Frazier, J. M., God, S. C., Goldberg, A. M. and McCulley, J. P. 1987. A critical evaluation of alternatives to acute ocular irritation testing. In *Alternative Methods in Toxicology,* Vol. 4, ed. A. M. Goldberg. New York: Mary Ann Liebert.

Gabriels, J. E., Van Buskirk, R. G. and MacDonald, C. 1989. A fluorescent in vitro toxicity assay which monitors acute plasma membrane damage of epithelial cells. *Abstr. 2nd Int. Conf. Practical In Vitro Toxicology* 15.

Gordon, V. C. and Bergmen, H. C. 1986. EYTEX, an in vitro method for evaluation of optical irritancy. National Testing Corporation Report.

Gordon, V. C., Kelly, C. P. and Bergman, H. C. 1989. SKINTEX, an in vitro method for determining dermal irritation. *Abstr. V. Int. Congress Toxicology* 123.

Jacaruso, R. B., Barlett, M. A., Carson, S. and Trombetta, L. D. 1985. Release of histamine from rat peritoneal cells in vitro as an index of irritation potential. *J. Toxicol. Cut. Ocular Toxicol.* 4:39–48.

Jackson, E. M., Hume, R. D. and Wallin, R. F. 1988. The agarose diffusion method for ocular irritancy screening: Cosmetic products, part II. *J. Toxicol. Cut. Ocular Toxicol.* 7(3):187–194.

Jumblatt, M. M. and Neufeld, A. H. 1985. A tissue culture model of the human corneal epithelium. In *In Vitro Toxicology. Alternative Methods in Toxicology,* ed. A. M. Goldberg, pp. 393–404. New York: Mary Ann Liebert.

Jumblatt, M. M. and Neufeld, A. H. 1986. A tissue culture assay of corneal epithelial wound closure. *Invest. Opthalmol. Vis. Sci.* 27:1986.

Kato, S., Itagaki, H., Chiyoda, I., Hagino, S., Kobayashi, T. and Fujiyama, Y. 1988. Liposomes as an in vitro model for predicting the eye irritancy of chemicals. *Toxicol. In Vitro* 6:125–130.

Kemp, R. B., Meredith, R. W. J., Gamble, S. and Frost, M. 1983. A rapid cell culture technique for assaying the toxicity of detergent based products in vitro as a possible screen for eye irritancy in vivo. *Cytobiology* 36:153–159.

Kercso, K. M., Muir, V. C., Owicki, J. E. and Parce, J. W. 1989. Rapid in vitro toxicology with a silicon based biosensor. *Toxicologist* 9:259.

Knox, P., Uphill, P. F., Fry, J. R., Benford, D. J. and Balls, M. 1986. The FRAME multicenter project on in vitro cytotoxicity. *Food Chem. Toxicol.* 24:457–464.

Koeter, H. B. W. M. and Prinsen, M. K. 1985. Introduction of an in vitro eye irritation test as a possible contribution to the reduction of the number of animals in toxicity teting. CIVO Institutes TNO Report No. V 85.188/140322.

Kong, B. M., Viau, C. J., Rizvi, P. Y. and DeSalva, S. J. 1987. The development and evaluation of the chorioallantoic membrane (CAM) assay. In *In Vitro Toxicology—Approaches to Validation. Alternative Methods in Toxicology,* vol. 5, ed. A. M. Goldberg, pp. 59–73. New York: Mary Ann Liebert.

Lamont, G. S., Bagley, D. M., Kong, B. M. and De Salva, S. J. 1989. Developing an alternative to the Draize skin test: Comparison of human skin cell responses to irritants in vitro. In *In Vitro Toxicology: New Directions—Alternative Methods in Toxicology,* vol. 7, ed. A. M. Goldberg, New York: Mary Ann Liebert.

Lawrence, R. S., Groom, M. H., Ackroyd, D. M. and Parish, W. E. 1986. The chorioallantoic membrane in irritation testing. *Food Chem. Toxicol.* 24:497–502.

Leighton, J., Nassauer, J., Tchao, R. and Verdone, J. 1983. Development of a procedure using the chick egg as an alternative to the Draize rabbit test. In *Product Safety Evaluation. Alternative Methods in Toxicology,* vol. 1, ed. A. M. Goldberg, pp. 165–177. New York: Mary Ann Liebert.

Leighton, J., Nassauer, J. and Tchao, R. 1985a. The chick embryo in toxicology: An alternative to the rabbit eye. *Food Chem. Toxicol.* 23:291–298.

Leighton, J., Tchao, R., Verdone, J. and Nassauer, J. 1985b. Microscopic assay of focal injury in the chorioallantoic membrane. In *In Vitro Toxicology. Alternative Methods in Toxicology,* vol. 3, ed. A. M. Goldberg, pp. 357–3703. New York: Mary Ann Liebert.

Leupke, N. P. 1985a. Hen's egg chorioallantoic membrane test for irritation potential. *Food Chem. Toxicol.* 23:287–291.

Leupke, N. P. 1985b. HET— Chorioallantoic test: An alternative to the Draize rabbit eye test. In *In Vitro Toxicology. Alternative Methods In Toxicology,* vol. 3, ed. A. M. Goldberg, pp. 591–606. New York: Mary Ann Liebert.

McCormick, J. F., Nassauer, J., Bielunas, J. and Leighton, J. 1984. Anatomy of the chick chorioallantoic membrane relevant to its use as a substrate. In *Bioassay Systems. Scanning Electron Microscopy,* pp. 2023–2030. Chicago: SEM.

Mol, M. A. E., Von Genderen, J. and Wolthus, O. L. 1986. Cultured human epidermal cells as tool in skin toxicology. *Food Chem. Toxicol.* 24:519–520.

More, K. G., Schofield, B. H., Higuchi, K., Kajiki, A., Au, K-W, Pula, P. J., Bassett, D. P. and Dannenberg, A. M., Jr. 1986. Two sensitive in vitro monitors of chemical toxicity to human and animal skin (in short-term organ culture): I. Para-nuclear vacuolization, in glycol methacrylate tissue sections, II. Interference with ^{14}C-leucine incorporation. *J. Toxicol. Cut. Ocular Toxicol.* 5:285–302.

Muir, C. K. 1984. A single method to assess surfactant-induced bovine corneal opacity in vitro. Preliminary findings. *Toxicol. Lett.* 22:199–203.

Muir, C. K. 1985. Opacity of bovine cornea in vitro induced by surfactants and industrial chemicals compared with ocular irritancy in vivo. *Toxicol. Lett.* 24:157–162.

Muir, C. K., Flower, C. and Van Abbe, N. J. 1983. A novel approach to the search for in vitro alternatives to in vivo eye irritancy testing. *Toxicol. Lett.* 18:1–5.

Muir, C. K., Flower, C. and Van Abbe, N. J. 1986. The effect of shampoos on rabbit ileum in vitro compared to eye irritancy in vivo. *J. Am. College Toxicol.* 5:2–113.

Naughton, G. K., Jacop, L. and Naughton, B. A. 1989. A physiological skin model for in vitro toxicity studies. In *In Vitro Toxicology: New Directions—Alternative Methods in Toxicology,* vol. 7, ed. A. M. Goldberg, pp. 183–189. New York: Mary Ann Liebert.

North-Root, H., Yakcovich, F., Demetrulias, J., Gacula, N. and Heinze, J. E. 1982. Evaluation of an in vitro cell toxicity test using rabbit corneal cells to predict the eye irritancy potential of surfactants. *Toxicol. Lett.* 14:207–212.

North-Root, H., Yackovich, F., Demetrulias, J., Gacula, N. and Heinze, J. E. 1985. Prediction of the eye irritation potential of shampoos using the in vitro SIRC toxicity test. *Food Chem. Toxicol.* 23:271–273.

Oliver, G. J. A. and Pemberton, M. A. 1985. An in vitro epidermal slice technique for identifying chemicals with potential for severe cutaneous effects. *Food Chem. Toxicol.* 23:229–232.

Price, J. B. and Andrews, I. J. 1985. The in vitro assessment of eye irritation using isolated eyes. *Food Chem. Toxicol.* 23:313–480.

Price, J. B., Barry, M. P. and Andrews, I. J. 1986. The use of chick chorioallantoic membrane to predict eye irritants. *Food Chem. Toxicol.* 24:503–506.

Reinhardt, C. A., Pelli, D. A. and Zbinden, G. 1985. Interpretation of cell toxicity data for the estimation of potential irritation. *Food Chem. Toxicol.* 23:247–252.

Scaife, M. C. 1982. An investigation of detergent action on cells in vitro and possible correlations with in vivo data. *Int. J. Cosmet. Sci.* 4:179–193.

Selling, J. and Ekwall, B. 1985. Screening for eye irritancy using cultured HeLa cells. *Xenobiotica* 15:713–717.

Shadduck, J. A., Everitt, J. and Bay, P. 1985. Use of in vitro cytotoxicity to rank ocular irritation of six surfactants. In *In Vitro Toxicology. Alternative Methods in Toxicology,* vol. 3, ed. A. M. Goldberg, pp. 643–649. New York: Mary Ann Liebert.

Shadduck, J. P., Render, J., Everitt, J., Meccoli, R. A. and Essex-Sorlie, D. 1987. An approach to validation. In *In Vitro Toxicology—Approaches to Validation. Alternative Methods in Toxicology,* vol. 5, ed. A. M. Goldberg, pp. 75–78. New York: Mary Ann Liebert.

Shopsis, C. 1984. Inhibition of uridine uptake and cultured cells: A rapid, sublethal cytotoxicity test. *J. Tissue Culture Methods* 9:19–22.

Shopsis, C. and Eng, B. 1985. Rapid cytotoxicity using a semi-automated protein determination on cultured cells. *Toxicol. Lett.* 26:1–8.

Shopsis, C. and Sathe, S. 1984. Uridine uptake inhibition as a cytotoxicity test: Correlation with the Draize test. *Toxicology* 29:195–206.

Shopsis, C., Borenfreund, E., Walburg, J. and Stark, D. M. 1985. A battery of potential alternatives to the Draize test: Uridine uptake inhibition, morphological cytotoxicity, macrophage cytotoxicity, macrophage chemotaxis and exfoliative cytology. *Food Chem. Toxicol.* 23:259–266.

Silverman, J. 1983. Preliminary findings on the use of protozoa (*Tetrahymena ther-*

mophila) as models for ocular irritation testing in rabbits. *Lab. Anim. Sci.* 33:56–59.

Soto, R. J., Servi, M. J. and Gordon, V. C. 1989. Evaluation of an alternative method for ocular irritation. In *In Vitro Toxicology: New Directions—Alternative Methods In Toxicology*, vo. 7, ed. A. M. Goldberg, pp. 289–296. New York: Mary Ann Liebert.

Stark, D. M., Shopsis, C., Borenfreund, E. and Babich, H. 1986. Progress and problems in evaluating and validating alternative assays in toxicology. *Food Chem. Toxicol.* 24:449–455.

Tchao, R. 1988. Trans-epithelial permeability of fluorescein in vitro as an assay to determine eye irritants. In *Progress in In Vitro Toxicology: Alternative Methods in Toxicology*, vol. 6, ed. A. M. Goldberg, pp. 271–283. New York: Mary Ann Liebert.

Thomson, M. A., Hearn, L. A., Smith, K. T., Teal, J. J. and Dickens, M. S. 1989. Evaluation of the Neutral Red cytotoxicity assay as a predictive test for ocular irritancy potential of cosmetic products. In *In Vitro Toxicology: New Directions—Alternative Methods in Toxicology*, vol. 7, ed. A. M. Goldberg, pp. 297–305. New York: Mary Ann Liebert.

Triglia, D., Wegener, P. T., Harbell, J., Wallace, K., Matheson, D. and Shopsis, C. 1989. Interlaboratory validation study of the keratinocyte neutral red bioassay from clonetics corporation. In *In Vitro Toxicology: New Directions—Alternative Methods in Toxicology*, vol. 7, ed. A. M. Goldberg, pp. 357–365. New York: Mary Ann Liebert.

U. S. Environmental Protection Agency. 1981. Eye irritation testing: An assessment of methods and guidelines for testing materials for eye irritancy: EPA-50/11-82-001.

Wallin, R. F., Hume, R. D. and Jackson, E. M. 1987. the agarose diffusion method for ocular irritancy screening: Cosmetic products. Part I. *J. Toxicol. Cut. Ocular Toxicol.* 6(4):239–250.

York, M., Lawerence, R. S. and Gibson, G. B. 1982. An in vitro test for the assessment of eye irritancy in consumer products—Preliminary findings. *Int. J. Cosmet. Sci.* 4:223–234.

33

cosmetics: substantiating safety

■ **Edward M. Jackson** ■

INTRODUCTION

The cosmetics industry is a multi-billion-dollar industry providing consumers with decorative cosmetics, hair care products, oral hygiene products, moisturizers, and soaps (Layman, 1988; Anonymous, 1990). These products are marketed in three ways: mass market outlets, department stores and door-to-door sales.

There are numerous ways to define and describe cosmetics. The Food, Drug and Cosmetic Act, which the Food and Drug Administration (FDA) administers, defines cosmetics in the following manner [CFR 21§201(i) paragraph 40, 1986]:

> The term "cosmetic" means [1] articles intended to be rubbed, poured, sprinkled, or sprayed on, introduced into, or otherwise applied to the human body or any part thereof for cleansing, beautifying, promoting attractiveness, or altering the appearance, and [2] articles intended for use as a component of any such articles; except the term shall not include soap.

There are two important aspects of this legal definition of cosmetics the reader should keep in mind. First, in the United States cosmetics do not contain active drug entities of any type nor can they be promoted as altering any physiological state either in disease or health. As the cosmetics industry resolves into a few multinational conglomerates in the 1990s, the tension associated with this aspect of the legal definition in the United States will increase. Other countries do not recognize this legal distinction. For example, Japan has classified consumer products into cosmetics, quasi-drugs, and drugs, versus the U.S. classification of cosmetics, OTC (over-the-counter) drugs, and prescription drugs. A product type exemplifying this legal difference is antiperspirants. By the U.S. definition, antiperspirants are OTC drug products regulated by the FDA through the OTC drug monograph system. In Japan, antiperspirants are quasidrugs, or cosmetics that perform a function. This example demonstrates how a product that contains an active ingredient that alters a bodily function can be regulated differently in a world-wide market. To add to this confusion, deodorants are cosmetics in both systems. Interestingly, the consumer is rarely knowledgeable of such legal distinctions.

The second aspect of the U.S. definition of cosmetics is the so-called soap exemption. Soap in the classic sense, as made from natural ingredients, is the type of soap that is exempted in the above definition. However, if the soap product is made of detergent chemicals (synthetic surfactants), the product is regulated by the Consumer Product Safety Commission under the Federal Hazardous Substances Act, as a household product. If the soap contains an antibacterial ingredient, the product is regulated as an OTC drug. If the soap contains a therapeutic ingredient for a medical condition, it is regulated as a prescription drug.

The classifying of cosmetics is equally complex. The FDA uses a product list approach as detailed in Table 1.

The cosmetics industry itself divides the products into more general categories oriented to their purpose as exemplified in the first paragraph of this chapter.

Formulators use a pharmaceutical formulation classification. Liquid make-ups are pigmented emulsions, while moisturizers are nonpigmented emulsions (the white color is technically a color, but is not referred to as such in this classification system). These emulsion type formulas can be either oil-in-water types, which predominate, or water-in-oil types, which are becoming more numerous in the marketplace. Many mascaras are suspensions. Fine fragrances and toners are solutions, either aqueous or hydroalcoholic solutions. Pressed powder products or loose powder products are physical mixtures, as are lipsticks. Products delivered as sprays are, of course, compressed gases (Jackson, 1990).

THE CONSUMER'S PERSPECTIVE OF COSMETIC SAFETY

Consumers expect cosmetics to be safe. This elementary fact is perhaps more true of cosmetic products than any other type of consumer product because of the physical and psychological benefits from cosmetic products.

The psychological benefits of cosmetics have been researched and described not only by the cosmetics industry itself (Project Associates, Inc. 1978) but by independent researchers (Graham and Kligman, 1985).

A more dramatic demonstration of these benefits is the immediate and

TABLE 1 Food and Drug Administration Classification of Cosmetics

1. Bath product
2. Eyebrow pencil
3. Eyeliner
4. Eye shadow
5. Eye makeup remover
6. Mascara
7. Cologne and toilet water
8. Perfume
9. Dusting and talcum powder
10. Hair conditioner
11. Hair spray
12. Permanent wave
13. Shampoo
14. Hair dye, tint, rinse, bleach
15. Blusher and rouge
16. Face powder
17. Liquid makeup (foundation)
18. Lipstick
19. Nail polish and enamel
20. Base coat and undercoat
21. Cuticle softener
22. Dentifrice
23. Mouthwash
24. Bath soap
25. Deodorant
26. Douche
27. Shaving preparation
28. Preshave and aftershave preparation
29. Cleansing creams and cold creams
30. Depilatory
31. Foot powder and spray
32. Moisturizing creams and lotions
33. Mask

[a]*Note.* Adapted from FDA Form 2706, Summary Report of Cosmetic Product Experience by Product Categories.

overwhelming acceptance of a new cosmetics industry program for cancer patients undergoing specific treatments such as chemotherapy called "Look Good . . . Feel Better." This industry-funded and industry-sponsored program combines appropriate products, educational materials, and qualified expert help in resolving serious cosmetic problems such as skin tone changes and hair loss (Cosmetic, Toiletry and Fragrance Association, 1988).

Physically, no other class of consumer product is applied in such quantities, at such high frequencies, over such continuing time frames as cosmetics. This translates toxicologically into the classic parameters of dose over time. The fact that the actual number of reactions per million product units sold is so very low is a function of the inherent safety of cosmetic products.

THE DERMATOLOGIST'S PERSPECTIVE ON COSMETIC SAFETY

There are two factors that provide insight into the dermatologist's perspective on cosmetic product safety. First, the dermatologist is a physician, and therefore trained in the diagnosis of a medical problem. This factor in and of itself means that the mindset of the practicing dermatologist must be to identify the offending agent, which often is a cosmetic ingredient or product. The patient may either have had a reaction to a cosmetic ingredient or product or have a medical condition or skin type that has been aggravated by a cosmetic ingredient or product.

Second, the dermatologist sees patients with problems caused by cosmetic ingredients or products and inherently builds a catalogue of offending ingredients and product types, which may be helpful in diagnosing a subsequent patient problem.

Recognizing the need for basic information on cosmetic product safety, the American Academy of Dermatology (AAD) has taken several educational steps to alleviate this. The AAD has established a symposium on cosmetics at its annual meetings in December of each year. These symposia have contributed not only to a basic understanding of cosmetic ingredients and products, but also indirectly to a better working relationship between the practicing dermatologist and the cosmetics industry scientists. The AAD is also providing information to the dermatology resident in the form of *A Primer on Cosmetics for Dermatology Residents* (American Academy of Dermatology, 1991). This primer is the result of both dermatologists and industry scientists working together to provide the residents with information during their residency training.

Reactions to cosmetic ingredients or products include dermatitis (both irritant and allergic contact dermatitis), contact urticaria, hypopigmentation and hyperpigmentation effects, paronychia or onycholysis or nail discoloration, split or broken hair shafts and acneform eruptions.

The actual etiologic agents in cosmetic products has been researched by the North American Contact Dermatitis Group (Eiermann et al., 1982; Adams and Maibach, 1985). This 5-yr study identified skin care products, hair preparations, including colors, and facial makeup as the cosmetic products most likely to cause dermatological problems. Fragrances, preservatives, *para*-phenylenediamine, and glyceryl monothioglycolate were the most frequently identified allergic sensitizers.

The AAD has also provided dermatologists' offices with a pamphlet for patient information on the subject of reactions to cosmetics (American Academy of Dermatology, 1987).

Acneform eruptions from using cosmetic products has long been an area of concern for both dermatologists and their patients. In 1988, the AAD held a consensus conference on comedogenicity that included both dermatology researchers and clinicians as well as cosmetics industry scientists (Strauss and Jackson, 1989). The conference concluded that the comedogenic potential of cosmetic products was somewhat exaggerated; in fact, the majority of cosmetic products currently in the marketplace can be considered noncomedogenic because of the cosmetic industry's safety testing practices and programs. Finally, the consensus conference coined the clinical designation "non-acnegenic" to identify products that have been demonstrated not to cause acneform eruptions under normal conditions of use.

To help the clinician in either identifying or eliminating cosmetics as the offending agent in a skin reaction, the cosmetics industry has provided the AAD with a directory of appropriate individuals in cosmetics companies to provide both information and patch test materials (Cosmetic, Toiletry and Fragrance Association, 1987). In addition, alleged adverse reactions can be discussed and help in diagnosing the problem can be provided by industry physicians and scientists (Jackson, 1986).

Often patients require help in camouflaging dermal defects. Many products are now available from the cosmetics manufacturers for this purpose, and some manufacturers will often provide both products and services free of charge.

In concluding this section on the dermatologist's perspective on cosmetic product safety, we would be remiss without briefly describing some of the more significant contributions in this area. Maibach and Engasser's chapter on cosmetic dermatitis in Fisher's classic book on contact dermatitis is simply required reading (Maibach and Engasser, 1986). A catalogue of cosmetic product effects is provided by Nater et al. (1985).

On the more positive side of the subject is Kligman and Leyden's work on the safety and efficacy of cosmetics (Kligman and Leyden, 1982), and Schoen and Lazar's (1990) recent revision of the AMA's book of skin and hair care.

OCCUPATIONAL DERMATITIS FROM COSMETICS

An often overlooked source of information about reactions or effects from cosmetic ingredients or products is the occupational parameter. We often forget that the manufacture of cosmetic ingredients by the chemical industry or major consumer product manufacturers, as well as the processing of cosmetic products themselves, exposes individuals to maximum concentrations of both ingredients and products. The practicing clinician and the industry toxicologist both can benefit from the information gained in the manufacturing setting. In the former case, this information can be helpful in diagnosing a patient reaction. In the latter, such information can help in the projection of the safety of the cosmetic ingredient or product.

Malten (1975) determined the theoretical impact of such information in 1973. He identified the types of reactions that can occur and the methods for determining the relationship between the reaction and the etiologic agent in the industrial manufacturing setting, which often is not the ingredient or product being manufactured.

Certain professions such as hairdressers often provide settings for occupational dermatitis. Stovall et al. (1983) have provided an excellent perspective on this particular occupation. Stovall correctly concludes that the etiology of dermatitis in hairdressers is both real and very complex, often made more complex by a confused view of what actually constitutes skin irritation, exogenous contact with other chemical agents, personal habits, and hygiene, not to mention the inherent potential for dermatitis based on previous exposure before becoming a hairdresser as well as genetic constitution.

Marks (1990) recently reviewed occupational dermatitis from cosmetic ingredients and products. He provides a comprehensive survey of cosmetic products and individual ingredients that have either the potential or have been demonstrated to be the causative agents in occupational dermatitis.

Once again, the above information is indirect evidence for the overall safety of cosmetic ingredients and products.

SUBSTANTIATING THE SAFETY OF COSMETIC PRODUCTS

In contrast to the dermatologist diagnosing a skin condition, the cosmetics industry toxicologist generates data on both cosmetic ingredients and products to determine their safety. This prognostic approach is not so much in marked contrast to the physician's diagnostic approach, but rather complimentary to it. Dermatologists and toxicologists realize they are better able to diagnose a skin condition or determine the potential safety of a cosmetic ingredient or product.

Substantiating the safety of cosmetic ingredients and products is required under the Food, Drug and Cosmetic Act, which the FDA administers. Unlike drugs and foods, however, specific toxicological tests, either preclinical or clinical, are not written into the law for cosmetics. This is actually a more comprehensive approach to the safety of cosmetic products because it permits the development of new test methodologies and encompasses the necessarily ever changing and developing understanding of the skin and its reactions to topical products such as cosmetics.

Safety testing of cosmetics begins with substantiating the safety of the ingredients themselves. The single most important program for reviewing both unpublished and published information about these ingredients is the cosmetics industry's Cosmetic Ingredient Review (CIR) program. A panel of independent physicians and scientists who have neither worked for nor consulted with companies in the cosmetics industry review this extensive data base prior to issuing two types of ingredient safety documents: a Cosmetic Ingredient Scientific Literature Review and a Cosmetic Ingredient Safety Analysis. The latter is actually a cosmetic ingredient safety monograph, which must provide a conclusion as to the safety or lack thereof of the ingredient under review. This program was founded by the cosmetics industry in 1976, and to date has produced safety monographs on cosmetic product ingredients that cover the vast majority of the formulations currently in the marketplace.

Once the safety of the individual ingredients has been established, the cosmetic product itself must be assessed for safety. This assessment begins with the safety assessment of the fragrance in the product, if any. Fragrances in cosmetic products really represent a product within a product. Fragrances in products are composites of between 50 and 300 natural and synthetic fragrance ingredients chosen from some 6000 natural and synthetic formulating ingredients (Johnson Publications, Ltd., 1984). If the cosmetic product is a soap, the number of ingredients typically range between 50 and 150, and if the cosmetic product is a fine fragrance, the range of ingredients can actually exceed 700. Flavors are more simple, ranging between 5 and 30 individual ingredients. The safety of these fragrance and flavor ingredients is supported through an ongoing safety evaluation by the fragrance industry's own expert panel of the Research Institute for Fragrance Materials (RIFM) and the technical and advisory committees of the International Fragrance Association (IFRA). In addition to their complexity, fragrances are confidential and proprietary in that they are formulated specifically for a cosmetic company's product by a fragrance manufacturer (Jackson, 1986).

Preservatives in cosmetic products are, of course, biologically active materials that have a large body of scientific literature describing reactions as well as patch test concentrations and vehicles.

Toxicologically, dermatitis translates to irritation and sensitization. Irritation, which is dose and time dependent, can be either subjective (stinging, burning, itching) or objective (erythema, edema, pain, and heat). Sensitization is dose and time independent. Photosensitization has unfortunately been accepted as an all-encompassing light-mediated reaction term that includes both phototoxicity (light-mediated irritation) and photoallergenicity (light-mediated sensitization).

Acneform eruptions include comedone formation (whiteheads or open comedones, and blackheads or closed comedones). These are noninflammatory lesions. Inflammatory lesions in acne include papules, pustules, and nodules.

All of these are the end points of the toxicological assessment of cosmetic products.

The target organs are primarily the skin, but secondarily the eye. The primary focus of this chapter is, then, the skin. The reader is directed elsewhere for a more complete treatment of the toxicity of cosmetic products and the eye (Jackson, 1984, 1987; Wortzman, 1987).

There are also sources for more detailed treatments of test methods to assess the toxicological endpoints already discussed (Cosmetic, Toiletry and Fragrance Association, 1981; Jackson, 1983). Here we will discuss the preclinical and clinical safety testing that has become routine in the cosmetics industry for new cosmetic products.

Preclinical testing or testing cosmetic products in animals is the first assessment of safety after a thorough review of the ingredients in the new cosmetic product, the fragrance formula, if the product is fragranced, and the formulation itself. This is true only if there is not enough information to support the initial testing of this new product in humans from this trio of reviews. The issue of using animals in safety testing has been a controversial one for the cosmetics industry for over a decade now. Research into alternatives to animal testing for the initial safety assessment of new cosmetic products, computerization of product safety data bases by individual companies, and the continuing work of the industry's Cosmetic Ingredient Review program have permitted many companies to move to human testing more quickly with an equivalent set of safety information that previously only animal testing yielded.

The clinical assessment of new cosmetic products includes patch testing and controlled use testing.

Patch testing as a prognostic tool often includes the short patch test or prophetic patch test (PPT), which dermatologists use diagnostically. There are several good references for the prophetic patch test, whether it is for prognostic or diagnostic purposes (Schwartz and Peck, 1944; Brunner and Smiljanic, 1952; Traub et al., 1954; North American Contact Dermatitis Group, 1982; American Academy of Dermatology, 1988).

The repeat insult patch test (RIPT) yields more detailed and complete information about the irritation or sensitization potential of a product. The RIPT can be modified for detecting photosensitization potential as well, although phototesting in small panels of individuals is another approach to producing this important safety information. Again, there are several references for the RIPT which the reader is referred to for more details (Shelanski and Shelanski, 1953; Draize, 1955; Shelanski, 1982; Lanman et al., 1968).

Many toxicologists conclude the clinical assessment of the safety of new cosmetic products with a controlled use test (Jackson and Robillard, 1982). The controlled use test usually lasts 4 wk, with daily product use as intended. This test yields valuable information about the subjective or objective irritation potential of a new cosmetic product.

Recently, a modification of the controlled use test has been proposed to assess the acnegenic (includes the comedogenic and inflammatory lesion potential of a product) potential of a new cosmetic product (Jackson, 1989).

Ancillary clinical information can be garnered from panelist testing of new cosmetic products during the product development cycle, as well as the numerous market research tests that are often a part of new product introductions.

The final phase of the safety assessment of new cosmetic products is through an industry–government (FDA) sponsored voluntary program for reporting alleged adverse reactions to cosmetic products. The Product Experience Reporting (PER) program is a vehicle for manufacturers to report on an annual basis the alleged adverse reactions to the FDA. There are two companion voluntary programs the cosmetics industry participates in: the Cosmetic Product

Ingredient Statement (CPIS) Program, which is a filing of cosmetic formulas with the FDA, and the Cosmetic Establishment Registration Program (CERP), which is a cosmetic plant registration program.

CONCLUSIONS

Substantiating the safety of cosmetic ingredients and cosmetic products has developed into a true prognostic science over the past decade. This tremendous growth in predicting cosmetic safety is mirrored in the marked increase in both clinical and scientific publications on both cosmetic ingredients and products.

A second change, perhaps even more important, over the past decade has been the breaking down of the walls of contention between the dermatology community and the cosmetics industry. New bonds of cooperation have been forged by a few key individuals on both sides initially, and now this type of relationship between the dermatology community and the cosmetics industry has become more the norm than the exception.

The result has been cosmetic products for the consumer that are more completely and thoroughly substantiated for their safety. As our knowledge of the skin has grown, new test methods have been developed to provide the safest cosmetic products to the consumer in history. This is the kind of benefit that results from cooperation rather than contention.

REFERENCES

Adams, R. M. and Maibach, H. I. 1985. A five-year study of cosmetic reactions. *J. Am. Acad. Dermatol.* 13:1062–1069.

American Academy of Dermatology. 1987. *Reactions to Cosmetics.* Evanston, Ill.: AAD.

American Academy of Dermatology. 1988. Diagnostic Patch Test Technique, CME video tape. Evanston, Ill.

American Academy of Dermatology. 1991. *A Primer on Cosmetics for Residents in Dermatology.* Evanston, Ill.: AAD.

Anonymous. 1990. Cosmetics shipments valued at $16.7 billion by commerce department. *Soap and Cosmet. Chem. Specialties* 66(2):36.

Brunner, M. J. and Smiljanic, B. 1952. Procedure for the evaluation of the skin sensitizing power of new materials. *Arch. Dermatol.* 66:703.

Code of Federal Regulations. 1986. 21§201(i) paragraph 40.

Cosmetic, Toiletry and Fragrance Association. 1981. Safety Testing Guidelines. Washington, D.C.

Cosmetic, Toiletry and Fragrance Association. 1987. *The Cosmetic Industry on Call,* (2nd ed.) Washington, D.C.: CTFA.

Cosmetic, Toiletry and Fragrance Association. 1988. "Look Good . . . Feel Better" video and booklet. Washington, D.C.: CTFA.

Draize, J. H. 1955. Dermal toxicity. *Food Drug and Cosmet. J. Law* 10:722.

Eiermann, H. J., Larsen, W. G., Maibach, H. I. and Taylor, J. S. 1982. Prospective study of cosmetic reactions: 1977–1980. *J. Am. Acad. Dermatol.* 6:909–917.

Graham, J. A. and Kligman, A. M. 1985. *The Psychology of Cosmetic Treatments.* New York: Praeger.

Jackson, E. M. 1983. Industrial safety testing practices. *Product Safety Evaluation,* ed. A. M. Goldberg, chap. 5. New York: Mary Ann Liebert.

Jackson, E. M. 1984. Ocular irritancy: The search for acceptable and humane test methods. *The Cosmetic Industry: Scientific and Regulatory Foundations,* ed. N. F. Estrin, chap. 28. New York: Marcel Dekker.

Jackson, E. M. 1986. Alleged adverse reactions: Cooperating with the dermatologist. *Cosmet. Toiletries* 101(2):33–38, 40.

Jackson, E. M. 1987. Eye irritation. In *Cosmetic Safety: A Primer for Cosmetic Scientists,* ed. J. H. Whittam, chap. 2. New York: Marcel Dekker.

Jackson, E. M. 1989. Clinical assessment of acnegenicity. *J. Toxicol. Cut. Ocular Toxicol.* 8(4):389.

Jackson, E. M. 1990a. Toxicological aspects of percutaneous absorption. *Cosmet. Toiletries* 105:135–147.

Jackson, E. M. 1990b. Irritation and sensitization. In *Clinical Safety and Efficacy Testing of Cosmetics,* ed. W. C. Waggoner, chap. 2. New York: Marcel Dekker.

Jackson, E. M. and Robillard, N. F. 1982. The controlled use test in a cosmetic safety substantiation program. *J. Toxicol. Cut. Ocular Toxicol.* 1(2):109.

Johnson Publications, Ltd. 1984. *The Haarman & Reimer Book of Perfumes,* vol. 1. London.

Kligman, A. M. and Leyden, J. J., eds. 1982. *Safety and Efficacy of Topical Drugs and Cosmetics.* New York: Grune & Stratton.

Lanman, B. M., Elvers, W. V. and Howard, C. S. 1968. The role of human patch testing in the product development program. *Proc. Joint Conf. Cosmet. Sci. Toilet Goods Assoc.* Washington, D.C.

Layman, P. L. 1988. Cosmetics. *Chem. Eng. News* April 4:21.

Maibach, H. I. and Engasser, P. G. 1986. Dermatitis due to cosmetics. In *Contact Dermatitis,* 3rd ed., ed. A. A. Fisher, chap. 21. Philadelphia: Lea & Febiger.

Malten, K. E. 1975. Cosmetics, the consumer, the factory worker and the occupational physician. *Contact Dermatitis* 1:16–26.

Marks, J. G. 1990. Cosmetics. In *Occupational Skin Disease,* 2nd ed., ed. R. M. Adams, pp. 326–348. Philadelphia: W. B. Saunders.

Nater, J. P., deGroot, A. C. and Liem, D. H., eds. 1985. *Unwanted Effects of Cosmetics and Drugs Used in Dermatology,* 2nd ed. Amsterdam: Elsevier.

North American Contact Dermatitis Group. 1982. *Patch Testing in Allergic Contact Dermatitis,* 6th ed. In conjunction with the American Academy of Dermatology. Evanston, Ill.: AAD.

Project Associates, Inc. 1978. The Cosmetic Benefit Study. For the Cosmetic, Toiletry and Fragrance Association (CTFA). Washington, D.C.

Schoen, L. A. and Lazar, P. 1990. *The Look You Like: Medical Answers to 400 Questions on Skin and Hair Care.* New York: Marcel Dekker.

Schwartz, L. and Peck, S. M. 1944. The patch test and contact dermatitis. *Public Health Rep.* 59:2.

Shelanski, M. V. 1982. The patch test: I, History and review of methods, capabilities and inherent limitations. *J. Toxicol. Cut. Ocular Toxicol.* 1(2):91.

Shelanski, H. A. and Shelanski, M. V. 1953. A new technique of human patch test. *Proc. Sci. Sect. Toilet Goods Assoc.* 19:46.

Stovall, G. K., Levin, L. and Osler, J. 1983. Occupational dermatitis among hairdressers: A multifactorial analysis. *J. Occup. Med.* 25(12):871–878.

Strauss, J. S. and Jackson, E. M. 1989. Consensus statement of the American Academy of Dermatology Invitational Symposium on Comedogenicity. *J. Am. Acad. Dermatol.* 20(2/1):272.

Traub, E. F., Tussing, T. W. and Spoor, H. J. 1954. Evaluating dermal sensitivity. *Arch. Dermatol.* 69:399.

Wortzman, M. S. 1987. Eye products. In *Cosmetic Safety: A Primer for Cosmetic Scientists,* ed. J. H. Whittam, chap. 7. New York: Marcel Dekker.

34

toxicity assessment
of dermal drugs

■ John M. Davitt ■

There are no specific methods of toxicity testing prescribed by statute or regulations for the approval of new drug products. What is required is adequate evidence that a candidate drug will be reasonably safe when used in accordance with a specific protocol for clinical investigation or as recommended in labeling once it is marketed.

Clearly, pharmaceuticals differ in some respects from the xenobiotics typically encountered in the environment, the diet, the workplace, or the home. Exposure to pharmaceuticals is deliberate; hence, dose and duration of exposure are relatively easy to control. Moreover, drugs other than the antiinfectives and antiparasitics are generally designed to have an effect on the structure and/ or function of the mammalian organism; accordingly, adverse effects may represent an extension of the desired pharmacologic activity.

The amount of risk considered acceptable for a specific drug is related to its potential therapeutic benefit. In assessing risk-to-benefit ratio, the benefit derived from a drug product is generally allotted far greater weight than that from a cosmetic. It should be understood, therefore, that included in the spectrum of topical products regulated as drugs in the United States are some with essentially only cosmetic utility, such as antiperspirants. Such products, like other cosmetics, are expected to be virtually risk free.

Generally, clinical investigation of a new drug proceeds along the lines of the phase 1, 2, and 3 scheme outlined in the new drug regulations (CFR 21, 1990), and the preclinical toxicological evaluation is similarly approached in a stepwise manner.

In most cases the rationale for trial of a candidate drug substance is based on a particular pharmacological activity it is known to possess. Preclinical investigations relating to this activity may yield preliminary information about the potential toxicity of a new drug entity. Toxicological information of a general nature is derived also from acute oral or parenteral toxicity studies at an early point in drug development.

New topical formations should be screened for primary dermal irritancy by the Draize method or a suitable modification thereof. Acute dermal toxicity studies (limit test) are also recommended; the routine procedure involves exposure of the animals to the test material for 24 h followed by an observation period of at least 2 wk.

Prior to entering phase 2 clinical trials or any clinical investigation involving multiple drug exposures, a drug should be tested for contact sensitization potential. The guinea pig is the preferred animal model; two widely used techniques, the Buehler test (Buehler, 1965) and the more sensitive Magnusson-Kligman maximization test (Magnusson and Kligman, 1969), are both currently acceptable. Normally, testing in guinea pigs precedes predictive tests of sensitization in humans (phase 1 clinical). In humans, the Draize-Shelanski 200-subject patch test (Shelanski and Shelanski) and the Kligman maximization test (Kligman, 1966) are two commonly employed methods.

Clinical studies involving repeated administration should be preceded by repeated dose toxicity studies in animals. While acute animal studies may support the dermal application of a single dose to humans in phase 1, repeated-dose animal studies are needed prior to phase 2 clinical trial. Studies in any phase of clinical investigation that involve repeated drug administration should not be initiated in the absence of adequate subchronic or chronic toxicity data. As a rule, the duration of animal studies considered necessary to provide these data equals or preferably exceeds the length of the projected clinical exposure.

Subacute dermal toxicity studies can be pivotal to a decision to proceed with short-term topical administration to humans. Formulated drug is applied daily to intact and abraded skin of the animals, usually rabbits, for 3–4 wk. In addition to assessment of local tolerance, these studies seek to identify systemic effects. Clinical chemistry and hematology parameters are monitored, and terminal examination includes complete gross necropsy and histopathology.

The duration of dermal toxicity studies needed to support phase 2 and/or 3 investigation depends to a large extent on the nature of the projected clinical trial. If it is to involve only one or two exposures to the drug in as many days, for example, additional more lengthy study may not be needed. Prediction of safety for long-term or unlimited clinical use, on the other hand, often requires animal toxicity studies of 3–6 mo duration. Commonly these studies involve daily application to the intact dorsal skin of rabbits. Alternative species are sometimes employed. For example, the rat has been used by some investigators in subchronic dermal toxicity studies of potent corticosteroids, since the rabbit's unusual vulnerability to typical corticosteroid effects has made some previous studies less than satisfactory.

It is useful to have, at a relatively early stage, quantitative data on percutaneous absorption of an active ingredient (or of a novel excipient in some cases). A study of target organ toxicity in a second (nonrodent) species may further elucidate the drug's toxicity profile and should be a requirement if significant systemic exposure is anticipated. (Significance depends on the substances absorbed as well as the degree of absorption.)

Percutaneous absorption also has to be taken into account in assessing the risk of treatment during pregnancy. Animal reproduction studies are routinely included in the toxicologic evaluation. Prior to treatment of women of childbearing potential, segment II (teratology) studies need to be completed. Segment I studies (fertility and general reproductive performance) are also desirable. Where topical application is not feasible, administration of the active ingredient by an alternate route should be considered.

Extrapolation from oral or parenteral studies in assessing the risks from dermal exposure requires careful consideration of differences in pharmacokinetics. Efficient absorption by the oral route is not always sufficient to recommend it, since first-pass metabolism is sometimes a complicating factor. The suitability of parenteral administration should be explored in such cases.

The possibility of carcinogenicity must always be considered. Animal studies should be carried out to explore carcinogenic potential if a new drug entity is suspect because of its pharmacological activity or its structural relationship to known carcinogens. The anticipated pattern of use must also be considered; even nonsuspect substances may be candidates for carcinogenicity bioassay if they are to be applied extensively over protracted periods. Likewise, some topical agents will require photocarcinogenicity assessment depending on suspicion of activity and/or pattern of use. Photocarcinogenicity testing methods employing hairless mice and a continuous-spectrum light source (solar simulator) are recommended (Forbes and Urbach, 1975).

Obviously, each and every drug product entering clinical trials does not require extensive preclinical testing in animals. A new drug entity formulated for topical application often needs rather thorough investigation. On the other hand, a new formulation of an established drug may require only a short-term irritancy test (and, if systemic toxicity is a concern, percutaneous absorption determination). Local tolerance is routinely evaluated clinically in 20-d cumulative irritancy tests, and of course, any evidence of local and/or systemic side effects encountered in phase 2 or 3 efficacy trials is considered in the final safety assessment.

REFERENCES

Buehler, E. V. 1965. Delayed contact hypersensitivity in the guinea pig. *Arch. Dermatol.* 91:171–175.
Code of Federal Regulations. 1990. Title 21, S 312.21.
Forbes, P. D. and Urbach, F. 1975. Experimental modification of photocarcinogenesis.

III. Simulation of exposure to sunlight and fluorescent whitening agents. *Fd. Cosmet. Toxicol.* 13:343–345.

Kligman, A. M. 1966. The identification of contact allergens by human assay. II The maximization test. A procedure for screening and rating contact sensitizers. *J. Invest. Dermatol.* 47:393–409.

Magnusson, B. and Kligman, A. M. 1969. The identification of contact allergens by animal assay. The guinea pig maximization test. *J. Invest. Dermatol.* 52:268–276.

Shelanski, H. A. and Shelanski, M. V. 1953. A new technique of human patch tests. *Proc. Sci. Sect. Toilet Goods Assoc.* 19:45–49.

35

systemic toxicity caused by absorption of drugs and chemicals through the skin

■ Susi Freeman ■ Howard I. Maibach ■

The skin forms an effective two-way barrier that controls the loss of chemicals from the body as well as the absorption of many foreign chemicals into the body. However, many chemicals do enter via the skin and some, when specifically applied to the skin, have been found to be sufficiently well absorbed to produce systemic toxicity.

FACTORS AFFECTING ABSORPTION

Many drugs for topical use on the skin and mucous membranes are capable of producing systemic side effects whose occurrence and severity depend largely on factors that affect the absorption of topically applied drugs. These are (1) the integrity of the barrier, (2) the physicochemical properties of the substance, (3) occlusion, (4) the vehicle containing the drug, (5) the site of application, (6) age, (7) temperature, and (8) metabolism.

The Integrity of the Barrier

The stratum corneum layer of the epidermis is the skin's main barrier to transepidermal absorption. Follicular orifices and sweat gland ducts may provide additional pathways for absorption. Anything that alters the structure or function of the stratum corneum will affect epidermal absorption. The integrity of this barrier, with resultant increase in percutaneous absorption, is reduced by

Reprinted from L. Haddad and J. Winchester, *Clinical Management of Poisoning and Drug Overdose*, 2nd ed. W. B. Saunders Co., Philadelphia, 1990.

any inflammatory process of the skin, such as any form of dermatitis or psoriasis. Similarly, removal of the stratum corneum by stripping or damage by alkalis, acids, etc. will increase percutaneous absorption.

The Physicochemical Properties of the Substance

Absorption decreases with increasing molecular size. It is affected by the relative water/lipid solubility of the drug and the relative solubility of the drug in its vehicle compared with its solubility in the stratum corneum.

Occlusion

The penetration of topical drugs may be increased by the use of an occlusive covering, by a factor of 10 or more. This is because of increased H_2O retention in the stratum corneum, increased blood flow, increased temperature, and increased surface area after prolonged occlusion (skin wrinkling).

The Vehicle Containing the Drug

The greater the affinity of a vehicle for the drug it contains, the less the percutaneous absorption of the drug.

Physical properties of vehicles, especially the degree of occlusion they produce, affect percutaneous absorption, as discussed under Occlusion above (e.g., greases).

Structural or chemical damage to the barrier layer can be caused by the vehicle used; vehicles such as dimethyl sulfoxide cause greatly increased percutaneous absorption.

In general, a higher concentration of the drug in its vehicle enhances penetration.

Site of Application

Regional differences in permeability of skin largely depend on the thickness of the intact stratum corneum. According to the findings of a study by Feldmann and Maibach (1967) the highest total absorption of hydrocortisone is that from the scrotum, followed (in decreasing order) by absorption from the forehead, scalp, back, forearms, palms, and plantar surfaces.

Age

The greatest toxicological response to topical administration has been seen in the infant. The preterm infant does not have intact barrier function and hence is more susceptible to systemic toxicity from topically applied drugs (Nachman and Esterly, 1971; Greaves et al. 1975).

A normal full-term infant probably has a fully developed stratum corneum with complete barrier function (Rasmussen, 1979). Yet according to Wester and Maibach (Wester et al., 1977a) topical application of the same amount of a compound to both adult and newborn results in a 2.7 times greater systemic availability in the newborn. This is because the ratio of surface area to body weight in the newborn is three times that in the adult. Therefore, given an equal area of application of a drug to skin of the newborn and adults, the proportion absorbed per kilogram of body weight is much more in the infant.

Temperature

Increased skin temperature usually enhances penetration.

Metabolism

Like the liver, the skin is capable of metabolizing drugs and foreign substances. It contains many of the enzyme systems of the liver, and its metabolizing potential has been estimated to be about 2% that of the liver (Pannatier et al., 1978).

SYSTEMIC SIDE EFFECTS CAUSED BY TOPICALLY APPLIED DRUGS AND COSMETICS

Topically applied drugs and cosmetics can cause allergic or irritant contact dermatitis. However, this type of side effect, usually limited to the skin, is outside the scope of the present article. The reader is referred to the textbooks of Cronin (1980b) and Fisher (1986) for references to contact dermatitis. Systemic side effects from topically applied chemicals can sometimes result from either a toxic (irritant) reaction or a hypersensitivity reaction. The latter can be an anaphylactic type of reaction, which is the extreme manifestation of the contact urticaria syndrome (Von Krogh and Maibach, 1987). Many topical drugs and cosmetics have reportedly caused anaphylactic reactions.

While anaphylactic reactions to topical medicaments are uncommon, their potentially serious nature warrants attention.

However, reports of toxic (as distinct from allergic) reactions to applied drugs and cosmetics are more numerous and include many medicaments that have been safely used for many years but that can be toxic under special circumstances.

TOPICALLY APPLIED DRUGS AND COSMETICS CAUSING SYSTEMIC SIDE EFFECTS

The following is a list in alphabetical order, followed by a detailed discussion of each chemical.

1. Antibiotics
   a. Chloromycetin
   b. Clindamycin
   c. Gentamycin
   d. Neomycin
2. Antihistamines

  a. Diphenyl pyraline hydrochloride
  b. Promethazine
 3. Antimicrobials
  a. Boric acid
  b. Castellani's paint
  c. Hexachlorophene
  d. Homosulfanilamide
  e. Iodine, povidone-iodine
  f. Phenol
  g. Resorcinol
  h. Silver sulfadiazine
  i. Trichlorocarbanilide
 4. Arsenic
 5. Carmustine
 6. Camphor
 7. Cosmetic agents
 8. Diethyltoluamide (DEET)
 9. Dimethyl sulfoxide (DMSO)
10. Dinitrochlorobenzene (DNCB)
11. Ethyl alcohol
12. Fumaric acid monoethyl ester
13. Local anesthetics
  a. Benzocaine
  b. Lidocaine
14. Mercurials
15. Monobenzone
16. 2-Naphthol
17. Insecticides
  a. Lindane
  b. Malathion
18. Podophyllum resin
19. Salicylic acid
20. Selenium sulfide
21. Silver nitrate
22. Steroids
  a. Corticosteroids
  b. Sex hormones
23. Tars
  a. Coal tar
  b. Dithranol

Antibiotics

Chloramphenicol. Oral administration of chloramphenicol may lead to aplastic anemia (Wilson and Mielke, 1983).

A case of marrow aplasia with a fatal outcome after topical application of chloramphenicol in eye ointment was described by Abrams et al. (1980). There have been three earlier reports of bone marrow aplasia after the use of chloramphenicol-containing eye drops.

Clindamycin. Topical clindamycin is widely used in the treatment of acne vulgaris. It is estimated that 4–5% clindamycin hydrochloride is absorbed systemically (Barza et al., 1982). The degree of absorption largely depends on the vehicle, ranging from 0.13% (acetone) to 13.92% (DMSO) (Franz, 1983). Several cases of topical clindamycin-associated diarrhea have been reported (Stoughton, 1979; Voron, 1978; Becker et al., 1981).

Pseudomembranous colitis is a well-recognized side effect of systemic administration of clindamycin. A case of pseudomembranous colitis has been reported after topical administration by Milstone et al. (1981). The authors conclude that all patients receiving topical clindamycin should be warned to discontinue therapy and consult their physician if intestinal symptoms occur.

Gentamycin. Ototoxicity is a well-known hazard of systemic gentamycin administration. However, topical application to large thermal injuries of the skin has similarly caused ototoxic effects, ranging from mild to severe hearing loss, with an associated decrease of vestibular function (Dayal et al., 1974). In the two patients described, serum levels of gentamycin measured were 1.0–3.0 and 3.3–4.3 μg/ml, respectively. Drake (1974) described a woman who developed tinnitus each time she treated her paronychia with gentamycin sulfate cream 0.1%. Use of gentamycin ear drops may also be associated with ototoxic reactions (Mittelman, 1972).

Neomycin. Just as ototoxicity is a well-known hazard of parenteral neomycin administration, so has deafness been reported after almost any form of local treatment, including treatment of skin infections and burns (Friedman, 1977; Anonymous, 1977; Bamford and Jones, 1978), application as an aerosol for inhalation, instillation into cavities (Masur et al., 1976), irrigation of large wounds (Kelly et al., 1969), and use of neomycin-containing eardrops (Goffinet, 1977). Kellerhals (1978) reported 13 cases of inner ear damage in which the use of eardrops containing neomycin and polymyxin was incriminated. All cases had perforated tympanic membranes, and the paper concludes that these drops (and also those containing chloromycetin, colistin, and polymyxin), should not be used in such cases for periods longer than 10 d.

Antihistamines

Diphenyl pyraline hydrochloride. Diphenyl pyraline hydrochloride has been used topically in Germany for the treatment of eczematous and other itching dermatoses. Symptomatic psychosis has been observed in 12 patients, 9 of whom were children. The amounts of the active drug applied ranged from 225 to 1350 mg. The first symptoms of intoxication were psychomotor restlessness in all cases, usually within 24 h. Other symptoms included disorientation, and optic and acoustic hallucinations. All symptoms disappeared 4 d after discontinuation of the topical medication. (Cammann et al., 1971).

Promethazine. Bloch and Beysovec (1982) reported a 16-mo-old male weighing 11.5 kg who was treated with 2% promethazine cream for generalized eczema. After approximately 15–20 g of the cream had been applied, the child fell asleep. He woke a few hours later with abnormal behavior, loss of balance, inability to focus, irritability, drowsiness, and failure to recognize his mother. One day later all symptoms had spontaneously disappeared. A diagnosis of promethazine toxicity through percutaneous absorption was made. Known symptoms of promethazine toxicity include disorientation, hallucinations, hyperactivity, convulsions, and coma.

Antimicrobials

Boric acid. The toxicity of this mildly bacteriostatic substance is dealt with elsewhere (Done, 1983). Undoubtedly the use of borates should be abandoned becuase of their limited therapeutic value and high toxicity. In recent times few cases of borate intoxication have been published, probably due to its disappearing use.

Castellani's solution. Castellani's solution (or paint) is an old medicament mainly used for the local treatment of fungal skin infections. It contains boric acid, 800 mg; magenta, 400 ml; phenol, 4g; resorcinol, 8g; acetone, 4 ml; alcohol, 8.5 ml; and water to 100 ml.

Lundell and Nordman (1973) reported a case in which 2 applications of Castellani's solution severely poisoned a 6-wk-old boy who became cyanotic with 41% methemoglobin. The authors state that this case demonstrates that the application of Castellani's to napkin eruptions and other areas where absorption is rapid may cause serious complications.

Another case report (Rogers et al., 1978) states that hours after the application of Castellani's paint to the entire body surface except the face of a 6-wk-old infant for severe seborrheic eczema, that child became drowsy and had shallow breathing. The authors state that phenol was detected in the urine of 4 out of 16 children treated with Castellani's paint.

Hexachlorophene. Hexachlorophene (Haddad, 1983b) has since 1961 been extensively used in hospital nurseries, mainly for reducing the incidence of staphylococcal infections among the newborn. In addition it has been an ingredient of many medical preparations, cosmetics, and other consumer goods.

Hexachlorophene readily penetrates damaged skin, and its absorption through intact skin has also been demonstrated (Tyrala et al., 1977; Curley et al., 1971; Alder et al, 1972).

In 1972 in France, as a result of the accidental addition of 6.3% hexachlorophene to batches of baby talcum powder, 204 babies fell ill and 36 died from respiratory arrest (Pine, 1972; Editorial, 1982). This report was followed by animal experiments with hexachlorophene confirming that the drug is neurotoxic.

Consequently in 1972 the U.S. Food and Drug Administration (FDA) banned use of hexachlorophene to prescription use only, or as a surgical scrub and hand wash for health care personnel. Hexachlorophene was excluded from cosmetics except as a preservative in levels not exceeding 0.1%.

Because of the high absorption through damaged skin and its proven neurotoxicity, hexachlorophene is contraindicated for the treatment of burns or application to otherwise damaged skin. Premature infants are also at risk. the safety of hexachlorophene for routine bathing of babies is still controversial. Plueckhahn et al. (1978) and Hopkins (1979) have reviewed the benefits and risks of hexachlorophene.

4-Homosulfanilamide (sulfamylon acetate). 4-Homosulfanilamide is a topical sulfonamide that was used for the treatment of large burns. It has now been largely replaced by silver sulfadiazine. Sulfamylon is a carbonic anhydrase inhibitor and caused hyperchloremic metabolic acidosis in patients with extensive burns treated with its topical application, caused by percutaneous absorptions of the drug (Otten and Plempel, 1975; Liebman et al., 1982). Reversible pulmonary complications (Albert et al., 1982) and methemoglobinuria (Ohlgisser et al., 1978) have also been reported.

Iodine and povidone-iodine. Povidone-iodine (Betadine) is a water-soluble complex that retains the broad-range microbiocidal activity of iodine without the undesirable effects of iodine tincture (Connell and Rousselo, 1964). However, toxicity still occurs from povidone iodine percutaneously absorbed, mainly when it is used on large areas of burnt skin or on neonates. This subject is comprehensively dealt with elsewhere (Mofenson et al., 1983b).

Phenol (carbolic acid). Phenol is no longer widely used as a skin antiseptic, but in dilutions of 0.5–2.0% it is sometimes prescribed as an antipruritic in topical medicaments and is used for phenol face peels.

It has been shown that as much as 25% of phenol is absorbed from 2 ml of a solution of 2.5 g phenol/l water applied to the skin of the forearm and left on for 60 min (Baranowski-Dutkiewicz, 1981). The toxic dose for adults has been estimated to be 8–15 g.

Phenol-induced ochronosis has been reported (Cullison et al., 1983) in patients who for many years treated leg ulcers with wet dressing containing phenol.

There have been several case reports of fatal reactions to percutaneously absorbed phenol. One was caused by accidental spillage of phenol (Johnstone, 1948), one due to treatment of burns with a phenol-containing preparation (Cronin and Brauer, 1949), and another due to the application of phenol to wounds (Deichmann, 1949). A 1-d-old child died after application of 2% phenol to the umbilicus (Von Hinkel and Kitzel, 1968).

Several cases of sudden death or intra- or postoperative complications have been reported after phenol face peels (Del Pizzo and Tonski, 1980).

Major cardiac arrhythmias were noted (Truppman and Ellerby, 1979) in 10 out of 43 patients during phenol face peels. However, this item is rather controversial, and some authors feel that when the procedure is done over more than 1 h, and when the dose applied is carefully monitored, phenol face peels are not risky (Tromovitch, 1982; Baker, 1979). Poisoning due to phenol ingestion is dealt with elsewhere (Haddad, 1983c).

Resorcinol. Resorcinol is used for its keratolytic properties in the treatment of acne vulgaris. It is also a constituent of the antifungal Castellani's solution. Formerly leg ulcers were treated with external applications of resorcinol–containing applications.

Resorcinol can penetrate human skin. It has an antithyroid activity similar to that of methyl thiouracil, although it is chemically unrelated to any of the known groups of antithyroid drugs. Consequently, several cases of myxoedema caused by percutaneous absorption of resorcinol, especially from ulcerated surfaces, have been described (Berthezene et al., 1973; Thomas and Gisburn, 1961).

Methemoglobinemia in children, caused by absorption of resorcinol applied to wounds, has been reported (Flandin et al., 1953, Murray, 1926). Cunningham (1956) reported a case in which an ointment containing 12.5% resorcinol applied to the napkin area of an infant produced cyanosis, hemolytic anemia, and hemoglobinemia. In the literature the author found seven cases of acute poisoning in babies as a consequence of topical resorcinol application, in some instances to limited areas; five fatalities were recorded.

A case of severe poisoning of a 6-wk-old infant due to two applications of Castellani's paint has been described (Lundell and Nordman, 1973).

Although the use of resorcinol in young children and for leg ulcers should be avoided, topical resorcinol, when used for acne vulgaris, appears to be safe (Yeung et al., 1983).

Silver sulfadiazine. Sulfadiazine silver cream is widely used for the topical treatment of burns. Intended primarily for the control of pseudomonas infections, this bactericidal agent acts on the cell membranes and cell walls of a variety of gram-positive and gram-negative bacteria, as well as on yeasts. Its relative freedom from appreciable side effects has contributed to its popularity.

Absorption of sulfonamide from burns to 17–46% body area treated with sulfadiazine silver showed 20–25% of the daily topical dose could be accounted for as conjugated sulfonamide. Unconjugated drug represented from 35 to 95% of the total output. Total plasma, sulfonamide concentration did not exceed 10 μg/ml (Gabrilove and Luria, 1978).

There has been one report of nephrotic syndrome following topical therapy (Owens et al., 1974). Several authors have reported leukopenia during treatment with silver sulfadiazine (Chan et al., 1976; Jarrett et al., 1978; Fraser and Beaulieu, 1979). Current evidence suggests a causal relationship of silver sulfadiazine with leukopenia, although the mechanism of this reaction is unknown. Examination of bone marrow aspirates show hyperplasia with no evidence of maturation arrest. The drug presumably affects the white blood cells peripherally (Fraser and Beaulieu, 1979). The sulfadiazine-induced leukopenia is at its nadir within 2–4 d of starting therapy. The leukocyte count returns to normal levels within 2–3 d and recovery is not affected by continuation of therapy. The erythrocyte count is not affected.

Triclocarban (trichlorocarbanilide, TCC). Triclocarban is a bacteriostatic agent used as an antimicrobial in toilet soap since 1956. The percutaneous absorption has been studied by Scharpf et al. (1975), who showed that after a simple shower employing a whole-body lather with approximately 6 g of soap containing 2% TCC, about 0.23% of the applied dose of TCC was recovered in feces after 6 d, and 0.16% of the dose in the urine after 2 d. At all sampling times, blood levels of radioactivity were below the detection limit of 10 ppb. There have been several reports (Ponte et al., 1974) of methemoglobinemia presumably induced by topical TCC in neonates.

Arsenic

The toxicity of ingested or inhaled arsenic is dealt with elsewhere (Robertson, 1983). Fowler's solution, long used orally in the treatment of psoriasis, contained arsenic. Arsenical keratoses and malignancies are well recognized long-term reactions to this.

Carmustine (BCNU)

Topical carmustine (BCNU) has been used for the treatment of mycosis fungoides, lymphomatoid papulosis, and parapsoriasis en plaques. Percutaneous absorption of BCNU has been demonstrated in man. Zackheim et al. (1983) treated 91 patients with mycosis fungoides and related disorders with topical BCNU. Mild to moderate reversible bone marrow depression occurred in three patients. Their data suggest that hematological toxicity arises primarily from the shorter intensive schedules; the prolonged use of up to 100 mg/wk appears to be safe. Although an occasional mild elevation in the blood urea nitrogen or serum glutamic oxaloacetic transaminases (SGOT) was noted in patients treated with courses exceeding 600 mg, no such changes were seen with lower doses. In the study of Zackheim et al. there were no apparent long-term harmful effects on the hematopoietic system or internal organs.

Camphor

Camphor is a pleasant-smelling cyclic ketone of the hydroaromatic terpene group. When rubbed on the skin, camphor is a rubefacient but, if not vigorously applied, produces a feeling of coolness. It is an ingredient of a large number of over-the-counter remedies (with a camphor content of 1/20%), taken especially for symptomatic relief of "chest congestion" and muscle aches, but its effectiveness is rather dubious.

Camphor is readily absorbed from all sites of administration, including topical application to the skin.

The compound is classified as a Class IV chemical, that is, a very toxic substance. Hundreds of cases of intoxications have been reported, usually after accidental ingestion in children (Skoglund et al., 1977; Gossweiler, 1982; Committee on Drugs, 1978; Kopelman, 1983).

Cosmetic Agents

The use of a henna dye is traditional in Islamic communities. The dye is used on nails, skin, and hair by married ladies, and traditionally it is also used by the major participants in marriage ceremonies, when the bridegroom and best man also apply henna to their hands.

Henna consists of the dried leaves of *Lawsonia alba* (family Lythraceae), a shrub cultivated in North Africa, India, and Sri Lanka. The coloring matter, lawsone, is a hydroxynapthoquinone and is associated with fats, resin, and henna-tannin in the leaf. Dyeing hair or skin with powdered henna is a somewhat lengthy procedure, and to speed up this process, Sudanese ladies mix a "black powder" with henna; this accelerates the fixing process of the dye merely to a matter of minutes. This black powder is *p*–phenylenediamine. The combination of henna and "black powder" is particularly toxic, and over 20 cases of such toxicity, some fatal, have been noted in Khartoum alone in a 2-y period. Initial symptoms are those of angioedema with massive edema of the face, lips, glottis, pharynx, neck, and bronchi. These occur within hours of the application of the dye mix to the skin. The symptoms may then progress on the second day to anuria and acute renal failure, with death occurring on the third day. Dialysis has helped some patients, but others have died from renal tubular necrosis (D'Arcy, 1982). Whether this toxicity is due to *p*-phenylenediamine per se (probably grossly impure) or whether its toxicity is potentiated in its combination with henna powder is unknown. Systemic administration of the "black powder" leads to similar symptoms, and several deaths due to ingestion with suicidal intent have been reported (El-Ansary et al., 1983; Cronin, 1980a).

Diethyltoluamide

This has been used as an insect repellent since 1957. Although diethyltoluamide has an overall low incidence of toxic effects, prolonged use in children has been discouraged because of reports of toxic encephalopathy (Grybowsky et al., 1961; Zadicoff, 1979). In one case the bedding, nightclothes, and skin of a 3 1/2-yr-old girl were sprayed for 2 wk with a total amount of 180 ml of 15% diethyltoluamide. Shaking and crying spells, slurred speech, and confusion developed. Improvement occurred after vigorous medical treatment including anticonvulsants. In another report, one of two children displaying signs of severe toxic encephalopathy died after prolonged hospitalization. At autopsy, edema of the brain and congestion of the meninges was found.

Dimethyl sulfoxide

The toxicology of topical dimethyl sulfoxide (DMSO) has been investigated by Kligman (1965). In this study, 9 ml of 90% dimethyl sulfoxide was applied twice daily to the entire trunk of 20 healthy volunteers for three weeks. The following laboratory tests were done: complete blood count, urinalysis, blood sedimentation rate, serum glutamic oxaloacetic transaminase (SGOT), blood urea nitrogen (BUN), and fasting blood sugar dermination. At the end of the study, all laboratory values had remained normal. Except for the appearance of cutaneous signs as erythema, scaling, contact urticaria, stinging, and burning sensations, the drug was tolerated well by all but two individuals, who developed systemic symptoms. In one, a toxic reaction developed on d 12 characterized by a diffuse erythematous and scaling rash accompanied by severe abdominal cramps; the other had a similar rash and complained of nausea, chills and chest pains. These signs, however, abated in spite of continued administration of the drug.

To investigate possible side effects of *chronic* exposure to dimethyl sulfoxide another 20 volunteers were painted wtih 9 ml of 90% dimethyl sulfoxide applied to the entire trunk, once daily for a period of 26 wk. Neither clinical nor laboratory investigations showed adverse effects of the drug. However, most subjects did experience the well-known DMSO-induced disagreeable oyster-like breath odor, to which they eventually became insensitive. One fatality due to a hypersensitivity reaction has been reported (Bennett, 1980).

Dinitrochlorobenzene

Dinitrochlorobenzene (DNCB), a potent contact allergen, has been used with some success for the treatment of recalcitrant alopecia areata; today, however, its use has been discouraged because suspicion has been aroused that DNCB may be mutagenic. Another drawback for its use is its ability to potentiate epicutaneous sensitization to nonrelated allergens (DeGrott et al., 1981). DNCB is absorbed in substantial amounts through the skin, and about 50% of the applied dose is ultimately recoverable in the urine (Feldmann and Maibach, 1970).

A possible systemic reaction to DNCB has been reported (McDaniel et al., 1982): a 25-yr-old man was treated with 0.1% DNCB in an absorbent ointment base for alopecia areata after prior sensitization. After 2 mo of daily applications the patient experienced generalized urticaria, pruritus, and dyspepsia; discontinuance of the drug led to cessation of all symptoms, which recurred after reintroduction of DNCB therapy.

Ethyl Alcohol

Twenty-eight children with alcohol intoxication from percutaneous absorption were described by Gimenez et al. (1968) from Buenos Aires, Argentina. Apparently, in that area it is (or was) a popular procedure to apply alcohol-soaked cloths to the abdomens of babies as a home remedy for the treatment of disturbances of the gastrointestinal tract such as cramps, pain, vomiting, and diarrhea, or because of crying, excitability, and irritability. The children were of both sexes and ranged in age from 33 mo to 1 yr (mean: 12 mo, 27 d). Alcohol-soaked cloths had been applied on the babies' abdomens under rubber panties, and the number of applications varied from one to three; it was estimated that each application contained approximately 40 cm^3 ethanol. Medical consultation took place from 1 to 23 h after application. Alcoholic breath and abdominal erythema were valuable clues to the diagnosis.

All 28 children showed some degree of CNS depression, 24 showed miosis, 15 hypoglycemia, 5 convulsions, 5 respiratory depression, and 2 died. Eleven cases showed blood alcohol from 0.6 to 1.49 g %. Of the two who died, one was autopsied: the findings were consistent with ethyl alcohol intoxication.

More recently a case of acute ethanol intoxication in a preterm infant of 1800 g due to local application of alcohol-soaked compresses on the legs as a treatment for puncture hematomas was reported (Castot et al., 1980).

Topically applied ethanol in tar gel (Ellis et al., 1979) and beer-containing shampoo (Stoll and King, 1980) have caused Antabuse effects in patients on disulfiram for alcoholism, through percutaneous absorption.

Fumaric Acid Monethyl Ester

The effect of systemically and/or topically administered fumaric acid monethyl ester (ethyl fumarate) on psoriasis was studied by Dubiel and Happle (1972) in six patients. Two patients who had been treated with locally applied ointments, consisting of 3 or 5% ethyl fumarate in petrolatum, developed symptoms of renal intoxication.

Local Anesthetics

Benzocaine. Methemoglobinemia has been reported following the topical application of benzocaine to both skin and mucous membranes (Haggerty, 1962; Meynadier and Peyron, 1982; Steinberg and Zepernick, 1962; Olson and McEvoy, 1981). However, this is an uncommon occurrence (American Medical Association, 1977); most cases occurred in infants.

Lidocaine. Lidocaine hydrochloride is widely used for both topical and local injection anesthesia. When the drug is applied to mucous membranes, blood levels simulate those resulting from intravenous injection (Adriani and Zepernick, 1964). Serum lidocaine concentrations higher than 6 μg/ml are associated with toxicity (Seldon and Sasahara, 1987) whose signs are central nervous system stimulation followed by depression and later inhibition of cardiovascular function. Systemic toxicity from viscous lidocaine applied to the oral cavity in two children has been described (Giard et al., 1983; Mofenson et al., 1983a). In one, the mother had been applying lidocaine hydrochloride 2% solution to the infant's gums with her finger 5–6 times daily for a week; the child experienced two generalized seizures within an hour. Urine examined by thin-layer chromatography revealed a large amount of lidocaine, and a blood level of 10 μg/ml was determined (Mofenson et al., 1983a). The other child had a seizure after having received 227.8 mg/kg oral viscous lidocaine for stomatitis herpetica over a 24-h period. In this case, however, ingestion and resorption from the gastrointestinal tract may have contributed to the clinical picture. It has been suggested that for pediatric patients viscous lidocaine should be applied with an oral swab to individual lesions, thus limiting buccal absorption by decreasing the surface area exposed to lidocaine (Giard et al., 1983).

Mercurials

The toxicology of mercury is comprehensively dealt with elsewhere (Aronow, 1983). With a few exceptions, the use of mercury in medicine is considered to be outdated. However, attention should be paid to the possibility of mercurial poisoning even nowadays, as mercury may still be present in many drugs, and in many countries even in over-the-counter remedies, often without mention on the label.

Although there are considerable differences between various mercurials regarding the rate of absorption through the skin, all mercurial preparations are a potential hazard and may cause intoxication. Metallic mercury is readily absorbed through intact skin; absorption of ammoniated mercury chloride in psoriatic patients was demonstrated by Bork et al. (1973).

Young (1960) examined 70 psoriatic patients treated wtih an ointment containing ammoniated mercury before, during, and after treatment. Symptoms and signs of mercurial poisoning could be detected in 33 of them.

Nephrotic syndrome has been reported in a 24-yr-old man using an ammoniated mercury-containing ointment for psoriasis (Silverberg et al., 1967; Turk and Baker, 1968). Nephrotic syndrome due to topical mercury was also reported by Lyons et al., 1975).

There have been two case reports (Stanley-Brown and Frank, 1971; Clark et al., 1982) of children who died following the treatment of an omphalocele with merbromin (an organic mercurial antiseptic).

In view of the risks of both systemic side effects and contact allergic reactions to mercurials, there hardly seems to be any justification for continuing the use of these drugs in dermatological therapy.

Monobenzone

Monobenzone (monobenzyl ether of hydroquinonel) is used topically by patients with extensive vitiligo to depigment their remaining normally pigmented skin. A patient who had been applying the drug for 1 yr had an anterior linear deposition of pigment on both corneas. In 11 additional patients with vitiligo who were using monobenzone, acquired conjuctival melanosis occurred in two patients and pingueculae in three (Hedges et al., 1983).

2-Naphthol(β-Naphthol)

2-Naphthol is used in peeling pastes for the treatment of acne, and between 5 and 10% of a cutaneous dose has been recovered from the urine (Harkness and Beveridge, 1966; Hemels, 1972).

The extensive application of 2-naphthol ointments has been responsible for systemic side effects, including vomiting and death (Osol and Farrar, 1947; Merck Index, 1976). Hemels (1972) concludes that 2-naphthol-containing pastes should be applied only for short periods of time and to a limited area not exceeding 150 cm².

Insecticides

Lindane. Lindane is the δ isomer of benzene hexachloride and is widely used in the treatment of scabies and pediculosis, usually in a 1% lotion, which is applied to the entire body and left on for 24 h (in the case of scabies). The percutaneous absorption of the drug has been studied (Feldmann and Maibach, 1974; Ginsburg et al., 1977; Hosler et al., 1980). The general toxicology is dealt with elsewhere (Haddad, 1983a).

Intoxication from excessive topical therapeutic application of Lindane has been documented (Lee and Groth, 1977; Telch and Jarvis, 1982; Davies et al., 1983).

The issue of possible toxic reactions to a single therapeutic application of Lindane, notably CNS toxicity, has not been settled yet (EDA Drug Bulletin, 1976; Lee and Groth, 1977; Matsuoka, 1981; Pramanik and Hansen, 1979).

Most authors seem to agree that the benefits to be derived from the use of Lindane as a scabicide and pediculicide outweigh the risks involved (Solomon et al., 1977; Schacter, 1981; Rasmussen, 1981; Kramer et al., 1980). The risk of toxicity appears minimal when Lindane is used properly according to directions.

Solomon et al. (1977) in their review on Lindane toxicity give the following observations and recommendations:

1. Lindane should not be applied after a hot bath.
2. The regimen of application for 24 h may be unnecessarily long; 8-12 h may be sufficient (Rasmussen 1981).
3. A concentration weaker than 1.0% may suffice, particularly for badly excoriated patients.
4. Lindane 1% should be used with extreme caution if at all in pregnant women, very small infants, and people with massively excoriated skin. Rassmussen (1981) does not agree on this point.
5. Lindane treatment should not be repeated within 8 d, and then only if necessary.

Malathion. The detailed toxicity of malathion is dealt with elsewhere (Haddad, 1983d). Malathion is used in the treatment of lice, a single application of 0.5% in a solution being customary. Used in this way, it is generally safe.

Ramu et al. (1973) reported on 4 children with an intoxication following hair washing with a solution containing 5% malathion in xylene for the purpose of louse control. Malathion is also a weak but definite skin sensitizer (Milby and Epstein, 1964).

Podophyllum

The toxicity of podophyllum was reviewed in 1982 (Cassidy et al., 1982). Although there have been a significant number of case reports describing serious neurologic illness or death following the application of podophyllum, these are generally related to its use in widespread lesions. Podophyllum 20% in tincture of benzoin is still indicated for isolated venereal warts (Chamberlain et al., 1972). Its use is contraindicated in pregnancy. Following application it should be washed off after a specific period of time.

Salicylic Acid

The general toxicology of salicylates is dealt with elsewhere (Proudfoot, 1983), including its absorption through the skin. Salicylic acid is widely used in dermatology as a topical application for its keratolytic properties. Cases of salicylate poisoning after topical use of salicylic acid have been reported several times. Taylor and Halprin (1975) used 6% salicyclic acid in a gel base under plastic suit occlusion in adults with extensive psoriasis. During their 5-d study, serum salicylates never exceeded 5 mg/100 ml and no patient developed toxicity. However, toxicity was noted by von Weis and Lever (1964); they found serum salicylate levels ranging from 46–64 mg/100 ml. Salicylic acid therapy for extensive lesions may be especially dangerous for children. An unpublished review (U. S. Department of Health, Education and Welfare, 1979) revealed 13 deaths associated wtih the widespread use of salicylic acid preparations, and all but 3 occurred in children. This compound should not be used on large areas (more than 25%) of the skin of a child.

In 1952 Young collected eight fatal cases of salicylate poisoning with symptoms of vomiting, tinnitus, stupor, Cheyne–Stokes respiration, and nuchal rigidity.

Von Weiss and Lever (1964) reported three adults with extensive psoriasis who were treated with an ointment containing 3% or 6% salicylic acid 6 times daily. Between the second and fourth days, symptoms of salicylism developed in all three patients.

The levels of salicylic acid in the serum ranged from 46 to 64 mg/100 ml. Within 1 d after discontinuation of the ointment, the symptoms had largely disappeared. The serum salicylic acid in the serum decreased to zero within a few days.

The same authors also recorded 13 deaths resulting from intoxication with salicylic acid following the application of salicylic ointment to the skin, reported in literature up to 1964, and several nonfatal intoxications. The 13 deaths included 3 patients with psoriasis, 5 cases of scabies, 3 of dermatitis, 1 of lupus vulgaris, and 1 of congenital ichthyosiform erythroderma. Ten of the fatal cases occurred in children, 3 of them being under 3 yr of age.

The most dramatic account in the literature is that of two plantation workers in Bougainville, in the Solomon Islands, who were painted twice a day with an alcoholic solution of 20% salicylic acid to tinea imbricata involving about 50% of the body. The victims were comatose within 6 h and dead within 28 h (Lindsey, 1968).

Wechelsberg (1969) reported a 3-mo-old baby with scaly erythroderma treated in a hospital with 1% salicylic acid in soft paraffin. After 10 d, the child began to vomit and lose weight. Later hyperpnea developed and an increasing somnolence. When the treatment was stopped, the child recovered rapidly.

Recently, a case of salicylic acid intoxication leading to coma in an adult patient with psoriasis who had been treated with 20% salicylic acid in petrolatum was described (Treguer et al., 1980).

Selenium Sulfide

Ransone et al. (1973) reported a case of systemic selenium toxicity in a woman who had been shampooing her hair 2 or 3 times weekly for 8 mo with selenium sulfide suspension.

Silver Nitrate

Ternberg and Luce (1968) observed fatal methemoglobinemia in a 3-yr-old girl suffering from burns involving 82% of the body surface, who was treated with silver nitrate solution.

Another complication of the use of silver nitrate in the treatment of large burns is electrolyte disturbance, especially in children. Due to the hypotonicity of the silver nitrate dressings hyponatremia, hypokalemia, and hyperchloremia may develop (Editoral, 1965; Connely, 1970). Also, loss of other water-soluble minerals and vitamins may occur. Postmortem examinations of patients treated with silver nitrate have revealed that silver has been deposited in internal organs, showing that absorption of silver from topical preparation does occur (Bader, 1966). It should be mentioned that the excessive use of silver-containing drugs has led to local and systemic argyria (Marshall and Schneider, 1977) and to renal damage involving the glomeruli and proteinuria (Zech et al., 1973).

Steroids

Corticosteroids. It has been amply documented that topically applied glucocorticosteroids are absorbed through the skin (Feldmann and Maibach, 1965). Systemic absorption in quantities sufficient to replace endogenous production is not uncommon. However, iatrogenic Cushing's syndrome resulting from the use of topical steroids is rare. Pascher (1978) summarized the relevant data of 12 cases.

Systemic side effects of topical corticosteroids occur more frequently in children than adults (Feiwell et al., 1969) and occur in patients with liver disease because of retarded degradation of the drug (Burton et al., 1976). The two main causes of systemic side effects are hypercorticism leading to an iatrogenic Cushing's syndrome and suppression of the hypothalamic–pituitary–adrenal axis (May et al., 1976).

It is not easy to provide data on "safe" uses of topical corticosteroids, but as for the potent corticosteroid clobetasol 17-propionate 0.05% the dose is recommended to be limited to 45 g per week (van der Harst et al. 1978).

Sex hormones. Estrogens. Topical application of estrogen-containing preparations may lead to resorption of these hormones and systemic estrogenic effects.

Beas et al. (1969) reported on seven children with pseudoprecocious puberty due to an ointment containing estrogens. The common fact found in every patient was the use of the same ointment for treatment or prevention of ammoniacal dermatitis for a period of 2–18 mo with 2–10 daily applications. Endocrinological and radiological studies had excluded other possible causes of sexual precocity. The most important clinical signs were intense pigmentation of mammillary areola, linea alba of the abdomen and the genitals, mammary enlargement, and the presence of pubic hair. Three female patients also had vaginal discharge and bleeding. Estrogenic contamination of the ointment was suspected and confirmed by a biological test of the vaginal opening of castrated female guinea pigs. After discontinuation of the incriminated topical drug, all symptomatology progressively disappeared in every patient.

Pseudoprecocious puberty has also been observed in young girls after contact with hair lotions and other substances containing estrogens (Bertaggia, 1968; Landolt and Murset, 1968; Ramos and Bower, 1969). Such contact has led to gynecomastia in young boys (Stoppelman and van Valkenburg, 1955; Edidin and Levitsky, 1982). Gynecomastia in a 70-yr-old man from exposure to 0.01% dienestrol cream used by his wife for atrophic vaginitis and as a lubricant before intercourse has been reported (DiRaimondo et al., 1980).

Estrogen cream for the treatment of baldness has also caused gynecomastia, which was persistent in the reported case (Gabrilove and Luria, 1978). In adult males both oral and topical administration of estrogens may result first in pigmentation of the areola and then in gynecomastia (Bazex et al. 1967; Goebel, 1969).

Tars

Coal tar. A case of methemoglobinemia in an infant following the 5-d application of an ointment containing 2.5% crude coal tar and 5% benzocaine to about half the body surface has been reported (Goluboff and MacFadyen, 1955).

Dithranol. Dithranol has been used since 1916 for the treatment of psoriasis. Although it causes irritant dermatitis and discoloration of the skin, its use is generally considered to be devoid of systemic side effects. (Gay et al., 1972; Farber and Harris, 1970).

COMMENT

This chapter summarizes literature citations and the basic aspects of percutaneous penetration. The purpose is to alert the reader to the potential for systemic toxicity from topical exposure. Demonstrating causality (rather than association) requires careful documentation. Combining knowledge of the inherent molecular and animal toxicology, cutaneous penetration, and metabolism with the adverse human reaction literature permits a more precise determination of causality. With each of the examples presented here, the original citations combined with the further documentation noted here should permit more discriminate causality judgements.

REFERENCES

Abrams, S. M., Degnan, T. J. and Vinciguerra, V. 1980. Marrow aplasia following topical application of chloramphenicol eye ointment. *Arch. Intern. Med.* 140:576.

Adriani, J. and Zepernick, R. 1964. Clinical effectiveness of drugs used for topical anesthesia. *J. Am. Med. Assoc.* 118:711.

Albert, T. A., Lewis, N. S. and Warpeha, R. L. 1982. Late pulmonary complications with use of mafenide acetate. *J. Burn Care Rehab.* 3:375.

Alder, V. D., Burman, D., Coroner-Beryl, D. and Gillespie, W. A. 1972. Absorption of hexachlorophene from infant's skin. *Lancet* 2:384.

American Medical Association. *Drug Evaluations.* 1977. 3rd ed. p. 269. Littleton, Mass.: Publishing Sciences Group.

Anonymous. 1977. Warning on aerosols containing neomycin. *Lancet* 1:1115.

Aronow, R. 1983. Mercury. In *Clinical Management of Poisoning and Drug Overdose,* eds. L. M. Haddad and J. F. Winchester, p. 637. Philadelphia: W. B. Saunders.

Bader, K. F. 1966. organ deposition of silver following silver nitrate therapy of burns. *Plast. Reconstr. Surg.* 37:550.

Baker, T. J. 1979. The voice of polite dissent. *Plast. Reconstr. Surg.* 63:262.

Bamford, M. F. M. and Jones, L. F. 1978. Deafness and biochemical imbalance after burns treatment with topical antibiotics in young children. *Arch. Dis. Child.* 53:326.

Baranowski-Dutkiewicz, B. 1981. Skin absorption of phenol from aqueous solutions in men. *Int. Arch. Environ. Health* 49:99.

Barza, M., Goldstein, J. A., Kane, A., Feingold, D. S. and Pochi, P. E. 1982. Systemic absorption of clindamycin hydrochloride after topical application. *J. Am. Acad. Dermatol.* 7:208.

Bazex, A., Salvader, R., Dupre, A. and Christol, B. 1967. Gynecomastie et hyperpigmentation areolaire apres oestrogenotherapie locale antiseborrheque. *Bull. Soc. Fr. Dermatol. Syphiligr.* 74:466.

Beas, F., Vargas, L., Spada, R. P. and Merchak, N. 1969. Pseudoprecocious puberty in infants caused by a dermal ointment containing estrogens. *J. Pediat.* 75:127.

Becker, L. E., Bergstresser, P. R., Whiting, D. A., et al. 1981. Topical clindamycin therapy for acne vulgaris: A cooperative clinical study. *Arch. Dermatol.* 117:482.

Bennett, C. C. 1980. Dimethyl sulfoxide. *J. Am. Med. Assoc.* 244:2768.

Bertaggia, A. 1968. A case of precocious puberty in a girl following the use of an estrogen preparation on the skin. *Pediatria (Napoli)* 76:579.

Berthezene, F., Fournier, M., Bernier, E. and Mornex, R. 1973. L'Hypothyroidie induite par la resorcine. *Lyon Med.* 230:319.

Bloch, R. and Beysovec, L. 1982. Promethazine toxicity through percutaneous absorption. *Contin. Practice* 9:28.

Bork, K., Morsches, B. and Holzmann, H. 1973. Zum Problem der Quecksilber-Resorption aus weisser Prazipatatsalbe. *Arch. Dermatol. Forsch.* 248:37.

Burton, T. T., Cunliffe, W. J., Holti, G. and Wright, W. 1974. Complications of topical corticosteroid therapy in patients with liver disease. *Br. J. Dermatol.* 9(suppl. 10):22.

Cammann, R., Hennecke, H. and Beier, R. 1971. Symptomatische Psychosen nach Kolton-Gelee-Applikation. *Psychiatr. Neurol. Med. Psychol.* 23:426.

Cassidy, D. E., Drewry, J. and Fanning, J. P. 1982. Podophyllum toxicity: A report of a fatal case and a review of the literature. *J. Toxicol. Clin. Toxicol.* 19:35.

Castot, A., Garnier, R., Lanfranchi, E., et al. 1980. Effects systematiques indesirables des medicaments appliques sur la peau chez l'enfant. *Therapie* 35:423.

Chan, C. K., Jarrett, F. and Moylan, J. A. 1976. Acute leukopenia as an allergic reaction to silver sulfadiazine in burn patients. *J. Trauma* 16:395.

Chamberlain, M. J., Reynolds, A. L. and Yeoman, W. V. 1972. Toxic effect of podophyllum application in pregnancy. *Br. J. Med.* 3:391.

Clark, J. A., Kasselberg, A. G., Glick, A. D. and O'Neill, J. A., Jr. 1982. Mercury poisoning from merbromin (Mercurochrome[R]) therapy of omphalocele. *Clin. Pediatr.* 21:445.

Committee on Drugs. 1978. Camphor—Who needs it? *Pediatrics* 62:404.

Connell, J. F., Jr. and Rousselot, L. M. 1964. Povidone-iodine, extensive surgical evaluation of a new antiseptic. *Am. J. Surg.* 108:849.

Connely, D. M. 1970. Silver nitrate—Ideal burn wound therapy? *NY State J. Med.* 70:1642.

Cronin, E. 1980a. Immediate-type hypersensitivity to henna. *Contact Dermatitis* 5:198.

Cronin, E. 1980b. *Contact Dermatitis.* Edinburgh: Churchill Livingstone.

Cronin, T. D. and Brauer, R. O. 1949. Death due to phenol contained in Foille[R]. *J. Am. Med. Assoc.* 139:777.

Cullison, D., Abele, D. C. and O'Quinn, J. L. 1983. Localized exogenous ochronosis. Report of a case and review of the literature. *J. Am. Acad. Dermatol.* 8:882.

Curley, A., Hawk, R. E., Kimbrough, R. D., Nathenson, G. and Finberg, L. 1971. Dermal absorption of hexachlorophane infants. *Lancet* 2:296.

Cunningham, A. A. 1956. Resorcin poisoning. *Arch. Dis. Child.* 31:173.

Davies, J. E., Dedhia, H. V., Morgade, C. et al. 1983. Lindane poisonings. *Arch. Dermatol.* 119:142.

Dayal, V. S., Smith, E. L. and McCain, W. G. 1974. Cochlear and vestibular gentamycin toxicity: A clinical study of systemic and topical usage. *Arch. Otolaryngol.* 100:338.

DeGroot, A. C., Nater, J. P., Bleumink, K. and de Long, M. C. J. M. 1981. Does DNCB therapy potentiate epicutaneous sensitization to non-related contact allergens? *Clin. Exp. Dermatol.* 6:139.

Deichmann, W. B. 1949. Local and systemic effects following skin contact with phenol—A review of the literature. *J. Ind. Hyg.* 31:146.

Del Pizzo, A. and Tanski, E. L. 1980. Chemical face peeling—Malignant therapy for benign disease? (Editorial). *Plast. Reconstr. Surg.* 66:121.

DiRaimondo, C. V., Roach, A. C. and Meador, C. K. 1980. Gynecomastia from exposure to vaginal estrogen cream (Letter). *N. Engl. J. Med.* 302:1089.

Done, A. K. 1983. Borates. In *Clinical Management of Poisoning and Drug Overdose,* eds. L. M. Haddad and J. F. Winchester, p. 929. Philadelphia: W. B. Saunders.

Drake, T. E. 1974. Reaction to gentamycin sulfate cream. *Arch. Dermatol.* 110:638.

Dubiel, W. and Happle, R. 1972. Behandlungsversuch mit Fumarsaure mono-athylester bei Psoriasis vulgaris. *Z. Haut. Geschlechtskr.* 47:545.

D'Arcy, P. F. 1982. Fatalities with the use of a henna dye. *Pharm. Int.* 3:217.

Edidin, D. V. and Levitsky, L. L. 1982. Prepubertal gynecomnastia associated with estrogen-containing hair cream. *Am. J. Dis. Child.* 136:587.

Editorial. 1965. Burns and silver nitrate. *J. Am. Med. Assoc.* 193:230.

Editorial. 1982. Hexachlorophene today. *Lancet* 1:500.

Ellis, C. N., Mitchell, A. J. and Beardsley, G. R., Jr. 1979. Tar gel interaction with disulfiram. *Arch. Dermatol.* 115:1367.

El-Ansary, E. H., Ahmed, M. E. K. and Clague, H. W. 1983. Systemic Toxicity of *para*-phenylenediamine. *Lancet* 1:1341.

Farber, E. M. and Harris, D. R. 1970. Hospital treatment of psoriasis. *Arch. Dermatol.* 101:381.

FDA Drug Bulletin. 1976. Gamma benzene hexachloride (Kwell) and other products alert. 6:28.

Feiwell, M., James, V. H. T. and Barnett, E. S. 1969. Effect of potential topical steroids on plasma-cortisol levels of infants and children with eczema. *Lancet* 1:485.

Feldmann, R. J. and Maibach, H. I. 1965. Penetration of 14C hydrocortisone through normal skin. *Arch. Dermatol.* 91:661.

Feldmann, R. J. and Maibach, H. I. 1967. Regional variation in percutaneous penetration of 14C cortesol in man. *J. Invest. Dermatol.* 48:181.

Feldmann, R. J. and Maibach, H. I. 1970. Absorption of some organic compounds through the skin in man. *J. Invest. Dermatol.* 54:399.

Feldmann, R. J. and Maibach, H. I. 1974. Percutaneous penetration of some pesticides and herbicides in man. *Toxicol. Appl. Pharmacol.* 28:126.

Fisher, A. E. 1986. *Contact Dermatitis,* 3rd ed. Philadelphia: Lea and Febiger.

Flandin, C., Rabeau, H. and Ukrainczyk, M. 1953. Intolerance a la resorcine. Test cutane. *Soc. Dermatol. Syph.* 12:1804.

Franz, T. J. 1983. On the bioavailability of topical formulations of clindamycin hydrochloride. *J. Am. Acad. Dermatol.* 9:66.

Fraser, G. L. and Beaulieu, J. T. 1979. Leukopenia secondary to sulfadiazine silver. *J. Am. Med. Assoc.* 241:1928.

Friedmann, I. 1977. Aerosols containing neomycin. *Lancet* 1:1662.

Gabrilove, J. L. and Luria, M. 1978. Persistent gynecomastia resulting from scalp inunction of estradiol: A model for persistent gynecomastia. *Arch. Dermatol.* 114:1672.

Gay, M. W., Moore, W. J., Morgan, J. M. and Montes, L. F. 1972. Anthralin toxicity. *Arch. Dermatol.* 105:213.

Giard, M. J., Uden, D. L. and Whitelock, D. J. 1983. Seizures induced by oral viscous lidocaine. *Clin. Pharm.* 2:110.

Gimenez, E. R., Vallejo, N. E., Roy, E., Lis, M., Izurieta, E. M., Rossi, S. and Capuccio, M. 1968. Percutaneous alcohol intoxication. *Clin. Toxicol.* 1:39.

Ginsburg, C. M., Lowry, W. and Reisch, J. S. 1977. Absorption of lindane (gamma benzene hexachloride) in infants and children. *J. Pediat.* 91:998.

Goebel, M. 1969. Mamillenhypertorphie mit Pigmentierung nach lokaler Oestrogentherapie im Kindesalter. *Hautarzt* 20:521.

Goffinet, M. 1977. A propos de la toxicite cliniquement presumable de certaintes gouttes otiques. *Acta Oto-rhino-laryngol. Belg.* 31:585.

Goluboff, N. and MacFadyen, D. J. 1955. Methemoglobinemia in an infant. *J. Pediatr.* 47:222.

Gossweiler, B. 1982. Kampfervergiftungen heute. *Schweiz. Rundschau Med. (PRAXIS)* 71:1475.

Greaves, S. J., Ferry D. G., McQueen, E. G., et al. 1975. Serial hexachlorophene blood levels in the premature infant. *N. Z. Med. J.* 81:334–336.

Grybowsky, J., Weinstein, D. and Ordway, N. 1961. Toxic encephalopathy apparently related to the use of an insect repellent. *N. Engl. J. Med.* 264:289.

Haddad, L. M. 1983a. The carbamate, organochlorine and botanical insecticides; insect repellants. In *Clinical Management of Poisoning and Drug Overdose,* eds. L. M. Haddad and J. F. Winchester, p. 711. Philadelphia: W. B. Saunders.

Haddad, L. M. 1983c. Phenol, dinotrophenol and pentachlorophene. In *Clinical Management of Poisoning and Drug Overdose,* eds. L. M. Haddad and J. F. Winchester, p. 810. Philadelphia: W. B. Saunders

Haddad, L. M. 1983b. Miscellany. In *Clinical Management of Poisoning and Drug Overdose,* eds. L. M. Haddad and J. F. Winchester, Chap. 101, p. 929. Philadelphia: W. B. Saunders.

Haddad, L. M. 1983d. The Organophosphate insecticides. In *Clinical Management of Poisoning and Drug Overdose,* eds. L. M. Haddam and J. F. Winchester, p. 704. Philadelphia: W. B. Saunders.

Haddad, L. M. 1983e. Miscellany. In *Clinical Management of Poisoning and Drug Overdose,* eds. L. M. Haddad and J. F. Winchester, p. 965.

Haggerty, R. J. 1962. Blue baby due to methemoglobinemia. *N. Engl. J. Med.* 267:13303.

Harkness, R. A. and Beveridge, G. W. 1966. Isolation of β-naphthol from urine after its application to skin. *Nature (Lond.)* 211:413.

Hedges, T. R. III, Kenyon, K. R., Hanninen, L. A. and Mosher, D. B. 1983. Corneal and conjunctival effects of monobenzone in patients with vitiligo. *Arch. Ophthalmol.* 101:64.

Hemels, H. G. W. M. 1972. Percutaneous absorption and distribution of 2-naphthol in man. *Br. J. Dermatol.* 87:614.

Hopkins, J. 1979. Hexachlorophene: More bad news than good. *Food Cosmet. Toxicol.* 17:410.

Hosler, J., Tschanz, C., Higuite, C. *et al.* 1980. Topical application of Lindane cream (Kwell) and antipyrine metabolism. *J. Invest. Dermatol.* 74:51.

Jarrett, F., Ellerbe, S. and Demling, R. 1978. Acute leukopenia during topical burn therapy with silver sulfadiazine. *Am. J. Surg.* 135:818.

Johnstone, R. T. 1948. *Occupational Medicine and Industrial Hygiene,* p. 216. St. Louis, MO: C. V. Mosby.

Kellerhals, B. 1978. Horschaden durch ototoxische Ohrtropfen. Ergebnisse einer Umfrage. *HNO (Berl.)* 26:49.

Kelly, D. R., Nilo, E. N. and Berggren, R. B. 1969. Deafness after topical neomycin wound irrigation. *N. Engl. J. Med.* 280:1338.

Kligman, A. M. 1965. Dimethyl sulfoxide—Part 2. *J. Am. Med. Assoc.* 193:151.

Kopelman, R. 1983. Camphor. In *Clinical Management of Poisoning and Drug Overdose,* eds. L. M. Haddad and J. F. Winchester, p. 926. Philadelphia: W. B. Saunders.

Kramer, M. S., Hutchinson, T. A., Rudnick, S. A. et al. 1980. Operational criteria for adverse drug reactions in evaluating suspected toxicity of a popular scabicide. *Clin. Pharmacol. Ther.* 27:149.

Landolt, R. and Murset, G. 1968. Vorzeitige Pubertatsmerkmale als Folge unbeabsichtigter Ostrogenverabreichung. *Schweiz. Med. Wochenschr.* 98:638.

Lee, B. and Groth, P. 1977. Scabies: Transcutaneous poisoning during treatment. *Pediatrics* 59:643.

Liebman, P. R., Kennelly, M. M. and Hirsch, E. F. 1982. Hypercarbia and acidosis associated with carbonic anhydrase inhibition: A hazard of topical mafenide acetate use in renal failure. *Burns* 8:395.

Lindsey, C. P. 1968. Two cases of fatal salicylate poisoning after topical application of an antifungal solution. *Med. J. Aust.* 1:353.

Lundell, E. and Nordman, R. 1973. A case of infantile poisoning by topical application of Castellani's solution. *Ann. Clin. Res.* 5:404.

Lyons, T. J., Christer, C. N. and Larsen, F. S. 1975. Ammoniated mercury ointment and the nephrotic syndrome. *Minn. Med.* 58:383.

Masur, H., Whelton, P. K. and Whelton, A. 1976. Neomycin toxicity revisited. *Arch. Surg.* 3:822.

Marshall, J. P. and Schneider, R. P. 1977. Systemic argyria secondary to topical silver nitrate. *Arch. Dermatol.* 113:1072.

Matsuoka, L. Y. 1981. Convulsions following application of gamma benzene hexachloride. *J. Am. Acad. Dermatol.* 5:98.

May, P., Stern, E. J., Ryter, R. J., Hirsch, F. S., Michel, B. and Levy, R. P. 1976. Cushing syndrome from percutaneous absorption of triamcinolone cream. *Arch. Intern. Med.* 136:612.

McDaniel, D. H., Blatchley, D. M. and Welton, W. A. 1982. Adverse systemic reaction to dinitrichlorobenzene (Letter). *Arch. Dermatol.* 118:371.

Merck Index. 1976. 9th ed., p. 291. Rahway, N.J.: Merck.

Meynadier, J. and Peyron, J.-L. 1982. Resorption transcutanee des medicaments. *Rev. Pract. (Paris)* 32:41.

Milby, T. H. and Epstein, W. L. 1964. Allergic sensitivity to malathion. *Arch. Environ. Health* 9:434.

Milstone, E. B., McDonald, A. J. and Scholhamer, C. F. 1986. Pseudomembranous colitis after topical application of clindamycin. *Arch. Dermatol.* 117:154.

Mittelman, H. 1972. Ototoxicity of 'ototopical' antibiotics: Past, present, and future. *Trans. Am. Acad. Ophthal. Otolaryngol.* 76:1432.

Mofenson, H. C., Caraccio, T. R., Miller, H. and Greensher, J. 1983a. Lidocaine toxicity from topical mucosal application. *Clin. Pediatr.* 22:190.

Mofenson, H. C., Caraccio, T. R. and Greensher, J. 1983b. Iodine. In *Clinical Management of Poisoning and Drug Overdose,* eds. L. M. Haddad and J. F. Winchester, p. 697. Philadelphia: W. B. Saunders.

Murray, M. C. 1926. An analysis of sixty cases of drug poisoning. *Arch. Pediatr.* 43:193.

Nachman, R. L. and Esterly, N. B. 1971. Increased skin permeability in pre-term infants. *J. Pediatr.* 89:628–632.

Ohlgisser, M., Adler, M. N., Ben-Dov, B., Taitelman, U., Birkhan, H. J. and Burzstein, S. 1978. Methemoglobinaemia induced by mafenide acetate in children. A report of two cases. *Br. J. Anaesth.* 50:299.

Olson, M. L. and McEvoy, G. K. 1981. Methemoglobinemia induced by local anesthetics. *Am. J. Hosp. Pharm.* 38:89.

Osol, A. and Farrar, G. E., Jr. 1947. *The Dispensatory of the United States of America,* 24th ed. Philadelphia: Lippincott.

Otten, H. and Plempel, M. 1975. Antibiotika und Chemotherapeutika in Einzeldarstellungen. Chemotherapeutika mit braitem Wirkungsbereich. Sulfon-amide. In *Antibiotika-Fibel,* eds. H. Otten, M. Plempel and Siegenthaler, G. pp. 110–145. Stuttgart: Thieme Verlag.

Owens, C. J., Yarbrough, D. R. and Brackett, N. R. 1974. Nephrotic syndrome following topically applied solfadiazine therapy. *Arch. Intern. Med.* 134:332.

Pannatier, A., Jenner, B., Testa, B., et al. 1978. The skin as a drug-metabolizing organ. *Drug Metab. Rev.* 8:319–343.

Pascher, F. 1978. Systemic reactions to topically applied drugs. *Int. J. Dermatol.* 17:768.

Pines, W. I. 1972. Hexachlorophene: Why FDA concluded that hexachlorophene was too potent and too dangerous to be used as it once was? *FDA Consumer* 6:24.

Plueckhahn, V. C., Ballard, B. A., Banis, J. M., Collins, R. B. and Flett, P. T. 1978. Hexachlorophene preparations in infant antiseptic skin care: Benefit, risk and the future. *Med. J. Aust.* 2:555.

Ponte, C., Richard, J., Bonte, C., Lequien, P. and Lacombe, A. 1974. Methemoglobinemies chez le nouveau-nie. Discussion du role etiologique du trichlorcarbanilide. *Ann. Pediatr.* 21:359.

Pramanik, A. K. and Hansen, R. C. 1979. Transcutaneous gamma benzene hexachloride absorption and toxicity in infants and children. *Arch. Dermatol.* 115:1224.

Proudfoot, A. T. 1983. Salicylates and salicylamide. In *Clinical Management of Poisoning and Drug Overdose,* eds. L. M. Haddad and J. F. Winchester, p. 575. Philadelphia: W. B. Saunders.

Ramos, A. S. and Bower, B. F. 1969. Pseudosexual precocity due to cosmetics ingestion. *J. Am. Med. Assoc.* 207:369.

Ransone, J. W., Scott, N. M. and Knoblock, E. C. 1973. Selenium sulfide intoxication. *N. Engl. J. Med.* 9:631.

Ramu, A., Slonim, E. A. and Egal, F. 1973. Hyperglycemia in acute malathion poisoning. *Israel J. Med. Sci.* 9:631.

Rasmussen, J. E. 1979. Percutaneous absorption in children. In *1979 Year Book of Dermatology,* ed. R. L. Dobson, pp. 15–38. Chicago: Year Book Medical.

Rasmussen, J. E. 1981. The problem of lindane. *J. Am. Acad. Dermatol.* 5:507.

Robertson, W. O. 1983. Arsenic and other heavy metals. In *Clinical Management of Poisoning and Drug Overdose,* eds. L. M. Haddad and J. F. Winchester, p. 656, Philadelphia: W. B. Saunders.

Rogers, S. C. F., Burrows, D. and Neill, D. 1978. Percutaneous absorption of phenol and methylalcohol in magenty paint B. P. C. *Br. J. Dermatol.* 98:559.

Scharpf, L. G., Hill, I. D. and Maibach, H. I. 1975. Percutaneous penetration and disposition of tricarban in man. *Arch. Environ. Health* 30:7.

Seldon, R. and Sasahara, A. A. 1987. Central nervous system toxicity induced by lidocaine. *J. Am. Med. Assoc.* 202:908.

Shacter, B. 1981. Treatment of scabies and pediculosis with lindane preparations: An evaluation. *J. Am. Acad. Dermatol.* 5:517.

Silverberg, D. S., McCall, J. T. and Hunt, J. C. 1967. Nephrotic syndrome with use of ammoniated mercury. *Arch. Intern. Med.* 120:581.

Skoglund, R. R., Ware, L. L., Jr. and Schanberger, J. E. 1977. Prolonged seizures due to contact and inhalation exposure to camphor. *Clin. Pediatr.* 16:901.

Solomon, L. M., Fahrner, L. and West, D. P. 1977. Gamma benzene hexachloride toxicity. A review. *Arch. Dermatol.* 113:353.

Stanley-Brown, E. G. and Frank. J. E. 1971. Mercury poisoning from application to ompohalocele. (Letter to the editor.) *J. Am. Med. Assoc.* 216:2144.

Steinberg, J. B. and Zepernick, R. G. L. 1962. Methemoglobinemia during anesthesia. *J. Pediatr.* 61:885.

Stoll, D. and King, L. E., Jr. 1980. Disulfiram—alcohol skin reaction to beer-containing shampoo. (Letter). *J. Am. Med. Assoc.* 244:2045.

Stoppelman, M. R. H. and Van Valkenburg, R. A. 1955. Pigmentaties en gynecomastie ten gevolge van het gebruik van stilboestrol bevattend haarewater bij kinderen. *Ned. Tijdschr. Geneesk.* 99:3925.

Stoughton, R. B. 1979. Topical antibiotics for acne vulgaris: Current usage. *Arch. Dermtaol.* 115:486.

Taylor, J. R. and Halprin, K. 1975. Percutaneous absorption of salicylic acid. *Arch. Dermatol.* 106:740.

Telch, J. and Jarvis, D. A. 1982. Acute intoxication with lindane (gamma benzene hexachloride). *Can. Med. Assoc. J.* 126:662.

Ternberg, J. L. and Luce, E. 1968. Methemoglobinemia: A complication of the silver nitrate treatment of burns. *Surgery* 63:328.

Thomas, A. E. and Gisburn, M. A. 1961. Exogenous ochronosis and myxoedema from resorcinol. *Br. J. Dermatol.* 73:378.

Treguer, G. L., Le Bihan, G., Coloignier, M., Le Roux, P. and Bernard, J. P. 1980. Intoxication salicylee par application locale de vaseline salicylee a 20% chez un psoriasique. *Nouv. Presse Med.* 9:192.

Tromovitch, T. A. 1982. Safety of chemical face peels. (Letter.) *J. Am. Acad. Dermatol.* 7:137.

Truppman, E. S. and Ellerby, J. D. 1979. Major electrocardiographic changes during chemical face peeling. *Plast. Reconstr. Surg.* 63:44.

Turk, J. L. and Baker, H. 1968. Nephrotic syndrome dur to ammoniated mercury. *Br. J. Dermatol.* 80:623.

Tyrala, E. E., Hillman, L. S., Hillman, R. E. and Dodson, W. E. 1977. Clinical pharmacology of hexachlorophene in newborn infants. *J. Pediatr.* 91:481.

U.S. Department of Health, Education and Welfare, Food and Drug Administration, OTC Antimicrobial II Advisory Panel. Cited by Rasmussen, J. E. 1979. Percutaneous absorption in children. In *Year Book of Dermatology,* ed. R. L. Dobson, p. 28. Chicago: Year Book Medical.

Van der Harst, L. C. A., Smeenk, G., Burger, P. M., Van der Rhee, J. H. and Polano, M. K. 1978. Waardebepaling en risicoschatting van de uitwendige behandeling met clobetasol-17-propionaat (Dermovate). *Ned. Tijdschr. Geneesk.* 122:219.

Von Hinkel, G. K. and Kitzel, H. W. 1968. Phenolvergiftungen bei Neugeborenen durch kutane Resorption. *Dtsch. Gesundheitwes.* 23:240.

Von Krogh, G. and Maibach, H. I. 1987. The contact curticaria syndrome. In *Dermatotoxicology,* 3rd ed., eds. F. N. Marzulli and H. I. Maibach, chap. 15, p. 341. Washington, D.C.: Hemisphere.

Von Weiss, J. F. and Lever, W. F. 1964. Percutaneous salicylic acid intoxication in psoriasis. *Arch. Dermatol.* 90:614.

Voron, D. A. 1978. Systemic absorption of topical clindamycin. *Arch. Dermatol.* 114:798.

Wechselberg, K. 1969. Salizylsaure-Vergiftung durch perkutane Resorption 1%-iger Salizylvaseline. *Anasth. Prax.* 4:103.

Wester, R. C., Noonan, P. K., Cole, M. P. and Maibach, H. I. 1977a. Percutaneous absorption of testosterone in the newborn rhesus monkey: Comparison to the adult. *Pediatr. Res.* 11:737–739.

Wilson, A. J. and Mielke, C. H. 1983. Haematological consequences of poisoning. In *Poisoning and Drug Overdose,* eds. L. M. Haddad and J. F. Winchester, chapter 96, p. 893. Philadelphia: W. B. Saunders.

Yeung, D., Kanto, S., Nacht, S. and Gans, E. H. 1983. Percutaneous absorption, blood levels and urinary excretion of resorcinol applied topically in humans. *Int. J. Dermatol.* 22:321.

Young, E. 1960. Ammoniated mercury poisoning. *Br. J. Dermatol.* 72:449.

Zackheim, H. S., Feldman, R. J., Lindsay, E. and Maibach H. I. 1977. Percutaneous absorption of 1,3-bis(2-chloro-ethyl)-l-nitrosurea (cbcnu, carmustine) in mycosis fungoides. *Br. J. Dermatol.* 97:65.

Zadicoff, C. 1979. Toxic encephalopathy associated with use of insect repellant. *J. Pediat.* 95:140.

Zech, P., Colon, S., Labeeuw, R., Blanc-Brunat, N., Richard, P. and Porol, M. 1973. Syndrome nephrotique avec depot d'argent dans les membranes glomerulaires au cours d'une argyrie. *Nouv. Presse Med.* 2:161.

appendixes

oecd guidelines
for testing of chemicals[1]

PREFACE

General

1. This publication contains the official OECD[2] Guidelines for Testing of Chemicals as adopted by the OECD Council.

2. The Test Guidelines have been developed initially under the OECD Chemicals Testing Programme (see paragraphs 10-16 below), and subsequently, since 1981, as provided by the council under the OECD Updating Programme for Test Guidelines.

3. Whenever testing of chemicals is contemplated, the OECD Test Guidelines should be consulted. Since the Test Guidelines have been endorsed by the OECD Member countries, their use in the generation of data provides a common basis for the acceptance of data internationally, together with the opportunity to reduce direct and indirect costs to governments and industry associated with testing and assessment of chemicals.

4. Other methods and guidelines not included in this publication may be judged to be appropriate in testing chemicals in certain scientific, legal, and administrative contexts.

5. The OECD Council Decision on Mutual Acceptance of Data [12th May, 1981; C(81)30] affirms that data generated in one country in accordance with the OECD Test Guidelines—and additionally in accordance with the OECD Principles of Good Laboratory Practice—should be accepted in OECD countries for purposes of assessment and other uses relating to protection of

man and the environment. The full text of this Decision and the OECD Principles of Good Laboratory Practice may be found in the Appendix to the OECD Guidelines for Testing of Chemicals.

6. The OECD Test Guidelines contain generally formulated procedures for the laboratory testing of a property or effect deemed important for the evaluation of health and environment hazards of a chemical. The Guidelines vary somewhat in respect of detail, but include all the essential elements which, assuming good laboratory practice, should enable an operator to carry out the required test.

7. OECD Test Guidelines are not designed to serve as rigid test protocols. They are instead designed to allow flexibility for expert judgment and adjustment to new developments.

8. It is intended that the OECD Test Guidelines be used by experienced laboratory staff familiar with the type(s) of testing involved. Proper conduct of testing and associated interpretation of results can only be achieved by appropriately trained personnel with access to equipped laboratory facilities.

9. The loose-leaf system chosen for the Guidelines allows for additions and changes to be made when necessary. Information will be circulated when such changes occur resulting from work under the Updating Programme.

OECD Chemicals Testing Programme

10. The OECD Chemicals Testing Programme was launched by the Chemicals Group in November, 1977. It comprised six Expert Groups under the leadership of individual Member countries. One of these Groups, the Step System Group, worked on phased approaches to testing and assessment of chemicals (see paragraphs 30–32 below).

11. Five of the groups reviewed the state-of-the-art of methods and produced draft Test Guidelines. The following areas were covered:
   i. Physical-chemical properties (Lead country—Germany).
   ii. Effects on biotic systems other than man (Lead country—the Netherlands).
   iii. Degradation/accumulation (Lead countries—Japan/Germany).
   iv. Long term health effects (Lead country—the United States).
   v. Short term health effects (Lead country—the United Kingdom).

12. Some 300 experts, drawn from academia, government, industry, international organizations, and other sectors, took part in the Programme. In all, some 50 meetings were held during 1978–1979 under the auspices of the OECD Chemicals Testing Programme.

13. In order to improve the international validation of tests, several methods were subjected to laboratory intercomparison exercises in the Chemicals Testing Programme. This work is being continued under the OECD Updating Programme.

14. In December 1979, the five Expert Groups working on test methods submitted their reports to the OECD. The two Groups on health effects submitted a combined report. The reports contained draft Test Guidelines and an analysis of approaches to testing within the respective areas.

15. During 1980, the draft Test Guidelines were subjected to an extensive commentary and review process. Member countries were invited to submit comments to the OECD which were subsequently taken into account by a Review Panel, established to finalise the product for adoption and printing. The Panel worked in close collaboration with the Chairman of the Expert Groups.

16. The review process was concluded by the Chemicals Group and the Environment Committee of the Organisation, which endorsed these Test Guidelines prior to their formal submission to the OECD Council.

17. The subject areas covered by the Expert Groups under the Chemicals Testing Programme have largely been kept separate in this publication. Thus, OECD Test Guidelines are presented under four different sections:

- physical-chemical properties
- effects on biotic systems other than man
- degradation/accumulation
- health effects

18. Each section is preceded by a summary of considerations raised in the individual expert group reports. These summaries reflect some of the major observations and explanations made at the scientific level during the preparatory process. Further, major portions of the expert group reports have been absorbed into the on-going activities of OECD on chemicals.

OECD Updating Programme for Test Guidelines

19. In 1981, the OECD Updating Programme for Test Guidelines was established by Member countries in consultation with the Commission of the European Communities. The aim was to ensure that OECD Test Guidelines will not become outdated as a result of major changes in the state-of-the-art or scientific advances.

20. The Updating Programming is considering:

a. Proposals for new or modified tests which offer conspicuous advantages over those already adopted.
b. New guidelines which are being developed in areas not yet covered.
c. Incorporation of results from the Chemicals Testing Programme into OECD Test Guidelines.
d. Those matters which need further investigation and research.

OECD Principles for Testing and Assessment of Chemicals

21. The OECD Test Guidelines are but one component in an OECD strategy to make testing of chemicals more systematic, relevant, and cost effective within an international framework which could lead to increased exchange and acceptance of test data between countries. This strategy has been developed with vigour in the Organisation during the 1970s leaving several important questions yet to be resolved.

22. While the OECD Test Guidelines can properly be used in establishing one effect or property, the Guidelines were developed under programmes directed towards an integrated and comprehensive approach to testing and assessment. Thus, the OECD Council, in 1974 and 1977, developed recommendations which deal respectively with "The Assessment of the Potential Environmental Effects of Chemicals" [C(74)215] and "Guidelines in Respect to Procedures and Requirements for Anticipating the Effects of Chemicals on Man and in the Environment" [C(77)97(Final)].

23. In 1974, the OECD Council recommended that prior to marketing of chemicals their potential effects on man and his environment should be assessed.

24. This concern, that assessments should encompass both man and his environment, was reflected in the subject areas chosen for the OECD Chemicals Testing programme, and is also reflected in the disposition of the Test Guidelines into sections.

25. Some outstanding features with respect to testing and assessment which derive from the 1977 OECD Council Recommendations can be summarised as follows:

  i. Chemical substances—with special emphasis on new substances—should be subjected to systematic assessment for potential effects, in relation to both human and environmental hazard.
  ii. It is possible to determine no more than the likelihood of adverse effects from chemicals, and this can only be done through the application of expert judgment based on methods that are technically practicable, as well as economically acceptable.
  iii. Responsibility for generating and assessing the data necessary to determine the potential effects of chemicals must be part of the overall function and liability of industry.
  iv. A phased approach should be applied in data gathering and assessments.

26. These four principles also provided guidance to the Expert Groups in their work in the Chemicals Testing Programme.

27. The need for expert judgment in testing and assessment has been emphasised throughout the work on chemicals in OECD. The Expert Groups under the OECD Chemicals Testing Programme reaffirmed this need when they

selected methods that were regarded as technically practicable and economically acceptable for inclusion into OECD Test Guidelines.

28. The question of a phased approach to testing and assessment is an important concept which is under continuing active consideration in OECD within the Chemicals Testing Programme. All the expert groups have contributed to the framework of an overall scheme for testing and assessment of chemicals.

29. In their work the five Expert Groups on test methods identified steps in which testing and assessment might proceed. The early steps were usually simple in character with the objective of establishing a first indication of hazard. Further steps brought the testing and assessment into a sophisticated and time-consuming range of tests, characterised by increased confidence in the assessments.

30. The Step Systems Group, the sixth Expert Group established under the Chemicals Testing Programme, draws upon the work of the other Expert Groups and is currently developing an integrated stepwise approach to testing and assessment of chemical hazard to man and his environment.

31. An important outcome of the work of the Step Systems Group is the OECD Minimum Pre-marketing set of Data (MPD).

32. MPD lists some thirty-five individual data components that normally would be sufficient to perform a meaningful first assessment of the potential hazard of a chemical.

33. Finally, it should be recognized that elaboration of principles for testing and assessment of chemicals is a continuing process within OECD. This process has been, and remains, possible only through the generous provision of time, knowledge, and enthusiasm from the participating experts, and the active support of Member countries.

ACUTE DERMAL TOXICITY
(GUIDELINE #402)

1. Introductory Information

Prerequisites

- Solid or liquid test substance
- Chemical identification of test substance
- Purity (impurities) of test substance
- Solubility characteristics
- Melting point/boiling point
- pH (where appropriate)

Standard Documents

There are no relevant international standards.

2. Method

A. Introduction, Purpose, Scope, Relevance, Application and Limits of Tests;

In the assessment and evaluation of the toxic characteristics of a substance, determination of acute dermal toxicity is useful where exposure by the dermal route is likely. It provides information on health hazards likely to arise from a short term exposure by the dermal route. Data from an acute dermal toxicity study may serve as a basis for classification and labelling. It is an initial step in establishing a dosage regimen in subchronic and other studies and may provide information on dermal absorption and the mode of toxic action of a substance by this route.

Definitions

Acute dermal toxicity is the adverse effects occurring within a short time of dermal application of a single dose of a test substance.

Dose is the amount of test substance applied. Dose is expressed as weight (g, mg) or as weight of test substance per unit weight of test animal (e.g., mg/kg).

---

[1]Adopted February 24, 1987. Users of this Test Guideline should consult the Preface, in particular, paragraphs 3, 4, 7, and 8.

The LD50 (median lethal dose), dermal, is a statistically derived single dose of a substance that can be expected to cause death in 50 per cent of treated animals when applied to the skin. The LD50 value is expressed in terms of weight of test substance per unit weight of test animal (mg/kg).

Dosage is a general term comprising the dose, its frequency and the duration of dosing.

Dose-response is the relationship between the dose and the proportion of a population sample showing a defined effect.

Dose-effect is the relationship between the dose and the magnitude of a defined biological effect either in an individual or in a population sample.

Principle of the Test Method

The test substance is applied to the skin in graduated doses to several groups of experimental animals, one dose being used per group. Subsequently, observations of effects and deaths are made. Animals which die during the test are necropsied, and at the conclusion of the test the surviving animals are sacrificed and necropsied. Animals showing severe and enduring signs of distress and pain may need to be humanely killed. Dosing test substances in a way known to cause marked pain and distress due to corrosive or irritating properties need not be carried out.

Description of Test Procedures

Preparations

Healthy young adult animals are acclimated to the laboratory conditions for at least 5 days prior to the test. Before the test, animals are randomised and assigned to the treatment groups. Approximately 24 hours before the test, fur should be removed from the dorsal area of the trunk of the test animals by clipping or shaving. Care must be taken to avoid abrading the skin which could alter its permeability.

Not less than 10 per cent of the body surface area should be clear for the application of the test substance. The weight of the animal should be taken into account when deciding on the area to be cleared and on the dimensions of the covering.

When testing solids, which may be pulverised if appropriate, the test substance should be moistened sufficiently with water or, where necessary, a suitable vehicle to ensure good contact with the skin. When a vehicle is used, the influence of the vehicle on penetration of skin by the test substance should be taken into account. Liquid test substances are generally used undiluted.

Experimental Animals

Selection of species. The adult rat, rabbit or guinea pig may be used. Other species may be used but their use would require justification. The following weight ranges are suggested to provide animals of a size which facilitates the conduct of the test: rats, 200 to 300 g; rabbits, 2.0 to 3.0 kg; guinea pigs, 350 to 450 g. Animals with healthy intact skin are required. (*Note:* In acute toxicity tests with animals of a higher order than rodents, the use of smaller numbers should be considered. Doses should be carefully selected, and every effort should be made not to exceed moderately toxic doses. In such tests, administration of lethal doses of the test substance should be avoided.)

Number and sex. At least 5 animals are used at each dose level. They should all be of the same sex. If females are used, they should be nulliparous and non-pregnant. The use of a smaller number of animals may be justified in some cases. Where information is available demonstrating that a sex is markedly more sensitive, animals of this sex should be dosed.

Housing and feeding conditions. Animals should be caged individually. The temperature of the experimental animal room should be 22 °C (± 3 °) for rodents, 20 °C (± 3 °) for rabbits, and the relative humidity 30–70 per cent. Where the lighting is artificial, the sequence should be 12 hours light, 12 hours dark. For feeding, conventional laboratory diets may be used with an unlimited supply of drinking water.

Test Conditions

Dose levels. These should be sufficient in number, at least three, and spaced appropriately to produce test groups with a range of toxic effects and mortality rates. The data should be sufficient to produce a dose-response curve and, where possible, permit an acceptable determination of the LD50.

Limit test. A limit test at one dose level of at least 2000 mg/kg bodyweight may be carried out in a group of 5 male and 5 female animals, using the procedures described above. If compound-related mortality is produced, a full study may need to be considered.

Observation period. The observation period should be at least 14 days. However, the duration of observation should not be fixed rigidly. It should be determined by the toxic reactions, rate of onset and length of recovery period, and may thus be extended when considered necessary. The time at which signs of toxicity appear and disappear, their duration and the time of death are important, especially if there is a tendency for deaths to be delayed.

Performance of the Test

The test substance should be applied uniformly over an area which is approximately 10 per cent of the total body surface area. With highly toxic substances the surface area covered may be less, but as much of the area should be covered with as thin and uniform a film as possible.

Test substances should be held in contact with the skin with a porous gauze dressing and non-irritating tape throughout a 24-hour exposure period. The test site should be further covered in a suitable manner to retain the gauze dressing and test substance and ensure that the animals cannot ingest the test substance. Restrainers may be used to prevent the ingestion of the test substance, but complete immobilisation is not a recommended method.

At the end of the exposure period, residual test substance should be removed, where practicable using water or an appropriate solvent.

Clinical Examinations

Observations should be recorded systematically as they are made. Individual records should be maintained for each animal. Following application of the test substance, the animals should be observed frequently during the first day and then a careful clinical examination should be made at least once each day. Additional observations should be made directly with appropriate actions taken to minimise loss of animals to the study, e.g., necropsy or refrigeration of those animals found dead and isolation or sacrifice of weak or moribund animals. Cageside observations should include changes in fur, eyes and mucous membranes, and also respiratory, circulatory, autonomic and central nervous system, and somatomotor activity and behavior pattern. Particular attention should be directed to observations of tremors, convulsions, salivation, diarrhea, lethargy, sleep and coma. The time of death must be recorded as precisely as possible.

Individual weights of animals should be determined shortly before the test substance is applied, weekly thereafter, and at death; changes in weight should be calculated and recorded when survival exceeds one day. At the end of the test surviving animals are weighed and then sacrificed.

Pathology

Necropsy of all animals should be carried out and all gross pathological changes should be recorded. Microscopic examination of organs showing evidence of gross pathology in animals surviving 24 or more hours should also be considered because it may yield useful information.

Assessment of Toxicity in the Other Sex

After completion of the study in one sex, at least one group of 5 animals of the other sex is dosed to establish that animals of this sex are not markedly more sensitive to the test substance. The use of fewer animals may be justified in individual circumstances. Where adequate information is available to demonstrate that animals of the sex tested are markedly more sensitive, testing in animals of the other sex may be dispensed with.

Data and Reporting

Treatment of Results

Data may be summarised in tabular form, showing for each test group the number of animals at the start of the test, time of death of individual animals at different dose levels, number of animals displaying other signs of toxicity, description of toxic effects and necropsy findings.

Animals which are humanely killed due to compound-related distress and pain are recorded as compound-related deaths.

The LD50 may be determined by any accepted method, e.g., Bliss (4), Litchfield and Wilcoxon (3), Finney (5), Weil (6), Thompson (7), Miller and Tainter (8).

Evaluation of Results

The dermal LD50 value should always be considered in conjunction with the observed toxic effects and the necropsy findings. The LD50 value is a relatively coarse measurement, useful only as a reference value for classification and labelling purposes, and an expression of the lethal potential of the test substance following dermal exposure.

Reference should always be made to the experimental animal species in which the LD50 value was obtained. An evaluation should include an evaluation of relationships, if any, between the animals' exposure to the test substance and the incidence and severity of all abnormalities, including behavioural and clinical abnormalities, gross lesions, body weight changes, effect on mortality, and any other toxic effects.

Test Report

The test report should include the following information:

- species/strain/source used; environmental conditions
- sex of animals dosed;
- tabulation of response data by dose level (i.e., number of animals that died or were killed durng the test, number of animals showing signs of toxicity, number of animals exposed);
- time of dosing and time of death after dosing;
- LD50 value for the sex dosed (intact skin) determined at 14 days with the method of determination specified;
- 95 per cent confidence interval for the LD50 (where this can be provided);
- dose-mortality curve and slope (where permitted by the method of determination);
- pathology findings; and
- results of any test on the other sex.

Interpretation of the Results

A study of acute toxicity by the dermal (percutaneous) route and determination of a dermal LD50 provides an estimate of the relative toxicity of a substance by the dermal route of exposure.

Extrapolation of the results of acute dermal toxicity studies and dermal

LD50 values in animals to man is valid only to a limited degree. The results of an acute dermal toxicity study should be considered in conjunction with data from acute toxicity studies by other routes.

Literature

(1) WHO Publication: Environmental Health Criteria 6, *Principles and Methods for Evaluating the Toxicity of Chemicals.* Part I, Geneva, 1978.

(2) National Academy of Sciences, Committee for the Revision of NAS Publication 1138, *Principles and Procedures for Evaluating the Toxicity of Household Substances,* Washington, 1977.

(3) Litchfield, J. T., and Wilcoxon, F., *J. Pharmacol., Exp. Ther., 96,* 99–113, 1949.

(4) Bliss, C. I., *Quart. J. Pharm. Pharmacol., 11,* 192–216, 1938.

(5) Finney, D. G., *Probit Analysis.* (3rd Ed.) London, Cambridge University Press, 1971.

(6) Weil, C. S., *Biometrics, 8, 249–263,* 1952.

(7) Thompson, W., *Bact. Rev., 11,* 115–141, 1947.

(8) Miller, L. C. and Tainter, M. L., *Proc. Soc. Exp. Biol. Med. NY, 57,* 261–264, 1944.

ACUTE DERMAL IRRITATION/CORROSION
(GUIDELINE #404)[1]

Introductory Information

Prerequisites

- Solid or liquid test substance
- Chemical identification of test substance
- Purity (impurities) of test substance
- Solubility characteristics
- pH (where appropriate)
- Melting point/boiling point

Standard Documents

There are no relevant international standards.

Method

Introduction, Purpose, Scope, Relevance, Application and Limits of Test

In the assessment and evaluation of the toxic characteristics of a substance, determination of the irritant or corrosive effects on skin of mammals is an important initial step. Information derived from this test serves to indicate the existence of possible hazards likely to arise from exposure to the skin.

Definitions

Dermal irritation is the production of reversible inflammatory changes in the skin following the application of a test substance.

Dermal corrosion is the production of irreversible tissue damage in the skin following the application of a test substance.

Principle of the Test Method

The substance to be tested is applied in a single dose to the skin of several experimental animals, each animal serving as its own control. The degree of

---

[1]Adopted May 12, 1981. Users of this Test Guideline should consult the Preface, in particular paragraphs 3, 4, 7, and 8.

irritation is read and scored at specified intervals and is further described to provide complete evaluation of the effects. The duration of the study should be sufficient to evaluate fully the reversibility or irreversibility of the effects observed.

Description of the Test Procedure

Preparations

Approximately 24 hours before the test, fur should be removed by clipping or shaving from the dorsal area of the trunk of the animals. Care should be taken to avoid abrading the skin. Only animals with healthy intact skin should be used.

When testing solids (which may be pulverised if considered necessary) the test substance should be moistened sufficiently with water or, where necessary, a suitable vehicle, to ensure good contact with the skin. When vehicles are used, the influence of the vehicle on irritation of skin by the test substance should be taken into account. Liquid test substances are generally used undiluted.

Strongly acidic or alkaline substances, for example with a demonstrated pH of 2 or less or 11.5 or greater, need not be tested for primary dermal irritation, owing to their predictable corrosive properties. The testing of materials which have been shown to be highly toxic by the dermal route is unnecessary.

Experimental Animals

Selection of species. Although several mammalian species may be used, the albino rabbit is recommended as the preferred species.

Number of animals. At least 3 healthy adult animals should be used. Additional animals may be required to clarify equivocal response.

Housing and feeding conditions. Animals should be individually housed. The temperature of the experimental animal room should be 22 °C (± 3°) for rodents, 20 °C (± 3°) for rabbits, and the relative humidity 30 to 70 per cent. Where the lighting is artificial, the sequences should be 12 hours light, 12 hours dark. Conventional laboratory diets are suitable for feeding and an unrestricted supply of drinking water should be available.

Test Conditions

Dose level. A dose of 0.5 ml of liquid or 0.5 g of solid or semisolid is applied to the test site. Separate animals are not required for an untreated control group. Adjacent areas of untreated skin of each animal serve as control for the rest.

Observation period. The duration of the observation period should not be fixed rigidly but should be sufficient to evaluate fully the reversibility or irreversibility of the effects observed. It need not normally exceed 14 days after application.

Procedure

The test substance should be applied to a small area (approximately 6 cm^2) of skin and covered with a gauze patch; which is held in place with nonirritating tape. In the case of liquids or some pastes it may be necessary to apply the test substance to the gauze patch and then apply that to the skin. The patch should be loosely held in contact with the skin by means of a suitable semi-occulsive dressing for the duration of the exposure period. However, the use of occlusive dressing may be considered appropriate in some cases. Access by the animal to the patch and resultant ingestion/inhalation of the test substance should be prevented.

Exposure duration is four hours. Longer exposures may be indicated under certain conditions, e.g., expected pattern of human use and exposure. At the end of the exposure period, residual test substance should be removed, where practicable, using water or an appropriate solvent, without altering the existing response or the integrity of the epidermis.

Clinical Observations and Scoring

Animals should be examined for signs of erythema and oedema and the responses scored at 30–60 minutes, and then at 24, 48, and 72 hours after patch removal.

Dermal irritation is scored and recorded according to the grades in Table 1. Further observations may be needed, as necessary to establish reversibility.

TABLE 1 Evaluation of Skin Reaction

Reaction	Value
Erythema and eschar formation	
No erythema	0
Very slight erythema (barely perceptible)	1
Well-defined erythema	2
Moderate to severe erythema	3
Severe erythema (beet redness) to slight eschar formation (injuries in depth)	4
Maximum possible	4
Oedema formation	
No oedema	0
Very slight oedema (barely perceptible)	1
Slight oedema (edges of area well defined by definite raising)	2
Moderate oedema (raised approximately 1 millimetre)	3
Severe oedema (raised more than 1 millimetre and extending beyond area of exposure)	4
Maximum possible	4

In addition to the observation of irritation, any serious lesions and other toxic effects should be fully described.

Data and Reporting

Treatment of Results

Data may be summarised in tabular form, showing for each individual animal the irritation scores for erythema and oedema at 30–60 minutes, 24, 48, and 72 hours after patch removal, any serious lesions, a description of the degree and nature of irritation, corrosion or reversibility, and any other toxic effects observed.

Evaluation of Results

The dermal irritation scores should be evaluated in conjunction with the nature and reversibility or otherwise of the responses observed. The individual scores do not represent any absolute standard for the irritant properties of a material, and they should be viewed as reference values which are only meaningful when supported by a full description and evaluation of the observation(s). The use of an occlusive dressing is a severe test and the results are relevant to very few likely human exposure conditions.

Test Report

The test report must include the following information:

* Species/strain used
* Physical nature and, where appropriate, concentration and pH value for the test substance
* Tabulation of irritation response data for each individual animal for each observation time period (e.g., 30–60 minutes, 24, 48, and 72 hours after patch removal)
* Description of any serious lesions observed
* Narrative description of the degree and nature of irritation observed
* Description of any toxic effects other than dermal irritation

Interpretation of the Results

Extrapolation of the results of dermal irritancy/corrosivity studies in animals to man is valid only to a limited degree. The albino rabbit is more sensitive than man to irritant substances in most cases. The finding of similar results in tests on other animal species may give more weight to extrapolation from animal studies to man.

Literature

(1) WHO Publication: Environmental Health Criteria 6, *Principles and Methods for Evaluating the Toxicity of Chemicals*. Part II, (in preparation).

(2) United States National Academy of Sciences, Committee for the Review of NAS Publication 1138, *Principles and Procedures for Evaluating the Toxicity of Household Substances*, Washington, 1977.

(3) Draize, J. H., Woodard, G. and Calvery, H. O., *J. Pharmacol. Exp. Ther.*, 83, 377–390, 1944.

(4) Draize, J. H. *The Appraisal of Chemicals in Foods, Drugs, and Cosmetics*, pp. 46–48. Association of Food and Drug Officials of the United States, Austin, Texas. 1959.

(5) *Advances in Modern Toxicology*, Vol. 4, Dermatotoxicology and Pharmacology, (Eds. Marzulli, F. N., and Maibach, H. I.), Hemisphere Publ. Co., Washington-London, 1977.

(6) Draize, J. H. *Appraisal of the Safety of Chemicals in Foods, Drugs and Cosmetics:* pp. 46–59. Assoc. of Food and Drug Officials of the United States, Topeka, Kansas, 1965.

ACUTE EYE IRRITATION/CORROSION
(GUIDELINE #405)[1]

Introductory Information

Prerequisites

- Solid or liquid test substance
- Chemical identification of test substance
- Purity (impurities) of test substance
- Solubility characteristics
- pH (where appropriate)
- Melting point/boiling point

Standard Documents

There are no relevant international standards.

Method

Introduction, Purpose, Scope, Relevance, Application and Limits of Test

In the assessment and evaluation of the toxic characteristics of a substance, determination of the irritant and/or corrosive effects on eyes of mammals is an important initial step. Information derived from this test serves to indicate the existence of possible hazards likely to arise from exposure of the eyes and associated mucous membranes to the test substance.

Definitions

Eye irritation is the production of reversible changes in the eye following the application of a test substance to the anterior surface of the eye.

Eye corrosion is the production of irreversible tissue damage in the eye following application of a test substance to the anterior surface of the eye.

Principle of the Test Method

The substance to be tested is applied in a single dose to one of the eyes in

---

[1]Adopted May 12, 1981. Users of this Test Guideline should consult the Preface, in particular, paragraphs 3, 4, 7, and 8.

each of several experimental animals; the untreated eye is used to provide control information. The degree of irritation/corrosion is evaluated and scored at specific intervals and is further described to provide a complete evaluation of the effects. The duration of the study should be sufficient to evaluate fully the reversibility or irreversibility of the effects observed.

Description of the Test Procedure

Preparations

Both eyes of each experimental animal provisionally selected for testing should be examined within 24 hours before testing starts. Animals showing eye irritation, ocular defects or pre-existing corneal injury should not be used. Strongly acidic or alkaline substances, for example with a demonstrated pH of 2 or less or 11.5 or greater, need not be tested owing to their probable corrosive properties.

Materials which have demonstrated definite corrosive or severe irritation in a dermal study need not be further tested for eye irritation. It may be presumed such substances will produce similarly severe effects in the eyes.

Experimental Animals

Selection of species. A variety of experimental animals have been used, but it is recommended that testing should be performed using healthy adult albino rabbits.

Number of animals. At least 3 animals should be used. Additional animals may be required to clarify equivocal responses.

Housing and feeding conditions. Animals should be individually housed. The temperature of the experimental animal room should be 22 °C ($\pm$ 3 °) for rodents, 20 °C ($\pm$ 3 °) for rabbits, and the relative humidity 30 to 70%. Where the lighting is artificial, the sequence should be 12 hours light, 12 hours dark. Conventional laboratory diets are suitable for feeding and an unrestricted supply of drinking water should be available.

Test Conditions

Dose level. For testing liquids, a dose of 0.1 ml is used. In testing solids, pastes, and particulate substances, the amount used should have a volume of 0.1 ml, or a weight of not more than 100 mg (the weight must always be recorded). If the test material is solid or granular it should be ground to a fine dust. The volume of particulates should be measured after gently compacting them, e.g., by tapping the measuring container. To test a substance contained in a pressurised aerosol container the eye should be held open and the test substance administered in a single burst of about one second from a distance of 10 cm directly in front of the eye. The dose may be estimated by weighing the container before and after use. Care should be taken not to damage the eye. Pump sprays should not be used but instead the liquid should be expelled and 0.1 ml collected and instilled into the eye as described for liquids.

Observation period. The duration of the observation period should not be fixed rigidly but should be sufficient to evaluate fully the reversibility or irreversibility of the effects observed. It normally need not exceed 21 days after instillation.

Procedure

The test substance should be placed in the conjunctival sac of one eye of each animal after gently pulling the lower lid away from the eyeball. The lids are then gently held together for about one second in order to prevent loss of the material. The other eye, which remains untreated, serves as a control. If it is thought that the substance could cause extreme pain, a local anaesthetic may be used prior to instillation of the test substance. The type and concentration of the local anaesthetic should be carefully selected to ensure that no significant differences in reaction to the test substance will result from its use. The control eye should be similarly anesthetised.

The eyes of the test animals should not be washed out for 24 hours following instillation of the test substance. At 24 hours a washout may be used if considered appropriate.

For some substances shown to be irritating by this test, additional tests using rabbits with eyes washed soon after instillation of the substance may be indicated. In these cases it is recommended that 6 rabbits be used. Four seconds after instillation of the test substance, the eyes of 3 rabbits are washed, and 30 seconds after instillation the eyes of the other 3 rabbits are washed. For both groups, the eyes are washed for 5 min using a volume and velocity of flow which will not cause injury.

Clinical Observations and Scoring

The eyes should be examined at 1, 24, 48, and 72 hours. If there is no evidence of irritation at 72 hours the study may be ended. Extended observation may be necessary if there is persistent corneal involvement or other ocular irritation in order to determine the progress of the lesions and their reversibility or irreversibility. In addition to the observations of the cornea, iris and conjunctivae, and other lesions which are noted should be recorded and reported. The grades of ocular reaction (Table 1) should be recorded at each examination.

Examination of reactions can be facilitated by use of a binocular loupe, hand slit-lamp, biomicroscope, or other suitable devices. After recording the observations at 24 hours, the eyes of any or all rabbits may be further examined with the aid of fluoroscein.

TABLE 1   Grades for Ocular Lesions

Lesions	Grade
Cornea	
Opacity: degree of density (area most dense taken for reading).	
No ulceration or opacity	0
Scattered or diffuse areas of opacity (other than slight dulling of normal lustre), details of iris clearly visible	1^a
Easily discernible translucent area, details of iris slightly obscured	2^a
Nacreous area, no details of iris visible, size of pupil barely discernible	3^a
Opaque cornea, iris not discernible through the opacity	4^a
Conjunctivae	
Redness (refers to palpebral and bulbar conjunctivae, cornea, and iris).	
Blood vessels normal	0
Some blood vessels definitely hyperaemic (injected)	1
Diffuse, crimson colour, individual vessels not easily discernible	2^a
Diffuse beefy red	3^a
Chemosis; lids and/or nictating membranes	
No swelling	0
Any swelling above normal (includes nictitating membranes)	1
Obvious swelling with partial eversion of lids	2^a
Swelling with lids about half closed	3^a
Swelling with lids more than half closed	4^a
Iris	
Normal	0
Markedly deepened rugae, congestion, swelling, moderate circumcorneal hyperaemia, or injection, any of these or combination of any thereof, iris still reacting to light (sluggish reaction is positive)	1^a
No reaction to light, haemorrhage, gross destruction (any or all of these)	2^a

[a]Indicates positive effect.

Data and Reporting

Treatment of Results

Data may be summarized in tabular form, showing for each individual animal the irritation scores at the designated observation time; a description of the degree and nature of irritation; the presence of serious lesions and any effects other than ocular which were observed.

Evaluation of the Results

The ocular irritation scores should be evaluated in conjunction with the nature and responsibility or otherwise of the responses observed. The individual scores do not represent an absolute standard for the irritant properties of a material. They should be viewed as reference values and are only meaningful when supported by a full description and evaluation of the observations.

Test Report

The test report should include the following information:

- Species/strain used
- Physical nature and, where applicable, concentration and pH value for the test substance
- Tabulation of irritant/corrosive response data for each individual animal at each observation time (e.g., 1, 24, 48, and 72 hours)
- Description of any serious lesions observed
- Narrative description of the degree and nature of irritation of corrosion observed
- Description of the method used to score the irritation at 1, 24, 48, and 72 hours (e.g., hand slit-lamp, biomicroscope, fluorescein)
- Description of any non-ocular topical effects noted

Interpretation of the Results

Extrapolation of the results of eye irritation studies in animals to man is valid only to a limited degree. The albino rabbit is more sensitive than man to ocular irritants or corrosives in most cases. Similar results in tests on other animal species can give more weight to extrapolation from animal studies to man.

Care should be taken in the interpretation of data to exclude irritation resulting from secondary infection.

Literature

(1) WHO Publication: Environmental Health Criteria 6, *Principles and Methods for Evaluating the Toxicity of Chemicals.* Part II, (in preparation).

(2) United States National Academy of Science, Committee for the Revision of NAS Publication 1138, *Principles and Procedures for Evaluating the Toxicity of Household Substances,* Washington, 1977.

(3) Draize, J. H., Woodard, G. and Calvery, H. O., *J. Pharmacol. Exp. Ther.,* 83, 377–390, 1944.

(4) Draize, J. H. *Appraisal of the Safety of Chemicals in Foods, Drugs, and Cosmetics-Dermal Toxicity,* pp. 49–52. Assoc. of Food and Drug Officials of the United States, Topeka, Kansas, 1965.

(5) Draize, J. H. *The Appraisal of Chemicals in Foods, Drugs, and Cosmetics,* pp. 36–45. Association of Food and Drug Officials of the United States, Austin, Texas, 1965.

Appendix

(6) United States Federal Hazardous Substances Act Regulations. Title 16, Code of Federal Regulations, 38 FR 27012, Sept. 27, 1973; 38 FR 30105, Nov. 1, 1973.

(7) Loomis, T. A. *Essentials of Toxicology,* 2d ed., pp. 207–213. Lea & Febiger, Philadelphia, 1974.

SKIN SENSITISATION
(GUIDELINE #406)[1]

Introductory Information

Prerequisites

- Solid or liquid test substance
- Chemical identification of test substance
- Purity (impurities) of test substance
- Solubility characteristics
- pH (where appropriate)
- Melting point/boiling point

Standard Documents

There are no relevant international standards.

Method

Introduction, Purpose, Scope, Relevance, Application and Limits of Test

In the assessment and evaluation of the toxic characteristics of a substance, determination of its potential to provoke skin sensitisation reactions is important. Information derived from tests for the skin sensitisation serves to identify the possible hazard to a population repeatedly exposed to the substance.

While the desirability of this type of safety evaluation is recognised, there are some real differences of opinion about the best method of testing for skin sensitising properties of a new substance. The test selected should be a reliable screening procedure which should not fail to identify substances with significant allergenic potential, while at the same time avoiding false negative results.

Definitions

Skin sensitisation (allergic contact dermatitis) is an immunologically mediated cutaneous reaction to a substance. In the human, the responses may be characterized by pruritis, erythema, oedema, papules, vesicles, bullae or a

---

[1]Adopted May 12, 1981. Users of this Test Guideline should consult the Preface, in particular, paragraphs 3, 4, 7, and 8.

combination of these. In other species the reactions may differ and only erythema and oedema may be seen.

Induction period. A period of at least one week following a sensitisation exposure during which a hypersensitive state is developed.

Induction exposure. An experimental exposure of a subject to a test substance with the intention of inducing a hypersensitive state.

Challenge exposure. An experimental exposure of a previously treated subject to a test substance following an induction period, to determine if the subject will react in a hypersensitive manner.

Principle of the Test Method

Following initial exposure(s) to a test substance, the animals are subsequently subject, after a period of not less than one week, to a challenge exposure with the test substance to establish whether a hypersensitive state has been induced. Sensitisation is determined by examining the reaction to the challenge exposure.

Description of the Test Procedure

Any of the following seven methods is considered to be acceptable. However, it is realised that the methods differ in their probability and degree of reaction to sensitising substances. Periodic uses of a positive control substance with an acceptable level of response in test animals is recommended to assess the reliability of a test system.

- Draize Test
- Freund's Complete Adjuvant Test
- Guinea Pig Maximisation Test
- Split Adjuvant Technique
- Buehler Test
- Open Epicutaneous Test
- Mauer Optimization Test

An additional method which has not, however, been widely used is described in the Annex.

Preparations

Healthy young adult animals are acclimatised to the laboratory conditions for at least 5 days prior to the test. Before the test, animals are randomised and assigned to the treatment groups. Removal of hair is by clipping, shaving or possibly by chemical depilation, depending on the test method used.

Experimental Animals

Selection of species. The guinea pig is the generally recommended species. If other species are used this should be justified.

Number and sex. The number and sex of animals used will depend on the method employed. If females are used, they should be nulliparous and nonpregnant. Animals may act as their own controls of groups if induced animals can be compared to groups which have received only a challenge exposure.

Housing and feeding conditions. The temperature of the experimental animal room should be 22 °C (± 3 °) and the relative humidity 30–70 %. Where the lighting is artificial, the sequence should be 12 hours light, 12 hours dark. For feeding, conventional laboratory diets may be used with an unlimited supply of drinking water. It is essential that guinea pigs receive an adequate amount of ascorbic acid.

Test Conditions

Dose levels. Depending on the method, the concentration used should produce skin reaction following the induction exposure and should be non-irritating following the challenge exposure. These concentrations can be determined by a small scale (2 or 3 animals) pilot study. The use of a control group is recommended.

Observation period. Skin reactions should be recorded 24 hours and 48 hours after the pertinent exposures. These exposures will vary depending on the method used.

Procedures

The principle features of the seven methods mentioned above are given in Table 1.

Data and Reporting

Treatment of Results

Data may be summarised in tabular form, showing for each individual animal the skin reaction results of the induction exposure(s) at 1 and 24 hours, and the challenge exposure(s) at 24 and 48 hours after exposure. As a minimum, the erythema and oedema should be graded. Any unusual finding should be recorded.

Evaluation of the Results

Evaluation of the results will provide information on the proportion of each group that became sensitised and the extent (slight, moderate, severe) of the sensitisation reaction in each individual animal.

Test Report

The test report should contain the following information:

- A description of the method used (and commonly accepted name)
- Species/strain used
- The number and sex of the animals
- Individual weights of the animals at the start of the test

TABLE 1. Principal Features of Test Methods

	Draize	Freund's complete adjuvant (FCA)	Mauer optimisation	Buehler	Open epicutaneous test	Maximisation	Split adjuvant
Species	Guinea pig	Guinea pig	Guinea pig	Guinea pig	Guinea pig	Guiea pig	Guinea pig
Route	id[a]	id	id	ec[b]	ec	id and ec	id and ec
Number in test group	20	8–10	10–10	10–20	6–8	20–25	10–20
Number of test group	—	—	—	—	up to 6	—	—
Number in control group	20	8–10	10–10	10–20	6–8	20–25	10–20
Induction exposure route	id	id	id	dermal	dermal	id and dermal	id and dermal
Number of exposures	10	5	9	3	20 or 21	1 id, 1 dermal	4
Exposure period	—	—	24 hr	6 hr each	continuous	48 hr	48 hr each
Patch type	—	—	—	closed	open	closed	closed
Test group(s)	TS	TS in FCA	TS in FCA	TS	TS	TS, TS + FCA, FCA FCA, FCA + V. V	TS
Control group	—	FCA only	—	—	vehicle (v) only	vehicle	—
Site	L. flank	R. flank	Back	L. flank	R. flank	shoulder	shoulder
Frequency	every 2nd day	every 2nd day	every other day	every 7 days	daily	0 (id), 7d (dermal)	0, 2, 4, 7d
Duration	0–18d	0–8d	0–21d	0–14d	0–20d	0–7d	0–7d
Concentration	2–10 times that of first	same throughout	0.1 ml of 0.1%	same throughout	same per group different between groups	—	same throughout
Challenge exposure route	id	dermal	id	dermal	dermal	dermal	dermal
Number of exposure	—	—	2	—	2	1	1
Day(s)	35	22 & 35	14 & 28	28	21 & 35	21	20
Exposure period	—	—	24 hr	6hr	—	24 hr	24 hr
Patch type	—	open	—	closed	open	closed	closed
Test group(s)	TS	TS	TS	TS	TS	TS	TS
Control group	TS	TS	TS	TS	TS	TS	TS
Site	R. flank	L. flank	back, new site	R. flank	L. flank	L. flank TS R. flank vehicle	shoulder
Concentration	same as first	4 different	0.1 ml of 0.1%	same as induction	4 different	same as 2nd induction	half induction
Evaluation (hr after challenge)	24, 48	24, 48, 72	24	24, 48	24, 48, and/ or 72	24, 48	24, 48
Reference	(2)	(3)	(7)	(4)	(3)	(5)	(6)

[a]Intradermal.
[b]Epicutaneous.

904

- Individual weights of the animals at the conclusion of the test
- A brief description of the grading system
- Each reading made on each individual animal

Interpretation of the Results

The test results should provide an estimate of the overall sensitisation potential of the test substance, i.e., essentially a non-sensitiser, a weak sensitiser, a moderate sensitiser, or a potent sensitiser.

A skin sensitisation study thus provides an assessment of whether or not a test substance could be a likely sensitiser. Extrapolation of these results to man is valid only to a very limited degree. The only generalisation that can be made is that substances which are strong sensitisers in guinea pigs also cause a substantial number of sensitisation reactions in man, whereas weak sensitisers in guinea pigs may or may not cause reactions in man.

Literature

(1) Klecak, G., Chapter 9 in *Advances in Modern Toxicology,* Vol. 4, *Dermatology and Pharmacology* (eds. Marzulli, F. N. and Maibach, H)., publ.: Hemisphere Publishing Corporation, Washington and London, 1977.

(2) Draize, J. H., Food Drug Cosmets. Law J., 10, 722, 1955.

(3) Klecak, G., et al., *J. Soc. Cosm. Chem.,* 28, 53, 1977.

(4) Buehler, E. V., *Toxicol. Appl. Pharmacol.* 6, 341, 1964, also *Arch. Dermatol.* 91, 171, 1965.

(5) Magnusson, B. and Kligman, A. M., *J. Invest. Dermatol.,* 52, 268, 1969; also *Allergic Contact Dermatitis in the Guinea Pig,* publ. Thomas, Springfield, Illinois, 1970.

(6) Maguire, A. C., Immunol. Commun., 1973, 1, 239, *J. Soc. Cosm. Chem.* 24, 151, 1973; also *Animals Models in Dermatology,* (ed. Maibach), publ. Churchill Livingstone, Edinburgh, 1975.

(7) Mauer, T., et al., *Agents and Actions,* 5, 174–179, 1975; also Int. Cong. Series Excerpts Medica No. 376.203, 1975.

Annex to Skin Sensitisation Test

Introductory Information

Prerequisites

- Solid or liquid test substance
- Chemical identification of test substance
- Purity (impurities) of test substance
- Solubility characteristics
- pH (where appropriate)
- Melting point/boiling point

Standard Documents
There are no relevant standards.

Method

Skin sensitisation (allergic contact dermatitis) is a condition occurring in man and some other animals in which skin reactions are exacerbated after two or more exposures to sensitising materials.

Footpad Technique for Evaluating
Sensitisation Potential in Guinea Pigs

A 1.0% mixture (w/v) of the test material is prepared in Freund's Complete Adjuvant (FCA) and stirred gently at room temperature for three hours.

After being allowed to settle for a few minutes, 0.05 ml of the mixture is injected into the front footpad of ten white guinea pigs which have not previously been exposed to test materials by any route.

One week later the test material is dissolved at a concentration of 1.0% in a solvent system of guinea pig fat[2] :dioxane:acetone, 1:2:7. Each previously injected animal is challenged by dropping 0.3 ml on the clipped (not depilated) skin of the lower back. (If a 1.0% solution produces moderate irritation, an 0.1% solution is used.)

An equal number of control guinea pigs which have not been previously exposed to test material, but were injected with FCA, are challenged in an identical manner.

Twenty-four hours after the "drop on" exposure, the stubble of the ex-

---

[2]Method of Preparing Guinea Pig Fat: Any method that produces clean guinea pig fat should be suitable. The following method has consistently provided an adequate product.
1. Strip fat from large, preferably obese, guinea pigs.
2. Freeze.
3. Grind frozen fat with a kitchen-style meat grinder.
4. Add acetone to ground fat (approximately 10:1, acetone:fat). Stir well and heat by placing flask in a hot water bath.
5. Filter (Whatman No. 4 paper or similar, through a Buchner funnel).
6. Add and stir with Norite—warmed.
7. Filter through Whatman No. 4 and Super Cell, pour into beaker.
8. Freeze, fat will solidify on bottom of beaker.
9. Decant acetone and discard.
10. Gently warm fat and vacuum distill off acetone.
11. Pour warmed fat into vials of a size which allow use of one vial per group of sensitisations.
12. Freeze all vials and use as needed. Frozen fat will remain acceptable for at least one year.

posed are is removed with a suitable depilatory[3] followed by a wash with warm (approximately 37 °C) tap water.

Approximately three hours after depilation, the challenged skin site is scored under uniform fluorescent lighting for irritation (erythema and oedema) compared to untreated skin areas.

The grading of redness is as follows: 0 = normal; 1 = slight, just detectable; 2 = moderate, easily seen; 3 = definite deep red, usually hot, not haemorrhagic; 4 = dark red, may show haemorrhagic areas, usually accompanied by marked swelling and increase in temperature of the skin.

The degree of swelling of the skin is determined by picking up a fold of skin about 1 cm in length, feeling it between thumb and forefinger, and grading as follows: 0 = normal; 1 = slight, just detectable; 2 = moderate, easily felt; 3 = marked, difficult to pick up a fold of skin, often visible without feeling the skin.

The total irritation score for each animal equals the sum of redness and swelling and ranges from zero for no irritation to seven for severe irritation.

The exposed skin sites are again graded 24 hours later (48 hours after the "drop on").

The difference between the control guinea pigs (primary irritation) and the injected guinea pigs (sensitisation response) is considered to be a measure of the degree of skin sensitisation.

---

[3]Depilatory: Any depilatory can, if misused, cause serious skin burns and death and therefore should be handled and used correctly. The following depilatory is preferred because of easy handling and excellent results: 6 parts soluble starch, 6 parts talc, 6 parts barium sulphide, 2.7 parts of a granular nonirritant anionic surfactant.

Add the parts in the order listed and mix well. Add cold water to make a viscous paste. Apply to the clipped skin of guinea pigs and allow to remain for about four minutes. Rinse off all traces of depilatory.

REPEATED DOSE DERMAL TOXICITY: 21/28-DAY STUDY (GUIDELINE #410)[1]

Introductory Information

Prerequisites

- Solid or liquid test substance
- Chemical identification of test substance
- Purity (impurities) of test substance
- Solubility characteristics
- pH (where appropriate)
- Stability, including stability in vehicle when so applied
- Melting point/boiling point

Standard Documents

There are no relevant international standards.

Method

Introduction, Purpose, Scope, Relevance, Application and Limits of Test

In the assessment and evaluation of the toxic characteristics of a chemical the determination of subchronic dermal toxicity may be carried out after initial information on toxicity has been obtained by acute testing. It provides information on possible health hazards likely to arise from repeated exposures by the dermal route over a limited period of time.

There is sufficient similarity between the considerations involved in the conduct of a 21-day or 28-day repeated dose dermal study to allow one Guideline to cover both test durations. The main difference lies in the time over which dosing takes place (indicated in the text).

[1]Adopted May 12, 1981. Users of this Test Guideline should consult the Preface, in particular, paragraphs 3, 4, 7, and 8.

Definitions

Dose in a dermal test is the amount of test substance applied to the skin. Dose is expressed as weight (g, mg) or as weight of test substance per unit weight of test animal (e.g., mg/kg).

No-effect level/No-toxic-effect level/No-adverse-effect level is the maximum dose used in a test which produces no adverse effects. A no-effect level is expressed in terms of the weight of a substance given daily per unit weight of test animal (mg/kg).

Cumulative toxicity is the adverse effects of repeated doses occurring as a result of prolonged action on, or increased concentration of the administered substance or its metabolites in, susceptible tissues.

Principles of the Test Method

The test substance is applied daily to the skin in graduated doses to several groups of experimental animals, one dose per group, for a period of 21/28 days. During the period of application the animals are observed daily to detect signs of toxicity. Animals which die during the test are necropsied, and at the conclusion of the test the surviving animals are sacrificed and necropsied.

Description of the Test Procedure

Preparations

Healthy young adult animals are acclimatised to the laboratory conditions for at least 5 days prior to the test. Before the test, animals are randomised and assigned to the treatment and control groups. Shortly before testing fur is clipped from the dorsal area of the trunk of the test animals. Shaving may be employed but it should be carried out approximately 24 hours before the test. Repeat clipping or shaving is usually needed at approximately weekly intervals. When clipping or shaving the fur care must be taken to avoid abrading the skin, which could alter its permeability, unless a requirement for abraded skin is part of the test design. Not less than 10% of the body surface area should be clear for the application of the test substance. The weight of the animal should be taken into account when deciding on the area to be cleared and on the dimensions of the covering. When testing solids, which may be pulverised if appropriate, the test substance should be moistened sufficiently with water or, where necessary, a suitable vehicle to ensure good contact with the skin. When a vehicle is used, the influence of the vehicle on penetration of skin by the test substance should be taken into account. Liquid test substances are generally used undiluted.

Experimental Animals

Selection of species. The adult rat, rabbit, or guinea pig may be used. Other species may be used but their use would require justification.

The following weight ranges at the start of the test are suggested in order to provide animals of a size which facilitates the conduct of the test: rats, 200 to 300 g; rabbits, 2.0 to 3.0 kg; guinea pigs, 350 to 450 g.

Where a repeated dose dermal study is conducted as a preliminary to a long term study, the same species and strain should be used in both studies.

Number and sex. At least 10 animals (5 female and 5 male) with healthy skin should be used at each dose level. The females should be nulliparous and non-pregnant. If interim sacrifices are planned the number should be increased by the number of animals scheduled to be sacrificed before the completion of the study. In addition, a satellite group of 10 animals (5 animals per sex) may be treated with the high dose level for 21/28 days and observed for reversibility, persistence, or delayed occurrence of toxic effects for 14 days post-treatment.

Housing and feeding conditions. Animals should be caged individually. The temperature in the experimental animal room should be 22 °C (± 3 °) for rodents or 20 °C (± 3 °) for rabbits and the relative humidity 30–70 %. When the lighting is artificial, the sequence should be 12 hours light, 12 hours dark. For feeding, conventional laboratory diets may be used with an unlimited supply of drinking water.

Test Conditions

Dose levels. At least three dose levels, with a control and, where appropriate, a vehicle control, should be used. Except for treatment with the test substances, animals in the control group should be handled in an identical manner to the test group subjects. The highest dose level should result in toxic effects but not produce an incidence of fatalities which would prevent a meaningful evaluation. The lowest dose level should not produce any evidence of toxicity. Where there is a usable estimation of human exposure the lowest level should exceed this. Ideally, the intermediate dose level(s) should produce minimal observable toxic effects. If more than one intermediate dose is used the dose levels should be spaced to produce a gradation of toxic effects. In the low and intermediate groups and in the controls the incidence of fatalities should be low, in order to permit a meaningful evaluation of the results.

If application of the test substance produces severe skin irritation, the concentration may be reduced although this may result in a reduction in, or absence of, other toxic effects at the high dose level. However, if the skin has been damaged badly early in the study it may be necessary to terminate the study and undertake a new study at lower concentrations.

Limit test. If a test at one dose level of at least 1000 mg/kg body weight (but expected human exposure may indicate the need for a higher dose level), using the procedures described for this study, produces no observable toxic effects and if toxicity would not be expected based upon data from structurally related compounds, then a full study using three dose levels may not be considered necessary.

Observations. A careful clinical examination should be made at least once each day. Additional observations should be made daily with appropriate actions taken to minimise loss of animals to thè study, e.g., necropsy or refrigeration of those animals found dead and isolation or sacrifice of weak or moribund animals.

Procedure

The animals are treated with the test substance, ideally for at least 6 hours per day on a 7-day per week basis, for a period of 21/28 days. However, based primarily on practical considerations, application on a 5-day per week basis is considered to be acceptable. Animals in a satellite group scheduled for follow-up observations should be kept for a further 14 days without treatment to detect recovery from, or persistence of, toxic effect.

The test substance should be applied uniformly over an area which is approximately 10 per cent of the total body surface area. With highly toxic substances the surface area covered may be less but as much of the area should be covered with as thin and uniform a film as possible.

Between applications the test substance is held in contact with the skin with a porous gauze dressing and non-irritating tape. The test site should be further covered in a suitable manner to retain the gauze dressing and test substance and ensure that the animals cannot ingest the test substance. Restrainers may be used to prevent ingestion of the test substance but complete immobilisation is not a recommended method.

Signs of toxicity should be recorded as they are observed including the time of onset, the degree and duration. Cage-side observations should include, but not be limited to, changes in skin and fur, eyes and mucous membranes and also respiratory, circulatory, autonomic and central nervous system, somatomotor activity and behaviour pattern. Measurements should be made of food consumption weekly and the animals weighed weekly. Regular observation of the animals is necessary to ensure that animals are not lost from the study due to causes such as cannibalism, autolysis of tissues or misplacement. At the end of the study period all survivors in the non-satellite treatment groups are sacrificed. Moribund animals should be removed and sacrificed when noticed.

Clinical Examinations

The following examinations should be made on all animals:

a. Haematology, including haematocrit, haemoglobin concentration, erythrocyte count, total and differential leucocyte count, and a measure of clotting potential such as clotting time, prothrombin time, thromboplastin time, or platelet count should be investigated at the end of the test period.

b. Clinical biochemistry determination on blood should be carried out at the end of the test period. Blood parameters of liver and kidney function are appropriate. The selection of specific tests will be influenced by observations on the mode of action of the substance. Suggested determinations are: calcium, phosphorus, chloride, sodium, potassium, fasting glucose (with period of fasting appropriate to the species), serum glutamic-pyruvic transaminase,[2] serum glutamicoxaloacetic transaminase,[3] ornithine decarboxylase, gamma glutamyl transpeptidase, urea nitrogen, albumen, blood creatinine, total bilirubin and total serum protein measurements. Other determinations which may be necessary for an adequate toxicological evaluation include analyses of lipids, hormones, acid/base balance, methaemoglobin, and cholinesterase activity. Additional clinical biochemistry may be employed, where necessary, to extend the investigation of observed effects.

c. Urinalysis is not required on a routine basis, but only when there is an indication based on expected or observed toxicity.

If historical baseline data are inadequate, consideration should be given to determination of haematological and clinical biochemistry parameters before dosing commences.

Pathology

Gross necropsy. All animals in the study should be subjected to a full gross necropsy which includes examination of the external surface of the body, all orifices, and the cranial, thoracic and abdominal cavities and their contents. The liver, kidneys, adrenals and testes must be weighed wet as soon as possible after dissection to avoid drying. The following organs and tissues should be preserved in a suitable medium for possible future histopathological examination: normal and treated skin, liver, kidney and target organs, that is, those organs showing gross lesions or changes in size.

Histopathology. Histological examination should be performed on the preserved organs and tissues of the high dose group and the control group. These examinations may be extended to animals of other dosage groups, if considered necessary to investigate the changes observed in the high dose group. Animals in the satellite group should be examined histologically with particular emphasis on those organs and tissues identified as showing effects in the other treated groups.

Data and Reporting

Treatment of Results

Data may be summarised in tabular form, showing for each test group the number of animals at the start of the test, the number of animals showing lesions, the type of lesions and the percentage of animals displaying each type of lesion.

All observed results, quantitative and incidental, should be evaluated by

[2]Now known as serum alanine aminotransferase.
[3]Now known as serum aspartate aminotransferase.

an appropriate statistical method. Any generally accepted statistical method may be used; the statistical method should be selected during the design of the study.

Evaluation of the Results

The findings of a repeated dose dermal toxicity study should be considered in terms of the observed toxic effects and the necropsy and histopathological findings. The evaluation will include the relationship between the dose of the test substance and the presence or absence, the incidence and severity, of abnormalities, including behavioural and clinical abnormalities, gross lesions, identified target organs, body weight changes, effects on mortality and any other general or specific toxic effects. A properly conducted 21/28-day study will provide information on the effects of repeated dermal application of a substance and can indicate the need for further longer term studies. It can also provide information on the selection of dose levels for longer term studies.

Test Report

The test report must include the following information:

- Species/strain used
- Toxic response data by sex and dose
- Time of death during the study or whether animals survived to termination
- Toxic or other effects
- The time of observation of each abnormal sign and its subsequent course
- Food and body weight data
- Haematological tests employed and results with relevant baseline data
- Clinical biochemistry tests employed and results with relevant baseline data
- Necropsy findings
- A detailed description of all histopathological findings
- Statistical treatment of results where appropriate

Interpretation of the Results

A repeated dose dermal study will provide information on the effects of repeated dermal exposure to a substance. Extrapolation from the results of the study to man is valid to a limited degree, but it can provide useful information on the degree of percutaneous absorption of a substance.

Literature

(1) WHO Publication: Environmental health Criteria. No. 6, *Principles and Methods for Evaluating the Toxicity of Chemicals. Part I.* Geneva, 1978.

SUBCHRONIC DERMAL TOXOCITY: 90-DAY STUDY (GUIDELINE #411)[1]

Introductory Information

Prerequisites

- Solid or liquid test substance
- Chemical identification of test substance
- Purity (impurities) of test substance
- Solubility characteristics
- pH (where appropriate)
- Stability, including stability in vehicle when so applied
- Melting point/boiling point

Standard Documents

There are no relevant international standards.

Method

Introduction, Purpose, Scope, Relevance, Application and Limits of Test

In the assessment and evaluation of the toxic characteristics of a chemical the determination of subchronic dermal toxicity may be carried out after initial information on toxicity has been obtained by acute testing. It provides information on possible health hazards likely to arise from repeated exposure by the dermal route over a limited period of time.

Definitions

Subchronic dermal toxicity is the adverse effects occurring as a result of the repeated daily dermal application of a chemical to experimental animals for part (not exceeding 10%) of a life span.

Dose in a dermal test is the amount of test substance applied to the skin

---

[1]Adopted May 12, 1981. Users of this Test Guideline should consult the Preface, in particular, paragraphs 3, 4, 7, and 8.

(applied daily in subchronic tests). Dose is expressed as weight (g, mg) or as weight of the test substance per unit weight of test animal (e.g., mg/kg).

No-effect level/No-toxic-effect level/No-adverse-effect level is the maximum dose used in a test which produces no adverse effects. A no-effect level is expressed in terms of the weight of a substance given daily per unit weight of test animal (mg/kg).

Cumulative toxicity is the adverse effects of repeated doses occurring as a result of prolonged action on, or increased concentration of the administered substance or its metabolites in, susceptible tissues.

Principle of the Test Method

The test substance is applied daily to the skin in graduated doses to several groups of experimental animals, one dose per group, for a period of 90 days. During the period of application the animals are observed daily to detect signs of toxicity. Animals which die during the test are necropsied, and at the conclusion of the test the surviving animals are sacrificed and necropsied.

Description of the Test Procedure

Preparations

Healthy young adult animals are acclimatised to the laboratory conditions for at least 5 days prior to the test. Before the test, animals are randomised and assigned to the treatment and control groups. Shortly before testing fur is clipped from the dorsal area of the trunk of the test animals. Shaving may be employed but it should be carried out approximately 24 hours before the test. Repeat clipping or shaving is usually needed at approximately weekly intervals. When clipping or shaving the fur care must be taken to avoid abrading the skin, which could alter its permeability. Not less than 10% of the body surface area should be clear for the application of the test substance. The weight of the animal should be taken into account when deciding on the area to be cleared and on the dimensions of the covering. When testing solids, which may be pulverised if appropriate, the test substance should be moistened sufficiently with water or, where necessary, a suitable vehicle to ensure good contact with the skin. When a vehicle is used, the influence of the vehicle on penetration of skin by the test substance should be taken into account. Liquid test substances are generally used undiluted.

Experimental Animals

Selection of species. The adult rat, rabbit, or guinea pig may be used. Other species may be used but their use would require justification.

The following weight ranges at the start of the test are suggested in order to provide animals of a size which facilitates the conduct of the test: rats, 200 to 300 g; rabbits, 2.0 to 3.0 kg; guinea pigs, 350 to 450 g.

Where a subchronic dermal study is conducted as a preliminary to a long term study, the same species and strain should be used in both studies.

Number and sex. At least 20 animals (10 female and 10 male) with healthy skin should be used at each dose level. The females should be nulliparous and non-pregnant. If interim sacrifices are planned the number should be increased by the number of animals scheduled to be sacrificed before the completion of the study. In addition, a satellite group of 20 animals (10 animals per sex) may be treated with the high dose level for 90 days and observed for reversibility, persistence, or delayed occurrence of toxic effects for a post-treatment period of appropriate length, normally not less than 28 days..

Housing and feeding conditions. Animals should be caged individually. The temperature in the experimental animal room should be 22 °C (± 3°) for rodents or 20 °C (± 3°) for rabbits and the relative humidity 30–70%. When the lighting is artificial, the sequence should be 12 hours light, 12 hours dark. For feeding, conventional laboratory diets may be used with an unlimited supply of drinking water.

Test Conditions

Dose levels. At least three dose levels, with a control and (where appropriate) a vehicle control should be used. Except for treatment with the test substances, animals in the control group should be handled in an identical manner to the test group subjects. The highest dose level should result in toxic effects but not produce an incidence of fatalities which would prevent a meaningful evaluation. The lowest dose level should not produce any evidence of toxicity. Where there is a usable estimation of human exposure the lowest level should exceed this. Ideally, the intermediate dose level(s) should produce minimal observable toxic effects. If more than one intermediate dose is used the dose levels should be spaced to produce a gradation of toxic effects. In the low and intermediate groups and in the controls the incidence of fatalities should be low, in order to permit a meaningful evaluation of the results.

If application of the test substance produces severe skin irritation, the concentration may be reduced although this may result in a reduction in, or absence of, other toxic effects at the high dose level. However, if the skin has been badly damaged early in the study, it may be necessary to terminate the study and undertake a new study at lower concentrations.

Limit test. If a test at one dose level of at least 1000 mg/kg body weight (but expected human exposure may indicate the need for a high dose level), using the procedures described for this study, produces no observable toxic effects and if toxicity would not be expected based upon data from structurally related compounds, then a full study using three dose levels may not be considered necessary.

Observations. A careful clinical examination should be made at least once each day. Additional observations should be made daily with appropriate actions taken to minimise loss of animals to the study, e.g., necropsy or refrigeration of those animals found dead and isolation or sacrifice of weak or moribund animals.

Procedure

The animals are treated with the test substance, ideally for at least 6 hours per day on a 7-day per week basis, for a period of 90 days. However, based primarily on practical considerations, application on a 5-day per week basis is considered to be acceptable. Animals in a satellite group scheduled for follow-up observations should be kept for at least a further 28 days without treatment to detect recovery from, or persistence of, toxic effect.

The test substance should be applied uniformly over an area which is approximately 10 per cent of the total body surface area. With highly toxic substances the surface area covered may be less, but as much of the area should be covered with as thin and uniform a film as possible.

Between applications the test substance is held in contact with the skin with a porous gauze dressing and non-irritating tape. The test site should be further covered in a suitable manner to retain the gauze dressing and test substance and ensure that the animals cannot ingest the test substance. Restrainers may be used to prevent ingestion of the test substance, but complete immobilisation is not a recommended method.

Signs of toxicity should be recorded as they are observed, including the time of onset, the degree and duration. Cage-side observations should include, but not be limited to, changes in skin and fur, eyes and mucous membranes, as well as respiratory, circulatory, autonomic and central nervous system, somatomotor activity and behaviour pattern. Measurements should be made of food consumption weekly and the animals weighed weekly. Regular observation of the animals is necessary to ensure that animals are not lost from the study due to causes such as cannibalism, autolysis of tissues or misplacement. At the end of the study period all survivors in the non-satellite treatment groups are sacrificed. Moribund animals should be removed and sacrificed when noticed.

Clinical Examinations

The following examinations should be made on all animals:

a. Ophthalmological examination, using an ophthalmoscope or equivalent suitable equipment, should be made prior to exposure to the test substance and at the termination of the study, preferably in all animals but at least in the high dose and control groups. If changes in the eyes are detected all animals should be examined.

b. Haematology, including haematocrit, haemoglobin concentration, erythrocyte count, total and differential leucocyte count, and a measure of clotting potential, such as clotting time, prothrombin time, thromboplastin time, or platelet count, should be investigated at the end of the test period.

b. Clinical biochemistry determinations on blood should be carried out at the end of the test period. Test areas which are considered appropriate to all studies are electrolyte balance, carbohydrate metabolism, liver and kidney function. The selection of specific tests will be influenced by observations on the mode of action of the substance. Suggested determinations are: calcium, phosphorus, chloride, sodium, potassium, fasting glucose (with period of fasting appropriate to the species), serum glutamicpyruvic transaminase,[2] serum glutamic oxaloacetic transaminase,[3] ornithine decarboxylase, gamma glutamyl transpeptidase, urea nitrogen, albumen, blood creatinine, total bilirubin and total serum protein measurements. Other determinations which may be necessary for an adequate toxicological evaluation include analyses of lipids, hormones, acid/base balance, methaemoglobin, cholinesterase activity. Additional clinical biochemistry may be employed, where necessary, to extend the investigation of observed effects.

c. Urinalysis is not required on a routine basis, but only when there is an indication based on expected or observed toxicity.

If historical baseline data are inadequate, consideration should be given to determination of haematological and clinical biochemistry parameters before dosing commences.

Pathology

Gross necropsy. All animals in the study should be subjected to a full gross necropsy which includes examination of the external surface of the body, all orifices, and the cranial, thoracic and abdominal cavities and their contents. The liver, kidneys, adrenals and testes must be weighed wet as soon as possible after dissection to avoid drying. The following organs and tissues should be preserved in a suitable medium for possible future histopathological examination: all gross lesions, brain—including sections of medulla/pons, cerebellar cortex and cerebral cortex, pituitary, thyroid/parathyroid, thymus, (trachea), lungs, heart, aorta, salivary glands, liver, spleen, kidneys, adrenals, pancreas, gonads, accessory genital organs, gall bladder (if present), esophagus, stomach, duodenum, jejunum, ileum, caecum, colon, rectum, urinary bladder, representative lymph node, (female mammary gland), (thigh musculature), peripheral nerve, (eyes), (sternum with bone marrow), (femur—including articular surface), (spinal cord at three levels—cervical, midthoracic and lumbar), and (extraorbital lachrymal glands). (The tissues mentioned in parentheses need only be examined if indicated by signs of toxicity or target organ involvement.).

Histopathology. (a) Full histopathology should be carried out on normal

[2]Now known as serum alanine aminotransferase.
[3]Now known as serum aspartate aminotransferase.

and treated skin and on organs and tissues of all animals in the control and high dose groups. (b) All gross lesions should be examined. (c) Target organs in other dose groups should be examined. (d) Where rats are used lungs of animals in the low and intermediate dose groups should be subjected to histopathological examination for evidence of infection, since this provides a convenient assessment of the state of health of the animals. Further histopathological examination may not be required routinely on the animals in these groups but must always be carried out in organs which showed evidence of lesions in the high dose group. (e) When a satellite group is used histopathology should be performed on tissues and organs identified as showing effects in other treated groups.

Data and Reporting

Treatment of Results

Data may be summarised in tabular form, showing for each test group the number of animals at the start of the test, the number of animals showing lesions, the type of lesions and the percentage of animals displaying each type of lesion.

All observed results, quantitative and incidental, should be evaluated by an appropriate statistical method. Any generally accepted statistical method may be used; the statistical method should be selected during the design of the study.

Evaluation of the Results

The findings of a subchronic dermal toxicity study should be evaluated in conjunction with the findings of preceding studies and considered in terms of the observed toxic effects and the necropsy and histopathological findings. The evaluation will include the relationship between the dose of the test substance and the presence or absence, the incidence and severity, of abnormalities, including behavioural and clinical abnormalities, gross lesions, identified target organs, body weight changes, effects on mortality and any other general or specific toxic effects. A properly conducted subchronic test should provide a satisfactory estimation of a no-effect level.

Test Report

The test report must include the following information:

- Species/strain used
- Toxic response data by sex and dose
- Time of death during the study or whether animals survived to termination
- Toxic or other effects
- The time of observation of each abnormal sign and its subsequent course

- Food and body weight data
- Haematological tests employed and results with relevant baseline data
- Clinical biochemistry tests employed and results with relevant baseline data
- Necropsy findings
- A detailed description of all histopathological findings
- Statistical treatment of results where appropriate

Interpretation of the Results

A subchronic dermal study will provide information on the effects of repeated dermal exposure to a substance. Extrapolation from the results of the study to man is valid to a limited degree, but it can provide useful information on the degree of percutaneous absorption of a substance, no-effect levels and permissible human exposure.

Literature

(1) WHO Publication: Environmental Health Criteria. No. 6, *Principles and Methods for Evaluating the Toxicity of Chemicals. Part I.* Geneva, 1978.

(2) United States National Academy of Sciences, Committee for the Revision of NAS Publication 1138, *Principles and Procedures for Evaluating the Toxicity of Household Substances,* Washington, 1977.

(3) Draize, J. H., *The Appraisal of Chemicals in Food, Drugs and Cosmetics,* 26–30. Association of Food and Drug Officials of the United States, Austin, Texas, 1959.

(4) Hagan, E. G., *Appraisal of the Safety of Chemicals. Appraisal of Chemicals in Foods, Drugs and Cosmetics,* 17–25. Association of Food and Drug Officials of the United States, Topeka, Kansas, 1965.

DERMAL TESTS REQUIRED
BY THE U.S. ENVIRONMENTAL PROTECTION AGENCY

The *Code of Federal Regulations* (40 CFR; 1989), parts 150 to 189, describes the U.S. Environmental Protection Agency's (EPA) pesticides programs. The Pesticide Assessment Guidelines (40 CFR §158.108) "contain the standards for conducting acceptable tests, guidance on evaluation and reporting of data, definition of terms, further guidance on when data are required, and examples of acceptable protocols." They can be obtained from the National Technical Informations Service, 5284 Port Royal Road, Springfield, VA 22161 (703-487-4650). They include Subdivision F (Hazard Evaluation: Humans and Domestic Animals; PB83-153916) and Subdivision M (Biorational Pesticides and Microbial & Biochemical Pest Control Agents; PB83-153965). The EPA recently asked the public for proposed changes in the Subdivision F Guidelines, and the scientific rationale and documentation for the changes (*Federal Register,* Vol. 55, #182, 1990).

Part 158 (40 CFR) gives the data requirements for registration, and includes the following tables:

Submitted by Van Seabaugh.

§158. 340 Toxicology data requirements. (a) Table. Sections 158.50 and 158.100 through 158.102 describe how to use this table to determine the toxicology data requirements and the substance to be tested.

Kind of data required	(b) Notes	Terrestrial Food crop	Terrestrial Nonfood crop	Aquatic Food crop	Aquatic Nonfood crop	Greenhouse Food crop	Greenhouse Nonfood crop	Forestry	Domestic outdoor	Indoor	Test substance Data to support MP	Data to support EP	Guidelines reference No.
Acute testing													
Acute oral toxicity—rat	(1)	[R]	[R]	[R]	[R]	[R]	[R]	[R]	[R]	[R]	MP and TGAI	EP* or EP dilution* and TGAI	81-1
Acute dermal toxicity	(1), (2)	[R]	[R]	[R]	[R]	[R]	[R]	[R]	[R]	[R]	MP and TGAI	EP* or EP dilution* and TGAI	81-2
Acute inhalation toxicity—rat.	(16)	[R]	[R]	[R]	[R]	[R]	[R]	[R]	[R]	[R]	MP and TGAI	EP* and TGAI	81-3
Primary eye irritation—rabbit.	(2)	[R]	[R]	[R]	[R]	[R]	[R]	[R]	[R]	[R]	MP	EP*	81-4
Primary dermal irritation	(1), (2)	[R]	[R]	[R]	[R]	[R]	[R]	[R]	[R]	[R]	MP	EP*	81-5
Dermal sensitization	(3)	[R]	[R]	[R]	[R]	[R]	[R]	[R]	[R]	[R]	MP	EP*	81-6
Acute delayed neurotoxicity—hen.	(4)	[R]	[R]	[R]	[R]	[R]	[R]	[R]	[R]	[R]	TGAI	TGAI	81-7
Subchronic testing													
90-day feeding studies—rodent and nonrodent.	(17)	[R]	CR	CR	CR	CR	CR	CR	CR	CR	TGAI	TGAI	82-1
21-day dermal	(18)	CR	CR	CR	CR	CR	CR	CR	CR	CR	TGAI	TGAI and EP*	82-2
90-day dermal	(5), (19)	CR	CR	CR	CR	CR	CR	CR	CR	CR	TGAI	TGAI	82-3
90-day inhalation—rat	(6)	CR	CR	CR	CR	CR	CR	CR	CR	CR	TGAI	TGAI	82-4
90-day neurotoxicity:													
Hen	(7)	CR	CR	CR	CR	CR	CR	CR	CR	CR	TGAI	TGAI	82-5
Mammal	(8)	CR	CR	CR	CR	CR	CR	CR	CR	CR	TGAI	TGAI	82-5
Chronic testing													
Chronic feeding—2 spp.	(9), (13)	[R]	CR	[R]	CR	CR	CR	CR	CR	CR	TGAI	TGAI	83-1

924

Data requirement	Notes	1	2	3	4	5	6	7	8	Test substance	Test substance	Guideline
Oncogenicity study—2 Spp. rat and mouse preferred.	(9), (21)	R	CR	R	CR	CR	CR	CR	CR	TGAI	TGAI	83-2
Teratogenicity—2 species	(10), (15)	[R]	CR	[R]	CR	CR	CR	CR	CR	TGAI	TGAI	83-3
Reproduction, 2-generation.	(11), (14)	[R]	CR	[R]	CR	CR	CR	CR	CR	TGAI	TGAI	83-4
Mutagenicity testing												
Gene mutation	(22)	[R]	R	[R]	R	R	R	R	R	TGAI	TGAI	84.2
Structural chromosomal aberration.	(22)	[R]	R	[R]	R	R	R	R	R	TGAI	TGAI	84.2
Other genotoxic effects Special testing	(22)	[R]	R	[R]	R	R	R	R	R	TGAI	TGAI	84.4
General metabolism	(23)	R	CR	R	CR	CR	CR	CR	CR	PAI or PAIRA	PAI or PAIRA	85-1
Dermal penetration	(24)	CR	CR	CR	CR	CR	CR	CR	CR	Choice	Choice	85-2
Domestic animal safety	(12)	CR	CR	CR	CR	CR	CR	CR	CR	Choice	Choice	86-1

Key: R = Required data; CR = Conditionally required. [ ] = Brackets (ie [R], [CR] indicate date requirements that apply when an experimental use permit is being sought; MP = manufacturing-use product; EP* = End-Use Product; (asterisk identifies those data requirements that end-use applicants (i.e. "formulators") must satisfy, provided that their active ingredient(s) is (are) purchased from a registered source); TGAI = Technical grade of the active ingredient; PAI = "Pure" active ingredient; PAIRA = "Pure" active ingredient, radio-labeled; Choice = choice of several test substances, depending on studies required.

(b) Notes—The following notes are referenced in column two of the table contained in paragraph (a) of this section.

(1) Not required if test material is a gas or highly volatile.

(2) Not required if test material is corrosive to skin or has pH less than 2 or greater than 11.5; such a product will be classified as toxicity category I on the basis of potential eye and dermal irritation effects.

(3) Required unless repeated dermal exposure does not occur under conditions of use.

(4) Not required unless test material, is an organophosphate, or a metabolite or degradation product thereof which causes acetyl cholinesterase depression or is structurally related to a substance that causes delayed neurotoxicity.

(5) Required if use involves purposeful dermal application to, or prolonged exposure of, human skin.

(6) Required if use may result in repeated inhalation exposure at a concentration likely to be toxic. A test with duration of 21 days is required if pesticide is used on tobacco.

(7) Required if acute delayed neurotoxicity test showed neuropathy or neurotoxicity or if closely related structural to a compound which can induce these effect.

(8) Required if acute oral, dermal, or inhalation studies showed neuropathy or neurotoxicity.

(9)(i) Studies designed to simultaneously meet the requirements of both the chronic feeding and oncogenicity studies (i.e., a combined study) can be conducted.

(continued on next page)

(ii) Minimum acceptable test durations for chronic feeding and oncogenicity studies are as follows:

(A) Chronic rodent feeding study (food use pesticides)—24 months.

(B) Chronic rodent feeding study (non-food pesticides)—12 months.

(C) Chronic nonrodent (i.e., dog) feeding study—12 months.

(D) Mouse oncogenicity study—18 months.

(E) Rat oncogenicity study—24 months.

(10) Required to support products intended for food uses and to support products intended for non-food uses if significant exposure of human females of child bearing age may reasonably be expected.

(11) Required to support products intended for food uses and to support products intended for non-food uses if use of the product is likely to result in human exposure over a portion of the human lifespan which is significant in terms of the frequency of exposure, magnitude of exposure, or the duration of exposure (for example; pesticides used in treated fabrics for wearing apparel, diapers, or bedding; insect repellents applied directly to human skin; swimming pool additives; constant-release indoor pesticides which are used in aerosol form).

(12) Required on a case by case basis.

(13) In most cases, where theoretical maximum residue contribution (TMRC) exceeds 50 percent of the maximum permitted intake (MPI), a one year (or longer) interim report on a chronic feed study is required to support a temporary tolerance.

(14) In most cases, where theoretical maximum residue contribution (TMRC) exceeds 50 percent of the maximum permitted intake (MPI), a first generation (or longer) interim report on multigeneration reproduction study is required to support a temporary tolerance.

(15) A teratology study in one species is required to support a temporary tolerance.

(16) Required if the product consists of, or under conditions of use will result in, an inhalable material (e.g. gas volatile substances, or aerosol/particulate).

(17) Required if intended use(s) of the pesticide product is expected to result in human exposure to the product, under the following conditions:

(i) Human exposure is via the oral route.

(ii) Expected human exposure is over a limited portion of the human lifespan, yet is significant in terms of the frequency of exposure, magnitude of exposure, or the duration of exposure (for example, products requiring a temporary tolerance to support an experimental use permit or emergency exemption).

(18) Required if intended use(s) of the pesticide product is expected to result in human exposure to the product, under the following conditions:

(i) Human exposure is via skin contact.

(ii) Expected human skin contact is not purposeful, and such exposure is of limited frequence and duration (for example, such exposure could result from use of certain disinfectant, liquid fumigant or agricultural or home/garden pesticide products, and other circumstances where the Agency determines that more than acute dermal exposure is involved).

(iii) Data from a subchronic 90-day dermal toxicity study are not required.

(19) Required if pesticide use will involve purposeful application to the human skin or will result in comparable human exposure to the product, (e.g, swimming pool algaecides, pesticides for impregnating clothing), and if either of the following criteria are met:

(i) Data from a subchronic oral study are not required.

(ii) The active ingredient of the product is known or expected to be metabolized differently by the dermal route of exposure than by the oral route, and metabolite of the active ingredient is the toxic moiety.

(20) Required if either of the following criteria are met:

(i) Use of the pesticide product is likely to result in repeated human exposure to the product, over a significant portion of the human life-span (for example, products intended for use and around residences, swimming pools, and enclosed working spaces or their immediate vicinity).

(ii) The use requires a tolerance for the pesticide or an exemption from the requirement to obtain a tolerance, or requires issuance of a food additive regulation.

(21) Required if any of the following criteria are met:

(i) The active ingredient(s) or any of its (their) metabolites, degradation products, or impurities.

(A) Is structurally related to a recognized carcinogen.

(B) Is a substance that causes mutagenic effect as demonstrated by *in vitro* or *in vivo* testing.

(C) Produces in subchronic studies a morphologic effect (e.g., hyperplasia, metaplasia) in any organ that may lead to neoplastic change.

(ii) The use requires a tolerance for the pesticide or exemption from the requirement to obtain a tolerance, or requires the issuance of a food additive regulation.

(iii) Use of the pesticide product is likely to result in human exposure over a portion of the human lifespan which is significant in terms of either the time the exposure occurs or the duration of exposure (for example; pesticides used in treated fabrics for wearing apparel, diapers, or bedding; insect repellents applied directly to human skin, swimming pool additives; constant release indoor pesticides which are used in aerosol form).

(22)(i) The required battery of mutagenicity tests must include tests appropriate to address the following three categories in accordance with the objectives set forth in §158.202.

(A) Gene mutations.

(B) Structural chromosomal aberrations.

(C) Other genotoxic effects as appropriate for the test substance, e.g., numerical chromosome aberrations, direct DNA damage and repair, mammalian cells transformation, target organ/cell analysis.

(ii) Currently recognized tests for each of these categories are listed with the National Technical Information Service (NTIS). Applicants shall explain their reasons for selecting specific tests from the battery of currently recognized tests. Because of the rapid improvements in this field, applicants are encouraged to discuss with the Agency: test selection, protocol design, and results of preliminary testing.

(iii) Not required if the pesticide use pattern precludes human exposure (e.g., nonvolatile pesticides packaged and used in enclosed bait boxes).

(23) Required if chronic feeding or oncogenicity studies are required.

(24) Dermal absorption studies required for compounds having a serious toxic effect as identified by oral or inhalation studies, for which a significant route of human exposure is dermal and for which the assumption of 100 percent absorption does not produce an adequate margin of safety. Registrants should work closely with the Agency in developing an acceptable protocol and performing dermal absorption studies.

(Approved by the Office of Management and Budget under control numbers 2000-0483 and 2000-0468) [49 FR 42881, Oct. 24, 1984. Redesignated and amended at 53 FR 15993, 15999, May 4, 1988]

927

(A) The subchronic effect levels established in the Tier subchronic oral toxicity studies, the Tier I subchronic dermal toxicity studies or the Tier I subchronic inhalation toxicity study.

(B) The pesticide use pattern (e.g., rate, frequency, and site of application).

(C) The frequency and level of repeated human exposure that is expected.

(xiii) Required if the product meets either of the following criteria:

(A) The active ingredient(s) or any of its (their) metabolites, degradation products, or impurities produce(s) in Tier I subchronic studies a morphologic effect (e.g., hyperplasia, metaplasia, and any organ that potentially could lead to neoplastic change.

(B) If adverse cellular effects suggesting oncogenic potential are observed in Tier I or Tier II immune response studies or in Tier II mammalian mutagenicity assays.

(xiv) Required if the product consists of, or under conditions of use results in, an inhalable material (e.g., gas, volatile substance, or aerosol/particulate).

(c) *Microbial pesticides-toxicology data requirements (in part)*—(1) Table. Sections 158.50 and 158.100 through 158.102 describe how to use this table to determine the microbial pesticides-toxicology data requirements and the substance to be tested.

Kind of data required	(b) Notes	Terrestrial Food crop	Terrestrial Nonfood	Aquatic Food crop	Aquatic Nonfood	Greenhouse Food crop	Greenhouse Nonfood	Forestry	Domestic outdoor	Indoor	Data to support MP	Data to support EP	Guidelines reference No.
Tier I:													
Acute oral		[R]	[R]	[R]	[R]	[R]	[R]	[R]	[R]	[R]	MP and TGAI	EP* or EP* dilution and TGAI.	152-30
*Acute dermal		[R]	[R]	[R]	[R]	[R]	[R]	[R]	[R]	[R]	MP and TGAI	EP* or EP dilution and TGAI.	152-31
Acute inhalation	(i)	[R]	[R]	[R]	[R]	[R]	[R]	[R]	[R]	[R]	MP and TGAI	EP* or EP dilution and TGAI.	152-32
I.V., I.C., I.P. injection	(ii)	[R]	[R]	[R]	[R]	[R]	[R]	[R]	[R]	[R]	TGAI	TGAI 152-33	
*Primary dermal		[R]	[R]	[R]	[R]	[R]	[R]	[R]	[R]	[R]	MP	EP*	152-34

Data requirement											MP	EP*	No.
Primary eye	(iii)	[R]	[R]	[R]	[R]	[R]	[R]	[R]	[R]		MP	EP*	152-35
Hypersensitivity study	(iv)	R	R	R	R	R	R	R	R		MP	EP*	152-36
Hypersensitivity incidents.		CR	CR	CR	CR	CR	CR	CR	CR		CR		152-37
Immune response		R	R	R	R	R	[R]	[R]	[R]		TGAI	TGAI	152-38
Tissue culture	(v)	R	R	R	R	R	[R]	[R]	[R]		TGAI	TGAI	152-39
Tier II:													
Acute oral	(vi)	CR	CR	CR	CR	CR	CR	CR	CR		MP	EP*	152-40
Acute inhalation	(vii)	CR	CR	CR	CR	CR	CR	CR	CR		MP	EP*	152-41
Subchronic oral	(viii)	CR	CR	CR	CR	CR	CR	CR	CR		TGAI	TGAI	152-42
Acute I.P., I.C.	(ix)	CR	CR	CR	CR	CR	CR	CR	CR		TGAI	TGAI	152-43
Primary dermal	(x)	CR	CR	CR	CR	CR	CR	CR	CR			EP*	152-44
Primary eye	(xi)	CR	CR	CR	CR	CR	CR	CR	CR			EP*	152-45
Immune response	(xii)	CR	CR	CR	CR	CR	CR	CR	CR		TGAI	TGAI	152-46
Teratogenicity	(xii)	CR	CR	CR	CR	CR	CR	CR	CR		TGAI	TGAI	152-47
Virulence enhancement.	(xiv)	CR	CR	CR	CR	CR	CR	CR	CR		TGAI	TGAI	152-48
Mammalian mutagenicity.	(xv)	CR	CR	CR	CR	CR	CR	CR	CR		TGAI	TGAI	152-49
Tier III:													
Chronic feeding	(xvi)			CR	CR	CR	CR	CR	CR		TGAI	TGAI	152-50
Oncogenicity	(xvii)			CR	CR	CR	CR	CR	CR		TGAI	TGAI	151-51
Mutagenicity	(xviii)	CR	CR	CR	CR	CR	CR	CR	CR		TGAI	TGAI	152-52
Teratogenicity	(xix)	CR	CR	CR	CR	CR	CR	CR	CR		TGAI	TGAI	152-53

Key: R = Required data; CR = Conditionally required; MP = manufacturing-use product; EP* = End-Use Product; (asterisk identifies those data requirements that end-use applicants (i.e. "formulators") must satisfy, provided that their active ingredient(s) is (are) purchased from a registered source); TGAI = Technical grade of the active ingredient; [ ] = Brackets (i.e., [R], [CR]) indicate data requirements that apply when an experimental use permit is being sought.

(2) Notes—The following notes are referenced in column two of the table contained in paragraph (c)(1) of this section.

(i) Required if 20 percent or more of the aerodynamic equivalent of the product (as registered or under conditions of use) is composed of particulates less than 10 microns in diameter.

(ii) Data required for products as follows:

(A) Intravenous ("IV") infectivity study for bacterial, and viral agents:

(continued on next page)

(B) Intracerebral ("IC") infectivity study for viral and protozoan agents; and

(C) Intraperitoneal ("IP") infectivity study for fungal and protozoan agents.

(iii) Required if commonly recognized use practices will result in repeated human contact by inhalation or dermal routes.

(iv) Hypersensitivity incidents must be reported, if they occur.

(v) Data required for products whose active ingredient is a virus.

(vi) Required if survival, replication, infectivity, toxicity, or persistence of the microbial agent (virus or protozoa) is observed in the test animals treated in the Tier I acute oral infectivity tests or the intraperitoneal or intracerebral injection test for protozoa.

(vii) Required if survival, replication, infectivity, toxicity, or persistence of the microbial agent (virus or protozoa) is observed in the test animals treated in the comparable Tier I acute inhalation tests.

(viii) Required if there is evidence of survival, replication, infectivity, or persistence of the protozoan agent in the Tier I oral infectivity test.

(ix) Required if in Tier I acute oral infectivity testing. Tier I dermal toxicity/infectivity testing, or Tier I intracerebral injection testing, the test microorganism (bacteria, fungi, or protozoa) survived for more than 2 weeks, caused toxic effects, or caused a severe illness response in an experimental animal as evidenced by irreversible gross pathology, severe weight loss, toxemia, or death.

(x) Required if infectivity or if marked edema or broad erythema was observed in the Tier I dermal irritation study.

(xi) Required if infectivity or if severe ocular lesions are observed in the Tier I primary eye irritation study.

(xii) Required if results of the Tier I immune response test indicate abnormalities.

(xiii) Required when Tier I tests on viral agents show replication of the virus in mammalian hosts and significant damage to mammalian cells.

(xiv) Required when Tier I infectivity tests on bacteria or fungi indicate prolonged survival (including presence of viable microbial agents in test animal excreta) and/or multiplication (infectivity) of the bacteria or fungal agent, respectively.

(xv) Required if any of the following criteria are met:

(A) Acute infectivity tests are positive in Tier I studies.

(B) Adverse effects are observed in immune response studies.

(C) Positive results are obtained in tissue culture tests with viral agents.

(xvi) Required when the potential for chronic adverse effects (e.g., replication or persistence of viral or subviral constituents, protozoans, fungi, or bacteria) are demonstrated by any of the Tier II tests (except primary dermal, primary ocular, and mammalian mutagenicity tests).

(xvii) Required when the potential for oncogenic effects is indicated (e.g., adverse cellular effects due to presence, replication, or persistence of viral or subviral constituents, or bacteria, or protozoans; or mutagenic effects) by any of the Tier II tests except the primary dermal and primary ocular studies.

(xviii) Required when the potential for mutagenic effects is indicated (e.g., adverse cellular effects due to presence, replication, or persistence of viral or subviral constituents, bacteria, fungi, or protozoa) by any of the Tier II tests except primary dermal or primary ocular studies.

(xix) Required when the potential for teratogenic effects is expected based on the presence or persistence of fungi, bacteria, viruses, or protozoa in mammalian species as a result of testing performed in Tier II, except primary dermal and primary ocular studies.

930

(c) *Biochemical pesticides toxicology data requirements (in part)*—(1) Table. Sections 158.50 and 158.100 through 158.102 describe how to use this table to determine the biochemical pesticides-toxicology data requirements and the substance to be tested.

Kind of data required	(b) Notes	Terrestrial Food crop	Terrestrial Nonfood	Aquatic Food crop	Aquatic Nonfood	Greenhouse Food crop	Greenhouse Nonfood	Forestry	Domestic outdoor	Indoor	Test substance Data to support MP	Test substance Data to support EP	Guidelines reference No.
Tier I:													
Acute oral toxicity	(i)	[R]	[R]	[R]	[R]	[R]	[R]	[R]	[R]	[R]	MP and TGAI	EP* or EP dilution* and TGAI.	152-10
Acute dermal toxicity	(i), (ii)	[R]	[R]	[R]	[R]	[R]	[R]	[R]	[R]	[R]	MP and TGAI	EP* or EP dilution* and TGAI.	152-11
Acute inhalation	(xiv)	[R]	[R]	[R]	[R]	[R]	[R]	[R]	[R]	[R]	MP and TGAI	EP8 and TGAI	152-12
Primary eye irritation	(ii)	[R]	[R]	[R]	[R]	[R]	[R]	[R]	[R]	[R]	MP	EP	152-13
Primary dermal irritation	(i), (ii)	[R]	[R]	[R]	[R]	[R]	[R]	[R]	[R]	[R]	MP	EP	152-14
Hypersensitivity study	(iii)	CR	CR	CR	CR	CR	CR	CR	CR	CR	MP	EP	152-15
Hypersensitivity	(iv)	CR	CR	CR	CR	CR	CR	CR	CR	CR	MP		152-16
Studies to detect genotoxicity	(v)	[R]	[CR]	[R]	[CR]	[R]	[CR]	[CR]	[CR]	[CR]	TGAI	TGAI	152-17
Immune response		[R]	R	[R]	R	[R]	R	R	R	R	TGAI	TGAI	152-18
90-day feeding (1 spp.)	(vi)	CR	CR	CR	CR	CR	CR	CR	CR	CR	TGAI	TGAI	152-20
90-day dermal (1 spp.)	(vii)	CR	CR	CR	CR	CR	CR	CR	CR	CR	TGAI	TGAI	152-21
90-day inhalation (1 spp.)	(viii)	CR	CR	CR	CR	CR	CR	CR	CR	CR	TGAI	TGAI	152-22
Teratogenicity (1 spp.)	(ix)	CR	CR	CR	CR	CR	CR	CR	CR	CR	TGAI	TGAI	152-23

Tier II:										
Mammalian mutagenicity tests	(x)	CR	CR	CR	CR	CR	CR	CR	CR	TGAI	152-19
Immune response	(xi)	CR	CR	CR	CR	CR	CR	CR	CR	TGAI	152-24
Tier III:										
Chronic exposure	(xii)	CR	CR	CR	CR	CR	CR	TGAI	TGAI	152-26
Oncogenicity	(xiii)	CR	CR	CR	CR	CR	CR	TGAI	TGAI	152-29

Key: R = Required data; CR = Conditionally required; MP = manufacturing-use product; EP* = End-Use Product; (asterisk identifies those data requirements that end-use applicants (i.e. "formulators") must satisfy, provided that their active ingredient(s) is (are) purchased from a registered source); TGAI = Technical grade of the active ingredient; [ ] = Brackets (i.e., [R], [CR]) indicate data requirements that apply when an experimental use permit is being sought.

(2) Notes—The following notes are referenced in column two of the table contained in paragraph (c)(1) of this section.

(i) Not required if test material is a gas or is highly volatile.

(ii) Not required if test material is corrosive to skin or has pH less than 2 or greater than 11.5; such a product will be classified toxicity category I on the basis of potential eye and dermal irritation effect.

(iii) Required if repeated contact with human skin results under condition of use.

(iv) Incidents must be reported, if they occur.

(v) Required to support non-food uses if use is likely to result in significant human exposure; or the active ingredient or its metabolites is (are) structurally related to a known mutagen, belongs(s) to any chemical class of compounds containing known mutagens.

(vi) Required if the use requires a tolerance or an exemption from the requirement for a tolerance, or its use requires a food additive regulation; or the use of the product is otherwise likely to result in repeated human exposure by the oral route.

(vii) Required if pesticidal use will involve purposeful application to the human skin or will result in comparable prolonged human exposure to the product, (e.g., swimming pool algaecide pesticides for impregnating clothing), and if either of the criteria are met:

(A) Data from a subchronic oral study are not required.

(B) The active ingredient of the product is known or expected to be metabolized differently by the dermal route of exposure than by the oral route, and a metabolite of the active ingredient is the toxic moiety.

(viii) Required if pesticidal use may result in repeated inhalation exposure at a concentration which is likely to be toxic.

(ix) Required if any of the following criteria are met:

(A) Use of the product under widespread and recognized practice may reasonably be expected to result in significant exposure to female humans.

(B) Its use requires a tolerance or an exemption from the requirement for a tolerance, or its use requires issuance of a food additive regulation.

(x) Required if results from any one of the Tier I mutagenicity tests were positive.

(xi) Required if adverse effects are observed in the Tier I immune response studies.

(xii) Required if the potential for adverse chronic effects are indicate based on:

(continued on next page)

932

§81-2 ACUTE DERMAL TOXICITY STUDY

(a) *When required.*

(1) *Routine testing.* Data on the single-dose dermal toxicity are required by 40 CFR Part 158 to support the registration of each manufacturing-use product and end-use product, unless the substance which would be tested under paragraph (e) of this section is corrosive or a gas or highly volatile substance that cannot be administered dermally.

(2) *Use dilution testing.* Data from tests performed with the use-dilutions of a product may be required if the use dilution is intended for non-domestic application as a mist or spray. Applicants should consult with the Agency to determine the principles for such testing, if required.

(3) See, specifically, 40 CFR §158.50 and §158.135 to determine whether these data must be submitted. Section II-A of this subdivision contains an additional discussion of the "Formulators' Exemption" and who must submit the required data as a general rule.

(b) *Purpose.*

In the assessment and evaluation of the toxic characteristics of a substance, determination of acute dermal toxicity is usually an initial step. It provides information on health hazards likely to arise from short-term exposure by the dermal route. Data from an acute study may serve as a basis for classification and labeling. It is traditionally a step in establishing a dosage regime in subchronic and other studies and may provide initial information on dermal absorption and the mode of toxic actions of a substance. An evaluation of acute toxicity data should include the relationship, if any, between the animals' exposure to the test substance and the incidence and severity of all abnormalities, including behavioral and clinical abnormalities, the reversibility of observed abnormalities, gross lesions, body weight changes, effects on mortality, and any other toxic effects.

(c) *Definitions.*

(1) "Acute dermal toxicity" is the adverse effect occurring during or following a 24-hour dermal exposure to a single dose of a test substance.

(2) "Dosage" is a general term comprising the dose, its frequency and the duration of dosing.

933

(3) "Dose" is the amount of test substance applied. Dose is expressed as weight of test substance (g, mg) per unit weight of test animal (e.g., mg/kg).

(4) "Dose-effect" is the relationship between the dose and the magnitude of a defined biological effect either in an individual or in a population sample.

(5) "Dose-response" is the relationship between the dose and the proportion of a population sample showing a defined effect.

(d) *Approaches to the determination of acute toxicity.*

At present, the evaluation of chemicals for acute toxicity is necessary for the protection of public health and the environment. When animal testing is required for this purpose, this testing should be done in ways that minimize numbers of animals used and that take full account of their welfare.

EPA recommends the following means to reduce the number of animals used to evaluate acute effects of chemical exposure while preserving its ability to make reasonable judgments about safety:

- Attempt the use of existing structurally related chemicals.
- If data for calculating an LD50 are needed, perform an acute toxicity study whereby the value of the data derived from the investment of animal lives is enhanced. EPA does not encourage the use of animals *solely* for the calculation of an LD50.
- Use methods that minimize the numbers of animals in the test.

The following provides an expanded discussion of these principles and their application to the evaluation of acute toxicity of chemicals.

Using Data from Structurally Related Chemicals. In order to minimize the need for animal testing, the Agency encourages the review of existing acute toxicity information on chemical substances that are structurally related to the agent under investigation. In certain cases, one may be able to glean enough information from these surrogate chemicals to make preliminary safety evaluations that may obviate the need for further animal testing.

"Limit" Test. When acute lethality data are desirable, EPA's test guideline encourages the use of methods that minimize the requirement for animals, sometimes by a factor of 90% as compared to the more traditional LD50 test. In the "limit" test, a single group of animals receives a large dose (2 g/kg body weight) of the agent by the dermal route. If no lethality is demonstrated, no further testing for acute dermal toxicity is pursued.

Estimation of Lethal Dose. For those substances demonstrating lethality in a "limit" test or for substances for which there are data on structurally related chemicals that indicate potential acute toxicity below 2 g/kg, the Agency can use estimates of the dose associated with some level of acute lethality that are derived from a study comprising three doses as described in this guideline. With such an approach, use of greater numbers of animals or increased numbers of dose levels are not necessary.

Multiple Endpoint Evaluation. The Agency stresses the simultaneous monitoring of several endpoints of toxicity in animals in a single acute study including sublethal effects as well as lethality. Dosed animals are observed for abnormal behavioral manifestations such as increased salivation or muscular incoordination, in addition to the recovery from these effects during the observation period. Both dead and surviving animals are autopsied to evaluate gross anatomical evidence of organ toxicity. In selected cases, additional testing may be justified to characterize better the kinds of abnormalities that have been found in the organs of the autopsied animals.

These sound, scientific practices represent some of the means which maximize the utility of the data obtained from a limited number of test animals to achieve a balance between protecting humans and the environment, and the welfare and utilization of laboratory animals. When animal testing is, nonetheless, determined to be necessary to achieve this balance, the following test method incorporates the principles discussed above.

(e) *Principle of the test method.*

When conducting acute toxicity testing, exposure by dermal application is recommended for chemicals where exposure of humans by the dermal route is likely. A single exposure and a 14-day observation period are used. The test substance is applied dermally in graduated doses to several groups of experimental animals, one dose being used per group. For the limit test, however, only one group is tested at a single (high) dose. Subsequent to exposure, systematic daily observations of effects and deaths are made. Based on the results of cage-side observations or gross necropsy, the tester may decide to initiate histopathological review of certain organs, and/or additional clinical laboratory tests. Animals that die during the test are necropsied, and at the conclusion of the observation period, the surviving animals are sacrificed and are necropsied.

(f) *Substance to be tested.*

(1) The manufacturing-use product and, if different, the technical grade of each active ingredient shall be tested to support the registration of a manufacturing-use product.

(2) The end-use product shall be tested to support the registration of an end-use product.

(3) If the toxicity of the end-use product can be established from tests performed on other end-use products, the end-use product for which registration is sought need not be separately tested.

(g) *Limit test.*

If a test dose of at least 2000 mg/kg body weight, using the procedures described for this study, produces no compound-related mortality, then a full study using a minimum of three dose levels might not be necessary.

(h) *Test procedures.*

(1) *Animal selection.* (i) *Species and strain.* The rat, rabbit or guinea pig may be used. The albino rabbit is preferred because of its size, ease of handling, skin permeability and extensive data base. Commonly used laboratory strains should be employed. If a species other than the three indicated above is used, the tester should provide justification/reasoning for its selection.

(ii) *Age.* Adult animals should be used. The following weight ranges are suggested to provide animals of a size which facilitates the conduct of the test: rats, 200 to 300 g; rabbits, 2.0 to 3.0 kg; guinea pigs, 350 to 450 g.

(iii) *Sex.* (A) Equal numbers of animals of each sex with healthy intact skin are recommended for each dose level.

(B) The females should be nulliparous and non-pregnant.

(iv) *Numbers.* At least 10 animals (5 females and 5 males) at each dose level should be used.

(2) *Control groups.* A concurrent untreated control is not necessary. A vehicle control group should be run concurrently except when historical data are available to determine the acute toxicity of the vehicle.

(3) *Dosing.* (i) *Dose levels and dose selection.* Three dose levels should be used and spaced appropriately to produce test groups with a range of toxic effects and mortality rates. The data should be sufficient to produce a dose-response curve and permit an acceptable estimation of the median lethal dose. Range finding studies using single animals may help to estimate the positioning of the dose groups so that no more than three dose levels will be necessary.

(ii) *Vehicle.* Where necessary, the test substance is dissolved or suspended in a suitable vehicle. It is recommended that wherever possible the usage of an aqueous solution be considered first, followed by consideration of a solution in oil (e.g., corn oil) and then by possible solution in other vehicles. For non-aqueous vehicles the toxic characteristics of the vehicle should be known, and if not known should be determined before the test.

(4) *Exposure duration.* The duration of exposure should be approximately 24 hours.

(5) *Observation period.* The observation period should be at least 14 days. However, the duration of observation should not be fixed rigidly. It should be determined by the toxic reactions, rate of onset and length of recovery period, and may thus be extended when considered necessary. The time at which signs of toxicity appear and disappear, their duration and the time of death are important, especially if there is a tendency for deaths to be delayed.

(6) *Preparation of animal skin.* (i) Approximately 24 hours before the test, fur should be removed from the dorsal and ventral area of the trunk of the test animals by clipping or shaving. Care must be taken to avoid abrading the skin which could alter its permeability.

(ii) Not less than 10% of the body surface area should be clear for the application of the test substance. The weight of the animal should be taken into account when deciding on the area to be cleared and on the dimensions of the covering.

(iii) When testing solids, which may be pulverized if appropriate, the test substance should be moistened sufficiently with water or, where necessary, a suitable vehicle to ensure good contact with the skin. When a vehicle is used, the influence of the vehicle on penetration of skin by the test substance should be taken into account.

(7) *Application of test substance.* (i) The test substance should be applied uniformly over an area which is approximately 10% of the total body surface area. With highly toxic substances the surface area covered may be less, but as much of the area should be covered with as thin and uniform a film as possible. In the case where less that 10% of the surface area is covered an approximation of the exposed areas should be determined.

(ii) Test substance should be held in contact with the skin with a porous gauze dressing and non-irritating tape throughout a 24-hour exposure period. The test site should be further covered in a suitable manner to retain the gauze dressing and test substance and ensure that the animals cannot ingest the test substance. Restrainers may be used to prevent the ingestion of the test substance, but complete immobilization is not a recommended method.

(iii) At the end of the exposure period, residual test substance should be removed, where practicable using water or an appropriate solvent.

(8) *Observation of animals.* (i) A careful clinical examination should be made at least once each day.

(ii) Additional observations should be made daily with appropriate actions taken to minimize loss of animals to the study, e.g., necropsy or refrigeration of those animals found dead and isolation of weak or moribund animals.

(iii) Cage-side observations should include, but not be limited to, changes in:

(A) Skin and fur;

(B) Eyes and mucous membranes;

(C) Respiratory system;

(D) Circulatory system;

(E) Autonomic and central nervous system;

(F) Somatomotor activity; and

(G) Behavior pattern.

(H) Particular attention should be directed to observations of tremors, convulsions, salivation, lethargy, sleep and coma.

(iv) Individual weights of animals should be determined shortly before the test substance is applied, weekly thereafter, and at death. Changes in weight should be calculated and recorded when survival exceeds one day.

(v) The time of death should be recorded as precisely as possible.

(vi) At the end of the test, surviving animals should be weighed and sacrificed.

(9) *Gross pathology.* Consideration should be given to performing a gross necropsy of all animals where indicated by the nature of the toxic effects observed. All gross pathological changes should be recorded.

(i) *Data and reporting.*

(1) *Treatment of results.* Data shall be summarized in tabular form, showing, for each test group;
  (i) The number of animals and their body weight at the start of the test;
  (ii) Time of death of individual animals at different dose levels;
  (iii) Number of animals displaying other signs of toxicity;
  (iv) Description of toxic effects; and
  (v) Necropsy findings.

(2) *Evaluation of results.* An evaluation of results should include the relationship, if any, between the dose of the test substance and the incidence, severity and reversibility of all abnormalities, including behavioral and clinical effects, gross lesions, body weight changes, effects on mortality, and any other toxicological effects.

(3) *Test report.* In addition to the information required by §80-4, and as specified in the EPA Good Laboratory Practice Standards [Subpart J, Part 160, Chapter I of Title 40, Code of Federal Regulations] the following specific information should be reported:
  (i) Tabulation of response data by sex and dose level (i.e., number of animals exposed; number of animals showing signs of toxicity; number of animals dying);
  (ii) Dose-response curves for mortality and other toxic effects (when permitted by the method of determination);
  (iii) Description of toxic effects including their time of onset, duration, reversibility, and relationship to dose;
  (iv) Time of death after dosing;
  (v) Body weight data;
  (vi) Gross pathology findings; and
  (vii) Histopathology findings and any additional clinical chemistry evaluations, if performed.
  (viii) The approximate amount of test material applied per unit of skin exposed (calculated in mg per square cm of skin).

§81-5 PRIMARY DERMAL IRRITATION

(a) *When required.*

Data on primary dermal irritation are required by 40 CFR Part 158 to support the registration of each manufacturing-use product and each end-use product. See, specifically, 40 CFR §158.50 and §158.135 to determine whether these data must be submitted. Section II-A of this subdivision contains an additional discussion of the "Formulators' Exemption" and who must submit the required data as a general rule.

(b) *Purpose.*

In the assessment and evaluation of the toxic characteristics of a substance, determination of the irritant and/or corrosive effects on skin of mammals is an important initial step. Information derived from this test serves to indicate the existence of possible hazards likely to arise from exposure of the skin to the test substance.

(c) *Definitions.*

(1) "Dermal corrosion" is the production of irreversible tissue damage in the skin following the application of the test substance.

(2) "Dermal irritation" is the production of reversible inflammatory changes in the skin following the application of the test substance.

(d) *Principles of the test method.*

(1) The substance to be tested is applied in a single dose to the skin of several experimental animals, each animal serving as its own control. The degree of irritation is read and scored at specified intervals and is further described to provide a complete evaluation of the effects. The duration of the study should be sufficient to permit a full evaluation of the reversibility or irreversibility of the effects observed but need not exceed 14 days.

(2) When testing solids (which may be pulverized if considered necessary), the test substance should be moistened sufficiently with water or, where necessary, a suitable vehicle, to ensure good contact with the skin. When vehicles are used, the influence of the vehicle on irritation of skin by the test substance should be taken into account. Liquid test substances are generally used undiluted.

(3) Strongly acidic or alkaline substances, for example with a demonstrated pH of 2 or less or 11.5 or greater, need not be tested for primary dermal irritation, owing to their predictable corrosive properties.

(4) The testing of materials which have been shown to be highly toxic (LD50 less than 200 mg/kg) by the dermal route is unnecessary.

(e) *Substance to be tested.*

(1) *Test substance.* (i) The manufacturing-use product shall be tested to support the registration of a manufacturing-use product.

(ii) The end-use product shall be tested to support the registration of an end-use product.

(2) *Condition of test substance.* (i) If the substance is a liquid, it should be applied undiluted.

(ii) If the test substance is a solid, it should be slightly moistened with water or, where necessary, a suitable vehicle before application.

(3) *Corrosive pesticides.* Data which demonstrate that the test substance specified by paragraph (e)(1) of this section has a pH of 1-2 or 11.5-14 may be submitted in lieu of data from a primary dermal irritation study conducted in accordance with paragraph (f) of this section. For all regulatory purposes, the Agency will assume that such a substance is corrosive.

(f) *Test procedures.*

(1) *Animal selection.* (i) *Species and strain.* The albino rabbit is recommended as the preferred species. If another mammalian species is used, the tester should provide justification/reasoning for its selection.

(ii) *Number of animals.* At least six healthy adult animals should be used, unless justification/reasoning for using fewer animals is provided.

(2) *Dose level.* (i) A dose of 0.5 ml of liquid or 0.5 g of solid or semi-solid is applied to the test site.

(ii) Separate animals are not recommended for an untreated control group. Adjacent areas of untreated skin of each animal serve as control for the test.

(3) *Preparation of animal skin.* Approximately 24 hours before the test, fur should be removed from the test area by clipping or shaving the dorsal area of the trunk of the animals. Care should be taken to avoid abrading the skin. Only animals with healthy intact skin should be used.

(4) *Application of the test substance.* (i) Exposure duration is for four hours. Longer exposures may be indicated under certain conditions, e.g., expected pattern of human use and exposure. At the end of the exposure period, residual test substance should generally be removed, where practicable, using water or an appropriate solvent, without altering the existing response or the integrity of the epidermis.

(ii) The test substance should be applied to a small area (approximately 6 cm^2) of skin and covered with a gauze patch, which is held in place with non-irritating tape. In the case of liquids or some pastes, it may be necessary to apply the test substance to the gauze patch and then apply that to the skin. The patch should be loosely held in contact with the skin by means of a suitable semi-occlusive dressing for the duration of the exposure period. However, the use of occlusive dressing may be considered appropriate in some cases. Access by the animal to the patch and resultant ingestion/inhalation of the test substance should be prevented.

(5) *Observation period.* (i) The duration of the observation period is at least 72 hours, but should not be fixed rigidly. It should be sufficient to evaluate fully the reversibility or irreversibility of the effects observed. It need not normally exceed 14 days after application.

(6) *Clinical examination and scoring.* (i) After removal of the patch, animals should be examined for signs of erythema and edema and the responses scored within 30–60 minutes, and then at 24, 48, and 72 hours after patch removal.

(ii) Dermal irritation is scored and recorded according to the grades in Table 2, below. Further observations may be needed, as necessary, to establish reversibility. In addition to the observation of irritation, any lesions and other toxic effects should be fully described.

TABLE 2. Evaluation of Skin Reaction

	Value
Erythema and Eschar Formation	
No erythema	0
Very slight erythema (barely perceptible)	1
Well-defined erythema	2
Moderate to severe erythema	3
Sever erythema (beet redness) to slight eschar formation (injuries in depth)	4
Maximum possible	4
Edema Formation	
No edema	
Very slight edema (barely perceptible)	1
Slight edema (edges of area well defined by definite raising)	2
Moderate edema (raised approximately 1 millimeter)	3
Severe edema (raised more than 1 millimeter and extending beyond area of exposure	4
Maximum possible	4

(g) *Data and reporting.*

(1) Data shall be summarized in tabular form, showing, for each individual animal:

(i) The irritation scores for erythema and edema at 30 and 60 minutes, 24, 48, and 72 hours after patch removal;

(ii) Any lesions;

(iii) A description of the degree and nature of irritation, corrosion, or reversibility; and

(iv) Any other toxic effects observed.

(2) *Evaluation of results.* The dermal irritation scores shall be evaluated in conjunction with the nature and reversibility or otherwise of the responses observed. The individual scores do not represent an absolute standard for the irritant properties of a material. They should be viewed as reference values which are only meaningful when supported by a full description and evaluation of the observations. The use of an occlusive dressing is a severe test and the results are relevant to very few likely human exposure conditions.

(3) *Test report.* In addition to the information recommended by §80-4, the test report should include the following information:

(i) Physical nature and, where appropriate, concentration and pH value for the test substance;

(ii) Species and strain used;

(iii) Tabulation of irritation response data for each individual animal for each observation time period (e.g., 30 to 60 minutes, 24, 48, and 72 hours after patch removal);

(iv) Description of any toxic effects other than dermal irritation.

§81-6 DERMAL SENSITIZATION STUDY

(a) *When required.*

Data from a dermal sensitization study are required by 40 CFR Part 158 to support the registration of each manufacturing-use product and of each end-use product which will result in repeated human skin contact under conditions of use.

(1) See, specifically, 40 CFR §158.50 and §158.135 to determine whether these data must be submitted. Section II-A of this subdivision contains an additional discussion of the "Formulators' Exemption" and who must submit the required data as a general rule.

(b) *Purpose.*

In the assessment and evaluation of the toxic characteristics of a substance, determination of its potential to provoke skin sensitization reactions is important. Information derived from tests for skin sensitization serves to identify the possible hazard to a population repeatedly exposed to the test substance. While the desirability of skin sensitization testing is recognized, there are some real differences of opinion about the best method to use. The test selected should be a reliable screening procedure which should not fail to identify substances with a significant allergenic potential, while at the same time avoiding false negative results.

(c) *Definitions.*

(1) "Challenge exposure" is an experimental exposure of a previously treated subject to a test substance following an induction period, to determine whether the subjects will react in a hypersensitive manner.

(2) "Induction exposure" is an experimental exposure of a subject to a test substance with the intention of inducing a hypersensitive state.

(3) "Induction period" is a period of at least one week following a sensitization exposure during which a hypersensitive state is developed.

(4) "Skin sensitization" ("allergic contact dermatitis") is an immunologically-mediated cutaneous reaction to a substance. In the human, the responses may be characterized by pruritis, erythema, edema, papules, vesi-

cles, bullae, or a combination of these. In other species, the reactions may differ and only erythema and edema may be seen.

(d) *Principle of the test method.*

Following initial exposure(s) to a test substance, the animals are subsequently subjected, after a period of not less than one week, to challenge exposure with the test substance to establish whether a hypersensitive state has been induced. Sensitization is determined by examining the reaction to the challenge exposure and comparing this reaction to that of the initial induction exposure.

(e) *Substance to be tested.*

(1) *Test substance.* (i) The manufacturing-use product shall be tested to support the registration of a manufacturing-use product.

(ii) The end-use product shall be tested to support the registration of an end-use product.

(2) *Conditions of test substance.* The test substance should be applied at a concentration in accordance with the test methods. If the test substance causes marked irritation, it should be diluted with physiological saline until a concentration is found which produces only slight irritation. If the test substance is a solid to be injected intradermally, it should be dissolved in a minimum amount of physiological saline or suspended in a suitable agent.

(f) *Test procedures.*

(1) Any of the following seven test methods is considered to be acceptable. It is realized, however, that the methods differ in their probability and degree of reaction to sensitizing substances.

(i) Freund's complete adjuvant test;
(ii) Guinea pig maximization test;
(iii) Split adjuvant technique;
(iv) Buehler test;
(v) Open epicutaneous test;
(vi) Mauer optimization test; and
(vii) Footpad technique in guinea pig.

(2) Removal of hair is by clipping, shaving, or possibly by depilation, depending on the test method used.

(3) *Animal selection.* (i) *Species and strain.* The young adult guinea pig is the preferred species. Commonly used laboratory strains should be employed. If other species are used, the tester should provide justification/ reasoning for their selection.

(ii) *Number and sex.* (A) The number and sex of animals used should depend on the method employed.

(B) The females should be nulliparous and non-pregnant.

(4) *Control animals.* (i) Periodic use of a positive control substance with an acceptable level of reliability for the test system selected is recommended.

(ii) Animals may act as their own controls or groups of induced animals can be compared to groups which have received only a challenge exposure.

(5) *Dose levels.* (i) The dose level will depend upon the method selected.

(6) *Observation of animals.* (i) Skin reactions are to be graded and recorded after the challenge exposures at the time specified by the methodology selected. This is usually 24, 48, and 72 hours. Additional notations should be made as necessary to fully describe unusual responses.

(ii) Regardless of method selected, initial and terminal body weights are to be recorded.

(7) *Procedures.* (i) The procedures to be used are those described by the methodology chosen.

(g) *Data and reporting.*

(1) *Data summary.* Data should be summarized in tabular form, showing, for each individual animal:

(i) The skin reaction; and

(ii) Results of the induction exposure(s) and the challenge exposure(s) at the times indicated by the method chosen.

(2) *Grading information.* As a minimum, the erythema and/or edema should be graded and any unusual findings should be recorded.

(3) *Evaluation of the results.* The evaluation of results will provide information on the proportion of each group that becomes sensitized and the extent (slight, moderate, severe) of the sensitization reaction in each individual animal.

(4) *Test report.* In addition to the information required by §80-4, the test report shall include the following information:

(i) A description of the method used and the commonly accepted name;

(ii) Information on positive control study, including:

(A) Positive control used;

(B) Method used; and

(C) Time conducted.

(iii) The number, species, strain and sex of the test animals;

(iv) Individual weights of the animals at the start of the test and at the conclusion of the test;

(v) A brief description of the grading system; and

(vi) Each reading made on each individual animal.

§82-2 REPEATED DOSE DERMAL TOXICITY: 21-DAY STUDY

(a) *When required.*

Data from a subchronic 21-day dermal toxicity study are required by 40 CFR Part 158 to support the registration of each manufacturing-use product and each end-use product whose pesticidal use is likely to result in repeated human skin contact with the product, its active ingredients, or their breakdown products. Data from this study are not required when data from a subchronic 90-day dermal toxicity study (see §82-3) are required.

(i) See, specifically, 40 CFR §158.50 and §158.135 to determine whether these data must be submitted. Section II-A of this subdivision contains an additional discussion of the "Formulators' Exemption" and who must submit the required data as a general rule.

(b) *Purpose.*

In the assessment and evaluation of the toxic characteristics of a chemical, the determination of subchronic dermal toxicity may be carried out after initial information on toxicity has been obtained by acute testing. It provides information on possible health hazards likely to arise from repeated exposures by the dermal route over a limited period of time.

(c) *Definitions.*

(1) "Cumulative toxicity" is the adverse effects of repeated doses occurring as a result of prolonged action on, or increased concentration of the administered substance or its metabolites in susceptible tissues.

(2) "Dose" in a dermal test is the amount of test substance applied to the skin. Dose is expressed as weight of test substance (g, mg) per unit weight of test animal (e.g., mg/kg).

(3) "No-effect level"/"No-toxic-effect level"/"No-adverse-effect level"/"No-observed-effect level" is the maximum dose used in a test which produces no adverse effects. A no-effect level is expressed in terms of the weight of a substance given daily per unit weight of test animal (mg/kg).

(d) *Principle of the test method.*

The test substance is applied daily to the skin in graduated doses to several groups of experimental animals, one dose per group, for a period of 21 days. During the period of application the animals are observed daily to detect signs of toxicity. Animals which die during the test are necropsied, and at the conclusion of the test the surviving animals are sacrificed and necropsied and appropriate histopathological examinations carried out.

(e) *Substance to be tested.*

The technical grade of each active ingredient in the product shall be tested. The end-use product is likely to increase dermal absorption of the test substance or potentiate toxic and pharmacologic effects.

(f) *Limit test.*

If a test at one dose level of at least 1000 mg/kg body weight (but expected human exposure may indicate the need for a higher dose level), using the procedures described for this study, produces no observable toxic effects, and if toxicity would not be expected based upon data of structurally related compounds, then a full study using three dose levels might not be necessary.

(g) *Test procedures.*

   (1) *Animal selection.*
   (i) *Species and strain.* The adult rat, rabbit or guinea pig may be used. Other species may be used but their use would require justification.
   (ii) *Age.* Adult animals should be used. The following weight ranges at the start of the test are suggested in order to provide animals of a size which facilitates the conduct of the test:
   (A) Rats, 200 to 300 g.
   (B) Rabbits, 2.0 to 3.0 kg.
   (C) Guinea pigs, 350 to 450 g.
   (iii) *Sex.* (A) Equal numbers of animals of each sex with healthy skin should be used at each dose level.
   (B) The females should be nulliparous and non-pregnant.
   (iv) *Numbers.* At least 10 animals (5 females and 5 males) should be used at each dose level.
   (2) *Control groups.* A concurrent control group is recommended. This group should be an untreated or sham treated control group, or, if a vehicle is used in administering the test substance, a vehicle control group. If the toxic properties of the vehicle are not known or cannot be made available, both untreated and vehicle control groups are recommended.
   (3) *Satellite group.* A satellite group of 10 animals (5 animals per sex) may be treated with the high dose level for 21 days and observed for reversibility, persistence, or delayed occurrence of toxic effects for 14 days post-treatment.
   (4) *Dose levels and dose selection.* (i) At least three dose levels, with a control and, where appropriate, a vehicle control, should be used.
   (ii) The highest dose level should result in toxic effects but not produce an incidence of fatalities which would prevent a meaningful evaluation.
   (iii) The lowest dose level should not produce any evidence of toxicity. Where there is a usable estimation of human exposure the lowest level should exceed this.
   (iv) Ideally, the intermediate dose level(s) should produce minimal observable toxic effects. If more than one intermediate dose is used the dose levels should be spaced to produce a gradation of toxic effects.
   (v) In the low and intermediate groups and in the controls the incidence of fatalities should be low, to permit a meaningful evaluation of the results.
   (vi) If application of the test substance produces severe skin irritation, the concentration may be reduced although this may result in a reduction in, or absence of, other toxic effects at the high dose level. However, if the skin has been badly damaged early in the study it may be necessary to terminate the study and undertake a new study at lower concentrations.

(5) *Exposure conditions.* The animals are treated with the test substance, ideally for at least 6 hours per day on a 7-days-per-week basis, for a period of 21 days. However, based primarily on practical considerations, application on a 5-days-per-week basis is considered to be acceptable.

(6) *Observation period.* Duration of observation should be for at least 21 days.

(7) *Preparation of animal skin.* (i) Shortly before testing, fur is clipped from the dorsal area of the trunk of the test animals. Shaving may be employed but it should be carried out approximately 24 hours before the test. Repeat clipping or shaving is usually needed at approximately weekly intervals. When clipping or shaving the fur, care must be taken to avoid abrading the skin which could alter its permeability.

(ii) Not less than 10 percent of the body surface area should be clear for the application of the test substance. The weight of the animal should be taken into account when deciding on the area to be cleared and on the dimensions of the covering.

(iii) When testing solids, which may be pulverized if appropriate, the test substance should be moistened sufficiently with water or, where necessary, a suitable vehicle to ensure good contact with the skin. When a vehicle is used, the influence of the vehicle on penetration of skin by the test substance should be taken into account.

(8) *Application of the test substance.* (i) The test substance should be applied uniformly over an area which is approximately 10% of the total body surface area. With high toxicity substances the surface area covered may be less, but as much of the area should be covered with as thin and uniform a film as possible.

(ii) During the exposure period the test substance is held in contact with the skin with a porous gauze dressing and nonirritating tape. The test site should be further covered in a suitable manner to retain the gauze dressing and test substance and ensure that the animals cannot ingest the test substance. Restrainers may be used to prevent the ingestion of the test substance but complete immobilization is not a recommended method.

(9) *Observation of animals.* (i) A careful cage-side examination should be made at least once each day.

(ii) Additional observations should be made daily with appropriate actions taken to minimize loss of animals to the study, e.g., necropsy or refrigeration of those animals found dead and isolation or sacrifice of weak or moribund animals, to ensure that not more than 10% of the animals in any test group are lost from the test due to cannibalism, analysis of tissues, misplacement, and similar management problems.

(iii) Signs of toxicity should be recorded as they are observed including the time of onset, the degree and duration.

(iv) Cage-side observations should include, but not be limited to, changes in:

(A) Skin and fur;

(B) Eyes and mucous membranes;

(C) Respiratory system;

(D) Circulatory system;

(E) Autonomic and central nervous system;

(F) Somatomotor activity; and

(G) Behavior pattern.

(v) Animals should be weighed weekly. Food consumption data should be collected weekly.

(vi) At the end of the study period all survivors in the non-satellite treatment groups are sacrificed. Moribund animals should be removed and sacrificed when noticed.

(10) *Clinical examinations.* The following examinations should be made on all animals:

(i) Hematology, including:

(A) Hematocrit;

(B) Hemoglobin concentration;

(C) Erythrocyte count;

(D) Total and differential leucocyte count; and

(E) A measure of clotting potential such as clotting time, prothrombin time, thromboplastin time, or platelet count, at the end of the test period.

(ii) Clinical biochemistry determinations on blood should be carried out at the end of the test period. Blood parameters of liver and kidney function are appropriate. The selection of specific tests will be influenced by observations on the mode of action of the substance. Suggested determinations are:

(A) Calcium;

(B) Phosphorus;

(C) Chloride;

(D) Sodium;

(E) Potassium;

(F) Fasting glucose (with period of fasting appropriate to the species);

(G) Serum glutamic-pyruvic transaminase (also known as serum alanine aminotransferase);

(H) Serum glutamic-oxaloacetic transaminase (also known as serum aspartite aminotransferase);

(I) Urea nitrogen;

(J) Albumen;

(K) Blood creatinine;

(L) Total bilirubin; and

(M) Total serum protein measurements.

(N) Other determinations which may be necessary for an adequate toxicological evaluation include analyses of lipids, hormones, acid/base balance, methemoglobin, cholinesterase activity.

(O) Additonal clinical biochemistry may be employed, where necessary, to extend the investigation of observed effects.

(iii) Urinalysis is not required on a routine basis, but only when there is an indication of obtaining useful data based on expected or observed toxicity.

(11) *Gross necropsy.*

(i) All animals should be subjected to full gross necropsy which includes examination of:

(A) The external surface of the body;

(ii) The liver, kidneys and testes should be weighed wet as soon as possible after dissection to avoid drying.

(12) *Tissue preservation.* The following organs and tissues, or representative samples thereof, should be preserved in a suitable medium for possible future histopathological examination:

(i) Normal and treated skin;

(ii) Liver;

(iii) Kidney; and

(iv) Target organs (i.e., those organs showing gross lesions or changes in size, which are suspected to be related to the treatment of the test substance).

(13) *Histopathology.* Histological examination should be performed on the preserved organs and tissues of the high dose group and the control group. These examinations should be extended to animals of other dosage groups, if considered necessary to investigate the changes observed in the high dose group. Animals in the satellite group if included should be examined histologically with particular emphasis on those organs and tissues identified as showing effects in the other treated groups.

(h) *Data and reporting.*

(1) *Treatment of results.* (i) Data shall be summarized in tabular form, showing for each test group:

(A) The number of animals at the start of the test;

(B) The number of animals showing lesions;

(C) The type of lesions; and

(D) The percentage of animals displaying each type of lesion.

(ii) All observed results, quantitative and incidental, shall be evaluated by an appropriate statistical method. Any generally accepted statistical method may be used; the statistical method shall be selected during the design of the study.

(2) *Evaluation of results.* The findings of a subchronic dermal toxicity study shall be considered in terms of the observed toxic effects and the necropsy and histopathological findings.

(i) The evaluation should include the relationship between the dose of the test substance and the presence or absence, the incidence and severity, of abnormalities, including:

(A) Behavioral abnormalities;

(B) Clinical abnormalities;

(C) Gross lesions;

(D) Identified target organs;

(E) Body weight changes;

(F) Effects on mortality; and

(G) Any other general or specific toxic effects.

(ii) A properly conducted 21-day study should provide information on the effects of repeated dermal application of a substance and can indicate the need for further longer term studies.

(iii) It can also provide information on the selection of dose levels for longer term studies.

(3) *Test report.* In addition to the information required by §80-4, the test report summary shall include the following information:

(i) Toxic response and other effects data by sex and dose.

(ii) Species and strain.

(iii) Individual animal data for the following:

(A) Time of death during the study or whether animals survived to termination;

(B) The time of the observation of each abnormal sign and its subsequent course;

(C) Body weight data;

(D) Hematological tests employed and results;

(E) Clinical biochemistry tests employed and results;

(F) Necropsy findings;

(G) Detailed description of all histopathological findings; and

(iv) Statistical treatment of results, where appropriate.

§82-3 SUBCHRONIC DERMAL TOXICITY: 90-DAY STUDY

(a) *When required.*

Data from a subchronic 90-day dermal toxicity study are required by 40 CFR Part 158 to support the registration of each manufacturing-use product and end-use product whose use will involve purposeful application to the human skin or whose pesticidal use will result in comparable human exposure to the product, its active ingredients, or their breakdown products (e.g., swimming pool algaecides, pesticides for impregnating clothing), and which meets either of the following criteria:

(1) Data from a subchronic oral study (see §82-1) are not required; or

(2) The active ingredient of the product is known or expected to be metabolized differently by the dermal route of exposure than by the oral route, and a metabolite of the active ingredient is the toxic moiety.

(3) See, specifically, 40 CFR §158.50 and §158.135 to determine

whether these data must be submitted. Section II-A of this subdivision contains an additional discussion of the "Formulators' Exemption" and who must submit the required data as a general rule.

(b) *Purpose.*

In the assessment and evaluation of the toxic characteristics of a chemical the determination of subchronic dermal toxicity may be carried out after initial information on toxicity has been obtained by acute testing. The subchronic dermal study has been designed to permit the determination of the toxic effects associated with continuous or repeated exposure to a test substance for a period of 90 days. The test is not capable of determining those effects that have a long latency period for development (e.g., carcinogenicity and life shortening).

(c) *Definitions.*

(1) "Cumulative toxicity" is the adverse effects of repeated doses occurring as a result of prolonged action on, or increased concentration of the administered substance or its metabolites, in susceptible tissues.

(2) "Dose" in a dermal test is the amount of test substance applied to the skin (applied daily in subchronic tests). Dose is expressed as weight of the test substance (g, mg) per unit weight of test animal (e.g., mg/kg).

(3) "No-effect level"/"No-toxic-effect level"/"No-adverse-effect level"/"No-observed-effect level" is the maximum dose used in a test which produces no adverse effects. A no-effect level is expressed in terms of the weight of a substance given daily per unit weight of test animal (mg/kg).

(4) "Subchronic dermal toxicity" is the adverse effects occurring as a result of the repeated daily dermal application of a chemical to experimental animals for part (approximately 10%) of a life span.

(d) *Principle of the test method.*

The test substance is applied daily to the skin in graduated doses to several groups of experimental animals, one dose per group, for a period of 90 days. During the period of application the animals are observed daily to detect signs of toxicity. Animals which die during the test are necropsied, and at the conclusion of the test the surviving animals are sacrificed and necropsied, and appropriate histopathological examinations carried out.

(e) *Substance to be tested.*

The technical grade of each active ingredient in the product shall be tested. In addition, the end-use product shall be tested if any component of the end-use product is likely to increase dermal absorption of the test substance and potentiate toxic or pharmacologic effects.

(f) *Limit test.*

If a test at one dose level of at least 1000 mg/kg body weight (expected human exposure may indicate the need for a high dose level), using the procedures described for this study, produces no observable toxic effects and if toxicity would not be expected based upon data of structurally-related compounds, then a full study using three dose levels might not be necessary.

(g) *Test procedures.*

(1) *Animal selection.* (i) *Species and strain.* The adult rat, rabbit or guinea pig may be used. Other species may be used but their use would require justification.

(ii) *Age.* Adult animals should be used. The following weight ranges at the start of the test are suggested in order to provide animals of a size which facilitates the conduct of the test:

(A) Rats, 200 to 300 g.

(B) Rabbits, 2.0 to 3.0 kg.

(C) Guinea pigs, 350 to 450 g.

(iii) *Sex.*

(A) Equal numbers of animals of each sex with healthy skin should be used at each dose level.

(B) The females should be nulliparous and non-pregnant.

(iv) *Numbers.* (A) At least 20 animals (10 females and 10 males) should be used at each dose level.

(B) If interim sacrifices are planned the number should be increased by the number of animals scheduled to be sacrificed before completion of the study.

(C) The number of animals at the termination of the study should be adequate for a meaningful evaluation of toxic effects.

(2) *Control groups.* A concurrent control group is recommended. This group should be an untreated or sham treated control group or, if a vehicle is used in administering the test substance, a vehicle control group. If the toxic properties of the vehicle are not known or cannot be made available, both untreated and vehicle control groups are recommended.

(3) *Satellite group.* A satellite group of 20 animals (10 animals per sex), if included, may be treated with the high dose level for 90 days and observed for reversibility, persistence, or delayed occurrence, of toxic effects for a post-treatment period of appropriate length, normally not less than 28 days.

(4) *Dose levels and dose selection.* (i) In subchronic toxicity tests, it is desirable to have a dose response relationship as well as a no-observed-toxic effect level. Therefore, at least three dose levels with a control and, where appropriate, a vehicle control (corresponding to the concentration of vehicle at the highest exposure level) should be used.

(ii) The highest dose level should result in toxic effect but not produce severe skin irritation or an incidence of fatalities which would prevent a meaningful evaluation.

(iii) The lowest dose level should not produce any evidence of toxicity. Where there is a usable estimation of human exposure the lowest level should exceed this.

(iv) Ideally, the intermediate dose level(s) should produce minimal observable effects. If more than one intermediate dose is used the dose levels should be spaced to produce a gradation of toxic effects.

(v) In the low and intermediate groups, and in the controls, the incidence of fatalities should be low to permit a meaningful evaluation of the results.

(5) *Exposure conditions.* The animals are treated with test substance, ideally for at least 6 hours per day on a 7-days-per-week basis, for a period of 90 days. However, based primarily on practical considerations, application on a 5-days-per-week basis is considered to be acceptable.

(6) *Observation period.* Duration of observation should be for at least 90 days.

(7) *Preparation of animal skin.* (i) Shortly before testing, fur is clipped from the dorsal area of the trunk of the test animals. Shaving may be employed, but it should be carried out approximately 24 hours before the test. Repeat clipping or shaving is usually needed at approximately weekly intervals. When clipping or shaving the fur, care must be taken to avoid abrading the skin, which could alter its permeability.

(ii) Not less than 10% of the body surface area should be clear for the application of the test substance. The weight of the animal should be taken into account when deciding on the area to be cleared and on the dimensions of the covering.

(iii) When testing solids, which may be pulverized if appropriate, the test substance should be moistened sufficiently with water or, where necessary, a suitable vehicle to ensure good contact with the skin. When a vehicle is used, the influence of the vehicle on penetration of skin by the test substance should be taken into account.

(8) *Application of the test substance.* (i) The test substance should be applied uniformly over an area which is approximately 10% of the total body surface area. With highly toxic substances the surface area covered may be less, but as much of the area should be covered with as thin and uniform a film as possible.

(ii) During the exposure period the test substance is held in contact with the skin with a porous gauze dressing and non-irritating tape. The test site should be further covered in a suitable manner to retain the gauze dressing and test substance and ensure that the animals cannot ingest the test substance. Restrainers may be used to prevent the ingestion of the test substance, but complete immobilization is not a recommended method.

(9) *Observation of animals.* (i) A careful cage-side examination should be made at least once each day.

(ii) Additional observations should be made daily with appropriate actions taken to minimize loss of animals to the study, e.g., necropsy or refrigeration of those animals found dead and isolation or sacrifice of weak or moribund animals, to ensure that not more than 10% of the animals in any test group are lost from the test due to cannibalism, analysis of tissues, misplacement, and similar management problems.

(iii) Signs of toxicity should be recorded as they are observed, including the time of onset, the degree, and duration.

(iv) Cage-side observations should include, but not be limited to, changes in skin and fur, eyes and mucous membranes, respiratory, circulatory, autonomic and central nervous system, somatomotor activity and behavior pattern.

(v) Animals should be weighed weekly. Food consumption data should be collected weekly.

(vi) At the end of the study period all survivors in the non-satellite treatment groups are sacrificed. Moribund animals should be removed and sacrificed when noticed.

(10) *Clinical examinations.* (i) The following examinations should be made on all animals of each sex in each group:

(A) Hematology determinations should be investigated at the end of the test period. Test areas which are considered to be appropriate to all studies are:

(1) Hemocrit;

(2) Hemoglobin concentration;

(3) Erythrocyte count;

(4) Total and differential leucocyte count; and

(5) A measure of clotting potential, such as clotting time, prothrombin time, thromboplastin time, or platelet count.

(B) Certain clinical biochemistry determinations on blood should be carried at the end of the test period. Test areas which are considered appropriate to all studies are:

(1) Electroyte balance;

(2) Carbohydrate metabolism; and

(3) Liver and kidney function.

(C) The selection of specific tests will be influenced by observations of the mode of action of the substance. Suggested determinations are:

(1) Calcium;

(2) Phosphorus;

(3) Chloride;

(4) Sodium;

(5) Potassium;

(6) Fasting glucose (with period of fasting appropriate to the species);

(7) Serum glutamic-pyruvic transaminase (also known as serum alanine aminotransferase)

(8) Serum glutamic-oxaloacetic transaminase (also known as serum aspartite aminotransferase);

(9) Urea nitrogen;

(10) Albumen;

(11) Blood creatinine;

(12) Total bilirubin; and

(13) Total serum protein measurements.

(14) Other determinations which may be necessary for an adequate toxicological evaluation include analyses of lipids, hormones, acid/base balance, methemoglobin, cholinesterase activity.

(15) Additional clinical biochemistry may be employed, where necessary, to extend the investigation of observed effects.

(ii) The following examinations should be made on all animals of each sex in each group:

(A) Ophthalmological examination, using an ophthalmoscope or equivalent suitable equipment. This examination should be made prior to exposure to the test substance and at the termination of the study, preferably in all animals but at least in the high dose and control groups. If changes in the eyes are detected, all animals should be examined.

(B) Urinalysis, but only when there is an indication of obtaining useful data based on expected or observed toxicity.

(11) *Gross necropsy.* (i) All animals shall be subjected to a full gross necropsy which includes examination of:

(A) The external surface of the body.

(ii) The liver, kidneys, and testes should be weighed wet, as soon as possible after dissection to avoid drying.

(12) *Preservation of tissues.* (i) The following organs and tissues, or representative samples thereof, should be preserved in a suitable medium for possible future histopathological examination:

(A) Normal and treated skin;

(B) All gross lesions;

(C) Brain—including sections of medulla/pons, cerebellar cortex and cerebral cortex;

(D) Pituitary;

(E) Thyroid/parathyroid;

(F) Thymus;

(G) Lungs;

(H) Heart;

(I) Salivary glands;

(J) Liver;

(K) Spleen;

(L) Kidneys;

(M) Adrenals;

(N) Pancreas

(O) Testes;

(P) Accessory genital organs; uterus;

(Q) Aorta;

(R) Gall bladder (if present);

(S) Esophagus;

(T) Stomach;

(U) Duodenum;

(V) Jejunum;

(W) Ileum;

(X) Caecum;

(Y) Colon;

(Z) Rectum;

(AA) Urinary bladder;

(BB) Representative lymph node;

(CC) Peripheral nerve; and

(DD) Aorta.

(ii) The following tissues need to be preserved only if indicated by signs of toxicity or target organ involvement:

(A) Trachea;

(B) Sternum with bone marrow;

(C) Mammary gland;

(D) Thigh musculature;

(E) Eyes;

(F) Femur—including articular surface;

(G) Spinal cord at three levels—cervical, midthoracid, and lumbar; and

(H) Extraorbital lachrymal glands.

(13) *Histopathology.* (i) The following histopathology should be performed:

(A) Full histopathology on normal and treated skin and on organs and tissues, listed in paragraphs (e)(12)(i) and (ii) of this section, of all animals in the control and high dose groups.

(B) All gross lesions in all animals.

(C) Target organs in all animal groups.

(ii) The following histopathology should be performed:

(A) Lungs of animals (rats) in the low and intermediate dose groups should be subjected to histopathological examination for evidence of infection, since this provides a convenient assessment of the state of health of the animals.

(B) When a satellite group is used, histopathology should be performed on tissues and organs identified as showing effects in other treated groups.

(h) *Data and reporting.*

(1) *Treatment of results.* (i) Data shall be summarized in tabular form, showing for each test group the number of animals at the start of the test, the number of animals showing lesions, the types of lesions and the percentage of animals displaying each type of lesion.

(ii) All observed results, quantitative and incidental, shall be evaluated by an appropriate statistical method. Any generally accepted statistical method may be used; the statistical method should be selected during the design of the study.

(2) *Evaluation of results.* The findings of a subchronic dermal toxicity study shall be evaluated in conjunction with the findings of preceding studies and considered in terms of the observed toxic effects and the necropsy and histopathological findings.

(i) The evaluation will include the relationship between the dose of the test substance and the presence or absence, the incidence and severity, of abnormalities, including:

(A) Behavioral abnormalities;

(B) Clinical abnormalities;

(C) Gross lesions;

(D) Identified target organs;

(E) Body weight changes;

(F) Effect on mortality; and

(G) Any other general or specific toxic effects.

(ii) A properly conducted subchronic test should provide a satisfactory estimation of a no-effect level.

(3) *Test report.* In addition to the information required by §80-4, the test report summary shall include the following information:

(i) Toxic response and other effects data by sex and dose;

(ii) Species and strain; and

(iii) Individual animal data for the following:

(A) Time of death during the study or whether animals survived to termination;

(B) Time of observation of each abnormal sign and its subsequent course;

(C) Body weight data;

(D) Hematological tests employed and results, with relevant baseline data, if available;

(E) Clinical biochemistry tests employed and results, with relevant baseline data, if available;

(F) Necropsy findings;

(G) Detailed description of all histopathological findings; and

(iv) Statistical treatment of results, where appropriate.

PESTICIDE ASSESSMENT GUIDELINES FOR HUMANS AND DOMESTIC ANIMALS: DERMAL IRRITATION DATA REPORTING

Introduction

A. Purpose

The purpose of this guideline is to provide a data reporting format for dermal irritation studies.

B. Objective

This data reporting guideline is designed to aid the registrant in the preparation and submission of reports which are compatible with the Agency's review process. While following this guideline is not mandatory except to the extend of compliance with the PR Notice 86-5, registrants are strongly encouraged to submit reports in this format.

Response to Public Comments

The Agency received three responses on dermal irritation to its request for public comments published in the FEDERAL REGISTER of March 25, 1987 (52 FR 9536). The comments concerning purpose, objective, guideline, and summary were taken under advisement and the document changed to conform better to the PR Notice 86-5. Comments on changes in the appendices were considered, but not adopted. The singular comment concerning the primary irritation index was noted and the number of scoring time points was corrected to 4 from the 8 in the document available for public comment.

Guideline

The Final Report should contain the following items.

Cover Page

The title page and additional documentation (i.e., requirements for data submission, Good Laboratory Practices statement, and statement of data confidentiality claims), if relevant to the study report, must preceed the content of the study format below. These requirements are described in PR Notice 86-5.

Subdivision F, Series 81-5.

Table of Contents

This item should be a concise listing of the essential elements of the Final Report including the page numbers for each. Essential elements should include the following: summary, introduction, materials and methods, results, discussion, bibliography, tables, figures, appendices, and key subsections as appropriate.

Body of Report

This item shall include all information required in §80-4 (b)(2), §80-4 (c), and §81-5. Additional recommendations are provided in paragraphs identified as III and IV of this addendum.

I. Summary

As per §80-4 (b)(1) of this Subdivision, this section of the test report shall contain a summary and analysis of the data and a statement of the conclusions drawn from the analysis. This summary should highlight any and all positive data or observations and any deviations from control data which may be indicative of toxic effects.

II. Introduction (include the objectives of this study).

Materials/Methods

This section of the Final Report shall include information required by §80-4 of this Subdivision. See also the Standard Evaluation Procedure (SEP)[1] and §81-5 for details.

IV. Results

Further reporting see Subdivision F: Pesticide Assessment Guidelines, Hazard Evaluation Division—Human And Domestic Animals; §81-5. See also other pertinent parts of the guideline in addition to the SEP. The results shall be summarized in tabular form.

A. *"Evaluation of results.* The dermal irritation scores shall be evaluated in conjunction with the nature and reversibility or otherwise of the responses observed. The individual scores do not represent an absolute standard for the irritation properties of a material. They should be viewed as reference values which are meaningful when supported by a full description and evaluation of the observations. The use of an occlusive dressing is a severe test and the results are relevant to very few likely human exposure conditions."

---

[1]The Standard Evaluation Procedure for Dermal Irritation is to be published. It aids the Agency reviewer in evaluating a Dermal Irritation report submitted in the registration of a pesticide.

C. *Score sheet (example): Dermal Irritation (Intact Skin)*

Test Substance: Date: _____ .

# & sex	Erythema/Eschar						Edema						Scores
	Observations (hrs.)*												
	1	24	48	72	168	336	1	24	48	72	168	336	
M/F 1002	2	3	3	3	0	—	2	2	2	2	0	—	19/4 = 4.75
M/F 1003	2	3	3	2	0	—	2	2	2	1	0	—	17/4 = 4.25
M/F 1004	3	3	3	3	0	—	2	2	1	1	0	—	18/4 = 34.50
M/F 1005	2	2	2	2	0	—	1	2	2	2	0	—	15/4 = 3.75
M/F 1006	0	2	2	2	0	—	0	2	2	2	0	—	12/4 = 3.00
M/F 1007	0	2	1	1	0	—	0	2	0	0	0	—	6/4 = 1.50

Primary irritation index (P.I.I.)** = 21.75/6 = 3.6.
* Only use 1, 24, 48, and 72 hour observations for calculations. The other observed times are for reversibility.
** P.I.I.: slight < 2, moderate 2–5, severe >5.

D. *Dermal Irritation Toxicity Categories (40 CFR §162.10)*

I	II	III	IV
Corrosive	Severe irritation at 72 hrs.	Moderate irritation at 72 hrs.	Mild or slight irritation at 72 hrs.

B. *"Test report.* In addition to the information recommended by §80-4, the test report should include the following information: physical nature and, where appropriate, concentration and pH value for the test substance; species and strain used; tabulation of irritation response data for each individual animal for each observation time period (e.g., 30 to 60 minutes, 24, 48 and 72 hours after patch removal), description of any lesions observed; narrative description of the degree and nature of irritation observed; and description of any toxic effects other than dermal irritation."

V. Discussion

VI. Bibliography

VII. Verification

This item shall contain information required by §80-4 (b)(2). Each test report shall be:

A. Signed by each of the senior scientific personnel, including the laboratory director, responsible for performing and supervising the testing, preparing, reviewing, and approval of the test report.

B. Certified by the applicant or an authorized agent of the applicant as a complete and unaltered copy of the report provided by the testing laboratory whether independent or owned, operated, or controlled by the applicant.

VIII. Archives

This section of the Final Report shall contain all information required in 40 CFR Part 160.185.

IX. Tables/Figures

X. Appendix(es)

PESTICIDE ASSESSMENT GUIDELINES FOR HUMANS AND DOMESTIC ANIMALS: DERMAL SENSITIZATION DATA REPORTING

Introduction

A. Purpose

The purpose of this guideline is to provide a data reporting format for dermal sensitization studies.

B. Objective

This data reporting guideline is designed to aid the registrant in the preparation and submission of reports which are compatible with the Agency's review process. While following the guideline is not mandatory except to the extent of compliance with the PR Notice 86-5, but registrants are strongly encouraged to submit reports in this format.

Response to Public Comments

The Agency received one response on dermal sensitization to its request for public comments published in the FEDERAL REGISTER of March 25, 1987 (52 FR 9536). The general comments concerning purpose, objective, guideline, and summary were taken under advisement, and changes were made to better conform to the PR Notice 86-5. Comments on changes in the appendices were considered but not adopted.

Subdivision F, Series 81-6.

Guideline

The Final Report should contain the following items.

Cover Page

The title page and additional documentation (i.e., requirements for data submission, Good Laboratory Practices statement, and statement of data confidentiality claims), if relevant to the study report, must preceed the content of the study format below. These requirements are described in PR Notice 86-5.

Table of Contents

This item should be a concise listing of the essential elements of the Final Report including the page numbers for each. Essential elements should include the following: Summary, Introduction, Materials and Methods, Results, Discussion, Bibliography, Tables, Figures, Appendices, and key subsections as appropriate.

Body of Report

This item shall include all information required in §80-4 (b)(2), §80-4 (c), and §81-6. Additional recommendations are provided in paragraphs identified as III and IV of this addendum.

I. Summary

As per §80-4 (b)(1) of this Subdivision, this section of the test report shall contain a summary and analysis of the data and a statement of the conclusions drawn from the analysis. This summary should highlight any and all positive data or observations and any deviations from control data which may be indicative of toxic effects.

II. Introduction (include the objectives of this study).

Materials/Methods

This section of the Final Report shall include information required by §80-4 of this Subdivision, and it may also contain the following descriptions specific to dermal sensitization.

A. See §81-5 and the Standard Evaluation Procedure (SEP)[1] for details.
B. Since any of seven tests are acceptable, we do not provide examples of data formats. In general, follow §81-5 and §80-4 in addition to the other requirements [49 FR (188) 37596 (9/26/84)]. §81.5 ". . . the test report shall include the following information: A description of the method used and the commonly accepted name; information on positive control study, including pos-

---

[1]The Standard Evaluation Procedure for Dermal Irritation is to be published. It aids the Agency reviewer in evaluating a Dermal Irritation report submitted in the registration of a pesticide.

itive control used, method used, and time conducted; the number, species, strain and sex of the test animals; individual weights of the animals at the start of the test and at the conclusion of the test; a brief description of the grading system; and each reading made on each individual animal."

IV. Results

Summary Tables. Paragraph 81-6 and §80-4 require results to be summarized in tabular form.

V. Discussion

VI. Bibliography

VII. Verification

This item shall contain information required by §80-4 (b)(2). Each test report shall be:

A. Signed by each of the senior scientific personnel, including the laboratory director responsible for performing and supervising the testing, preparing, reviewing, and approval of the test report.

B. Certified by the applicant or an authorized agent of the applicant as a complete and unaltered copy of the report provided by the testing laboratory whether independent or owned, operated, or controlled by the applicant.

VIII. Archives

This section of the Final Report shall contain all information required in 40 CFR Part 160.185.

IX. Tables/Figures

X. Appendix(es)

These should include individual animal data, histopathology (if indicated), source of animals, diet, animal weights, protocol, and other information as appropriate.

PESTICIDE ASSESSMENT GUIDELINES FOR HUMANS AND DOMESTIC ANIMALS: ACUTE DERMAL TOXICITY DATA REPORTING

Introduction

A. Purpose

The purpose of this addendum to the guideline is to provide a data reporting format for acute dermal toxicity studies. Subpart F, Series 81-2 provides guidelines for carrying out the acute dermal toxicity study.

Subdivision F, Series 81-2.

B. Objective

The objective of the Data Reporting Guidelines (DRGs) is to provide an example of an acceptable general reporting format that can be reviewed effectively and expeditiously in accordance with the Agency's review process. The recommendations are intended to be consistent with the guidelines for data reporting as described in Sections 80-4 and 81-2 and those described in the Agency's Good Laboratory Practice Standards (40 CFR Part 160).

While following this Guideline is not mandatory, data submitters are encouraged to submit complete reports which can be effectively reviewed by the Agency. 40 CFR Part 158 pertains to the physical formatting of reports (which are referred to as "studies") and submitted packages. Some of its requirements are mandatory.

Response to Public Comments

The Agency received one response to its request for public comments on these documents published in the FEDERAL REGISTER of March 8, 1989 (54 FR 9886). These comments were considered in the final form of this DRG.

Guideline

The Final Report should contain the following items.

Cover Page

The title page and additional documentation (i.e., requirements for data submission, Good Laboratory Practices statement and statement of data confidentiality claims), if relevant to the study report, must precede the content of the study format below. These requirements are described in 40 CFR Part 158.

Table of Contents

The table of contents should include a listing of the elements of the final report such as the Summary, an Introduction, the Materials and Methods, Results, Discussion, Bibliography, Tables, Figures, Appendices and key subsections as appropriate.

Body of the Report

This item shall include all information required in §80-4(b)(2), 80-4(c) and 81-2(h) of this subdivision and should be provided in such detail that the reviewer can assess the quality of the study and conformity to the acute dermal toxicity Guideline. It should contain the following sections.

I. Summary

As per §80-4(b)(1) of this subdivision, the test report shall contain a summary including a brief description of the study protocol, chemical used, the animals tested and the highlights of the results of the study relative to the positive findings. Any deviations from the intended protocols should be noted.

II. Introduction

Include the objectives of the study and the Guideline reference. The overall experimental design should be explained.

III. Materials and Methods

A. Test substance

test material (chemical name)
form (technical, manufacturing-use product or formulation)
source
lot number
CAS No.
purity
state
Ionization constant (if applicable)
pH (if applicable)
octanol/water partition coefficient (if known)
vapor pressure at 20 °C (if known)

vehicles used

B. Test animals

species and strain
source
sex
body weight
number of test animals
number of control animals
pre-test condition
housing conditions
test environment

C. Experimental design

dose and duration of exposure
number and sex of animals per dose group
application site, preparation and method(s) of protection
observations, type and time
termination

D. Evaluation procedures

The final report should describe the types of observations of the animals for toxic signs, body weights, the frequency of observations, the gross pathological examination procedures and any other observations performed. The statistical methods used for calculation of the LD50, the 95% confidence limits and the slope of the dose-response curve should be specified and referenced.

E. Deviations from protocol

Deviations from the protocol recommended in §81-2 should be described along with the rationale for the changes.

IV. Results

This section should provide a summary of the toxic signs, mortality, body weight changes, gross pathology and other observations performed associated with the doses tested. Typically, these results are summarized in tabular form.

V. Discussion

This section should provide an assessment of the results of the study, an interpretation of the toxicity observed, the consistency of the dose-response effects and should try to explain unexpected findings. The impact of any deviation from the Guideline protocol should be discussed.

VI. Bibliography

This item should contain a list of references cited in the body of the report.

VII. Verification

This item shall contain information required by §80-4(b)(2). Each test report shall be:

A. Signed by each of the senior scientific personnel, including the laboratory director responsible for performing and supervising the testing, preparing, reviewing and approving the test report and
B. Certified by the applicant or an authorized agent of the applicant as a complete and unaltered copy of the report provided by the testing laboratory whether independent or owned, operated or controlled by the applicant.

VII. Archives

This section of the final report shall contain all information required in 40 CFR 160.185.

IX. Tables/Figures

X. Appendix(es)

These should include individual animal data, historical control data, pathology report, analytical methods and results of analysis of the test substance, details of statistical analysis, protocol and other information as appropriate.

PESTICIDE ASSESSMENT GUIDELINES FOR HUMANS AND DOMESTIC ANIMALS: REPEATED DOSE DERMAL TOXICITY (21 DAYS and 90 DAYS) DATA REPORTING

Introduction

A. Purpose

The purpose of this addendum to the guideline is to provide a data reporting format for repeated dose dermal toxicity studies. Subpart F, Series 82-2 and 82-3 provide guidelines for carrying out the repeated dose dermal toxicity studies.

B. Objective

The objective of the Data Reporting Guidelines (DRGs) is to provide an example of an acceptable general reporting format that can be reviewed effectively and expeditiously in accordance with the Agency's review process. The recommendations are intended to be consistent with the guidelines for data reporting as described in Sections 80-4, 82-2 and 82-3 and those described in the Agency's Good Laboratory Practice Standards (40 CFR Part 160).

While following this Guideline is not mandatory, data submitters are encouraged to submit complete reports which can be effectively reviewed by the Agency. 40 CFR Part 158 pertains to the physical formatting of reports (which are referred to as "studies") and submitted packages. Some of its requirements are mandatory.

Response to Public Comments

The Agency received one response to its request for public comments on these documents published in the FEDERAL REGISTER of March 8, 1989 (54 FR 9886). These comments were considered in the final form of this DRG.

Guideline

The Final Report should contain the following items.

Cover Page

The title page and additional documentation (i.e., requirements for data submission, Good Laboratory Practices statement and statement of data confi-

Subdivision F, Series 81-5.

dentiality claims), if relevant to the study report, must precede the content of the study format below. These requirements are described in 40 CFR Part 158.

Table of Contents

The table of contents should include a listing of the elements of the final report such as the Summary, an Introduction, the Materials and Methods, Results, Discussion, Bibliography, Tables, Figures, Appendices and key subsections as appropriate.

Body of the Report

This item shall include all information required in §80-4(b)(2), 80-4(c), 82-2(h) and 82-3(h) of this subdivision and should be provided in such detail that the reviewer can assess the quality of the study and conformity to the repeated dose dermal toxicity Guideline. It should contain the following sections.

I. Summary

As per §80-4(b)(1) of this subdivision, the test report shall contain a summary including a brief description of the study protocol, chemical used, the animals tested and the highlights of the results of the study relative to the positive findings. Any deviations from the intended protocols should be noted.

II. Introduction

Include the objectives of the study and the Guideline reference. The overall experimental design should be explained.

III. Materials and Methods

A. Test substance.

• test material (chemical name)
• source
• lot number
• CAS No.
• purity
• state
• ionization constant (if applicable)
• pH (if applicable)
• octanol/water partition coefficient (if known)
• vapor pressure at 20 °C (if known)
• vehicles used

B. Test animals.

• species and strain
• source

- sex
- body weight
- number of test animals
- number of control animals
- pre-test condition
- housing conditions
- test environment

C. Experimental design.

- doses and duration of exposure
- number and sex of animals per dose group
- application site, preparation and method(s) of protection
- observations, type and time
- termination

D. Evaluation procedures.

The final report should describe the types of observations of the animals for toxic signs, body weights, the frequency of observations, the gross pathological examination procedures, histopathology and any other observations performed.

E. Deviation from protocol.

Deviations for the protocol recommended in §82-2 or 82-3 should be described along with the rationale for the changes.

IV. Results

This section should provide a summary of the toxic signs, mortality, body weight changes, gross pathology and other observations performed associated with the doses tested. Typically, these results are summarized in tabular form.

V. Discussion

This section should provide an assessment of the results of the study, an interpretation of the toxicity observed, and the dose-response effects and should try to explain unexpected findings. The impact of any deviation from the Guideline protocol should be discussed.

VI. Bibliography

This item should contain a list of references cited in the body of the report.

VII. Verification

This item shall contain information required by §80-4(b)(2). Each test report shall be:

A. Signed by each of the senior scientific personnel, including the laboratory director responsible for performing and supervising the testing, preparing, reviewing and approving the test report and

B. Certified by the applicant or an authorized agent of the applicant as a complete and unaltered copy of the report provided by the testing laboratory whether independent or owned, operated or controlled by the applicant.

VII. Archives

This section of the final report shall contain all information required in 40 CFR 160.185.

IX. Tables/Figures

X. Appendix(es)

These should include individual animal data, historical control data, pathology report, analytical methods and results of analysis of the test substance, details of statistical analysis, protocol and other information as appropriate.

152A-11 ACUTE DERMAL TOXICITY STUDY WITH MICROBIAL PEST CONTROL AGENTS [(MPCA)s]: TIER I.

(a) *When required.*

Acute dermal toxicity data are required by 40 CFR 158.740 to support the registration of each manufacturing-use product and each end-use product, and the technical grade of each active ingredient.

(b) *Purpose.*

Acute dermal toxicity data provide information on health hazards likely to arise from a single dermal application of soluble or particulate chemicals associated with a preparation of the MPCA, and/or associated with other ingredients in formulations of the MPCA, and/or associated with products from genetic material intentionally introduced in the MPCA.

(C) *Definitions.*

(1) "Acute dermal toxicity" is the adverse effect occurring during or following a 24-hour dermal exposure to a single dose of a test substance.

(2) "Dose level" is based on the amount of MPCA administered. It is expressed as:

Subdivision M Of The Pesticide Testing Guidelines Microbial And Biochemical Pest Control Agents (EPA-540/9-8-82-028). Includes the test required to support the field testing and registration of naturally occurring or genetically altered microbial pest control agents. *Tier I Testing*, 152A-11: Acute Dermal Toxicity Study.

(i) units of the microorganism applied at each test site on the test animal, and as;

(ii) dry weight of applied test substance at a single test site per kilogram body weight of test animal.

(3) "Units of MPCAs." One unit of representative MPCA groups usually would be defined as follows:

(i) vegetative bacterium: a single, viable organism, and usually the entity that produces a single colony forming unit (CFU) on an appropriate semisolid growth medium.

(ii) bacterial or fungal spore, bacterial aor protozoan cyst: an intact individual spore or cyst as determined microscopically, and usually the entity that produces a single CFU on appropriate germination medium.

(iii) fungal mycelium: 10^{-9} gram dry weight or, after standardization preparatory procedures, a mycelium-producing entity on semi-solid growth medium.

(iv) virus; an intact, complete virion or a polyhedral body as determined by electron microscopy, and, usually the entity that produces an infective unit (IU) on appropriate host cells or tissues.

(v) protozoa: an intact vegetative organism, spore, or cyst of the members in the various classes of this phylum.

Due to the wide diversity of forms among microorganisms, other definitions of a unit of a MPCA may be equally appropriate.

(d) *Principles of the test method.*

The MPCA in each formulation to be tested is applied in a single high dose to the skin of experimental animals. Subsequently, observations of effects and deaths are made. Animals that die during the test are necropsied, and at the conclusion of the test, the surviving animals are sacrificed and necropsied as indicated by the nature of the toxic effects observed.

(e) *Substance to be tested.*

(1) The manufacturing-use product shall be tested to support the registration of each manufacturing-use product.

(2) The end-use product shall be tested to support the registration of each end-use product.

(3) The form (e.g., vegetative cell, spore, cyst, virion) of the MPCA used for preparation of the dosing material should be equivalent to the form that is intended for registration or application. To the extent possible, the test MPCA also should be equivalent to the MPCA intended for registration or application with respect to stage of growth, possession of organelles and appendages, and appendages, and expression of phenotypic traits (including products from intentionally introduced genes). If significant exposure to other forms of the MPCA are expected, then these forms also may have to be tested.

(f) *Characteristics of the test MPCA.*

The test MPCA should be thoroughly characterized as required in section 151A of these guidelines.

(g) *Test procedures.*

(1) *Animal selection.*

(i) *Species and strain.* Although several mammalian test species may be used, the albino rabbit is the preferred species. Commonly used laboratory strains should be employed. If another species is used, the investigator should provide justification/reasoning for the alternative selection. All test animals should be free of parasites or pathogens. Females should be nulliparous and non-pregnant.

(ii) *Age.* Young adults should be used. The weight variation of animals used in a test should not exceed ±20% of the mean weight for each sex.

(iii) *Sex.* Equal numbers of animals of each sex with healthy intact skin are recommended.

(iv) *Numbers.* At least 10 animals (five animals of each sex) should be used.

(2) *Control groups.* (i) Neither a concurrent untreated nor vehicle control group are required except when the toxicity of the vehicle is unknown.

(3) *Dosing.* (i) *Dose level.* The test substance should be applied at 2 grams/test animal. If a dose level of less than 2 grams/test animal is used, then a justification/explanation must be provided.

(ii) *Vehicle.* Where necessary, the formulation to be tested is suspended in a suitable vehicle. An aqueous solution should be used. The recommended vehicle for the end-use product usually is the same material in which the MPCA will be mixed, suspended, or diluted for application.

(iii) *Volume.* The moisture content of the test material should not be excessive, but should be sufficient to prevent significant drying of the test material during the exposure period, and to ensure good contact with the skin.

(iv) *MPCA quantification.* The numbers of MPCAs in the dose material should be enumerated. Techniques used to quantify the units of MPCA in any dose will depend on the group of microorganisms to which the MPCA belongs. Where possible, determinations of viable, or potentially viable, or ineffective units in each dose should be made. A measurement of metabolism associated with a defined biomass may be the preferred technique for quantification of mycelial forms of MPCAs. Quantification should be done concurrently with testing.

(4) *Exposure duration.* The exposure duration should be for approximately 24 hours.

(5) *Observation period.* The observation period should be at least for 14 days, but should not be fixed rigidly. It should be determined by the toxic reactions, rate of onset and length of recovery period, and thus may be ex-

tended when considered necessary. The time at which toxicity signs appear and disappear, and their duration are important.

(6) *Preparation of animal skin.*

(i) Approximately 24 hours before the test, fur should be removed from the dorsal and ventral area of the trunk of each test animal by clipping or shaving.

(ii) Not less than 10% of the body surface area should be cleared for application of the test substance. The weight of the animal should be taken into account when deciding on the area to be cleared and on the dimensions of the covering.

(7) *Application of the test substance.*

(i) The test substance should be applied uniformly over an area which is approximately 10% of the total body surface area.

(ii) The test substance should be held in contact with the skin with porous gauze and a non-irritating tape throughout a 24-hour exposure period. The test site further should be covered in a suitable manner to retain the gauze dressing and test substance and ensure that the animals cannot ingest the test substance. Restrainers may be used to prevent the ingestion of the test substance, but complete immobilization is not recommended.

(iii) At the end of the exposure period, residual test substance should be removed, where practical, using water.

(8) *Observation of animals.*

(i) A careful clinical examination should be made at least once each day.

(ii) Cage-side observations should include, but not be limited to, changes in:

(A) the skin (including signs of irritation) and fur;

(B) eyes and mucous membranes;

(C) circulatory system;

(E) autonomic and central nervous system;

(F) somatomotor activity; and,

(G) behavior pattern.

(H) Particular attention should be directed to observation of tremors, convulsions, diarrhea, lethargy, salivation, sleep and coma.

(iv) Individual weights of animals should be determined shortly before the test material is administered, weekly thereafter, and at death or at final sacrifice. Changes in weight should be calculated and recorded when survival exceeds one day.

(v) The time of death should be recorded as precisely as possible.

(vi) At the end of the 24-hour exposure period, and daily thereafter, any signs of skin irritation should be recorded and scored.

(9) *Gross pathology.* Consideration should be given to performing a gross necropsy of all animals if indicated by the appearance of toxic effects. If done, all gross pathological changes should be recorded.

(i) *Data and reporting.*

(1) *Treatment of results.* In addition to the information recommended by 150A-4, the test report should include the following information:
(i) number of animals at the start of the test;
(ii) time of death of individual animals;
(iii) number of animals displaying other signs of toxicity;
(iv) description of toxic effects;
(v) definition for one unit of the MPCA used, and the units in the dosing material;
(vi) dry weight and net weight determinations of the test material applied per kilogram body weight of the test animal;
(vii) body weights and time taken;
(viii) necropsy findings, when performed; and,
(ix) pathology findings, when performed;
(2) *Evaluation of results.* An evaluation should include the relationship if any, between the animals exposed to the test substance and the incidence and severity of all abnormalities, including;
(i) behavioral abnormalities;
(ii) clinical abnormalities;
(iii) skin lesions and skin irritation;
(iv) body weight changes;
(v) mortality; and
(vi) toxicity.

(j) *Tier progression.*

(1) If evidence of significant and/or persistent toxicity are observed, then the toxic component(s) of the dosing material are to be identified, and to a practical extent, isolated.
(i) An acute toxicity study (152A-20) is to be conducted with the toxic components.
(2) If no toxic effects are observed, then no further testing is required.

PESTICIDE ASSESSMENT GUIDELINES SUBDIVISION M[1]

This section includes the following tests (listed below) to support the registration of biorational pesticide products.

- *Group A-1: Tier I Testing*
  152-11: Acute Dermal Toxicity.
  152-14: Primary Dermal Irritation.
  152-15: Hypersensitivity Study
  152-16: Hypersensitivity Incidences

[1]Biorational Pesticides (EPA-540/9-820028).

- *Group A-2: Tier II Testing*
  152-21: Subchronic Dermal Toxicity Study.

  152-31: Acute Dermal Toxicity/Infectivity Study With Microbial Pest Control Agents.
  152-34: Primary Dermal Irritation Study With Microbial Pest Control Agents.
  152-36: Hypersensitivity Study With Microbial Pest Control Agent.
  152-37: Hypersensitivity Incidious With Microbial Pest Control Agents.
- *Group B-2: Tier II Testing*
  152-44: Primary Dermal Irritation Study With Microbial Agents.

§152-11 ACUTE DERMAL TOXICITY STUDY: TIER I

(a) *When required.*

Data on the single-dose dermal LD_{50} are required by 40 CFR 158.165 to support the registration of each manufacturing-use product and each end-use formulated product, unless the substance to be tested under paragraph (b) of this section is a gas or highly volatile substance that cannot be administered dermally.

(b) *Test Standards.*

The test standards set forth in §150-3 of this subdivision and §82-2(d) through (g) of Subdivision F should be met with the following exceptions:

(1) *Test species.* A generally recognized strain of laboratory rat, mouse, or rabbit should be tested.

(2) *Number of animals and selection of dose levels.* (i) A trial test is recommended for the purpose of establishing a dosing regimen which shall include one dose level higher than the expected LD50 and at least one dose level lower than the expected LD50. If data based on testing with at least 5 animals per sex with abraded skin are submitted showing that the LD50 is greater than 2 g/kg for the 24-hour contact period, no further testing at other dose levels is necessary. If mortality occurs, the recommendations of paragraph (b)(ii) of this section apply.

(ii) The number of animals per dose level, and the number and spacing of dose levels should be chosen such that mortality rates between 10% and 90% are produced, in order that calculation of the LD50 (abraded skin and intact skin) of males and females with a 95% confidence interval of 20% or less can be made. At least 3 dose levels of the test substance, in addition to controls, should be tested; test groups shall contain approximately equal numbers of male and female animals.

(c) *Reporting.*

In addition to the information required by §150-4, the following recommendations should be met:
(1) Information on the gross pathology of animal tissues, organs, and fluids;
(2) Pathological changes to the skin receiving the initial challenge dose;
(3) Clinical signs of illness or toxicity such as elevated temperature, unkempt appearance, altered feeding habits, weight loss, and other forms of distress or physical depression; and
(4) Any signs of recovery from these symptoms.

(d) *Tier progression.*

(1) If acute adverse effects are observed, then subchronic dermal toxicity tests (§152-21) shall be required as specified in 40 CFR §158.165 when pesticide use is likely to result in repeated human skin contact with the product, its active ingredients, or their breakdown products.
(2) If no acute effects are observed (e.g., during testing, greater than 2 g/kg), then no further testing is recommended.

§152-14 PRIMARY DERMAL IRRITATION STUDY: TIER I

(a) *When required.*

(1) *General requirement.* Data on primary dermal irritation are required by 40 CFR §158.165 to support the registration of each manufacturing-use product and each end-use product.
(2) *Corrosive pesticides.* Data which demonstrate that the test substance specified by paragraph (a) of this section has a pH of 1–3 or 12–14 may be submitted in lieu of data from a primary dermal irritation study conducted in accordance with paragraph (b) of this section. For all regulatory purposes, the Agency will assume that such a substance is corrosive.

(6) *Test standards.*

The test standards set forth in §150-3 of this subdivision and §81-5(e) and (f) of Subdivision F should be met, with the following exceptions:
(1) *Test species.* Testing should be performed on either the albino rabbit or the guinea pig. Selection of other mammalial species may be acceptable, but should be justified.

(c) *Reporting.*

The reporting requirements set forth in §150-4 of this subdivision and §81-5(g) of Subdivision F should be met.

§152-15 HYPERSENSITIVITY STUDY: TIER I

(a) *When required.*

Data on hypersensitivity are required by 40 CFR §159.165 to support the registration of each manufacturing-use product and of each end-use product whose use will result in repeated human skin contact under conditions of use.

(b) *Test standards.*

The test standards set forth in §150-3 of this subdivision and §81-6(e) and (f) of Subdivision F shall be met, with the following exceptions:
(1) *Species.* The test should be performed on at least one mammalian species. The albino guinea pig and hamster are the preferred species.
(2) *Age and sex.* Young adult males should be used when albino guinea pigs are tested. Young adults of either sex may be used when hamsters are tested.

(c) *Reporting.*

The reporting requirements are the same as those set forth in §150-4 of this subdivision and §81-6(g) of Subdivision F.

§152-6 HYPERSENSITIVITY INCIDENTS: TIER I

(a) *When required.*

Data on incidents of hypersensitivity to humans or domestic animals that occur during the production or testing of the technical chemical, the manufacturing-use product, or end-use product shall be reported as required by 40 CFR §158.165 with the toxicology data supplied in support of an application for registration. For reporting of incidents taking place after registration, refer to the requirements in sec. 6(a)(2) of FIFRA.

(b) *Reporting.*

The reporting provisions for these incidents shall be the same as those for conventional chemical pesticides, as specified in the Pesticide Incident Report form (EPA form number 8550-5, OMB number 158-R0008). The following information shall be provided, if available:
(1) The name of the biochemical agent;
(2) The length of exposure to the agent;
(3) The time, date, and location of exposure to the agent;
(4) The situation or circumstances under which exposure to the agent occurred.
(5) Clinical observations.
(1) The use for which registration application is made requires a tolerance

for the pesticide or an exemption from the requirement to obtain a tolerance, or requires issuing a food additive regulation; or

(2) The use of the pesticide product is likely to result in repeated human exposure to the product, its active ingredient(s), or degradation product(s) through the oral route.

(b) *Test standards.*

The test standards are set forth in §150-3 of this subdivision and §82-1(c) of Subdivision F.

(c) *Reporting.*

The reporting provisions are the same as those required in §82-1(h) of Subdivision F.

(d) *Tier progression.*

(1) Data on a chronic exposure study (§152-26) are required by 40 CFR 158.165 if the potential for adverse chronic effects is indicated based on:
(i) The subchronic effect level established in this study;
(ii) The pesticide use pattern (e.g., rate, frequency, and location of application); and
(iii) The frequency and level of repeated human exposure that is expected.
(2) Data on an oncogenicity study (§152-29) are required by 40 CFR 158.165 if the test results of this study reveal a morphologic effect (e.g., hyperplasia, metaplasia) in any organ that potentially could lead to neoplastic change.
(3) If the potential for chronic adverse effects is not indicated by paragraph (d)(1)(i), (ii), and (iii) of this section, and no morphological effects are noted (in any organ) that potentially could lead to neoplastic change, then no additional testing is recommended.

§152-21 SUBCHRONIC DERMAL TOXICITY STUDY: TIER II

(a) *When required.*

Data from the subchronic dermal toxicity studies are required by 40 CFR §158.165 to support the registration of each end-use product for which acute adverse effects were observed during acute dermal toxicity studies (§152-11) and each manufacturing-use product which may legally be used to formulate such an end-use product and when the pesticide use is likely to result in repeated human skin contact with the product, its active ingredients, or its breakdown products. See 40 CFR §158.50 and §158.165 to determine whether these data must be submitted;

Section II-B of this subdivision contains an additional discussion of the formulators' exemption and who, as a general rule, is responsible for submission of the required data.

(b) *Test standards.*

The test standards are set forth in §150-3 of this subdivision and §82-2(b) of Subdivision F.

(c) *Reporting.*

The reporting provisions are the same as those for testing conventional chemical pesticides as set forth in §82-2(h) of Subdivision F.

(d) *Tier progression.*

(1) Data on a chronic exposure study (§152-26) are required by 40 CFR 158.165 if a potential for adverse chronic effects is indicated, based on:
(i) The subchronic effect levels established in this study;
(ii) The pesticide use pattern (e.g., rate, frequency, and site of application); and
(iii) The site, frequency, and level of repeated human exposure that is expected.

(2) Data on an oncogenicity study (§152-29) are required by 40 CFR §158.165 if the test results of this study reveal a morphologic effect (e.g., hyperplasia, metaplasia) in any organ that potentially could lead to neoplastic change.

(3) If the potential for chronic adverse effects is not indicated based on paragraph (d)(1)(i), (ii), and (iii), and no morphologic effects are noted (in any organ) that potentially could lead to neoplastic change, then no further testing is recommended.

§152-31 ACUTE DERMAL TOXICITY/INEFFECTIVITY STUDY WITH MICROBIAL PEST CONTROL AGENTS: TIER I

(a) *When required.*

Data on acute dermal infectivity are required by 40 CFR §158.165 to support the registration of each manufacturing-use and each end-use product.

(b) *Test standards.*

In addition to the applicable standards set forth in §150-3 of this subdivision and §80-3 and §81-2(d) through (g) of Subdivision F, an acute dermal infectivity study should meet the following standards:
(1) *Species.* Testing should be performed with at least one mammalian species, preferably the rat or mouse.
(2) *Sex and age.* Young adult male and female animals should be used.
(3) *Number of animals and selection of dose levels.*
(i) A trial test is recommended for the purpose of establishing a dosing regimen which should include one dose level higher than the expected LD50. If data from abraded skin tests on at least 5 animals of each sex are submitted

showing that the dermal LD50 is greater than 2 g/kg for the 24-hour contact period, no further testing at other dose levels is necessary. If mortality is produced, the provisions of paragraph (b)(3)(ii) of this section apply.

(ii) At least 3 dose levels spaced appropriately should be tested using adequate numbers of animals to form test groups with mortality rates in the 10 to 90% range in order to permit LD50 determinations (abraded skin and intact skin) for males and for females with a 95% confidence interval of 20% or less. In addition, the requirements of paragraph (b)(3)(iii) of this section may apply.

(iii) Data from tests performed with the use dilutions of a product may be necessary if the use dilution is intended for application as a mist or spray.

(4) *Control animals.* A concurrent untreated control group of animals should be included in the test. A concurrent vehicle control group is recommended if a vehicle or dilutent used in administering the test substance is expected to elicit an important toxicologic response, or if insufficient data exists on the acute effects of the vehicle.

(5) *Dose quantification.* Titers of microbial suspensions to test animals should be performed by plating dilutions on laboratory surface or other suitable media or host organisms for enumeration of viable organisms.

(6) *Conduct of test.*

(i) Application. In all animals, the application site should be as free of hair as possible. In addition, the application sites in abraded-skin groups should be abraded in such a way as to penetrate the stratum corneum but not the dermis. The test substance must be kept in contact with skin covering at least 10 percent of the body surface for at least 24 hours. [See Draize (1944) for equivalent sq. cm. of body surface.] The preferred application site is a band around the trunk of the test animal. A wrapping material such as gauze covered by an impervious nonreactive rubberized or plastic material should be used to retard evaporation and to keep the test substance in contact with the skin. At the end of the exposure period, the wrapping should be removed and the skin wiped (but not washed) to remove remaining test substance.

(ii) *Duration of observation.* Animals should be observed for at least 14 days after dosing or until all signs of reversible infectivity or toxicity in survivors subside, whichever occurs later.

(iii) *Observations.* The animals should be observed frequently during the day of dosing and checked at least once each morning and late afternoon thereafter. The following should be recorded even though the animals recover completely from the exposure: nature and onset of all gross or visible clinical signs of illness such as elevated temperature, unkempt appearance, altered feeding habits, weight loss, various forms of physical distress, depression, and similar responses.

(iv) *Assay for specific antibody production.* If test duration exceeds 14 days, then an assay for antibody production should be performed.

(v) *Sacrifice and necropsy.* All test and control animals surviving at the end of the observation period (14 days) are sacrificed. All test animals, whether dying during the test or sacrificed, are subjected to a complete gross necropsy. In addition to gross pathology, microorganism dissemination, replication, survival in animal tissue, organs, and fluids should be determined, including survival in the skin. Samples should be cultured on laboratory surface or other suitable media or host organisms to provide qualitative and quantitative measurements of survival and multiplication of the microorganism.

(vi) *Histopathology.* Examination of skin should include histological examination of treated tissues in accordance with §80-3(b)(11) of Subdivision F.

(c) *Data reporting and evaluation.*

In addition to the applicable general information required by §80-4 of Subdivision F, the test report should include the following information:

(1) Tabulation of response data by sex and dose level (number of animals dying per number of animals showing signs of infectivity per number of animals exposed);

(2) Time of death after dosing;

(3) Observations of signs and symptoms;

(4) Gross pathological findings;

(5) Evidence of microorganism dissemination, replication, and survival in animal tissues, organs, and fluids, including survival in skin;

(6) LD50 determinations for each sex and for each test substance for animals with abraded skin and for animals with intact skin calculated at the end of the observation period (with method of calculation specified) expressed in numbers of viable microorganisms per kg body weight and mg of test substance per kg body weight;

(7) 95% confidence interval for the LD50;

(8) Dose-response curve and slope; and

(9) Identification of the test microorganism, including:

(i) Genus, species, serotype, and strain (to the extent possible), according to current acceptable taxonomy; and

(ii) The percent of unknown fermentation solids or other materials present to account for 100% of the sample.

(10) Results of assays for specific antibody production, when applicable.

(d) *Tier progression.*

No further testing is require by 40 CFR 158.165 for viruses or protozoa.

(2) If evidence of infectivity, organism persistence or replication, or toxic effects is observed following acute dermal studies with bacteria or fungi, then acute intraperitoneal or intracerebral tests shall be conducted in two animal species other than those used in Tier I (§152-43) as specified by 40 CFR 158.165. Half of the test animals should be immunodepressed.

(e) *References.*

(1) Draize, J. H., G. Woodard, and H. O. Calvery. 1944. Methods for study of irritation and toxicity of substances applied topically to skin and mucous membranes. *J. Pharmacol. Exp. Ther.* 83:377–390.

(2) Draize, J. H. 1965. Appraisal of the safety of chemicals in foods, drugs and cosmetics—Dermal toxicity. Assoc. of Food and Drug Officials of the United States. Topeka, Kansas. Pp. 46–59.

(3) Lamanna, C., and L. Jones. 1963. Lethality for mice of vegetative and spore forms of Bacillus cereus and Bacillus cereus-like insect pathogens injected intraperitoneally and subcutaneously. *J. Bacteriol.* 85:532–535.

(4) Leise, J. M., C. H. Carter, H. Friedlander, and S. W. Freed. 1959. Criteria for the identification of *Bacillus anthracis*. *J. Bacteriol.* 77:655–660.

§152-34 PRIMARY DERMAL IRRITATION STUDY WITH MICROBIAL PEST CONTROL AGENTS: TIER I

(a) *When required.*

Data on primary dermal irritation are required by 40 CFR §158.165 to support the registration of each manufacturing-use product and each end-use product.

(b) *Test standards.*

The general standards set forth in §150-3 of this subdivision and §80-3 of Subdivision F should apply. In addition to these general test standards, a primary dermal irritation study should meet the following standards:

(1) *Substances to be tested.*

(i) The manufacturing-use product shall be tested to support the registration of a manufacturing-use product.

(ii) The end-use product shall be tested to support the registration of an end-use product.

(2) *Species and age.* Testing should be performed with young adult guinea pigs or rabbits.

(3) Condition of test substances.

(i) If the substance is a liquid, it should be applied undiluted.

(ii) If the test substance is a solid, it should be slightly moistened with physiological saline before application.

(4) *Number of animals.* At least six animals shall be used.

(5) *Number and selection of dose levels.* A dose of 0.5 ml of liquid or 0.5 g of solid or semi-solid microbial preparation is to be applied to each application site.

(6) *Dose quantification.* Titers of microbial suspension administered to test animals should be performed by plating dilutions on laboratory surface

media or other suitable media or host organism for enumeration of viable organisms.

(7) *Control groups.*

(i) A vehicle control group is recommended if the vehicle is known to cause any toxic dermal reactions or if there is insufficient information concerning the dermal effects of the vehicle.

(ii) Separate animals are not necessary for an untreated control group. Each animal serves as its own control.

(8) *Conduct of test.* The test substance is introduced under one-inch square gauze patches. The patches should be applied to two intact and two abraded skin sites on each animal. In all animals, the application sites should be clipped free of hair. The abrasion should penetrate the stratum corneum, but not the dermis. A wrapping material such as gauze covered by an impervious, nonreactive rubberized or plastic material should be used to retard evaporation and to keep the test substance in contact with the skin. The animals should be restrained. The test substance must be kept in contact with the skin for 24 hours. At the end of the exposure period, the wrapping should be removed and the skin wiped (but not washed) to remove any test substance still remaining. It may be necessary to rinse off the material if colored test substances are used.

(9) *Observation and scoring.* Animals shall be observed and signs of erythema and edema shall be scored at 24 hours and 72 hours after application of the test substance. The irritation is to be scored according to the technique of J. H. Draize (1959). Observation for irritation and scoring of any irritation shall continue daily until all irritation subsides or is obviously irreversible.

(c) *Data reporting and evaluation.* In addition to the applicable general information required by §80-4 of Subdivision F [excepting paragraphs 2)(iii)(A) and (b)(2)(vii)], the test report shall include the following information.

(1) In tabular form, the following data for each individual animal and averages and ranges for each test group:

(i) Scores for erythema and edema at 24 hours, at 72 hours, and at any subsequent observation, and;

(ii) Primary skin irritation scores according to the techniques of Draize.

(d) *Tier progression.*

(1) No further testing is necessary for manufacturing-use products.

(2) If evidence of primary dermal irritation is observed (marked edema or broad erythema) in tests conducted on the end-use formulated product, then:

(i) Primary dermal irritation studies in the guinea pig shall be required by 40 CFR 158.165 using use dilutions of the end-use product (§152-44).

(3) If no evidence of primary dermal irritation is observed, then further testing is not necessary.

§152-36 HYPERSENSITIVITY STUDY WITH MICROBIAL PEST CONTROL AGENTS: TIER I

(a) *When required.*

Data from a hypersensitivity study are required by 40 CFR §158.165 to support the registration of each end-use product for which commonly recognized use practices will result in repeated human contact by inhalation or dermal routes and each manufacturing-use product which legally may be used to formulate such and end-use product.

(b) *Test standards.*

In addition to the applicable general standards set forth in §150-3 of this subdivision and §80-3 of Subdivision F, a hypersensitivity study shall meet the following standards.

(1) *Substance to be tested.*
(i) The manufacturing-use product shall be tested to support the registration of a manufacturing-use product.

(ii) The end-use product shall be tested to support the registration of an end-use product.

(2) *Condition of test substance.* The test substance should be applied undiluted. If the test substance causes marked irritation, it should be diluted with physiological saline until a concentration is found which produces only slight irritation. If the test substance is a solid to be injected intradermally, it should be dissolved in a minimum amount of physiological saline.

(3) *Species.* The test should be performed in the hamster or guinea pig.

(4) *Age and sex.* Young adult males should be used when albino guinea pigs are tested. Young adults of either sex may be used when hamsters are tested.

(5) *Number of animals.* At least 10 animals should be used.

(6) *Dose quantification.* Titers of microbial suspensions should be determined by plating dilutions on laboratory surface or other suitable media or a host organism for enumeration of viable organisms.

(7) *Number and selection of dose levels.* (i) An initial dose of 0.05 ml should be injected intradermally. This dose shall be followed by injection of 0.1 ml three times weekly on alternate days for three weeks, so that a total of ten treatments is administered. Two weeks after the tenth sensitizing treatment, the animals should be challenged by a final injection (Landsteiner and Jacobs, 1935);

(8) *Controls.* (i) A positive control, using a known sensitizing agent, is recommended; and

(ii) A concurrent vehicle control group is not required.

(9) *Conduct of test.*

(1) *Preparation of test animals.* Hair is removed first by clipping and then by shaving to form a strip running from flank to trunk along each side of each animal. This procedure should be repeated as necessary.

(ii) *Intradermal injection.* After preparation of the test animal, the test substance is injected intradermally. The first sensitizing injection is to be made at one end of one strip. The succeeding injections should be made by moving along the shaved strip choosing a new location for each treatment.

(10) *Observation and scoring.* Erythema, edema, and other lesions are scored at 24 hours and 48 hours following each application, according to the standard method (Draize, 1959).

(c) *Data reporting and evaluation.*

In addition to the applicable basic information in §80-4 of Subpart F, the following information should be reported:

(1) Tabulated scores for each animal for erythema and edema at 24 and 48 hours post-application or post-injection; and

(2) Tabulated average scores from all sensitizing treatments, and the score of the challenge treatment.

(d) *Tier progression.*

No tier progression from the hypersensitivity study is necessary.

§152-37 HYPERSENSITIVITY INCIDENTS WITH MICROBIAL PEST CONTROL AGENTS: TIER I

(a) *When required.*

Data on incidents of hypersensitivity of humans or domestic animals that occur during the production or testing of the technical grade of the active ingredient, the manufacturing-use product, or the end-use product should be reported with the toxicology data supplied in support of an application for registration. For reporting of incidents taking place after registration, refer to the requirements in connection with sec. 6(a)(2) of FIFRA.

(b) *Reporting.*

The reporting requirements for these incidents should be the same as those for conventional chemical pesticide incident reports as specified in the Pesticide Incident Report form (EPA form number 8550-5, OMB form number 158-R0008). The following information should be provided if available:

(1) The name of the microbial agent;

(2) The length of exposure to the agent;

(3) The time, data and location of exposure to the agent;

(4) The situation or circumstances under which exposure to the agent occurred; and

(5) Any clinical observations.

§152-44 PRIMARY DERMAL IRRITATION STUDY WITH MICROBIAL AGENTS: TIER II

(a) *When required.*

Data from a primary dermal irritation study (Tier II) are required by 40 CFR §158.165 to support the registration of each end-use product for which marked edema or broad erythema was observed in the Tier I dermal irritation study (§152-34).

(b) *Test standards.*

The test standards set forth in §152-34 apply, except that the use-dilution of the end-use product should be tested.

(c) *Data reporting and evaluation.*

The provisions of §152-34 apply.

(d) *Tier progression.*

No additional tests are necessary.

§152-45 PRIMARY EYE IRRITATION STUDY WITH MICROBIAL AGENTS: TIER II

(a) *When required.*

Data on primary eye irritation (Tier II) are required by 40 CFR §158.165 to support the registration of each end-use product for which severe ocular lesions are observed in the Tier I primary eye irritation study (§152-35 of this subdivision).

(b) *Test standards.*

The test standards set forth in §152-35 apply except that the use-dilution of the end-use formulated product should be tested.

(c) *Data reporting and evaluation.*

The provisions of §152-35 apply.

(d) Tier progression.

No additional testing is required.

PRIMARY DERMAL IRRITATION

Purpose

In the assessment and evaluation of the toxic characteristics of a substance, determination of the irritant and/or corrosive effects on skin of mammals is an important initial step. Information derived from this test serves to indicate the existence of possible hazards likely to arise from exposure of the skin to the test substance.

II. Definitions

    A. Dermal irritation is the production of reversible inflammatory changes in the skin following the application of a test substance.

    B. Dermal corrosion is the production of irreversible tissue damage in the skin following the application of the test substance.

III. Principle of the Test Method

    A. The substance to be tested is applied in a single dose to the skin of several experimental animals, each animal serving as its own control. The degree of irritation is read and scored at specified intervals and is further described to provide a complete evaluation of the effects. The duration of the study should be sufficient to permit a full evaluation of the reversibility or irreversibility of the effects observed but need not exceed 14 days.

    B. When testing solids (which may be pulverized if considered necessary), the test substance should be moistened sufficiently with water or, where necessary, a suitable vehicle, to ensure good contact with the skin. When vehicles are used, the influence of the vehicle on irritation of skin by the test substance should be taken into account. Liquid test substances are generally used undiluted.

    C. Strongly acidic or alkaline substances, for example with a demonstrated pH of 2 or less, or 11.5 or greater, need not be tested for primary dermal irritation, owing to their predictable corrosive properties.

    D. The testing of materials which have been shown to be highly toxic by the dermal route is unnecessary.

IV. Test Procedures

    A. *Animal selection*

    1. Species and strain '
The albino rabbit is recommended as the preferred species. If another mammalian species is used, the tester should provide justification/reasoning for its selection.

U.S. Environmental Protection Agency (1985) Toxic Substances Control Act Testing Guidelines 40 CFR, Part 798, Subpart G, Section 798.6050. *Federal Register,* Vol. 50, No. 188, Friday, September 27, 1985 (pp. 39, 458–39, 460).

2. *Number of animals*

At least 6 healthy adult animals should be used unless, justification/reasoning for using fewer animals is provided.

B. *Control animals*

Separate animals are not recommended for an untreated control group. Adjacent areas of untreated skin of each animal may serve as a control for the test.

C. *Dose level*

A dose of 0.5 ml of liquid or 5 mg of solid or semi-solid is applied to the test site.

D. *Preparation of animals' skins*

Approximately 24 hours before the test, fur should be removed from the test area by clipping or shaving from the dorsal area of the trunk of the animals. Care should be taken to avoid abrading the skin. Only animals with healthy intact skin should be used.

E. *Application of the test substance*

1. The recommended exposure duration is 4-hours. Longer exposure may be indicated under certain conditions (e.g., expected pattern of human use and exposure). At the end of the exposure period, residual test substance should generally be removed, where practicable, using water or an appropriate solvent, without altering the existing response or the integrity of the epidermis.

2. The test substance should be applied to a small area (approximately 6 cm^2) of skin and covered with a gauze patch, which is held in place with non-irritating tape. In the case of liquids or some pastes, it may be necessary to apply the test substance to the gauze patch and then apply that to the skin. The patch should be loosely held in contact with the skin by means of a suitable semi-occlusive dressing for the duration of the exposure period. However, the use of an occlusive dressing may be considered appropriate in some cases. Access by the animal to the patch and resultant ingestion/inhalation of the test substance should be prevented.

F. *Observation period*

The duration of the observation period should be at least 72 hours, but should not be rigidly fixed. It should be sufficient to fully evaluate the reversibility or irreversibility of the effects observed. It need not exceed 14 days after application.

G. Clinical examination and scoring

After removal of the patch, animals should be examined for signs of erythema and edema and the responses scored within 30–60 minutes, and then at 24, 48, and 72 hours after patch removal.

Dermal irritation should be scored and recorded according to the grades in Table 1, below. Further observations may be needed, as necessary, to establish reversibility. In addition to the observation of irritation, any lesions and other toxic effects should be fully described.

V. Data and Reporting

A. Data should be summarized in tabular form, showing for each individual animal the irritation scores for erythema and edema at 30 to 60 minutes, 24, 48, and 72 hours after patch removal, any lesions, a description of the degree and nature of irritation, corrosion or reversibility, and any other toxic effects observed.

B. Evaluation of results

The dermal irritation scores should be evaluated in conjunction with the nature and reversibility or otherwise of the responses observed. The individual scores do not represent an absolute standard for the irritant properties of a material. They should be viewed as reference values which are only meaningful when supported by a full description and evaluation of the observations. The

TABLE 1 Evaluation of Skin Reaction

	Value
Erythema and Eschar Formation	
No erythema	0
Very slight erythema (barely perceptible)	1
Well-defined erythema	2
Moderate to severe erythema	3
Severe erythema (beet redness) to slight eschar formation (injuries in depth)	4
Maximum possible	4
Edema Formation	
No edema	0
Very slight edema (barely perceptible)	1
Slight edema (edges of area well defined by definite raising)	2
Moderate edema (raised approximately 1 millimeter)	3
Severe edema (raised more than 1 millimeter and extending beyond area of exposure	4
Maximum possible	4

use of an occlusive dressing is a severe test and the results are relevant to very few likely human exposure conditions.

C. *Test report*

In addition to the reporting recommendations as specified in the EPA Good Laboratory Practice Standards [Subpart J, Part 792, Chapter I of Title 40. Code of Federal Regulations] the following specific information should be reported.

1. Physical nature and, where appropriate, concentration, and pH value for the test substance;
2. Species and strain;
3. Tabulation of irritation response data for each individual animal for each observation time period (e.g., 30 to 60 minutes, 24, 48, 72 hours after patch removal);
4. Description of any lesions observed;
5. Narrative description of the degree and nature of irritation observed; and
6. Description of any toxic effects other than dermal irritation.

VI. References

The following references may be helpful in developing acceptable protocols, and provide a background of information on which this section is based. They should not be considered the only source of information on test performance, however.

1. Draize, J. H. 1959. Third Printing: 1975. "Dermal Toxicity," *in* "Appraisal of the Safety of Chemicals in Foods, Drugs and Cosmetics." Association of Food and Drug Officials of the United States. pp. 46–59.
2. Draize, J. H. Woodard, G., Calvery, H. O. 1944. Methods for the Study of Irritation and Toxicity of Substances Applied Topically to the Skin and Mucous Membranes. Journal of Pharmacology Experiment Therapeutics. 83:377–390.
3. Marzulli, F. N., Maibach, H. I. 1977. "Dermatoxicology and Pharmacology," *in* "Advances in Modern Toxicology." Vol. 4. New York: Hemisphere Publishing Corporation.
4. NAS. 1978. National Academy of Sciences. Principles and Procedures for Evaluating the Toxicity of Household Substances. Washington, D.C.: A report prepared by the Committee for the Revision of NAS Publication 1138, Under the auspices of the Committee on Toxicology, National Research Council, National Academy of Sciences. 130 pp.
5. WHO. 1978. World Health Organization. Principles and Methods for Evaluating the Toxicity of Chemicals. Part I. Environmental Health Criteria 6. Geneva: World Health Organization. 272 pp.

DERMAL SENSITIZATION

I. Purpose

In the assessment and evaluation of the toxic characteristics of a substance, determination of its potential to provoke skin sensitization reactions is important. Information derived from the tests for skin sensitization serves to identify the possible hazard to a population repeatedly exposed to a test substance. While the desirability of skin sensitization testing is recognized, there are some real differences of opinion about the best method to use. The test selected should be a reliable screening procedure which should not fail to identify substances with significant allergenic potential, while at the same time avoiding false negative results.

II. Definitions

A. Skin sensitization (allergic contact dermatitis) is an immunologically mediated cutaneous reaction to a substance. In the human, the responses may be characterized by pruritis, erythema, edema, papules, vesicles, bullae or a combination of these. In other species the reactions may differ and only erythema and edema may be seen.

B. Induction period is a period of at least one week following a sensitization exposure during which a hypersensitive state is developed.

C. Induction exposure is an experimental exposure of a previously treated subject to a test substance following an induction period, to determine whether the subject will react in a hypersensitive manner.

III. Principle of the Test Method

Following initial exposure(s) to a test substance, the animals are subsequently subjected, after a period of not less than one week, to a challenge exposure with the test substance to establish whether a hypersensitive state has been induced. Sensitization is determined by examining the reaction to the challenge exposure and comparing this reaction to that of the initial induction exposure.

IV. Test Procedures

A. Any of the following seven test methods is considered to be acceptable. It is realized, however, that the methods differ in their probability and degree of reaction to sensitizing substances.

    1. Freund's complete adjuvant test.
    2. Guinea pig maximization test;
    3. Split adjuvant technique;
    4. Buehler test;
    5. Open epicutaneous test;
    6. Mauer optimization test.
    7. Footpad technique in guinea pig.

B. Removal of hair is by clipping, shaving, or possibly by depilation, depending on the test method used.

C. *Animal selection*

1. Species and strain

The young adult guinea pig is the preferred species. Commonly used laboratory strains should be employed. If other species are used, the tester should provide justification/reasoning for their selection.

2. *Number and sex*

a. The number and sex of animals used will depend on the method employed.
b. The females should be nulliparous and nonpregnant.

D. *Control animals*

1. Periodic use of a positive control substance with an acceptable level of reliability for the test system selected is recommended;
2. Animals may act as their own controls or groups of induced animals can be compared to groups which have received only a challenge exposure.

E. *Dose levels*

The dose level will depend upon the method selected.

F. *Observation of animals*

1. Skin reactions should be graded and recorded after the challenge exposures at the time specified by the methodology selected. This is usually 24, 48, and 72 hours. Additional notations should be made as necessary to fully describe unusual responses;
2. Regardless of method selected, initial and terminal body weights should be recorded.

G. *Procedures*

The procedures to be used are those described by the methodology chosen.

V. Data and Reporting

A. Data should be summarized in tabular form, showing for each individual animal the skin reaction, the results of the induction exposure(s) and the challenge exposure(s) at times indicated by the method chosen. As a minimum, the erythema and edema should be graded and any unusual findings should be recorded.

B. *Evaluation of the results*

The evaluation of results will provide information on the proportion of each group that became sensitized and the extent (slight, moderate, severe) of the sensitization reaction in each individual animal.

C. *Test report*

In addition to the reporting requirements as specified in the EPA Good Laboratory Practice Standards [Subpart J, Part 792, Chapter I of Title 40. Code of Federal Regulations] the following specific information should be reported:

1. A description of the method used and the commonly accepted name;
2. Information on the positive control study; including positive control used, method used and time conducted;
3. The number and sex of the test animals;
4. Species and strain;
5. Individual weights of the animals at the start of the test and at the conclusion of the test;
6. A brief description of the grading system; and
7. Each reading made on each individual animal.

VI. References

The following references may be helpful in developing acceptable protocols, and provide a background of information on which this section is based. They should not be considered the only source of information on test performance, however.

1. Buehler, E. V. 1965. Delayed Contact Hypersensitivity in the Guinea Pig. Archives Dermatology. 91:171.

2. Draize, J. H. 1955. Dermal Toxicity. Food Drug Cosmetic Law Journal. 10:722–732.

3. Klecak, G. 1977. Identification of Contact Allergens: Predictive Tests in Animals," *in* "Advances in Modern Toxicology: Dermatology and Pharmacology." Edited by F. N. Marzulli and H. I. Maibach. Washington, D.C.: Hemisphere Publishing Corporation. 4:305–339.

4. Klecak, G., Geleick, H., Grey, J. R. 1977. Screening of Fragrance Materials for Allergenicity in the Guinea Pig. 1. Comparison of Four Testing Methods. Journal of the Society of Cosmetic Chemists. 28:53–64.

5. Magnusson, B., Kligman, A. M. 1973. The Identification of Contact Allergens by Animal Assay. The Guinea Pig Maximization Test. The Journal of Investigative Dermatology. 52:268–276.

6. Maguire, H. C. 1973. The Bioassay of Contact Allergens in the Guinea Pig. Journal of the Society of Cosmetic Chemists. 24:151–162.

7. Maurer, T., Thomann, P., Weirich, E. G., Hess, R. 1975. "The Optimization Test in the Guinea Pig. A Method for the Predictive Evaluation of the

Contact Allergenicity of Chemicals. Agents and Actions. Basel: Birkhauser Verlag. Vol 5/2. pp. 174–149.

8. Maurer, T., Thomann, P., Weirich, E. G., Hess, R. 1975. "The Optimization Test in the Guinea Pig: A Method for the Predictive Evaluation of the Contact Allergenicity of Chemicals," *In* "International Congress Series Excerpta Medica No. 376. Vol. 203." pp. 203–205.

SUBCHRONIC EXPOSURE DERMAL TOXICITY

Purpose

In the assessment and evaluation of the toxic characteristics of a chemical, the determination of subchronic dermal toxicity may be carried out after initial information on toxicity has been obtained by acute testing. The subchronic dermal study has been designed to permit the determination of the no-observed-effect level and toxic effects associated with continuous or repeated exposure to a test substance for a period of 90 days. The test is not capable of determining those effects that have a long latency period for development (e.g., carcinogenicity and life shortening). It provides information on health hazards likely to arise from repeated exposure by the dermal route over a limited period of time. It will provide information on target organs, the possibilities of accumulation, and can be of use in selecting dose levels for chronic studies and for establishing safety criteria for human exposure.

II. Definitions

A. Subchronic dermal toxicity is the adverse effects occurring as a result of the repeated daily exposure of experimental animals to a chemical by dermal application for part (approximately 10%) of a life span.

B. Dose in a dermal test is the amount of test substance applied to the skin (applied daily in subchronic tests). Dose is expressed as weight of the substance (g, mg) per unit weight of test animal (e.g., mg/kg).

C. No-effect level/No-toxic-effect level/No-adverse-effect level/No-observed-effect level is the maximum dose used in a test which produces no observed adverse effects. A no-observed-effect level is expressed in terms of the weight of a test substance given daily per unit weight of test animal (mg/kg).

D. Cumulative toxicity is the adverse effects of repeated doses occurring as a result of prolonged action on, or increased concentration of the administered test substance or its metabolites in susceptible tissues.

Principle of the Test Method

The test substance is applied daily to the skin in graduated doses to several groups of experimental animals, one does level per unit group, for a period of 90 days. During the period of application the animals are observed daily to detect signs of toxicity. Animals which die during the test are necropsied, and at the conclusion of the test the surviving animals are sacrificed and necropsied and appropriate histopathological examinations carried out.

IV. Limit Test

If a test at one dose level of at least 1000 mg/kg body weight (expected human exposure may indicate the need for a higher dose level), using the procedures described for this study, produces no observable toxic effects and if toxicity would not be expected based upon data of structurally related compounds, then a full study using three dose levels might not be necessary.

V. Test Procedures

A. *Animal selection*

1. *Species and strain*
The rat, rabbit or guinea pig may be used although the albino rabbit is preferred. The albino rabbit is preferred because of its size, skin permeability and extensive data base. Commonly used laboratory strains should be employed. If another mammalian species is used, the tester should provide justification/reasoning for its selection.

2. *Age*

Young adult animals should be used. The following weight ranges at the start of the test are suggested in order to provide animals of a size which facilitates the conduct of the test: rats, 200 to 300 g; rabbits, 2.0 to 3.0 kg; guinea pigs, 350 to 450 g.

3. *Sex*

a. Equal numbers of animals of each sex with healthy skin should be used at each dose level.
b. The females should be nulliparous and non-pregnant.

4. *Numbers*

a. At least 20 animals (10 females and 10 males) should be used at each dose level.
b. If interim sacrifices are planned, the number should be increased by the number of animals scheduled to be sacrificed before completion of the study.

B. *Control groups*

A concurrent control group is recommended. This group should be an untreated or sham treated control group or, if a vehicle is used in administering the test substance, a vehicle control group. If the toxic properties of the vehicle are not known or cannot be made available, both untreated and vehicle control groups are recommended.

C. *Satellite group*

A satellite group of 20 animals (10 animals per sex) may be treated with the high dose level for 90 days and observed for reversibility, persistence, or delayed occurence, of toxic effects for a post-treatment period of appropriate length, normally not less than 28 days.

D. *Dose level and dose selection.*

1. In subchronic toxicity tests, it is desirable to have a dose-response relationship as well as a no-observed-toxic-effect level. Therefore, at least three dose levels with a control and, where appropriate, a vehicle control (corresponding to the concentration of vehicle at the highest exposure level) should be used. Doses should be spaced appropriately to produce test groups with the range of toxic effects and mortality rates. The data should be sufficient to produce a dose-response curve.

2. The highest dose level should result in toxic effects but not produce severe skin irritation or an incidence of fatalities which would prevent a meaningful evaluation.

3. The lowest dose level should not produce any evidence of toxicity. Where there is a usable estimation of human exposure, the lowest dose level should exceed this.

4. Ideally, the intermediate dose level(s) should produce minimal observable toxic effects. If more than one intermediate dose is used, the dose levels should be spaced to produce a gradation of toxic effects.

5. In the low and intermediate groups and in the controls the incidence of fatalities should be low, to permit a meaningful evaluation of the results.

E. *Exposure conditions*

The animals are treated with test substance, ideally for at least 6 hours per day on a 7-day per week basis, for a period of 90 days. However, based primarily on practical considerations, application of a 5-day per week basis is considered to be acceptable.

F. *Observation period*

1. Duration of observation should be for at least 90 days.

2. Animals in the satellite group schedules for follow-up observations should be kept for a further 28 days without treatment to detect recovery from, or persistence of, toxic effects.

G. *Preparation of animal skin*

1. Shortly before testing, fur should be clipped from the dorsal area of the trunk of the test animals. Shaving may be employed, but it should be carried out

approximately 24 hours before the test. Repeat clipping or shaving is usually needed at approximately weekly intervals. When clipping or shaving the fur, care should be taken to avoid abrading the skin, which could alter its permeability.

2. Not less than 10% of the body surface area should be clear for the application of the test substance. The weight of the animal should be taken into account when deciding on the area to be cleared and on the dimensions of any covering used.

3. When testing solids, which may be pulverized if appropriate, the test substance should be moistened sufficiently with water or, where necessary, a suitable vehicle to ensure good contact with the skin. When a vehicle is used, the influence of the vehicle on penetration of skin by the test substance should be taken into account.

H. *Application of the test substance.*

1. The test substance should be applied uniformly over an area which is approximately 10% of the total body surface area. With highly toxic substances, the surface area covered may be less, but as much of the area should be covered with as thin and uniform a film as possible.

2. During the exposure period, the test substance should be held in contact with the skin with a porous gauze dressing and non-irritating tape. The test site should be further covered in a suitable manner to retain to gauze dressing and test substance and ensure that the animals cannot ingest the test substance. Restrainers may be used to prevent the ingestion of the test substance, but complete immobilization is not a recommended method.

I. *Observation of animals*

1. A careful clinical examination should be made at least once each day.

2. Additional observations should be made daily with appropriate actions taken to minimize loss of animals to the study (e.g., necropsy or refrigeration of those animals found dead and isolation or sacrifice of weak or moribund animals).

3. Signs of toxicity should be recorded as they are observed, including the time of onset, the degree and duration.

4. Cage-side observations should include, but not be limited to, changes in skin and fur, eyes and mucous membranes, respiratory, circulatory, autonomic and central nervous systems, somatomotor activity and behavior pattern.

5. Animals should be weighted weekly. Food consumption should also be determined weekly if abnormal body weight changes are observed.

6. At the end of the study period, all survivors in the non-satellite treatment groups are sacrificed. Moribund animals should be removed and sacrificed when noticed.

J. Clinical examinations

1. The following examinations should be made on at least 5 animals of each sex in each group:

a. Certain hematology determinations should be carried out at least three times during the test period: just prior to initiation of dosing (baseline data), after approximately 30 days on test and just prior to terminal sacrifice at the end of the test period. Hematology determinations which should be appropriate to all studies: hematocrit, hemoglobin concentration, erythrocyte count, total and differential leucocyte count, and a measure of clotting potential such as clotting time, prothrombin time, thromboplastin time, or platelet count.

b. Certain clinical biochemistry determinations on blood should be carried out at least three times: just prior to initiation of dosing (baseline data), after approximately 30 days on test and just prior to terminal sacrifice at the end of the test period. Test areas which are considered appropriate to all studies: electrolyte balance, carbohydrate metabolism, and liver and kidney function. The selection of specific tests will be influenced by observations on the mode of action of the substance. Suggested determinations: calcium, phosphorus, chloride, sodium, potassium, fasting glucose (with the period of fasting appropriate to the species), serum glutamic-pyruvic transaminase*, serum glutamic oxaloacetic transaminase**, ornithine decarboxylase, gamma glutamyl transpeptidase, urea nitrogen, albumen, blood creatinine, total bilirubin and total serum protein measurements. Other determinations which may be necessary for an adequate toxicological evaluation include: analyses of lipids, hormones, acid/base balance, methemoglobin and cholinesterase activity. Additional clinical biochemistry may be employed, where necessary, to extend the investigation of observed effects.

*Now known as serum alanine aminotransferase.

**Now known as serum aspartate aminotransferase.

2. The following examinations should be made on at least 5 animals of each sex in each group:

a. Ophthalmological examination, using an ophthalmoscope or equivalent suitable equipment, should be made prior to exposure to the test substance and at the termination of the study. If changes in the eyes are detected all animals should be examined.

b. Urinalysis is not suggested on a routine basis, but only when there is an indication based on expected or observed toxicity.

K. Gross necropsy

1. All animals should be subjected to a full gross necropsy which includes examination of the external surface of the body, all orifices, and the cranial, thoracic and abdominal cavities and their contents.

2. The liver, kidneys, adrenals, brain and gonads should be weighed wet, as soon as possible after dissection, to avoid drying.

3. The following organs and tissues, or representative samples thereof, should be preserved in a suitable medium for possible future histopathological examination: normal and treated skin; all gross lesions; brain—including sections of medulla/pons, cerebellar cortex and cerebral cortex; pituitary; thyroid/parathyroid; thymus; trachea; lungs; heart; (sternum with bone marrow); salivary glands; liver; spleen; kidneys; adrenals; pancreas; gonads; uterus; accessory genital organs; aorta; gall bladder (if present); esophagus; stomach; duodenum; jejunum; ileum; cecum; colon; rectum; urinary bladder; representative lymph node; (mammary gland); (thigh musculature); peripheral nerve; (eye); (femur—including articular surface); (spinal cord at three levels—cervical; midthoracic and lumbar); and (extraorbital lachrymal glands).

L. *Histopathology*

The following histopathology should be performed:

1. Full histopathology on normal and treated skin and on organs and tissues; listed above, of all animals in the control and high dose groups.

2. All gross lesions in all animals.

3. Target organs in all animals.

4. The tissues mentioned in brackets (listed above) if indicated by signs of toxicity or expected target organ involvement.

5. Lungs of animals (rodents) in the low and intermediate dose groups should be subjected to histopathological examination for evidence of infection, since this provides a convenient assessment of the state of health of the animals.

6. When a satellite group is used, histopatholgy should be performed on tissues and organs identified as showing effect in other treated groups.

VI. Data and Reporting

A. *Treatment of results*

1. Data should be summarized in tabular form, showing for each test group the number of animals at the start of the test, the number of animals showing lesions, the types of lesions and the percentage of animals displaying each type of lesion.

2. All observed results, quantitative and incidental, should be evaluated by an appropriate statistical method. Any generally accepted statistical method may be used; the statistical methods should be selected during the design of the study.

B. *Evaluation of results*

The findings of a subchronic dermal toxicity study should be evaluated in conjunction with the findings of preceding studies and considered in terms of the observed toxic effects and the necropsy and histopathological findings. The evaluation should include the relationship between the dose of the test substance and the presence or absence, the incidence and severity, of abnormalities, including behavioral and clinical abnormalities, gross lesions, identified target organs, body weight changes, effect on mortality and any other general or specific toxic effects. A properly conducted subchronic test should provide a satisfactory estimation of a no-effect level.

C. *Test report*

In addition to the reporting requirements as specified in the EPA Good Laboratory Practice Standards [Subpart J, Part 792, Chapter I of Title 40. Code of Federal Regulations] the following specific information should be reported.

1. *Group animal data*

Tabulation of toxic response data by species, strain, sex and exposure level for:
a. Number of animals dying;
b. Number of animals showing signs of toxicity; and
c. Number of animals exposed.

2. *Individual animal data*

a. Time of death during the study or whether animals survived to termination;
b. Time of observation of each abnormal sign and its subsequent course;
c. Body weight data;
d. Food consumption data when collected;
e. Hematological tests employed and all results;
f. Clinical biochemistry tests employed and all results;
g. Necropsy findings;
h. Detailed description of all histopathological findings; and
i. Statistical treatment of results where appropriate.

VII. References

The following references may be helpful in developing acceptable protocols, and provide a background of information on which this section is based. They should not be considered the only source of information on test performance, however.

1. Draize, H. H. 1959. Third Printing: 1975. "Dermal toxicity," *in* "Appraisal of Chemical in Food, Drugs, and Cosmetics." The Association of Food and Drug Officials of the United States. pp. 46–59.
2. Fitzhugh, O. G. 1959. Third Printing: 1975. "Subacute toxicity," *in* "Appraisal of the Safety of Chemicals in Foods, Drugs and Cosmetics." The Association of Food and Drug Officials of the Untied States. pp. 26–35.
3. NAS. 1977. National Academy of Sciences. Principles and Procedures for Evaluating the Toxicity of Household Substances. Washington, D.C.: A

report prepared by the Committee for the Revision of NAS Publication 1138, under the auspices of the Committee on Toxicology, National Research Council, National Academy of Sciences. 140 pp.

4. WHO. 1978. World Health Organization. Principles and Methods for Evaluating the Toxicity of Chemicals, Part I. Environmental Health Criteria 6. Geneva: World Health Organization. 272 pp.

ACUTE EXPOSURE DERMAL TOXICITY

I. Purpose

In the assessment and evaluation of the toxic characteristics of a substance, determination of acute dermal toxicity is useful where exposure by the dermal route is likely. The purpose of an acute dermal study is to determine the median lethal dose (LD50), its statistical limits and slope using a single exposure up to a 24-hour period and a 14-day post-exposure observation period. This purpose can be accomplished by performing the provisions contained in this guideline. Data from an acute dermal toxicity study serves as a basis for classification and labelling. It is also an initial step in establishing a dosage regimen in subchronic and other studies. With the addition of certain other test elements this guideline may provide information on dermal absorption and the mode of toxic action of a substance by this route.

II. Definitions

A. Acute dermal toxicity is the adverse effects occurring within a short time period following a dermal application of single dose of a test substance.

B. Dosage is a general term comprising the dose, its frequency and the duration of dosing.

C. Dose is the amount of test substance applied. Dose is expressed as weight of test substance (g, mg) per unit weight of test substance (g, mg) per unit weight of test animal (e.g., mg/kg).

D. Dose-effect is the relationship between the dose and the magnitude of a defined biological effect either in an individual or in a population sample.

E. Dose-response is the relationship between the dose and the proportion of a population sample showing a defined effect.

F. LD50 (median lethal dose), dermal, is a statistically derived single dose of a test substance that can be expected to cause death in 50% of treated animals when applied to the skin. The LD50 value is expressed in terms of weight of test substance (g, mg) per unit weight of test animals (e.g., mg/kg).

III. Principle of the Test Method

The test substance is applied to the skin in graduated doses to several groups of experimental animals, one dose being used per group. Subsequently, observations of effects and deaths are made. Animals which die during the test are necropsied, and at the conclusion of the test the surviving animals are sacrificed and necropsied.

IV. Limit Test

If a test at a dose of at least 2000 mg/kg body weight, using the procedures described for this study, produces no compound-related mortality, then a full study using three dose levels might not be necessary.

Test Procedures

A. *Animal selection*

1. Species and strain

The rat, rabbit or guinea pig may be used. The albino rabbit is preferred because of its size, skin permeability and extensive data base. Commonly used laboratory strains should be employed. If a species other than the three indicated above is used, the tester should provide justification and reasoning for its selection.

2. *Age*

Young adult animals should be used. The following weight ranges are suggested to provide animals of a size which facilitates the conduct of the test: rats, 200 to 300 g; rabbits 2.0 to 3.0 kg; guinea pigs 350 to 450 g.

3. *Sex*

a. Equal numbers of animals of each sex with healthy intact skin should be used for each dose level.

b. The females should be nulliparous and non-pregnant.

4. *Numbers*

At least 10 animals (5 females and 5 males) at each dose level should be used.

B. *Control groups*

Neither a concurrent untreated nor vehicle control group is recommended except when the toxicity of the vehicle is unknown.

C. *Dose levels and dose selection*

1. At least three dose levels should be used and spaced appropriately to produce test groups with a range of toxic effects and mortality rates. The data should be sufficient to produce a dose-response curve and, where possible, permit an acceptable determination of the LD50.

2. *Vehicle*

a. When necessary, the test substance is dissolved or suspended in a suitable vehicle. It is recommended that whenever possible the usage of an aqueous solution be considered first, followed by consideration of a solution in oil (e.g., corn oil) and then by possible solution in other vehicles. For non-aqueous vehicles the toxic characteristics of the vehicle should be known, and if not known should be determined before the test.

b. When testing solids, which may be pulverized if appropriate, the test substances should be moistened sufficiently with water or, where necessary, a suitable vehicle to ensure good contact with skin. When a vehicle is used, the influence of the vehicle on penetration of skin by the test substance should be taken into account.

D. *Exposure duration*

The duration of exposure should be 24 hours.

E. *Observation period*

The observation period should be at least 14 days. However, the duration of observation should not be fixed rigidly. It should be determined by the toxic reactions, rate on onset and length of recovery period, and may thus be extended when considered necessary. The time at which signs of toxicity appear and disappear, their duration and the time of death are important, especially if there is a tendency for deaths to be delayed.

F. *Preparation of animal skin*

1. Shortly before testing, fur should be clipped from the dorsal area of the trunk of the test animals. Shaving may be employed, but it should be carried out approximately 24 hours before the test. Care must be taken to avoid abrading the skin which could alter its permeability.

2. Not less than 10 percent of the body surface area should be clear for the application of the test substance. The weight of the animal should be taken into account when deciding on the area to be cleared and on the dimensions of any covering used.

G. *Application of test substance*

1. The test substance should be applied uniformly over an area which is approximately 10 percent of the total body surface area. With highly toxic substances the surface area covered may be less, but as much of the area should be covered with as thin and uniform a film as possible.

2. The test substance should be held in contact with the skin with a porous gauze dressing and non-irritating tape throughout a 24-hour exposure period. The test site should be further covered in a suitable manner to retain the gauze dressing and test substance and ensure that the animals cannot ingest the test substance. Restrainers may be used to prevent the ingestion of the test substance, but complete immobilization is not a recommended method.

3. At the end of the exposure period, residual test substance should be removed, where practicable using water or an appropriate solvent.

H. *Observation of animals*

1. A careful clinical examination should be made at least once each day.

2. Additional observations should be made daily with appropriate actions taken to minimize loss of animals to the study (e.g., necropsy or refrigeration of those animals found dead and isolation of weak or moribund animals).

3. Cage-side observations should include, but not be limited to, changes in skin and fur, eyes and mucous membranes, respiratory, circulatory, autonomic and central nervous systems, somatomotor activity and behavior pattern. Particular attention should be directed to observations of tremors, convulsions, salivation, diarrhea, lethargy, sleep and coma.

4. Individual weights of animals should be determined shortly before the test substance is applied. Individual weights should also be taken weekly thereafter and at death. Changes in weight should be calculated and recorded when survival exceeds one day.

5. The time of death should be recorded as precisely as possible.

6. At the end of the test, surviving animals should be weighed and sacrificed.

I. *Gross pathology*

Consideration should be given to performing a gross necropsy of all animals where indicated by the nature of the toxic effects observed. All gross pathological changes should be recorded.

J. *Histopathology*

Microscopic examination of organs showing evidence of gross pathology in animals surviving 24 hours or more should also be considered because it may yield useful information.

VI. Data and Reporting

A. *Treatment of results*

Data should be summarized in tabular form, showing for each test group the number of animals at the start of the test, time of death of individual animals at different dose levels, number of animals displaying other signs of toxicity, description of toxic effects and necropsy findings.

D. *Evaluation of results*

The dermal LD50 value should always be considered in conjunction with the observed toxic effects and any necropsy findings. The LD50 value is a relatively coarse measurement, useful only as a reference value for classification and labelling purposes, and expressing the possible lethal potential of the test substance following dermal exposure. Reference should always be made to the experimental animal species in which the LD50 value was obtained. An evaluation should include the relationships, if any, between the animals' exposure to the test substance and the incidence and severity of all abnormalities, including behavioral and clinical abnormalities, gross lesions, body weight changes, effects on mortality, and any other toxicological effects.

C. *Test report*

In addition to the reporting requirements as specified in the EPA Good Laboratory Practice Standards [Subpart J, Part 792, Chapter I of Title 40. Code of Federal Regulations] the following specific information should be reported.

1. Tabulation of response data by sex and dose level (i.e., number of animals dying, number of animals showing signs of toxicity, number of animals exposed);

2. Description of toxic effects;

3. Time of death after dosing;

4. LD50 value for each sex (intact skin) determined at 14 days (with the method of determination specified);

5. Ninety-five percent confidence interval for the LD50;

6. Dose-mortality curve and slope (where permitted by the method of determination);

7. Body weight data; and

8. Pathology findings, when performed.

sot position paper

COMMENTS ON THE LD50 AND ACUTE EYE
AND SKIN IRRITATION TESTS

SOT Position Paper-Comments on the LD50 and Acute Eye and Skin Irritation
Tests (Prepared by the Animals in Research Committee of The Society of Toxicology and Approved by the SOT Council) (1989). *Fundam. Appl. Toxicol.* 13, 621–
623. Conduct of any form of testing of potentially hazardous materials in animals,
including lethality or eye and skin irritation testing, should be undertaken only
after careful consideration of the necessity for, the objectives behind, and the
possible alternatives to, such testing. Acute toxicity testing to determine an approximate lethal dose provides a basis for a comparison of the relative toxicities
of different materials. These data are used to classify materials for transportation
and labeling, to provide information for treatment of acute intoxications, to aid in
dose selection for subsequent toxicity studies, and to provide comparison data for
evaluation and validation of alternative methods in toxicology. Although the classical LD50 test provides a general estimate of the quantity of chemical likely to
cause death, much of the same information can be provided by other forms of
testing in which significantly fewer number of animals are employed. Acute eye
and skin irritation tests on chemical substances are conducted in order to characterize the hazards associated with ocular or dermal exposure. At present, tests in
intact animals are the only means of assessing the potential hazard from such
exposure other than direct testing in man. Although validated *in vitro* alternatives

Prepared by the Animals in Research Committee of The Society of Toxicology and Approved
by the SOT Council.
Received June 26, 1989; accepted July 24, 1989.

to eye and skin irritation tests in animals are not available currently, many tests under development show promise and may be useful as initial screening techniques. Complete validation of these alternate forms of testing for irritation may reduce the need to use whole animals. Until these procedures have been thoroughly tested and validated, the investigator will have to rely on conventional methods. In each case, however, attention should be given to the design and conduct of the study to reduce the number of animals and to minimize animal discomfort. © 1989 Society of Toxicology.

THE LD50 TEST

Origin of the LD50. Many years ago, the use of plants or extracts of plant or animal tissues in medicine created a need for a means of comparing the therapeutic potency of different lots of materials. This led to the development of bioassay procedures which estimated the ED50 (effective dose/50% response or median effective dose) of similar materials so that comparisons could be made. If the effect measured was death, such as the stopping of a frog heart in systole by digitalis, the ED50 became an LD50 (median lethal dose). Thus, LD50 is one of the specialized variants of the more general term, ED50. Later, the LD50 became a measurement by which the relative toxicities of different materials could be compared.

Utility of the LD50. If conducted appropriately, LD50 determinations provide information on the types of toxic effects a chemical produces, the onset of acute toxicity, and an estimate of the quantity of a chemical that is lethal (Klaassen, 1986). This information is also used in the design of other toxicity tests, and it serves as a basis for the design of rational treatment regimens for cases of human poisoning. Chemicals that are lethal in low doses, i.e., having an oral LD50 of 50 mg/kg or less, are classified as poisons and are so labeled in the United States. In general use, LD50 data refer to lethality resulting from a single high-level exposure; other procedures are necessary to characterize the hazards associated with chronic low-level exposure.

Precision of the LD50. As the LD50 became more widely used as a comparative measure of the hazards associated with acute exposure to different substances, it became evident that the derived values varied from experiment to experiment. In an attempt to decrease this variability, a minimum number of animals was specified (most often 10 of each sex in each of five dose groups) to attain the desired levels of precision. In bioassays for drug potency, the control of this variable was properly given a very high priority. For most purposes this high degree of precision is not necessary or appropriate for the LD50 test. An estimate of an approximate lethal dose will meet most needs for this type of information: these data can be obtained using fewer animals than the standard test procedure.

Regulatory uses of the LD50. The amount of chemical exposure required to produce lethality (traditionally measured as the LD50) determines whether a substance is classified as a poison, i.e., a highly toxic material which requires special precautions during its transportation and handling. Among the agencies regulating the transportation or use of poisons are the Department of Transportation, The U.S. Coast Guard, the Environmental Protection Agency, and the Consumer Product Safety Commission. Some estimate of the LD50 is required for registration, use, and transportation. Most of these agencies have modified their requirements to permit procedures other than the classical LD50 test to be used to fulfill this requirement.

Alternative lethality tests. Some common procedures which use fewer animals than the standard LD50 determination are the limit test (Gad et al., 1984) and a modified LD50 test using as few as three dose groups (British Toxicology Society, 1984). Many other designs have been proposed (Gad and Chengelis, 1988), but none are currently in common use. To place materials into categories according to hazard, some laboratories use a "classification" approach in which animals in groups are treated in a series of sequential experiments using predesignated dose levels. The study is completed when the criteria for an appropriate category are reached. This is a variation of the limit test and, if a material has a low order of toxicity, may be done with only 10 animals, if most or all survive treatment at the highest dose in the classification scheme. Other proposed alternatives in study design emphasize the evaluation of toxicity, rather than lethality, as an endpoint. The "up-and-down" study, described by Bruce (1985), permits the estimation of lethal and nonlethal doses with as few as 6 animals.

Some guidelines, i.e., the Organization for Economic Cooperation and Development (OECD) acute toxicity guidelines (draft revision, April 1986), suggest that acute studies be performed using animals of one sex only and only five animals per dose. Administration of one dose to the opposite sex is recommended to confirm the absence of sex-related differences. This approach essentially halves the number of animals that are conventionally required.

Although some government agencies still require precise numerical values for lethal and nonlethal doses, a number of the newer regulatory guidelines permit or even encourage the design of studies from which one obtains only an estimation of the lethal dose. For example, the OECD draft suggests that doses "known to cause marked pain and distress . . . need not be administered, even when no mortality has been observed at tolerated doses."

ACUTE IRRITATION TESTS

The traditional tests for evaluating the potential of chemicals and other agents to cause eye or skin irritation have been *in vivo* tests in the rabbit, often referred to as Draize tests. These have been employed for almost 50 years and are regarded as standard requirements for estimating the hazards associated with human skin and eye exposure to test materials. Since 1980, the validity and propriety of these tests have been increasingly questioned. Much more attention has been given to the search for alternative test procedures with the hope that methods could be developed that would be both more humane and more predictive of human response. As a part of ongoing test programs many investigators have also refined and modified existing *in vivo* techniques to include:

1. The use of prescreens to identify those materials that may be corrosive or severely irritating. This would include, for example, the practiced exclusion of materials with very acidic or alkaline properties (which would impart a high potential for irritation). In addition, knowledge of the outcome of the skin irritation test before the test for ocular irritation permits a decision on the utility of the latter test: it is reasonable to conclude that severe skin irritants will also be severe eye irritants without actual test data.
2. The reduction of the volume of material instilled into the eye of the test animal during eye irritation tests.
3. The reduction of the number of animals required for each test (OECD guidelines accept three rather than six rabbits for skin and eye irritation testing).
4. The sequential exposure of only one or a few animals at a time to preclude the need for further testing if an extreme reaction results.
5. The use of anesthesia during testing.

There are currently more than 60 proposed tests for predicting eye irritation which do not employ intact animals (Frazier et al., 1987). These can be divided into six different categories, depending upon the test measure employed:

1. Cell toxicity
2. Inflammation or immune system response
3. Effects on recovery or repair processes
4. Effects on cellular or tissue physiology
5. Cell morphology
6. Other measures, such as biochemical endpoints or structure-activity analysis.

None of these proposed models are yet validated or evaluated for a broad range of chemical moieties, and none can be relied upon to provide the scientific reliability of predictive accuracy which would be required of a new test for regulatory or legal acceptability. Many hold promise for this and may be suitable, at least, as screens as further validation studies are being conducted.

REFERENCES

British Toxicology Society (1984). A new approach to the classification of substances and preparations on the basis of their acute toxicology. *Human Toxicol.* 3, 85–92.

Bruce, R. D. (1985). An up-and-down procedure for acute toxicity testing. *Fundam. Appl. Toxicol.* 5, 151–157.

Frazier, J. M., Gad, S. C., Goldberg, A. M., and McCalley, J. P. (1987). *A Critical Evaluation of Alternatives to Acute Irritation Testing.* Mary Ann Liebert, New York.

Gad, S. C. and Chengelis, C. P. (1988). *Acute Toxicology Testing: Perspectives and Horizons.* The Telford Press, Caldwell, NJ.

Gad, S. C., Smith, A. C., Cramp, A. L., Gavigan, F. A., and Derelanko, M. J. (1984). Innovative designs and practices for acute systemic toxicity studies. *Drug Chem. Toxicol.* 7, 423–434.

Klaassen, C. D. (1986). Principles of toxicology. In *Casarett and Doull's Toxicology: The Basic Science of Poisons,* 3rd ed., Chap. 2, pp. 11–32.

contents of the first edition

1013

contents of the second edition

contents of the third edition

index